# Occupational Therapy Essentials for Clinical Competence

# Occupational Therapy Essentials for Clinical Competence

Karen Sladyk, PhD, OTR/L, FAOTA
Bay Path College
Longmeadow, MA

Karen Jacobs, EdD, OTR/L, CPE, FAOTA
Boston University
College of Health & Rehabilitation Sciences: Sargent College
Boston, MA

Nancy MacRae, MS, OTR/L, FAOTA
Westbrook College of Health Professions
University of New England
Portland, ME

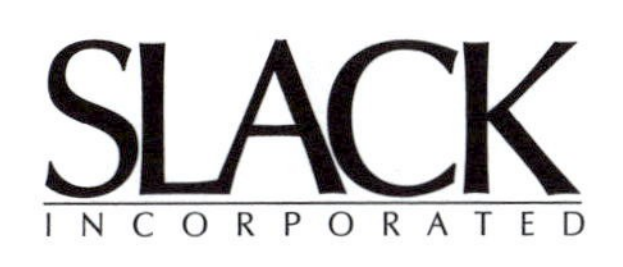

www.slackbooks.com

ISBN: 978-1-55642-819-7



The Instructor's Manual is also available from SLACK Incorporated. Don't miss this important companion to *Occupational Therapy Essentials for Clinical Competence*. To obtain the Instructor's Manual, please visit http://www.efacultylounge.com.



The procedures and practices described in this book should be implemented in a manner consistent with the professional standards set for the circumstances that apply in each specific situation. Every effort has been made to confirm the accuracy of the information presented and to correctly relate generally accepted practices. The authors, editor, and publisher cannot accept responsibility for errors or exclusions or for the outcome of the material presented herein. There is no expressed or implied warranty of this book or information imparted by it. Care has been taken to ensure that drug selection and dosages are in accordance with currently accepted/recommended practice. Due to continuing research, changes in government policy and regulations, and various effects of drug reactions and interactions, it is recommended that the reader carefully review all materials and literature provided for each drug, especially those that are new or not frequently used. Any review or mention of specific companies or products is not intended as an endorsement by the author or publisher.

SLACK Incorporated uses a review process to evaluate submitted material. Prior to publication, educators or clinicians provide important feedback on the content that we publish. We welcome feedback on this work.

Published by: SLACK Incorporated
6900 Grove Road
Thorofare, NJ 08086 USA
Telephone: 856-848-1000
Fax: 856-853-5991
www.slackbooks.com

Contact SLACK Incorporated for more information about other books in this field or about the availability of our books from distributors outside the United States.

Library of Congress Cataloging-in-Publication Data

Occupational therapy essentials for clinical competence / [edited by] Karen Sladyk, Karen Jacobs, Nancy MacRae.
p. ; cm.
Includes bibliographical references and index.
ISBN 978-1-55642-819-7 (alk. paper)
1. Occupational therapy. 2. Clinical competence. I. Sladyk, Karen, 1958- II. Jacobs, Karen, 1951- III. MacRae, Nancy, 1944-
[DNLM: 1. Occupational Therapy. 2. Accreditation--standards. 3. Clinical Competence--standards. WB 555 O1495 2010]
RM735.O323 2010
615.8'515--dc22

2009024728



Printed in the United States of America

Last digit is print number: 10 9 8 7 6 5 4 3 2 1

# Dedication

To occupational therapy leaders and mentors of the past and present; our past, present, and future occupational therapy students; and the uniquely simple and complex concept of occupation.

# Contents



*The numbers after the chapter titles represent the 2006 ACOTE Accreditation Standards for a Master's-Degree-Level Educational Program for the Occupational Therapist (effective January 2008).

## Section VI: Context of Service Delivery



## Section VII: Management of Occupational Therapy Services



## Section VIII: Research



## Section IX: Professional Ethics, Values, and Responsibilities

# Acknowledgments

Our gratitude is extended to all of the contributors to this textbook. Thank you for sharing your professional expertise with us. A special thanks to Kayla Hinkley for help in devising a number of the PowerPoint presentations.

To our friends at SLACK—John, Peter, Brien, Amy, Jenn, Debra, and Dani—thank you for your support.

# About the Editors

*Karen Sladyk, PhD, OTR/L, FAOTA* has been an occupational therapy educator in New England for 18 years—first at Quinnipiac University and currently at Bay Path College. She "accidentally" fell into writing when she was a substitute at a focus group at an American Occupational Therapy Association (AOTA) annual meeting and conference, offering suggestions of what she thought students wanted to know. Since that time, she has edited or authored 9 textbooks targeted specifically at occupational therapy/occupational therapy assistant students' specific needs. Known as a "hard and demanding" teacher, she cares very deeply about students getting an intense and meaningful education.

Like every occupational therapist/occupational therapy assistant, she has a difficult time balancing her life, but she enjoys travel, quilting, crafts, and writing. She recently visited all 50 states before turning 50 herself. Karen spends time with her sisters and nephews in Connecticut and Utah and continues to collect vintage jewelry at flea markets. Lately, she has been hunting for Disney Lanyard pins. When developing this newest book, she had the good fortune of teaming up with Karen and Nancy.

*Karen Jacobs, EdD, OTR/L, CPE, FAOTA* is a past president and vice president of the AOTA and a 2005 recipient of a Fulbright Scholarship to the University of Akuryeri in Akuryeri, Iceland. Dr. Jacobs is a clinical professor and the program director of distance education post-professional programs in occupational therapy at Boston University, Boston, MA. She earned a doctoral degree at the University of Massachusetts, a master of science degree in occupational therapy at Boston University, and a bachelor of arts degree at Washington University in St. Louis, MO.

Dr. Jacobs' research examines the interface between the environment and human capabilities. In particular, she examines the individual factors and environmental demands associated with increased risk of functional limitations among populations of university- and middle school-aged students, particularly in notebook computing and backpack use (http://people.bu.edu/kjacobs/index.shtml).

In addition to being an occupational therapist, Dr. Jacobs is also a certified professional ergonomist (CPE) and the founding editor of the international journal *WORK: A Journal of Prevention, Assessment, and Rehabilitation* (IOS Press, The Netherlands).

Dr. Jacobs is a faculty-in-residence and lives in an apartment in one of the dormitories at Boston University. She is the mother of 3 children—Laela, Joshua, and Ariel; and the amma (grandma in Icelandic) to Sophie Redd. She balances work with occupations such as cross country skiing, kayaking, photography, yoga, and travel.

*Nancy MacRae, MS, OTR/L, FAOTA* is an associate professor, graduate coordinator, and academic fieldwork coordinator at the University of New England (UNE) in Portland, ME, where she has taught for nearly 20 years. She is a past president of the Maine Occupational Therapy Association.

Nancy's work experience has been within the field of developmental disabilities, primarily mental retardation, across the lifespan. Her graduate degree is in adult education, with a minor in educational gerontology. Involvement in the Interprofessional Geriatric Education Program at UNE allows her to mentor and learn from future health care practitioners. Ms. MacRae is the proud mother of 2 sons and a 10-year-old granddaughter. Occupational balance is maintained through participation in reading, yoga, walking, baking, and basket-making.

# Contributing Authors

*Diane P. Bergey, MOT, OTR/L (Chapter 23)*
Belfast, ME

*Roxie M. Black, PhD, OTR/L, FAOTA (Chapter 2)*
Professor and Program Director
Master of Occupational Therapy Program
University of Southern Maine
Lewiston, ME

*Gail M. Bloom, OTD, MA, OTR/L (Chapter 40)*
Andover, MA

*Alfred G. Bracciano, EdD, OTR/L, FAOTA (Chapter 27)*
Associate Professor and Coordinator, Entry Level Distance Programs
Creighton University at University of Alaska Anchorage
School of Pharmacy and Health Professions
Creighton University
Department of Occupational Therapy
Creighton University Medical Center
Omaha, NE

*Lisa L. Clark, MS, OTR/L (Chapters 34 and 38)*
Clinical Faculty, Master of Occupational Therapy Program
University of Southern Maine, Lewiston-Auburn
Lewiston, ME
Mid Coast Hospital
Rehabilitation Services
Brunswick, ME

*Marilyn B. Cole, MS, OTR/L, FAOTA (Chapter 8)*
Professor Emerita, Occupational Therapy
Quinnipiac University
Hamden, CT

*Jeffrey L. Crabtree, MS, OTD, FAOTA (Chapter 33)*
Department of Occupational Therapy
School of Health & Rehabilitation Sciences
Indiana University, Purdue University of Indianapolis
Indianapolis, IN

*William R. Croninger, MA, OTR/L (Chapters 24, 25, and 32)*
Associate Professor, Occupational Therapy
College of Health Sciences
University of New England
Portland, ME

*Betsy DeBrakeleer, COTA/L, ROH (Chapters 24 and 25)*
Clinical Fieldwork Supervisor
University of New England
Portland, ME

*Mary V. Donohue, PhD, OTL, FAOTA (Chapter 14)*
Co-Editor, *Occupational Therapy in Mental Health*
Stony Brook University
New York University Retiree
Stony Brook, NY

*Thomas F. Fisher, PhD, OTR, CCM, FAOTA (Chapter 45)*
Associate Professor and Chair
Department of Occupational Therapy
School of Health & Rehabilitation Sciences
Indiana University, Purdue University of Indianapolis
Indianapolis, IN

*Erica A. Flagg, OT (Chapter 23)*
Union, ME

*Kathleen Flecky, OTD, OTR/L (Chapter 5)*
Assistant Professor
Department of Occupational Therapy
School of Pharmacy and Health Professions
Creighton University
Omaha, NE

*Jan Froehlich, MS, OTR/L (Chapters 22 and 30)*
Associate Professor; Advising Coordinator
Department of Occupational Therapy
University of New England
Portland, ME

*Tara J. Glennon, EdD, OTR/L, FAOTA (Chapter 10)*
Professor, Occupational Therapy
Department of Occupational Therapy
Quinnipiac University
Hamden, CT

*Heather Goertz, OTD, OTR/L (Chapter 5)*
Director of Ministry
St. John's Lutheran Church
Bennington, NE

*Kristin B. Haas, OTD, OTR/L (Chapter 7)*
Assistant Professor, Occupational Therapy
College of Saint Mary
Omaha, NE

*Dory E. Holmes, MPH, OTR/L (Chapter 34)*
Director, Rehabilitation Services
Mid Coast Hospital
Brunswick, ME

*Bevin J. Journey, MS, OTR/L (Chapter 18)*
Occupational Therapy Department
University of New England
Biddeford, ME

*Jennifer Kaldenberg, MSA, OTR/L, SCLV, CLVT (Chapter 36)*
Director, Occupational Therapy Services
New England Eye
Adjunct Assistant Professor, Vision Rehabilitation
New England College of Optometry
Boston, MA

*Rosalie M. King, DHS, OTR/L (Chapter 1)*
Assistant Professor
Occupational Therapy Program
The University of Findlay
Findlay, OH

*Lisa J. Knecht-Sabres, DHS, OTR/L (Chapter 11)*
Assistant Professor
Occupational Therapy Program
Midwestern University
Downers Grove, IL

*Cheryl Kuczynski, MOT, OTR/L (Chapter 3)*
Genesis Rehabilitation
Florence, MA

*Amy Jo Lamb, OTD, OTR (Chapter 37)*
AOTPAC Chair
Outpatient Coordinator
Brookdale Senior Living
Denver, CO

*John E. Lane, Jr., OTR/L (Chapter 24)*
Owner, WorkFit Rehabilitation Services
Lancaster, NH

*Barbara Larson, MA, OTR/L, FAOTA (Chapter 12)*
Occupational Health Consultant
Adjunct Faculty, The College of Saint Scholastica
Duluth, MN

*Kathryn M. Loukas, MS, OTR/L, FAOTA (Chapters 18, 26, 28, and 29)*
Associate Clinical Professor
University of New England
Portland, ME
Doctoral Candidate
Creighton University
Omaha, NE

*James Marc-Aurele, MBA, OTR/L (Chapter 38)*
Clinical Supervisor, Occupational Therapy
Department of Rehabilitation Services
Mid Coast Hospital
Brunswick, ME

*Elisa Marks, MS, OTR/L, CEAS, CHT (Chapter 47)*
Senior Occupational Therapist, Rehabnet Outpatient Center
President, Fearless Seminars
Santa Monica, CA

*Penelope A. Moyers, EdD, BCMH, OTR/L, FAOTA (Chapter 44)*
Chair and Professor, Department of Occupational Therapy
University of Alabama at Birmingham
Birmingham, AL

*Jim Murray, SPHR (Chapter 46)*
Arlington, VA

*Jane O'Brien, PhD, OTR/L (Chapters 15 and 19)*
Associate Professor
Department of Occupational Therapy
Westbrook College of Health Professions
University of New England
Portland, ME

*Beth O'Sullivan, MPH, OTR/L (Chapter 4)*
Easter Seals Rehabilitation
Center of Greater Waterbury
Meriden, CT

*Claudia E. Oakes, OTR/L, PhD (Chapter 6)*
Assistant Professor, Health Science
University of Hartford
Department of Health Science
West Hartford, CT

*Celeste M. Richard, MOT, OTR/L (Chapter 3)*
Memorial Hospital of Rhode Island
Pawtucket, RI

*Michael E. Roberts, MS, OTR/L (Chapter 16)*
Academic Fieldwork Coordinator and Lecturer
Tufts University
Medford, MA

*Regula H. Robnett, PhD, OTR/L (Chapter 21)*
Associate Professor
Director, Department of Occupational Therapy
University of New England
Portland, ME

*Jan Rowe, Dr. OT (Chapter 42)*
Associate Professor
Department of Occupational Therapy
University of Alabama
Birmingham, AL

*Diane Sauter-Davis, MA, OTR/L (Chapter 41)*
Kennebec Valley Community College
Fairfield, ME

*Julie Savoyski, MS, OTR/L (Chapter 31)*
Jamaica Plain, MA

*Barbara J. Steva, MS, OTR/L (Chapter 17)*
Clinical Supervisor
University of New England
Community Occupational Therapy Clinic
Biddeford, ME

*Roseanna Tufano, MFT, OTR/L (Chapter 9)*
Quinnipiac University
Department of Occupational Therapy
Hamden, CT

*Lori Vaughn, OTD, OTR/L (Chapter 13)*
Assistant Professor of Occupational Therapy
Bay Path College
Longmeadow, MA

*Callie Watson, OTD, OTR/L (Chapter 7)*
Associate Professor, Occupational Therapy
College of Saint Mary
Omaha, NE

*Kristin Winston, PhD, OTR/L (Chapter 28)*
Assistant Professor
Master of Occupational Therapy Program
University of Southern Maine
Lewiston, ME

# Foreword

The process of health care fascinates me. Lately, the word *process*, when linked with health care in the United States, calls to mind the formidable problems that beset the system and the growing discourse around the topic of structural reform. But I am less interested in the larger structures that define health care than in the daily interactions between patients and providers. In the end, this is where health care occurs.

Years ago, perhaps well before most readers of this book had been born, my mother was grooming me to become interested in medicine. Even then, as now, there was a widespread public fascination with health care, but the system at that time was economically viable, much more patient friendly, and far less driven by profit and high technology.

As I contemplated career choices in high school, quite by coincidence, (or perhaps not, in the grander cosmic scheme of things) I went to a movie featuring 2 popular stars of the era, Warren Beatty and Jean Seberg. The movie was based on a novel about a relationship between a patient and a provider. In this case, the setting was a private sanitarium, (a polite term used in those days for a private mental health facility), of the variety less frequently seen today. As they often were, the sanitarium inhabited a setting defined by manicured lawns, spreading trees, and recreational areas where patients could get their lives back in order away from the overwhelming demands of life beyond the hospital's gated entrance.

Warren Beatty played an occupational therapist who was assigned to provide structure and engagement to Lilith, a patient[1] portrayed by actress Jean Seberg. Although the storyline was deeply psychological, and remains a great study in the phenomenon of transference, I was less interested in those aspects of the movie than with the field being depicted. I had previously not heard of nor contemplated occupational therapy prior to viewing the movie on that fateful day.

The idea that people could be helped through guided engagement in the activities of everyday life seemed so logical and natural to me (and so full of possibility) that as soon as the movie ended, I resolved to visit the library and learn more about the profession to which I had been introduced. As it turned out, occupational therapy has been my calling now for nearly 40 years.

Of course, the world has changed dramatically during that time. Occupational therapy has largely squandered its respected role in mental health through neglect and has pursued a series of preoccupations with trendier opportunities—too often failing to recognize that the magic of the process lies in connecting people with and enabling them to participate fully in lives of meaning.

A brilliant historian, philosopher, physician, and observer of occupational therapy, Tristram Englehardt, Jr., once observed "people are healthy or diseased in terms of the activities open to them or denied them."[2] This is such a profoundly important observation that it should be chiseled above the doorways through which every occupational therapy student passes. Yet, despite this, the larger health care system continues to define health in a manner that ignores this central point.

Clearly, (as my colleague Joan Rogers brilliantly observed[3]), it is folly to assume, as the health care system and medical practice so frequently do, that when a patient's symptom or part is fixed the problem is solved. To use a mechanical metaphor, repaired cars only matter when they enable us to arrive at destinations of choice. This applies equally well to "repaired" bodies.

And just as we expect our car mechanics to be technically competent in what they do, people seeking services in health care also expect their providers to be technically proficient—to know the what and how of interventions. But, they also expect providers to know why—an essential feature of ethical practice. To borrow from that wonderful play on words: When we receive health care, we expect competent professionals to do things right and to do the right thing. In the case of occupational therapy, doing the right thing begins with considering who the patient is, and what the patient wants to do.

---

1 Despite contemporary usage in the field (and in healthcare generally) that describes those receiving care as "clients or consumers," I prefer the term *patient* because I think it reinforces the idea of a caring relationship rather than purely a business one. Health care may be viewed nowadays as a business, but seeking health care is a far different proposition than purchasing a lawnmower or a pair of shoes. In the latter instances, the customer has a choice, so the transaction is done without the coercion of necessity or urgency that so often characterizes health care.

2 Englehardt, T. H. Jr. (1983). Occupational therapists as technologist and custodians of meaning. In G. Kielhofner (Ed.), *Health through occupation: Theory and practice in occupational therapy* (pp. 139-145). Philadelphia, PA: F.A. Davis.

3 Rogers, J. (1982). Order and disorder in medicine and occupational therapy. *American Journal of Occupational Therapy, 36*, 29-35.

This textbook, edited by leading educators in the field (my friends Karen Sladyk, Karen Jacobs, and Nancy MacRae), benefits from numerous expert contributors, and is printed under the banner of one of occupational therapy's leading publishers. It is appropriately and cleverly organized around the essentials of competence in the occupational therapy process. It begins by setting the proper context for therapy, discussing the ideas of meaningful engagement, history and the founding principles, and beliefs of the field. It proceeds with informed and useful contributions about reasoning and screening and evaluation as vital constituents of the intervention plan. I prefer calling this a "plan of care."

The term *health care* can be an oxymoron, especially when it is disconnected with the lives of patients in a manner that suggests anything but caring. Or, it can represent an occasion to cooperatively and competently guide and enable individuals to contend with or overcome the barriers to participation that their life circumstances have served up. At its best, therapy engenders a belief by the receiver of care that that the provider is acting in that person's best interest. This is the ethical, caring dimension of competent therapeutic practice.

Long after these chapters have been read, the reader who aspires to provide effective occupational therapy services must not forget to step back and view the therapeutic encounter as a relationship characterized by competence and care. Careful attention to the essentials of clinical competence contained in this volume should make such an outcome much more likely.

Charles H. Christiansen, EdD, OTR, OT(C), FAOTA
American Occupational Therapy Foundation
Bethesda, MD

# Introduction

Welcome! You are holding a one-of-a-kind textbook never yet seen in occupational therapy education. This book begins with the 2006 ACOTE Accreditation Standards for a Master's-Degree-Level Educational Program for the Occupational Therapist (effective January 2008), and links these with current practice in organized chapters for students and their faculty educators. The book has been intentionally arranged to follow the order of the ACOTE Accreditation Standards as much as possible. However, it is unlikely that you will read the book from start to finish. Realistically, you will read what is relevant to your current learning.

Designed as a comprehensive overview of the ACOTE Standards relative to curriculum, this book is helpful in introducing every topic needed for a competent, entry-level occupational therapy practitioner. In most chapters, examples are provided that can be viewed from multiple perspectives. For instance, the student example in Chapter 7 can be analyzed as a student-to-peer or as an advanced practitioner-to-student. Such examples enrich the content and its application to practice.

Based on adult learning theory, it is easier to understand concepts if they are "chunked" together or if they utilize "scaffolding" techniques to reinforce and facilitate learning. This is the case for many chapters. For example, the content and application of theory are covered between two chapters. Both chapters cover theory. However, Chapter 8 introduces the development and organization, while Chapter 9 applies theory to evaluation and intervention.

When appropriate, chapters include evidence-based practice reviews that provide the beginning resources to help the student explore the topic in depth. Further, there are student application and self-assessment exercises in each chapter for the students to evaluate their mastery.

The second edition of *The Occupational Therapy Practice Framework: Domain and Process* (2008) has been integrated into the book. To simplify reading, we are using the word *framework* when referring to this document, and using *occupational therapy practitioners* when referring to occupational therapists and occupational therapy assistants.

The reader may notice that some chapters are longer and more comprehensive than others, and that the book has multiple expert contributors. These were mindful decisions of the co-editors. Although no chapter is meant to stand independent of other resources, some chapters were more appropriately comprehensive. This is the case for the chapters on ethics and physical agent modalities. Fifty authors contributed their specific expertise to enhance your learning experience, leading to our decision to include multiple voices. An Instructor's Manual is also available, with multiple choice questions and simple power points to assist the occupational therapy educator.

We want to set the stage with two foundational concepts vital to the study of occupation: flow and culture. Occupational therapy practitioners and students are concerned with identifying occupations meaningful to clients in order to provide the "just right challenge." The use of valued, goal-directed activities promotes health and well-being, and it contributes to satisfaction and quality of life. Csikszentmihalyi's construct of flow shares many of the same tenets held by occupational therapy.

Although there is not a specific ACOTE Standard on culture, the concept of culture is woven throughout the standards, indicating the need for occupational therapy practitioners and students to have a sound understanding of culture and its importance in occupational choice and performance, and in culturally competent care.

The remainder of the chapters address specific assigned standards in the following sections:

- I: Setting the Stage
- II: Basic Tenets of Occupational Therapy
- III: Occupational Therapy Theoretical Perspectives
- IV: Screening, Evaluation, and Referral
- V: Intervention Plan: Formulation and Implementation
- VI: Context of Service Delivery
- VII: Management of Occupational Therapy Services
- VIII: Research
- IX: Professional Ethics, Values, and Responsibilities

Enjoy, as this book is dedicated to you and your lifelong learning!

Karen, Karen, & Nancy

# Section I
## Setting the Stage

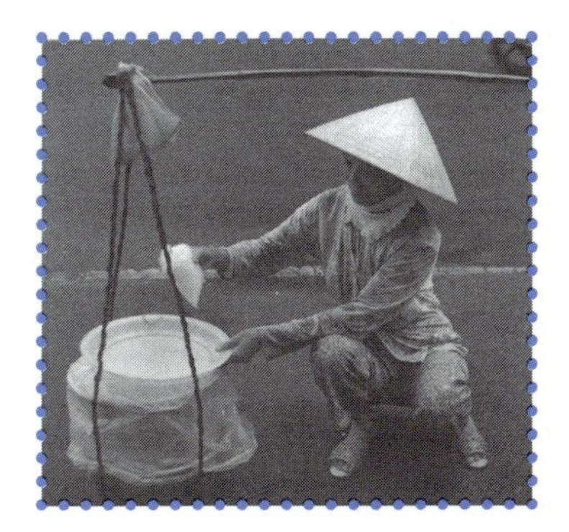

# 1

# The Experience of Flow and Meaningful Occupation

*Rosalie M. King, DHS, OTR/L*

**ACOTE Standard Explored in This Chapter**

B.3.6

**Key Terms**

Experience Sampling Method
Flow experience
Meaningful occupation
Occupational therapy
Well-being

## Introduction

A review of the literature indicates a relationship between the characteristics of meaningful occupation and the experience of flow. Current literature within the occupational therapy profession frequently emphasizes the importance of using occupation, and in doing so, practicing in a client-centered, holistic manner. Although there is a strongly held belief in the profession about the value of occupation, the need to provide supporting evidence still exists. There is also a paucity of evidence available to assist occupational therapy practitioners in determining what is meaningful and enjoyable to the client and the assignment of value and meaning to occupations is very subjective (Csikszentmihalyi, 1997; Persson, Erlandsson, Eklund, & Iwarsson, 2001). People are not always able to articulate what is of particular value to them when asked directly. This review of the literature is an attempt to examine the characteristics of the concept of flow experiences and of occupations that contribute to the well-being of those we serve. In addition, because the flow construct is well established in the field of psychology, finding parallels would support the validity of the use of occupation and afford occupational therapists a larger body of knowledge upon which to build.

Flow, or optimal experience, is a construct studied in the discipline of social psychology and developed by Mihaly Csikszentmihalyi (1990). Flow describes a subjective state of consciousness in which one becomes totally immersed in the occupation or task at hand and from which the individual derives satisfaction and a sense of well-being. The theory has been well researched and clearly delineates the conditions that must be present in order for the flow experience to occur. A more thorough explanation of the construct will be developed to increase understanding of the prerequisite conditions for flow and the benefits to the person experiencing this state.

Occupational therapy has identified the importance of using meaningful occupation in interventions with client populations in order to increase motivation and success in



K. Sladyk, K. Jacobs, & N. MacRae (Eds.).
*Occupational Therapy Essentials for Clinical Competence* (pp. 3-10).

achieving client goals. Cristiansen, Backman, Little, and Nguyen (1999) spoke of the predominant perception within the field that engagement in daily occupations serves to meet intrinsic and extrinsic needs and contributes to satisfaction and quality of life. Founders of the profession of occupational therapy equated health and life satisfaction with balance in daily activities, a tenet we still espouse today. Yet it is true that a healthy balance varies from person to person, as does the idea of which activities and occupations are considered meaningful.

Because there are activities and occupations an individual may consider important that do not result in optimal experience, the idea of examining and determining occupations that do result in flow for a given person does not provide a complete recipe for successful intervention. However, exploration of the concept of flow in relation to meaningful occupation bears consideration in terms of its potential to support the philosophical belief of occupational therapy and to learn more about how we might enable our clients to achieve a greater sense of well-being and life satisfaction.

## Methodology for Searching the Literature

A search of databases including CINAHL, PsycINFO, OT Search, and the American Occupational Therapy Association's (AOTA) journal holdings was conducted using the key terms *meaningful occupation, occupational therapy,* and *flow experience.* To increase responses, the key word *well-being* was also added. A Google search was also conducted using the same key words. Retrieved abstracts and articles, as well as references cited in some of the literature, led to an additional search using the term *experience sampling method.* The search yielded 35 articles, which were narrowed down to 24 for this review. Information that did not come from a peer-reviewed source was discarded.

## Review of the Literature

In order to address this topic, a review of the occupational therapy literature was conducted regarding the use of occupation and its role in contributing to life experience and satisfaction. While the idea of participation in life through the activities and engagement in the occupations people take part in every day is not new, its importance has been emphasized in the past decade as the occupational therapy profession attempts to reconnect with its roots. The psychology literature was consulted to examine optimal experience or flow. The search yielded examples of studies conducted using the flow construct, which have been done by researchers in various fields to include psychology, leisure, education, occupational therapy, and business. While flow is not particularly a novel concept in the discipline of psychology, little emphasis has been placed on it in the occupational therapy literature since the 1990s. Therefore, an exploration of both constructs seems to have merit, followed by an examination of the literature looking at a possible correlation between the two.

## The Importance of Meaningful Occupation

There has been a shift in the global view of health from that of absence of disease or impairment to one that supports the idea that true health has more to do with satisfaction, quality of life, and the pursuit of health (Zemke, 2004). Numerous accounts exist of individuals who have found new meaning in life after the onset of a traumatic illness or life-altering event, which has contributed to a greater sense of purpose and well-being. Dossey (1991, as cited in Bridle, 1999) talked about individuals not only seeking meaning in their lives and in their doing, but in their debility. Celebrities such as Michael J. Fox, Christopher Reeve, and countless others have openly talked about finding a new sense of purpose and meaning as a result of injury and illness. Finding meaning in everyday occupations is important for all human beings. As occupational therapy practitioners, we are faced with the challenge of not only discerning which occupations a client values, but also aiding the individual in discovering new sources of meaning when previously valued occupations are no longer possible.

Christiansen (1999) highlighted the importance of occupations in contributing to one's sense of identity. He discussed the need human beings have to express themselves in a unique way that gives meaning to life and sees engagement in occupations as a vehicle to fulfill that need. He also talked about the relationship between self and others in influencing this sense of identity, stating that we both affect others and are affected by them. Our identities are closely related to the things we do, as well as how we interpret what we do in the social context. In our analysis of events, human beings look for personal meaning, and if these events are deemed significant, we respond in an emotional way and are shaped by them. Our perceptions of life are subsequently formed as well. Therefore, Christiansen stated that identity plays an important role in promoting well-being and satisfaction in life. Having a sense of control and purpose gives meaning to individuals. Bridle (1999) also discussed identity in terms of the relationship between being and doing as a dimension of holism.

In a qualitative study examining the relationship between occupation and its contribution to competence and identity, persons with serious mental illness engaged in woodworking occupations in two community settings (Mee, Sumsion, & Craik, 2004). All participants identified engagement in occupation as the mechanism to acquire skills, a sense of competence and purpose, and a personal sense of self-worth and identity. Hvalsøe and Josephsson (2003) found that their subjects with mental illness felt it was essential that occupations met their need to be engaged in various roles and that these occupations matched their personal preferences and interests in order for them to be of value. Using occupations that are meaningful to people and that contribute to their sense of identity only underscores the importance of employing this in our intervention strategies with clients, because in doing so, practitioners will be facilitating the fulfillment of a common basic need experienced by all human beings.

Yerxa (1998) examined the relationship between health and engagement in occupation, bringing in the idea of the importance of the human spirit. She cited some of the early theorists of the occupational therapy profession, such as Reilly and Meyer, who clearly espoused the connection between involvement in everyday occupations and health. She cited research that has studied some of the creative thinkers of the world and that revealed how little attention has been paid to the idea of work being a contributor to happiness, even if a given individual lacks close personal relationships. The point is made that the drive for autonomy is just as important as the impetus to get closer to other people. What is of greater significance is that the interests pursued are those that contribute to well-being and life satisfaction.

For many individuals, the occupation of work is a source of great meaning and satisfaction, regardless of health status (Kennedy-Jones, Cooper, & Fossey, 2005). In addition to the obvious practical benefits of working for a wage to sustain one's livelihood and one's family, the occupation of work is seen as an avenue to establish one's place in society, help form self-identity, and utilize and increase skills. In numerous studies conducted to determine which everyday occupations resulted in optimal experiences, positive feelings, and satisfaction, work was more frequently cited than leisure (Csikszentmihalyi, 1997; Csikszentmihalyi & LeFevre, 1989; Gerhardsson & Jonsson, 1996; Rebeiro & Polgar, 1998). Because many clients referred for occupational therapy services experience limitations in their ability to work, it is important to recognize the importance of changes negatively affecting this meaningful role. Occupational therapy intervention may involve helping clients to make adaptations so they can resume the worker role or can discover meaning through different occupations.

Effective occupational therapy intervention may require drawing upon past occupations that once provided meaning for an individual. When asked why certain occupations were preferred, subjects in a study eliciting the perspectives of persons with mental illness identified occupations that had evoked positive feelings in the past (Hvalsøe & Josephsson, 2003). Knowledge of occupations that have been valued by the client may serve as an impetus to continue involvement or to reintroduce that occupation into one's life. Recently during a Level II fieldwork placement in the community mental health system, my student discovered that one of her clients used to derive satisfaction from needlework, but had stopped engaging in this leisure occupation. Inspired by that knowledge, the student provided materials for the client to participate in a similar occupation, which proved to be meaningful and, therefore, motivating.

The founders of occupational therapy strongly believed that health and well-being could be influenced by engagement in occupation (Schwartz, 2005). Schwartz gave the following examples of the meaning occupation held for these historical figures in occupational therapy. William Rush Dunton found crafts had a therapeutic effect on him personally and went on to further the arts and crafts movement as part of the intervention of children and adults with mental illness. Meyer and Slagle espoused the importance of habits and involvement in occupations as a way to deal with problems in living. Hall focused on the importance of work, rather than rest, as an avenue toward improved health. The profession, in some respects, has come full circle in recognizing the power of occupation. Thus, it is imperative that we continue to learn how to unleash that power.

## The Concept of Flow

The theory of optimal experience based on the concept of "flow" was developed in the 1970s by Mihaly Csikszentmihalyi: "Flow [autotelic experience] is the way people describe their state of mind when consciousness is harmoniously ordered, and they want to pursue whatever they are doing for its own sake" (1990, p. 6). The experience is so enjoyable and absorbing it becomes autotelic, meaning it is worth doing even if there is no tangible outcome (Csikszentmihalyi, 1999). Csikszentmihalyi wanted to understand the internal feeling state of individuals when they were doing what they enjoyed the most and to determine why they felt that way. He viewed this construct as a possible avenue to help improve quality of life. In addition, Csikszentmihalyi believed that the ability to experience flow, as well as hope and optimism, could be learned, which would in turn affect one's level of happiness (Csikszentmihalyi & Hunter, 2003). While research has gathered information about the kinds of experiences (e.g., leisure, work, athletics, music, religious rituals, and creative activities) that may result in flow, Csikszentmihalyi discussed the possibility of ordering one's consciousness so any activity could result in flow and, thereby, enhance well-being (Csikszentmihalyi, 1990).

Regardless of the activity generating the flow experience, people describe flow similarly across all cultures (Carlson & Clark, 1991; Moneta, 2001). When in optimal flow, individuals become so immersed that they lose a sense of time and feel joyful, motivated, creative, and intensely focused. There is a lack of self-consciousness, an escape from problems, and a clear sense of one's goal (Carlson & Clark, 1991; Csikszentmihalyi, 1990, 1999; Csikszentmihalyi & LeFevre,

1989; Gerhardsson & Jonsson, 1996; Jacobs, 1994; Rebeiro & Polgar, 1998). Process becomes more important than any outcome of this expenditure of psychic energy (Rebeiro & Polgar). It is also true that stress is an aspect of flow, the degree depending on the level of the challenge involved.

Certain conditions must exist in order for flow to occur (Csikszentmihalyi, 1990; Gerhardsson & Jonsson, 1996; Jacobs, 1994; Persson, 1996; Rebeiro & Polgar, 1998):

- There must be a match between one's skills and the challenge of the activity
- There must be clear short-term goals
- The individual needs to feel he or she has control
- The activity must provide immediate feedback

Csikszentmihalyi identified challenge and skills contexts: anxiety, flow, boredom, and apathy (Jacobs, 1994; McCormick, Funderburk, Lee, & Hale-Fought, 2005). In the anxiety context, the individual perceives the challenge of the activity as beyond one's capacity as compared with the skills the person possesses. Flow occurs when challenges and skills are equal, with the caveat that the activity or experience requires that the individual stretch beyond usual performance. Boredom occurs when the challenges are less than skill level as perceived by the individual. Apathy occurs when both skills and challenges are perceived as below that of the individual's perception of his or her average capability and challenge (Jacobs, 1994).

The Experience Sampling Method (ESM) was developed as an alternative to qualitative interviews to gather data about the flow experience of individuals as they occurred in natural contexts over time (Carlson & Clark, 1991; Csikszentmihalyi, 2003; Csikszentmihalyi & LeFevre, 1989; Farnworth, Mostert, Harrison, & Worrell, 1996; Jacobs, 1994). The instrument asks about challenges the subject is experiencing in the here and now in order to identify flow, and gathers information about the subjective experience of the individual regarding the quality of experience and kind of activity in which he or she is engaged. Subjects wear an electronic device that beeps randomly throughout the day, and they are asked to complete an Experience Sampling Form (ESF) addressing pertinent questions regarding what activities they were engaged in at the time as well as perceived challenges and skills related to the task. This methodology for studying the experience of flow was seen as an improvement on other means of gathering this data (Farnworth et al). Time diaries have been used to collect similar data, but they do not necessarily provide direct access to the individual's internal experience, nor the intensity of it. Interviews also have their limitations due to selective remembering as well as the possibility that the subjects may skew their reports based on a desire to please the researcher in some way (Farnworth et al.). Carlson and Clark (1991) highlighted the merits of this methodology as a valid way to record data to increase our knowledge of how human beings are affected by ordinary activities.

To exemplify the use of the flow construct and the ESM of gathering data, some examples are given. Studies outside of the discipline of occupational therapy and within the profession are described.

In a study designed to predict boredom and anxiety in the lives of community mental health clients, McCormick et al. (2005) discovered that states of boredom and anxiety interfered with social and cognitive functioning. Through the use of the ESM, he learned that individuals with severe mental illness (SMI) tend to have fewer challenges in their lives and spend most of their time engaged in activities below their skill level, which would be thought to result in boredom. However, that was not the subjective experience of the participants. While his research indicated there is little in the way of stimulating activity in the lives of persons with SMI, it may well be that these individuals avoid anxiety by not seeking out more challenging situations. He concluded that for this population, understimulation and overstimulation could be problematic. Either way, his findings speak to the importance of balance between skills and challenge in order to promote well-being and quality of life.

Csikszentmihalyi and Hunter (2003) conducted a study of American youth using the ESM in order to examine behaviors and habits that could be associated with happiness. As a premise, it was understood that events occurring outside of oneself have an impact on personal happiness, but one's values and interpretation of events also have an effect. Given the age of the subjects, weekdays were consumed with school or work activities. In regard to the time of day, the teens indicated a higher level of happiness at lunch and after school when their time was more free. The activities the subjects were involved in at a given time, as well as their companions, also had an effect on perceived happiness. The final results indicated younger teens of lower socio-economic stature were happier—they tended to spend less time alone and more time in high-challenge/high-skill activities, which resulted in flow. The ESM allowed researchers to capture information about what was meaningful and fulfilling to this population.

Jacobs (1994) used the ESM to examine optimal flow experiences and job satisfaction in occupational therapy practitioners. Most of her subjects worked in physical rehabilitation settings and reported experiencing flow a relatively small percentage of time (average of 5.24 times per week) (Jacobs). As expected, flow experiences occurred most often during the intervention process. Her intent was to gain information to enable practitioners to develop and apply strategies to enhance flow experiences for occupational therapists while at work, as well as to enable them to facilitate this experience for their clients. In her article, she reiterates the suggestions made by Csikszentmihalyi (1990) regarding how this might be accomplished.

Persson (1996) used the concepts of play and flow theories in examining the occupational process through a creative activity group with chronic pain patients. The aim was to look at theory that would emphasize a doing perspective and to see if the chosen theories could be used to study this process. Many of the components of both theories are congruent. The results indicated that the concepts of play and flow are useful in this context. Subjects experienced the creative activities as both serious and playful, as well as enjoyable though frustrating at times (Persson). Some typical characteristics of flow experiences were reported by the subjects while engaged in the activity, including statements that pain was sometimes forgotten. Persson gave an example describing "how a meaningful activity and its possibilities and demands can arouse the energy and intention for the actor when he/she at first enters into it with skepticism" (p. 40).

Subjects with schizophrenia were engaged in a study by Gerhardsson and Jonsson (1996) designed to explore intrinsic motivation and flow experience. The participants were observed during selected activities of personal interest at three different times, followed by a semi-structured interview immediately after each session. The content of the interview was designed to learn about the subject's experience of the activity and to compare his or her report with the observation report, which was based on elements of the flow experience. If the participant had experienced the activity previously, the chances of flow increased. Overall, the results suggested that the elements of the flow theory are useful in describing which aspects of a particular occupation have a therapeutic effect on an individual (Gerhardsson & Jonsson).

Csikszentmihalyi and LeFevre (1989) used the ESM in a study with adult workers to discern any differences in the quality of experience for these individuals while engaged in work versus leisure. Quality was measured in terms of the match of challenges and skills, as well as level of happiness, satisfaction, creativity, and motivation. While it might seem unlikely, more subjects appeared to experience flow-like conditions while at work as opposed to when engaged in leisure pursuits. The researchers hypothesized it may be that during free time, people just need to relax and recuperate from an intense work day, or they are unable to direct their psychic energy when time is not organized and structured. It was suggested that if people realized they actually derived more benefits from work than they had previously thought, it might result in a reevaluation of any negative perceptions they held about their jobs. Also, it might be that a more conscious use of leisure activities could result in experiences more conducive to flow during free time.

## Discussion

Early theorists as well as current scholars in the field of occupational therapy discuss skill acquisition and providing the "just right challenge" when planning and implementing interventions for those we serve (Carlson & Clark, 1991; Mee et al., 2004; Yerxa, 1998). One of the most important criterions in producing flow is that skills must match the challenge of the activity and that there should be a certain degree of tension. An individual should have to stretch his or her capacity in order to expand, grow, and actualize potential. Csikszentmihalyi's (1989) work in breaking down the ratio of skills to challenge into the contexts of anxiety, boredom, flow, and apathy provides a lens through which the occupational therapist might analyze occupational choices and occupational behavior when designing effective interventions for clients (Carlson & Clark).

Another important requirement to facilitate flow is that the goals of the activity or occupation must be clear and distinct. Christiansen (1999) equated occupation to "goal-directed activity in the context of living" (p. 553), and elaborated by saying that because an individual imagines the outcome if a goal is met, that goal becomes a source of motivation. Setting achievable goals based on client input to increase motivation is inherent in occupational therapy practice.

The concept of balance in life as a determinant of health has been germane to the field of occupational therapy since its inception. Yerxa (1998) cited leaders in the profession, to include Meyer and Reilly, as espousing the merits of a healthy balance. Csikszentmihalyi, too, saw the value of balance when he discussed the need for a match between perceived skills and the challenge of activities in the environment (Yerxa).

Christiansen (1999), in discussing the power of occupation, proposed that we create life meaning through the things we do. Csikszentmihalyi (1990) devoted a chapter to the subject of meaning, stating that "creating meaning involves bringing order to the contents of the mind by integrating actions into a unified flow experience" (p. 216). Meaningful lives require challenging goals of significance which must be pursued with resolve in order to produce harmony (Csikszentmihalyi). Englehart (1986) echoed the perspective of founders of the profession by describing occupational therapists as custodians of meaning. Studies designed to validate the importance of meaningful occupation, including some cited in this paper, have provided evidence that what we do in everyday life has a profound effect on life satisfaction and well-being. However, what is meaningful to one individual may not be to another (Persson et al., 2001). In order for occupational therapy interventions to be successful, we must learn which occupations are of value to clients because the concepts of purpose and meaning are central to therapeutic outcomes (Farnworth et al., 1996). To underscore the powerful effect the discovery of a meaningful occupation can have on an individual, Csikszentmihalyi (1997) described a woman with chronic schizophrenia who had been hospitalized for over 10 years. In a period of study using the ESM, she reported having positive moods several times, which occurred when she was caring for her fingernails. Based on those findings, the staff in the facility enlisted the aid of a professional manicurist to teach the patient skills that resulted in the woman giving manicures to other patients. Not only did her mood improve, but she was able to be discharged to the community where she eventually took up the trade and became self-sufficient within a year.

Despite the similarities between the concept of flow and the philosophy of occupational therapy regarding the value of meaningful occupation, Csikszentmihalyi's work has not been utilized to provide evidence supporting our work. The flow construct has been researched and utilized in the fields of psychology, leisure, education, and business. However, there was little to be found in the occupational therapy literature that referenced flow, and much of the evidence produced took place over 10 years ago, primarily outside of the United States. It would appear we have not taken advantage of a well-researched body of work that has considerable merit, but we have the opportunity to do so. On a macro level, the flow construct could serve to validate the importance of occupational therapy's role in facilitating health, well-being, and quality of life. On a micro level, Csikszentmihalyi's theory could enable us to determine what is, in fact, meaningful occupation as we intervene with clients on a day-to-day basis.

## Summary

The literature clearly indicates a relationship between meaningful occupation and the concept of flow. The studies described exemplify how one might use Csikszentmihalyi's work and methodology to provide further evidence on the value of occupation. Flow "is highly relevant to occupational science because it documents an everyday phenomenon that importantly relates to, among other things, happiness, self-esteem, work productivity, the enjoyment of leisure, and life satisfaction" (Carlson & Clark, 1991, p. 239).

Embracing Csikszentmihalyi's theory and capitalizing on the extensive body of evidence that has been produced primarily outside of the occupational therapy profession would lend credence to our own body of knowledge. The degree to which the relationship between these two constructs needs to be investigated is beyond the scope of this chapter. Occupational therapists need to engage in the meaningful occupation of producing evidence to validate what we do and increase our understanding of how we can best intervene to facilitate successful outcomes for our clients who are depending on us to assist them in improving quality of life.

## Student Self-Assessment

1. List some of your favorite occupations. What are some of your usual feelings when engaged in these pursuits?
2. Do you think you experience flow when participating in any of these occupations? Which ones?
3. Evaluate your favorite occupations in terms of Csikszentmihalyi's conditions of flow listed on p. 5. Do any of these pursuits meet his criteria for flow? If so, which ones? If not, which ones? Why or why not?
4. Review the challenge and skills contexts discussed on pp. 5-6. Identify an activity or occupation in which you experience (a) anxiety, (b) boredom, and (c) apathy. How do these subjective feelings affect your motivation and sense of well-being?
5. Discuss any parallels you see between the experience of flow and occupations that are meaningful to individuals. How could you apply this to occupational therapy practice?
6. Do you think it is possible to experience flow while engaged in an activity or occupation even if all of Csikzentmihalyi's conditions are not met?

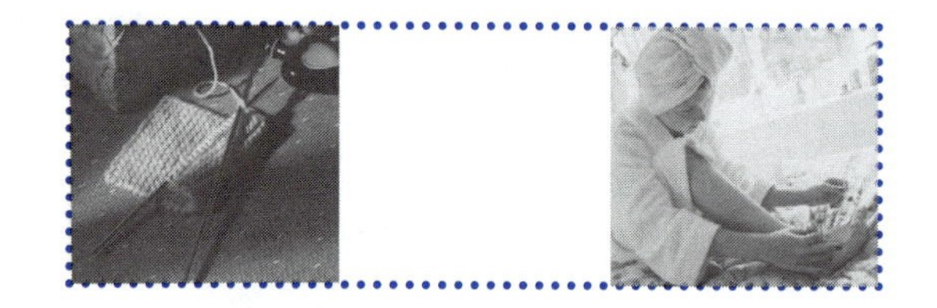

## References


Bridle, M. J. (1999). Are doing and being dimensions of holism? *American Journal of Occupational Therapy, 53*(6), 636-639.

Carlson, M. E., & Clark, F. A. (1991). The search for useful methodologies in occupational science. *American Journal of Occupational Therapy, 45*(3), 235-241.

Christiansen, C. H. (1999). The 1999 Eleanor Clarke Slagle lecture: Defining lives: Occupation as identity: An essay on competence, coherence, and the creation of meaning. *American Journal of Occupational Therapy, 53*(6), 547-558.

Christiansen, C. H., Backman, C., Little, B. R., & Nguyen, A. (1999). Occupations and well-being: A study of personal projects. *American Journal of Occupational Therapy, 53*(1), 91-100.

Csikszentmihalyi, M. (1990). *Flow: The psychology of optimal experience.* New York, NY: HarperCollins.

Csikszentmihalyi, M. (1997). *Finding flow: The psychology of engagement with everyday life.* New York, NY: Basic Books.

Csikszentmihalyi, M. (1999). If we are so rich, why aren't we happy? *American Psychologist, 54*(10), 821-827.

Csikszentmihalyi, M. (2003). Happiness in everyday life: The uses of experience sampling. *Journal of Happiness Studies, 4*(2), 185-199.

Csikszentmihalyi, M., & Hunter, J. (2003). Happiness in everyday life: The uses of experience sampling. *Journal of Happiness Studies, 4*, 185-199.

Csikszentmihalyi, M., & LeFevre, J. (1989). Optimal experience in work and leisure. *Journal of Personality and Social Psychology, 56*(5). 815-822.

Englehardt, T. (1986). Occupational therapists as technologists and custodians of meaning. In G. Kielhofner (Ed.), *Health through occupation* (pp. 139-144). Philadelphia, PA: F.A. Davis.

Farnworth, L., Mostert, E., Harrison, S., & Worrell, D. (1996). The experience sampling method: Its potential use in occupational therapy research. *Occupational Therapy International, 3*(1), 1-17.

Gerhardsson, C., & Jonsson, H. (1996). Experience of therapeutic occupations in schizophrenic subjects: Clinical observations organized in terms of the flow theory. *Scandinavian Journal of Occupational Therapy, 3*(4), 149-155.

Hvalsøe, B., & Josephsson, S. (2003). Characteristics of meaningful occupations from the perspective of mentally ill people. *Scandinavian Journal of Occupational Therapy, 10*(2), 61-71.

Kennedy-Jones, M., Cooper, J., & Fossey, E. (2005). Developing a worker role: Stories of four people with mental illness. *Australian Occupational Therapy Journal, 52*(2), 116-126.

Jacobs, K. (1994). Flow and the occupational therapy practitioner. *American Journal of Occupational Therapy, 48*(11), 989-996.

McCormick, B. P., Funderburk, J. A., Lee, Y. K., & Hale-Fought, M. (2005). Activity characteristics and emotional experience: Predicting boredom and anxiety in the daily life of community mental health clients. *Journal of Leisure Research, 37,* 236-253.

Mee, J., Sumsion, T., & Craik, C. (2004). Mental health clients confirm the value of occupation in building competence and self-identity. *British Journal of Occupational Therapy, 67*(5), 225-233.

Moneta, G. (2004). The flow experience across cultures. *Journal of Happiness Studies, 5*(4), 115-121.

Persson, D. (1996). Play and flow in an activity group—A case study of creative occupations with chronic pain patients. *Scandinavian Journal of Occupational Therapy, 3*(1), 33-42.

Persson, D., Erlandsson, L., Eklund, M., & Iwarsson, S. (2001). Value dimensions, meaning, and complexity in human occupation—A tentative structure for analysis. *Scandinavian Journal of Occupational Therapy, 8*(1), 7-18.

Rebeiro, K. L., & Polgar, J. M. (1999). Enabling occupational performance: Optimal experiences in therapy. *Canadian Journal of Occupational Therapy, 66*(1), 14-22.

Schwartz, K. (2005). The history and philosophy of psychosocial occupational therapy. In E. Cara & A. MacRae (Eds.), *Psychosocial occupational therapy: A clinical practice* (2nd ed., pp. 61-68). Florence, KY: Delmar Cengage Learning.

Yerxa, E. J. (1998). Health and the human spirit for occupation. *American Journal of Occupational Therapy, 52*(6), 412-418.

Zemke, R. (2004). The 2004 Eleanor Clarke Slagle lecture: Time, space, and the kaleidoscopes of occupation. *American Journal of Occupational Therapy, 58*(6), 608-620.

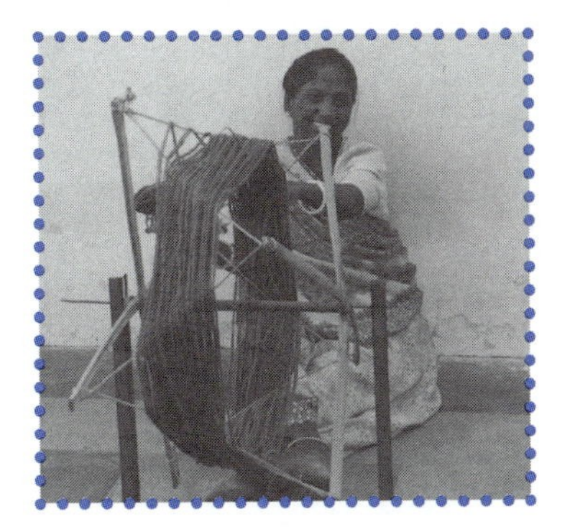

# 2

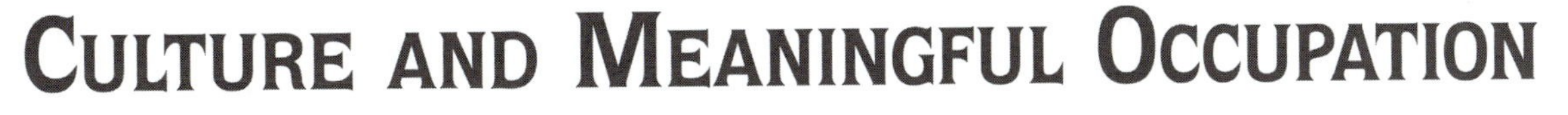

# Culture and Meaningful Occupation

Roxie M. Black, PhD, OTR/L, FAOTA

**ACOTE Standards Explored in This Chapter**

B.1.7, 2.10, 4.2, 4.4, 4.7, 5.0, 5.2

**Key Terms**

| | |
|---|---|
| Client-centered care | Culture |
| Cultural competence | Occupational justice |
| Culturally competent care | |

## Introduction

The concept of culture is embedded in multiple ACOTE educational standards and implied in several others that address the social issues and social factors related to the context of service delivery (B.6.1, 6.2, 6.3). It is clear that understanding culture is not only important in occupational therapy, but that it is a foundation upon which other skills and knowledge are built. Therefore, it is a vital aspect of occupational therapy education.

The concept of culture, however, is complex. This chapter will define culture, discuss its relevance to occupational therapy practitioners and culturally competent care, introduce the readers to the characteristics of cultural competence, and identify some of the related research.

## Culture Defined

Iwama (2004) described culture as a "slippery concept, taking on a variety of definitions and meanings depending on how it has been socially situated and by whom" (p. 1). This is understandable when you think about the fact that "having culture" might mean being sophisticated and knowledgeable to some people, while the term *culture* might connote racial and ethnic difference to others. A much broader concept of culture is defined in this way: "The sum total of a way of living, including values, beliefs, standards, linguistic expression, patterns of thinking, behavioral norms, and styles of communication that influence the behavior(s) of a group of people that is transmitted from generation to generation. [Culture] includes demographic variables such as age, gender, and place of residence; status variables such as social, educational, and economic levels; and affiliation variables" (Wells & Black, 2000, p. 279). Because it is transmitted to following generations, culture is learned, and therefore, aspects of it such as attitudes, values, and behaviors may be unlearned.

As can be discerned by this complex definition, culture is all-encompassing, influencing all aspects of someone's life. The culture in which each of us lives influences the time we rise in the morning, the breakfast we eat (or don't eat), the utensils we use (or don't use), what time of the day we eat, how much time we take to have a meal, the clothes and accessories (such as jewelry or hair adornments) we wear, the job we hold, our mode of transportation to that



K. Sladyk, K. Jacobs, & N. MacRae (Eds.).
*Occupational Therapy Essentials for Clinical Competence* (pp. 11-22).

job, the style of home in which we live, the chores in which we engage in that home, and on and on. Additionally, culture defines gender roles, relationships, and the multiple ways we express ourselves.

Not only are we influenced by the culture in which we are born (family, community, society), we are also impacted by the subcultures to which we often choose to belong. These may include groups from our church, synagogue, or temple; our college and program; our cohort of friends; our biking or hiking group; or our gym companions. Because each of these subgroups holds certain values and expectations for us, they also influence our behaviors and choices. Sometimes the expectations of these subcultures are in conflict with one another. For example, your occupational therapy educational program faculty may expect you to study for several hours a day/night, while your family or roommates may have expectations that you will be home for dinner each evening. You will resolve this conflict, making an occupational choice based on what is most important to you at that time (your values) given the context of the situation.

If what is meaningful and important to us is culturally determined, and given that our values are evident through our actions, culture influences what we do including our occupational choices, occupational behaviors, and occupational performance. Because of this fact, "culture represents one of the most important issues facing occupational therapy today" (Iwama, 2004, p. 1).

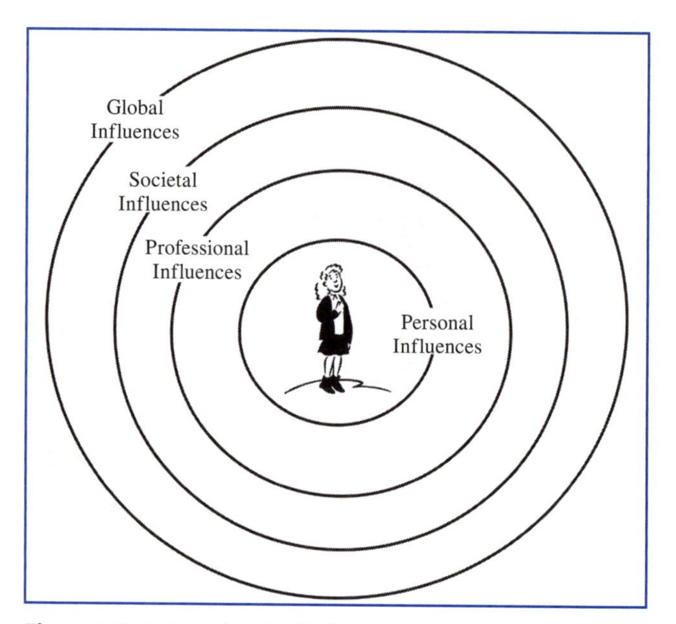


**Figure 2-1.** Cultural levels of influence.

# Multiple Levels of Cultural Influence

As occupational therapy students and practitioners, culture influences us and our occupational choice on many levels, just as it does for the people with whom we work. These levels begin at the personal level and move through several levels to the global level (Figure 2-1). We'll briefly examine each of these levels in this section of the chapter.

## Personal Influences

Each of us develops from a particular social location. This means that our place of birth, the year of our birth, birth order, gender, sexual identity, class, family structure, ability, religion, and ethnicity all influence who we are at birth, and in many cases, who we will become as adults. All of these cultural characteristics influence our behavior or what we do (our occupations). For example, I was born just after the end of World War II and raised in a rural state by working-class parents. I was raised to believe in hard work, the importance of education (which my parents were unable to achieve, yet knew the value of), the importance of helping others, and the love of family and nature. All of these values influence what I choose to do today, from teaching in an occupational therapy program to spending important time with family and friends, or to one of my favorite pastimes—gardening.

Most of us are taught our cultural values by members of our families, friends, mentors, teachers, and spiritual leaders. We also learn cultural lessons from the media such as the standard of feminine beauty, the importance of wealth, and the value of commodities. Often, the messages learned from these various groups/people conflict and we have to choose what best meets our needs. For example, we may come from a large Italian family where the message of *mangia, mangia* (eat! eat!) rings in our ears, yet the print and electronic media constantly tell us that being painfully thin is the true vision of beauty in our country. Or our peer group enjoys playing at the beach, lying in the sun, and developing a deep, rich tan, while the message from the health community is that getting too much sun can lead to health issues. What do we do? Each of us is a unique and complex cultural being, so we will make occupational choices based on what we value, or what is important to us at that time. For these reasons, each person must be viewed as an individual.

This is also true of the people with whom we work as occupational therapy practitioners. Although there may be cultural similarities between members of a particular group, we cannot assume that each member of the group holds the same beliefs, values, and occupational interests, and we cannot treat each member of a group in the same way. Certainly not all of the students in an academic program perform the same, learn in the same manner, study the same way, or enjoy the same topics, even though they may all be Caucasian and all female. Therefore, it is imperative that the faculty understand each student as an individual.

One reason there is such individuality within a group or subgroup is that culture can be learned as well as unlearned. Although we are taught certain values as children, as we develop and experience more of life, we sometimes reject those earlier teachings and assume other values. For instance, we may have been taught negative things about a certain race or ethnicity, that older people are cranky and helpless, that women are emotional and weak, or that motorcyclists are all hoodlums, but our life experiences or education have refuted those lessons and we may now perceive members of those groups in different ways. As we mature, we may choose a different spiritual path or lifestyle from that of our parents or cultural group, or we may move into a different socioeconomic class that may change our perception of our world and the people in it. These changing beliefs and values will alter our occupational choices and patterns, indicating the dynamic nature of our cultural influences and reemphasizing the importance of learning about people's individual and personal cultures as we work with them.

**Student Activity**

Identify three meaningful activities in which you engage. Reflect on which aspects of your main culture or any of your subcultures may influence your activity choice. Think about why you choose to engage in these activities, who or what impacts your decision, and what meaning the activities have for you. Write these down. Now, try to imagine whether you would still be engaged in these activities if you lived in another country or community, or if you had a different family. Think about why you would or would not still be engaged in the same activities.

# Professional Influences: Culture and Occupational Therapy

The concept of culture is embedded in our profession and has been since we first began recognizing clients as individuals with unique needs. The very first set of standards for occupational therapy emphasized the importance of providing intervention to each client as an individual (Dunton, 1925). Although a client's "cultural influences" may not have been the language used at that time, as we sought to understand each unique person's interests, beliefs, and needs, we were actually examining aspects of his or her culture. Over the past 9 decades, we have continued to view each recipient of occupational therapy services as an individual, although many concepts within the field have developed and changed. Some of the more current notions and language related to occupational therapy and culture are identified next.

## Culture and the Occupational Therapy Practice Framework

Several of the educational standards written at the beginning of this chapter refer to culture as being part of the context of a client's life. That language derives from the framework (AOTA, 2008), which describes the domain of occupational therapy practice as an outline of the "profession's purview and the areas in which its members have an established body of knowledge and expertise" (pp. 625-626).

Occupational therapy recognizes the importance of the context of a person's life to support engagement in occupation. The framework states that "context refers to a variety of interrelated conditions within and surrounding the client" (AOTA, 2008, p. 645). This document identifies six contextual conditions that an occupational therapy practitioner must consider when working with a client, one of which is culture. The framework defines culture as the "customs, beliefs, activity patterns, behavior standards, and expectations accepted by the society of which the individual is a member...includes political aspects, such as laws that affect access to resources and affirm personal rights...also includes opportunities for education, employment, and economic support" (AOTA, p. 645).

The framework (AOTA, 2008) not only identifies the domain of occupational therapy practice and the process by which we provide interventions, but it also guides practice. Therefore, this document highlights the importance of considering the culture of the people with whom we work, and in some ways it mandates that we consider the clients' cultural influences.

## Client-Centered Care

Another important concept in occupational therapy practice that supports cultural consideration of clients is client-centered care. This notion arose from Rogers' (1951) theoretical belief that a client is a partner in the client/therapist dyad and should/must be part of the decision-making process regarding his or her own intervention. The therapist or practitioner must respect the client, recognize the client as the first authority on what he or she needs, and must try to see the world through the client's eyes as well as through those of the authoritative health professional. Since the early 1990s, occupational therapists have adopted Rogers' ideas and have been redefining them to support and frame occupational therapy practice (Law, 1998; Law, Baptiste, & Mills, 1995; Pollock, 1993; Sumsion, 1993, 1999). Many of these authors suggest that for client-centered care to occur, the occupational therapy practitioner must understand the client's medical, social, and occupational history as well as his or her beliefs and values so that together, the client and practitioner can collaboratively determine an intervention approach that is meaningful to the client. In other words, the practitioner must understand the client's culture and the cultural influences on his or her performance. Understanding another's culture is one aspect of cultural competence and part of culturally competent care. I have previously made the argument that client-centered care must, by its definition, be culturally competent care (Black, 2005).

## Cultural Competence and Culturally Competent Care

In order to provide culturally competent care, occupational therapists and occupational therapy assistants must be culturally competent. In today's health and human services practices, "cultural competence is increasingly seen as important to quality of care" (Chin, 2000). Although cultural competence is often used when talking about race and ethnicity, the changing demography of the United States assures a greater increase in the multiple diversities of our clients. Diversity is apparent in race and ethnicity, in class and socioeconomic levels, in age and ability, in religion and political views, and in gender and sexual identity. If we understand culture to incorporate all of the above and more, then cultural competence is appropriate when working with all people, not just those who are racially or ethnically different from ourselves (Black, 2005).

Within the occupational therapy literature, cultural competence is described as "the process of actively developing and practicing appropriate, relevant, and sensitive strategies and skills in interacting with culturally different persons" (AOTA Multicultural Task Force, 1995). An often-used definition from Cross, Bazron, Dennis, and Isaacs (1989) states that cultural competence is "a set of congruent behaviors, attitudes, and policies that come together in a system, agency, or among professionals and enable that system, agency, or those professionals to work effectively in cross-cultural situations" (p. 13). As might be extrapolated from these definitions, cultural competence is more than just understanding the culture of our clients. It incorporates three distinct characteristics that include cultural self-awareness, cultural knowledge, and cross-cultural skill (Black & Wells, 2007).

- *Cultural self-awareness*: Cultural self-awareness may be the most important of the three characteristics of cultural competence (Harry, 1992; Lynch & Hanson, 1998; Weaver, 1999; Wells & Black, 2000). It means recognizing yourself as a cultural being who sees the world through a unique cultural lens. This awareness helps us to understand ourselves as having special "unearned" privileges if we are white-skinned or male (McIntosh, 1988), or assists us in knowing where we fit in the sociocultural matrix of the dominant culture if we are a person of color, female, poor, old, physically or mentally impaired, or have a sexual identity other than heterosexuality. Being culturally self-aware means recognizing our biases and prejudices and knowing how and from where and whom we learned these. It is extremely important to do the hard work of cultural self-exploration because knowing ourselves in this way will make us much more aware when working with a client who is culturally different from ourselves. Without that awareness, unexplored biases may become a barrier when working with certain culturally diverse clients and may lead to ineffective or inappropriate interventions. In the worst case, it might lead to discriminatory behaviors that might harm the client in some way.
- *Cultural knowledge*: Cultural knowledge is the information we gather about a client's culture, which includes customs, traditions, body language, values, beliefs about health and wellness, and the meaning of illness. It may mean learning a little of their language if it differs from our own. Trying to speak to people in their own language connotes respect for them and, in my experience, is always appreciated. Additionally, cultural knowledge includes understanding the sociocultural "status" of this person's culture, and his or her understanding of oppression and discrimination. Taking the time to learn about a client's culture is vital in establishing rapport and providing client-centered care.
- *Cross-cultural skill*: Cross-cultural skill is what differentiates cultural competence from cultural sensitivity. To develop skill, you must actively engage in communicating and interacting with others who differ from yourself. You must be willing to "put yourself out there," to be open to differing ideas and beliefs, and to make mistakes (Black, 2002). You must also learn how to recover from those mistakes. Successful cross-cultural communication means understanding nonverbal communications as well as negotiating conflict.

All three of these characteristics must either be developing or in place in order to provide culturally competent care. More than a decade ago, Abney (1996) argued for its importance when she stated,

> Cultural identification has a crucial impact on an individual's response to traumatic stress. Therefore cultural identification must be considered carefully when addressing practice issues...It determines the individual's view and disclosure of the trauma, expression of symptoms, and attitude toward treatment and recovery (pp. 409-410).

These words are as relevant today as they were when they were first written, and the ideas can be expanded to include all people with whom we work, not just those who have experienced traumatic stress. In order for us to understand the client's perspective of his or her illness or condition, we need to learn to ask the right questions through a culturally sensitive assessment approach, and to listen well to the answers. We cannot assume that a culturally diverse client believes and thinks the same way we do. Therefore, we must constantly ask for clarification of ideas and meaning. Assuming that we understand what the client means without clarification is a recipe for miscommunication and inadequate or poor intervention. The antithesis of culturally competent care is cultural incompetence, which may result in the following ("Cultural competence practice," n.d.):

- Client-practitioner relationships, which are negatively affected when clear understanding of each other's expectations is missing
- Miscommunication between the client and practitioner
- Client may not follow instructions
- Client may reject the practitioner because of nonverbal cues that do not fit expectations
- Inadequate or poor intervention occurs

### Cultural Competence and Occupational Justice

*Occupational justice* is a fairly new term found in occupational therapy literature that connotes that individuals have a right to access and engage in meaningful occupations. "Occupational injustices exist when, for example, participation is barred, confined, segregated, prohibited, undeveloped, disrupted, alienated, marginalized, exploited, or otherwise devalued" (Townsend & Whiteford, 2005). Much of the literature on occupational justice and injustice has been written outside of the United States about groups of people who are socially oppressed. However, the terminology and ideas are increasingly and appropriately used in this country as well, as many individuals and groups in the United States also are barred from engaging in activities that have meaning for them. Many of these folks come from a sociocultural background that differs from the occupational therapy practitioners who work with them; the majority of whom are white, middle-class, and highly educated women. In order to recognize occupational injustices and to provide the best interventions, occupational therapy practitioners will have to provide effective client-centered and culturally competent care as meaningful occupations are culturally defined.

## Societal Influences

The next level of cultural influence is that of the societal level. Every society has its own cultural beliefs and customs. Lewis (2002) wrote that "culture is constructed by humans in order to communicate and create community" (p. 13). In the United States, we are guided by the principles of the U.S. Constitution, which extol freedom, equality, and the pursuit of happiness for all. However, those of us who fall within the dominant categories may have more privileges than others and more access to the goods and services of our country.

Therefore, although all citizens of the United States may be governed by the same principles and beliefs, our experiences and perceptions of our world may differ because of our cultural characteristics and the societal hierarchy within our country. Our opportunities will differ from one another, leading to varied choices and occupational behaviors. For example, the daily activities of a widowed 79-year-old Caucasian woman living in low-income housing in a small city in the northeast section of the United States may differ significantly from that of a Puerto Rican woman of the same age living with her daughter and her family in the northeast. The first woman may be far more isolated, especially in the winter. Her occupations may include watching favorite television shows, doing crossword puzzles, reading biographies and non-fiction literature, talking on the telephone with family and friends, and doing light housework. Because she cannot afford a car, this woman rarely leaves her housing development, having to rely on others to take her grocery shopping or to do other errands. Her children and grandchildren see her regularly every few weeks or so. Nevertheless, she keeps busy and, although sometimes lonely, is fairly satisfied with her life (Figure 2-2).

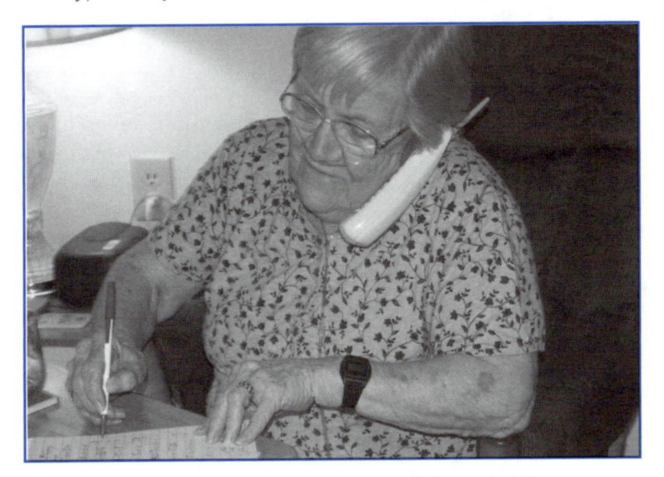

**Figure 2-2.** Enjoying the solitary occupation of doing a crossword puzzle while socially interacting with a friend on the telephone.

The second woman comes from a cultural background where it is common to live with extended family and where being a senior has value. She continues to have an important place in this family and her occupations reflect that. She often cooks and helps to clean up meals, assists with laundry and babysitting for the older children, and has become a confidante to her granddaughter. She watches favorite television shows with the family in the evenings and is included in family excursions on the weekends. She reads to the younger children and tells them stories of their parents and grandparents, and of times in the "old country." Although she goes to bed fairly exhausted in the evening and sometimes wishes for a little more time to herself, this woman is also quite satisfied with her life (Figure 2-3).

Both of these women live full, but very different lives. If we were to receive them as clients in our practice, we could not effectively work with them in the same way, nor expect their occupations to be alike just because they are women in their seventies living in the same region of the United States. Each is influenced by societal expectations, yet their personal and family cultures allow them to be individuals, and they must be respected as such.

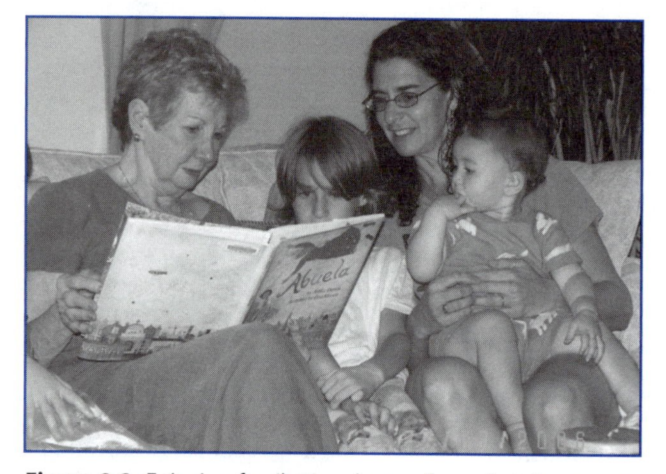


**Figure 2-3.** Enjoying family time by reading a favorite story to grandchildren.

Within the health professions, our behaviors are impacted not only by societal expectations, but also by federal and state rules and regulations. Among these are the National Standards for Culturally and Linguistically Appropriate Services (CLAS) in Health Care (U.S. Department of Health and Human Services [HHS], 2000). This collective set of 14 mandates, guidelines, and recommendations were developed to inform, guide, and facilitate required and recommended practices related to culturally and linguistically appropriate health services for health care organizations and their employees. As occupational therapy practitioners, these standards will help guide our work with people and groups who are culturally diverse.

## Global Influences

The broadest level (and, perhaps, the least apparent for many) of cultural influence on occupations comes from the larger, global world. Oftentimes, many people are ethnocentric and exclusionary, and do not seem interested in what is going on outside of the country, nor do they believe they are impacted by events beyond our shores. Yet, there is an impact on each of us. There is an old saying that goes something like the flutter of a butterfly's wings in one part of the world can spawn a hurricane in another. Our occupations may change in significant or subtle ways due to events happening around the world.

The wars in Iraq and Afghanistan, for instance, have changed the occupations of not only the men and women from this country who are fighting overseas, but also those of their families and friends who spend more time writing letters or emails, or searching for gifts and sending them, or in the worst case, spending time in hospitals or funeral homes. Others who did not have friends or family members engaged in war may have spent more time watching news casts, reading newspapers and news magazines, or campaigning for favorite politicians as a result of the conflicts. Many of us engaged in new occupations as a direct result of the war.

When the tsunami hit Indonesia and Sri Lanka in 2005, many from the United States traveled there to help, or began campaigns to send supplies or money as aid, or again, stayed glued to their television sets to watch the latest news or increased the amount of time they spent reading papers and other news magazines.

Before the prevalence of technology, people could ignore what was happening outside of their own communities or country, but with television, radio, and print media in most homes in the United States, and with email, instant messaging, and other technological advances in communication, people not only know what is going on around the world, but we know it as it happens (Black & Wells, 2007). And, because we are more aware of world events, we become a more active part of our global culture and may choose to act on those events.

In summary, the multiple levels of cultural influences impact each of us in unique ways, shaping our identities, the identities of the people with whom we work, and the manner in which we engage in occupational pursuits. How we understand and use this important information informs and guides our occupational therapy practice.

# Cultural Characteristics That Impact Effective Cross-Cultural Interactions

There are many unique characteristics and beliefs that various cultures hold that, if not examined, may interfere with effective client-centered and culturally competent care. As a point of illustration, this chapter will briefly examine three: self-concept, perceptions of power and authority, and temporal issues.

## Self-Concept

In Western societies, the notion of self-concept was thought to be about the individual, where identity is developed as something unique and differentiated from others, often called individualism (Brewer & Gardner, 2004). Cross-cultural research, however, identified another approach to the development of self-concept and identity, one that relied on a social identity that "reflects internalizations of the norms and characteristics of important reference groups and consists of cognitions about the self that are consistent with that group identification" (Brewer & Gardner, p. 68). This type of identity is called collectivism.

Although very few people develop a sense of self apart from others (Brewer & Gardner, 2004), and every person is unique, there are many cultures whose belief system and ideals strongly emphasize one or the other of these approaches.

### Individualism

Banks (1997) stated that "individualism as an ideal is extreme in the U.S. core culture" (p. 9). In an individualistic society, the focus is on "I" rather than on the family, group, or community. People are taught to be strong and tough and take care of themselves, and seeking out help or advice from others is sometimes seen as weakness. Consider the icons in American culture such as the strong, independent heroes like John Wayne. Independence and autonomy are valued, and people who are ill or disadvantaged should "tough it out" or "pull themselves up by the bootstraps." The Protestant work ethic, with the belief that hard work is morally good and that sloth is sinful, has contributed to the individualistic ideal (Banks). Doing something is more important than talking, and practicality and efficiency are important values. The individualist is often future-oriented, resulting in comfort with change (Lattanzi & Purnell, 2006).

When working with someone who holds individualistic beliefs, the occupational therapy practitioner must remember the following concepts:

- Illness is a major threat to this person's independence.
- It is important to consult the person on every decision so he or she will have some sense of control.
- This person will appreciate "working hard" toward recovery.
- Respect the person's privacy.
- Ask permission before entering this person's space.
- Set individual goals to increase independence.

Because many of the values of occupational therapy were developed from a Western, individualistic ideal (Iwama, 2006), working with a client with these values should not cause much conflict with U.S. practitioners.

### Collectivism

Many Eastern cultures, including the Chinese and Japanese, have more of a collectivist worldview. People from these cultures develop the identity of the larger society and self-concept, and identity focuses on the "we." One is expected to be committed first to the family and group, and then to self (Banks, 1997). Interdependence is valued, and decisions are usually made by group consideration rather than individually. Health may be measured by one's ability to function within the group. Human interaction is valued over time, and cooperation is important. The past and tradition are important and authority is respected (Lattanzi & Purnell, 2006).

When working with people with a collectivist viewpoint, practitioners will want to consider the following:

- They may view the health care provider as an outsider, and not trust easily.
- You may want to find someone who knows the client to introduce you.
- On the other hand, they may expect you to provide the answers since you are the authority figure.
- It will be important to work closely with family and group members regarding decisions about the client's interventions.
- Emphasize the team approach to effective and safe care.

## Perceptions of Power and Authority

The way in which people view authority figures and the power inherent within those positions often influences relationships and occupational behaviors. The perception of personal power is the sense of our ability to impact our environment, which allows us to feel good about ourselves and believe that we're important and others recognize our worth (Glasser, 1984). Personal power impacts our own sense of authority and our ability to control others. It is often internalized and unconscious.

The perception of power informs one's degree of acceptance of inequality. For instance, if I accept the inequality of power, authority, and privilege as a given, then I will not see myself as having the need or power to change it. If I do not accept inequality as a given, and instead believe that everyone should be equal to me, I perceive a need for change in an unequal context. Geert Hofstede's (1981, 2001) research with people from 40 different nations resulted in a description of Power Distance, which is "the extent to which the less powerful members of organizations and institutions (like the family) accept and expect that power is distributed unequally" ("Clearly Cultural," n.d., para. 1). Hofstede identified the difference in High Power Distance (HPD) and Low Power Distance (LPD) cultures, stating that "the basic issue involved, which different societies handle differently, is human inequality" (p. 79).

### High Power Distance Cultures

HPD defines a culture where inequality is accepted. Members of the culture believe that each person has a rightful place, and that superiors and subordinates treat each other differently and don't mix socially. Members of these cultures do not challenge power and authority (Hofstede, 1981, 2001).

It is important to recognize these cultural characteristics in occupational therapy practice, as they will impact the relationship practitioners have with diverse clients. When working with people from HPD cultures, one must consider the following:

- They are more conscious of the hierarchy in the health care system.
- They will want to know their place in that hierarchy and how the health care facility works.
- They may relate to people differently based on age, gender, and professional role.

- Authority is important to them and they will tend to look to the professional for decisions and directions.
- It may be important for the practitioner to share their credentials and accomplishments with the client so that authority may be established.
- It may be more difficult to provide a client-centered approach to interventions.
- It may be more difficult to develop an empowered or participatory power relationship with the client.

### Low Power Distance Cultures

In LPD cultures, the majority of the members feel that any inequality in the society should be minimized. Members believe in equal rights and that the existence of hierarchy is only for the convenience of accomplishing tasks in an organization. The belief is that education increases power and that people can move within this fluid system (Hofstede, 1981).

With the client from a LPD culture, consider the following:

- This person will expect to be treated on an equal basis, and may want to be treated as a peer when not in a professional role.
- He may challenge authority, and in turn, expect to be challenged. This is seen as a sign of respect.
- Keep this client apprised of the progress of therapy.
- This client is usually a good candidate for client-centered occupational therapy.

Hofstede developed a Power Distance Index (PDI), which determined the relative power distance of various nations (Clearly Cultural, n.d.). Interestingly, Austria has a PDI of 11 (very low), while Malaysia's PDI is 104 (very high). Many Central American countries and the Philippines fall in the 90s, Arab nations' PDI is 80, and the United States has a PDI of 40 (Clearly Cultural). Occupational therapy practitioners must recognize this important cultural characteristic in their clients for effective cross-cultural interactions.

## Temporal Issues: The Concept of Time

Although the characteristics identified above are culturally defined and important to recognize, one aspect that causes a tremendous amount of difficulty in business and health care is the differences in the concept of time between the employer and employee and therapist and client. All cultures have unique concepts of time and much has been written about this cultural characteristic. Although several authors discuss the difference between future, present, and past temporal orientations (Bonder, Martin, & Miracle, 2002; Lattanzi & Purnell, 2006) and its impact on health care, this section of the chapter will address the relationship of monochronic and polychronic time and how it may impact cross-cultural interactions.

### Monochronic Time

There are cultures and people who perceive time as linear, and can only do one thing at a time. These monochronic people are schedule-dominated and tend to live by the clock. They see the world in segmented compartments, and even tend to sequence communications as well as tasks (O'Hara-Devereaux & Johansen, 1994). According to O'Hara-Devereaux and Johansen, these folks would be disinclined to interrupt a telephone conversation to greet a third person. Efficiency and convenience are important factors for monochronic people (Table 2-1).

Within a therapeutic relationship with a monochromic client, consider:

- The client may not be interested in a holistic approach.
- The client will be interested in information about schedules, interventions, time of discharge, etc.

**Table 2-1. Common Time Differences**

| Monochronic People | Polychronic People |
|---|---|
| Do one thing at a time | Do many things at once |
| Concentrate on a task | Highly distractible; Accept interruptions |
| Time commitments such as deadlines and schedules are taken seriously | Time commitments to be achieved only if possible |
| Low context: Needs information | High context: Has information |
| Committed to the task | Committed to people |
| Religious adherence to plans | Change plans often and easily |
| Follow rules of privacy and consideration: Doesn't want to disturb others | More concerned with relations (families, friends, colleagues) than with privacy |
| Emphasize promptness | Base promptness on the relationship |

Adapted from Hall, E. T., & Hall, M. R. (1990). *Understanding cultural differences: Germans, French, and Americans*. Yarmouth, ME: Intercultural Press and from O'Hara-Devereaux, M., & Johansen, R. (1994). *Globalwork: Bridging distance, culture, and time*. San Francisco, CA: Jossey-Bass.

- The practitioner must follow the schedules as closely as possible; inform the client if you must be late to the appointment.
- If the client is highly stressed, give him or her permission to relax; schedule time for relaxation.

#### Polychronic Time

In contrast to the above characteristics, a polychronic person can accomplish multiple activities at the same time and won't cut a discussion short if he or she is "out of time." "Polychronic time is open-ended: completing the task or communication is more important than adhering to a schedule" (O'Hara-Devereaux & Johansen, 1994, p. 37). These people can and often will carry on several conversations simultaneously. Polychronic people are relation-dominated—their strength is an emphasis on interactions with others and they enjoy non-linear, creative tasks (see Table 2-1).

Within a therapeutic setting, remember:

- Developing rapport and a comfortable relationship with the client is primary.
- Always relate to the person in some way before and during the intervention.
- Expect there to be family and friends in the intervention room.
- You may have to remind the client about the schedule and follow-up home activities.

### Summary

As occupational therapy practitioners, providing effective cross-cultural care is vitally important when working with diverse clients. Being aware of the characteristics identified above and addressing them with the client in an effort to minimize misunderstandings will move the practitioner toward cultural competence and the client to a place of trust, both of which will result in effective and respectful care.

## Research on Culture and Culturally Competent Care

There has been a significant increase in the occupational therapy literature in the past few years on issues of culture, diversity, and cultural competence (Black, 2005; Black & Wells, 2007; Bonder, 2004; Fisher, 2005; Fitzgerald, 2004; Froehlich & Nesbit, 2004; Iwama, 2003; Kondo, 2004; Wittman, 2002). However, many of the articles written have been concept papers or descriptions of programs. Although this body of literature provides significant value in developing dialogue in this area, there is limited reported research on the importance of the knowledge of culture, on aspects of cultural competence, and on the effectiveness of culturally competent care in occupational therapy practice. Some notable exceptions are the case study by Odawara (2005), which examined the stories about the therapeutic process between Japanese clients and their therapists; Awaad's (2003) published literature search on culture, cultural competency, and occupational therapy, examined in order to provide evidence for good practice; Scott's (1997) qualitative study that explored British occupational therapists' perceptions of cross-cultural practices; and Whiteford and Wilcock's (2000) longitudinal study of occupational therapy students in Auckland, New Zealand that focused on the students' perceptions of their experiences as they learned to work with people who were culturally different from themselves.

There is a need for further research in occupational therapy practice to provide the evidence that supports culturally competent care. According to the Center on an Aging Society, "cultural competence is not an isolated aspect of medical care, but an important component of overall excellence in health care delivery" (2004, p. 11). Providing excellence in health care delivery is an important goal of occupational therapy practice, but we must increase the amount of research that is completed and published in order to further support aspects of our practice.

There are multiple research articles supporting aspects of cultural competence and culturally competent care in the fields of medicine, social work, and nursing, however, and several of these sources are included in the evidence-based practice chart at the end of the chapter.

## Summary

Understanding the impact of culture on values, beliefs, perceptions, occupational choice, and occupational behaviors for ourselves and the people with whom we work is vital for occupational therapy students and practitioners. Understanding clients' cultural context has been identified as part of the domain of occupational therapy practice (AOTA, 2008), and providing culturally competent care has been noted as an aspect of excellence in health care delivery. This chapter has introduced and discussed the concepts of culture, the multiple levels of cultural influence on occupational choice, selected cultural characteristics that impact cross-cultural interactions, cultural competence, and culturally competent care to its readers. I have emphasized the value of these constructs in occupational therapy practice, and have argued for increased research to provide support and evidence of their impact on practice. It is my hope that this introduction will provide the foundation for continued study and practice in the areas of culture and diversity in occupational therapy.

## Student Self-Assessment

1. How does your dominant culture affect your occupational choices?
2. List some of your subcultures and reflect on whether the values inherent within these subcultures conflict with one another or with your dominant culture.
3. Define culture in your own words.
4. In what ways does culture affect occupational therapy practice?
5. How would you recognize culturally competent care?
6. Describe the three characteristics of cultural competence. Which of these do you feel confident in? Which do you need to do more work with?
7. What is the relationship between client-centered care and culturally competent care?
8. How might you recognize occupational injustice?
9. How might differing concepts of time impact a therapist/client relationship?

## Electronic Resources

- American Association of University Professors (AAUP) diversity bibliography: http://aaup.org/AAUP/issues/diversity/Diversitybib.htm
- Boston Center for Refugee Health and Human Rights: www.glphr.org/refugee/library.htm
- Center for Cross-Cultural Health: www.crosshealth.com
- Cultural Competence Resources: www.med.yale.edu/library/education/culturalcomp
- Cultural Competence Resources for Health Care Providers: http://hrsa.gov/culturalcompetence
- Cultural Competency Web page: http://cecp.air.org/cultural/default.htm
- Global Health Source: www.globalhealth.gov
- Minority Health Concerns and Cultural Competence Resources (National Network of Libraries of Medicine, Midcontinental Region): http://nnlm.gov/mcr/resources/community/competence.html
- National Center for Cultural Competence: www11.georgetown.edu/research/gucchd/nccc
- Office of Minority Health: www.omhrc.gov/templates/browse.aspx?lvl=2&lvlID=11
- Provider's Guide to Quality and Culture: http://erc.msh.org/qualityandculture
- U.S. Department of Health and Human Services, Office of Minority Health: www.omhrc.gov

### Evidence-Based Research Chart

| Topic | Issue | Evidence |
|---|---|---|
| Cultural Competence | Perceptions and skills of students and practitioners regarding cultural competence | Black, 2002; Forwell, Whiteford, & Dyck, 2001; Kim, 1996; D. Pope-Davis, Prieto, Whitaker, & S. Pope-Davis, 1993; Weaver, 1999; Whiteford & Wilcock, 2000 |
| | Impact of education for cultural competency | Vaughan, 2005 |
| | Research on cultural competence assessment tools | Arthur et al., 2005; D'Andrea & Heck, 1991; Schim, Doorenbos, Miller, & Benkert, 2003; Smith, 1998; Vinh-Thomas, Bunch, & Card, 2003 |
| | Assessment of culturally competent scholarship | Mendias & Guevara, 2001; Price et al., 2005 |
| Culturally Competent Care | Efficacy—Improvements in health and well-being | Callister, 2005; Health Resources and Service Administration, 2001 |
| | Efficacy—Improvements in client satisfaction | Beach et al., 2005 |
| | Examination of perceptions and skills of culturally competent care | Austin, Gallop, McCay, Peternelj-Taylor, & Bayer, 1999; Schilder et al., 2001; Scott, 1997 |

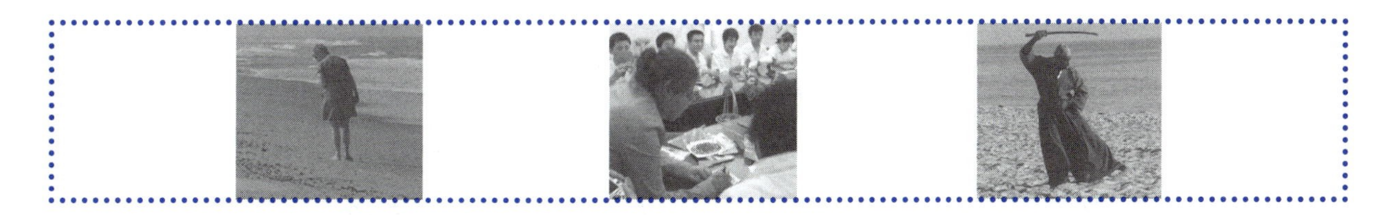

# References


Abney, V. D. (1996). Cultural competency in the field of child maltreatment. In J. Briere, L. Berliner, J. A. Bulkley, C. Jenny, & T. Reid (Eds.), *The APSAC handbook on child maltreatment* (pp. 409-419). Thousand Oaks, CA: Sage Publications.

American Occupational Therapy Association. (2008). Occupational therapy practice framework: Domain and process, second edition. *American Journal of Occupational Therapy, 62*, 625-683.

American Occupational Therapy Association, Multicultural Task Force. (1995). *Definition and terms*. Bethesda, MD: AOTA Press.

Arthur, T. E., Reeves, I., Morgan, O., Cornelius, L. J., Booker, N. C., Brathwaite, J., et al. (2005). Developing a cultural competence assessment tool for people in recovery from racial, ethnic, and cultural backgrounds: The journey, challenges, and lessons learned. *Psychiatric Rehabilitation Journal, 28*(3), 243-250.

Austin, W., Gallop, R., McCay, E., Peternelj-Taylor, C., & Bayer, M. (1999). Culturally competent care for psychiatric clients who have a history of sexual abuse. *Clinical Nursing Research, 8*(1), 5-25.

Awaad, T. (2003). Culture, cultural competency and occupational therapy: A review of the literature. *British Journal of Occupational Therapy, 66*(8), 356-362.

Banks, J. A. (1997). Multicultural education: Characteristics and goals. In J. A. Banks & C. A. M. Banks (Eds.), *Multicultural education: Issues and perspectives* (3rd ed., pp. 3-31). Hoboken, NJ: John Wiley & Sons Inc.

Beach, M. C., Price, E. G., Gary, T. L., Robinson, K. A., Gozu, A., Palacio, A., et al. (2005). Cultural competence: A systematic review of health care provider educational interventions. *Medical Care, 43*(4), 356-373.

Black, R. M. (2002). *The essence of cultural competence: Listening to the voices of occupational therapy students*. Unpublished dissertation. Cambridge, MA: Lesley University.

Black, R. M. (2005). Intersections of care: An analysis of culturally competent care, client-centered care, and the feminist ethic of care. *WORK: A Journal of Prevention, Assessment & Rehabilitation, 24*(4), 409-422.

Black, R. M., & Wells, S. A. (2007). *Cultural & occupation: A model of empowerment in occupational therapy.* Bethesda, MD: AOTA Press.

Bonder, B. R., Martin, L., & Miracle, A. W. (2002). *Culture in clinical care.* Thorofare, NJ: SLACK Incorporated.

Bonder, B. R., Martin L., & Miracle, A. W. (2004). Culture emergent in occupation. *American Journal of Occupational Therapy, 58*(2), 159-168.

Brewer, M. B., & Gardner, W. (2004). Who is this 'we?' Levels of collective identity and self representations. In M. J. Hatch & M. Schultz (Eds.), *Organizational identity: A reader.* New York, NY: Oxford University Press.

Callister, L. C. (2005). What has the literature taught us about culturally competent care of women and children? *American Journal of Maternal Child Nursing (MCN), 30*(6), 380-388.

Center on an Aging Society. (2004). Cultural competence in health care: Is it important for people with chronic conditions? Issue Brief No. 5. Georgetown University. Retrieved May 30, 2008, from http://ihcrp.georgetown.edu/agingsociety/pubhtml/cultural/cultural.html

Chin, J. L. (2000). Culturally competent health care. *Public Health Reports, 115*(1), 25-33.

Clearly Cultural. (n.d.). Making Sense of Cross Cultural Communication. Retrieved June 6, 2008, from http://www.clearlycultural.com/geert-hofstede-cultural-dimensions/power-distance-index

Cross, T., Bazron, B., Dennis, K., & Isaacs, M. (1989). *Towards a culturally competent system of care* (Vol. 1). Washington, DC: Georgetown University Child Development Center.

Cultural competence practice and training: Overview. (n.d.) Retrieved February 22, 2000, from http://www.diversityrx.org/HTML/MOCPT1.htm

D'Andrea, M., Daniels, J., & Heck, R. (1991). Evaluating the impact of multicultural counselor training. *Journal of Counseling and Development, 70*, 143-150.

Dunton, W. R. (1925). *Standards of the National Society for the Promotion of Occupational Therapy*. Bethesda, MD: American Occupational Therapy Association, Archives in Wilma L. West Library.

Fisher, S. (2005). The Canadian Occupational Performance Measure: Does it address the cultural occupations of ethnic minorities? *British Journal of Occupational Therapy, 68*(5), 224-234.

Fitzgerald, M. H. (2004). A dialogue on occupational therapy, culture, and families. *American Journal of Occupational Therapy, 58*(5), 489-498.

Forwell, S. J., Whiteford, G., & Dyck, I. (2001). Cultural competence in New Zealand and Canada: Occupational therapy students' reflections on class and fieldwork curriculum. *Canadian Journal of Occupational Therapy, 68*(2), 90-103.

Froehlich, J., & Nesbit, S. G. (2004). The aware communicator: Dialogues on diversity. *Occupational Therapy in Health Care, 18*(1), 171-184.

Glasser, W. (1984). *Take effective control of your life.* New York, NY: HarperCollins.

Hall, E. T., & Hall, M. R. (1990). *Understanding cultural differences: Germans, French, and Americans*. Yarmouth, ME: Intercultural Press.

Harry, B. (1992). Developing cultural self awareness: The first step in values clarification for early interventionists. *Topics in Early Childhood Special Education, 12*(3), 333-350.

Health Resources and Services Administration, U.S. Department of Health and Human Services. (2001). *Cultural competency works: Using cultural competency to improve the quality of health care for diverse populations and add value to managed care arrangements.* Washington, DC: Author.

Hofstede, G. (1981). *Culture's consequences: Comparing values, behaviors, institutions.* Thousand Oaks, CA: Sage Publications.

Hofstede, G. (2001). *Culture's consequences: Comparing values, behaviors, institutions* (2nd ed.). Thousand Oaks, CA: Sage Publications.

Iwama, M. (2003). Toward culturally relevant epistemologies in occupational therapy. *American Journal of Occupational Therapy, 57*(5), 582-588.

Iwama, M. (2004). Meaning and inclusion: Revisiting culture in occupational therapy. [Guest editorial]. *Australian Occupational Therapy Journal, 51*(1), 1-2.

Iwama, M. (2006). *The KAWA model: Culturally relevant occupational therapy.* Toronto, Ontario: Churchill Livingstone.

Kim, B. M. (1996). *The impact of cross-cultural practice on multicultural competence among occupational therapists*. Unpublished master's thesis. Chicago, IL: Rush University.

Kondo, T. (2004). Cultural tensions in occupational therapy practice: Considerations from a Japanese vantage point. *American Journal of Occupational Therapy, 58*(2), 174-184.

Lattanzi, J. B., & Purnell, L. D. (2006). *Developing cultural competence in physical therapy practice*. Philadelphia, PA: F.A. Davis.

Law, M. (1998). *Client-centered occupational therapy*. Thorofare, NJ: SLACK Incorporated.

Law, M., Baptiste, S., & Mills, J. (1995). Client-centred practice: What does it mean and does it make a difference? *Canadian Journal of Occupational Therapy, 62*(5), 250-257.

Lewis, J. (2002). *Cultural studies: The basics*. Thousand Oaks, CA: Sage Publications.

Lynch, E. W., & Hanson, M. J. (Eds.). (1998). *Developing cross-cultural competencies: A guide for working with children and their families* (2nd ed.). Baltimore, MD: Brookes Publishing Company.

McIntosh, P. (1988). *White privilege and male privilege: A personal account of coming to see correspondences through work in women's studies*. (Working paper No. 189). Wellesley, MA: Wellesley College Center for Research on Women.

Mendias, E. P., & Guevara, E. B. (2001). Assessing culturally competent scholarship. *Journal of Professional Nursing, 17*(5), 256-266.

Odawara, E. (2005). Cultural competency in occupational therapy: Beyond a cross-cultural view of practice. *American Journal of Occupational Therapy, 59*(3), 325-334.

O'Hara-Devereaux, M., & Johansen, R. (1994). *Globalwork: Bridging distance, culture and time*. San Francisco, CA: Jossey-Bass. Excerpt retrieved June 7, 2008, from http://www.csub.edu/TLC/options/resources/handouts/fac_dev/culturalbarries.html

Pollock, N. (1993). Client-centered assessment. *American Journal of Occupational Therapy, 47*(4), 298-301.

Pope-Davis, D. B., Prieto, L. R., Whitaker, C. M., & Pope-Davis, S. A. (1993). Exploring multicultural competencies of occupational therapists: Implications for education and training. *American Journal of Occupational Therapy, 47*(9), 838-844.

Price, E. G., Beach, M. C., Gary, T. L., Robinson, K. A., Gozu, A., Palacio, A., et al. (2005). A systematic review of the methodological rigor of studies evaluating cultural competence training of health professionals. *Academic Medicine: Journal of the Association of American Medical Colleges, 80*(6), 578-586.

Rogers, C. R. (1951). *Client-centered therapy*. Boston, MA: Houghton-Mifflin.

Schilder, A. J., Kennedy, C., Goldstone, I. L., Ogden, R. D., Hogg, R. S., & O'Shaughnessy, M. V. (2001). "Being dealt with as a whole person." Care seeking and adherence: The benefits of culturally competent care. *Social Science & Medicine, 52*(11), 1643-1659.

Schim, S. M., Doorenbos, A. Z., Miller, J., & Benkert, R. (2003). Development of a Cultural Competence Assessment instrument. *Journal of Nursing Measurement, 11*(1), 29-40.

Scott, R. (1997). Investigation of cross-cultural practice: Implications for curriculum development. *Canadian Journal of Occupational Therapy, 64*(2), 89-96.

Smith, L. S. (1998). Cultural competence for nurses: Canonical correlation of two culture scales. *Journal of Cultural Diversity, 5*(4), 120-126.

Sumsion, T. (1993). Client-centered practice: The true impact. *Canadian Journal of Occupational Therapy, 60*(1), 6-8.

Sumsion, T. (Ed.). (1999). *Client-centered practice in occupational therapy: A guide to implementation*. New York, NY: Churchill Livingstone.

Townsend, E., & Whiteford, G. (2005). A participatory occupational justice framework. In F. Kronenberg, S. Algado, & N. Pollard (Eds.), *Occupational therapy without borders: Learning from the spirit of survivors* (pp. 110-126). Edinburgh, Scotland: Churchill Livingstone.

U.S. Department of Health and Human Services, Office of Minority Health. (2001). *National standards for culturally and linguistically appropriate services in health care*. Washington, DC: Author.

Vaughan, W. (2005). Educating for diversity, social responsibility and action: Preservice teachers engage in immersion experiences. *Journal of Cultural Diversity, 12*(1), 26-30.

Vinh-Thomas, P., Bunch, M. M., & Card, J. J. (2003). A research-based tool for identifying and strengthening culturally competent and evaluation-ready HIV-AIDS prevention programs. *AIDS Education & Prevention, 15*(6), 481-498.

Weaver, H. N. (1999). Indigenous people and the social work profession: Defining culturally competent services. *Social Work, 44*(3), 217-225.

Wells, S. A., & Black, R. M. (2000). *Cultural competency for health professionals*. Bethesda, MD: AOTA Press.

Whiteford, G. E., & Wilcock, A. A. (2000). Cultural relativism: Occupation and independence reconsidered. *Canadian Journal of Occupational Therapy, 67*(5), 324-336.

Wittman, P., & Velde, B. P. (2002). Attaining cultural competence, critical thinking, and intellectual development: A challenge of occupational therapists. *American Journal of Occupational Therapy, 56*(4), 454-456.

# Section II

## Basic Tenets of Occupational Therapy

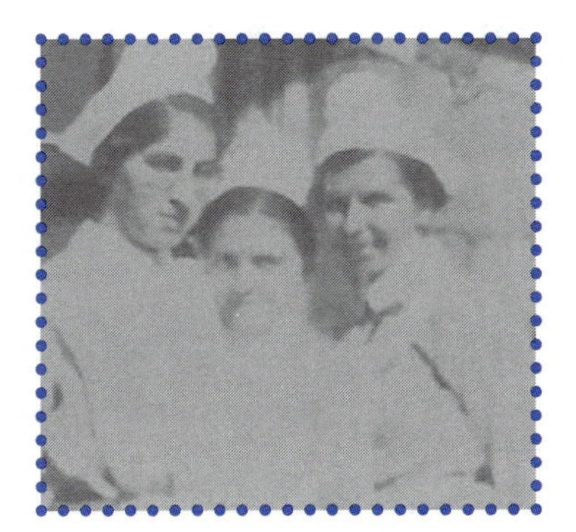

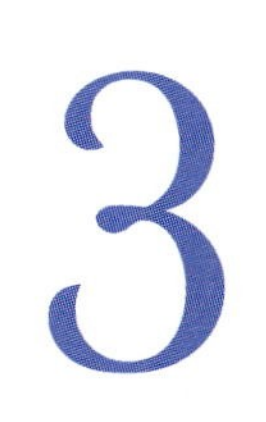

# History and Philosophy

Cheryl Kuczynski, MOT, OTR/L and Celeste M. Richard, MOT, OTR/L

**ACOTE Standard Explored in This Chapter**

B.2.1

**Key Terms**

| | |
|---|---|
| Arts and Crafts movement | Deinstitutionalization |
| Certified occupational therapy assistant | Moral Treatment movement |
| | Rehabilitation movement |

## Introduction

Occupational therapy has a deep and rich history—one that can be traced back as early as the 1800s. It is believed that occupational therapy's deepest roots can be found in the Moral Treatment movement. Many believe the history of moral treatment in America is not only synonymous with but is the history of occupational therapy before it acquired its 20th century name of "occupational therapy" (Bockoven, 1971). Similar to occupational therapy, the philosophy of moral treatment is based on the respect and dignity for all humans and their need to participate in daily occupations.

Philippe Pinel, a French physician, is often credited with being the first to coin the term *moral treatment* in 1801. Pinel, based on his own beliefs, established practices that led to a more human approach to treating persons with mental illnesses (Sladyk & Ryan, 2001). Pinel's beliefs were heavily influential throughout Europe; however, he did not have a distinct following in America.

Samuel Tuke, grandson of William Tuke, was responsible for popularizing moral treatment within the English Quaker society. The Tuke family was among the most influential leaders in England (Sladyk & Ryan, 2001). In the late 1700s, William Tuke founded the York Retreat in York, England. Tuke, like Pinel, believed chains and punishment would not help a person with a mental illness recover. Rather, he encouraged the client to learn self-control, and engaged him or her in a variety of employment or amusements best adapted to him or her (Sladyk & Ryan, 2001). During this time, American Quakers began to visit retreats in England and returned with the concepts of "occupation and non-restraint." In 1817, American Quakers, based on their beliefs of moral treatment, constructed the Friend's Asylum for the Insane in Pennsylvania. The Friend's Asylum was the first mental health hospital in America used solely for the purpose of providing moral treatment (Peloquin, 1989).

Throughout the early 19th century, moral treatment hospitals continued to come into existence. Within these hospitals, physicians altered the client's environment to include humane treatment, a routine of work and recreation, an appeal to reason, and the development of desirable moral traits (Peloquin, 1989). Goals of mental wellness were met through recreational and craft shops. Moral treatment was an effective means to recovery from mental illness, and its effectiveness may be attributed to the comprehensive occupational recreational program (Bockoven, 1971).



K. Sladyk, K. Jacobs, & N. MacRae (Eds.).
*Occupational Therapy Essentials for Clinical Competence* (pp. 25-32).

The Arts and Crafts movement was an extreme transformation of the American lifestyle and was created in response to workers and their working environments. In its beginning years, the Arts and Crafts movement was widespread and deeply influential (Levine, 1987). Prior to the establishment of the Arts and Crafts movement, employees were required to work in less-than-satisfactory environments with poor ventilation and exposure to toxic agents (Rayback, 1966). It was believed that these conditions and the machinery used contributed to the deterioration of the workers' general health and happiness. Many felt as though the focus of the American civilization was shifting. It was believed that machines were replacing hardworking individuals. John Ruskin, an early pioneer of the movement, felt as though humans were being perceived as an extension of their machines, only present to assist machines in making the final merchandise (Levine). Detecting a decline in workers' general health, Ruskin set forth to change what our civilization was becoming. He believed the sole solution was to return to an authentic lifestyle.

Americans began to feel the effects of the Arts and Crafts movement in the early 20th century. Advocates of the movement urged fellow Americans to return to a genuine lifestyle, which included farming, using natural materials, and producing and purchasing items that were simple in design (Levine, 1987). For many, the Arts and Crafts movement was not only about authenticity resurfacing, but human dignity and quality of life resurfacing.

In the 1900s, Dr. Herbert James Hall and several other physicians developed sheltered workshops. Sheltered workshops had a significant purpose of returning clients to an authentic lifestyle and increasing their quality of life. Clients were responsible for designing and producing products that were to be sold in local shops. Dr. Hall believed that the producing and selling of the products had three important purposes (Levine, 1987):

1. Employing talented people who could earn a living by making authentic objects
2. Providing spiritual support to craftspeople who pursued crafts as an avocation
3. Helping employ the persons with mental and physical challenges

It was soon revealed that the role of craft work on clients was significant for improving both physical and mental health (Kielhofner, 2004), and rehabilitation goals could be attained by applying the concepts of the Arts and Crafts movement to the persons with physical and mental challenges. Arts and crafts became a central focus of the early occupational therapy practice as demonstrated by several early founders, including George Edward Barton, Susan E. Tracy, and Eleanor Clarke Slagle (Cole & Tufano, 2008).

# Early Pioneers of Occupational Therapy

When reviewing history, it is evident that many of the founders of occupational therapy were the doctors, nurses, and craftsmen engaged in using activities to help clients with mental illness experience the feeling of productivity (Woodside, 1971). Dr. William Rush Dunton, Jr., a physician, believed that occupation served as a means of restoring a person's way of thinking, feeling, and acting normal. Dunton believed that the hospital environment should be modeled after normal living so the client could learn appropriate behaviors for functioning in daily life. According to Dunton:

> The client should be taught sportsmanship in sports and craftsmanship in workshop activities. Learning with these activities provided a basis upon which the client could progress toward workmanship and citizenship in the community (Kielhofner & Burke, 1977, p. 680).

Based on his beliefs and interests in occupation as a means for intervention, Dunton published the text *Occupational Therapy, A Manual for Nurses* in 1915. Dunton is also credited for first proposing the establishment of a national association of occupational therapists, for which he served as President from 1917 to 1919 (Dunton, 1967).

Mr. George Edward Barton, an architect, was one of the many forefathers of occupational therapy. Having suffered from tuberculosis, Barton had his own personal experience with a disability. As a result of having frequent and recurrent attacks of tuberculosis, Barton was a victim of left hemiparesis. Realizing he would not be able to return to architectural work, he assisted in his own recovery by performing manual work—primarily carpentry and gardening (Licht, 1967). Being so successful with his recovery, he became determined to devote the rest of his life to the reclamation of the "sick and disabled" (Licht).

Soon after his recovery, Barton became highly interested in occupation as therapy. In 1914, Barton purchased a house, which he named the Consolation House. The Consolation House was a school, a workshop, and a vocational bureau (Licht, 1967) where clients could return to occupations as a means for recovery. While at the Consolation House, Barton began to study the effects of occupation on the clients referred to him by local physicians.

It has been considered on several occasions that Barton was the first to coin the term *occupational therapy*, having first made reference to occupational therapy as "occupational nursing" in his early literature. According to Barton, a proper occupation promoted physical improvement, clarified and strengthened the mind, and could become the basis or the corollary of a new life upon recovery (Peloquin, 1991a). Barton believed that occupational therapy services should be provided from a skilled and highly trained nurse—one who understood both medicine and occupations. According to Barton, the role of the nurse/therapist was to ensure harmony between occupational and medical interventions and to use a frame of reference for intervention broader than but parallel to medicine (Peloquin, 1991a). Nurses were instructed when developing an intervention to be aware of the person's mental, physical, and spiritual strengths, goals, and ambitions (Peloquin, 1991a).

Susan E. Tracy, a nurse, valued occupation for the happiness and changed attitude it produced and for that attitude's curative effect on disabilities (Peloquin, 1991a). Licht (1967) believed that no one did more in this country to resurrect and establish occupational therapy than did Tracy. During her formal training at Massachusetts Homeopathic Hospital, Tracy made several clinical observations that the clients on the surgical wards who passed the time working were usually happier than those who remained idle (Licht). With this hypothesis, she began to view occupation as a means for the nursing profession to help care for the whole person (Peloquin, 1991a). As director of the nurses' training school at the Adams Nervine Asylum in Boston, Massachusetts, Tracy intertwined her observations and beliefs into her students' coursework. In 1906, Tracy's program became the first course in the United States designed to prepare instructors for clients' activities (Licht, 1948).

In 1910, Tracy published the first American book on occupational therapy, *Studies in Invalid Occupations: A Manual for Nurses and Attendants* (Levine, 1987; Licht, 1967; Peloquin, 1991a). Based on Tracy's 1906 training course, the manual was geared toward nurses. However, it was also extended to those competent persons (attendants) who had not been formally trained in nursing (Peloquin). Levine described Tracy's work as a craft book that offered teaching strategies, supply lists, and intervention rationales for a variety of settings, including the homes of advantaged and disadvantaged clients.

One of the most influential physicians to contribute to the promotion of occupational therapy was Dr. Herbert James Hall. Hall was well known within the Harvard University community for his studies on treating clients with neurasthenia. Persons with neurasthenia presented severe weakness when performing any work activity (Kielhofner, 2004). Influenced by the Arts and Crafts movement and not satisfied with the recovery of clients treated with bed rest, Hall began using occupations as intervention. After receiving a grant from Harvard University, Hall began performing his study on the correlation between occupation and neurasthenia. During his study, clients performed progressive and graded manual occupations such as needlework (Dunton, 1967). Significant findings were reported, and great attention was given from the medical society. In total, Hall wrote 3 books on occupational therapy and trained nearly 60 women (Dunton).

Adolph Meyer's greatest contribution to the field of occupational therapy was his presentation of the first organized model of occupational therapy in 1921. His lecture, "The Philosophy of Occupation Therapy," was not only thought provoking, but it was also the first article in *Archives of Occupational Therapy.* Throughout his lecture, Meyer engaged his audience to continually think of what occupation really means and its benefits to persons throughout the country. Meyer also challenged the audience to think about what their role was in treating clients. Meyer (1977) believed that the main role was not to give prescriptions but rather to give opportunities to work; to do, plan, and create; and to learn to use material. According to Meyer, providing clients with opportunities was necessary to maintain a balance between work and play, and rest and sleep. A balance between these four factors helped promote achievement in healthy harmony with human nature (Meyer).

## National Society for the Promotion of Occupational Therapy

The idea of developing an association for those interested in occupational therapy was formulated shortly after Dunton published *Occupational Therapy, A Manual for Nurses.* Having been influenced by reading the text, Barton developed the idea of creating an organization for persons interested in occupational therapy. Barton wrote to Dunton, expressing his ideas on developing a national society. Dunton replied with great enthusiasm. Recognizing a need for occupational therapists to unite, Dunton and Barton sought to establish a national society for occupational therapy (Woodside, 1971). Soon after, Dunton and Barton selected several individuals to attend the association's first meeting, which was to be held at Barton's Consolation House.

According to Licht (1967), Barton lost interest in the association in an early meeting, but Dunton persisted in the belief that there should be a national society. Not only did Barton lose interest, but he was in disbelief that a national society could be formed. Barton felt as though many workers were interested in arts and crafts, not therapy (Licht).

Dunton is credited with establishing the National Society for the Promotion of Occupational Therapy (Woodside, 1971) based on his persistence and motivation to hold the first initial meeting on October 17, 1917. The six attendees and contributors of the first meeting included Susan Cox Johnson, George Edward Barton, Eleanor Clarke Slagle, William Rush Dunton, Jr., Isabel Gladwin Newton, and Thomas B. Kidner. Four of the six founders are numbered among its presidents, including Barton (1917), Dunton (1917-1919), Slagle (1919-1920), and Kidner (1923-1928) (Dunton, 1967).

The purpose of the Society was "to provide information and assistance to all who are desirous of teaching the work, or who are interested in it" (Dunton, 1967, p. 288). Dunton stated, "Let us all unite to make this society a success and promote the cause of occupation therapy" (p. 289). The association surprisingly expanded. By 1921 there were 450 members; in 1928, there were 803 (Woodside, 1971). These practitioners were diverse, coming from the mental health field, the military, and from newly trained students (Woodside, 1971). In 1924, the organization changed its name to the American Occupational Therapy Association (AOTA). Each of the founding members, in addition to Dunton, provided his or her own unique perspective of occupational therapy.

Eleanor Clarke Slagle was born in New York in 1876. She graduated from the Chicago School of Civics and Philanthropy. In 1913, she became director of the occupational therapy department in the Henry Phipps Psychiatric Clinic of the Johns Hopkins Hospital (Licht, 1967). As time passed, Slagle held every office in the National Society for the Promotion of Occupational Therapy and held those offices for a longer period of time than any other individual, holding the presidency from 1919 to 1920 and serving as secretary-treasurer for 15 years (Licht). As a founder, she was very influential in establishing the policies and procedures of the organization, seeking high standards and professional recognition ("Presidents of the American Occupational Therapy Association," 1976). With such an impact on the profession, the Eleanor Clarke Slagle Lectureship—the highest award given to any member of the AOTA—was created in her honor in 1955, 13 years after her death.

Thomas B. Kidner was born in England where he received an education in architecture and building construction. Kidner went to Canada in 1900 to promote the reform of education in schools and improvement of school buildings. He joined the National Tuberculosis Association with an expertise in hospital operation, construction, and remodeling for individuals with disabilities ("Presidents," 1976). Kidner was president of the Society from 1923 to 1928, working to make further gains to establish occupational therapy as a profession. As a founder, Kidner began as chair of the International Committee. Dunton believed that his "chief objects in life...[were] to prevent the convalescent soldier from falling into habits of idleness and self indulgence..." (1967, p. 288).

Susan Cox Johnson was born in Texas in 1876. She was educated in Berkeley, California where she studied arts and crafts. She later taught the subject in both the United States and Asia. As the Society formed, she was invited by Columbia University to teach occupational therapy. As a founder, she began as the chair of the Committee on Admissions and Positions (Licht, 1967). When speaking of Johnson, Dunton stated, "Besides the general humanitarian interest in making her clients better by making them more contented, she believes that the work which they turn out should have both artistic and commercial value" (1967, p. 288).

Isabel Gladwin Newton was born in 1891 in New York, where she was educated and became a secretary. She worked for Barton in 1916 and, due to convenience, became the secretary of the Society. She married Barton in 1918 (Licht, 1967). In 1921, with Hall as president, the name "National Society for the Promotion of Occupational Therapy" was changed to the "American Occupational Therapy Association" (Peloquin, 1991a). With the increase in membership, a new constitution was established to include a Board of Managers and a House of Delegates. With the rise of members and the leadership of the six founders, occupational therapy expanded into the 1920s.

## Educational Standards Over the Years

As the new profession of occupational therapy became more recognized and respected, the educational standards started to change. The first documented course to train practitioners was Susan Tracy's "Invalid Occupations for Student Nurses," held at the Massachusetts General Hospital. Prior to Susan Tracy's training course, programs were supervised by physicians and carried out by craftsmen or untrained individuals (Woodside, 1971). "Invalid Occupations" replaced craftsmen with nurses as trained occupational therapy practitioners. Several other courses, such as Dr. Dunton's "Occupation Therapy" lectures held at the Sheppard and Enoch Pratt Hospital, were becoming very popular throughout the country.

With the demand for practitioners increasing, professional schools began opening. The first occupational therapy school within an academic setting to open was the Milwaukee-Dower College in 1918. Soon after, many other occupational therapy schools began to develop. Early occupational therapy schools included the Philadelphia School of Occupational Therapy, the St. Louis School for Reconstruction Aides, and the Boston School of Occupational Therapy (Woodside, 1971).

After the establishment of the first occupational therapy schools, it was recognized that there was a need for organization between the national association and the educational schools. In 1923, two actions were established: the *Essentials for Professional Education* by the AOTA and the *Council on Medical Education of the American Medical Association* were published, and the process of registration by examination administered by the professional association was created (Woodside, 1971).

## Effects of World War I

Prior to World War I, occupational therapy's philosophy was primarily applied to clients with illnesses. Afterward, however, emphasis was placed more on clients with physical limitations as a result of war casualties. World War I created a forceful movement in occupational therapy by providing a new and exciting opportunity for practice.

Dr. Frankwood Williams, a military psychiatrist, was the first to bring occupations to the battle grounds during World War I. Having been familiar with the benefits of occupation therapy, Williams repeatedly asked his superiors for occupational workers to accompany his hospital unit Base Hospital 117 in France (Punwar, 1994). His request for occupational workers was denied, but Williams remained confident as he searched for women to fulfill his request. Finally, he convinced a small group of women with some training in arts and crafts to join the hospital unit team as "scrubwomen" (Punwar).

With little to no money or supplies, this small group of "scrubwomen" traveled to France to assist Williams in creating the craft shop he had envisioned. Long days eventually paid off when the craft shop opened its doors. Soldiers flocked to the craft shop, first out of curiosity and then out of interest in the craft work available (Low, 1992). The craft shop was so successful that scrubwomen became a recognized category of hospital worker (Punwar, 1994).

The greatest effect World War I had on the profession of occupational therapy was the population of individuals being treated. After seeing the positive results of using occupations on clients with physical limitations, the emphasis of occupational therapy shifted gears. Army and Navy hospitals expanded, and the Veterans' Bureau began in 1922 with 57 hospitals and a caseload of 1 million (Woodside, 1971).

The 1920s were associated with the post-World War I boom. This economic boom resulted in an increase in the number of hospitals and, in turn, a greater need for occupational therapists whose services were finally recognized. Between 1917 and 1920, the number of hospitals more than doubled (Cole & Tufano, 2008). Rehabilitation services were being seen as a right for all individuals. The Smith-Bankhead Bill of 1920 established the basis for federal vocational rehabilitation. The bill emphasized vocation as a way to reclaim individuals who were unemployed by educating them vocationally regardless of their disability (Woodside, 1971). This bill led the way for further legislation and public acceptance of rehabilitation and occupational therapy (Woodside). With the expanding field, the need for standardizing occupational therapy and its education was recognized.

In the early 1920s, Susan Cox Johnson and Elizabeth Upham Davis, as chairs of the Committee on Admissions and Positions, felt that their duties included standardizing education requirements, developing a laddering of practitioners, and researching information about then-current medical conditions common in occupational therapy. Johnson believed that training schools should be placed in educational institutions because a certified system would eliminate independent emergency schools associated with the war. Many felt that by raising the educational standards, those practitioners who were educated in war emergency schools would lose their credibility. Johnson felt that all occupational therapists should hold college degrees to gain further acceptance by other professions. In 1923, the "Minimum Standards for Courses of Training in Occupational Therapy" was adopted by the AOTA by a unanimous vote (Quiroga, 1995).

The standards covered three major areas: prerequisites for admission to training programs, length of courses, and content of courses (Quiroga, 1995). These requirements changed through the years, and by 1930, the age requirement was to be 21 years old by graduation with students having at least 2 years of training in arts and crafts, education, nursing, or social service. The minimum length of course work was 15 months in 1927, which was extended to 18 months by 1930. The standards stated a required time for medical lectures, which increased from 75 hours in 1923 to 165 hours in 1930. Hospital practice and craft training also increased from 1,080 hours in 1923 to 2,300 hours in 1930 (Quiroga). Instruction was required in areas of psychology, anatomy, kinesiology, orthopedics, mental diseases, tuberculosis, and general medical cases (Peloquin, 1991b). By 1925, a committee of physicians, including Dunton, created an outline to be used for lectures given to medical students, which was accepted as a guide for the AOTA. The outline illustrated that occupational therapy is a form of educating the physically or mentally ill by way of training and service in productive tasks (Bing, 1981). The outline also exemplified that the activities be selected with the consideration of the client's interests and capabilities (Bing). With a change toward standardization, many believed that a push toward the medical model would further enhance the profession.

In 1923, the Federal Industrial Rehabilitation Act required every hospital that dealt with industrial accidents or illness to employ occupational therapists to treat affected individuals (Rerek, 1971). With an increase of occupational therapy services in the hospital setting, an alliance with physicians was seen as beneficial. The 1920s showed a shift in the profession from women's volunteer work to medicine. Occupational therapy was being required by physicians' prescriptions and was adopting medical standards for recordkeeping (Quiroga, 1995). The AOTA looked toward the American Medical Association (AMA) to assist in establishing standards for training institutions and to accredit the new educational facilities, which also helped to enforce the new standards being put into place. By the end of the 1920s, occupational therapy was formally considered a medical ancillary service (Rerek). The expansion and gains of occupational therapy were halted with the stock market crash of 1929 and the Depression to follow.

## The Great Depression and World War II

The Great Depression affected the United States from 1929 to 1941, and health care experienced setbacks along with all fields. Even though physicians and hospitals lowered their fees between 1929 and 1933, spending on health care decreased 33% (Rerek, 1971). The Depression and the National Economy Act of 1933 were causes of the budget cuts affecting occupational therapy, resulting in a decrease in personnel and the closing of clinics and even schools of occupational therapy (Hopkins & Smith, 1993). With cutbacks, the profession of occupational therapy was not prepared for the onset of World War II.

World War II was responsible for bringing the United States out of the Depression, but the effects of the Depression on health care were lasting. Services to meet the needs of the returning wounded veterans were inadequate. During World War I, occupational therapists failed to receive military status, and without status, funding was not guaranteed in World War II, leading to a shortage of services. There were only 12 people in the United States army working in occupational therapy, only 8 of whom were actual registered therapists (Hopkins & Smith, 1993). As veterans began to return home, it became evident that there were few facilities available to them in the areas of rehabilitation and long-term care. Families and educational institutions were not able to provide the care these veterans needed to reintegrate into the community. The medical field pushed to fix the physical problems, not recognizing the need for long-term care. The families and the veterans soon sought the right for the care they deserved, and the government responded (Rerek, 1971).

In 1947, occupational therapists finally achieved military status (Messick, 1947). With newfound military status; the New Deal, which provided social security income for those with disabilities; and the GI Bill, which provided funding for vocational training, there was now adequate funding for occupational therapy services (Cole & Tufano, 2008). Along with the Vocational Rehabilitation Act and amendments of 1943, which allowed for the payment of medical services, occupational therapy was covered (Harvey-Krefting, 1985). Recognizing the health care system's inability to respond to the number of wounded vets returning from the war, society pushed for a rehabilitation movement.

## Rehabilitation Movement

The Rehabilitation movement began with a change in the way society viewed those with disabilities. Society was beginning to believe that with the proper care, individuals with disabilities could become independent and contributing members of the community (Mosey, 1971). Rehabilitation was believed to have not just physical advantages, but also economical as the number of people with disabilities grew due to medical advances (Mosey). At this time, occupational therapists functioned on a technical level. Intervention focused on ambulation, reconditioning exercises, and fitting and training in prosthetics and orthotics (Mosey). Therapists received training in activities of daily living, progressive resistive exercise, and neuromuscular facilitation and inhibition (Kielhofner, 2004). Intervention was done without a connection to theory or frames of reference. During this period, occupational therapy was recognized as a valuable service, but the profession still failed in recruiting and training enough professionals to meet the demands of the growing populations in need of services.

In 1956, occupational therapy made a move toward increasing the manpower of its profession. In this year, a report was created to recognize nonprofessional personnel in the career of occupational therapy. These individuals were trained to work alongside registered occupational therapists and given the title "occupational therapy assistant" (Hopkins & Smith, 1993). In 1958, a 3-month educational program was created to educate personnel in the area of mental health, and by 1960, programs began to educate personnel to assist with general practice as well (Punwar, 1994). The first programs created to educate occupational therapy assistants were found in hospitals and later expanded to technical and community colleges. Occupational therapy assistants were employed to enhance and expand current occupational therapy services by providing additional assistance (Sladyk & Ryan, 2001). The need for and the creation of the occupational therapy assistant marked an important milestone for occupational therapy as the profession moved into the 1960s.

The 1960s was a time of protest and social reform. Society protested everything from the Vietnam War, civil rights, and racial integration, to institutions such as prisons and mental hospitals (Cole & Tufano, 2008). Society believed the rights of the individuals in these institutions were being violated. It was felt that they would lead more productive lives in the community. These feelings lead to the deinstitutionalization of mental hospitals and residential institutions for persons with retardation. As individuals were discharged, it became evident that community programs did not exist to provide these individuals with the support they needed (Torrey, 1988). Occupational therapy itself soon began to move to a more community-based model.

## Community Versus Medical Model

Occupational therapists began to believe that their profession might fit better with an educational or social model rather than the medical model, which emphasized pathology. Clients' problems could not simply be explained in medical terms, leading to the concept of a multidisciplinary approach (Diasio, 1971). People began to take responsibility about their own health, which lead to an increase in prevention and wellness. Occupational therapists began to take on roles in education, prevention, screening, and health maintenance (Punwar, 1994). Technological advances allowed for a higher survival rate and specialization in the medical field. Some occupational therapists began to specialize in areas such as hand therapy, spinal cord injuries, burns, and sensory integration. More children with disabilities were surviving birth, the elderly were living longer, and stress was on an increase along with drug and alcohol abuse, all adding to the populations with whom occupational therapists already worked (Punwar). With the growing and changing populations, health care services legislation was soon created in an attempt to make services available to all who needed them.

In 1963, the Community Mental Health Act required mental health services be provided on a variety of levels, including inpatient, outpatient, emergency services, and community and educational programs. Increased services in the 1970s aided the transition from institutions to the community (Cole & Tufano, 2008). In 1965, new legislation was created as Medicare became law. With Medicare, occupational therapy services were now covered for inpatient and limited outpatient. Medicaid soon followed, both providing health care to persons with disabilities and who were poor (Coombs, 2005). As occupational therapy transitioned into the 1970s, the AOTA sought to find the common thread connecting all of the newly specialized areas of occupational therapy.

During this time, many leaders of the profession created frames of reference to reflect the diversity of the profession (Cole & Tufano, 2008). By the end of the 1970s, the AOTA created the Representative Assembly, and in 1979, *Uniform Terminology* sought to unify the practice under one set of guidelines of documentation (Cole & Tufano). In 1975, legislation continued to increase as the Education of Handicapped Children Act (Cengage Learning, n.d.) was passed. The law mandated that children with disabilities receive free and appropriate education (Cengage). With this act and its future amendments, occupational therapy moved into the school systems. In 1989, with the publication of *Uniform Terminology for Occupational Therapy, Second Edition*, a common language and definition of the practice was found. As the 1980s approached, occupational therapy found a need to support the profession through research.

## Setting the Stage for Research

The 1970s and 1980s showed a steady increase in the number of graduate programs available to occupational therapists and the number of individuals entering those programs. The need for further education and research was found necessary as the profession sought to gain acceptance. Research was needed to determine the reliability of assessments and intervention techniques and the cost effectiveness of occupational therapy (Punwar, 1994). By the 1990s, research was being published by scholars and doctoral-level students, providing evidence of the effectiveness of occupational therapy services and intervention.

The profession was beginning to gain respect in the medical community. With the Americans With Disabilities Act (ADA) of 1990, the need for occupational therapists grew, creating a booming job market and a need for occupational therapy education. The ADA made any discrimination of people with disabilities illegal in all settings. The ADA addressed architectural barriers that prevented an individual from participating or using a facility, as well as environmental modifications that would allow for the buildings' use (U.S. Equal Employment Opportunity Commission, n.d.). Occupational therapists served as an advocate for those individuals. The late 1990s also brought attempts to control runaway Medicare spending, resulting in downsizing many rehabilitation programs. At the same time, AOTA passed a resolution to mandate that the profession move to an entry-level master of science degree, done in part to compete with the other health care fields such as physical therapy (Cole & Tufano, 2008). Today, the profession continues to make gains—it is in demand and services have become diverse.

Occupational therapy has continued to move away from the medical model and focus on a client-centered approach. Occupational therapists look at clients' needs and wants to create intervention plans especially tailored to them. The importance of cultural diversity has been recognized and put into practice. The health care system continues to change, as does the reimbursement system for services. Fee-for-services gave way to managed care and a third-party payer who determined what was covered (Punwar, 1994). With the influence of the pioneers and early founders of the profession, occupational therapy has advanced to be an accepted and admired health care profession.

## Summary

Our early leaders would have never thought about evidence-based practice, the concept of the Internet supporting best practice, or even the diverse settings in which occupational therapy practitioners work. To fully honor those practitioners who worked so hard to form the foundations of occupational therapy, current practitioners must understand and respect what came ahead of their work. Understanding the history of our past allows us to plan better for our future.

## Student Self-Assessment

1. Describe the Moral Treatment movement and key figures.
2. Explain the shift to the Arts and Crafts movement.
3. Name the six founders of the National Society for the Promotion of Occupational Therapy and one key contribution of each.

4. How did World War I impact the field of occupational therapy?
5. Describe the Rehabilitation movement.
6. Describe the shift from a medical model to a community model.
7. Explain the need for research.

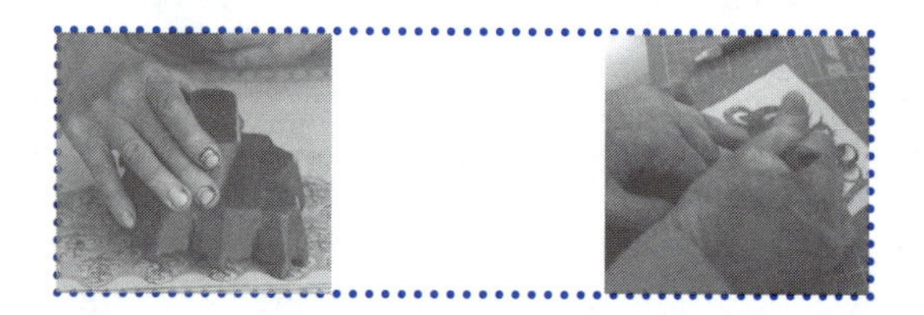

# References


Bing, R. K. (1981). Eleanor Clarke Slagle Lectureship—1981. Occupational therapy revisited: A paraphrastic journey. *American Journal of Occupational Therapy, 35*(8), 499-517.

Bockoven, J. S. (1971). Occupational therapy—a historical perspective. Legacy of moral treatment—1800s to 1910. *American Journal of Occupational Therapy, 25*(5), 223-225.

Cengage Learning. (n.d.). The Education For All Handicapped Children Act (PL 94-142) 1975. Retrieved July 31, 2009, from http://college.cengage.com/education/resources/res_prof/students/spec_ed/legislation/pl_94-142.html

Cole, M. B., & Tufano, R. (2008). *Applied theories in occupational therapy: A practical approach.* Thorofare, NJ: SLACK Incorporated.

Coombs, J. G. (2005). *The rise and fall of HMOs: An American health care revolution.* Madison, WS: The University of Wisconsin Press.

Diasio, K. (1971). The modern era—1960-1970. *American Journal of Occupational Therapy, 25*(5), 237-242.

Dunton, W. R. (1967). Occupations and amusements: Organization of the National Society for Promotion of Occupational Therapy. Reprinted in *American Journal of Occupational Therapy, 21*(5), 287-289.

Harvey-Krefting, L. (1985). The concept of work in occupational therapy: A historical review. *American Journal of Occupational Therapy, 39*(5), 301-307.

Hopkins, H. L., & Smith, H. D. (Eds.). (1993). *Willard & Spackman's occupational therapy* (8th ed.). Philadelphia, PA: J. B. Lippincott.

Kielhofner, G., & Burke, J. P. (1977). Occupational therapy after 60 years: An account of changing identity and knowledge. *American Journal of Occupational Therapy, 31*(10), 675-689.

Kielhofner, G. (2004). *Conceptual foundations of occupational therapy* (3rd ed.). Philadelphia, PA: F.A. Davis Company.

Levine, R. (1987). The influence of the arts-and-crafts movement on the professional status of occupational therapy. *American Journal of Occupational Therapy, 41*(4), 248-254.

Licht, S. (1948). *Occupational therapy sourcebook.* Baltimore, MD: Williams & Wilkins.

Licht, S. (1967). The founding and founders of the American Occupational Therapy Association. *American Journal of Occupational Therapy, 21*(5), 269-277.

Low, J. F. (1992). The reconstruction aides. *American Journal of Occupational Therapy, 46*(1), 38-43.

Messick, H. E. (1947). The new women's medical specialist corps. *American Journal of Occupational Therapy, 1*(5), 298-300.

Meyer, A. (1977). The philosophy of occupation therapy. *American Journal of Occupational Therapy, 31*, 639-642.

Mosey, A. C. (1971). Involvement in the rehabilitation movement—1942-1960. *American Journal of Occupational Therapy, 25*(5), 234-236.

Peloquin, S. M. (1989). Moral treatment: Contexts considered. *American Journal of Occupational Therapy, 43*(8), 537-544.

Peloquin, S. M. (1991a). Occupational therapy service: Individual and collective understandings of the founders, part 1. *American Journal of Occupational Therapy, 45*(4), 352-360.

Peloquin, S. M. (1991b). Occupational therapy service: Individual and collective understandings of the founders, part 2. *American Journal of Occupational Therapy, 45*(8), 733-744.

Presidents of the American Occuaptional Therapy Assocation (1917-1967). (1976). *American Journal of Occupational Therapy, 21*(5), 290-298.

Punwar, A. J. (1994). *Occupational therapy: Principles and practice* (2nd ed.). Baltimore, MD: Williams & Wilkins.

Quiroga, V. A. M. (1995). *Occupational therapy: The first 30 years, 1900 to 1930.* Bethesda, MD: AOTA Press.

Rayback, J. G. (1966). *A history of American labor.* New York, NY: Free Press.

Rerek, M. D. (1971). The depression years—1929-1941. *American Journal of Occupational Therapy, 25*(5), 231-233.

Sladyk, K., & Ryan, S. E. (2001). *Ryan's occupational therapy assistant* (3rd ed.). Thorofare, NJ: SLACK Incorporated.

Torrey, E. F. (1988). *Nowhere to go: The tragic odyssey of the homeless mentally ill.* New York, NY: HarperCollins.

U.S. Equal Employment Opportunity Commission. (n.d.). American with Disabilities Act (ADA): 1990–2002. Retrieved July 31, 2009, from http://www.eeoc.gov/ada

Woodside, H. H. (1971). The development of occupational therapy 1910-1929. *American Journal of Occupational Therapy, 25*(5), 226-230.

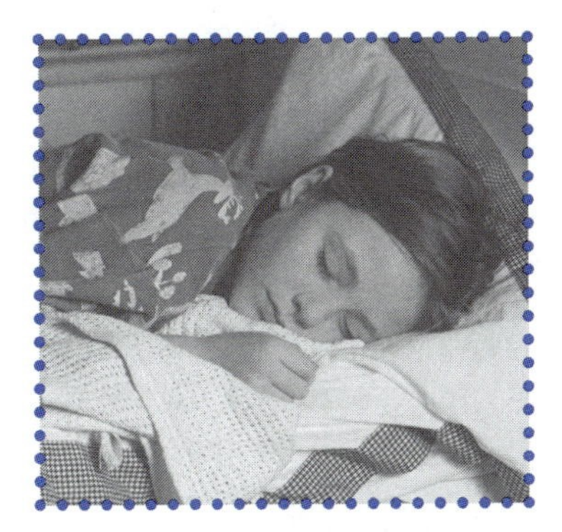

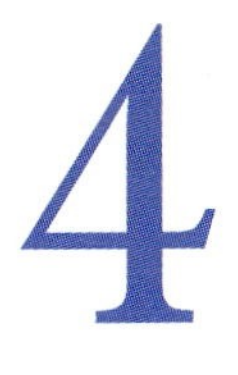

# Occupation, Activity, Skills, Patterns, Demands, Context, and Balance

*Karen Sladyk, PhD, OTR/L, FAOTA and Beth O'Sullivan, MPH, OTR/L*

**ACOTE Standards Explored in This Chapter**

B.2.2-2.4, 2.7

**Key Terms**

Activity demands
Client factors
Contexts
Occupation
Performance in areas of occupation
Performance patterns
Performance skills

## Introduction

This chapter will explore the critical significance of the role of occupation as it is used in the foundation of the occupational therapy profession. Occupational functioning is at the nature of every individual regardless of age, and it impacts our daily functional performance in the areas of skills, patterns, and contexts. The nature of a human being as an occupational being also allows us to participate in meaningful activities that maintain and promote both the physical and mental well-being of an individual and reinforce participation within society.

## Meaning and Dynamics of Occupation

From the development of the profession, the term *occupation* has been a basic construct. Dr. Adolph Meyer (1922, reprinted 1977), a founding father of the profession, wrote about the foundation of occupation in *Archives of Occupational Therapy.* Our conception of man is that of an organism that maintains and balances itself in the world of reality and actuality by being in active life and active use (i.e., using, living, and acting its time in harmony with its own nature and the qualities about it). It is the use that we make of ourselves that gives the ultimate stamp on every organ. Meyer and another founding father of our profession, William Rush Dunton, Jr., stated that the process of being involved in an occupation consists of a person alternating between modes of existing, thinking, and acting. At this time of writing, it was also noted that individuals should have a self-determined balance of daily pursuits, including creative, leisure, and daily activities and productive work, in order to remain healthy. The consistent incorporation of these activities tends to provide the individual with a typical daily rhythm and, in turn, a balance of life.



K. Sladyk, K. Jacobs, & N. MacRae (Eds.).
*Occupational Therapy Essentials for Clinical Competence* (pp. 33-42).

In the most basic sense, an occupation is anything an individual does that provides meaning and value in his or her daily life. According to Christiansen and Baum (2005), occupations all have specific characteristics such as being goal directed, having a purpose, and being performed within certain environments or contexts. These contextual factors include the areas of cultural, physical, social, personal, temporal, spiritual, and virtual domains (American Occupational Therapy Association [AOTA], 2008). Christiansen and Baum also stated that occupations can be identified by both the individual involved in the occupation as well as observers of the occupation, and they will provide meaning to the individual performing the occupation as well as to others. Occupations also allow the individual to establish and define specific roles, habits, and routines within their daily life.

When occupational therapists and occupational therapy assistants observe individuals performing daily occupations, they can analyze occupations and categorize them into specific areas. According to the framework (AOTA, 2008), documented areas of occupation include activities of daily living (ADL), instrumental activities of daily living (IADL), education, rest/sleep, work, play, leisure, and social participation. Every area should be evaluated and explored for relevance and meaning to the client on an individual basis.

# The Occupational Therapy Practice Framework: Domain and Process

The framework is an official document produced for the AOTA by the Commission on Practice (2008). This document was designed to bring a common language and consistency to practice in the profession. It also provides a clear description of occupational therapy's unique contribution and focus on an individual's ADL and occupations as they can become impacted by his or her performance abilities.

## History

The revised framework was approved by the Representative Assembly and published by AOTA in 2008. This document was created after extensive input and research from educators, practitioners, and theorists within the field of occupational therapy. Acceptance of the document replaced the original framework developed in 2002. In creating this new updated framework, the Commission on Practice strove to clearly articulate that occupational therapy is consistently grounded in occupation with the terminology clearly understood and current in practice.

## Organization of Document

The framework document first describes the domain of occupational therapy and describes occupational therapy as the ability to allow individuals to engage in occupation that supports participation in contexts. Occupation is the main purpose of occupational therapy and its intervention. This engagement in occupations allows individuals to participate in their own life roles. The ability to engage in occupation also includes a variety of contextual areas such as cultural, physical, social, personal, temporal, spiritual, and virtual domains. One cannot look at an individual or a task without looking at these factors (O'Sullivan, 2003).

The framework also identifies the domain of concern occupational therapy practitioners address during their assessment and provision of services. These terms are identified as performance in areas of occupation, performance skills and patterns, the contextual factors, activity or task demands, and the individual client's factors, which can also influence intervention approaches and outcomes.

# Performance in Areas of Occupation

The framework identifies seven kinds of life activities in which individuals participate. These include ADL and IADL: rest, sleep, education, work, play, leisure, and social participation. See Tables 4-1 and 4-2 for specific examples.

ADL include the ability to take care of one's self, while IADL are more complex activities and involve an individual interacting with the environment. These activities can be delegated to other individuals for assistance if necessary, but most individuals want to be independent in ADL and IADL.

## Rest and Sleep

Rest and sleep involve the ability to partake in a period of being inactive in which one may or may not suspend consciousness and the ability to recognize that a regular period of rest and sleep results in deep rejuvenation of energy and mental health (AOTA, 2008). Examples of rest and sleep roles are as follows (AOTA):

- *Rest*: The ability to have a period of quiet and decrease in effort, which could include relaxing, decreasing one's participation in physical, mental, or social activities that could be taxing.
- *Sleep*: One's ability to go to sleep and maintain a period of sleep.
- *Sleep preparation*: Completing the routines and tasks, such as donning and doffing one's clothes, getting one's bed prepared for sleep, and turning out the lights.
- *Sleep participation*: Allowing one's self to take the time and need for personal sleep. Also having the ability to understand and identify the need of those also sleeping in the same area, such as small children and their need for assistance during the night.

**Table 4-1. Activities of Daily Living**

| Activity | Description |
|---|---|
| Bathing/showering | The competency to obtain and use bathing supplies such as soap, shower gel, and towels. Of prime importance is the ability to maintain the safe water temperature and the proper bathing position; to transfer in and out of the tub or shower; and to soap, rinse, and dry one's body. |
| Bowel/bladder management | The ability to have control of bowel and bladder function and use equipment for bladder control if needed. |
| Dressing | The proficiency to select appropriate clothing with the time of day, weather, and occasion in mind. Also included in dressing is the ability to dress and undress one's self. |
| Eating | The ability to manipulate food in one's mouth, to chew, and to swallow. |
| Feeding | The ability to bring food to one's mouth by choosing the appropriate utensils. |
| Functional mobility | The skill to move from one position to another or from one place to another, as in transferring from bed or chair to walker or wheelchair. |
| Personal device care | The capacity to clean and properly maintain items such as hearing aids, contact lenses, glasses, orthotics, prosthetics, adaptive equipment, and contraceptive and sexual devices. |
| Personal hygiene and grooming | The proficiency to obtain and use the necessary supplies for the care of skin, ears, eyes, and nails. Also included is the ability to obtain the necessary supplies for the removal of body hair using razors, tweezers, or lotions, as well those products for the control of body odor (e.g., deodorants). Other requirements are the management of one's hairstyle and the daily application and removal of makeup, as well as the ability to obtain and use cleansing supplies for good oral hygiene, including toothpaste, mouthwash, and dental floss. Many persons need to develop the ability to cleanse and insert dentures or prosthetics. |
| Sexual activity | The ability to recognize sexual desires and to engage in intimate expressions of those desires that provide sexual satisfaction. |
| Toilet hygiene | The skill to obtain and use bathroom supplies. Also included is the ability to adjust clothing in preparation to toilet, to transfer on and off the toilet, to cleanse one's self, and to care for menstrual/continence needs, including sanitary pads, suppositories, catheters, or supplies for colostomies. |

Reprinted with permission from O'Sullivan, B. (2003). Practice framework and activity analysis. In K. Sladyk (Ed.), *OT study cards in a box*. Thorofare, NJ: SLACK Incorporated.

## Education and Work

Education is the ability to complete the activities needed to be an active participant in the learning environment, and work is activities in which one engages that encourage self-development in order to be a productive member of society. In many arenas, education is completed in early life in preparation for work in adulthood. However, learning is lifelong for many clients (AOTA, 2008). Examples of educational and work roles include the following (O'Sullivan, 2003):

- *Formal educational participation*: The proficiency to participate in a variety of activities related to formal education, including academic work such as reading and math, and nonacademic responsibility such as lunch or recess, extracurricular activities, or prevocational/vocational work activities.
- *Informal personal educational needs or interests exploration*: The capacity to obtain information related to personal interests.
- *Informal personal education participation*: The competency to participate in classes or programs of an individual's area of interest.
- *Employment interests and pursuits*: The proficiency to identify and choose work opportunities that support one's personal strengths, weaknesses, likes, and dislikes.
- *Employment seeking and acquisition*: The ability to pursue employment by being able to complete job application forms, to perform well in interviews, and to obtain a job.
- *Job performance*: The capacity to complete on-the-job tasks to the satisfaction of those in charge and, in doing so, contribute to a positive work environment.
- *Retirement preparation and adjustment*: The capability to recognize one's own interests, talents, and skills that can be carried into the years after active employment and, consequently, find meaningful outlets for those attributes.
- *Volunteer exploration*: The ability to identify organizations and opportunities within one's own local community to contribute one's talents and skills as a volunteer.
- *Volunteer participation*: The accomplishment to contribute one's talents and skills as a volunteer in the aid of individuals or groups within the community who depend on the work of unpaid supporters.

**Table 4-2. Instrumental Activities of Daily Living**

| Activity | Description |
|---|---|
| Care of others | The capability to foster the care of others, including arranging for that care, supervision, and/or providing the care. |
| Care of pets | The capability to foster the care of pets or service animals, including arranging for care, supervision, and/or providing care. |
| Child rearing | The proficiency to foster and provide supervision and care of a child, which includes fostering his or her developmental needs. |
| Communication management | The ability to utilize equipment used in sending and receiving information, including writing pens and pads, telephones, computers, call lights, and other emergency systems. |
| Community mobility | The skill to move through the community via public or private transportation. |
| Financial management | The capacity to handle one's finances, including planning and living within a budget, paying bills, and understanding banking procedures and various methods of completing transactions. |
| Health management and maintenance | The competency to maintain a healthy lifestyle that promotes wellness. |
| Home establishment and management | The proficiency to maintain a home, both the interior and the exterior, including the yard, garden, tools, appliances, and vehicles. Included in this task is the ability to maintain personal clothing and possessions. |
| Sexual activity | The ability to recognize sexual desires and to engage in intimate expressions of those desires that provide sexual satisfaction. |
| Meal preparation/clean-up | The ability to plan and prepare nutritious meals and to prepare leftover food for storage. |
| Religious observance | The ability to participate, acknowledge, and understand specific beliefs, practices, or rituals related to the religious practice. |
| Safety procedures and emergency procedures | The proficiency to understand and perform within the bounds of safety measures, including emergency procedures when necessary. |
| Shopping | The ability to complete the entire shopping activity, including writing a list of products needed, finding them in a store, and paying for the purchases. |

Reprinted with permission from O'Sullivan, B. (2003). Practice framework and activity analysis. In K. Sladyk (Ed.), *OT study cards in a box*. Thorofare, NJ: SLACK Incorporated.

## Play and Leisure

Play and leisure are activities that provide amusement, relaxation, or enjoyment and also foster internal motivation in children or adults. Typically, *play* is the term used for children, while *leisure* describes adult activities. However, the word *play* is also currently used in adulthood especially around unstructured play for play's sake. Examples of play and leisure include the following (O'Sullivan, 2003):

- *Play exploration*: The ability to identify areas of interests, skills, or play activities. This includes play exploration, practice, and participating within or learning the rules of play, whether it is pretend play, symbolic play, or structured games.
- *Play participation*: The accomplishment in play that includes obtaining the proper equipment and supplies, and maintenance of the same.
- *Leisure exploration*: The ability to identify interests, skills, or leisure activities.
- *Leisure participation*: The accomplishment to plan and participate in a variety of activities that provide and support leisure interests, including the ability to use the necessary equipment or supplies for the activity chosen.

## Social Participation

Social participation is being adept at participation in activities or behaviors that allow the individual to engage within his or her society. One could argue that social skills are an ADL activity, but the experts developing the framework felt social participation is more complex than simply communicating. Social participation needs to be assessed in all contexts and across the life span as social skills are developmental. Examples of social participation include the following (O'Sullivan, 2003):

- *Community*: The ability to participate within one's community or community environment, neighborhood, work, or school.
- *Family*: The proficiency to participate and be successful with family roles.
- *Peer, friend*: The capability to participate in relationships at varying degrees of intimacy.

Areas of ocupation are typically easy to articulate to clients, families, society, and funding sources because these people are active in their own occupations. Many other professions believe they can treat clients in these areas because of their own life experiences. What makes occupational therapy different from these other professions is its understanding of performance patterns, performance skills, and the environment in which occupations are performed. The following sections will address these important aspects of occupational therapy.

Performance patterns of occupation are very important to assess and provide intervention when there is a disruption of these patterns. Patterns of performance provide a day-in-and-day-out routine. This predictability of routine can be utilized as a way of grounding us and providing us with consistency in our occupations. Performance patterns include habits, roles, and routines. Habits are the skills and patterns that one will engage in on a day-to-day basis. Habits tend to become very automatic and are typically performed at a preconscious brain level of functioning. In doing so, they are actually conserving our energy and allowing us to focus on higher-level thinking tasks. Habits can be useful to assist individuals. They also may be impoverished; if so, occupational therapy practitioners will then identify this as a performance pattern in need of intervention services.

Routines are one's occupations typically performed in a particular sequence. Routines provide a sense of order and provide an individual or group of individuals with structure for daily living tasks. Studies have shown that routines are performed at specific times of the day and in some ways assist an individual in maintaining his or her biological or circadian rhythm internal clock. Routines are also structured by society and culture. An example of this is when children return to school, they must perform certain tasks according to the school demands.

Both habits and routines provide an individual with predictable activities on a daily basis. Habits and routines help an individual comprise a particular lifestyle. Lifestyles can be predictive of health and wellness. Individuals who use preventative measures, habits, and routines such as walking daily and not smoking will have a healthier lifestyle. Occupational therapy practitioners must become aware of their individual client's occupations and their particular meaning to the individual. In addition, they must be able to articulate the importance of occupations to the client, family, society, and reimbursement funders (O'Sullivan, 2003).

Performance skills identify specific skills and qualities that one typically incorporates to complete a functional skill. These include sensory, motor, emotional regulation, cognition, and communication/interaction skills. Specific examples are as follows.

- *Motor and praxis skills*: The skills that one typically utilizes to interact with one's environment and the tasks or objects within that environment (O'Sullivan, 2003).
  - *Posture*: The ability to maintain an upright position when one's equilibrium and balance are challenged. This skill incorporates the stabilization of one's trunk, alignment of one's body in an upright position, and the positioning of one's self in a safe and controlled manner when completing an activity.
  - *Mobility*: The ability to move one's body to complete an activity or task. This skill incorporates the ability to walk on uneven surfaces without stumbling, scuffing one's feet, or using an assistive device such as a cane, walker, or wheelchair. Once an individual is able to walk, the skill also incorporates the ability to successfully reach for an object with one's arm or long-handled reacher and bend one's trunk to appropriately orient one's self to the task.
  - *Coordination*: The capacity to utilize more than one body part in relationship to a task object or activity. This skill incorporates the utilization of two or more body parts to stabilize and manipulate an object. An individual must incorporate the utilization of small muscle groups for controlled movements such as object manipulation or speed and dexterity.
  - *Strength and effort*: The amount of muscle power utilized to resist movement, or the power to move objects, including the ability to move against gravity, as in lifting an object from its position on the floor. One must incorporate the proper grip or pinch techniques to grasp objects and regulate their speed, extent, or force placed on an object during a task.
  - *Energy*: The capability to maintain and sustain a proper endurance and pace throughout the entire task without showing signs of fatigue.
- *Process skills*: The skills that one typically uses to manage the actions required to complete daily living skills (O'Sullivan, 2003).
  - *Energy*: The capability to focus a continued effort over the time frame of a task. This skill includes the ability to pace one's self and maintain focused attention over the period of the task.
  - *Knowledge*: The proficiency to seek, gain, and utilize knowledge in regard to the task at hand. This skill includes one's ability to select, utilize, and protect appropriate tools and materials related to a task. One must also require gaining further information by asking questions of others or reading directions in order to efficiently complete the task.
  - *Temporal organization*: The ability to plan, organize, and carry out the steps involved in a task in the proper sequential order. The skill includes

the ability to initiate, continue a task in sequential order, and discontinue or stop an activity at the proper time.

- *Organizing space and objects*: The capacity to organize work or task spaces and supplies. This skill includes one's ability to search for tools, to gather the items necessary for the task, and to position the tools in a logical and organized manner for successful task performance. Once the task is completed, one must clean the work area and return tools or materials to appropriate storage places. Incorporated in this skill is the ability to negotiate and move one's body or wheelchair around any environmental object.
- *Adaptation*: The ability to learn from one's mistakes during the task performance. This includes the ability to recognize a problem and accommodate or modify one's actions or task objects in response to or in advance of a problem. This skill also requires one to adapt or adjust one's work environment in response to or in advance of a problem that is present in the workspace or environment. An example would be to change to a quiet room if the room in which one is studying is too noisy. Once an individual is able to adapt to the task or environment, one would see the benefits and continue with the adaptive style in the future.

- *Sensory perceptual skills*: The ability to identify, interpret, and respond to sensory information. These skills also require an individual to recall and remember sensory events. Sensory information can be interpreted by a variety of sensory pathways, including auditory, visual, tactile, olfactory, gustatory, proprioceptive, and vestibular (AOTA, 2008).
  - *Positioning of the body*: The ability to set one's body in the appropriate position for a motor act.
  - *Hearing*: The ability to receive auditory information and discriminate the information.
  - *Visualizing*: The ability to use vision to interpret information.
  - *Locating*: This skill is utilized when one uses sensory information to retrieve objects. This is the ability to utilize stereognosis to retrieve a quarter from one's pocket and not use visual skills.
  - *Timing*: The ability to position one's self and use the appropriate speed and force to carry out a controlled motor task or activity.
  - *Discerning*: The ability to use sensory skills to identify differences between items. An example of this skill would be when one can tell the difference between temperatures of food.
- *Emotional regulation skills*: The ability to use actions or behavior to express or manage feelings when interacting with individuals or groups.
  - *Responding*: The ability to identify feelings of others and react appropriately.
  - *Persisting*: Having the capability to continue a task despite having difficulty.
  - *Controlling*: The ability to maintain emotions or anger in relation to other individuals.
  - *Recovering*: This skill is utilized when an individual can experience disappointment or hurt feelings and not retaliate.
  - *Displaying*: Having the ability to express the appropriate emotions in relation to a situation or experience.
  - *Utilizing*: The ability to use skills or techniques to deal with emotional situations.
- *Cognitive skills*: Utilizing thoughts or behaviors to plan and perform an activity or task.
  - *Judging*: The skill to identify what is important or necessary for task completion. An example of this skill is when one makes a decision to prioritize job tasks with deadlines.
  - *Selecting*: The ability to choose the appropriate tools for a specific task.
  - *Organizing*: Having an ability to complete activities within the appropriate order and timing.
  - *Prioritizing*: One's ability to identify steps or solutions necessary to complete a task.
  - *Creating*: Being able to participate in activities that are fun and enjoyable.
  - *Multitasking*: Having the ability to do more than one activity at the same time. An example of this would be when one can talk on the phone and cook a meal at the same time.
- *Communication/social skills*: The competency to explain and describe one's needs and ideas to others in a socially acceptable manner (O'Sullivan, 2003).
  - *Physicality*: The ability to use one's physical body, or body language, to communicate. This skill includes the ability to physically touch others, use one's eyes to make eye contact, and move one's body in a position or in a direction that is in relation to others.
  - *Information exchange*: The skill to give and receive information to and from others. This skill includes the ability to articulate clearly, assert one's self, ask for information, and engage in meaningful conversation. In doing so, one can express his or her feelings, sharing information through speech.
  - *Relations*: The ability to maintain relationships. This skill requires one to have the ability to interact with other people, bond, or form connections with people with common interests, or maintain appropriate relationships in day-to-day interactions.

# Contexts and Environments

This area considers other outside factors in the environment that can influence or impact upon an individual's functioning. Occupational therapists must keep cultural, physical, social, personal, spiritual, temporal, and virtual contexts in mind when choosing the appropriate intervention program and therapeutic activities. Examples are (O'Sullivan, 2003):

- *Cultural*: Refers to the expectations of the society in which one lives, considering customs and behavioral patterns. Regardless of cultural setting, state and national legislation will affect the funding of basic programs, including education, employment, and transportation. Consequently, these will impact upon the availability of services to those in need. Every effort should be made to protect the personal rights of individuals.
- *Physical*: Includes factors that may affect one's ability to function within a specific environment such as the outdoor physical terrain; the indoor surroundings, including furniture, rugs, and pets; and the need for specific tools to cope with each setting.
- *Social*: Requires the evaluation of the social support system, in each case noting the availability and expectations of a variety of caregivers, spouses, other family members, friends, community health aides, and support groups.
- *Personal*: Includes individual attributes or factors that are not related to one's current physical health condition. These factors include contexts such as an individual's age, extent of education, and social or economic status.
- *Spiritual*: Can be both defined by our culture and be socially motivated. The definition includes one's individual values, individual motivators, and experiences. Spirituality can be found by one's ability to bring peace into their world.
- *Temporal*: Refers to the time aspect of occupational performance, such as the time of day or stage of an individual's life.
- *Virtual*: Refers to an individual utilizing technology and tools such as computers or radios for communication.

In addition to factors specific to the individual, the activity the person wishes to participate in also has demands. Occupational therapists use activity analysis to study the unique demands of a specific activity. Activity analysis (Lamport, Coffey, & Hersch, 2001) breaks down an activity into simple steps and looks at simplifying the activity (grading down) and making the activity more challenging (grading up).

Activity demands are specific components of an activity necessary for completion of an activity or task. Included in the category are the objects, physical space demands, social requirements, sequencing, and timing of an activity. Also included are specific body requirements or underlying body functions required to complete the task successfully. These are client factors that address what any human would need to complete an activity. The occupational therapist would need to understand both the activity demands and the required client demands before adjusting an activity for a specific client (Table 4-3).

# Occupational Therapy Intervention Approaches

This section of the framework describes a variety of intervention approaches and variation of intervention focus. Intervention may include creating/promoting, establishing/restoring, and maintaining (O'Sullivan, 2003).

- *Creating/Promoting*: This approach is founded in a health promotion model and believes that occupational therapy can assist in improving and enriching an activity or the context in which it is performed. In doing so, there are opportunities for enhancement of performance within one's daily life. In this model, intervention focuses on performance skills, performance patterns, activity demands, and client factors.
- *Establishing/Restoring*: This approach focuses on the remediation or restoration of client factors to assist with a current skill, develop a new skill, or restore an impaired skill. In this model, intervention focuses on performance skills, performance patterns, and body functions/body structures.
- *Maintaining*: This approach is designed to establish routines or supports that will focus on maintaining one's capabilities.

Intervention can include therapeutic use of self, therapeutic use of occupations/activities, purposeful activity, or preparatory methods (such as moist heat). Intervention may be a direct treatment model or use consultation or education models. The occupational therapist would choose these models based on desired outcomes of occupational performance, client satisfaction, role competence, adaptation, health/wellness, prevention, and/or quality of life. After considering all of these factors, the occupational therapist would specifically select meaningful activities and occupations for each specific client.

## Choice of Activities

In trying to choose the appropriate task for a client in order to achieve the most effective intervention, one must keep several factors in mind (O'Sullivan, 2003):

- *Activities should be goal directed.* Activities should always have a specific reason or purpose for their use. They are not chosen to fill idle time. Typically,

**Table 4-3. Activity Demands**

| Activity Demands | Client Factors |
|---|---|
| • *Objects used and their properties*: The tools, equipment, or materials necessary to complete the task.<br>• *Space demands*: Looking at the physical environment in which the activity must take place or will be taking place. One must look at several environmental factors such as lighting, surface of the work area, temperature, and noise.<br>• *Social demands*: The demands that society expects that are required for the activity. An example is when a child is expected to start sharing toys.<br>• *Sequence and timing*: The specific steps and order that one must complete to carry out the task.<br>• *Requires actions*: The typical skills or demands that one must perform to complete the task. These demands would be required of any person who was trying to attempt the activity.<br>• *Required body functions*: The body functions and requirements that are needed to complete the activity or task.<br>• *Required body structures*: The specific anatomical parts or body system usage, such as vision, required to do the task. | • *Body functions*: The physiological and psychological functions of one's body.<br>• *Mental functions*: Global mental, consciousness, orientation, temperament, and personality functions; the role of sleep, energy, and specific mental functions. The practitioner should consider attention, memory, perception, thought, higher-level cognitive functions, psychomotor and sensory demands, as well as the voice and speech requirements and bodily functions on general and specific organs. |

Reprinted with permission from O'Sullivan, B. (2003). Practice framework and activity analysis. In K. Sladyk (Ed.), *OT study cards in a box*. Thorofare, NJ: SLACK Incorporated.

therapists validate their choices of activity by relating that activity to address a deficit in a performance area or performance component according to the framework.

- *Activities should be of interest.* Activities should have some level of interest or significance to the client. This may be in the form of being an important step in assisting the client to reach a larger goal in the future or to have a relationship to his or her required life roles.
- *Activities should require involvement.* Activities require mental and/or physical involvement, meaning that the client can be part of the selection process; the client may determine a chosen task or activity before actually performing the same.
- *Activities should be adaptable and gradeable.* Several factors must be kept in mind when selecting an activity, including age and developmental appropriateness. There must also be the potential to break the activity into various grades of complexity or competence in order to grade participants of different ages and abilities.

## Summary

A person learning to become an occupational therapy practitioner must have a complete and competent understanding of the framework as it is the foundation to everything done in occupational therapy. Sadly, some practitioners do not use the framework in their practice of occupational therapy because of complacency or ignorance. Our history as occupational therapists and occupational therapy assistants is in occupation-based practice with a holistic approach to individual client needs. To avoid integrating the framework into every day practice is to do disservice to our consumers.

## Student Self-Assessment

These assignments are given to allow the student to test his or her own knowledge and incorporate the framework document into activities.

1. Take a case study from a textbook and analyze it according to the framework document.
2. Interview a family member or friend and complete an occupational profile.
3. Record your daily activities, then evaluate your activities. Are they a role, habit, or routine?
4. Interview a family member, classmate, or friend. Ask him or her to describe his or her daily activities and occupations. Then choose one or two areas of occupation and try to identify client factors involved.

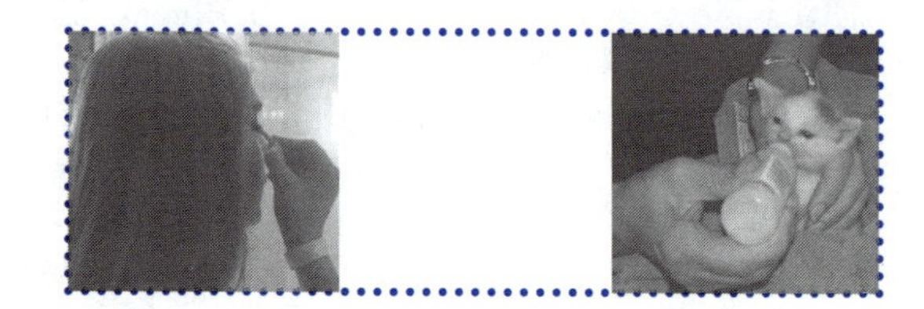

# References

American Occupational Therapy Association. (2008). Occupational therapy practice framework: Domain and process, second edition. *American Journal of Occupational Therapy, 62*, 625-683.

Christiansen, C. H., Baum, C. M., & Haugen, J. B. (2005). *Occupational therapy: Performance, participation, and well-being* (3rd ed.). Thorofare, NJ: SLACK Incorporated.

Lamport, N. K., Coffey, M. S., & Hersch, G. I. (2001). *Activity analysis & application* (4th ed.). Thorofare, NJ: SLACK Incorporated.

Meyer, A. (1977). The philosophy of occupation therapy. *American Journal of Occupational Therapy, 31*, 639-642.

O'Sullivan, B. (2003). Practice framework and activity analysis. In K. Sladyk, *OT study cards in a box* (2nd ed.; 2/1–2/32). Thorofare, NJ: SLACK Incorporated.

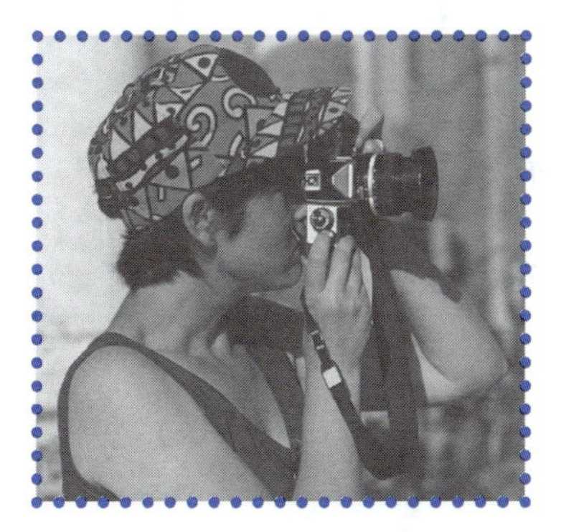

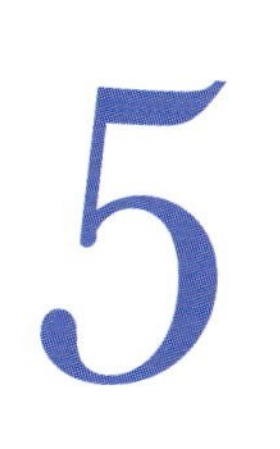

# Occupational Performance: Analyzing Occupational Perspectives on Health and Disease

*Kathleen Flecky, OTD, OTR/L and Heather Goertz, OTD, OTR/L*

**ACOTE Standards Explored in This Chapter**

B.2.5-2.6

**Key Terms**

Activity
Areas of occupation
Body functions and structures
Disability
Disease
Environmental factors
Function
Health
Health promotion
Impairments
*International Classification of Diseases* (ICD-10)
*International Classification of Functioning, Disability, and Health* (ICF)
Occupational performance
Participation
Partnerships in health
Personal factors
Wellness

## Introduction

What does it mean to be healthy and well? Occupational therapy professionals generally view persons as more than their disease processes. Two people can have the same disease or condition and differ widely in terms of physical, mental, social, and spiritual well-being. An individual's state of health is considered within the context of the ability to participate in needed and desired roles and to meet occupational lifestyle goals and tasks. Disease, illness, injury, and trauma can create occupational disruption that may lead to conditions of impairment, dysfunction, and disability. Occupational therapy professionals analyze information about diseases, impairments, and other health conditions in terms of how these health states impact performance in life's roles and routines (Hansen & Atchinson, 2000). We value a perspective of health that includes the consideration of one's ability to participate in meaningful occupations. According to Wilcock (2006), an occupational perspective of health encompasses "aiming for a balance of physical,



K. Sladyk, K. Jacobs, & N. MacRae (Eds.).
*Occupational Therapy Essentials for Clinical Competence* (pp. 43-54).

mental, and social well-being attained through valued occupation" (p. 112).

This chapter discusses health, disease, and disability within the context of occupational functioning and performance. Additionally, the effects of physical and mental health, inheritable diseases, predisposing genetic conditions, disability, disease processes, and injury on the individual will be analyzed in terms of health and health promotion.

Health perspectives from a sampling of occupational therapy students have been provided to begin this chapter. In 2006, the American Occupational Therapy Association (AOTA, 2007) reported an enrollment of 10,861 students in occupational therapy programs across America (AOTA, 2007). As occupational therapy students embrace concepts of health and disease, it is important to understand that health and disease are complex and there is much more information about these concepts that exists beyond the scope of this chapter. This section introduces the discussion by exposing students to different viewpoints of health and disease.

Let us begin this discussion by reviewing occupational therapy students who individually completed a survey about their opinions of health and disease characteristics. They were not given health definitions prior to completing the survey. The students granted permission to have their comments shared with others when asked the following questions:

- Describe health.
- Describe your own personal characteristics of occupational performance when you are healthy.
- Have you ever had a major disease or illness? If yes, explain.
- Describe your own personal characteristics of occupational performance when you were affected by disease or illness.

The following vignettes highlight four students' views related to health, disease, and occupational performance. Following these views is a description of several themes identified through analysis of the students' narratives.

As the student narratives reveal, health and wellness are multidimensional concepts that include physical, emotional, social, and spiritual aspects. Definitions of health vary individually depending on one's personal values, cultural beliefs, societal values, and experiences. Other factors that influence our conceptualizations of health, as well as what it means to be ill or disabled, may include age, gender, race, ethnicity, socioeconomic status, and current and past medical status. In summary, terms such as *health* and *well-being* are difficult to define because they are personally and socially constructed. They have evolved over time as society has revised notions of health, disease, and disability. For example, the constructs of health, as described by these occupational therapy students, represented the following characteristics as shown in Table 5-1.

**Shelly's View**

Health is mind, body, and spiritual wellness. I have balance in my life between work, school, friends, self-care, and leisure. When I let one take over, I usually stress about the others. If I allow time for everything, I feel I have a better handle on my life and I do a better job at each individual component. I have not experienced a major disease or illness.

**Elisa's View**

Health is a state of being at an optimal weight, not having high blood pressure, exercising, eating right, and having no illness or disease. When I am healthy, I can function at a high level, perform at my best, focus, be sweet to others, and feel good about myself. I had atrioventricular nodal reentrant tachycardia. I needed help getting out of bed. I felt dependent on others and paid closer attention to how everyone treated me.

**Joseph's View**

Health is physical, mental, and emotional balance and general wellness. I feel more productive, I can multitask, and I feel pretty confident in the work I am completing. I had chronic pain and depression. It was harder to complete schoolwork on time, and sometimes I just did the bare minimum. I slept a lot more, and sometimes my occupations didn't seem important. Reading, cooking, and exercise were discontinued in favor of sleep.

**Amber's View**

Health is the physical absence of disease or sickness with a mental balance and stability. I have more energy and motivation, I work toward goals, and I have a balance of occupations and leisure when I am healthy. I have Crohn's disease. The following are some characteristics of my occupational performance when I am ill: lack of energy and motivation, preoccupation with being physically ill and knowing that occupational performance is limited, difficulty focusing on working hard at school and balancing that with a social life, all while I feel that I physically and mentally can't perform up to my potential.

Table 5-1. Student Survey Responses

| Student Survey Categories | Disease Thematic Characteristics | Health Thematic Characteristics | Occupational Performance Characteristics |
|---|---|---|---|
| Responses from 24 occupational therapy students | • Difficulty completing work on time<br>• Increased sleep<br>• Occupations do not seem important<br>• Lack of energy and motivation<br>• Preoccupation with being physically ill<br>• Easily frustrated<br>• Dependent on others | • Wellbeing of physical or bodily, mental, spiritual, and emotional health<br>• An absence of disease<br>• All of the above<br>• A harmonious state | • Balanced life<br>• Alert<br>• Well rested<br>• Productive<br>• Energetic<br>• Active<br>• Motivated<br>• Goal oriented<br>• Happier<br>• Determined |

An awareness of your personal views of health constructs is vital to understanding how you will collaborate with your clients. Imagine standing in line at a grocery store behind a person in a wheelchair. Do you consider this person to be impaired? Why or why not? The answer to these questions is based largely on perceptions and life experiences and not necessarily on the unique lived experience of that person. An exploration of personal presuppositions and assumptions, beliefs, values, past experiences, and historical perspectives, as well as asking and clarifying client views, will enhance your professional skills at analyzing the effects of health and disease on occupational performance.

This chapter does not seek to examine every different view of health, but it introduces the concept of health by discussing historical perspectives of health, impairment, disease, and disability. For you to appreciate the complexity of health and disease, we have chosen to examine the historical views of impairments. Whether you have learned to recognize impairment as just a normal part of daily life or whether you feel sorry for the neighbor-lady next door because she walks so slowly and painfully, occupational therapy professionals recognize that society has classified and categorized persons who are different from the norm. The consequences of these categorizations is that experts have identified and defined who is impaired, diseased, or disabled rather than the people being categorized. Lack of attention to personal experiences of persons with impairments, diseases, and disabilities has led to marginalization, stigmatization, and exclusion (Depoy & Gilson, 2004; Oliver, 1996).

It is necessary to recognize that contemporary perceptions of health, impairments, diseases, and disabilities exist within a historical context—where we are today is based largely upon where we have been. Therefore, three predominant health models are described in the next section, which illustrates how persons have been viewed as different, atypical, or abnormal due to disease, impairment, and disability. Historical background is provided with these models of health in order to show how perspectives of health and disability are influenced by the cultural, social, spiritual, economic, and political contexts.

## Historical Perspectives on Health and Disability

Throughout the history of Western civilization, the predominant cultural and religious values along with social, political, and economic contexts influenced how persons with disease, impairment, and disability were viewed by society (Altman, 2001; Stiker & Sayers, 2000). A multitude of health perspectives have been advanced to define and describe health, but this section focuses on three predominant models: the religious, medical, and social perspectives as identified in Table 5-2.

Prior to the Enlightenment Era of the 1600s, disablement or abnormality in general, whether due to illness, injury, disease, or mental or physical impairment, was based on a religious model of disability (Stiker & Sayers, 2000). Within the religious approach, personal impairments and limitations were attributed to moral or supernatural causes. Illnesses and disease were manifestations of either sinfulness or a special spiritual relationship with higher powers or with God (Braddock & Parish, 2001).

With increased scientific and medical knowledge and with the influence of industrialization, atypicality was increasingly viewed as an individual affliction that limited one's ability to be a productive member of society. The impairment or disease required one to be fixed or restored through the care of others (Llewellyn & Hogan, 2000; Oliver, 1996). Charitable and medical care systems worked to either rehabilitate the disabled for the purpose of returning them to society or they confined them to custodial care within institutions (Braddock & Parish, 2001; Llewellyn & Hogan).

Initially, the occupational therapy profession was grounded in the social charitable movements of the early 20th century (Quiroga, 1995). The use of arts and crafts

| Table 5-2. Health Models | | | |
|---|---|---|---|
| **Features** | **Religious Model** | **Medical Model** | **Social Model** |
| Views of health | • Individual<br>• Based on spiritual or supernatural factors<br>• A reward for living a good life or a punishment for sinfulness | • Individual<br>• Based on intrinsic biological factors<br>• Biological interactions and processes lead to health or ill health | • Individual and environmental<br>• Based on interaction of intrinsic and extrinsic factors<br>• Social and physical environments influence health |
| Views of disability | Afflictions due to either sinfulness and deviancy, or impairments that indicated a special relationship with higher powers | Impairments and disability are a result of disease, illness, injury, and other abnormal health conditions; Impairments are the cause of disability | Social, economic, and political factors create disability along with individual characteristics |

activities and habit training were incorporated into the everyday lives of those persons considered unproductive due to physical and mental impairments. During World War I and II, occupational therapy flourished within the milieu of the medical model of disablement treating those with physical and mental disabilities (Quiroga). Our profession aligned with the medical model, which explained health, disease, and illness as bodily entities intrinsic to the person and treatable through either remediation or compensation for the effects of disease or injury (Kielhofner, 2004).

By the 20th century, medical diagnostic classification systems were created to categorize illnesses, diseases, and conditions based on health conditions, impairments, and limitations. Further advancement in medicine increased the survival rate for those with illness, injury, disease, impairment, and disability, which led to progressively more complex delineation of medical diagnoses and categories (Longmore & Umansky, 2001; Oliver, 1996). Health, ability, and disability became a function of one's individual health condition status rather than the capacity or opportunity to participate in desired life activities. Moreover, social, economic, and political policies based on these classifications created a climate of exclusion from participation from work and other valued life experiences for persons who had certain health conditions or impairments (Altman, 2001; Falk, 2001; Longmore & Umansky).

More recently, civil rights and social movements in Western societies advocating for self-determination and equal opportunity for all persons influenced both the development of a rights-based model of disability and the disability movement. Further, legislation and disability advocacy and activism promoted a conceptual shift in disability as a medical construct to disability as a social construct (Donoghue, 2003; Oliver, 1996). In contrast to the medical model of disability, an individual with a disability was considered impaired or limited not based upon individual attributes but by an unaccommodating environment and society (Barnes, Mercer, & Shakespeare, 1999; Gill, 2001). Through the advocacy effort to enhance opportunities for participation in society, provisions for protective legislation and resources were established to prevent discrimination based on disability (Albrecht, 2001; Hahn, 1993).

## World Health Organization Classifications

The need for a universal classification system for increasingly complex medical categorizations and consequences of health, disease, and disability led to the development of the family of World Health Organization (WHO) classifications. As part of this classification system, the *International Classification of Impairments, Disabilities, and Handicaps* (ICIDH) was developed in an effort to create a universal framework to describe the consequences of disease and disorders that included definitions of impairment, disability, and handicap (WHO, 2001).

In the new millennium, the WHO recognizes the importance of revisions to the ICIDH constructs of impairment, disability, and handicap to include a more comprehensive view of health that reflects both medical and social models of health and disability (WHO, 2001). It encompasses components of health for all persons, not just those with disease, illness, or disability. According to the *International Classification of Functioning, Disability, and Health* (ICF), elements of health, functioning, disease, and disability, termed *health conditions*, are organized according to two dimensions: body structures and function as one dimension, and activities and participation as a second dimension (WHO).

Moreover, contextual factors, including personal and environmental factors, are significant components of health, functioning, and disability. Health and functioning are impacted by contextual factors in an interactive and dynamic manner to impact health and functioning, and biological, personal, and sociocultural dimensions are included in a more holistic picture of health. In this way, these dimensions are linked to each other in a nonlinear manner to demonstrate the impact of change of one dimension on another (Figure 5-1) (WHO, 2001).

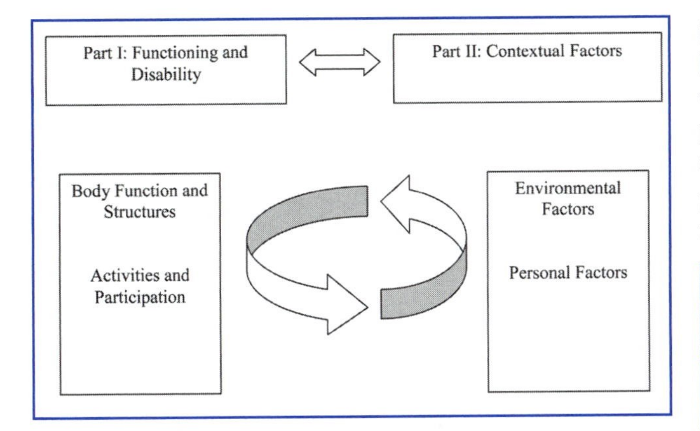


**Figure 5-1.** ICF: Multidimensional aspects of health and functioning. Adapted from World Health Organization. (2001). *ICF: International Classification of Functioning, Disability, and Health.* Geneva, Switzerland: Author.

Body functions and structures in ICF denote the anatomy, physiology, and psychology of the body systems in terms of degree of impairment or problems in body structure or function (WHO, 2001). The ICF recognizes that health and disability are not only internal to the individual, but also involve factors that define the ability to function and participate in life situations. Activities are defined as actions or tasks being executed by an individual, while participation comprises the level of involvement of an individual in performing actions and tasks in everyday life (WHO). Examples of activities and participation are shown in Table 5-3.

**Table 5-3. ICF Activities and Participation**

- Learning and applying knowledge (e.g., school occupations)
- General tasks and knowledge (e.g., coordinating multiple tasks)
- Communication
- Mobility
- Self care
- Domestic life (e.g., obtaining a place to live)
- Interpersonal interactions and relationships
- Major life areas (e.g., work occupations)
- Community, social, and civic life

Adapted from World Health Organization. (2001). *ICF: International Classification of Functioning, Disability, and Health.* Geneva, Switzerland: Author.

Contextual factors are recognized as an important aspect of health, functioning, and disability. The ICF was developed to blend a medical model of disability with a socioecological model. Instead of classifying health, disease, and disability only as intrinsic aspects of the individual, these domains are viewed as having intrinsic and extrinsic components that have multiple interactions with the environment (WHO, 2001). Therefore, contextual factors involve both environmental and personal factors. The ICF views environmental factors as extrinsic to the individual, such as the physical and social environment, but personal factors are considered intrinsic to the individual and include features such as age, gender, genetics, personality, education, sociocultural background, and past and current life experiences (WHO, 2001). Examples of personal and environmental factors from the ICF are shown in Table 5-4.

**Table 5-4. ICF Personal and Environmental Factors**

| Personal Factors | Environmental Factors |
|---|---|
| Gender, age, other health conditions, coping style, social background, education, profession, past experience, character style | Products, relationships, institutions, social norms, culture, built environment, political factors, nature |

Adapted from World Health Organization. (2001). *ICF: International Classification of Functioning, Disability, and Health.* Geneva, Switzerland: Author.

The interactions between body structures, body functioning, personal factors, and environmental factors are evident in the way genetics and the environment influence the nature of human disease. For example, in the United States, racial and ethnic groups display differences in incidence, progression, and severity of disease. Although there are differences in genetic frequencies that contribute to these disparities, most of the differences are due to the effects from the physical and social environment (Race, Ethnicity, and Genetics Working Group, 2005).

Disease and illness are components of health that reflect the interplay of factors intrinsic and extrinsic to the individual. Genetics, biology, personality, temperament, age, gender, etc. impact the potential to experience disease and illness. Environmental factors, including physical and sociocultural aspects, can interact with intrinsic factors in both positive and negative ways to tip the balance toward health and well-being or toward ill health (AOTA, 2008; Edelman & Mandle, 2006). Alternatively, having a disease, illness, or disability does not by necessity mean that an individual is disabled or has limited opportunities to engage in meaningful occupations (Altman, 2001; Brownson & Scaffa, 2001).

# ICF and Occupational Performance

The framework (AOTA, 2008) has much in common with the ICF with its emphasis upon health and functioning as related to participation in life tasks and activities. Both frameworks provide a shared language regarding the domains of health, functioning, disability, participation, and activity (AOTA; WHO, 2001). In the framework, body function and body structures as described in the ICF are situated within client factors. Additionally, the ICF conceptualizes activities and participation as centrally located within areas of occupation. Finally, ICF environmental factors are congruent with the framework constructs of context (AOTA; WHO). Both the framework and the ICF acknowledge the central role of participation and the environment as contributors to health and disability (AOTA; WHO). The framework further asserts that the essence of occupational engagement is a vital link to health and participation. Occupational performance becomes an interactive and dynamic engagement of an individual within environments that support and/or inhibit health and well-being (AOTA).

## Importance of Occupation in Relation to Health

In order to promote health, it is necessary to discover the occupations that are meaningful to the individual in the community. Personal motivation is reflective of an established meaning in life and the roles and routines of one's lifestyle. Referring back to the occupational therapy student narratives of health, the students who indicated that they were healthy used self-descriptors such as *active, motivated, energetic*, and *goal directed*. However, when students commented on disease characteristics, they used self-descriptors that included the terms *unmotivated, exhausted*, and *preoccupied*. It is possible for illness to be exacerbated or reduced depending on our ability to participate in meaningful occupations (Bridle, 1999). Also, it is possible for individuals with terminal illness to maintain well-being when they are actively engaged in doing occupations (Lyons, Orozovic, Davis, & Newman, 2002).

Consider how you feel when you are ill. How does being ill change your daily routines and your lifestyle? Occupational therapy professionals play a key role in health promotion with individuals in the community through promoting healthy lifestyles, incorporating occupation into existing health programs, and advocating for community and individual needs. It is important to remember that health promotion is an approach that "does not assume a disability is present or that any factors would interfere with performance" (Brownson & Scaffa, 2001, p. 657). AOTA identifies various interventions that may enhance the occupational therapist and occupational therapy assistant's role in health promotion. Examples of health promotion interventions include advocating for safe playgrounds, promoting policies that support economic self-determination for all persons, and training business personnel about disability etiquette (Brownson & Scaffa, 2001).

Health promotion is relevant within the context of occupational performance because the effects of illness and disease are influenced by environmental factors, and such factors influence personal health. Individuals rely on community supports and resources for optimal performance. Partnerships in health are critical for the overall well-being of individuals in community with others. Healthy People 2010, a joint document developed by the United States Public Health Service and United States Department of Health and Human Services (HHS), encourages partnerships in health and delineates core health objectives to increase quality and years of healthy life and to eliminate health disparities (HHS, 2000).

## Partnerships for Health: Health Promotion and Disease Prevention

Health promotion from an occupational perspective involves not only the prevention and reduction of illness, injury, trauma, and disability, but the enhancement of health and well-being of all persons through the promotion of healthy lifestyle practices and healthy communities (Brownson & Scaffa, 2001).

Acknowledging Wilcock's (1998) occupational perspective relating to health and occupational performance is essential. She articulated that for health and well-being to be present in individuals and communities alike, the following must occur for engagement in occupation (p. 123):

- Have meaning and be balanced between capacities
- Provide optimal opportunity for desired growth in individuals or groups
- Be flexible enough to develop and change according to context and choice
- Be compatible with sustaining ecology and sociocultural values

Occupational therapists and occupational therapy assistants should be mindful of the above qualities in order to improve the effects of health and disease on clients' performance. We also encourage practitioners to ask many questions until arriving at a comfortable knowledge of the occupational profile of your client. It is through such questioning or interviews that we develop a trusting relationship between the therapist and client. Mutual interview is preferred in order to honor collaboration with occupational therapists, occupational therapy assistants, and clients. Hence, the therapist is sharing stories and examples of his or her own experiences to guide the client toward sharing his or her experiences. Some other traits that we have found to be transforming in the therapist-client relationship are to recognize that health and/or disease is a normal part of the client's life and to look for the client's strengths and positive health indicators rather than focusing on disease specifics.

Occupational therapists and occupational therapy assistants are in a position to advocate for health promotion regardless of a person's current impairment. For instance, imagine that you are working with a client that has a wrist fracture and a long history of major depressive disorder. She is also obese and inactive. The physician referral calls for upper extremity rehabilitation, including strengthening, functional and home safety assessments, and a medication maintenance plan. However, you, the therapist, know that more services are necessary to improve this person's overall health. Thus, you request and are granted additional referrals for nutrition and activity planning that will promote healthy living at home. Partnering with other professionals and seeking external resources would be necessary for this client's well-being.

We have worked collaboratively with multiple organizations and agencies, including school systems, nonprofits, businesses, and institutions, as consultants and trainers in health promotion. We have chosen three case studies to help you better understand perspectives of health and disability. In these examples, composites of persons have been used and client names and identifying information have been removed. You will meet Carrie, Salvatore, and Thomas, who exemplify the effects of health, disease, and disability on occupational performance within their own cultural context.

### Carrie's Story

Carrie is an artist who experienced a stroke several years ago. She currently is not able to work as a mortgage broker at a bank due to frequent seizures and difficulties in speaking. Carrie uses her work as an artist as a means to support herself and as an expression for her feelings and experiences as a person with a disability. Carrie is a mentor and partner with occupational therapy students who are learning about environmental strengths and barriers to persons with disabilities participating in their local arts and entertainment venues. As Carrie and the students visit an art gallery to investigate physical and social barriers and make recommendations, they realize that the staff has not been trained in disability etiquette. Carrie also notes that the gallery brochure, labels for exhibits, and other signage would not be accessible to persons with visual concerns. The students and Carrie discussed with the staff that if disability etiquette staff training and minor signage changes were put in place, the gallery would be more welcoming to all persons, not just persons with disabilities. This case is an example of how the physical and social environments interact with individual capacities and abilities in a way that could disable an individual by limiting access and participation.

This case is an example of how the physical and social environments can interact with individual capacities and abilities in a way that promotes exclusion and marginalization by limiting access and participation to certain individuals. Due to her personal experiences, disability training, and previous interactions with persons with disabilities, Carrie had an increased awareness and knowledge of potential problems that persons might encounter in enjoying the gallery offerings. The occupational therapy students were skilled in analyzing client personal factors, environmental factors, and activity demands in terms of how these interact with client occupations. Together, Carrie and the students discussed how the contexts or interrelated environmental conditions, such as physical, personal, social, cultural, and attitudinal aspects of the gallery, impact a visitor's ability to both gain access and fully engage in desired activities.

### Salvatore's Story

Below is a letter that Salvatore wrote about his experience with West Nile virus. West Nile virus is spread by infected mosquitoes and can cause serious, life-altering, and even fatal disease.

Hello Family and Friends,

Get ready for this: I am now an official number at the CDC—one of over 30 cases this year. I have seen the West Nile virus and I have survived! Twenty days ago I began feeling a bit tired and my tummy was out of sorts. One morning I woke up with the worst headache I've ever had. It not only hurt inside but also the outside hurt! I had no desire to eat and the couple times I did it squirted right back out one end or the other. I was getting chills that had my teeth chattering. My mouth was desert-dry! My coffee cup felt so heavy! My weight had lessened and my thermal output was heightened to 101 degrees. On trip 2 to the doctor, I found out I had lost the ability to sign my name. Sonya, my wife, got me loaded into the car for another trip to the Emergency Room. They got me in quick while doctor #3 got me one of those glorious IV's heated to perfection. He ordered up a CAT and spinal tap, and then sent me home to wait for results. The weekend passed by and I began feeling a little bit better every day, but the external tenderness persisted. I came home at lunch and had to stay. My doctor finally called at 4:45 pm on Friday and said the results were positive for West Nile. She couldn't understand why I was so happy. I said, "Mystery finally solved. Now you can get me healed." I hadn't been out of the house in 2 weeks except for work, so I went and enjoyed watching high school football on a glorious late summer evening, played games on my computer, and then looked at emails around 1 am and stumbled upon these messages that Sonya "The Wise, Well-Connected, Always-By-My-Side, Fleet-of-Foot, Medically Savvy, Persistent, Morbid, Well-Stashed, and Truthful" had been circulating. I guess Salvatore "The Nightowl" is back!

Thanks for your prayers,

Salvatore

Salvatore's story exemplifies the need for external supports. In this case, his wife was his primary health advocate. There were many unknowns about his condition (i.e., diagnosis, unexplainable symptoms), along with many occupations that motivated him to heal. Health literacy, the degree to which individuals have the capacity to obtain, process, and understand basic health information and services needed to make appropriate health decisions, was a factor in this case (HHS, 2000).

Health and wellness services can be population specific. Many communities focus on population-specific care for cohorts including adolescents, refugees, or HIV/AIDS survivors. The following story comes from a class of occupational therapy students that served as mentors through a community-based course.

### Thomas' Story

Occupational therapy students participated in a service-learning experience that involved developing a health promotion program with teenagers. Their semester-long efforts resulted in the "Health Through Photography" project. This project's goal was to empower teenagers to develop a new skill of photography while learning about healthy lifestyles through a camera's lens. Thomas, a quiet, polite teen expressed some potential interest in photography. The teens took photos of numerous health objects and settings and brought this all together in an art portfolio of which they earned high-school art credit. The concentrated effort toward health promotion encouraged Thomas to develop a trusting relationship with a group of college students while exploring various environments. The neighborhood, the city's downtown, and a college fitness center were some examples of the locations visited. During such visits, Thomas learned the importance of nutrition, physical fitness, hygiene, and environments on healthy lifestyles. He increased his trust in others and developed confidence in acquiring new skills (i.e., photography). His school then acknowledged this new skill by asking him to be the photographer for a special event at the end of the semester. The following photographs are samples of this project (Figures 5-2 and 5-3).

For this project, the students chose an adolescent-specific population because there are numerous health risks facing youth (i.e., mental illness, asthma, sexually transmitted diseases, and obesity). The most common causes of disability, disease, and premature death may result from adolescents' individual choices and behaviors. Thomas is an example of the success that health promotion can have on an individual's occupational performance even in the absence of disease.

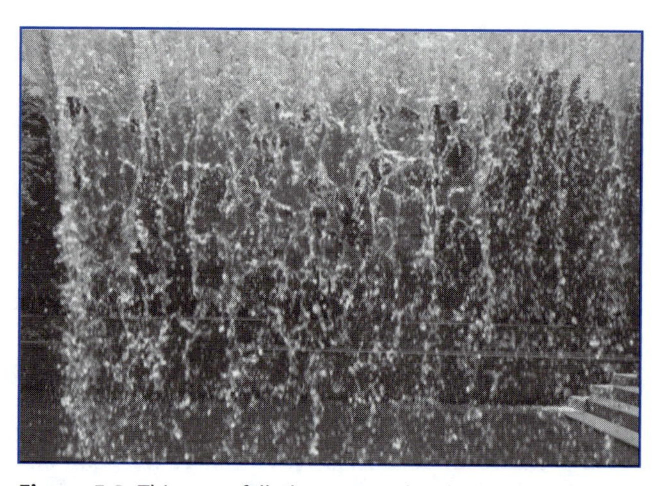

**Figure 5-2.** This waterfall photo was taken by a teen exploring environmental influences on health.

SCENERY
187
SMOKING IS NOT PERMITTED ANYWHERE ON SCHOOL PROPERTY

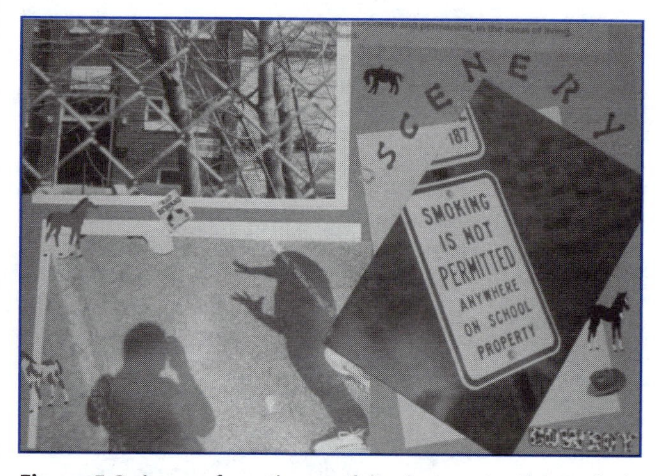

**Figure 5-3.** A page from the portfolio designed collaboratively by high school students and occupational therapy students.

## Summary

This chapter has examined health as a dynamic process that is everchanging based on the individual, his or her occupational performance, and the environment. You should be able to discuss the importance of health, disease, and disability from multiple perspectives both intrinsic and extrinsic to the person. Persons are more than their disease processes, as explained through the occupational therapy perspective and the WHO's ICF framework. We encourage occupational therapy students to continue learning about health promotion and disability along with the effects occupational performance can have on well-being. Understanding the role of occupation in health promotion is necessary early on in your education, such that you may appreciate the complexity of health when collaborating and advocating for and with clients.

## Student Self-Assessment

1. The ICF provides a framework that describes functioning as an interaction between health conditions and the environment. Compare and contrast an occupational perspective of health with perspectives within the ICF.
2. Going back to Carrie's case study, what are strategies that Carrie and the students could suggest to the gallery owners that have the potential to enhance participation and occupational engagement in this cultural venue? Many strategies can enhance participation for all persons, not just people with disabilities. How could the strategies you described in Question 1 be beneficial for others?
3. Going back to Salvatore's case study, how is the health status of Salvatore influenced by his occupations? If health and illness are dynamic and viewed as a continuum of interaction among many factors, which factors seem to facilitate health for Salvatore? Which are barriers to health?
4. Going back to Thomas' case study, explain the importance of population-specific interventions for the occupational therapy profession. How does health promotion benefit individuals that are not affected by a specific disease or impairment? If you were Thomas, how might your thinking about your abilities have changed through the "Health Through Photography" project?
5. As indicated in this chapter, student self-examination of their perceptions about health and disease enhances their understanding of occupational performance in relationship to health. Return to the student health survey. Compare and contrast your personal health experiences with the student responses. What interactions have you had with persons with different health conditions? How did you respond to these differences? How have the concepts discussed in this chapter enhanced your understanding about differences related to health, disease, and disability?
6. Encourage students to explore diversity in health, disease, and disability. Ask them to complete a health application in another language. For example, you may access a form for children's health insurance in Spanish by going to www.hhs.state.ne.us/med/spanish%20application.pdf.
7. Review concepts and definitions from the ICF framework and compare definitions of activity and participation to the AOTA practice framework's definitions of activity, occupation, and participation.
8. Give examples of personal and environmental factors that impact occupational performance, functioning, and participation.

## Electronic Resources

- Office of Disease Prevention and Health Promotion: www.odphp.osophs.dhhs.gov
- Community Campus Partnerships for Health: www.ccph.info
- Disability History Museum: www.disabilitymuseum.org
- Health Literacy Consulting: www.healthliteracy.com
- World Health Organization and ICF link: www.who.int/en or www.who.int/classifications/icf/en

### Evidence-Based Research Chart

| Issue | Evidence |
|---|---|
| Health, participation, and wellness | Baum, 2003; Goldworth, 2005; Shaw & MacKinnon, 2004; Suarez-Balcazar, 2005; Wilcock, 1993, 2005 |
| Health promotion and occupational therapy | AOTA, 2001, 2008; Duque, 2004; Matuska, Giles-Heinz, Flinn, Neighbor, & Bass-Haugen, 2003; Scriven & Atwal, 2004: Thibodaux, 2005 |
| Prevention of disease, injury, and disability | AOTA, 2001; Clark et al., 1997; Kroll, Jones, Kehn, & Neri, 2006; Michaud, Murray, & Bloom, 2001; Nakasato & Carnes, 2006; |
| Disability constructs | Donoghue, 2003; Gitlow & Flecky, 2005; Llewellyn & Hogan, 2000; Lutz & Bowers, 2005; Mitra, 2006; Taylor, 2005; Temple, McLeod, Gallinger, & Wright, 2001; Vrkljan, 2005 |
| *International Classification of Functioning and Disability* (ICF) | Battaglia et al., 2004; Grill Stucki, Boldt, Joisten, & Swoboda, 2005; Hemmingsson & Jonsson, 2005; Kuijer, Brouwer, Preuper, Groothoff, & Dijkstra, 2006; Stamm, Cieza, Machold, Smolen, & Stucki, 2006 |
| Health promotion and partnerships | Hemming & Langille, 2006; King, Tucker, Baldwin, & LaPorta, 2006; Suarez-Balcazar et al., 2005 |
| Occupational performance despite impairment | Bedell, Cohn, & Dumas, 2005; Chan, 2004; Kirsh, Cockburn, & Gewutz, 2005; Reid, 2002; Rice & Thomas, 2000; Schenker, Coster, & Parush, 2005; Wilkins, Jung, Wishart, Edwards, & Norton, 2003 |

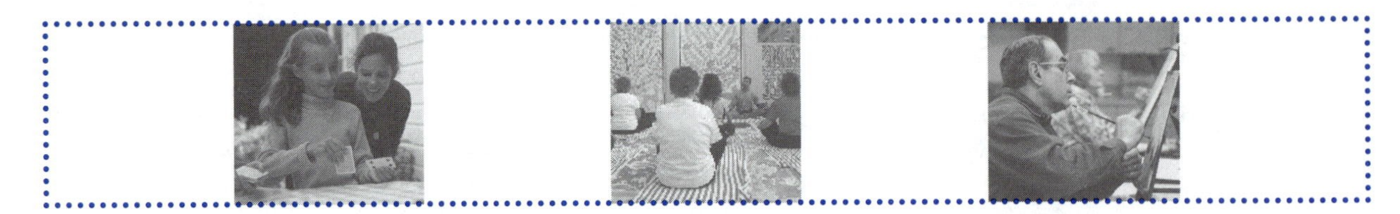

# References

Albrecht, G. L., Seelman, K. D., & Bury, M. (2003). Introduction: The formation of disabilities studies. In G. L. Albrecht, K. D. Seelman, & M. Bury (Eds.), *Handbook of Disabilities Studies* (pp. 1-8). Thousand Oaks, CA: Sage Publications.

Altman, B. M. (2001). Disability definitions, models, classification schemes, and application. In G. L. Albrecht, K. D. Seelman, & M. Bury (Eds.), *Handbook of disability studies* (pp. 97-122). Thousand Oaks, CA: Sage Publications.

American Occupational Therapy Association. (2007). Academic programs annual data: Academic year 2006-2007. Retrieved December 12, 2007, from http://www.aota.org/Educate/EdRes/OTEdDAta

American Occupational Therapy Association. (2008). Occupational therapy practice framework: Domain and process, second edition. *American Journal of Occupational Therapy, 62*, 625-683.

Barnes, C., Mercer, G., & Shakespeare, T. (1999). *Exploring disability: A sociological introduction*. Cambridge, UK: Polity Press.

Battaglia, M., Russo, E., Bolla, A., Chiusso, A., Bertelli, S., Pellegri, A., et al. (2004). International Classification of Functioning, Disability, and Health in a cohort of children with cognitive, motor, and complex disabilities. *Developmental Medicine and Child Neurology, 46*(2), 98-106.

Baum, C. M. (2003). Participation: Its relationship to occupation and health. *OTJR: Occupation, Participation and Health, 23*(2), 46-47.

Bedell, G. M., Cohn, E.S., & Dumas, H. M. (2005). Exploring parents' use of strategies to promote social participation of school-age children with acquired brain injuries. *American Journal of Occupational Therapy, 59*, 273-284.

Braddock, D. L., & Parish, S. L. (2001). An institutional history of disability. In G. L. Albrecht, K. D. Seelman, & M. Bury (Eds.), *Handbook of disability studies* (pp. 11-68). Thousand Oaks, CA: Sage Publications.

Bridle, M. J. (1999). Are doing and being dimensions of holism? *American Journal of Occupational Therapy, 53*(6), 636-639.

Brownson, C. A., & Scaffa, M. E. (2001). Occupational therapy in the promotion of health and the prevention of disease and disability statement. *American Journal of Occupational Therapy, 55*(6), 656-660.

Chan, S. C. C. (2004). Chronic obstructive pulmonary disease and engagement in occupation. *American Journal of Occupational Therapy, 58*, 408-415.

Clark, F., Azen, S. P., Zemke, R., Jackson, J., Carlson, M., Mandel, D., et al. (1997). Occupational therapy for independent-living older adults. A randomized controlled trial. *Journal of the American Medical Association, 278*(16), 1321-1326.

Department of Health and Human Services, Public Health Service. (2000). *Healthy people 2010: Volume 1: Understanding and Improving Health. Objectives for Improving Health* (2nd ed.). Washington, DC: U.S. Government Printing Office.

Depoy, E., & Gilson, S. F. (2004). *Rethinking disability: Principles for professional and social change*. Belmont, CA: Brooks/Cole.

Donoghue, C. (2003). Challenging the authority of the medical definition of disability: Analysis of the resistance to the social constructionist paradigm. *Disability and Society, 18*, 199-208.

Duque, R. L. (2004). Health promotion and the values of occupational therapy. *World Federation of Occupational Therapy Bulletin, 49*, 5-8.

Edelman, C. L., & Mandle, C. L. (Eds.). (2006). *Health promotion throughout the lifespan*. (6th ed.). St. Louis, MO: Elsevier Mosby.

Falk, G. (2001). *Stigma: How we treat outsiders*. Amherst, NY: Prometheus Books.

Gill, C. J. (2001). Divided understandings: The social experience of disability. In G. L. Albrecht, K. D. Seelman, & M. Bury (Eds.), *Handbook of disability studies* (pp. 351-372). Thousand Oaks, CA: Sage Publications.

Gitlow, L., & Flecky, K. (2005). Integrating disability studies concepts into occupational therapy education using service learning. *American Journal of Occupational Therapy, 59*(5), 546-553.

Goldworth, A. (2005). Disease, illness, and ethics. *Cambridge Quarterly of Healthcare Ethics, 14*(3), 346-351.

Grill, E., Stucki, G., Boldt, C., Joisten, S., & Swoboda, W. (2005). Identification of relevant ICF categories by geriatric patients in an early post-acute rehabilitation facility. *Disability and Rehabilitation, 27*(7-8), 467-473.

Hahn, H. (1993). The politics of physical differences: Disability and discrimination. In M. Nagler (Ed.), *Perspectives on disability* (2nd ed., pp. 37-42). Palo Alto, CA: Health Markets Research.

Hansen, R. A., & Atchinson, B. (2000). *Conditions in occupational therapy: Effect on occupational performance* (2nd ed.). Baltimore, MD: Lippincott Williams & Wilkins.

Hemming, H. E., & Langille, L. (2006). Building knowledge in literacy and health. *Canadian Journal of Public Health, 97*(suppl 2), S31-S36.

Hemmingsson, H., & Jonsson, H. (2005). An occupational perspective on the concept of participation in the International Classification of Functioning, Disability and Health—Some critical remarks. *American Journal of Occupational Therapy, 59*(5), 569-576.

Kielhofner, G. (2004). *Conceptual foundations of occupational therapy* (3rd ed.). Philadelphia, PA: F.A. Davis.

King, G. A., Tucker, M. A., Baldwin, P. J., & LaPorta, J. A. (2006). Bringing the Life Needs Model to life: Implementing a service delivery model for pediatric rehabilitation. *Physical and Occupational Therapy in Pediatrics, 26*(1-2), 43-70.

Kirsh, B., Cockburn, L., & Gewutz, R. (2005). Best practice in occupational therapy: Program characteristics that influence vocational outcomes for people with serious mental illness. *Canadian Journal of Occupational Therapy, 72*, 265-279.

Kroll, T., Jones, G. C., Kehn, M. E., & Neri, M. T. (2006). Barriers and strategies affecting the utilization of primary preventive services for people with physical disabilities: A qualitative inquiry. *Health & Social Care in the Community, 14*(4), 284-293.

Kuijer, W., Brouwer, S., Preuper, H. R., Groothoff, J. W., Geertzen, J. H., & Dijkstra, P. U. (2006). Work status and chronic low back pain: Exploring the International Classification of Functioning, Disability and Health. *Disability and Rehabilitation, 28*(6), 379-388.

Llewellyn, A., & Hogan, K. (2000). The use and abuse of models of disability. *Disability & Society, 15*(1), 157-165.

Longmore, P., & Umansky, L. (2001). *The new disability history: American perspectives (history of disability)*. New York, NY: New York University Press.

Lutz, B. J., & Bowers, B. J. (2005). Disability in everyday life. *Qualitative Health Research, 15*(8), 1037-1054.

Lyons, M., Orozovic, N., Davis, J., & Newman, J. (2002). Doing-being-becoming: Occupational experiences of persons with life-threatening illnesses. *American Journal of Occupational Therapy, 56*(3), 285-295.

Matuska, K., Giles-Heinz, A., Flinn, N., Neighbor, M., & Bass-Haugen, J. (2003). Outcomes of a pilot occupational therapy wellness program for older adults. *American Journal of Occupational Therapy, 57*(2), 220-224.

Michaud, C. M., Murray, C. J., & Bloom, B. R. (2001). Burden of disease: Implications for future research. *Journal of the American Medical Association, 285*(5), 535-539.

Mitra, S. (2006). The capability approach and disability. *Journal of Disability Policy Studies, 16*(4), 236-247.

Nakasato, Y. R., & Carnes, B. A. (2006). Health promotion in older adults: Promoting successful aging in primary care settings. *Geriatrics, 61*(4), 27-31.

Oliver, M.(1996). *Understanding disability: From theory to practice.* New York, NY: Palgrave Macmillan.

Quiroga, V. A. M. (1995). *Occupational therapy: The first 30 years: 1900 to 1930.* Bethesda, MD: AOTA Press.

Race, Ethnicity, and Genetics Working Group, National Human Genome Research Institute. (2005). The use of racial, ethnic, and ancestral categories in human genetics research. *American Journal of Human Genetics, 77*(4), 519-532.

Reid, D. T. (2002). Critical review of the research literature of seating interventions: A focus on adults with mobility impairments. *Assistive Technology, 14*, 118-129.

Rice, M. S., & Thomas, J. J. (2000). Perceived risk as a constraint on occupational performance during hot and cold water pouring. *American Journal of Occupational Therapy, 54*, 525-532.

Schenker, R., Coster, W. J., & Parush, S. (2005). Neuroimpairments, activity performance and participation in children with cerebral palsy mainstreamed in elementary schools. *Developmental Medicine and Child Neurology, 47*(12), 808-814.

Scriven, A., & Atwal, A. (2004). Occupational therapists as primary health promoters: Opportunities and barriers. *British Journal of Occupational Therapy, 67*(10), 424-429.

Shaw, L., & MacKinnon, J. (2004). A multidimensional view of health. *Education for Health, 17*(2), 213-222.

Stamm, T. A., Cieza, A., Machold, K. P., Smolen, J. S., & Stucki, G. (2005). An exploration of the link of conceptual occupational therapy models and the International Classification of Functioning, Disability and Health. *Australian Occupational Therapy Journal, 53*(1), 9-17.

Stiker, H. J., & Sayers, W. (Trans.). (2000). *A history of disabilities (Corporealities: Discourses of Disability).* Ann Arbor, MI: University of Michigan Press.

Suarez-Balcazar, Y. (2005). Empowerment and participatory evaluation of a community health intervention: Implications for occupational therapy. *OTJR: Occupation, Participation and Health, 25*(4), 133-142.

Suarez-Balcazar, Y., Hammel, J., Helfrich, C., Thomas, J., Wilson, T., & Head-Ball, D. (2005). A model of university-community partnerships for occupational therapy scholarship and practice. *Occupational Therapy in Health Care, 19*, 47-70.

Taylor, R. R. (2005). Can the social model explain all of disability experience? Perspectives of persons with chronic fatigue syndrome. *American Journal of Occupational Therapy, 59*(5), 497-506.

Temple, L. K., McLeod, R. S., Gallinger, S., & Wright, J. G. (2001). Essays on science and society. Defining disease in the genomics era. *Science, 293*(5531), 807-810.

Thibodaux, L. R. (2005). Habitus and the embodiment of disability through lifestyle. *American Journal of Occupational Therapy, 59*(5), 507-515.

Vrkljan, B. H. (2005). Dispelling the disability stereotype: Embracing a universalistic perspective of disablement. *Canadian Journal of Occupational Therapy, 72*(1), 57-59.

Wilcock, A. A. (1993). Biological and sociocultural aspects of occupation, health and health promotion. *British Journal of Occupational Therapy, 56*(6), 200-203.

Wilcock, A. A. (1998). *An occupational perspective of health.* Thorofare, NJ: SLACK Incorporated.

Wilcock, A. A. (2005). Occupational science: Bridging occupation and health. *Canadian Journal of Occupational Therapy, 72*(1), 5-12.

Wilcock, A. A. (2006). *An occupational perspective of health* (2nd ed.). Thorofare, NJ: SLACK Incorporated.

Wilkins, S., Jung, B., Wishart, L., Edwards, M., & Norton, S. G. (2003). The effectiveness of community-based occupational therapy education and functional training programs for older adults: A critical literature review. *Canadian Journal of Occupational Therapy, 70*, 214-225

World Health Organization. (2001). *International classification of functioning, disability, and health (ICF).* Geneva, Switzerland: Author.

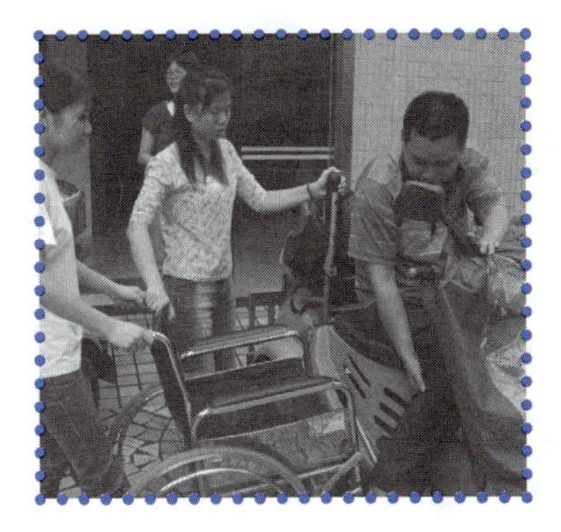

# 6

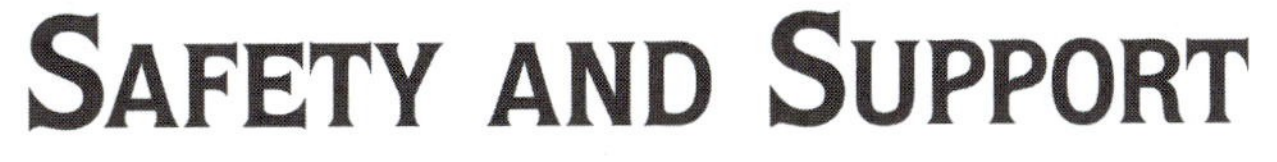

# SAFETY AND SUPPORT

*Claudia E. Oakes, OTR/L, PhD*

**ACOTE Standards Explored in This Chapter**

B.2.8-2.9

**Key Terms**

| | |
|---|---|
| Safety | Support |
| Standard precautions | |

## Introduction

This chapter will address ways in which occupational therapy practitioners can take steps to optimize their personal safety and the safety of their clients. It will also address ways in which practitioners support clients' occupational performance to promote satisfaction and well-being. While individual health care facilities provide routine training on safety issues, this chapter will provide an overview of the basic issues related to safety. It is not intended to serve as a replacement for individualized safety training specific to a particular setting. All practitioners have a responsibility to receive ongoing training and to adhere to institutional policies and procedures related to safety.

Safety and support, in the context of occupational therapy, are multifaceted concepts encompassing elements of the person, the environment, and the activity and the interaction between them (Holm, Rogers, & James, 1998). The "person" in the context of safety may refer to the occupational therapy practitioner or the client. Any activity may fall on a continuum of risk from "not safe at all" to "very safe." However, it is the interaction between the person, the activity, and the environment that largely dictates whether an activity is safe. For example, consider the activity of meal preparation. There is minimal safety risk for a person without impairments who is making a simple meal in an uncluttered kitchen using appliances that are in good working condition. However, meal preparation does present a safety risk for a person with impaired vision (interaction between the person and the activity) or for a person who is attempting to cook in a cluttered or inadequately lit work space (interaction between the person and the environment).

The framework identifies "safety and emergency maintenance" as instrumental activities of daily living (IADL) that involve "knowing and performing preventive procedures to maintain a safe environment as well as recognizing sudden, unexpected hazardous situations and initiating emergency action to reduce the threat to health and safety" (American Occupational Therapy Association [AOTA], 2008, p. 620). This definition can be applied to practitioners for use in their daily practice, as well as to clients who are addressing issues related to functional independence. Safety concerns are present across the continuum of settings in which occupational therapy practitioners work. Although the safety issues that emerge in acute care, rehabilitation, skilled nursing facilities, schools, or home care may differ, practitioners must be vigilant in their efforts to maximize safety. Practitioners support clients' independence by providing a safe context for the participant to explore and master his or her chosen occupations. Practitioners' efforts to support the



K. Sladyk, K. Jacobs, & N. MacRae (Eds.).
*Occupational Therapy Essentials for Clinical Competence* (pp. 55-64).

functional independence of clients must always be balanced with efforts to maintain their safety.

## General Safety Principles

When initiating contact with a client, practitioners must take steps to ensure that they are working with the correct client. For hospitalized clients, this may include checking their wrist band and/or confirming the identity with the client, a family member, or staff.

Occupational therapy practitioners must have accurate, up-to-date information about their clients. This may involve reading the medical chart or consulting with other staff members in preparation for the therapeutic encounter. If there is a question with respect to a client's status or his or her ability to engage in therapy (e.g., there may be conflicting information in a client's medical chart), clarification must be obtained before initiating contact with the client. Practitioners must be aware of any precautions or contraindications for intervention. For example, there may be the following:

- Orthopedic precautions (do not flex hips greater than 90 degrees)
- Cardiac precautions (stop activity if heart rate increases more than 20 beats per minute over baseline)
- Positioning precautions (do not raise head of bed greater than 30 degrees)
- Weight-bearing precautions (no more than toe-touch weight bearing on left lower extremity)
- Precautions related to feeding status (fluid restrictions, thickened liquids only)
- Supervision precautions (do not leave client unattended)

Practitioners must be aware of any procedures that the client may have undergone and whether any follow-up precautions must be observed. For example, clients may be required to remain on bed rest for a set amount of time following an angiography (Gall, Tarique, Natarajan, & Zaman, 2006). Additionally, practitioners must be aware of the effects of drugs and common side effects that might relate to occupational therapy. Practitioners should know how to interpret common laboratory values with respect to a client's ability to engage in therapy.

The practitioner should reduce physical hazards in the environment in order to support occupational performance. The space should be visually inspected to ensure that falling hazards have been eliminated, sharp objects from previous sessions have been stored, and potentially dangerous objects have been removed. Floors should be clear of liquid and debris.

The practitioner is required to make judgments about what is safe for each individual client. Judgments about materials such as sharp-edged scissors, needles, knives, ovens, and stoves need to be made on a case-by-case basis with each client. The dynamic nature of clients' status requires therapists to continually reassess clients' ability to safely engage in a particular occupation on a given day. Further, in order to fully support clients in performing their occupational roles and responsibilities, the practitioner must support the cultural, physical, social, personal, spiritual, temporal, and virtual contexts in which the clients are engaged. For example, some clients may need both safety education and social support to explore the Internet. The therapist must use clinical reasoning during the evaluation and intervention of both safety and support to enhance clients' quality of life.

Practitioners must consider the physical, cognitive, and emotional demands of activities to determine whether participation has the potential to compromise the client's safety. Ongoing activity analysis helps to ensure an appropriate "fit" between the client, the activity, and the materials that are needed. Adapting an activity in order to provide an appropriate challenge is a fundamental step in providing support for clients and in keeping them safe while allowing them to advance their functional status.

Impaired cognition presents serious safety concerns across intervention settings. Practitioners must be aware of clients' awareness of and ability to respond to potentially dangerous situations. In order to maintain safety, clients must demonstrate adequate attention, memory, judgment, temporal awareness, problem solving, decision making, and the ability to initiate actions in a timely manner. Occupational therapists are often called upon to determine if a client can safely perform an activity independently. Part of that decision making involves determining the client's ability to respond to unsafe conditions in an effective manner and what supports might be needed to maximize safe performance. Supports may be environmental (e.g., grab bars), social (e.g., "friendly visitors"), or virtual (e.g., daily e-mail contact).

Following intervention encounters, therapists must use judgment when making decisions about how and where to leave clients. For example, some clients may be left alone in their hospital room, while others must be supervised at all times. Some will need assistance with transport to another therapy session. It is important to know each client's status with respect to his or her ability to manage independently after a therapy session.

## Suicide Risk

As health care workers who treat clients with a wide range of diagnoses and stressors, occupational therapy practitioners must be alert to the risk of suicide. Practitioners must be able to accurately assess whether clients have made a suicide attempt, the risk of repetition, if suicidal ideation is present, and if the client feels hopelessness and/or impulsivity (Bruce & Borg, 2002). If a client makes indirect comments that suggest he or she has considered suicide, ask directly if there is a plan to commit suicide. Any statement about suicide should be taken seriously and shared with other members of the team.

A client who appears to be suicidal should not be left unattended. The practitioner should inform the client that he or she has a responsibility to alert the physician immediately. It is critical to document any statement the client has made relative to a suicide threat, as well as any action that has been taken.

# Infection Control

Infection control is a basic component of clinical practice for all practitioners regardless of the practice setting. Therapists must be vigilant in their efforts to curb the spread of infection and reduce their personal risk of becoming infected with contaminated materials. Practitioners must be aware of the risk of drug-resistant pathogens.

Methicillin-resistant *Staphylococcus aureus* (MRSA), vancomycin-resistant enterococci (VRE), and other gram-negative bacilli (GNB) are microorganisms that are resistant to one or more classes of antibiotics. Since there are limited intervention options if an infection develops from one of these organisms, it is critical that all health care workers take steps to reduce the spread of infection. The Centers for Disease Control and Prevention (CDC) has developed a campaign that is available online to help hospital workers reduce the risk of spreading drug-resistant pathogens (www.cdc.gov/drugresistance/healthcare/default.htm). Guidelines differ for hospitalized adults, adults receiving dialysis, hospitalized children, long-term care clients, and surgical clients (CDC, 2002).

Therapists should routinely follow standard precautions, which include thorough hand washing and the use of workplace procedures to reduce the risk of transmission of infectious agents. Workplace procedures, or the way tasks are performed, can minimize risk. Workplace procedures include proper waste disposal; appropriate laundry handling; and the proper use of personal protective equipment (PPE) such as gloves, eye protection, face shields, masks, and gowns.

Standard precautions are a combination of universal precautions and body substance isolation (BSI). Universal precautions were developed in the 1980s to prevent the transmission of blood-borne pathogens such as human immunodeficiency virus (HIV) (Occupational Safety and Health Administration [OSHA], 2002a). BSI precautions were developed to minimize the risk of transmission of pathogens from moist body substances such as infected respiratory secretions or urine. The CDC developed standard precautions based on the assumption that all blood, body fluids, secretions, excretions (other than sweat), nonintact skin, and mucous membranes may contain infectious agents that could be transmitted to other people (Siegel, Rhinehart, Jackson, Chiarello, & Healthcare Infection Control Practices Advisory Committee, 2007). Some standard precautions are below.

## Hand Hygiene

When properly performed, hand washing can be the single most important way to prevent the spread of disease (Potter & Perry, 2004). Hands should be washed before and after contact with every client. Additionally, hand washing should be completed after coming into contact with blood, body fluids, secretions, excretions, or any client care equipment. If contact with these substances takes place, practitioners should wash their hands even if gloves were worn.

The correct technique involves rubbing the hands together under running water for at least 15 seconds using a mild soap (Boyce, Pittet, Healthcare Infection Control Practices Advisory Committee, & HICPAC/SHEA/APIC/IDSA Hand Hygiene Task Force, 2002). Rub vigorously under the nails, in between the fingers, and on both surfaces of the hands. Rinse thoroughly under running water. Leave the water running while drying hands and use a clean paper towel to turn off the water. Waterless, alcohol-based, antiseptic rubs are acceptable substitutes for routine hand washing when no visible soil is present. Such rubs may be used when running water is not accessible or convenient, though hands should be washed under running water at the earliest opportunity. The CDC guidelines for hand washing are available online in an interactive video format at www.cdc.gov/handhygiene/training/interactiveEducation.

## Gloves

Gloves are a critical component of PPE used to reduce the risk of transmission of infectious agents. Therapists should don gloves before coming into contact with blood, body fluids, secretions, excretions, and contaminated items and before touching mucous membranes or nonintact skin. For occupational therapy practitioners, it is appropriate to don gloves during sessions involving wound care, oral hygiene, or toileting. Remove gloves immediately after use. The proper technique for removing gloves involves pulling the first glove off by grasping the outer surface of the glove to be removed (not the surface touching the skin) and slipping the glove inside out as it is pulled off the hand. To remove the second glove, slip a nongloved finger under the remaining glove and pull it off while turning it inside out. Dispose of both gloves by touching only the inner glove surface. Do not touch noncontaminated items before removing gloves. Hands should be washed immediately after removing gloves (Boyce et al., 2002).

## Masks, Eye Protection, and Face Shields

Masks, eye protection, and face shields may be needed if it is anticipated that blood, body fluids, secretions, or excretions will splash during interaction with the client.

These pieces of PPE protect the practitioner's eyes, nose, and mouth from exposure to sprayed microorganisms.

## Gowns

A nonsterile gown is used for protecting skin and clothing during interactions when splashes are likely to occur. The cuffs of the gown should be tucked into the top of the gloves. After the session, the gown should be untied, held away from the body while being removed, rolled inside out, then disposed of in an appropriate container. Hands should be washed immediately after the gown and gloves are removed.

## Client Care Equipment

Care must be taken to prevent the spread of microorganisms on equipment that is used by and with clients. Equipment should be cleaned after use with an approved solution according to institutional policy. Mat tables and adaptive equipment should be cleaned according to departmental policy. Single-use items should be discarded appropriately.

## Linens

Practitioners should take steps to minimize skin and mucous membrane exposure to soiled linens. Practitioners may encounter soiled linens when performing activities of daily living (ADL) with clients. Gloves should be worn to remove soiled linens, then soiled linens should be placed in an appropriate leak-proof container for transport to laundry.

## Other Precautions

Additional practices, including airborne infection isolation rooms, contact precautions, and droplet precautions, are used to prevent transmission of infectious agents spread by direct or indirect contact with a client or the client's environment (CDC, 2004). They reflect a higher standard of infection control than standard precautions. Private rooms, negative airflow pressure, and respiratory protection devices add extra levels of infection control for clients placed under these precautions. Appropriate signage will alert practitioners of the need to follow special precautions.

## Respiratory Hygiene/ Coughing Etiquette

This recent addition to standard precautions (Siegel et al., 2007) broadly applies to all people who enter health care settings, including visitors. For example, a client's family member may have a cough and should therefore use coughing etiquette (e.g., covering the mouth) to reduce the spread of undiagnosed infection. Respiratory hygiene requires people with coughs or respiratory discharge to cover their mouths when coughing, dispose of used tissues, and wash hands as soon as possible after doing so, wear masks if tolerated, and maintain greater than 3 feet distance from others.

## Vaccinations

The Hepatitis B virus (HBV) presents a serious risk of infection for health care workers (CDC, 1997). The HBV series reduces the risk of infection and is available, free of charge, to hospital employees who are at risk of exposure (OSHA, 2003). Health care workers may be asked to sign a declination if they choose not to receive the vaccine.

The CDC (1997) recommends that health care workers receive annual influenza vaccinations. The CDC (2004) also recommends periodic skin testing to detect the presence of tuberculosis for health care workers at risk of exposure.

# Basic First Aid

Occupational therapy practitioners should demonstrate competence with basic first aid. It is important to keep current with training, as the standards periodically change. Contact the American Red Cross (www.redcross.org) for the most up-to-date information and for information about training sessions.

## Burns

Therapists should take care to ensure that burns do not occur during the course of splinting, cooking, or bathing with clients. First-degree thermal burns, which result in reddened skin, should be treated by putting the burned area under cool, running water for five minutes. The burned area should be covered with a clean or sterile dressing. Creams or ointments should not be applied. Any more serious injury should be immediately reported and treated by other health care professionals (American Red Cross, 2005).

## Bleeding

In the event of bleeding, the practitioner should don gloves and then apply pressure with a sterile dressing. Tourniquets should not be used due to the risk of injury to nerves and/or muscles because of problems associated with ischemia. If a client has a laceration, running water should be applied for up to 5 minutes to clear the area of any foreign matter (American Red Cross, 2005). Professional judgment is necessary to determine if further medical assistance is necessary.

## Allergies

### Latex Allergy

Latex allergies emerged as a significant public health issue in the late 1980s and into the early 1990s. During the 1990s, some estimates suggested that 1 in 10 health care workers suffered from latex allergy, but a shift to powder-free, low-protein latex has resulted in a significant decline in the incidence (Beezhold & Sussman, 2005). However, even with this reduction, practitioners need to be aware of the symptoms of latex allergy, which include redness and itching (typically on hands); difficulty breathing; wheezing; swelling of skin, lips, and tongue; and shortness of breath. If a person exhibits these symptoms after exposure to latex products, emergency medical attention is required. Be aware that some supplies in the occupational therapy department may contain latex, such as gloves and resistance bands. Latex-free versions of many products are available for clients with latex sensitivities.

### Food Allergies and Anaphylaxis

It is estimated that 11 million Americans have food allergies; 5 million of which are children (Sicherer, 2006). It is important for occupational therapy practitioners to be aware of the presence of food allergies in their clients. Allergies should be taken into account when working with feeding, meal preparation, certain craft activities, or when going on food-related outings. Be aware of the symptoms of an allergic reaction: hives, swelling of lips or tongue, vomiting, trouble breathing, or a drop in blood pressure (anaphylaxis). Should these symptoms develop, emergency medical attention is required. To prevent accidental ingestion of allergens, always read labels when completing meal preparation activities. Avoid cross contamination when engaging in cooking activities by keeping utensils separate. For example, always use separate utensils for peanut better and jelly. Be aware of each client's emergency protocol in the event of accidental ingestion. Reactions to food allergies are commonly treated with an auto-injector of epinephrine (Epi-Pen; DEY, L. P., Napa, CA). It is important to know where the Epi-Pen is located and who is trained in its use.

## Orthostatic Hypotension

A client with orthostatic hypotension (OH) demonstrates a decrease in blood pressure of more than 20 mm Hg in systolic and of more than 10 mm Hg in diastolic, while also experiencing a 20% increase in heart rate (Goodman, Fuller, & Boissonnault, 2003). A client may experience confusion, dizziness, visual blurring, and possibly fainting when coming to stand. Practitioners must be aware of the potential causes of OH in order to prevent its onset. Some common causes include dehydration, venous pooling, side effects to medications, and prolonged immobility. To minimize the risk of orthostatic hypotension in a client who is coming to stand from a supine or seated position, instruct the client to rise slowly, flex and extend the ankles, and lift the arms overhead while tightening the abdominal muscles and exhaling through pursed lips. If symptoms develop, help the client into a supine position with the legs elevated, unless contraindicated. Monitor the client's vital signs, including pulse, blood pressure, and respiratory rate. This is particularly important in clients with chronic obstructive pulmonary disease who may not tolerate the "legs elevated" position.

Be aware of the risk of fainting for others in the health care environment. Visitors, including students and volunteers, may be at risk of fainting. This is due to emotional stress and the tendency of blood to pool in the lower extremities while standing with knees locked, as is often the case when observing intervention sessions. To prevent fainting, keep legs moving by marching in place or crossing legs. Warn visitors to alert a staff member if they feel lightheaded or dizzy. Provide assurance that they should feel free to leave the immediate area if they feel faint.

## Seizures

If a client has a generalized tonic-clonic or grand mal seizure during an occupational therapy session, the practitioner is responsible for ensuring the client is not injured and that an open airway is maintained. These types of seizures generally last approximately 2 minutes and are characterized by a loss of consciousness, rigidity, jerky movements, and shallow breathing. The client should be gently lowered to the ground, mat table, or bed. Do not make any attempt to prevent the client from biting his or her tongue. Loosen clothing around the client's neck to ensure adequate airflow. Do not restrain the client. After the seizure is complete, place the client in the recovery position, lying on his or her side with his or her hand in front. Call for medical assistance (American Red Cross, 2005).

A seizure that lasts for more than 15 minutes, or a series of seizures that lasts for 20 minutes without regaining consciousness in between may suggest status epilepticus. This is a medical emergency and assistance should be sought at once.

## Diabetes

When working with clients who have diabetes, it is important for practitioners to differentiate between signs and symptoms of low blood sugar (hypoglycemia) and high blood sugar (hyperglycemia). Low blood sugar occurs when blood glucose falls below optimal levels and can occur if a client is engaging in physical activity, if there is too much systemic insulin, or if the client has ingested too little food. Some oral medications used to treat diabetes can also cause low blood sugar. Symptoms are variable and may include shakiness, a sense of weakness, a feeling of anxiety and confusion, dizziness, headache, blurred vision, and/or sweating. Practitioners should be aware that therapy sessions may interrupt the usual meal or snack time and, therefore, result in hypoglycemia. If a client displays symptoms of hypoglycemia, he or she should have a small snack that has a fast-acting source of sugar, such as juice or hard candy. After the snack, the client should check his or her blood sugar level, then contact a nurse or physician if levels are not within the client's acceptable parameters.

High blood sugar may be caused by overeating, poor coordination of eating, medication, infection, or stress. Clients with hyperglycemia may experience fatigue, low energy levels, frequent urination, and/or excessive thirst. High blood sugar may lead to diabetic ketoacidosis, which is a medical emergency. It is caused by inadequate insulin, vast deviation from diet, fever, or infection. The client may have gradual-onset weakness, stomach pain, body aches, labored breathing, fruity breath, dry mouth, nausea, and/or vomiting. Should these symptoms occur, contact medical professionals at once, immediately test blood sugar, and provide the client with plain water (Ross, Boucher, & O'Connell, 2005).

### Cardiac Arrest and Choking

Occupational therapy practitioners should maintain cardiopulmonary resuscitation (CPR) certification to treat a person who is choking or who is experiencing cardiac arrest. Local chapters of the American Red Cross or the American Heart Association (www.americanheart.org) may be contacted for information about training courses. Protocols are constantly changing as best practices are updated. A thorough description of these procedures is beyond the scope of this chapter.

## Client Care Equipment

Clients may be connected to intravenous (IV) lines, arterial lines, central lines, feeding tubes, chest tubes, ventilators, catheters, and/or a variety of monitors. It is essential that the occupational therapy practitioner be aware of the purpose of various tubes and monitors. The practitioner should identify all lines and where they connect. In general, it is wise to avoid tugging, pulling, or occluding lines and to ensure adequate slack before moving the client. If any tension is felt, it is recommended that the practitioner stop and check to determine the cause.

Precautions for each tube, line, or monitor must be identified. For example, an arterial line is a catheter that is placed in the radial artery to continually measure blood pressure. Extra caution must be taken to prevent dislodging an arterial line as dislodging one will cause profuse bleeding (Potter & Perry, 2004). The practitioner must be aware of institutional policies regarding specific equipment and of any particular precautions for an individual client.

Additionally, it is important that the practitioner is aware of the parameters for any monitors that are providing information about a client's physiologic state. For example, it is generally recommended that activity be stopped if oxygen saturation is below 90%, as measured by a pulse oxymeter. The acceptable saturation may be lower in some clients with chronic pulmonary disease (Goodman et al., 2003).

## Hazardous Materials

Practitioners should be aware of the presence of hazardous materials in the occupational therapy department. It is important to know where the Material Safety Data Sheets (MSDS) are stored. These sheets are required by OSHA (www.osha.gov). They contain useful information about proper storage of hazards, ways in which products are toxic, and information on how to clean a spill, or how to administer first aid if accidental exposure occurs.

## Fire Safety

All institutionally-based practitioners must be familiar with the fire safety procedures at their facility. This includes knowing the floor map of the facility, the areas for zone evacuation, the location of fire pulls, and the specifics of any emergency plan (OSHA, 2002b). In general, the acronym RACE is helpful to recall in the event of a fire (Potter & Perry, 2004):

- *R*—Remove all persons who are in immediate danger.
- *A*—Activate the pull station and call 911.
- *C*—Close doors to prevent the spread of fire. This includes fire doors, smoke doors, and doors to client rooms.
- *E*—Extinguish the fire as dictated by department policy.

If a practitioner is called upon to use a fire extinguisher, the acronym PASS guides technique:

- *P*—Pull the pin to break the glass.
- *A*—Aim the extinguisher at the base of the fire.
- *S*—Squeeze the handles together.
- *S*—Sweep from side to side at the base of the fire.

It is essential that the correct extinguisher is used for the specific type of fire. Labels on extinguishers identify whether they are best used for combustibles, flammable liquids, or electrical fires. More information can be obtained on the OSHA Web site at: www.osha.gov/SLTC/etools/evacuation/portable_use.html.

### Fire Safety in Clients' Homes

Practitioners working in home care settings should ensure that clients have smoke detectors in their homes. There should be at least one smoke detector on each level of the home, including the basement. Batteries should be checked twice yearly, at a minimum. Smoke detectors should be replaced every 8 to 10 years.

Therapists should review fire plans with members of the household, which should include:

- How to exit the house
- Where to meet outside
- Who is responsible for any person who may need extra help

There should be two methods of egress in every dwelling, and this may include a window (U.S. Fire Administration, 2007). It is recommended that people with disabilities notify members of local fire departments in order to facilitate assistance in the event of an emergency.

## Safety During Transfers and Mobility

Practitioners should be familiar with the parts of hospital beds, mechanical lifts, and mobility aids before performing transfers or mobility with clients. It is critical to be aware of the procedure for locking bed and wheelchair locks to keep the objects in place. Each client should be positioned in a way that is consistent with precautions specific to his or her condition. Adjusting the height of the bed can ease transfers, requiring less effort for clients and ensuring safety for the practitioner who is assisting.

It is important to have adequate room to work, whether in clients' rooms, in the clinic, or in clients' homes. Practitioners should avoid working in small spaces as much as possible. They should also clear out unneeded equipment such as bedside tables, extra wheelchairs, or other mobility aides in order to have adequate room.

Any equipment belonging to an occupational therapy department should be properly maintained. This includes cleaning, ensuring that locks work, and ensuring that all working parts are intact. Routine checks to ensure that every piece of equipment works properly and is stable are important preventive steps to ensure client safety (Kangas, 2002).

The use of proper body mechanics when transferring clients minimizes the risk of injury to practitioners or others who are assisting in the transfer. In general, this involves positioning one's self close to the person being transferred, maintaining a wide base of support, using large muscle groups to move the person, and avoiding twisting movements (Pierson, 1999). Additionally, it is important to be aware of any conditions that may affect the client's performance during transfers such as fragile skin, orthostatic hypotension, amputations, pain, or spasms. Also, it is essential that the practitioner stay current with any precautions or contraindications related to transfers, as these are subject to change.

Practitioners must take the time to be aware of best practices regarding injury prevention. For example, research does not support a commonly held belief that back belts reduce injuries caused by lifting (Wassell, Gerdner, Landsittel, J. J. Johnston & J. M. Johnston, 2001). It is recommended, however, that practitioners use a gait belt with clients when performing transfers or ambulation, unless contraindicated (e.g., after abdominal surgery) (Pierson, 1999). A gait belt prevents the practitioner from having to grasp body parts or clothing when providing assistance with mobility. It can also be instrumental in controlling the speed and direction of a fall if the client cannot support his or her own body weight.

Working with clients who are extremely overweight poses potential safety concerns for health care workers and for the clients themselves. Of particular concern is the use of transfer devices and bathroom equipment. Special equipment designed for the bariatric population may be ordered to ensure safety when transferring, bathing, and toileting (Foti & Littrel, 2004). Typically, the weight capacity of durable medical equipment is listed in the ordering information. The practitioner should also consider the distribution of the client's weight, his or her preferred methods of movement, and any anxiety related to mobility.

## Fall Prevention and Restraint Use

Minimizing the incidence of client falls is an important safety consideration for occupational therapy practitioners. This is especially true for the elderly and persons with chronic illness who are at an elevated risk. The consequences of a serious fall may include head injury, hip fracture, psychological harm, or death. Falls may be caused by many factors, including medications; age-related changes (such as increased need to urinate at night); visual, balance, strength, or cognitive impairments; or environmental obstacles. Fall prevention efforts are context-specific, but generally include multiple interventions such as balance and gait training, medication management, environmental modifications, and attention to health concerns such as postural hypotension (American Geriatrics Society, British Geriatrics Society, & American Academy of Orthopedic Surgeons, 2001).

The Centers for Medicare and Medicaid Services (CMS) defines restraints as

> Any manual method, physical or manual device, material, or equipment that immobilizes or reduces the ability of a client to move his or her arms, legs, body, or head freely; a drug or medication when it is used as a restriction to manage the client's behavior or restrict the client's freedom of movement and is not a standard intervention or dosage for the client's condition (CMS & HHS, 2006).

Historically, restraints were thought to reduce the risk of falling, but research has shown that restraints are ineffective in reducing fall risk. In fact, they can pose serious threats to safety, including incontinence, physical injury, and in some cases, death (Evans & Strumpf, 1990; Miles & Irvine, 1992).

Physicians or other licensed independent practitioners are permitted to order physical restraints to treat medical symptoms. The client or surrogate decision makers must consent to their use. Physician's orders must include the circumstances and duration of restraint use, and clients must be carefully monitored while restraints are in use.

Occupational therapy practitioners can play an important part in carefully analyzing a client's fall risk to determine if there are less-restrictive options available. A variety of physical and social supports can minimize reliance on external restraints. In the event that physical restraints are in use, practitioners must ensure that the restraints are applied correctly each time they are fastened in order to prevent accidental injury. Restraints should be fastened to the frame of the bed or wheelchair rather than to a moveable part such as a bed rail or arm rest. A strap attached to a bed rail, for example, may tighten when the rail is lifted or lowered, causing injury to the client (Potter & Perry, 2004).

## Home Safety

Working in clients' homes provides an opportunity for the practitioner to make recommendations to enhance safety within the home. Every client presents with different safety needs due to the complex interaction between individual impairments, unique elements of the physical and social environment, and the range of activities performed (Clemson, 1997). Practitioners have the ability, when working in clients' homes, to observe how activities are performed in their own context, how their social supports influence participation in occupations, and how routines and habits enhance or impede safety.

The following list is a useful starting point for addressing physical safety in clients' homes:

- Ensure adequate lighting throughout the home. While assessing lighting, also consider blocking light to minimize the effects of glare.
- Ensure adequate support during mobility. This may include hand rails on stairs, grab bars in bathrooms, and/or bed mobility aids.
- Minimize tripping hazards such as obstacles on floor, unsecured rugs, unfastened sills/uneven flooring, and electrical cords.
- Ensure safe and simple access to commonly used items around the home.
- Reduce the risk of scalding injuries by setting the water heater thermostat to no more than 120 degrees.
- Prevent electrical injuries by covering outlets, using surge protectors, and keeping electrical cords intact by storing them out of the way of foot traffic.

## Personal Safety in Home Care Contexts

Working in clients' homes poses a unique set of safety concerns. Practitioners must take precautions to ensure personal safety when working in the home care environment. It is a safe practice to call before going to a client's home to confirm your arrival. Additionally, practitioners should use an escort if there is a perceived threat to personal safety. This is a common service available through many home care agencies. A mobile phone should be readily available (on your person, if possible) in the event of an emergency.

As a means of infection control, it is recommended that practitioners refrain from placing personal items or therapy equipment bags on the ground. Rather, they should be placed over a chair back. Therapy equipment should be appropriately disinfected after each client encounter.

### Areas of Competence

Therapists have a responsibility to "work within their areas of competence" (Reitz et al., 2006, p. 654) and to be aware of their personal limitations in knowledge or expertise. To maintain safe practices, assistance should be sought before performing an evaluation or intervention beyond one's skill set. Additional training, coursework, or education may be needed before working with certain groups of clients. For example, an *American Journal of Occupational Therapy* paper describes the advanced knowledge and skill for occupational therapy practice in neonatal intensive care units (Vergara et al., 2006). The complexity of this practice setting is compounded by the unique nature of the medical diagnoses, medication regimes, technology, and the family and team dynamics that are present. It is therefore not a recommended practice context for occupational therapy assistants, entry-level therapists, or therapists without prior pediatric experience.

It is imperative for practitioners to allow only authorized personnel to provide intervention. Family members, volunteers, or other unqualified persons should not assist with or carry out interventions they are not capable of completing. When providing caregiver education and training, the practitioner should document their competence before allowing the caregiver to complete a task independently. Additionally, occupational therapists have a duty to be clear about the roles and responsibilities of the occupational therapy assistant.

Occupational therapy practitioners should report any potentially unsafe practices to a supervisor and work within their means to ensure that the practices are not carried out in the interim. Careful documentation of adverse incidents is necessary. Proper reporting procedures dictated by your institution should be used.

## Summary

Occupational therapy practitioners are instrumental in ensuring that the physical and social environments provide support for client functioning while minimizing the risk of adverse events. Careful attention to the interaction between the person, the environment, and the activity allows practitioners to create situations in which clients can successfully engage in meaningful occupations and enhance their quality of life.

Practitioners must engage in lifelong learning to maintain competence in safety-related issues. It is critical to keep current regarding institutional policies and procedures, clients' conditions, and the physical and social environments in order to optimize safety.

# Student Self-Assessment

1. Become a keen observer of safety in a variety of contexts. Identify safety hazards in a variety of contexts:
   - In your own living environment
   - At the mall
   - In a waiting room
   - On a playground
   - On a road or sidewalk in your neighborhood.

   Attend to the interaction between different people in the environment (children, adults, older adults), the activities (walking, driving, cooking), and elements of the context (mobile phones, branches in the road, shoes on the floor). Identify the threats to safety and make recommendations to improve safety.

   Example (Figure 6-1):

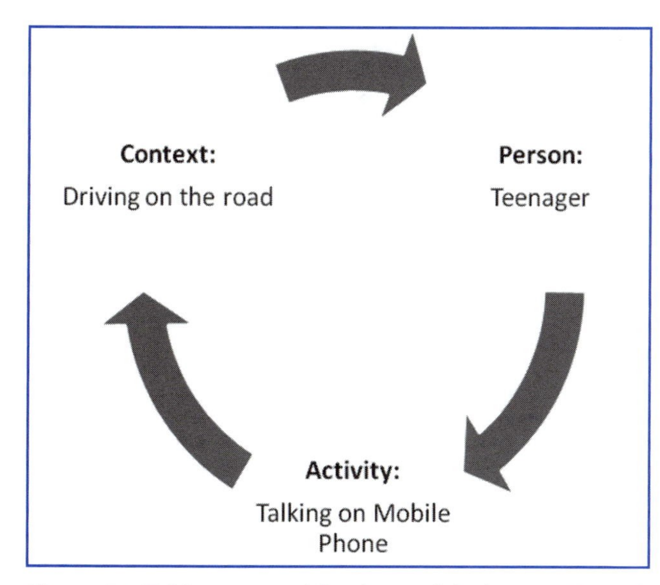


**Figure 6-1.** Talking on a mobile phone while driving is hazardous to the driver, other passengers in the car, and to others on the road. The solution is to pull off the side of the road to make or receive a phone call.

2. Practice washing your hands according to the CDC standards. Notice how long 15 seconds of scrubbing feels. Also practice donning and doffing PPE according to the standards.
3. Develop a fire escape plan for your current living conditions. Be sure to have two methods of egress. Be sure the dwelling has smoke detectors with intact batteries. If there is an extinguisher present, read the directions to identify the type of fire it can be used on and the procedure for use. Identify the actions suggested by the acronyms RACE and PASS.

# Electronic Resources

- Centers for Disease Control and Prevention: www.cdc.gov
- Occupational Safety and Health Administration: www.osha.gov
- American Red Cross: www.redcross.org
- American Heart Association: www.americanheart.org
- Joint Commission: www.jointcommission.org
- National Safety Council: www.nsc.org

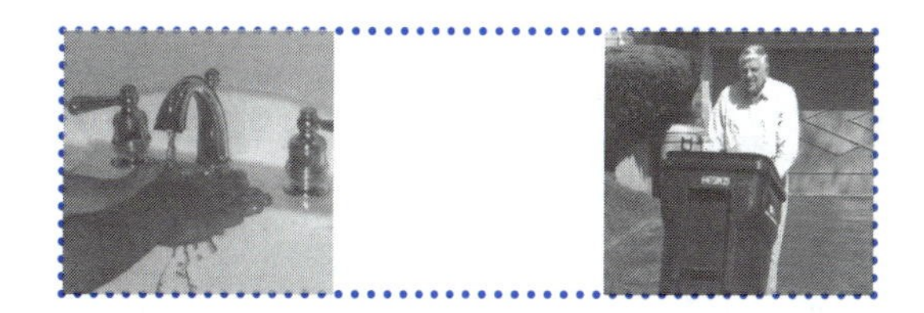

# References

American Geriatrics Society, British Geriatrics Society, & American Academy of Orthopedic Surgeons Panel on Falls Prevention. (2001). Guidelines for the prevention of falls in older persons. *Journal of the American Geriatrics Society, 49*(5), 664-672.

American Occupational Therapy Association. (2008). Occupational therapy framework: Domain and process, second edition. *American Journal of Occupational Therapy, 62*, 625-683.

American Red Cross. (2005). First aid. *Circulation, 112*(Supplement I), IV-196–IV-203. Retrieved June 30, 2007, from http://circ.ahajournals.org/cgi/reprint/112/24_suppl/IV-196

Beezhold, D., & Sussman, G. (2005). Lessons learned from latex allergy. *Business Briefing: Global Surgery and Future Directions*. Retrieved August 5, 2009, from http://www.touchbriefings.com/cdps/cditem.cfm?NID=1438

Boyce, J. M., Pittet, D., Healthcare Infection Control Practices Advisory Committee, & HICPAC/SHEA/APIC/IDSA Hand Hygiene Task Force. (2002). Guideline for hand hygiene in health-care settings: Recommendations of the Healthcare Infection Control Practices Advisory Committee and the HICPAC/SHEA/APIC/IDSA Hand Hygiene Task Force. *MMWR: Recommendations and Reports, 51*(RR-16), 1-45.

Bruce, M. A. G., & Borg, B. (2002). Suicidal behavior: Critical information for clinical reasoning. In M. A. G. Bruce & B. Borg. *Psychosocial frames of reference: Core for occupation-based practice* (3rd ed., pp. 323-324). Thorofare, NJ: SLACK Incorporated.

Centers for Disease Control and Prevention. (1997). Immunization of health-care workers: Recommendations of the Advisory Committee on Immunization Practices (ACIP) and the Hospital Infection Control Practices Advisory Committee (HICPAC). *MMWR: Recommendations and Reports, 46*(RR-18), 1-42.

Centers for Disease Control and Prevention. (2002). CDC's campaign to prevent antimicrobial resistance in health-care settings. *MMWR: Morbidity and Mortality Weekly Report, 51*(15), 343. Retrieved May 30, 2007, from http://www.cdc.gov/drugresistance/healthcare/default.htm

Centers for Disease Control and Prevention. (2004). Surveillance for tuberculosis infection in health care workers. *Worker Health Chartbook 2004. NIOSH Publication No. 2004-146.* Retrieved August 5, 2009, from http://www.cdc.gov/niosh/docs/2004-146/appendix/ap-a/ap-a-19.html

Centers for Medicare and Medicaid Services, Department of Health and Human Services. (2006). Medicare and Medicaid Programs; Hospital conditions of participation: Patients' rights: Final rule. *Federal Register, 71*(236), 71377-71428.

Clemson, L. (1997). *Home fall hazards: A guide to identifying fall hazards in the homes of elderly people and an accompaniment to the assessment tool, the Westmead Home Safety Assessment.* West Brunswick, Victoria, Australia: Coordinates Publication.

Evans, L. K., & Strumpf, N. E. (1990). Myths about elder restraint. *Image: Journal of Nursing Scholarship, 22*(2), 124-128.

Foti, D., & Littrel, E. (2004.) Bariatric care: Practical problem solving and interventions. *Physical Disabilities Special Interest Section Quarterly, 27,* 1-3, 6.

Gall, S., Tarique, A., Natarajan, A., & Zaman, A. (2006). Rapid ambulation after coronary angiography via femoral artery access: A prospective study of 1000 patients. *Journal of Invasive Cardiology, 18,* 106-108.

Goodman, C. C., Boissonnault, W. G., & Fuller, K. S.. (2003). *Pathology: Implications for the physical therapist* (2nd ed.). Philadelphia, PA: Saunders.

Holm, M. B., Rogers, J. C., & James, A. B. (1998). Treatment of occupational performance areas. In M. E. Neidstadt & E. B. Crepeau (Eds.), *Willard & Spackman's occupational therapy* (9th ed., pp. 323-390). Philadelphia, PA: Lippincott Williams and Wilkins.

Kangas, K. M. (2002). Managing transfers and lifting with the complicated patient. *Gerontology Special Interest Section Quarterly, 25,* 1-4.

Miles, S. H., & Irvine, P. (1992). Deaths caused by physical restraints. *Gerontologist, 32*(6), 762-766.

OSHA. (2002a). Fact Sheet: Bloodborne Pathogens. Retrieved June 30, 2007, from http://www.osha.gov/OshDoc/data_BloodborneFacts/bbfact01.pdf

OSHA. (2002b). Fact Sheet: Fire Safety in the Workplace. Retrieved June 30, 2007, from http://www.osha.gov/OshDoc/data_General_Facts/FireSafetyN.pdf

OSHA. (2003). Hospital eTool: Bloodborne Illnesses: Hepatitis B Virus. Retrieved June 30, 2007, from http://www.osha.gov/SLTC/etools/hospital/hazards/bbp/bbp.html#HepatitisBVirus

Pierson, F. M. (1999). *Principles and techniques of patient care* (2nd ed.). Philadelphia, PA: W.B. Saunders Company.

Potter, P. A., & Perry, A. G. (2004). *Fundamentals of nursing* (6th ed.). St. Louis, MO: Mosby.

Reitz, S. M., Austin, D. J., Brandt, L. C., DeBrakeller, B., Franck, L. G., Homenko, D. F., et al. (2006). Guidelines to the occupational therapy code of ethics. *American Journal of Occupational Therapy, 60*(6), 652-658.

Ross, T. A., Boucher, J. L., & O'Connell, B. S. (Eds.). (2005). *ADA guide to diabetes medical nutrition therapy and education.* Chicago, IL: American Dietetic Association.

Sicherer, S. H. (2006). *Understanding and managing your child's food allergies.* Baltimore, MD: The Johns Hopkins University Press.

Siegel, J. D., Rhinehart, E., Jackson, M., Chiarello, L., & Healthcare Infection Control Practices Advisory Committee. (2007). 2007 guideline for isolation precautions: Preventing transmission of infectious diseases in healthcare settings. Atlanta, GA: Centers for Disease Control. Retrieved July 10, 2007, from http://www.cdc.gov/ncidod/dhqp/pdf/guidelines/Isolation2007.pdf

U.S. Fire Administration. (2007). Home fire prevention. Retrieved May 25, 2007, from http://www.usfa.dhs.gov/citizens/all_citizens/home_fire_prev/

Vergara, E., Anzalone, M., Bigsby, R., Gorga, D., Holloway, E., Hunter, J., et al. (2006). Specialized knowledge and skills for occupational therapy practice in the Neonatal Intensive care unit. *American Journal of Occupational Therapy, 60*(6), 659-668.

Wassell, J. T., Gardner, L. I., Landsittel, D. P., Johnston, J. J., & Johnston, J. M. (2001). A prospective study of back belts for prevention of back pain and injury. *Journal of the American Medical Association, 284*(21), 2727-2732. Retrieved June 8, 2007, from www.cdc.gov/niosh/jamapapr.html

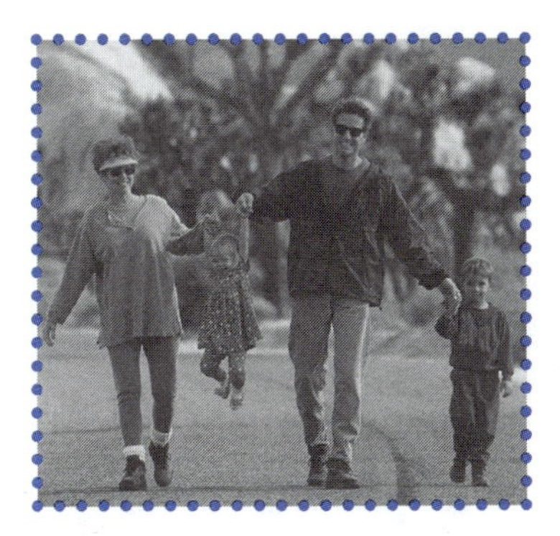

# 7

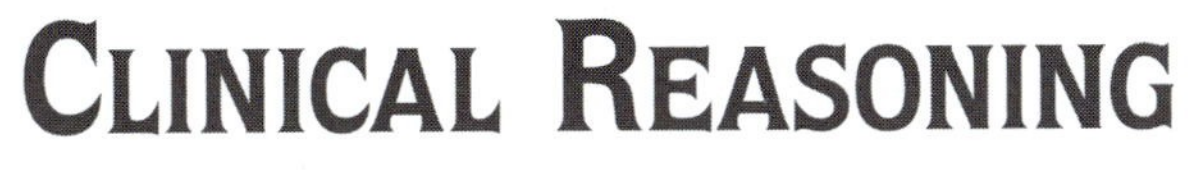

# Clinical Reasoning

*Callie Watson, OTD, OTR/L and Kristin B. Haas, OTD, OTR/L*

**ACOTE Standards Explored in This Chapter**

B.2.10-2.11

**Key Terms**

| | |
|---|---|
| Clinical reasoning | Pragmatic reasoning |
| Conditional reasoning | Procedural reasoning |
| Ethical reasoning | Reflection |
| Interactive reasoning | Scientific reasoning |
| Narrative reasoning | Tacit |

## Introduction

Occupational therapists and occupational therapy assistants make every effort to provide the best possible therapy to clients. In order to offer the best practice, to be able to influence policy and funding, and to better advocate for our clients, students and clinicians must understand clinical reasoning. For best practice, clinicians must make numerous decisions during the therapeutic process. These decisions and the processes by which one makes them can be referred to as clinical reasoning. Clinical reasoning is a complex process and can be difficult to describe secondary to its many tacit or unspoken methods.

Clinical reasoning is a concept that may be a challenge for students and new clinicians to fully grasp because experienced clinicians have a difficult time describing the complete process for their clinical reasoning and decision making. Research suggests that using a clinical reasoning thinking frame to organize clinical observations is an effective method to help entry-level occupational therapy students learn and apply clinical reasoning concepts (Neistadt, 1998). Rogers and Masagatani (1982) and Mattingly and Fleming (1994) had studied clinical reasoning in occupational therapy. The basis for their research involved the depiction of clinical reasoning as a cognitive process. The findings specifically from the American Occupational Therapy Association's (AOTA) Clinical Reasoning Study (Mattingly, 1991; Mattingly & Fleming) indicated that clinicians use several types of reasoning. The cognitive process includes narrative, procedural, interactive, and conditional reasoning. Mattingly and Fleming concluded that experienced practitioners seem to shift from one mode of thinking to another during the therapeutic intervention process. Other cognitive processes noted in clinical reasoning literature are conditional, scientific, pragmatic, and ethical reasoning.

### Narrative Reasoning

Narrative reasoning provides a way to learn about the person's life story. Developing an occupational profile on the client is a good example of narrative reasoning.



K. Sladyk, K. Jacobs, & N. MacRae (Eds.).
*Occupational Therapy Essentials for Clinical Competence* (pp. 65-72).

## Procedural Reasoning

Procedural reasoning involves thinking about the client's performance (Fleming, 1991). Clinicians and students use procedural reasoning to think about the disability level (diagnosis), focusing primarily on the body. Using this type of reasoning, one would next choose specific occupation-based intervention activities to maximize function while addressing the client's performance problems.

## Interactive Reasoning

Interactive reasoning is used to individualize the therapeutic approach and to understand the client as a human being. This type of reasoning suggests how clinicians may interpret and use verbal and nonverbal cues to engage the client (Crepeau, 1991). Interactive reasoning tries to understand the extent of limitation to occupational performance from the client's perspective and allows the clinician and client to collaborate for the best possible outcome(s).

## Conditional Reasoning

Conditional reasoning encompasses the holistic context of the person, his or her illness, and the possible and actual intervention. Scientific reasoning is used to understand the condition that may be affecting the person and family. Schell (1998) described scientific reasoning as the logical thinking about the nature of the client's problems and the optimal course of action in intervention. Scientific reasoning requires the clinician to consider the background knowledge that might help one to understand the characteristics of the condition better.

## Pragmatic Reasoning

Pragmatic reasoning is used to understand the practical issues that may have an impact on the situation with the person and family. Pragmatic reasoning enables clinicians to incorporate ideas into the situation this family is enduring, allowing one to identify practical strategies for intervention. Examples can include what are the family, caregiver, and community resources available to support intervention and follow-up recommendations? What materials and interdisciplinary support is available for intervention?

## Ethical Reasoning

Ethical reasoning is used to make sure one selects the morally justifiable choices. Ethical reasoning introduces the consideration of what "should" be done in the best interest of the person and family. To completely integrate all of these types of reasoning into best clinical reasoning, clinicians must utilize three methods of thinking. Figure 7-1 shows the overlap of these areas into best clinical reasoning. It is important that clinicians utilize their personal experience, evidence-based practice, and information about the client and his or her context. By incorporating these three areas with the various types of reasoning thought, clinicians can develop the best plan of care for their clients.

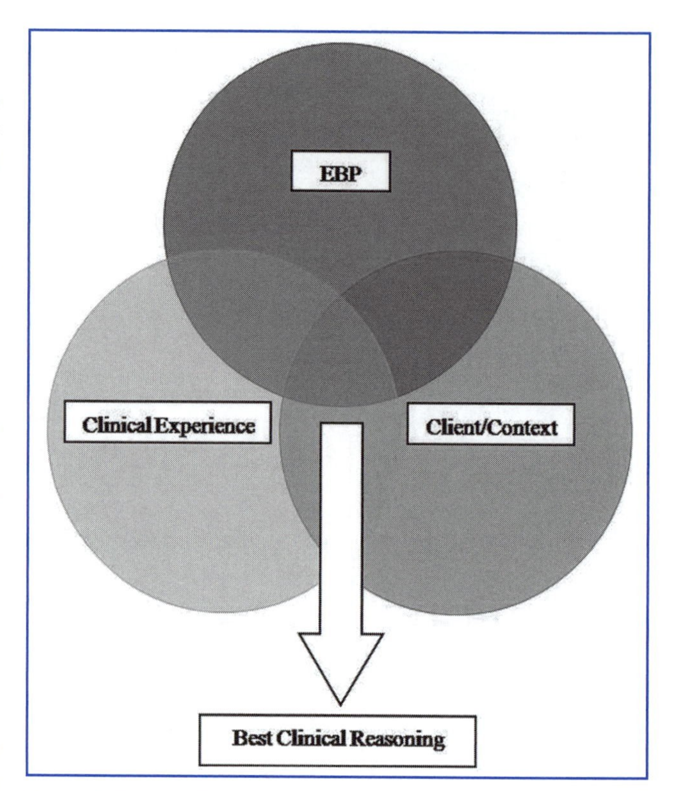


**Figure 7-1.** Best clinical reasoning.

# Case Study

The following case study, developed by occupational therapist Christa Hudson while she was a student, is utilized to illustrate the clinical reasoning process from a student perspective. The process focuses on framework (AOTA, 2008) and its application to real-life therapeutic situations.

For this case study, the student broke down each area in the framework and related those important aspects back to the client. In this case, the student lacked clinical experience, especially with this type of client. Therefore, she utilized reasoning skills to relate what she knew about the client to what she knows about occupational therapy based on the framework.

B. R. has been at a long-term care brain injury facility since September 2002, secondary to a traumatic brain injury (TBI) that occurred in a motor vehicle accident (MVA). B. R. is classified as being in a state of moderate coma, which was evaluated during his last Rappaport Coma Scale Assessment. His coma state and impairments have qualified him for neuro-specific skilled services at this facility.

### Areas of Occupation

For B. R., it is difficult to know what areas of occupation are important, as he is unable to communicate. From what I have seen when in B. R.'s room, it appears that his prior occupations include being independent in activities of daily living (ADL); participating in instrumental activities of daily living (IADL) such as child rearing, community mobility, home establishment, and management; being self-employed as a farmer; participating in sports and other play/leisure activities; and enjoying social participation within his family and community. His current occupations include spending time with his family during visits, enjoying his 2 children, watching television, participating in social/leisure activities planned by staff, and working with staff and therapy personnel on therapy goals. Caregiver staff and family were consulted to collaborate these findings.

### Performance Skills

The performance skills involved in occupational therapy include skills that one is able to do, not what a person has, in relation to actions with specific functional purposes (AOTA, 2008). Occupational therapy performance skills are classified as motor skills, process skills, and communication/interaction skills. In terms of the client, B. R., there are many difficulties associated with his ability to perform skills falling under the above categories.

Motor skills consist of skills related to "moving and interacting with tasks, objects, and the environment" (AOTA, 2008, p. 621). Difficult motor skills for B. R. include the following: posture, mobility, coordination, and strength/effort. However, I have seen that sustained energy is being attempted during therapeutic activities. The awareness and sensation required for postural changes, mobility, coordination, and strength/effort have been impaired secondary to the TBI and additional underlying factors. Due to B. R.'s level of consciousness (LOC), coma state, and physical condition, he is dependent on staff for the completion of necessary motor skills.

Process skills consist of skills "used in managing and modifying actions for the completion of daily life tasks" (AOTA, 2008, p. 621). The notion of B. R.'s ability to perform process skills is uncertain at this time. Skills require that B. R. be cognizant, aware, and understand the tasks involved in daily life. With B. R.'s impaired LOC and reduced capabilities for completing process skills (using knowledge, temporal organization, organizing space and objects, and adaptation), occupational therapists have decided not to focus on this area.

Communication skills consist of "conveying intentions and needs and coordinating social behavior to act with people" (AOTA, 2008, p. 622). With B. R. being unable to communicate using verbal or written methods, it is difficult to assess his skills. At this time, B. R. experiences difficulties with completing skills of physicality (use of physical body during communication), information exchange (giving and receiving information), and relations (maintaining relations within occupations) (AOTA, 2008, p. 623). Despite the weaknesses within these categories, B. R. is able to gaze with his eyes, use expressions to identify his emotions, and demonstrate respect by following requests during therapy sessions. The attempts may purely be reflexive, but you can see that he is trying his best. Consistency in eliciting responses is limited for the above skills, but B. R. is attempting to use communication methods that are available.

### Patterns

As a client at this facility, B. R. participates in daily and weekly routines that are arranged by appropriate staff members. For example, it is routine for B. R. to receive a daily bath, as well as receive hydrotherapy every Wednesday afternoon. In this type of environment, it is normal to have an established routine or "occupations with established sequences" and "patterns of behavior related to daily life activities" because a routine can help with the rehabilitation process (AOTA, 2008, p. 623). For any client faced with trauma, it is evident that developing a system of normalcy will ease the stress associated with that trauma. In a word, it means develop a routine.

### Contexts

Contexts can be viewed as "a variety of interrelated conditions within and surrounding the client" (AOTA, 2008, p. 623). For B. R., the contexts that influence his performance are personal, physical, cultural, and social. As far as I know, his personal context includes being a 31-year-old self-employed (prior to accident) male. Socioeconomic and educational status is unknown at this time. His physical context includes living in a long-term care facility in a small town in the Midwest, which consists of uncarpeted hallways, hospital-style rooms, a hydrotherapy pool, and a therapy clinic with mats and related equipment, that currently meets B. R.'s rehabilitative needs. Additional related contexts are cultural, including being of White heritage, growing up in a small community, and being raised in a White, middle-class household. On the other hand, social contexts include sharing relationships with his wife, two children, and other friends/family from his community. The remaining contexts do not apply to B. R.'s situation.

### Client Factors—Impaired

Following B. R.'s TBI, it is apparent that numerous client factors are impaired. The impairments occur within each category, so at this time I will only focus on the most serious areas of impairment. With client factors having an impact on overall performance, it is important to have an awareness of these impairments and their affect on the client. Under the body functions category, I want to focus on the following factors: global/specific mental function, sensory function/pain, and skin and related structure functions.

With B. R.'s impaired LOC, it is evident that his global/specific mental functions will also be impaired. In particular, he is unable to orient to person, place, or time in addition to demonstrating limited affective, cognitive, and perceptual abilities required for specific mental functions. At this time, B. R.'s LOC and awareness make it difficult to maintain attention, memory, perception, and thought processes. These basic processes must be mastered before higher-level activities can be attempted.

The level of response needed for adequate sensory function/pain stimuli is impaired. B. R. is unable to accurately respond to stimuli associated with the five senses. For example, his vision is highly impaired, he rarely responds to auditory stimuli, and he is inconsistent with response to tactile stimuli. It may be that B. R. is capable of a response, but his consistency in eliciting responses varies. His apparent level of understanding and consciousness makes it difficult to assess sensory function/pain, as he is unable to communicate.

Skin integrity and function is the next major factor for B. R. With his dependence on staff members for mobility, incontinence problems, and bed positioning, it is crucial to maintain his skin integrity. His key impairment is his protective skin function—he is at risk for pressure sores and skin shearing/tearing when staff transfer him. To improve this area, it is necessary to monitor his skin at regular intervals and train staff and caregivers on proper handling, transfering, and positioning techniques.

As you can see, the student completing this case study thoroughly analyzed the client utilizing the framework as her clinical guideline. In lieu of clinical experience, this student made the most of her skills sets learned in school while utilizing the framework as her basis. The above case study thoroughly analyzes B. R. from the perspective of occupational therapy. The student utilized a combination of narrative, procedural, and conditional reasoning to come to her conclusions. An occupational therapist or occupational therapy assistant with more clinical experience in these types of clients may have been able to make these assumptions about B. R. without directly relating them to the framework. For a student just learning and with limited clinical experience, utilizing the framework as a guide assists in looking at all clinical areas of concern for the client, thus employing procedural reasoning. The case of B. R. is difficult for any practitioner, especially a student, secondary to B. R.'s LOC. The clinician is unable to gain significant knowledge about B. R. from B. R. himself. However, by obtaining well-rounded information, narrative and conditional caregiver and family information was utilized. Many of the hypotheses are based on what is normally seen with a client of his LOC and moderate state of coma.

The student, under the supervision of a licensed occupational therapist, also worked with the other therapists treating B. R. In visiting with the physical therapist, speech therapist, nursing, and activities staff, it was determined that all involved were working toward similar client outcomes and addressing client difficulties. The student improved her own learning and provided best care for the client by co-treating with physical therapy when working on goals.

The student and supervising therapist next examined what the client's input would be in regard to therapy and the client's context attempting to draw upon pragmatic reasoning. As stated above, this is difficult to discern from B. R. Staff and family members were interviewed to obtain information on B. R.'s previous lifestyle. We know that B. R. is a young adult who worked independently on a farm and had an active family life with two children and a wife. The family visits at least once a week and affective changes can be noted in B. R. when his children and wife are around. Based on interviews with his wife, B. R.'s leisure interests included country music, hunting, poker, and playing with his kids. In addition, his wife stated that he enjoyed farming and living in a small Midwestern town. Staff reported that B. R. relaxes significantly during hydrotherapy, which was confirmed by the student during a therapy session in the pool. The staff also informed the student that B. R. appears more restless and agitated after his family visits. Family and staff also confirm the student's assertion that B. R. inconsistently responds to stimuli and requests for purposeful movement and activity. His family is concerned about the progress B. R. will or will not make in recovering from his TBI. They are hopeful B. R. will return to some level of independence and cognitive ability. His family is also concerned about maintaining health and preventing any further deterioration. From this information, the student, using narrative and interactive reasoning to the ability she was able, came up with ideas about how goals and intervention should be for B. R. This information will be helpful in planning goals and intervention for B. R.

Finally, the student examined the evidence for the intervention of clients such as B. R. The following questions were asked:

- What is the best type of intervention techniques for a client in a moderate coma?

- What outcomes are we attempting to elicit from B. R.?
- What data do I need to show that the intervention techniques I chose will benefit B. R.?
- What theory should back the intervention chosen?
- What are my hypotheses for the reasons behind B. R.'s difficulties?
- Did I clearly identify the clinical problems related to B. R.?

Based on these questions and the research the student completed to answer them, the student determined the following to be the occupational therapy intervention approach best suited for B. R., utilizing clinical reasoning from a procedural and scientific method and continuing to take into account both narrative and interactive reasoning. Again, the student went back to the framework to assist in formulating the best intervention approach.

The best occupational therapy intervention approach for B. R. is a combination of maintenance with a modified prevention focus. B. R. is currently receiving intervention focusing on maintaining his physical mobility, skin integrity, and muscle strength and function. This is appropriate for B. R. because his rehabilitation progress is uncertain—his impairments from his TBI might be too complex to overcome. With a maintenance program, the therapist will "provide the supports that will allow clients to preserve their performance capabilities that they have regained, while continuing to meet their occupational needs" (AOTA, 2008, p. 627). A maintenance program, in cooperation with prevention, will work to eliminate further impairments that may occur secondary to immobility, poor posture, poor skin integrity, and psychosocial well-being. This is the best approach because it provides intervention in a manner not traumatic to the client and meets the concerns of the family and caregivers.

The biomechanical frame of reference in conjunction with the Model of Human Occupation (MOHO) were chosen to drive intervention. This is based on the student's knowledge of these theories, client abilities and difficulties, and stated family/caregiver concerns. By utilizing the biomechanical frame of reference, the student can focus on the concerns related to range of motion (ROM) and positioning. In addition, by employing the MOHO, the student can utilize B. R.'s inconsistent performance in relation to requests made to him in therapy, volition by using activities that have meaning to the client, and B. R.'s previous and current habits and roles.

Finally, the student developed a list of interventions and outcomes to assist B. R., his family, and caregivers in achieving therapy goals.

During our weekly therapy sessions, I focused on maintaining B. R.'s upper extremity (UE) ROM through passive methods. During these therapy sessions, B. R. is encouraged to assist in ROM exercises with desired music/activities included to enhance client-centered practice. Additional interventions include maintaining head and neck control in midline, using manual massage on neck muscles to reduce muscle tightness, and assessing his responses to verbal and visual stimuli (through visual tracking). Again, visual stimuli of interest to B. R. were utilized such as pictures of his children or cards sent by family. The outcomes we hope to obtain when completing these interventions is to maintain or improve his joint mobility and ROM, to improve posture and positioning when in his wheelchair, and to maximize B. R.'s level of social awareness and interaction with various people and the environment (Cuff, 2004). A focus with maintaining his head/neck in midline is so his headrest can provide more efficacious use in order to prevent contractures and poor positioning. By working on these interventions, I hope to improve his occupational performance, prevent further impairment, and enhance his quality of life. In addition, training was completed with family and the facility caregivers to continually reinforce these techniques.

In selecting these intervention strategies, the student completed research to show the evidence that this type of intervention would be beneficial to B. R. An evidence-based practice review was done for passive range of motion (PROM) exercise, head/neck control, use of manual massage, and sensory stimuli on moderate-level coma clients. The literature that was found supports these efforts as intervention strategies with B. R. Therefore, the student completed scientific and ethical reasoning in this case.

In closing, this case study of a student's use of clinical reasoning to treat a client that is not typically seen is a short reflection by the student on this experience.

Through this assignment, it has become apparent that an occupational therapist must consider numerous aspects when treating a client. There is more to providing intervention than just going through the motions of exercise, ROM, and therapeutic activities. A therapist must consider the impaired factors and functions so appropriate interventions and methodology behind them can produce the outcomes necessary for client rehabilitation. In addition, the literature must be reviewed to provide evidence that intervention, methodology, and outcomes are sound. Clients, families, and caregivers should be consulted whenever decisions about intervention, goals, and outcomes are decided. Client-centered practice should stay at the focus of our intervention even if the client is unable to state wishes or goals via written or verbal methods. When all of the proper steps have been completed, an occupational therapist can truly know that he or she has done the best job possible.

Reflection is an important tool to assist students, occupational therapists, and occupational therapy assistants in making sure one is providing the best quality of care. By consciously looking at one's experience and asking, "What," "So what," and "Now what?" practitioners can examine one's beliefs, values, opinions, assumptions, judgments, and practices related to the experience; gain a deeper understanding of them; and construct meaning and significance for future practice.

## Summary

The use of clinical reasoning by the student in the preceding case study is shown in Table 7-1.

Clinical reasoning continues to be difficult secondary to the complexity of the issues that occupational therapy practitioners face. In utilizing their clinical reasoning skills, clinicians and students can link theory to practice and name, frame, and solve problems facing clients.

## Student Self-Assessment

Students should assess their clinical reasoning skills while on all levels of fieldwork affiliations. Research suggested many methods for fostering clinical reasoning skills for students. McKay and Ryan (1995) suggested that students share personal therapeutic stories (narrative reasoning) with peers and supervisor(s). Buchanan, Moore, and van Niekerk (1997) proposed using a revised case study guide format and reflective writing to improve reasoning. Cohn (1989) suggested that fieldwork supervisors use probing questions with students to help them develop a range of intervention strategies. Cohn also recommended that students tell intervention stories and use case studies to demonstrate consistent revision of intervention planning over time. Journaling or reflective writing is commonly used by supervisors for students and supervisors to observe just how much students have expanded their scope of practice and decision-making processes. Sladyk and Sheckley (2000) found seven activities that enhanced students' clinical reasoning skill development. These activities included journal writing, videotaping, reviewing case studies, probing questions, working with a consistent population, role modeling, and listening to supervisor stories. An assessment students can use to self-evaluate can be found on the next page.

As discussed previously, reflection is an important piece of learning clinical reasoning. By completing this self-assessment, a student should be able to determine areas of growth for clinical reasoning skills. During and after each level I fieldwork, students should reassess their progress toward advanced clinical reasoning skills using this assessment. Students should strive to apply all concepts consistently by the end of the level II fieldwork affiliations.

## Electronic Resources

- Critically appraised topics related to occupational therapy: www.otcats.com
- Evidence-based practice briefs related to occupational therapy: www.otseeker.com
- PubMed search engine from the National Library of Medicine and the National Institutes of Health: www.ncbi.nlm.nih.gov/entrez/query.fcgi
- Evidence-Based Practice Research Group: www.srs-mcmaster.ca

Table 7-1. How Clinical Reasoning is Applied in Practice

| Therapist/Student Action | Critical Reasoning Utilized |
|---|---|
| Choice of frame of reference | Ethical |
| Use of pool for intervention | Interactive |
| Observation of the client's environment | Interactive |
| Consultation with family and caregivers | Narrative, interactive |
| Use of the framework to guide decisions | Procedural |
| Choice of intervention approaches | Interactive |
| Sensory stimulation as an intervention modality | Interactive |
| Family/caregiver training activities | Pragmatic |
| Reflection | Conditional |
| Use of evidence-based practice in guiding intervention planning | Scientific, ethical |

| Skill | Consistently demonstrates | Demonstrates more than 50% of the time | Demonstrates less than 50% of the time | Never demonstrates |
|---|---|---|---|---|
| Using an inquiring or questioning approach in classroom or clinic settings. | | | | |
| Giving alternative solutions to complex issues and situations. | | | | |
| Seeks resources to address personal growth needs. | | | | |
| Able to identify ideas/theories/frames of reference that guide reasoning. | | | | |
| Giving and receiving constructive feedback. | | | | |
| Modifying performance in response to meaningful feedback. | | | | |
| Respectful of others. | | | | |
| Seeks feedback. | | | | |
| Engages in self-reflection. | | | | |
| Willing to ask questions of supervisor of how and why he or she does things. | | | | |
| Ability to analyze, synthesize, and interpret information. | | | | |
| Able to apply framework to clients. | | | | |
| Ability to observe relevant behaviors and apply to intervention planning | | | | |
| Creative problem solving to intervention planning. | | | | |
| Utilize questions and feedback as a way of learning. | | | | |
| Research the data to support the learning process. | | | | |
| Employ therapeutic use of self to get to know client's wishes and concerns. | | | | |
| Open mindedness. | | | | |
| Look to theory to assist with understanding client's problems and the intervention to support client independence. | | | | |
| Collaborate with other disciplines and caregivers. | | | | |
| Validate hypotheses about clients through EBP, experience, and client/context. | | | | |
| Cope well with change and uncertainty. | | | | |
| Given an intervention strategy, ask the questions, "What makes this work?" and "Will it work in this context?" | | | | |

# References


American Occupational Therapy Association. (2008). Occupational therapy practice framework: Domain and process, second edition. *American Journal of Occupational Therapy, 62*, 625-683.

Buchanan, H., Moore, R., & van Niekerk, L. (1998). The fieldwork case study: Writing for clinical reasoning. *American Journal of Occupational Therapy, 52*(4), 291-295.

Cohn, E. S. (1989). Fieldwork education: Shaping a foundation for clinical reasoning. *American Journal of Occupational Therapy, 43*(4), 240-244.

Crepeau, E. B. (1991). Achieving intersubjective understanding: Examples from an occupational therapy treatment session. *American Journal of Occupational Therapy, 45*(11), 1016-1025.

Cuff, J. (2004). *Occupational therapy plan of care*. Glenwood, IA: On With Life.

Fleming, M. H. (1991). The therapist with the three-track mind. *American Journal of Occupational Therapy, 45*(11), 1007-1014.

Mattingly, C. F. (1991). What is clinical reasoning? *American Journal of Occupational Therapy, 45*(11), 979-986.

Mattingly, C., & Fleming, M. H. (1994). *Clinical reasoning: Forms of inquiry in a therapeutic practice*. Philadelphia, PA: F.A. Davis.

McKay, E. A., & Ryan, S. (1995). Clinical reasoning through story telling: Examining a student's case story on a fieldwork placement. *British Journal of Occupational Therapy, 58*(6), 234-238.

Neistadt, M. E. (1998). Teaching clinical reasoning as a thinking frame. *American Journal of Occupational Therapy, 52*(3), 221-229.

Rogers, J. C., & Masagatani, G. (1982). Clinical reasoning of occupational therapists during the initial assessment of physically disabled clients. *Occupational Therapy Journal of Research, 2*, 195-219.

Sladyk, K., & Sheckley, B. (2000). Clinical reasoning and reflective practice: Implications of fieldwork activities. *Occupational Therapy in Health Care, 13*(1), 11-22.

Schell, B. B. (1998). Clinical reasoning: The basis of practice. In M. E. Neistadt & E. B. Crepeau (Eds.), *Willard & Spackman's occupational therapy* (9th ed., pp. 90-100). Philadelphia, PA: Lippincott Williams & Wilkins.

# Section III

## Occupational Therapy Theoretical Perspectives

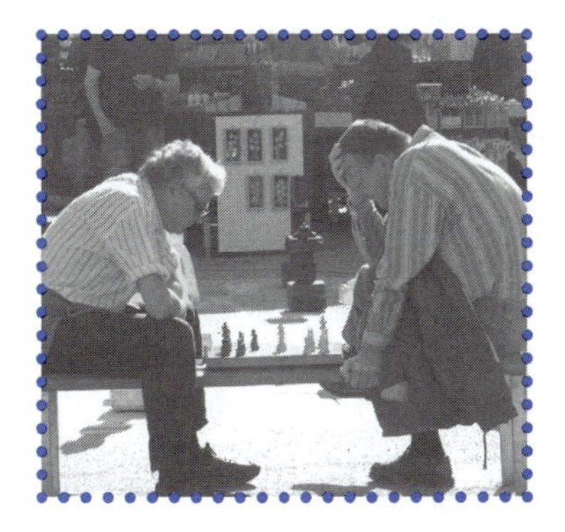

# 8

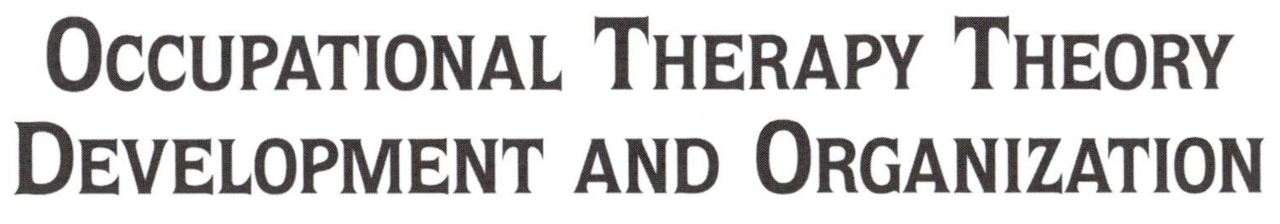

# Occupational Therapy Theory Development and Organization

*Marilyn B. Cole, MS, OTR/L, FAOTA*

**ACOTE Standards Explored in This Chapter**

B.3.1-3.2, 3.4, 3.6

**Key Terms**

| | |
|---|---|
| Applied research | Humanism |
| Applied theory | Occupation-Based Model |
| Assumptions | Occupational Performance Model |
| Basic research | Paradigm |
| Concept | Philosophy |
| Conceptual models in occupational therapy | Postulate |
| Construct | Pragmatism |
| Epistemology | Reductionistic approach |
| Frame of reference | Social participation |
| Holistic approach | Taxonomy |
| | Theory |

## Introduction

Most occupational therapy students and practitioners regard theory as the concern of academia and science, not practice. Although we know that all assessment tools and intervention strategies have their base in theory, practice focuses on the application of these tools with clients. Theory is elusive, influencing our behaviors, but often without our awareness. Most of us would be surprised at how often we use theory in our daily lives. For example, my dog, Blitzen, used to hide under the table whenever he heard thunder. A dog's hearing is better than a human's, and he could hear the thunder long before I. I could almost predict the weather by his behavior. What was Blitzen's theory about thunderstorms? What assumptions of cause and effect did his behavior reflect? I imagine it must have been something like, "Here comes trouble, I could get hurt. I'd better go where trouble can't find me." Humans use similar assumptions unconsciously when reacting to thunder. Although we may not think about the reasons, habitually we make certain predictions and take action to avoid unwanted consequences. We pick up our beach towels, cell



K. Sladyk, K. Jacobs, & N. MacRae (Eds.).
*Occupational Therapy Essentials for Clinical Competence* (pp. 75-86).

phones, and iPods (Apple Inc, Cupertino, CA) and move indoors to avoid getting wet; we get out of the pool to avoid the danger of lightning; and we take cover from the wind and rain to avoid discomfort, damage to our belongings, and threats to our health.

Whenever we make a decision or form an opinion on something, we are using theory in the reasoning process to justify or validate our thoughts and actions. Only through reflection can we become aware of the assumptions we are making—the theories behind our thoughts and actions. It is the same with the practice of occupational therapy. In the beginning of the 20th century, occupational therapists learned techniques and applied them without giving much thought to the theories or assumptions upon which they were based. However, current trends compel us to raise our awareness of frames of reference, to reflect upon the outcomes of our tools and techniques, and to read research studies that provide evidence that the theories behind our actions in practice are valid. These are the requirements of evidence-based occupational therapy practice in the 21st century.

In this chapter, we will define theory as it relates to occupational therapy, trace the evolution of theory from occupational therapy's founding in 1917 to the present, and discuss the paradigm shifts in health care within the context of historical events and trends. Finally, we will propose an organizational model for understanding and applying the various levels of theory in occupational therapy practice.

# What Is Theory?

Kerlinger's most-often quoted definition of theory is "a set of interrelated constructs (variables), definitions, and propositions that presents a systematic view of phenomena by specifying relations among variables, with the purpose of explaining natural phenomena" (1979, p. 64). In occupational therapy, this "scientific" view of theory assumes knowledge is derived from systematic, controlled, and empirical study of some aspect of human occupational behavior (Table 8-1).

Most of us recognize many theories that have been developed and validated through scientific research. Newton's gravitational theory and Einstein's theory of relativity are examples of scientific theories validated through basic research, while Skinner's theory of operant conditioning and Bandura's social learning theory are examples of applied research. This distinction parallels the difference between occupational science and occupational therapy. Occupational science is an academic discipline that is aligned with basic research. Occupational scientists study the form, function, and meaning of occupation without regard to the practical use of the theories generated. Occupational therapists are mainly concerned with the application of its theories in practice. While we may borrow from the theories of occupational science, occupational therapists look for ways to relate them to our understanding of occupational dysfunction, deprivation, restoration, and adaptation for the clients and populations we serve. The

**Table 8-1. Purposes Served by Theory and Examples**

| Purpose | Question Addressed/ Theory | Example |
|---|---|---|
| Define a concept | What is figure-ground perception? (sensory integration theory) | Ability to recognize shapes of objects in a cluttered line drawing. Ability to find two matching black socks in cluttered drawer. |
| Describe | What is good time management? (cognitive behavioral theory) | Ability to plan and execute daily activities to meet one's needs and obligations in an efficient and satisfying manner. |
| Correlate | How does exercise relate to successful aging? (biomechanical theory) | Studies show that 30 minutes of moderate exercise each day maintains both mental and physical fitness for older adults. |
| Explain why | What causes stress at work? (person, environment, occupational performance model) | Stress is produced when a worker's occupational performance does not match the demands or cultural/social expectations of the workplace. |
| Predict | What activities prevent cognitive decline in aging? (cognitive behavioral theory and cognitive theories of aging) | Practicing mentally challenging tasks such as crossword puzzles, and participating socially with others such as playing cards or chess helps to maintain an aging brain. |
| Evaluate | How does volunteering with the homeless help adolescents develop empathy and compassion? (attachment theory and social participation) | Informal personal interactions with persons different from one's self increases the likelihood of finding common ground and developing cultural awareness and sensitivity. |

framework (American Occupational Therapy Association [AOTA], 2008) defines five categories of occupational intervention as:

1. Create/promote
2. Establish/restore
3. Maintain
4. Modify through adaptation or compensation
5. Prevent occupational dysfunction

Occupational therapists need to develop and test theories that give us evidence about the best ways to enable occupational performance for our clients.

## How Are Theories Developed?

A theory begins with asking a question. Applied theories represent attempts to solve practical problems. Why do children misbehave in school? What causes people to get stressed out with their jobs? How do some elders manage to stay healthy and fit well into old age while others do not? The researcher next forms a hypothesis, a possible explanation for something observed. For example, A. Jean Ayres hypothesized that some school children misbehave because they cannot integrate sensory input, resulting in their inability to sit still and pay attention to the teacher. She tested this hypothesis by creating a way to measure the way children process different types of sensory input, mainly vestibular, proprioceptive, and tactile, but also incorporating auditory and visual systems. By evaluating many children, Ayres identified several patterns of sensory dysfunction. When she applied carefully graded sensory input through play activities, she found that children were able to better integrate sensations and both their classroom behavior and academic learning dramatically improved (Ayres, 1979). Her research resulted in the theory of sensory integration, a frame of reference used widely by occupational therapists working in school systems today.

Experimental research, such as the study just described, uses the scientific method to collect data according to specific criteria, ideally including a random selection of subjects, control of extraneous influences, and some form of manipulation such as an occupational therapy intervention. When a theory has been developed to a certain point, a good way to test the theory is to do an experiment. Two groups of subjects are randomly selected, and one group is treated in a designated way (experimental group) while the other group is not (control group). In order to control for bias, or unanticipated influences on the outcome, both groups should be the same in every aspect, except for the intervention being tested. Both groups are evaluated before and after the intervention interval in order to determine whether the experimental group has changed in a way that is different from the control group. Ayres studied a randomly selected sample of school-age children representative of the normal population, and developed age-equivalent norms for each sensory subtest in her sensory integration battery. This is called a norm-referenced assessment, which generated a theory of normal sensory integrative development (Ayres, 1979). Many occupational therapy researchers have tested different parts of Ayres' theory by using specific interventions such as scooter board play and spinning on a tire swing with groups of children who have sensory deficits. When the subjects are not randomly selected but chosen because of their disability status, this type of research is called quasi-experimental. Most clinical research falls into this category. The results give occupational therapists useful evidence about how well certain interventions work with disabled populations.

Qualitative research is the preferred method when a theory is not well developed. Qualitative research begins with a different question, one that is more descriptive rather than cause and effect. For example, a group of occupational therapists wondered how they could become better time managers. They designed a qualitative study, which involved in-depth interviews with six people they had identified as good time managers—women who successfully juggled marriage, child care, gainful employment, community involvement, and home maintenance. This is called a purposive sample. Their interviews included many questions about how the women planned their time, what tools they used, what motivated them, and what made them successful time managers. The results described the nature of good time management and identified some themes that helped us to better understand the concepts involved. It suggests some occupational therapy interventions, such as the practice of routines, the development of social networks that combine or exchange obligations, and the building of short-term memory and self-management strategies. If taken further, this research could form the basis for a theory of "time mastery" (Cole, 1998).

In occupational science, qualitative research has been cited as the preferred method for studying the form, function, and meaning of human occupation. When building theories of occupation's role in maintaining and restoring health and functional abilities, qualitative methods have been most useful in determining the outcomes related to client satisfaction and well-being. In general, qualitative methods relate best to theory development, while experimental research works best for theory testing. This description of research has been simplified for clarification purposes. In fact, there are many categories and variations of research not included here. Table 8-2 compares experimental and qualitative research methods in relation to theory in occupational therapy.

## Evolution of Theory in Science and Occupational Therapy

Occupational therapy theory did not develop in isolation. Historical trends and events have shaped the development of professional theory and practice from the

| Table 8-2. Experimental Versus Qualitative Research in Occupational Therapy | |
|---|---|
| **Experimental Research** | **Qualitative Research** |
| Includes manipulation, randomization, and control | Includes single cases, in-depth interviews, detailed descriptions |
| Theory testing | Theory development |
| Objective reality, correlation, cause and effect, use of quantitative statistics | Subjective reality, personal narratives and perceptions, multiple truths |
| Many subjects | Fewer participants |
| Standardized tests for dependent variables, surveys, controlled observations | Self-reports, attitudes and beliefs, the lived body, the illness experience |

beginning. Some of the trends of the early 1900s included industrialization, economic growth and prosperity, reconstruction after World War I, and a recognition of the need to preserve skilled craftsmanship. Humanism and pragmatism were the predominant philosophical trends influencing the profession's founding and early years. Breines (1987) recognized the predominance of pragmatism at the time of occupational therapy's founding, citing philosophers William James, George Herbert Meade, and John Dewey at the University of Chicago, colleagues of Adolph Meyer and William Dunton (1919), who later applied pragmatic principles to occupational therapy. Pragmatism, based in part on Darwin's theory of evolution, stressed the growth of knowledge and science through adaptation. The Hull House, in association with the University of Chicago, demonstrated pragmatic principles through the practice of arts and crafts and other activities, which served the needs of both individuals and the community. Occupational therapy founder Eleanor Clarke Slagle trained and later taught arts and crafts at the Hull House. Founders Susan Tracy and Susan Johnson, both from a nursing background, devoted most of their lives to practicing and teaching the application of occupations such as arts and crafts, work, and self-care tasks to the healing, rehabilitation, and adaptation of persons with disabilities. Although the assumptions of pragmatism were not clearly defined by occupational therapy founders, they were apparent in the focus on learning by doing, mind/body unity, and building health through engagement in occupation. Tracy is the only occupational therapy founder to publish the applied principles of pragmatism in occupational therapy (1918).

Most occupational therapy professionals today take a pragmatic approach. Knowledge, ideas, and methods are valued according to their practical usefulness. When we read research studies, we look for ways we can use or apply the results in our own lives and in those of our clients. In doing so, we are using the theory of pragmatism. Perhaps the reason the concept of occupation as therapy has withstood the test of time is because of its pragmatic nature. Occupation continues to unify time and space, mind, and body and to facilitate the growth and development of individuals and societies.

Kielhofner and Burke (1977) traced the history of epistemological changes that took place in occupational therapy and identified two distinct shifts in occupational therapy's professional paradigm (Figure 8-1). Epistemology is the nature of knowledge and the way it is developed and used. Occupational therapy knowledge through the 1930s was based on humanism and pragmatism. Humanism fueled the profession through its dedication to the betterment of the human condition and the right of each person to respect, dignity, and a meaningful and productive role in society. Professionals learned and collected knowledge about the use of occupations in therapy through extensive apprenticeship and practice of its practical (pragmatic) application with a variety of disabilities: mental illness, long-term infectious diseases such as polio and tuberculosis, and injuries due to industrial accidents or war. Kielhofner and Burke identified this period as the "Paradigm of Occupation" (1977, p. 679).

Paradigms reflect the theoretical base, views of phenomena, range and nature of problems addressed, problem-solving methods, and goals of a scientific discipline (Kuhn,

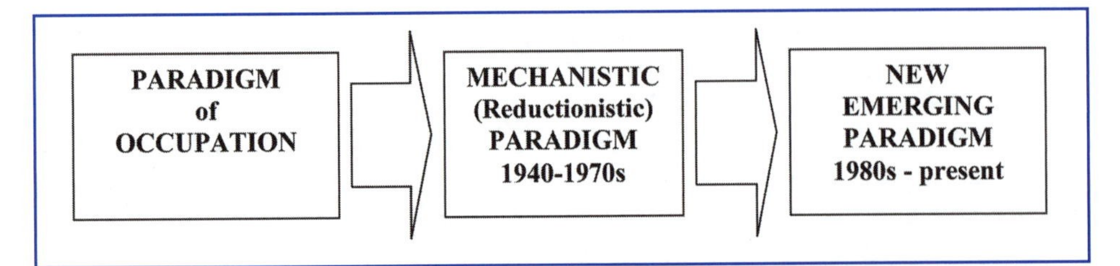


**Figure 8-1.** Paradigm shifts identified by Kielhofner and Burke. Adapted from Kielhofner, G. (2004). *Conceptual foundations of occupational therapy* (3rd ed.). Philadelphia, PA: F.A. Davis.

1970). According to Kuhn, paradigm shifts occur by revolution, not evolution. When new problems that cannot be solved with the old paradigm emerge, a crisis occurs within the discipline, which calls for fundamental and sweeping changes in both theoretical perspectives and methodology. Paralleling Kuhn's model of theoretical development in basic science, Kielhofner and Burke identify a crisis period in occupational therapy toward the end of the 1930s when the profession was challenged to become more scientific. Advances in technology and the predominance of the scientific method in basic science, social sciences, and in medicine challenged the philosophical validations of morality and social responsibility for the medical and allied medical professions, occupational therapy among them. The scientific method, viewed as the only way to discover basic truths and to substantiate theory, calls for the reduction of the focus of study into its component parts for the purpose of more precise examination and understanding. Reductionism directly opposes the holistic and systems perspective of the original paradigm of occupation.

In the mid-20th century, occupational therapy resolved this crisis by becoming more closely aligned with the medical profession. Courses in anatomy and physiology, neurology, psychiatry, and medical conditions were added to the requirements for occupational therapy education. Concurrently, a reductionistic view of illness and disability led to a focus on component parts, the diagnosis of specific problems, and the prescription of specific intervention strategies or methods. This approach views man and the world as machines; when they stop working, the method for restoring them is to locate the part that is broken (diagnosis) and fix or replace it (prescription, intervention). Later, Kielhofner renamed this reductionistic approach the "mechanistic paradigm" (2004, p. 56). According to Kielhofner and Burke (1977), the reductionistic paradigm generated three major theoretical models in occupational therapy: kinesiology (biomechanical, rehabilitative), psychoanalytic (psychodynamic), and sensory integrative (neuroscience, motor control).

Occupational therapy enjoyed a period of stability and growth in the 1950s and 1960s and benefited from its alliance with medicine with gains in respectability and status within the medical community; membership on health care teams; and inclusion in legislation, reimbursement, and social policy. For example, the passing of Public Law 91-142 (Education of Handicapped Act) in 1975, requiring children with disabilities to be educated in the least restrictive environment, opened up a whole new area of practice for occupational therapists treating children in public schools. Many useful assessment and intervention techniques were developed in occupational therapy throughout these decades in collaboration with other scientists and medical professionals (e.g., Bobath's [1990] neurodevelopmental treatment [NDT]). However, by the late 1970s, signs of the inadequacy of the mechanistic paradigm became apparent. In occupational therapy, reductionism had resulted in many extremes of specialization, leading some occupational therapy scholars to view this era as the profession's "identity crisis." The effects of the crisis identified by Kielhofner and Burke in 1977 continue to haunt us in the new millennium, especially in the areas of documentation and reimbursement. The medical profession, which once gave needed recognition to the occupational therapy profession, is itself suffering from cost-cutting measures, both public (Medicare reform and the Omnibus Budget Reconciliation Act [OBRA] of 1987), and private (managed care, malpractice, and health insurance costs) (Evanofski, 2003). Although many state licensure laws still require a doctor's prescription for occupational therapy intervention, doctors and other referral sources must choose between several competing service providers (nursing, physical therapy, speech/language therapy, home health aides) for a piece of the ever-shrinking reimbursement pie.

Within the profession, the AOTA initiated some remedial measures to resolve the identity crisis, beginning in 1979 with the publication of *Uniform Terminology* (AOTA, 1979), giving the profession a common language and defining the scope of practice. The Association further unified the profession by providing standards for the different areas of practice and by establishing the American Occupational Therapy Foundation (AOTF) dedicated to the support of research initiatives. Theory took the form of "Frames of Reference" in the 1970s (Mosey, 1970), "Clinical Reasoning" (Mattingly & Fleming, 1994; Rogers, 1983) in the 1980s, and "Occupational Performance Models" in the 1990s (Baum & Christiansen, 2005; Christiansen & Baum, 1997; Dunn, Brown, & McGuigan, 1994; Schkade & Schultz, 1992a, 1992b).

## Professional Trends in the New Millennium

The major trends of the profession may be summarized as holistic, client centered, and systems oriented. In becoming more holistic, occupational therapy must move away from a reductionistic medical model and instead partner with community organizations in the service of public health. Occupational therapy's method of reimbursement will remain under the umbrella of medicine unless we can demonstrate the value of our services in the broader spectrum of wellness and prevention. The client-centered focus gives occupational therapy a structure for making the transition from clinic to community, with an increased focus on collaborating with clients and establishing stronger therapeutic relationships. From the client-centered perspective, occupational therapists apply theoretical knowledge and evidence in partnership with clients to assist them in making informed choices and solving occupational problems and to enable occupational performance.

The trend toward a systems orientation is evident at many levels. Dynamical systems theories have impacted the basic and social sciences, and they are evident in the latest revisions of many occupational therapy frames of reference, providing evidence of the importance of environmental factors in facilitating or creating barriers to occupational performance. Occupational therapists need to help clients navigate the vast bureaucracy of the health care system, make use of community resources, and remove barriers to their inclusion in their life occupations. On a practice level, the client's social participation, the performance of roles and occupations in social groups such as families, classrooms, work teams, and the community, must become a part of occupational therapy services if we are to enable our clients to find and perform meaningful roles in society (Cole & Donohue, in press).

These trends have helped to define the current professional paradigm. The shift away from reductionism has occurred across many disciplines and professions. Evidence of this may be seen in the changes in the systems of health care, both nationally and globally.

# Medical Versus Client-Centered Models

The client-centered model, defined for occupational therapists by the Canadian Occupational Therapy Association in conjunction with Canadian national health care, gained prominence in the United States during the 1990s. For health care professionals, the term *client-centered* refers to the nature of the therapeutic relationship and implies roles for both professional and client that are clearly different from those of the medical model (Table 8-3). As occupational therapy moves away from the medical model, the client-centered model serves the purpose of structuring and clarifying our interactions with clients and gives greater importance to our therapeutic use of self. When clients seek occupational therapy services directly or through community agencies rather than being referred by a doctor, their satisfaction with the outcome surpasses the need for precise measurement of functional performance. Ideally, clients' progress in the performance of preferred occupations will lead to greater client satisfaction and will validate the value of occupational therapy in many new areas of practice.

# ICF Model of Global Health and Wellness

The World Health Organization (WHO) made significant revisions to its classification system that reflect the shift to a holistic and systems perspective of global health care. The *International Classification of Functioning, Disability, and Health* (ICF) encompasses all aspects of human health and some health-relevant components of well-being, and its intent is as a companion classification system for the 10th

**Table 8-3. Medical and Client-Centered Model Comparison**

| Medical Model | Client-Centered Model |
|---|---|
| Patient: Passive recipient of treatment; implies a sick role and a lack of participation or responsibility, requires compliance with doctor's orders | Client: Actively seeks assistance from medical and other professionals or experts; shifts responsibility for solving health problems onto the client |
| Health = Absence of disease | Health = Mental and physical fitness and a sense of well-being |
| Disease: Illness or injury affecting ability to perform activities of daily living (ADL) | Health condition: Any circumstance that interferes with full participation in life |
| Diagnosis: Identification of disease through analysis of signs, symptoms, and syndromes, which allows the doctor to predict the course of illness and to prescribe remedies | Disability: Experienced by the person, sometimes determined by the person's experience of illness; that which prevents the person from participating in life |
| Prescription: Medications or specific techniques or instructions intended to cure disease and/or manage symptoms | Enablement: Sharing expertise, which empowers the client to set reasonable goals and make informed choices regarding interventions to remove barriers to participation in life |
| Objective methods of study, based on experimental research, data gathering, and norms | Subjective methods of study based on qualitative research, looking at each individual's culture, perceptions, and situation |
| Progress is measured by objective measures applied by the medical professional | Outcome includes both objective measures and client satisfaction with results |
| Treatment: Specific medical or surgical procedures prescribed by a doctor or specialist in order to heal or cure a disease | Intervention: Procedures and strategies created by collaboration between client and professional to overcome barriers to occupational performance |
| Occupational therapy applies expertise to focus on using activities to relieve symptoms, to adapt task demands, or to compensate for disability. Rehabilitation ends when the patient has met functional goals established by the therapist and/or medical treatment team | Occupational therapist collaborates with client to identify occupational problems and priorities, to set goals, and to enable client participation through supporting skill development, and taking preventive actions and/or through adaptation of tasks and environments |

edition of the *International Classification of Disease* (ICD-10), which classifies all known diseases, both mental and physical. The stated purposes of ICF are as follows:

- To provide a scientific basis for studying health and health determinants
- To establish a common language
- To allow comparison across countries, disciplines, and time
- To provide systematic coding for purposes of record-keeping and research

Given the global nature of health care today, the fact that this international guideline confirms the central role of occupation (activity) in health has important implications for occupational therapy. ICF places "activity" at the center of its model and defines the goal of health care efforts as "participation in life" (WHO, 2001).

## Holistic Perspective

The initial publication was entitled *International Classification of Impairments, Disabilities, and Handicaps* (ICIDH) (WHO, 1980). Each of these terms has been replaced to reflect the shift to a holistic perspective:

- *Handicap* is changed to *participation restriction*
- *Disability* is changed to *activity limitation*
- *Impairment* is changed to *health condition*, an umbrella term for not only disease, disorder, injury, and trauma, but also for conditions such as pregnancy, aging, stress, congenital anomaly, and genetic predisposition.

In its 2001 revision, WHO broadens the horizons of health-related research, service provision, and policymaking beyond the constraints of the medical model. It states, "There is a widely held misunderstanding that ICF is only about people with disability; in fact, it is about all people" (WHO, 2001, p. 7).

## Systems Orientation

ICF conceives a person's functioning and/or disability as a "dynamic interaction" between a health condition and contextual factors. Contextual factors are those external factors, "features of the physical, social, and attitudinal world," that facilitate or hinder participation (WHO, 2001, p. 8). Accordingly, ICF is divided into two parts. The first lists the components of human functioning and disability, including both body systems and structures and activities and participation, denoting both an individual and a societal perspective. The systems of the human body and the activities represented closely resemble occupational therapy's domain of concern according to the framework (AOTA, 2008).

The second half of ICF lists and classifies contexts in the following categories:

- *Products and technology*: Includes foods, consumable goods, money, and the systems for distributing these, as well as objects and tools for other systems such as education, sports and recreation, and the practice of religion.
- *Natural and human-made environments*: Includes land and water, climate, population, light, noise, vibration, natural events such as an earthquake or tsunami, human-made events such as war, and time-related changes such as seasons.
- *Support and relationships*: Includes immediate and extended family, friends, acquaintances, authority figures, subordinates, care providers, domesticated animals, strangers, health care providers, and other professionals.
- *Attitudes*: Includes individual and societal views, biases, and stigmas, as well as norms, practices, and ideologies.
- *Services, systems, and policies*: Includes a vast range of systems such as economic, education, media, transportation, housing, utilities, communication, legal systems, labor, and employment, political, and civil protection systems. This category includes the system of health care as well as general social support.

The inclusion of so many external or environmental factors reflects the system's view of occupational performance as a product of the interaction between the person, the task, and the environment. The basic language of ICF is compatible with occupational therapy in this regard, stating "improvement of participation (can be encouraged) by removing or mitigating societal hindrances and encouraging the provision of social supports and facilitators" (WHO, 2001, p. 6). The model of functioning and disability also describes the interaction of ICF components: health conditions, body structures and functions, personal factors, contexts, activities, and participation in life. One can easily see the parallels with the framework, which uses similar terminology and an equally broad perspective of health (AOTA, 2008).

Occupational therapy's identity crisis in the 1970s and 1980s precipitated a search for theories to address common threads and unify occupational therapy practice. While many diverse frames of reference in the profession had been identified, we now needed to develop a systematic theoretical and scientific basis for occupation itself as intervention. Ironically, this is the same goal proposed by our founders (Dunton, 1919; Quiroga, 1995). By the 1990s, scholars had reflected upon the problem of professional identity considerably and had come to understand that the unifying concept for all of the areas of specialization within occupational therapy practice was, quite simply, occupation.

## Understanding Recent Changes in Occupational Therapy Theory Development

While the focus on the broader concepts of occupation seems simple and logical in retrospect, its implications for theory development are quite complex. The collective occupational therapy professional community—practitioners, researchers, scholars, and educators who have participated in the process of resolving the 1970s crisis—may recognize the fundamental nature of the recent theoretical shifts only through reflection. At first, we thought all that was needed was to articulate our frames of reference. In doing so, we moved from Mosey's three frames of reference to hundreds (Reed & Sanderson, 1999) with no more professional unity than we had before. We failed to recognize the true nature of the Model of Human Occupation (Kielhofner & Burke, 1980) as an occupation-based model, trying instead to define it as one more frame of reference. This worked as well as fitting the proverbial square peg into a round hole.

Then in the 1980s, Joan Rogers (1983) got us thinking about the clinical reasoning process, and this approach to unity proved to be a better fit. If occupational therapists did not all share a common frame of reference, at least they could share a common reasoning process. Mattingly and Fleming (1994) further defined the process of reasoning in occupational therapy, citing three tracks: procedural, interactive, and conditional. Herein lies the beginning of the real transformation—not in the theories of occupational therapy themselves, but the way we develop them. Procedural reasoning applies objective scientific knowledge, interactive reasoning combines this with the subjective reality of the individual client's experience (the lived experience) and conditional reasoning considers all of the contexts or systems within which persons exist, live, and perform occupations. Our professional understanding of the process of occupational therapy changed fundamentally as a result of these revelations. We had moved from an exclusively scientific view (procedures such as assessment and intervention), to one that also considered the personal perspective of the client (interactive or client-centered) and the contexts (conditional, systems) of occupational performance.

The 1990s focused on two major theoretical trends in occupational therapy: the development of occupation-based models and the movement toward client-centered practice. Occupation-based models moved occupational therapy away from the study of components of occupational performance, which viewed physical, sensory, psychosocial, emotional, and cognitive processes separately. Instead, they refocused our attention on occupation itself. Hooper (2006) explained it as an epistemological transformation, or a shift in the way we define knowledge and in the methods by which we acquire knowledge. The mid-century reductionistic approach led occupational therapists to develop and research many specific techniques, such as sensory integration for the intervention of children with learning disabilities, biomechanical strategies for the intervention of hand injuries, and cognitive rehabilitation for the intervention of traumatic brain injuries. These applied theories, while useful and valid, represented fragments of occupation developed in isolation of each other. Broader theories of occupation, such as the Model of Human Occupation (Kielhofner & Burke, 1980), and subsequent occupation-based models, served the purpose of defining the interconnections between the fragments or components of occupation. Furthermore, the application of dynamical systems theories influenced the newer occupation-based models in synthesizing much of the specific knowledge developed earlier within the multiple dimensions of occupation (Hooper, 2006).

The move toward client-centeredness represents a similar change in focus, one that questions the nature of reality itself. Creek put it simply as "...the truth is no longer out there" (1997, p. 50), suggesting truth is not objective, but subjective and therefore dependent upon personal perspectives and specific contexts. The scientific view of truth relies on accurate and objective observations inherent in the scientific method and without regard for human activity. Mosey identifies this view as "rational empiricism," which can serve as a way of thinking about practice, as well as a context for action (1992, p. 42). According to this view of truth, prominent in mid-20th century reductionism, theories are best tested through experimental research, such as the randomized controlled trials typical of medical research. As late as 1999, Holm (2000) referred to the randomized controlled trial as the most valid form of evidence supporting the theories occupational therapists use in practice. If we compare our research with that of other professions such as medicine, occupational therapy scholars must recognize that we have a lot of catching up to do. Citing a postmodernist perspective that is shared with science generally, Creek concluded that "truth is not external, universal, and eternal, but is personal, local, and ephemeral. Occupational therapists, with their concern for the personal experiences of individuals as they live their everyday lives, understand this" (p. 52).

Using a subjective view of truth, theories should not be tested using quantitative, experimental research methods, large samples, or statistical analysis. Rather, theories are built through qualitative or ethnographic methodology. While this method has been cited as the least valid from a scientific perspective (Holm, 2000), it has also been viewed as the most relevant method for occupational therapy (Clark, 1993; Zemke, 2004). Mosey (1992) has called this method "phenomenological" (p. 42), seeking knowledge through individual experiences (of clients and ourselves) and reflection. Within this approach, "knowledge is not used but rather created anew in the process of assisting each client" (Mosey, p. 42). If we accept this view of reality, using a client-centered approach is more than a new technique. It is the only valid way to build theory in practice. While occupational therapy practitioners may have knowledge of many scientific theories and evidence, they use this expertise differently in client-centered practice, recognizing that the client's perspective is paramount. Theories are only relevant as they relate to specific individuals in specific situations, and the tools and techniques they generate are only valid if they result in positive changes in occupational performance and client satisfaction.

Without this historical background, new students and graduates cannot possibly appreciate the enormity of what has occurred in the occupational therapy profession. Over the past 25 to 30 years, we have witnessed the elevation of occupational therapy from an "allied medical profession" to a profession in its own right, complete with its own body of knowledge and research, its unique theories of occupation, and with a masters degree entry level, the community of scholars needed to continue the quest for prominence as a profession.

# Organizing Occupational Therapy Knowledge

Currently, occupational therapy practitioners need both occupation-based models, using a top-down or occupation-first approach (Trombly Latham, 2008), and frames of reference, which address the components of performance using a bottom-up approach. Components such as range of motion or cognition can be targeted for assessment and intervention when these "client factors" are identified as barriers to engagement in occupation. It is comforting to learn that occupation-based models are not going to replace all of the collected wisdom of occupational therapy's more traditional frames of reference. However, as practitioners, occupational therapists will be expected to use specific techniques within the context of the broader occupation-based models, and this requires an understanding of both levels. In fact, occupational therapy students and practitioners need to develop an appreciation of all the levels of theory as necessary within our new paradigm of client-centered, holistic, and systems-oriented occupational therapy practice. Mosey (1992) identifies three levels of applied theory in occupational therapy as it had progressed to that point in time:

1. A fundamental body of knowledge, including philosophical assumptions, an ethical code, a theoretical foundation of both theories and empirical data, a domain of concern, and legitimate tools. Occupational therapy's professional paradigm and the framework fall into this category in our proposed taxonomy because these are common to all practice.
2. An applied body of knowledge that includes sets of guidelines for practice. The occupation-based models addressing the interrelationships of person, environment, and occupation fall into this category in our taxonomy.
3. Practice, which includes action sequences, use of applied knowledge, the clinical reasoning process, and the art of practice. Frames of reference, the most concrete level of theory, fall into this category by providing specific techniques and evidence for specific disabilities.

Taking these distinctions into account, we will clarify some different levels of theory as they currently appear to be understood by our scholars and/or defined by the American Occupational Therapy Association. Our proposed organization of theory for occupational therapy appears in Figure 8-2. It includes three levels: occupational therapy paradigm, occupation-based models, and frames of reference. Each of these terms will be defined.

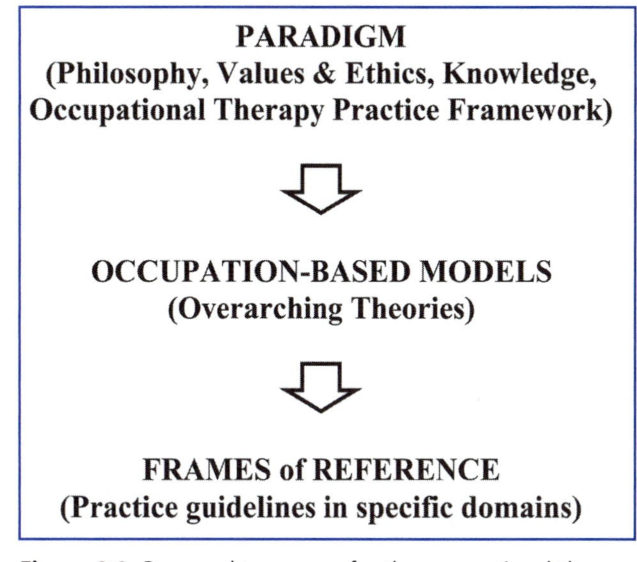


**Figure 8-2.** Proposed taxonomy for the occupational therapy profession. Reprinted with permission from Cole, M. B., & Tufano, R. (2008). *Applied theories in occupational therapy.* Thorofare, NJ: SLACK Incorporated.

Earlier we said that the paradigm in health care has shifted to one that is holistic, client-centered, and systems-oriented. These broad concepts represent the most general levels of theory. In an attempt to both broaden and unify today's practice, the framework has redefined some of the fundamental concepts of occupational therapy practice and has incorporated many of the concepts from occupation-based models as well. For example, patients are now called "clients," treatment is redefined as "intervention," and disease or illness has been replaced by "health condition" (AOTA, 2008). These changes in terminology reflect the shift in focus toward wellness and prevention of disability and imply fundamental changes in the way occupational therapists will practice in the 21st century.

The next level includes the occupation-based models, which have been called overarching frames of reference (Dunn, 2000), conceptual models (Reed & Sanderson, 1999), or occupation-based frameworks (Baum & Christiansen, 2005). In occupational therapy, occupation-based models help explain the relationship between the person, the environment, and occupational performance, forming the foundation for the profession's focus on occupation. However, they do not provide guidelines for application with specific populations or disability areas. For example, the Canadian Model of Occupational Performance (Townsend, 1997) defines the interactions of person, occupation, and environment, with each of these concepts further defined as the following:

- *Person*: Spirituality as the source of the affective, cognitive, and physical self
- *Occupation*: Consisting of productivity, self-care, and leisure
- *Environment*: Including physical, institutional, cultural, and societal systems

The Canadian model has generated a holistic, client-centered assessment tool, the Canadian Occupational Performance Measure, which can be applied in all areas of occupational therapy practice (Townsend, 1997). This may be understood as a top-down approach, beginning with a client's occupational priorities and goals, and working backwards to identify barriers to achieving them.

Theories that explain how therapy works in practice have been called practice models (Kielhofner, 2004; Reed & Sanderson, 1999) or frames of reference (Mosey, 1986, 1992). Frames of reference address specific areas of occupation and help occupational therapists to apply theory with individual clients in specific situations. Most frames of reference were developed to address particular areas of disability. For example, the Sensory Integration frame of reference was originally developed for the intervention of children with learning disabilities. This frame of reference has produced many specific assessment tools for measuring sensory systems and their motor and cognitive outcomes, as well as tools and techniques for providing specific types of sensory input. The assessment of specific sensory systems and application of remedial strategies demonstrates a bottom-up approach, beginning with foundation skills and working upwards toward using these skills during occupational performance. Frames of reference represent the most concrete level of occupational therapy theory.

Certified occupational therapy assistants, as well as master's level therapists, need to have a basic understanding of how the theories used in practice are developed and why. The knowledge gained from more traditional frames of reference, such as biomechanical, rehabilitative, sensory integrative, or psychodynamic, is still relevant and useful, but it needs to be applied within occupation-based models of practice. In particular, the client-centered approach has changed the way we approach evaluation and intervention, giving greater importance to therapeutic use of self in the therapeutic relationship. Therapeutic interventions become most meaningful when their relationship to the clients' important life roles is outwardly discussed and appreciated by the individuals and groups receiving service.

Chapter 9 will review some of the more prominent occupation-based models and frames of reference and will describe how they are used in practice.

# Summary

Theory development has been addressed in this chapter on two levels—general and specific. Generally, theory begins with a desire to better understand something in our own experience and develops through a continuum of qualitative (ethnographic), descriptive, and experimental research. In occupational therapy specifically, theories have evolved over the history of the profession in response to (or in tandem with) the changing nature of client problems with occupational performance resulting from illness, injury, or other cause, requiring occupational therapy intervention, together with occupational therapy's changing role in the overall system of health care service delivery. From occupational therapy's philosophical roots in humanism and pragmatism, the profession has developed many scientific theories to substantiate its unique focus and methods and has broadened into the holistic, client-centered, and systems-oriented practice of the 21st century. Accordingly, occupational therapy practitioners need to understand and use all of the collective levels of theory. This includes application of frames of reference, which guide occupational therapy's interventions with specific client occupational issues and priorities, within the context of occupation-based models that consider the interrelationships of the client's personal strengths and limitations, the environmental facilitators and barriers to social participation, and the social, cultural, physical, and spiritual nature of human occupation.

# Student Self-Assesment

1. How does theory help people make decisions? Give an example.
2. Explain how theory in occupational therapy differs from theory in occupational science.
3. What problems occurred in the occupational therapy profession in the 1930s that caused the paradigm to shift? What problems occurred in the 1970s that caused the professional paradigm to shift again?
4. What are two philosophical schools that influenced the founding of occupational therapy in the early 1900s? Explain each and give an example.
5. What is the purpose of theory? How does it help us with practical problems?
6. Describe two types of research that are used to develop and validate theory.
7. Using the medical model, describe the steps you would follow if you fell and broke your ankle.

8. Using the client-centered model in the broken ankle scenario, what areas of occupational performance would you evaluate in order to determine what theories should be applied?
9. How does the ICF relate to the professional paradigm of occupational therapy? Name three concepts that are similar.
10. What does the Canadian Model of Occupational Performance contribute to occupational therapy's current paradigm in the United States?
11. How is an occupation-based model in occupational therapy different from a frame of reference?
12. What three theoretical trends make up occupational therapy's current paradigm? Describe each briefly.
13. Describe the difference between a "top-down" approach and a "bottom-up" approach to the application of theory in occupational therapy practice.
14. How does a client's social participation impact the occupations that are addressed in therapy, and why is this important to consider?

# Case Study

Jeanette is a 75-year-old woman living alone who had a knee replacement and must learn to use a walker. Her apartment is all one level, but she has a flight of stairs to get from her garage up to her back door. She is able to drive but unable to climb the stairs without assistance. Although her husband died a decade ago and her son and daughter both have families and homes of their own, Jeanette still spends each morning cleaning her 3-room apartment and feels frustrated that she cannot continue to do this as before. Jeanette loves to cook but cannot easily reach the items she needs in her cramped kitchenette. Fatigue sets in quickly, preventing her from completing tasks. Although she had participated in several social activities prior to her surgery, she has avoided attending them because of her physical issues. She has no problems with toileting or dressing but fears she will fall while getting in and out of the tub. Jeanette's daughter and son-in-law live in the next town. Her daughter, Gail, calls several times each day and visits often even though she works full time. Her grandson, Rob, a college student, has offered to help Jeanette do her shopping on Saturdays.

1. Using the medical model, list five client factors to be addressed in occupational therapy.
2. Using a client-centered approach with Jeanette, write 10 questions you would ask the client or her family members in order to gain a "holistic" understanding of her occupational problems.
3. Identify three barriers to occupational performance and do an internet search to learn what theories and applications might be helpful to this case. For example, fear of falling, fatigue, and home adaptation might be relevant areas for Jeanette.

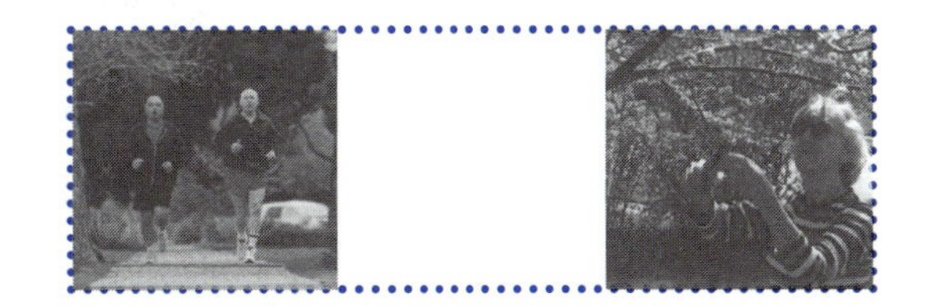

# References


American Occupational Therapy Association. (1979). Uniform terminology for reporting occupational therapy services. *Occupational Therapy News, 35*(11), 1-8.

American Occupational Therapy Association. (2008). Occupational therapy practice framework: Domain and process, second edition. *American Journal of Occupational Therapy, 62*, 625-683.

Ayres, A. J. (1979). *Sensory integration and the child.* Los Angeles, CA: Western Psychological Services.

Baum, C., & Christiansen, C. (2005). Person-environment-occupation-performance. In C. Christiansen, C. Baum, & J. B. Haugen (Eds.), *Occupational therapy: Performance, participation, and well-being* (pp. 242-267). Thorofare, NJ: SLACK Incorporated.

Bobath, B. (1990). *Adult hemiplegia: Evaluation and treatment* (3rd ed.). London, England: Butterworth-Heinemann.

Breines, E. (1987). Pragmatism as a foundation for occupational therapy curricula. *American Journal of Occupational Therapy, 41*(8), 522-525.

Christiansen, C., & Baum, C. (1997). Person-environment occupational performance. In C. Christiansen & C. Baum (Eds.), *Occupational therapy: Enabling function and well-being* (pp. 46-71). Thorofare, NJ: SLACK Incorporated.

Clark, F. (1993). Occupation embedded in a real life: Interweaving occupational science and occupational therapy. 1993 Eleanor Clarke Slagle Lecture. *American Journal of Occupational Therapy, 47*(12), 1067-1077.

Cole, M. B. (1998). Time mastery in business and occupational therapy. *Work: A Journal of Prevention, Assessment and Rehabilitation, 10*(2), 119-127.

Cole, M. B., & Donohue, M. V. (in press). *Social participation in occupational contexts: In schools, clinics, and communities*. Thorofare, NJ: SLACK Incorporated.

Cole, M. B., & Tufano, R. (2008). *Applied theories in occupational therapy.* Thorofare, NJ: SLACK Incorporated.

Creek, J. (1997). The truth is no longer out there. *British Journal of Occupational Therapy, 60*(2), 50-52.

Dunn, W. (2000). *Best practice occupational therapy: In community service with children and families*. Thorofare, NJ: SLACK Incorporated.

Dunn, W., Brown, C., & McGuigan, A. (1994). The ecology of human performance: A framework for considering the effect of context. *American Journal of Occupational Therapy, 48*(7), 595-607.

Dunton, W. R. (1919). *Reconstruction therapy.* Philadelphia, PA: W.B. Saunders.

Evanofski, M. (2003). Occupational therapy reimbursement, regulation, and the evolving scope of practice. In E. B. Crepeau, E. S. Cohn, & B. A. B. Schell (Eds.), *Willard & Spackman's occupational therapy* (10th ed., pp. 887-905). Philadelphia, PA: Lippincott Williams & Wilkins.

Holm, M. B. (2000). The 2000 Eleanor Clarke Slagle Lecture. Our mandate for the new millennium: Evidence-based practice. *American Journal of Occupational Therapy, 54*(6), 575-585.

Hooper, B. (2006). Epistemological transformation in occupational therapy: Educational implications and challenges. *OTJR: Occupation, Participation and Health, 26*(1), 15-24.

Kerlinger, F. N. (1979). *Behavioral research: A conceptual approach*. New York, NY: Holt McDougal.

Kielhofner, G., & Burke, J. P. (1977). Occupational therapy after 60 years: An account changing identity and knowledge. *American Journal of Occupational Therapy, 31*(10), 675-689.

Kielhofner, G., & Burke, J. P. (1980). A model of human occupation, part 1. Conceptual framework and content. *American Journal of Occupational Therapy, 34*(9), 572-581.

Kielhofner, G. (2004). *Conceptual foundations of occupational therapy* (3rd ed.). Philadelphia, PA: F.A. Davis.

Kuhn, T. S. (1970). *The structure of scientific revolutions* (2nd ed.). Chicago, IL: University of Chicago Press.

Mattingly, C., & Fleming, M. H. (1994). *Clinical reasoning: Forms of inquiry in a therapeutic practice.* Philadelphia, PA: F.A. Davis.

Mosey, A. C. (1970). *Three frames of reference for mental health*. Thorofare, NJ: SLACK Incorporated.

Mosey, A. C. (1986). *Psychosocial components of occupational therapy.* New York, NY: Lippincott Williams & Wilkins.

Mosey, A. C. (1992). *Applied scientific inquiry in the health professions: An epistemological orientation*. Rockville, MD: AOTA Press.

Quiroga, V. A. M. (1995). *Occupational therapy: The first 30 years 1900-1930*. Bethesda, MD: AOTA Press.

Reed, K. L., & Sanderson, S. N. (1999). *Concepts of occupational therapy* (4th ed.). Philadelphia, PA: Lippincott, Williams & Wilkins.

Rogers, J. C. (1983). 1983 Eleanor Clarke Slagle Lectureship—1983. Clinical reasoning: The ethics, science, and art. *American Journal of Occupational Therapy, 37*(9), 601-616.

Schkade, J. K., & Schultz, S. (1992a). Occupational adaptation: Toward a holistic approach to contemporary practice, part 1. *American Journal of Occupational Therapy, 46*(9), 829-837.

Schkade, J. K., & Schultz, S. (1992b). Occupational adaptation: Toward a holistic approach to contemporary practice, part 2. *American Journal of Occupational Therapy, 46*(10), 917-925.

Townsend, E. (1997). *Enabling occupation: An occupational therapy perspective*. Ottawa, Ontario: CAOT Publications.

Tracy, S. E. (1918). *Studies in invalid occupation: A manual for nurses and attendants*. Boston, MA: Whitcomb & Barrows.

Trombly Latham, C. A. (2008). Occupation: Philosophy and concepts. In M. V. Radomski & C. A. Trombly Latham (Eds.), *Occupational therapy for physical dysfunction* (6th ed., pp. 339-357). Philadelphia, PA: Lippincott Williams & Wilkins.

World Health Organization. (1980). *International classification of impairments, disabilities, and handicaps*. Geneva, Switzerland: Author

World Health Organization. (2001). *International classification of functioning, disability, and health*. Geneva, Switzerland: Author.

Zemke, R. (2004). The 2004 Eleanor Clarke Slagle Lecture—Time, space, and the kaleidoscopes of occupation. *American Journal of Occupational Therapy, 58*(6), 608-620.

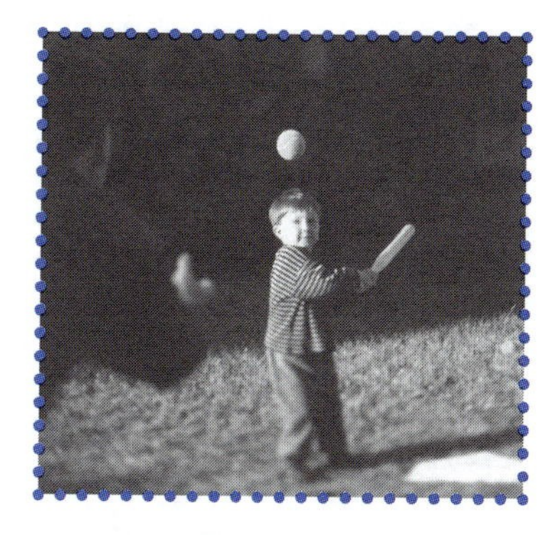

# 9

# Occupational Therapy Theory Use in the Process of Evaluation and Intervention

*Roseanna Tufano, MFT, OTR/L*

**ACOTE Standards Explored in This Chapter**

B.3.3, 3.5

**Key Terms**

| | |
|---|---|
| Analysis of occupational performance | Occupation-based models |
| Frames of reference | Occupational profile |
| Intervention plan | Theoretical constructs |
| | Therapeutic use of self |

## Introduction

Understanding how theories, models, and frames of reference are used in occupational therapy practice is a very complex phenomenon. Academicians and scholars tend to emphasize theory development as critical to establishing effective and meaningful practice. In other words, theory should serve as the foundation upon which occupational therapists make decisions regarding the best evaluation and intervention strategies for their clients. Loyal proponents of basic and scientific research will emphasize learning, understanding, and appreciating theory as a foundation for implementing practice. However, practitioners in the field often argue an opposite view. Practitioners often emphasize that solving problems for a client significantly depends on knowing what set of strategies to implement in the day-to-day life of a client. Some practitioners are of the opinion that theory does not always provide an explanation for why clients behave the way they do. These occupational therapists may carefully utilize a trial-and-error approach or implement a set of strategies observed to be effective for other clients with similar conditions. Most people would agree that understanding how and why a problem exists in therapy is very different from knowing what to do about it from a pragmatic point of view. Practitioners are often more interested in seeing what works for a given client. It is not that practitioners do not value theory or seek to understand the reasons why a problem does or does not exist for their client. Rather, practitioners will use this theoretical understanding to select a relevant intervention strategy for intervention purposes instead of researching whether their hypothesis about the problem is correct or not. Is it better to understand the complexities surrounding a client's behavior or is it more practical to figure out how to manage a problem so the client has a better occupational experience? These questions continue to be asked every day among occupational therapists who wear many hats in our profession, including academicians, researchers, consultants, and clinical staff.



K. Sladyk, K. Jacobs, & N. MacRae (Eds.).
*Occupational Therapy Essentials for Clinical Competence* (pp. 87-98).

Our standards of practice require that occupational therapists not only know and understand applicable theories, models, and frames of reference used in our profession but also be able to apply theoretical concepts to a variety of clients within different practice environments. Occupational therapy professional standards identify two distinct reasons for the integration of theoretical constructs to practice. Occupational therapists should rely on theory as an objective and valid base to make clinical decisions for relevant evaluation and intervention strategies across various domains of concern. Secondly, practitioners should apply theoretical constructs, and not one's opinion, to successfully analyze the effectiveness of occupation-based intervention outcomes, also known as evidence-based practice.

In this chapter, the reader will be introduced to a variety of models and frames of reference that serve as theoretical threads for practice and understand their importance to the evaluation and intervention process. Strategies meant to guide students on how to integrate these models and frames of reference for both practice delivery and the analysis of effective clinical outcomes will also be discussed.

## Understanding Occupation-Based Models and Frames of Reference

How does one begin to gather together and learn a repertoire of theories when there are so many from which to choose? This question has been asked by many occupational therapy students and practitioners. While there is no definitive answer to this question, the occupational therapy profession has recommended a set of guidelines in this complex decision-making process. The first step is to learn and study the models and frames of reference that are instrumental to occupational therapy practice. A review of current professional literature and trends in practice has resulted in the culminated list of models and frames of reference cited here. In the previous chapter written by Cole, a proposed taxonomy of occupational therapy theories was presented in Figure 8-2 (Cole & Tufano, 2008). One such level of theory is called *occupation-based models* and was defined as overarching theories that help to explain the relationship between the person, environment, and occupational performance. Another tier within this proposed taxonomy is *frames of reference,* defined as theories that explain how therapy works in practice. Frames of reference are designed to address a client's specific performance components within an occupational therapy practitioner's domain of practice. These performance components are currently represented in the framework document under the headings of performance skills and client factors. Frames of reference tend to have more of a disability focus, while the occupation-based models focus on the overall enhancement and promotion of health and well-being as related to occupational performance. The reader will be briefly introduced to these occupation-based models and frames of reference in this chapter. This author has identified a proposed list of occupational-based models and frames of reference that are pertinent for occupational therapy practice. Continued reading and study will undoubtedly be needed to promote a further depth of understanding and an analysis of these theories.

## A Summary of Occupation-Based Models

As previously discussed in the last chapter, the occupation-based models are designed to refocus the attention of practitioners on occupations and the interdependent relationship that ensues among person, occupation, and environment. Common features among these overarching theories include the following:

- All are founded by occupational therapists.
- All have their roots in broader theories, including humanism, holism, general systems, normal development, and behavioral and social psychology and anthropology.
- All are client centered.
- All provide guidelines for the evaluation and intervention process.
- All emphasize the promotion of health and well-being through occupational performance.

Table 9-1 represents an inventory of five such models in order of their formation. The list begins with Mary Reilly, who has been credited by many proponents in the occupational therapy field as the catalyst for the paradigm shift back to occupation (Cole & Tufano, 2008; Kielhofner, 1997). Reilly is famous for her quote, "Man, through the use of his hands as they are energized by his mind and will, can influence the state of his own health" (1962, p. 2). This statement is a good example of a construct that is included in all of the occupation-based models that followed her original work. Reilly believed that comprehensive theories were needed to guide the practice of occupational therapy (1958). She introduced her own model in 1969, called Occupational Behavior, as an attempt to promote a general theory for occupational therapy practice. As a direct result of Reilly's study and publications, Kielhofner and Burke, originally two students of Mary Reilly, incorporated the concepts of Occupational Behavior into a model of practice called the Model of Human Occupation (MOHO). Kielhofner and his colleagues published MOHO for the first time in 1980 (Kielhofner, 1980a, 1980b; Kielhofner & Burke, 1980; Kielhofner, Burke, & Igi, 1980). Since its original form in 1975, MOHO has continued to flourish as a practice model for occupational therapy. It proposes a theoretical systems view that supports engagement in occupational behaviors

Table 9-1. List of Occupation-Based Models

| Model | Author(s) | Focus of Concern for Occupational Therapy Practice |
|---|---|---|
| Occupational Behavior | Reilly, 1969 | To prevent and reduce the disruptions and incapacities in occupational behavior that result from injury and illness. Health and well-being are represented by a balance of occupational behavior in self-care, work, and play/leisure. |
| Model of Human Occupation | Kielhofner and Burke, 1980 | Conceptualized the interactive and cyclical nature of human interaction with one's environment; interplay between person and environment is critical to one's source of motivation, patterns of behavior, and performance. |
| Occupational Adaptation | Schkade and Schultz, 1992 | A framework that describes a normal human phenomenon called adaptation and its role in the interactive process between a person and his or her occupational environment. |
| Ecology of Human Performance | Dunn, Brown, and McGuigan, 1994 | Targeted area of concern is the role of context in task performance within the areas of activities of daily living (ADL), work, productive activities, education, leisure/play, and social participation. |
| Person, Environment, Occupation Performance | Christiansen and Baum, 1997 | The model's focus is on the interdependent relationship between occupations (consisting of valued roles, tasks, and activities) and performance. These occupations in turn influence one's life roles. |

intended to maintain, restore, reorganize, or develop one's capacities, motives, and lifestyle. MOHO attempts to show the complexities that exist within each person and the role of the environment in shaping one's occupational performance throughout the life span. "Through participation in therapeutic occupations, persons transform themselves into more adaptive and healthy beings" (Kielhofner, 1997, pp. 204-205).

Mary Reilly also identified another significant construct that has influenced how occupational therapists view practice concerns. Her belief was that as persons are challenged to deal with tasks of everyday life, engagement in occupation will allow for adaptation to occur naturally. While adaptation was not a new concept to the practice of occupational therapy, the occupation-based models that emerged in the 1990s analyzed the relationship between adaptation and occupation more closely. Schkade and Schultz first published their Occupational Adaptation model in 1992, reflecting an updated and comprehensive systems approach to occupational therapy practice. Persons with disrupted or inadequate occupational performance are assumed to need a change in the adaptation cycle, comprised of the various interdependent variables defined by the authors. This model's general intent is to explain 2 important phenomenons. The first is a normal human experience called adaptation. The second is the process that describes how occupational therapists can plan, guide, and implement interventions for persons in this state of transition (Schkade & McClung, 2001).

In 1994, Dunn, Brown, and McGuigan further identified several issues of concern among the current models of practice. Believing that there was not enough attention given to the role of context in occupational therapy practice, Dunn et al. also drew attention to the benefits of an interdisciplinary relationship among occupational therapy practitioners, educators within school systems, and rehabilitation specialists. Ecology of Human Performance was published by Dunn and her colleagues (1994) as a model that could be applied not only by occupational therapists but by rehabilitation specialists as well. Its conceptual emphasis is on the role of a person's context and how one's environment impacts a person and his or her task performance. Dunn's five intervention strategies have been directly integrated into the framework (American Occupational Therapy Association [AOTA], 2008). They include the following:

1. Creating and promoting health promotion
2. Establishing, remediating, and restoring skills or abilities
3. Maintaining performance capacities to meet occupational needs
4. Modifying contexts and/or activity demands as a form of compensation or adaptation
5. Preventing disability in persons who are at risk for occupational performance problems

The most recent occupation-based model to be published is the Person, Environment, Occupation Performance (PEOP) model. It was developed in 1985 and published for the first time in 1991 by Christiansen and Baum. It has since been updated in 1997. The PEOP model highlights the complexity of person-occupation-environment relationships. These authors were also greatly influenced by the Canadian guidelines for client-centered practice. In 1983, the Canadian Association of Occupational Therapists with the Department of Health and Welfare published the Model of Occupational Performance and Client-Centered Practice, two critical models that have significantly influenced the PEOP model and our current paradigm of occupational therapy practice today. These two Canadian therapeutic approaches both emphasized the reciprocal nature of persons and their occupations within social, cultural, and physical environments and led to the development of the Canadian Occupational Performance Measure (COPM) (Law et al., 1991), a well-accepted assessment tool for gathering a client's occupational profile. One of the unique features of PEOP is that it represents a top-down approach, meaning the client's view of the problem is of primary concern (Baum & Christiansen, 2005). The client's perceptions of occupational performance issues become the cornerstones for clinical intervention. PEOP also complements the current global health care trends that emphasize health and well-being as defined in the revised *International Classification of Functioning, Disability and Health* (ICF) system (World Health Organization [WHO], 2001).

# Summary of Frames of Reference

A frame of reference is defined as

> A set of interrelated, internally consistent concepts, definitions, and postulates derived from or compatible with empirical data (theory) that provides a systematic description of or prescription for particular designs of the environment for the purpose of facilitating evaluation and effecting change relative to a specified part of the profession's domain of concern (Mosey, 1986, p. 12).

Frames of reference are meant to be applied to specific areas of clinical concern and often highlight these problem areas by their titles. While each frame of reference is meant to be applied to a specific focus of occupational therapy concern, there are some common features that can be found among all of these practice theories. All frames of reference include the following:

- A clearly defined domain or focus of concern for occupational therapy application
- A listing of compatible concepts derived from broad or meta theories that explain possible causes and/or contributing factors for function and dysfunction patterns
- A definition of how persons demonstrate traits, behaviors, attitudes, and emotions that reflect function and dysfunction according to each theoretical perspective
- A listing of assumptions about how occupational therapy might assist clients in promoting therapeutic change as well as enhancing motivation for engagement in meaningful occupations
- A plan of action meant to guide occupational therapists in the evaluation and intervention process
- Evidence gathered by researchers about the validity of the theoretical concepts outlined and the effectiveness of the techniques used by occupational therapists according to its guidelines

The following brief descriptions of eight different frames of reference are among many theoretical resources for occupational therapy practice. This list is not meant to be all inclusive, however, as there are many useful and legitimate frames of reference that may have been omitted by this author. It is recommended that the reader further explore each of the frames of reference for a more comprehensive understanding by consulting Cole and Tufano (2008), as well as other original publications cited at the end of this chapter.

The psychodynamic frame of reference in occupational therapy encompasses concepts from object relations, ego psychology, humanism, and human spirituality (Bruce & Borg, 2002). Various occupational therapy theorists have integrated the concepts of psychodynamic theory into mental health practice. Examples include Diasio (1968), who explored the psychoanalytic view of motivation and the environment; G. S. Fidler and J. W. Fidler (1963), who emphasized the role of the unconscious in task completion and viewed activities as a means to effectively gratify instinctual needs; Mosey (1986), whose "analytical frame of reference" emphasized the "structure for linking psychoanalytic theories, the symbolic potential and reality aspects of activities, and the process of altering intrapsychic content in the direction of providing a more adaptive basis for interaction with the environment;" and Llorens and Johnson (1966), who emphasized how "socially acceptable, ego-adaptive functioning" needed for activity group participation could help to develop and strengthen the functions of the ego.

Behavioral frames of reference apply the scientific method to human behavior, focusing upon only the external features of human functioning that can be observed and measured. Concepts are based on such theorists as Skinner, Pavlov, and Bandura. Familiar interventions found within occupational therapy practice include behavior modification and social skills training. Ann Mosey (1970, 1986) also adapted behavioral principles for occupational therapy in her "acquisitional frame of reference." An offspring of its earlier proponents, the cognitive behavioral frame of reference builds upon preceding behavioral theory concepts with the addition of thoughts (cognition) as "behaviors" that can be modified. Related occupational therapy interventions include the psychoeducational group approach, Self-Regulation Model (Stein & Cutler, 2002), Social and Life Skills Training Model (Salo-Chydenius, 1996) and Coping Model (Williamson & Szczepanski, 1999).

The biomechanical frame of reference applies the principles of physics to human movement and posture with respect to the forces of gravity. It is a popular theoretical framework for many practicing occupational therapists in rehabilitation. Pertinent client factors and performance skill concerns include range of motion, strength, endurance, ergonomics, and the effects or avoidance of pain as related to occupational performance.

Toglia's Dynamic Interactional Model to Cognitive Rehabilitation (2005) has its foundation in neuroscience and its application guidelines within the theory of occupation. Occupational therapists can rely on this frame of reference when concerned with restoring functional performance for persons with cognitive dysfunction. Domains of concern and related client factors include orientation, attention, visual processing, motor planning, cognition, occupational behaviors, and effort.

Allen's cognitive disabilities frame of reference has been updated by Levy (2005) and renamed the Cognitive Disabilities Reconsidered Model (Levy, 2005; Levy & Burns, 2006). The six clinically defined cognitive levels and 52 cognitive modes, originally designed by Allen, offer occupational therapists some of the best detailed guidelines for assessing, assisting, and adapting environments for persons with cognitive disabilities. This frame of reference focuses on the role of cognition (a process skill), the role of habits and routines, the effect of physical and social contexts, and the analysis of activity demand.

Developmental theories continue to influence our practice. Common developmental theories that impact occupational therapy reflect childhood (Piaget, Kohlberg, Erikson, Gesell), while others focus on adulthood (Levinson, Gilligan) and aging (Laslett, Atchley, Havighurst, etc.). Occupational therapy theories based on neuromaturation include the works of Ayres, King, and Bobaths, while more generalist views were defined by Llorens and Johnson and Mosey. The framework (AOTA, 2008) cites age and "life stage" as an aspect of personal context. Occupational therapists who use a developmental frame of reference are concerned with establishing or restoring client-chosen, age-appropriate occupations within continued life roles and helping them to adapt to the changes brought on by health conditions within and across the lifespan developmental continuum (Cole & Tufano, 2008).

Sensory motor frames of reference in occupational therapy have been applied to children, adults with mental health conditions, and older adults. Three commonly used approaches include Ayres' "sensory integration" (Bundy, Lane, & Murray, 2002), Dunn's "sensory processing" (Dunn, 2001), and "sensory defensiveness" (J. Wilbarger & P. Wilbarger, 2002). Neuroscientists define sensory integration as the brain's ability to organize sensory information from the body and environment and to produce an adaptive response. Within each of these approaches, interventions are provided by occupational therapists through guided sensory input on a 1:1 or group activity basis.

The next grouping is referred to as motor control and motor learning frames of reference (Cole & Tufano, 2008). Traditional examples of motor control theories include Bobath's Neurodevelopmental Therapy (NDT) (1990), Rood's Sensorimotor Approach (1954), Knott and Voss' Proprioceptive Neuromuscular Facilitation (PNF) (1968), and Brunnstrom's Movement Therapy (1970). Principles of normal neurological development are considered in a reflex-hierarchical or neuromaturational sequence for establishing or restoring functional movement. More recent models have emerged with updated evidence, including the task-oriented frame of reference described by Horak (1991). Motor learning theories currently provide guidelines for restoring functional movement with clients having a broad range of health conditions. Task accomplishment is the ultimate goal. Occupational therapy intervention focuses on assisting clients in developing the optimal motor and cognitive strategies needed to achieve functional goals (Cole & Tufano, 2008).

## How to Use Models and Frames of Reference for Occupational Therapy Evaluation and Intervention

Most practitioners implement a variety of assessment tools and intervention strategies within their practice. What do theoretical models and frames of reference have to do with the day-to-day delivery of service? Is it OK to rely on more than one theoretical perspective at the same time? While it may appear comfortable for an occupational therapist to rely on familiar therapeutic approaches he or she may have used over and over again, new research data continue to provide evidence for best practice approaches. "Occupational therapists often exhibit an eclectic therapeutic style when assisting their individual clients, utilizing a variety of ideas and techniques based on different theories" (K. Jacobs & L. Jacobs, 2004, p. 72). Imagine if you only had five outfits in your closet to wear every day, regardless of weather conditions in the environment, your internal mood, your external body shape at the present time, or the dress occasion. Would you describe your choices as "familiar and comfortable" or "limiting and outdated?" While specializing in one theory approach may seem initially comfortable and less confusing, like wearing an old shoe, it can also limit the practitioner's ability to be most effective within today's complex health care demands. What if the frame of reference in which you feel some level of expertise turns out not to be an appropriate match for the client's needs and situation? Not every theory is an appropriate fit for every client. Not every theory will provide answers to every condition within occupational therapy's domain of practice. In like suit, not every theory may be a good match for every occupational therapist. Allowing one's self to have more choices from a theoretical repertoire rather than less in the selection of evaluation and intervention options will undoubtedly increase the likelihood of a satisfying and more suitable fit between the client, the therapist, and the desired outcomes.

The process of service delivery is challenging for anyone working in health care today. Creating the right fit among the practitioner him- or herself, the client, and the desired clinical outcomes is a dynamic process. How could we as a profession support the expansion of a theoretical closet that holds a wardrobe fitting to both the client and therapist, while also representing the most updated styles and looks of the day? The selection of the best plan for each client and his or her relevant occupational performance includes a multi-step decision-making process. As occupational therapists, we can look to the framework (AOTA 2008) for guidance on how to select and apply theory to practice. In other words, how does a practitioner create a closet that includes multiple styles of clothing for unique preferences and different occasions?

The framework (AOTA, 2008) gives some general expectations for how practitioners should include models and frames within the scope of occupational therapy practice. Occupational therapy standards of practice likewise state that students must learn how these theories are used in the evaluation and intervention process. Many principles assist the reader to link these two distinct aspects: knowledge and practice. The following statements represent an integration of ideas from both the framework and this author's practical experience in the field.

Occupational therapy models and frames of reference can assist the practitioner in the following ways:

- To understand data and formulate hypotheses about a client's occupational performance issues gathered initially from an occupational profile interview process
- To guide the practitioner in selecting relevant assessments for further data collection
- To create a therapeutic framework for interpreting data and forming initial conclusions about a person's occupational performance within this perspective
- To create collaborative goals with specific outcome measures that are based on sound and rational constructs from theory rather than one's opinion
- To develop an intervention plan for the client utilizing interventions based on best practice and evidence as supported by various models and frames of reference

In summary, the application of theory is a reasoning process that should fit the following (AOTA, 2008):

- The client's occupational needs and wants as determined from the occupational profile
- The practitioner's analysis of a client's occupational performance

While these two components are significant aspects of a collaborative therapeutic process, there are also other factors that will influence the final dress rehearsal. The delivery of occupational therapy services is as much an art as it is a science. It is the practitioner's personality, insights, perceptions, and judgments, also defined as therapeutic use of self (AOTA, 2008, p. 628), that allow the therapist to appreciate and regard a client's unique style. A practitioner's therapeutic use of self may be described as the ability to influence a client's total image through communication, modeling, intuition, and dress rehearsals. Therapeutic evaluation and intervention is as much a dynamic process as it is a cognitive and rational one. Occupational therapists are expected to use their own perceptions and insights to tailor a client's needs coupled with an objective and accurate evaluation process. A weaving of professional knowledge based on theory and a client-centered attitude will make for a well-made suit. A fashion-forward therapist can offer a variety of updated options for wear to please a client's preferences, fit one's body type, and promote a healthy lifestyle image.

# How to Apply Theoretical Constructs in the Evaluation and Intervention Process

Let us discuss the "how to" part here. So far, we have identified and introduced five common occupational therapy models and eight classifications of frames of reference. As previously noted, the process of integrating theory into practice is a multistep process. Each of the theories is complex with cumulative layers of concepts and its own set of terminology. It is common for students to struggle with such abstract concepts; after all, a theory cannot be seen, only understood.

The first step within this clinical reasoning process is to learn each of the models and/or frames of reference individually. A template designed by Cole and Tufano (2008) is provided to assist the reader in gathering key concepts about each model and frame of reference. The template is based on Mosey's original definition of a frame of reference and how knowledge is organized within this body of knowledge. Refer to Table 9-2 for a sample of this template design. Categories listed on the left side of the template reflect the various related parts, or constructs, commonly found in each theory. The student is encouraged to complete this template on each model and/or frame of reference being studied by filling in one section at a time. It will require further reading and study from references cited at the end of this chapter. Students will initially gather and identify the many concepts that comprise each theory as identified by each section of the template. The completed template can serve as a study guide and assist the student to comprehend the overall picture of the theory.

The next learning step is to be able to compare and contrast each outlined model and/or frame of reference. The process of distinguishing one theory from another simulates what practitioners are required to do in practice. Every occupational therapist must use clinical judgment in determining best practice interventions. This reasoning process begins by gathering client data and relying on theoretical explanations to form hypotheses about one's occupational performance.

Table 9-2. Template for Analysis of Occupation-Based Models and Frames of Reference

| Model or Frame of Reference | Analysis |
|---|---|
| Focus (Includes the population suited for and domains of practice according to framework) | |
| Theorists (Includes authors and related theorists who have contributed to this body of knowledge) | |
| Theoretical base (Includes defined compatible constructs that explain possible causes and/or contributing factors for function and dysfunction) | |
| Function (How does this theory define healthy or optimal functioning?) | |
| Dysfunction (How does this theory define incapacities or barriers to functioning?) | |
| Change (What are the concepts that define how change is likely to occur according to this theory?) | |
| Motivation (What motivates a client to change according to this theory?) | |
| Assessment (What formal or informal assessments are specifically created or recommended according to this theory?) | |
| Intervention guidelines (What specific therapeutic techniques or strategies have been developed and/or recommended based on this theory?) | |
| Research (To what extent has this theory been validated through research?) | |

Crepeau and Boyt Schell (2003) pointed out that the major theories in occupational therapy differ in purpose, scope, complexity, extent of development and validation through research, and usefulness in practice (p. 204). In fact, occupational therapists apply the various levels of theory at different stages of the evaluation, intervention, and outcomes continuum. The occupation-based models help occupational therapists develop a perspective about how the client, who engages within a particular environment, is participating in occupations. Constructs from these models relate well to aspects of the framework and the occupational profile because of their holistic and client-centered orientation. Constructs are also rooted in occupational therapy language and theory because each model is authored by an occupational therapist. These models help to identify the range of possibilities when setting collaborative goals for client engagement in occupations as well as identifying barriers to participation. In addition, occupation-based models help us think about ways in which our clients can find meaningful roles in society.

Frames of reference enter the clinical reasoning process as the occupational therapist thinks about problem areas observed and/or identified by a client. They specifically target selective aspects of the framework such as performance areas, skill patterns, and most often client factors. For example, Allen's Cognitive Disability Frame of Reference specifically addresses the following aspects within the framework: ADL performance areas; process performance skills; the performance patterns of habits, routines, and roles; and client factors defined as mental functions.

Crepeau and Boyt Schell (2003) suggested that practitioners tend to incorporate theory into their reasoning process in ways that allow them to use it automatically (i.e., without conscious awareness). Thus, practicing occupational therapists may not always be able to identify the frame of reference they are using. This does not mean they are not using theory but rather that its use has become habitual. Since occupational therapy students are in the beginning stages of clinical reasoning development, it is important to consciously think about the choices and to use objective information for the selection of various theoretical approaches (Cole & Tufano, 2008).

Occupational therapy assistants are expected to know the various occupation-based models and frames of reference used in occupational therapy practice. Understanding these theories will only benefit the occupational therapy assistants so they can have a more comprehensive view of working with a client. As part of their role delineation, occupational therapy assistants are not required to apply the theoretical constructs to practice. Rather, occupational therapy assistants will take direction from the occupational therapist about which model and/or frame of reference to employ when providing intervention strategies.

## Summary

The process of understanding relevant occupational therapy theories is often a challenge for students, academicians, and practitioners alike. This chapter attempts to de-mystify the process for learning about various theories by highlighting common occupation-based models and popular frames of reference found in current practice. The five occupational therapy models mentioned here can be appreciated for their holistic, client-centered, and universal application to persons across the life span and across all domains of practice. These models represent the current healthcare trend toward prevention of disease and promotion of health with emphasis on occupational performance. Each model provides a list of guidelines for the occupational therapy practitioner within the evaluation and intervention process. They pose a direct contrast to the frames of reference that are much more prescriptive and specific in nature however. Generally speaking, frames of reference are oriented toward restoring, adapting and/or compensating for the loss of occupational functioning. In their own unique way, they may be easier to apply because they are limited in their performance scope and are meant to be applied to a specific focus of concern in practice. Unlike the occupational therapy models, specific techniques and strategies are prescribed by each frame of reference for use in the evaluation and intervention process.

As a profession, we look to the framework for suggestions on how these occupational therapy models and frames of reference could assist the practitioner in the therapeutic process. The art and science of occupational therapy practice includes a two-prong evaluative approach. First we begin with regard for a client's overt and covert occupational needs while we also include the practitioner's objective analyses of a client's performance. The delivery of occupational therapy service for both evaluation and intervention is a dynamic interactive process impacted by both the practitioner's therapeutic use of self and the personality traits of his or her client. Occupational therapists need to balance their professional knowledge with the desires and needs of their clients in a highly reciprocal relationship.

It is common for professions such as occupational therapy to develop and consider multiple and often contrasting ideas about best practice. There are many theories from which to choose. For students, academicians, and practitioners inclusively, the process of becoming proficient at understanding and applying the various theoretical constructs for evaluation and intervention purposes takes time and effort. The process begins with learning the basics of each theory and understanding its intended therapeutic purpose. The ability to analyze and select the best theory option for a client requires that a practitioner have a repertoire of models and frames of reference to choose from. This decision-making process encompasses clinical reasoning—a process that is based on knowing what a theory says and how to use it. Understanding theoretical constructs combined with applying these components into simulated or real practical experience fosters the development of clinical synthesis. Just think, there are yet more theories to be modified and created with each passing experiment or study—it is an ongoing professional responsibility and one that we should all aspire to embrace. Evidence-based practice is in its young stages for the profession of occupational therapy. There is much to be learned, understood, and practically applied. Here's to our future!

## Student Self-Assessment

1. How do today's complex health concerns impact an occupational therapist's need for theoretical knowledge?
2. How do the occupation-based models support the trend toward health promotion and prevention of illness?
3. What are the pros and cons to practicing within a specialty area of occupational therapy versus practicing as a generalist?
4. What is your opinion about the following statement? Theory drives practice versus practice drives theory.
5. What are some similarities and differences among the two theoretical classifications of practice discussed in this chapter (occupation-based models and frames of reference)?
6. How has Mary Reilly influenced the profession of occupational therapy? Consider her quote, "Man, through the use of his hands as they are energized by his mind and will, can influence the state of his own health."
7. When is it appropriate to use more than one theoretical perspective for a given client in occupational therapy practice? Give a specific example.
8. In your opinion, what takes more priority—understanding the complexities of what makes someone behave the way he or she does by uncovering the cause for the dysfunction or showing someone how to correct and manage the problem behavior in order to improve his or her quality of life?

## Case Study

John is a 58-year-old divorced male with two adult children. He is employed at a naval base where he works as a chief engine engineer. He lives alone in a nearby apartment and reports that his favorite pastime is "hanging out" with his old naval buddies at the local pub. "We look out for each other," John tells the occupational therapist who notices missing teeth as he laughs out loud.

The client has been diagnosed with peripheral neuropathy due to chronic alcohol abuse. Recently hospitalized because he reported difficulty walking over a period of 4 months, John thought his "weak legs" were a result of a motorcycle fall that he sustained last year. "I never would have thought that a few beers a day would have given me sea legs!"

John is presently in a rehabilitation center. He is referred to occupational therapy for evaluation of ADL, IADL, work, and social/leisure participation. Due to the recent health concerns, John has decided to pursue retirement. He wants to return to his second floor apartment, but worries about his ability to climb stairs and care for himself. "What am I going to do all day long?" he questions. John tells the occupational therapist that he also notices that his "mind is not as sharp as it used to be…Last week, I left the oven on all night long."

1. After reading the above case, fill in as much information as you can gather about John's personal characteristics, his engagement in various occupations, and his present living environment. Make a point to identify both strengths and problem areas in each of the three categories. Based on your knowledge so far about the five occupation-based models, which one would you possibly consider as a theoretical base for evaluation and intervention strategies for John? Why?
2. Identify occupational therapy concerns for John by completing the following chart. Consult the framework for the definitions of each category as needed. Based on your knowledge so far about the different types of frames of reference, which ones would you possibly consider as a theoretical base for evaluation and intervention strategies for John? Why?

| | |
|---|---|
| Areas of occupation (ADL, IADL, education, work, play, leisure, social participation | |
| Performance skills (motor, process, communication) | |
| Performance patterns (habits, routines, roles) | |
| Context | |
| Body function categories | |

## Evidence-Based Research Chart

| Theoretical Construct | Evaluation and/or Intervention Focus | Evidence |
|---|---|---|
| Occupational performance | Both | Humphry & Wakeford, 2006; Rebeiro, 2001; Rebeiro & Polgar, 1999; Trombly, 1995 |
| Therapeutic use of self | Both | Goulet, Rousseau, & Fortier, 2007; Maitra & Erway, 2006; Restall, Ripat, & Stern, 2003; Wilkins, Pollock, Rochon, & Law, 2001 |
| PEOP Model | Both | Letts et al., 1994; Strong et al., 1999 |
| MOHO | Both | Lee, Taylor, Kielhofner, & Fisher, 2008; Pizzi, 1990 |
| Occupational Adaptation | Both | Schkade & Schultz, 1992; Schultz & Schkade, 1992 |
| Ecology of Human Performance | Both | Dunn et al., 1994 |
| Frames of reference | Intervention | Cicerone et al., 2000; Diller, 2005; Hart & Evans, 2006; Henderson, 1999; Laatsch et al., 2007; Leichsenring, Hiller, Weissberg, & Leibing, 2006; Mastos, Miller, Eliasson, & Imms, 2007; Roley, Clark, Bissell, Brayman, & Commission on Practice, 2003; Schaaf & Miller, 2005; Teasell, Foley, Bhogal, & Speechley, 2003; Watling & Dietz, 2007; Whedon, 2000 |

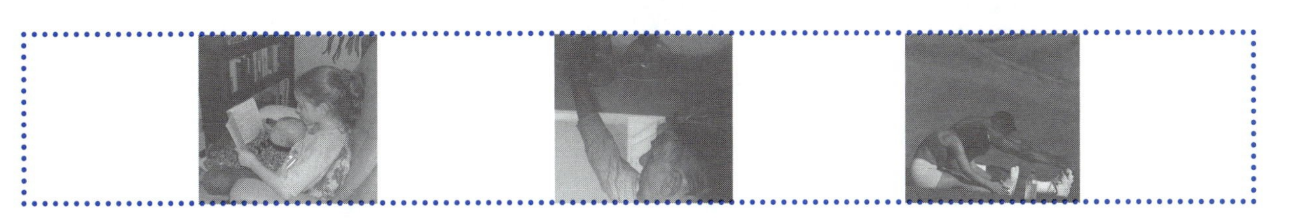

# References


American Occupational Therapy Association. (2008). Occupational therapy practice framework: Domain and process, second edition. *American Journal of Occupational Therapy, 62*, 625-683.

Baum, C. M., & Christiansen, C. H. (2005). Person-environment-occupation performance: An occupation based framework for practice. In C. H. Christiansen, C. M. Baum, & J. Bass-Haugen (Eds.), *Occupational therapy: Performance, participation, and well-being* (3rd ed., pp. 243-266). Thorofare, NJ: SLACK Incorporated.

Bobath, B. (1990). *Adult hemiplegia: Evaluation and treatment* (3rd ed.). London, England: Butterworth-Heinemann.

Bruce, M. A., & Borg, B. (2002). *Psychosocial frames of reference: Core for occupation-based practice*. Thorofare, NJ: SLACK Incorporated.

Brunnstrom, S. (1970). *Movement therapy in hemiplegia*. New York, NY: Harper & Row.

Bundy, A. C., Lane, S. J., & Murray, E. A. (2002). *Sensory integration: Theory and practice* (2nd ed.). Philadelphia, PA: F.A. Davis.

Canadian Association of Occupational Therapists. (1991). *Client-centered guidelines for the practice of occupational therapy*. Toronto, Ontario: Author.

Christiansen, C. H., & Baum, C. M. (1991). *Occupational therapy: Overcoming human performance deficits*. Thorofare, NJ: SLACK Incorporated.

Christiansen, C. H., & Baum, C. M. (1997). *Occupational therapy: Enabling function and well-being* (2nd ed.). Thorofare, NJ: SLACK Incorporated.

Cicerone, K. D., Dahlberg, C., Kalmar, K., Langenbahn, D. M., Malec, J. F., Bergquist, T. F., et al. (2000). Evidence-based cognitive rehabilitation: Recommendations for clinical practice. *Archives of Physical Medicine and Rehabilitation, 81*(12), 1596-1615.

Cole, M. B., & Tufano, R. (2008). *Applied theories in occupational therapy: A practical approach*. Thorofare, NJ: SLACK Incorporated.

Crepeau, E. B., & Boyt Schell, B. A. (2003). Theory and practice in occupational therapy. In E. B. Crepeau, E. S. Cohn, & B. A. Boyt Schell (Eds.), *Willard & Spackman's occupational therapy* (10th ed.). Philadelphia, PA: Lippincott Williams & Wilkins.

Diasio, K. (1968). Psychiatric occupational therapy: Search for a conceptual framework in light of psychoanalytic ego psychology and learning theory. *American Journal of Occupational Therapy, 22*(5), 400-414.

Diller, L. (2005). Pushing the frames of reference in traumatic brain injury rehabilitation. *Archives of Physical Medicine and Rehabilitation, 86*(6), 1075-1080.

Dunn, W. (2001). The sensations of everyday life: Empirical, theoretical, and pragmatic considerations. *American Journal of Occupational Therapy, 55*(6), 608-620.

Dunn, W., Brown, C., & McGuigan, A. (1994). The ecology of human performance: A framework for considering the effect of context. *American Journal of Occupational Therapy, 48*(7), 595-607.

Fidler, G. S., & Fidler, J. W. (1963). *Occupational therapy: A communication process in psychiatry*. New York, NY: Macmillan.

Goulet, C., Rousseau, J., & Fortier, P. (2007). A literature review on perception of the providers and clients regarding the use of the client centered approach in psychiatry. *Canadian Journal Occupational Therapy, 74*(3), 172-182.

Hart, T., & Evans, J. (2006). Self-regulation and goal theories in brain injury rehabilitation. *Journal of Head Trauma Rehabilitation, 21*(2), 142-155.

Henderson, S. (1999). Frames of reference utilized in the rehabilitation of individuals with eating disorders. *Canadian Journal Occupational Therapy, 66*(1), 43-51.

Horak, F. B. (1991). Assumptions underlying motor control for neurologic rehabilitation. In Foundation for Physical Therapy, *Contemporary management of motor control problems: Proceedings of the II STEP Conference* (pp. 11-27). Alexandria, VA: Author.

Humphry, R., & Wakeford, L. (2006). An occupation-centered discussion of development and implications for practice. *American Journal of Occupational Therapy, 60*(3), 258-267.

Jacobs, K., & Jacobs, L. (2004). *Quick reference dictionary for occupational therapy* (4th ed.). Thorofare, NJ: SLACK Incorporated.

Kielhofner, G. (1980a). A model of human occupation, part 2. Ontogenesis from the perspective of temporal adaptation. *American Journal of Occupational Therapy, 34*(10), 657-663.

Kielhofner, G. (1980b). A model of human occupation, part 3. Benign and vicious cycles. *American Journal of Occupational Therapy, 34*(11), 731-737.

Kielhofner, G. (1997). *Conceptual foundations of occupational therapy* (2nd ed.). Philadelphia, PA: F.A. Davis.

Kielhofner, G., & Burke, J. P. (1980). A model of human occupation, part 1. Conceptual framework and content. *American Journal of Occupational Therapy, 34*(9), 572-581.

Kielhofner, G., Burke, J. P., & Igi, C. H. (1980). A model of human occupation, part 4. Assessment and intervention. *American Journal of Occupational Therapy, 34*(12), 777-788.

Knott, M., & Voss, D. E. (1968). *Proprioceptive neuromuscular facilitation: Patterns and techniques* (2nd ed.). Philadelphia, PA: Harper & Row.

Laatsch, L., Harrington, D., Hotz, G., Marcantuono, J., Mozzoni, M. P., Walsh, V., et al. (2007). An evidence-based review of cognitive and behavioral rehabilitation treatment studies in children with acquired brain injury. *Journal of Head Trauma Rehabilitation, 22*(4), 248-256.

Law, M., Baptiste, S., Carswell-Opzoomer, A., McColl, M., Polatajko, H., & Pollock, N. (1991). *Canadian Occupational Performance Measure manual*. Toronto, Ontario: CAOT Publications.

Lee, S. W., Taylor, R., Kielhofner, G., & Fisher, G. (2008). Theory use in practice: A national survey of therapists who use the Model of Human Occupation. *American Journal of Occupational Therapy, 62*(1), 106-117.

Leichsenring, F., Hiller, W., Weissberg, M., & Leibing, E. (2006). Cognitive-behavioral therapy and psychodynamic psychotherapy: Techniques, efficacy, and indications. *American Journal Psychotherapy, 60*(3), 233-259.

Letts, L., Law, M., Rigby, P., Cooper, B., Stewart, D., & Strong, S. (1994). Person environment assessments in occupational therapy. *American Journal of Occupational Therapy, 48*(7), 608-618.

Levy, L. L. (2005). Cognitive disabilities reconsidered: Rehabilitation of older adults with dementia. In N. Katz (Ed.), *Cognition & occupation across the life span: Models for intervention in occupational therapy* (2nd ed.). Bethesda, MD: AOTA Press.

Levy, L. L., & Burns, T. (2006). Neurocognitive practice essentials in dementia: Cognitive disabilities-reconsidered model. *OT Practice, 11*(3) CE-1–CE-8.

Llorens, L., & Johnson, P. A. (1966). Occupational therapy in an ego oriented milieu. *American Journal of Occupational Therapy, 20*(4), 178-181.

Maitra, K. K., & Erway, F. (2006). Perception of client-centered practice in occupational therapists and their clients. *American Journal of Occupational Therapy, 60*(3), 298-310.

Mastos, M., Miller, K., Eliasson, A. C., & Imms, C. (2007). Goal-directed training: Linking theories of treatment to clinical practice for improved functional activities in daily life. *Clinical Rehabilitation, 21*(1), 47-55.

Mosey, A. C. (1970). *Three frames of reference for mental health*. Thorofare, NJ: SLACK Incorporated.

Mosey, A. C. (1986). *Psychosocial components of occupational therapy*. New York, NY: Raven Press.

Pizzi, M. (1990). The model of human occupation and adults with HIV infection and AIDS. *American Journal of Occupational Therapy, 44*(3), 257-264.

Rebeiro, K. L. (2001). Enabling occupation: the importance of an affirming environment. *Canadian Journal Occupational Therapy, 68*(2), 80-89.

Rebeiro, K. L., & Polgar, J. M. (1999). Enabling occupational performance; optimal experiences in therapy. *Canadian Journal Occupational Therapy, 66*(1), 14-22.

Reilly, M. (1958). An occupational therapy curriculum for 1965. *American Journal of Occupational Therapy, 12*(6), 293-299.

Reilly, M. (1962). Occupational therapy can be one of the great ideas of 20th century medicine. *American Journal of Occupational Therapy, 16*, 1-9.

Reilly, M. (1969). The educational process. *American Journal of Occupational Therapy, 23*, 299-307.

Restall, G., Ripat, J., & Stern, M. (2003). A framework of strategies for client-centered practice. *Canadian Journal Occupational Therapy, 70*(2), 103-112.

Roley, S. S., Clark, G. F., Bissell, J., Brayman, S. J., Commission on Practice. (2003). Applying sensory integration framework in educationally related occupational therapy practice (2003 statement). *American Journal of Occupational Therapy, 57*(6), 652-659.

Rood, M. S. (1954). Neurophysiological reactions as a basis for physical therapy. *Physical Therapy Review, 34*, 444-449.

Salo-Chydenius, S. (1996). Changing helplessness to coping: An exploratory study of social skills training with individuals with long-term mental illness. *Occupational Therapy in Mental Health, 8*(2), 21-30.

Schaaf, R. C., & Miller, L. J. (2005). Occupational therapy using a sensory integrative approach for children for children with developmental disabilities. *Mental Retardation and Developmental Disabilities Research Reviews, 11*(2), 143-148.

Schkade, J. K., & McClung, M. (2001). *Occupational adaptation in practice: Concepts and cases*. Thorofare, NJ: SLACK Incorporated.

Schkade, J. K., & Schultz, S. (1992). Occupational adaptation: Toward a holistic approach for contemporary practice, part 1. *American Journal of Occupational Therapy, 46*(9), 829-837.

Schultz, S., & Schkade, J. K. (1992). Occupational adaptation: Toward a holistic approach for contemporary practice, part 2. *American Journal of Occupational Therapy, 46*(10), 917-926.

Stein, F., & Cutler, S. K. (2002). *Psychosocial occupational therapy: A holistic approach* (2nd ed.). Clifton Park, NY: Delmar Thomson Learning.

Strong, S., Rigby, P., Stewart, D., Law, M., Letts, L., & Cooper, B. (1999). Application of the person-environment-occupation model: A practical tool. *Canadian Journal Occupational Therapy, 66*(3), 122-133.

Teasell, R. W., Foley, N. C., Bhogal, S. K., & Speechley, M. R. (2003). An evidence-based review of stroke rehabilitation. *Top Stroke Rehabilitation, 10*(1), 29-58.

Toglia, J. (2005).A dynamic interactional approach to cognitive rehabilitation. In N. Katz (Ed.), *Cognition and occupation in rehabilitation: Cognitive models for intervention in occupational therapy* (2nd ed.). Bethesda, MD: AOTA Press.

Trombly, C. A. (1995). Occupation: Purposefulness and meaningfulness as therapeutic mechanisms. 1995 Eleanor Clarke Slagle Lecture. *American Journal of Occupational Therapy, 49*(10), 960-972.

Watling, R. L., & Dietz, J. (2007). Immediate effect of Ayres's sensory integration-based occupational therapy intervention on children with autism spectrum disorders. *American Journal of Occupational Therapy, 61*(5), 574-583.

Whedon, C. A. (2000). Frames of reference that address the impact of physical environments on occupational performance. *Work, 14*(2), 165-174.

Wilbarger, J., & Wilbarger, P. (2002). The Wilbarger approach to treating sensory defensiveness. In A. C. Bundy, S. J. Lane, & E. A. Murray (Eds.), *Sensory integration: Theory and practice* (2nd ed.). Philadelphia, PA: F.A. Davis.

Wilkins, S., Pollock, N. Rochon, S., & Law, M. (2001). Implementing client-centered practice: Why is it so difficult to do? *Canadian Journal of Occupational Therapy, 68*(2), 70-79.

Williamson, G. G., & Szczepanski, M. (1999). Coping frame of reference. In P. Kramer & J. Hinojosa (Eds.), *Frames of reference for pediatric occupational therapy* (2nd ed.). Philadelphia, PA: Lippincott Williams & Wilkins.

World Health Organization. (2001). *International classification of functioning, disability and health (ICF)*. Geneva, Switzerland: Author.

# Section IV
## Screening, Evaluation, and Referral

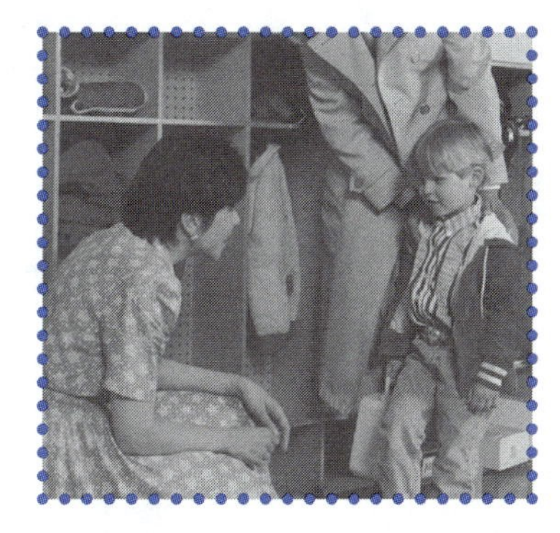

# 10

# Screening, Evaluation, and Referral

*Tara J. Glennon, EdD, OTR/L, FAOTA*

**ACOTE Standards Explored in This Chapter**

B.4.1-4.3, 4.5-4.10

**Key Terms**

| | |
|---|---|
| Assessment | Evaluation |
| Client | Norm referenced |
| Criterion referenced | Referral |
| Documentation | Screening |

## Introduction

The last decade has seen significant changes in the implementation and documentation of occupational therapy services. A variety of factors, both within and outside of our profession, have contributed to these changes. These factors include the view of health and disability in the *International Classification of Functioning, Disability, and Health* (ICF) by the World Health Organization (WHO, 2001), the need for evidence-based practice (American Occupational Therapy Association [AOTA], 2007a; Holm, 2000), the health care system's mandate for efficiency, and the publication and implementation of the framework (AOTA, 2008).

With regard to the evaluation process specifically, what is considered to be best practice has led to dramatic improvement in the assessment tools available to practitioners in order to meet the current responsibilities of an occupational therapy evaluation. In addition to the previously available performance, skill, client-centered, and daily living assessments, our profession now has assessments with focused attention related to occupation, social participation, work, activities of daily living (ADL), instrumental activities of daily living (IADL), environment/context, educational performance, and play/leisure. This section serves to identify important concepts related to the occupational therapy evaluation process, including information related to each of the above assessment areas.

## Terms and Definitions

This section is designed to familiarize occupational therapy practitioners with the terms and components of the evaluation process as currently understood within the occupational therapy profession. It is important, however, for clinicians to realize that other professions might use the terms interchangeably or might define them differently. In fact, older occupational therapy texts have offered differing definitions than those described in this chapter as the occupational therapy profession has revised and clarified its understanding of these components over the years. It is important to clarify the occupational therapy perspective when case conferencing, when sharing your occupational therapy evaluation results with other professions, or when



K. Sladyk, K. Jacobs, & N. MacRae (Eds.).
*Occupational Therapy Essentials for Clinical Competence* (pp. 101-114).

(as occurs in some instances) preparing a comprehensive evaluation report that includes the work of several disciplines. Screening, assessment, evaluation, and documentation are discussed next.

## Screening

Basically stated, a screening is a process by which the occupational therapy practitioner determines if further assessment is needed. Therefore, intervention planning can never occur with screening information alone. Screening methods can be formal (i.e., a standardized screening instrument or an organization's intake form) or informal (e.g., chart review, interview of a teacher, observation of a client).

While the framework does not specifically discuss the screening process, it is an important component in many institutions and, therefore, needs to be presented within this chapter. While the more experienced therapist might easily observe a client (informal) and determine if additional testing is required, the novice therapist might need more formalized methods to help determine if a potential difficulty is present. In fact, some might argue that when formalized methods of screening are utilized, the results factor into the therapist's clinical decision-making process, form the basis of the occupational therapy evaluation, and the screening results are included in the evaluation report as one of the processes utilized for obtaining information.

Mrs. Johnson, a second-grade teacher, ran into the occupational therapist in the teacher's lounge and indicated there were concerns about Mary's performance in the classroom. Mrs. Johnson asked if the occupational therapist could "just take a look" at Mary. Since the school district had a pre-referral program to assist children within the general education system prior to referral for special education services, the therapist asked Mrs. Johnson to complete the paperwork that would allow her to review Mary's educational history, observe Mary in the classroom, and send a questionnaire home to Mary's parents.

Upon record review, Mary has been having difficulty since preschool with her fine motor skills and how she organizes educational materials. This was also confirmed via the parent questionnaire. Within the classroom, Mary was observed to sit under her desk with her hands over her ears during morning announcements over the PA system, watch how other children were completing assignments before beginning herself, and rarely finished her workbook assignments within the allotted time. This screening information was sufficient for recommending a complete evaluation to determine Mary's specific difficulties so an effective intervention plan might be developed. The evaluation report ultimately included these occupational difficulties as examples of the client and contextual factors that interfered with Mary's successful engagement in school-related tasks.

## Assessment

Once the need for a comprehensive evaluation is determined, specific assessment tools are identified based on the data deemed necessary and the environment in which the client's occupations are limited. If a formalized screening was not completed, the informal methods of chart review and interview would be an appropriate starting point in the evaluation process. From this investigation, the appropriate assessment tools can be identified and implemented by the occupational therapist or the occupational therapy assistant. While the occupational therapist directs and initiates the evaluation process, the two practitioners can collaboratively determine which assessment(s) can be administered by the occupational therapy assistant based on professional experience, training, establishment of competency, and level of supervision provided. Per the *Guidelines for Supervision, Roles, and Responsibilities During the Delivery of Occupational Therapy Services* (Brayman et al., 2004) and AOTA's Standards of Practice (2005), the occupational therapy assistant "contributes to the evaluation process by implementing delegated assessments and by providing verbal and written reports of observations and client capacities to the occupational therapist" so the occupational therapist can interpret and integrate the information into the evaluation and decision-making process. While these are our professional guidelines, licensure regulations for each state have specific requirements with regard to service providers and supervision, which should be investigated prior to the implementation of service by the occupational therapy assistant. Additionally, relevant principles in the *Code of Ethics* (Reitz et al., 2005) and *Guidelines to the Occupational Therapy Code of Ethics* (Reitz et al., 2006) speak to appropriate delegation of tasks and supervision of occupational therapy assistants.

Assessments are the specific tests, tools, or methods used to collect the data needed for a comprehensive evaluation. Appendix B provides information related to commonly used assessment tools. Each assessment manual provides instructions for implementation, application, and interpretation, and it is each clinician's responsibility to be familiar and competent with each assessment tool utilized as part of his or her practice. Some assessment tools require advanced training and/or certification in order to implement, while some are only applicable to certain populations or age groups. In these cases, it is each professional's responsibility to meet the parameters set forth in the manual in order to assure ethical implementation in accordance with the test author's guidelines. Novice therapists can include the acquiring of these skills in their annual professional development plans and request time and financial resources to gain these skills.

There are times when an expert clinical decision is made to implement an assessment outside the boundaries set forth in the manual's implementation guidelines (e.g., not the intended population, procedures modified for language or physical limitations). This practice is frowned upon and should only occur when there are no other means of obtaining data to assist with intervention planning. With regard to reporting the assessment results, however, the data collected in these instances can only be used and reported informally, and scores cannot be reported as they are no longer valid or reliable as reported in the assessment manual.

As previously stated, great change in available assessment tools has occurred during the past decade. If, however, the setting within which you work requires standardized, client factor-focused assessments, it is the occupational therapist's role to determine how these specific pieces of information integrate with a more comprehensive, occupation-based perspective. For only with this clinical process can appropriate and effective interventions be planned so that occupational engagement, which is part of the continuum of care, will eventually be achieved.

## Standardized

An assessment tool manual can maximize consistency of professional implementation by outlining a formalized procedure to be followed. The formalized, or standardized, implementation and interpretation methods designed for best practice do not make a tool "standardized." Clinicians need to be clear: a standardized test requires rigorous analysis utilizing accepted psychometric procedures.

Standardization guarantees an assessment has psychometric characteristics, including statistical review of reliability and validity, established norms, standard error of measurement, and standardized administration (Cohen, Hinojosa, & Kramer, 2005). Understanding the psychometric properties of each assessment tool utilized allows the occupational therapist to have confidence in the fairness and consistency of the results. Verifying the assessment tool's reliability (accuracy and stability of the test; get the same test scores each time the test is given under the same conditions) and validity (measures the constructs, traits, or behaviors it says it will measure) via the test manual and professional literature allows the occupational therapist to speak with authority concerning professional recommendations.

Therapists sometimes determine that only portions of a standardized assessment are appropriate, or busy therapists sometimes try to focus only on certain sections of a standardized assessment. You cannot, however, administer a portion of the assessment tool and still consider the scores valid or reliable. If an assessment tool has several subtests implemented in a particular order or sequence during the standardization process and the therapist only implements some of those subtests, those scores cannot be fairly compared to the standardized population who completed all subtests in the same sequence. Therefore, if the therapist has broken the rules of the assessment administration, then the client is denied the full exploration of his or her issues, resulting in a biased assessment of his or her performance.

Although one might argue that standardized assessments are preferred given the evidence-based practice environment we are now in, this is not necessarily an accurate statement. Occupational therapy leaders have long argued the merits of utilizing a variety of assessment tools in order to gain the most comprehensive view of client preferences, habits, routines, skills, and occupational performance levels. In order to improve on the value of obtaining standardized assessments scores, the therapist's clinical reasoning, professional judgment, and review of evidence-based practice may lead to incorporating nonstandardized alternatives. Hinojosa, Kramer, and Crist (2005) argued that clinicians should question how best to get the needed information rather than what information is needed. Therefore, if nonstandardized methods (e.g., skilled observations, interviews, facility designed questionnaires, checklists, histories, and/or data collection on the frequency and duration of the identified behavior) are deemed necessary to assessing a client's performance, each therapist must know his or her own skill level for implementation and interpretation in order to minimize subjectivity and personal bias.

## Norm Referenced

Most tests are developed using a sample from the "normal" population. As a result, each client's scores can be compared to this "normal population." There are times when a test is developed from a group of persons with similar characteristics (i.e., age, gender, diagnosis). If this "normative" group matches your client's profile, the tool would be appropriate for implementation.

## Criterion Referenced

A criterion-referenced assessment tool outlines a set of objective criteria or skill components used to document what the client is and is not able to master. In this type of assessment, the client's score is then compared to the set of expected criteria rather than to the performance of other people in a normative group. For example, the components of eating with a fork would be visually locates fork on table, reaches for fork, grasps fork, brings fork to plate, scoops or spears, brings fork to mouth, opens mouth, inserts fork in mouth, closes lips around fork, removes food from fork, and removes fork from mouth. In this scenario, a client's skill level could be documented and future skills requiring intervention can be identified. These tools are particularly helpful for children with physical or mental difficulties where standardized assessment tools that compare a child to a typically developing child's scores are inappropriate or inapplicable.

## Culturally Sensitive Assessments

As previously stated, it is important for the occupational therapy practitioner to utilize assessment tools in the manner in which they were intended. If the standardization pool utilized during test development was homogeneous, the results for a client with differing characteristics will be limited and inadequate. For example, if the population sample included 500 men and 52 women, the results would be biased with regard to gender. While many standardized tests are based on the demographic profile provided by the United States Census Bureau and the tool's manual should identify the scope of the population sample used for standardization purposes, it is the clinician's responsibility to interpret the assessment results based on the cultural or ethnic differences of each specific client. For example, if the assessment requires a client to put pictures of his bedtime routine in order, and he places "brush his teeth" after he is in bed, this would be clinical data for the therapist. However, if he did not include the brushing the teeth picture, this might be cultural versus clinical. Taugher (2000) identified this cultural bias in our assessment tools as a primary issue as health care shifts from hospital or institution based to community based, and he posed several scenarios where decreased understanding of a client's cultural patterns might lead to inaccurate assessment of a person's skill level. The following examples could be culturally related or consistent with a diagnostic category:

- Talking fast (as with flight of ideas)
- Slow and laborious talk (as in depression and unable to pull thoughts together)
- Illogical syntax and thought (as in schizophrenia)

Lyons (2000) went on to include other examples such as not sharing during an interview, not following through on home programming, and that clutter in the house yields an unsafe walking environment. A multitude of cultural differences can affect the evaluation process. Wells and Black (2000) defined cultural competency as "lifelong learning designed to foster understanding, acceptance, knowledge, and constructive relations between persons of various cultures and differences" (p. 147). With this definition in mind, it is each clinician's responsibility to seek out the research information necessary to be efficient, effective, and ethical for the variety of cultural influences on one's specific caseload.

Cultural sensitivity is the last point to be discussed and perhaps the most important. Historically, healthcare workers have the motto, "Treat the client as I would want to be treated." Salimbene (2000) argued just the opposite in her *10 Tips for Successful Caregiver/Client Interaction*. The premise of how "you" want to be treated is based on your cultural background and experiences. If this is not your client's background and you do not recognize your interactions need to change based on the client's background, then you are not being culturally sensitive. With regard to the evaluation process, if you have not educated yourself on the routines, habits, traditions, and practices of a specific client's background, you are not being culturally sensitive. This is more than simply an insult; this leads to ineffective and inefficient information and inappropriate planning, and is professionally unethical (Reitz et al., 2005).

## Reassessment

In addition to the professional requirements of reassessment for discharge planning purposes, which includes documenting current performance level and planning for additional or follow-up intervention, the documentation of intervention outcomes itself often requires a reassessment. In today's healthcare environment of accountability, an assessment tool might be utilized pre- and post-intervention as a mechanism to provide evidence of intervention outcomes, to measure change from the initial evaluation period, and/or to plan for discharge. Although using the same assessment tool would be the easiest to detect change (i.e., by comparing the reassessment score with the initial assessment score and noting any change in score), many assessment tools are not designed to be reimplemented and, in fact, are not recommended for reimplementation. For example, if retested with the same standardized tool, the client might know what to expect, be comfortable with the format because he or she has been through it before (which is a difference from the first implementation), or become familiar with the test items from the first implementation. Additionally, different observers, testers, and raters should be factored into the reassessment process (termed *inter-rater reliability* in the test manual). Each of these factors would influence the reassessment score. Therefore, familiarity with the assessment tool manual is important in order for the clinician to fully understand the strengths and limitations of the assessment tool prior to reimplementation.

Once the assessment tool has been deemed appropriate to readminister, there are additional professional benefits to utilizing a pre- and post-administration of the tool. For example, utilizing pre- and post-assessment data for specific client groups allows the information to be used to compare or evaluate the outcomes for the client group as a whole, as well as provides the ability to compare each client's outcomes to the results found in more rigorous research studies completed on the same client group (Mandich, Miller, & Law, 2002).

A point of consideration, however, is the type and purpose of the reassessment. For example, administering a standardized tool before, during, and after intervention might not yield the information needed to alter or redefine a specific client-centered intervention plan. In fact, these tools might miss personal or environmental factors that need to be considered throughout the intervention process. However, ongoing measurements such as rating scales (criterion-referenced tools that identify objectively observable actions or behaviors) or skilled observations related to targeted goal areas would provide immediate feedback. This immediacy allows the clinician and client to determine if a change in plan is warranted to meet the specific goals for the individual client (Mandich et al., 2002).

## Summary

There are wide varieties of assessment tools available, and picking the appropriate tool for each specific client's profile requires great thought. The following list will help the practitioner pick the most appropriate tool while meeting professional standards:

- What is the credibility of the assessment tool, and is it commonly used in the profession?
- Does the occupational therapy literature support the use of this assessment tool as appropriate and applicable to occupational therapy practice?
- Is this tool appropriate, useful, and the best method to obtain the information I need?
- Am I adequately prepared and trained to implement and interpret this assessment?
- Are there any cultural (including education level, English as a first language, etc.) limitations for applicability?
- Does the tool have acceptable psychometric qualities (including reliability, validity, adequate specificity, and sensitivity) for my needs?

After choosing the assessment tool, the practitioner must be prepared to do the following:

- Follow the parameters outlined
- Administer in the manner and for the population which the tool was intended (i.e., if intended for clients with dementia, do not use with clients diagnosed with schizophrenia)
- Interpret as intended and outlined in the manual
- Provide a clinical rationale for any variance in established procedures, and provide a statement indicating that the results were not gained in the manner intended or outlined in the manual
- Utilize all necessary assessment tools to gather the needed data within the evaluation process in order to provide the most comprehensive picture of the facilitators of and barriers to participation in life's roles

# Evaluation

Evaluation refers to the process of obtaining and interpreting data in order to fully understand and appreciate the client's strengths and areas of concern. This includes information related to the client's ability to function in chosen occupations and roles; the contextual factors influencing this function; and client factors, routines, and habits (AOTA, 2008). While the process includes determining which assessment tools will best yield the necessary information and which pieces of information obtained are most important in understanding the client's needs, one cannot forget it is a "process" that is fluid.

After the initial phone intake, which identified that 7-year-old Harry had fine motor difficulties and the priority for the mother was for Harry to write, the occupational therapist chose two assessment tools that focused on handwriting and the underlying fine motor skills. Upon arrival, however, Harry was unable to sit up in the waiting room chair. This information prompted the occupational therapist to alter the table top assessment tools originally planned for the evaluation session as Harry would be unable to perform the tasks required on either assessment tool without the ability to sit up in the chair.

The evaluation process requires ongoing clinical reasoning and a combination of both standardized and nonstandardized assessment tools in order to obtain a comprehensive picture of the client (Strickland, 2005). In order to complete an evaluation, the therapist must understand the strengths and limitations of each assessment tool, identify information that must be obtained outside of standardized or formal methods of the assessment tools previously mentioned, and make effective decisions about how the evaluation needs to be adjusted based on the findings during the evaluation process.

# Evaluation Factors to Consider

In preparation for the evaluation process, several underlying issues need to be considered. Specifically, the influence of professional parameters and initiatives (AOTA, 2007a, 2008; Reitz et al., 2006), evidence-based practice mandates (AOTA, 2007a; Holm, 2000), and reimbursement constraints. Additionally, depending on the context in which the evaluation must occur, various factors might be more pertinent than others, while some factors are universal across domains and contexts. This section will discuss considerations that the occupational therapy practitioner must be aware of during the evaluation process.

## Professional

The framework (AOTA, 2008) provides parameters in which the occupational therapist and occupational therapy assistant must function. Specific information related to the components of this document related to evaluation will be presented in the next section, where the evaluation process is discussed. However, the influence of the ICF (WHO, 2001), from which the framework was created, has greatly changed how the evaluative process is implemented. Specifically, the focus on function, participation, and context have contributed to the development of the framework and are consistent with the longstanding philosophy of occupational therapy to identify the facilitators of and barriers to functional participation in meaningful occupations.

## Evidence-Based Practice

An underlying premise of practice, specifically evaluation, is that decisions need to be made based on evidence. Effective decisions made within the evaluation process yield valuable information, that, in turn, leads to appropriate intervention plans and, ultimately, improved outcomes. Muir Gray's (2004) "Doing the Right Things Right" outline for evidence-based medicine also applies to the occupational therapy evaluation process (Table 10-1). Additionally, evidence-based, clinical decision models emphasize clinical expertise and client preference as equally important to research/evidence within the clinical process. This triad allows for the clinician to utilize his or her expertise and understanding of client preferences to determine the applicability and appropriateness of the external research evidence. Implementing a client-centered evaluation process, as recommended in occupational therapy literature, fits within this more global model of evidence-based clinical/medical practice. In order to make these decisions correctly, the occupational therapy practitioner needs to understand the design, rationale, strengths, and limitations of various assessment tools and interface this information with client preferences and clinical reasoning for various client populations.

## Organizational

While the unique perspective on occupational engagement should always guide our evaluative choices, the scope of evaluative responsibilities and procedures is determined by each specific setting. Organizations focusing primarily on client factors or performance skills (e.g., acute rehabilitation, hand therapy) literally set the stage for engagement in meaningful occupations later in the continuum of care. Additionally, each practice setting has its own philosophy, and assuring a match with your own personal philosophy, including your own values and beliefs, would be important as they will factor into the evaluative decisions made. Understanding your scope of practice as defined within a specific organization and assuring it meets the scope of practice outlined by the professional credentialing body and state licensure laws is imperative prior to the implementation of any occupational therapy service.

The financial constraints of an organization will also influence the evaluative process. The assessment resources available; the time available in your schedule to complete the evaluation, including implementation, processing of information, and documentation; and the requirements of the funding source(s) greatly influence the methods chosen to obtain the necessary information. Therefore, it would be prudent for the practitioner to understand the unique attributes and limitations of the assessment methods within this section, develop a mentoring system to improve clinical reasoning skills related to evaluation implementation, and continually examine personal patterns of performance in order to meet the demands of current practice.

## Funding Source and Referral

Understanding the system in which you are working, and thus having specific knowledge of the funding source(s) or referral options, will also help to determine the appropriate assessment tool(s) to be utilized. First, the therapist needs to be sure the funding source's evaluation requirements to approve payment can be met. If there are requirements that cannot be completed (i.e., standardized scores are required but there is no tool available given the client's physical limitations), the therapist needs to contact the funding agency to clearly explain the limitations of the requirements and gain approval to continue in an alternative manner. Second, if the client has expressed concerns during the client profile that do not fall under the domain

**Table 10-1. Evidence-Based Evaluation Process**

| Performance | Outcome | Evaluation Implications |
|---|---|---|
| Doing the right things | Increasing effectiveness | • Choose appropriate evaluation methods and procedures to obtain the information critical to intervention planning and referral to others internal and external to the profession.<br>• Ask: How can I best obtain the needed information?<br>• Adhering to the established professional standards related to the role of the occupational therapist and occupational therapy assistant. |
| Doing things right | Efficiency; cost effectiveness | • Focus on occupational engagement throughout the process.<br>• Familiarity with, and knowledge of, specific evaluation methods and procedures yields efficient utilization of time and resources.<br>• Thorough documentation of the evaluative process results and plan of intervention. |
| Doing the right things right | Best; quality improvement | • Making effective decisions pertaining to the methods necessary to yield the best information for the evaluative purpose and determining the best or most efficient means of obtaining the needed information is both clinically appropriate and fiscally responsible |

of the funding agency or the intervention site, this needs to be discussed and alternative or additional arrangements need to be explored with the organization's administration. It may be necessary to refer the client to another discipline or intervention facility.

It is also important to remember that each funding source has rules on who can refer to occupational therapy. Typically for third-party payers, it is from a physician. Therefore, if the referral is not generated from the physician, as it is often from another professional, self-initiated by the client, or the client's parent after speaking to others in similar circumstances, having the client contact his or her physician for a prescription to occupational therapy would be necessary in order to assure proper and timely payment.

# Evaluation Components

With regard to an occupational therapy evaluation, AOTA (2007b) emphasizes the need to include client information, reason for referral, an occupational profile, the assessments utilized, the assessment results, summary and analysis, and recommendations. The first area, client information, will be dependent on the system in which the practitioner works, but it generally includes name, age, diagnoses, medical history, medications, precautions, and contraindications (Figure 10-1). There are instances, however, where the client is an organization, population, or community that supports the engagement of individuals in functional activities. In those instances, the client information would include demographics of the group and any other information that would influence the evaluative process necessary to develop an intervention, support, consultation, or education plan for the group.

The subsequent components of the evaluation process are as follows with additional information related to specific assessments, assessment results, and assessment analysis presented in the following chapters (Tables 10-2 and 10-3).

## Reason for Referral

First and foremost, it is imperative to understand the reason for referral so that appropriate assessment methods can be identified. While this may seem to be a basic concept, it is often overlooked. A referral for an occupational therapy evaluation can come from many sources, with varying levels of information for you to review and/or with specific outcomes expected. If the referral does not have the required information, it would be the therapist's responsibility to obtain the required documentation. This lack of information can range from no age on the referral form to the lack of written documentation of medical clearance for the evaluation of a client with a neck injury. Regardless of what information is missing, the importance of complete information is clear.

The following examples illustrate the diverse nature of referral information.

The hospital in which you work has a standard procedure for a referral to occupational therapy if the admission has any injury to the head. In this case, you would have access to files with intake information related to the personal and medical histories, initial medical findings by your organization, reports written by the professionals who have already evaluated the client, etc. In this scenario,

**Table 10-2. Engagement in Occupation to Support Participation in Context or Contexts**

- Performance in areas of occupation
  - Activities of daily living (ADL)
  - Instrumental activities of daily living (IADL)
  - Education
  - Work
  - Play
  - Leisure
  - Social participation
- Performance skills
  - Motor skills/habits
  - Process skills/routines
  - Communication/interaction skills/roles
- Performance patterns
  - Habits
  - Routines
  - Roles
- Context
  - Cultural
  - Physical
  - Social
  - Personal
  - Spiritual
  - Temporal
  - Virtual
- Activity demands
  - Objects used and their properties body functions
  - Space demands
  - Social demands
  - Sequencing and timing
  - Required actions
  - Required body functions
  - Required body structures
- Client factors
  - Body functions
  - Body structures

Adapted from American Occupational Therapy Association. (2008). Occupational therapy practice framework: Domain and process, second edition. *American Journal of Occupational Therapy, 62*, 625-683.

**Center for Pediatric Therapy**

◆ Executive Director: Tara J. Glennon, EdD, OTR/L, BCP, FAOTA

❑ Fairfield
❑ Wallingford
❑ Milford

INTAKE/CLIENT PROFILE

❑ In Network ❑ Out Of Network ❑ OT ❑ PT ❑ SPEECH

| | | |
|---|---|---|
| Child's Name: | | Date of Intake: |
| DOB: | | Date of Eval: |
| Diagnosis Code: | | Therapist: |
| Medications: | if applicable | |
| Precautions: | if applicable | |
| Parents' Names: | | Home: |
| | mother<br>father | Work: |
| Home Address: | | Cell: |
| | | |
| School Program: | | Grade: |
| Insurance Co.: | | Phone: |
| | | Group #: |
| Subscriber Name: | | ID #: |
| | | |
| MD Script: | ☐ bringing day of evaluation | ☐ faxing |
| Pediatrician: | Dr. | Phone: |
| MD Address: | | |
| Other Therapists: | | |
| Other Physicians: | | |
| Referred By: | psychologist<br>neurologist | pediatrician<br>other |
| Reason for Referral: | | |
| Parent-Family-Child Concerns (use back of page if necessary): | | |
| When, where, how do these issues interfere? What does the parent wish to get from evaluation and/or intervention? What is important to the parent and/or child? | | |
| | | |
| | | |
| | | |
| | | |
| | | |
| | | |
| | | |
| | | |
| | | |
| | | |
| Available evaluation times: | | TOTAL TIME: |
| Available intervention times: | | |

**CPT Locations:**

Therapy Offices:

CPT - Fairfield, Inc.
1300 Post Road
Suite 204
Fairfield, CT 06824
(203) 255-3669
Fax (203) 255-1173

CPT - Wallingford, LLC
101 N. Plains Industrial
Building 2
Wallingford, CT 06492
(203) 949-9337
Fax (203) 284-3779

Administrative Office:

CPT
203 Broad Street
Unit C-2
Milford, CT 06460
(203) 876-2000
Fax (203) 876-1545

www.centerforpediatrictherapy.com

**Figure 10-1.** Sample Intake/Client Profile Form.

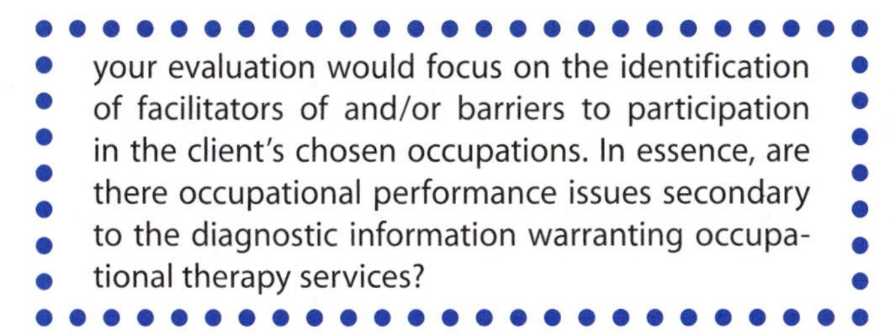
your evaluation would focus on the identification of facilitators of and/or barriers to participation in the client's chosen occupations. In essence, are there occupational performance issues secondary to the diagnostic information warranting occupational therapy services?

These types of "systems" referrals often have specific evaluative procedures, outlined via departmental or organizational review, that need to be followed in order for "eligibility" for occupational therapy services to be determined. Other systems might utilize this type of procedure, including federal or state programs (i.e., Birth-to-Three and Boards of Education). As a point of clarification, these types of eligibility evaluations were previously termed *diagnostic evaluations* but should not be interpreted to indicate that a simple medical or rehabilitative diagnosis alone would determine eligibility. Rather, identifying the unique, client-specific facilitators of and barriers to functional participation in meaningful activities, which might include a qualifying test/assessment score if mandated, would be the information that determines eligibility.

**Table 10-3. Components of an Occupational Therapy Evaluation**

| Category | Description |
|---|---|
| Client information | For recordkeeping purposes: Name; parent name if appropriate; age; client number if needed; funding identification number; contact information.<br>For planning purposes: Pertinent diagnoses; relevant medical history; medications; precautions; limitations; contraindications. |
| Reason for referral | Generated by whom; for what reason; what information is being requested and for what purpose; include date of request on documentation. |
| Occupational profile | The framework mandates clinicians utilize a client-centered approach; obtain information that allows the practitioner to understand what is meaningful for the client; client's desired outcomes; past experiences and history contributing to the client's desired outcomes; client priorities and preferences; factors influencing meaningful engagement in occupations. |
| Assessments methods/ tools utilized | Per the framework, the evaluation considers performance skills, performance patterns, context, activity demands, and client factors; an evaluation often requires the implementation of multiple assessment tools; implementation of multiple assessment tools is not often practical or feasible in certain organizations; minimum expectations are to have sufficient data to plan interventions; document which tools utilized (standardized, norm referenced, criterion referenced, formal, informal, etc.), why implemented, why and how established protocols were not followed if applicable, and how these tools contributed to a full understanding of the client's needs; chosen assessment tools are bias free with regard to cultural (in the broadest sense) issues; therapists must have required level of skill and knowledge to implement the assessment tool; occupational therapist and occupational therapy assistant mutually determine which tools can be administered by the occupational therapy assistant based on level of expertise, training, supervision, and pertinent regulations. |
| Assessment tool(s) results | Score and report all formalized assessment results according to the procedures outlined in the test manual; identify limitations with information obtained if exact testing protocols were unable to be followed; indicate if you believe the assessment results to be accurate or inaccurate for any external reason; make no other assumptions on the data at this time; include skilled, clinical observations, and other informal findings. |
| Analysis and summary | Interpret the assessment findings, summarize strengths and vulnerabilities, and identify the supports and barriers to successful engagement or performance; synthesize the information in a manner consistent with the presenting concerns identified in the referral and the client's life and environment; incorporate information from formal and informal tools, observations, clinical judgment, and how these findings interface with client's goals, interests, and preferences; do not over-interpret the data—report what you know from your clinical expertise and you can continue to investigate any unsubstantiated hypotheses during the intervention period; provide summary statement of findings. |
| Recommendation | Use clinical judgment to determine if services are warranted or additional referrals are necessary; these decisions must relate to the initial referral request, client preferences and priorities, potential intervention approach(es) based on best practice and evidence, and the feasibility of the intervention's success given the evaluative findings; identify the types of service that address the presenting concerns (i.e., education, consultation, direct, monitor); depending on the organization's funding source, this section may include goals, objectives, and specifics about the intervention recommended (i.e., frequency, duration)—otherwise, this information would belong in a plan of care. |

A parent calls your clinic to say her neighbor said to call as her baby is colicky and not eating well. In this case, with no other formal documentation available, and the parent potentially not even understanding what occupational therapy can offer, the clinician must obtain as much information as possible to help guide the decision-making process for the evaluation session. Equally important, however, is to remember that the therapeutic relationship begins during this initial conversation.

The conversation must be a forum to respond to, respect, and empathize with the parent who is now fearful there is something wrong with her child; educate the parent on the types of issues that could be impacting the child's patterns; and provide reassurance that the parent is doing the right thing by investigating any support he or she believes would make his or her child's interactions with the world more calm and joyful. While this may be non-billable therapeutic time, a full discussion with the parent/client at the time of the intake call would be critical for the process to move forward successfully. In fact, this is the beginning of the therapeutic relationship, and the implications of this concept should not be overlooked. The bottom section of the Intake/Profile Form provided in Figure 10-1 provides a framework for beginning this conversation.

The local psychologist has been working with an agitated client for the past 3 months. As the agitation has diminished, the psychologist realizes there are underlying difficulties related to home management, life skills, and ongoing issues with holding a job. While you may now have the psychologist's referral and report, which outlines some of the occupational challenges for the client, the underlying reason for these challenges needs to be investigated. This type of evaluation is intended to determine the most appropriate intervention plan rather than eligibility. In this case, the evaluation report might be more descriptive in nature versus simply stating scores from a standardized assessment tool. This scenario is similar to Harry's case study previously discussed as the evaluation could provide a poor score on a handwriting assessment, but this does not guide how best to support him. This support is best designed with a fuller understanding of the facilitators of and barriers (both client specific and environmental/contextual) to Harry's ability to successfully engage in handwriting activities.

It is important to recognize how these preliminary findings help you form an initial picture of the client in your mind. While this assists with designing your approach to the evaluation process, it should not limit your expectations of the client or eliminate the possibility of shifting your preliminary plans to accommodate for your own observations of performance with the unique perspective of occupation. Additionally, once the client's priorities and preferences are communicated, either by the client him- or herself or significant persons if the client is unable, alternative assessment tools may need to be incorporated.

## Occupational Profile

The occupational profile, defined in the framework as "information that describes the client's occupational history and experiences, patterns of daily living, interests, values, and needs" (AOTA, 2008), identifies and guides our understanding of the occupational issues that are important and meaningful to the client. Beginning the evaluation process with an occupational profile also supports the top-down approach to an occupational therapy evaluation as it begins with the client perspective of occupational performance and then works downward to investigate the factors (client specific or contextual) that contribute to the occupational limitations.

## Assessments Utilized and Assessment Analysis

As stated above and as illustrated in Appendix B, there are many assessment tools available. While the following chapters in this section of the text will discuss specific assessment tools focusing on occupational performance components, it is clear that the choice of assessment tool(s) needs to be guided by the occupational profile. Therefore, the occupational therapy evaluation report needs to identify which tools were utilized to obtain the data, the rationale for the decision, any alterations to the assessment's procedures required, and how each of these choices contribute to the overarching view of occupation being evaluated. Within the analysis section of the occupational therapy evaluation report, it would be important to discuss information from different assessment methods that support the evaluator's analysis as well as information considered to be a contradiction.

# Documentation

Documentation is necessary whenever professional services are provided to a client. Occupational therapists and occupational therapy assistants under the supervision of an occupational therapist determine the appropriate type of documentation and document the services provided with their scope of practice (AOTA, 2007b, p. 197).

Documentation, an important legal and professional component for all occupational therapy services, has an important function within the evaluation process. An evaluation report, which clearly, accurately, and comprehensively outlines the current level of functioning and concerns to be supported by occupational therapy, not only guides entrance into the health care arena but also offers a framework for communication with the client and other professionals; forms the basis for referral to specialists both internal and external to occupational therapy; establishes the rationale for financial support for services; and provides a mechanism to plan interventions moving forward, which will be compared to this original baseline of performance. Sames (2005) argued that the report of the initial evaluation is the most important document the occupational therapist will write. Components of documentation requirements can be found in Table 10-4, and additional information can be found in Chapter 32.

## Professional

As one begins the evaluation report, understanding the target audience or stakeholder will guide the presentation of results. For example, a report for a child's family for program planning purposes might look very different from a report for a third-party payer. Asking who needs the information and why (i.e., funding source, organization, external accrediting agency requirements) will assist the therapist in producing a report reflective of the practice setting. Despite the nuances, every occupational therapy report should have established components (see Table 10-2).

## Reimbursement

While documentation is important for the continuity of care and therapeutic intervention planning, it is also intricately linked to payment. No matter the payment source, documentation is a mechanism to obtain approval for payment. The type and frequency of documentation is generally determined by the payment source (e.g., federal or state programs, third-party payers, grant funding). Thus, the therapist needs to be fully aware of the rules and requirements, including any updates or revisions, prior to report completion in order to minimize the possibility of claim denial. Additionally, effectively communicating this information from the perspective of occupational engagement will help distinguish occupational therapy from other therapeutic services also requesting payment for services.

## Legal Requirements

Any written communication produced by occupational therapy personnel with regard to a client's care is considered a legal document and should be kept confidential in adherence to professional standards, state laws, and the Health Insurance Portability and Accountability Act (HIPPA) (United States Department of Health and Human Services, 2002). Not only does the paperwork substantiate that the services were delivered, but it also serves to provide

**Table 10-4. Documentation Requirements**

| | |
|---|---|
| **Professional** | • Identify and meet agency/organization expectations and ensure these expectations match professional guidelines, licensure, and ethical responsibilities.<br>• Write for the reader (target audience).<br>• Differentiate direct observations from opinions regarding the performance (i.e., client stated she is the mother of 13 children versus client is delusional as she believes she is the mother of 13 children).<br>• Information for referral to another specialist should be prompt and comprehensive.<br>• If using hardcopy format versus computerized, documentation should be legible and well organized.<br>• Complete required documentation in a timely manner. |
| **Legal** | • Remember, every piece of documentation is considered a legal document that can be subpoenaed.<br>• All documentation should meet employer, accrediting body, and funding sources requirements.<br>• All documentation should be complete and accurate (including dates of service and date of documentation of service if required).<br>• If hardcopy format is utilized, do not change, remove, or alter your documentation with erasures or white-out. Simply cross out the error with a single line and initial to indicate it was you who deleted the piece of information. Put a line through unused lines or spaces on any forms.<br>• Include only first hand information of what you see or hear versus what the client told you (i.e., client stated he completed the home program once per day versus client completed home program as designed).<br>• Avoid negative statements as, aside from being unprofessional, they can be interpreted as you disliked the client, then other information would be subject to interpretation.<br>• The treating therapist must sign all documentation, including co-signing as the supervising therapist as required with name, professional credentials, and date.<br>• Client name and identifying information should be on each page of documentation in case pages become separated. |

a history of what actually happened on behalf of the client. Even the screening, which led to a full evaluation, should be documented as a client contact in the chart because if it is not documented, it did not happen in the eyes of the law. Therefore, any errors, inconsistencies, or omissions can be used against you in a court of law. It is imperative for each clinician to understand the legal requirements of the funding source and the legal implications for the agency in which you work. Most employers will set the rules of how their staff should perform in terms of documentation, and once the practitioner is aware of the employer's expectations, it is important to be sure the expectations meet professional licensure, guidelines, and ethical expectations. It is the responsibility of the individual practitioner to assure all of these requirements are met and communicate any disparities to the employer.

Each agency/organization will have its own rules on the types of documentation required, as well as its own system of recording the information. If the system is computerized, thorough training for all occupational therapy personnel should be completed, and no other clinician should enter information into the client files of other therapists. If there are hardcopy files, there may be one formal/official/legal file where all pertinent information needs to be recorded. Thereafter, there may be a clinical file by each clinician for information related to intervention planning, copies of performance measures, and day-to-day information the therapist needs to monitor and track. While notes/documents/performance samples are not in the "official" file, they are still considered legal documents, should be kept in a locked file cabinet, and can be subpoenaed in a court of law.

# Summary

The occupational therapy evaluation process is a complicated procedure from a clinical perspective and an administrative process. As the initial evaluation is the entry into occupational therapy services, evaluation from an occupational perspective; competence in administration and interpretation of the assessment tools utilized; and efficient, accurate, and timely documentation are all necessary. Using the evidence-based medicine model previously discussed (Muir Gray, 2004), Table 10-1 provides a synopsis of this concept with regard to the evaluation process. The remainder of this section of the text will discuss specific assessment tools and their use in practice.

# Student Self-Assessment

1. From the information provided on Mary's case study on page 98, which assessment tools might be appropriate to administer and why? Which frame of reference do the chosen assessments follow? Identify a part of the assessment process an occupational therapy assistant might be able to complete.
2. Complete Appendix B, Assessment Tool Grid, with additional assessment tools from your coursework.
3. Identify various state, federal, and private funding sources that might influence the evaluative processes within a given practice setting.
4. Discuss how funding source limitations might influence the documentation of the full scope of your occupational therapy services.
5. Examine your own personal values and beliefs regarding service delivery, and identify how these might influence your approach to an occupational therapy evaluation.
6. Identify the assessment tools appropriate for Harry's case study given his inability to sit up in a chair and the influence on his fine and graphomotor skills.
7. Based on one occupational therapy setting you have observed, create an intake form you believe would be appropriate in that environment.
8. Based on one occupational therapy client you observed this semester, assume the observed session was the evaluation session and complete the information requested in Table 10-2.
9. Referring to Table 10-4, Documentation Requirements, create a list of situations that you have observed throughout your education that might be in conflict with the rules provided. Be prepared to discuss these observations in class.

# Electronic Resources

- The American Occupational Therapy Association for compliance with Standards of Practice: www.aota.org
- Department of Health and Human Services, Centers for Medicare & Medicaid Services: www.cms.hhs.gov

# References

American Occupational Therapy Association. (2005). Standards of practice for occupational therapy. *American Journal of Occupational Therapy, 59*, 663–665.

American Occupational Therapy Association. (2007a). *The Centennial Vision*. Bethesda, MD: Author. Retrieved August 15, 2009, from http://www.aota.org/News/Centennial.aspx

American Occupational Therapy Association. (2007b). Guidelines for documentation of occupational therapy. In American Occupational Therapy Association. *The reference manual of the official documents of the American Occupational Therapy Associations* (12th ed., pp. 197-201). Bethesda, MD: Author.

American Occupational Therapy Association. (2008). Occupational therapy practice framework: Domain and process, second edition. *American Journal of Occupational Therapy, 62*, 625-683.

Brayman, S. J., Clark, G. F., DeLany, J. V., Garza, E. R., Radomski, M. V., Ramsey, R., et al. (2004). Guidelines for supervision, roles, and responsibilities during the delivery of occupational therapy services. *American Journal of Occupational Therapy, 58*(6), 663-667.

Cohen, M. E., Hinojosa, J., & Kramer, P. (2005). Administration of evaluation and assessments. In J. Hinojosa, P. Kramer, & P. Crist (Eds.), *Evaluation: Obtaining and interpreting data* (2nd ed., pp. 81-99). Bethesda, MD: AOTA Press.

Hinojosa, J., Kramer, P., & Crist, P. (Eds.). (2005). *Evaluation: Obtaining and interpreting data*. Bethesda, MD: AOTA Press.

Holm, M. B. (2000). The 2000 Eleanor Clarke Slagle Lecture. Our mandate for the new millennium: Evidence-based practice. *American Journal of Occupational Therapy, 54*(6), 575-585.

Lyons, A. (2000). Cultural competence in occupational therapy practice. *Home & Community Health Special Interest Section Quarterly, 7*, 1-2.

Mandich, A., Miller, L., & Law, M. (2002). Outcomes in evidence-based practice. In M. Law (Ed.), *Evidence-based rehabilitation: A guide to practice* (pp. 49-69). Thorofare, NJ: SLACK Incorporated.

Muir Gray, J. A. (2004). *Evidence-based healthcare: How to make health policy and management decisions*. Upper Saddle River, NJ: Pearson Prentice Hall.

Reitz, S. M., Arnold, M., Franck, L. G., Austin, D. J, Hill, D., McQuade, L. J., et al. (2005). Occupational Therapy Code of Ethics (2005). *American Journal of Occupational Therapy, 59*(6), 639-642.

Reitz, S. M., Austin, D. J., Brandt, L. C., DeBrakeller, B., Franck, L. G., Homenko, D. F., et al. (2006). Guidelines to the Occupational Therapy Code of Ethics. *American Journal of Occupational Therapy, 60*(6), 652-658.

Salimbene, S. (2000). *What language does your patient hurt in? A practical guide to culturally competent patient care*. Amherst, MA: Diversity Resources.

Sames, K. M. (2005). *Documenting occupational therapy practice*. Upper Saddle River, NJ: Prentice Hall.

Strickland, L. S. (2005). Evaluation issues in today's practice. In J. Hinojosa, P. Kramer, & P. Crist (Eds.), *Evaluation: Obtaining and interpreting data* (2nd ed., pp. 51-58). Bethesda, MD: AOTA Press.

Taugher, M. (2000). Persons with limited English proficiency: A challenge for home and community practitioners. *Home & Community Health Special Interest Section Quarterly, 7*, 2-4.

United States Department of Health and Human Services. (2002). *Standards for Privacy of Individually Identifiable Health Information*. Retrieved August 15, 2009, from http://www.hhs.gov/ocr/privacy/hipaa/news/2002/combinedregtext02.pdf

Wells, S. A., & Black, R. M. (2000). *Cultural competency for health professionals*. Bethesda, MD: AOTA Press.

World Health Organization. (2001). *International classification of functioning, disability, and health*. Geneva, Switzerland: Author

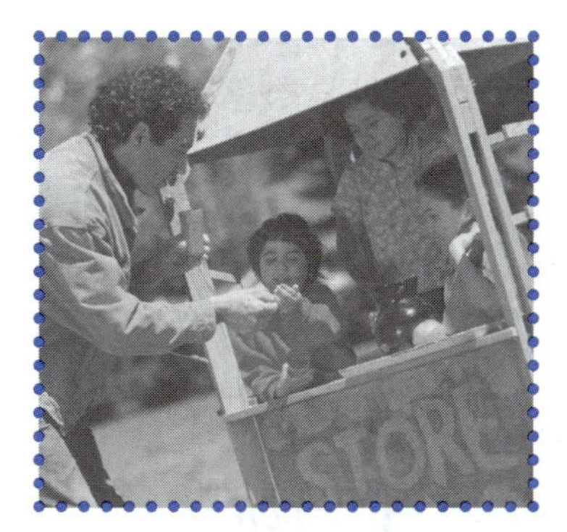

# 11

# Evaluation of Activities of Daily Living and Instrumental Activities of Daily Living

*Lisa J. Knecht-Sabres, DHS, OTR/L*

**ACOTE Standard Explored in This Chapter**

B.4.4

**Key Terms**

- Activities of daily living
- Activity
- Client-centered approach
- Instrumental activities of daily living
- Occupation
- Occupational profile
- Performance skills

## Introduction

Occupational therapy practitioners have a unique perspective of their clients. That is, the expertise of an occupational therapy practitioner lies in his or her ability to appreciate the broad range of human occupations and activities that make up peoples' lives (American Occupational Therapy Association [AOTA], 2008). Since occupational therapy practitioners focus on enabling people to engage (or re-engage) in the everyday activities that bring meaningfulness and purposefulness to their lives, the occupational therapy practitioner's evaluation process must include an assessment of the daily activities the person either needs or wants to perform. According to the framework (AOTA, 2008), the types of activities people engage in each day consist of activities of daily living (ADL), instrumental activities of daily living (IADL), education, work, play, leisure, and social participation.

The framework defines occupations as activities that have unique meaning and purpose in one's life, are central to one's identity, and influence how one spends time and makes decisions.

Similarly, Fisher, Bryze, and Hume (2002) defined occupations as the purposeful and meaningful task performances people engage in that support the social and personal roles that define each person. In contrast, the framework asserted that activities are the tasks or actions in which an individual may participate in order to achieve a goal. Thus, one of the key differences between occupations and activities is that, even though certain activities may be vital to the completion of an occupation, activities do not hold a place of central importance or meaning to the individual. For instance, one of the occupations I value most in my life is my role as a mother. However, even though this occupation is central to my identity and influences how I spend my time, it entails numerous activities I might not perceive as



K. Sladyk, K. Jacobs, & N. MacRae (Eds.).
*Occupational Therapy Essentials for Clinical Competence* (pp. 115-126).

possessing central importance to me. Another way to look at the difference between an occupation and an activity is with an example related to cooking. For instance, one person may view cooking as a mandatory activity that needs to be done on a daily basis to sustain life. However, another person may view cooking as an occupation, whether it is because the person is the head chef in an Italian restaurant or because the person finds enormous pleasure and a sense of fulfillment from making gourmet meals for family and friends.

This chapter focuses on how occupational therapy practitioners should approach the evaluation of ADL and IADL with their clients (Table 11-1). The framework (AOTA, 2008) defined ADL as the activities that are oriented toward taking care of one's own body. They include the following (AOTA, 2008):

- Bathing/showing
- Bowel and bladder management
- Dressing
- Eating
- Feeding
- Functional mobility
- Personal device care
- Personal hygiene and grooming
- Sexual activity
- Sleep/rest
- Toilet hygiene

The framework defined IADL as the activities that are oriented toward interacting with the environment, are often complex, and include the following (AOTA, 2008):

- Care of others
- Care of pets
- Child rearing
- Use of communication devices
- Community mobility
- Financial management
- Health management and maintenance
- Home establishment and maintenance
- Meal preparation and clean-up
- Safety procedures and emergency responses
- Shopping

Each ADL and IADL activity listed above is individually defined in the framework.

The first critical step in any occupational therapy evaluation is to obtain an understanding of the client's occupational profile (AOTA, 2008). In other words, it is imperative for the occupational therapy practitioner to gain a deep understanding of the person's occupational history and experiences, patterns of daily living, interests, values, and needs. Furthermore, it is essential to ascertain the person's concerns about performing his or her occupations and daily life activities, as well as his or her priorities for occupational performance. After obtaining the occupational profile, the next vital step in the evaluation process is the analysis of occupational performance, which requires the therapist to observe the person's occupational performance, ideally within the natural context, in order to determine what supports and hinders performance (AOTA, 2008).

# Obtaining the Client's Occupational Profile

Since the first essential step in the occupational therapy evaluation process is to obtain an understanding of the person's occupational profile, the occupational therapy practitioner needs to decide how he or she is going to gather this vital information. Utilizing a client-centered approach to evaluate one's ADL and IADL provides a natural means for the client to identify his or her own unique occupational performance problems that are pertinent to his or her unique circumstances and context (Law, Baum, & Dunn, 2005). There are a few occupational therapy evaluations that evaluate occupational performance in a client-centered manner. The Canadian Occupational Performance Measure (COPM) (Law, Baptiste, et al., 2005) appears to be a widely used and clinically sound client-centered occupational therapy evaluation tool. The COPM is a semi-structured interview designed to have the client do the following (Law, Baptiste, et al., 2005):

1. Identify concerns regarding his or her performance during self-care, productivity, and leisure activities
2. Evaluate his or her performance and satisfaction relative to the identified problematic occupational performance areas
3. Prioritize his or her problems in occupational performance
4. Measure changes in his or her perception of his or her occupational performance over the course of occupational therapy intervention

The COPM can be used with virtually any client regardless of his or her age or diagnosis since this tool can be administered to a family member or caregiver if the client is unable to participate in the interview. Not only is the COPM an excellent tool to gain critical information about the client's occupational profile, but equally important is the plethora of research on the COPM, which has repeatedly demonstrated the reliability and validity of this tool, as well as the usefulness of this tool as an outcome measure (Carswell et al., 2004; Dedding, Cardol, Eyssen, Dekker, & Beelen, 2004; Gilbertson & Langhorne, 2000; Harper, Stalker, & Templeton, 2006; Kjeken et al., 2005; Pan, Chung, & Hsin-Hwei, 2003; Persson, Rivano-Fischer, & Eklund, 2004; Verkerk, Wolf, Louwers, Meester-Delver, & Nollet, 2006; Wressle, Lindstrand, Neher, Marcusson, & Henricksson, 2003).

**Table 11-1. Role of the Occupational Therapist Versus Role of the Occupational Therapy Assistant With ADL/IADL Evaluation**

| Model | Premises |
|---|---|
| Administer standardized and nonstandardized screening and assessment tools to determine the need for occupational therapy intervention including but limited to (1) specific screening tools; (2) assessments; (3) skilled observation; (4) checklists; (5) histories; (6) interviews with the client, family, and significant others; and (7) consultations with other professionals. | Gather and share data for the purposes of screening and evaluation by implementing delegated assessments including but not limited to (1) specific screening tools; (2) assessments; (3) skilled observation; (4) checklists; (5) histories; (6) interviews with the client, family, and significant others; and (7) consultations with other professionals. |
| Select appropriate assessment tools based on client need, contextual factors, and psychometric properties of tests. The assessment tools must be relevant to the individual client, based on available evidence, and incorporate occupational performance in the assessment process. Use appropriate procedures and protocols when administering assessments. | Administer selected assessments using appropriate procedures and protocols, including standardized formats and use of occupation for the purpose of assessment. |
| Evaluate client's occupational performance in ADL, IADL, education, work, play, leisure, and social participation, including:<br>• Client factors<br>• Performance patterns<br>• Contextual factors<br>• Activity demands affecting performance<br>• Performance skills | Gather and share data for the purposes of evaluating client's occupational performance in ADL, IADL, education, work, play, leisure, and social participation, including:<br>• Client factors<br>• Performance patterns<br>• Contextual factors<br>• Activity demands affecting performance<br>• Performance skills |
| Determine the client's goals and priorities. Establish intervention priorities. Determine additional assessment needs. Determine specific assessment tasks that can be delegated to the occupational therapy assistant. | |
| Interpret criterion-referenced and norm-referenced standardized test scores based on an understanding of sampling, normative data, standard and criterion scores, reliability, and validity. | |
| Consider factors that might bias assessment results such as culture, disability status, and situational variables related to the individual and context. | |
| Interpret the evaluation data in relation to accepted terminology of the profession and relevant theoretical frameworks | |
| Evaluate the appropriateness and discuss mechanisms for referring clients for additional evaluation to specialists internal and external to the profession. | Identify when to recommend to the occupational therapist the need for referring clients for additional evaluation. |
| Document occupational therapy services to ensure accountability of service provision and to meet standards for reimbursement of services, adhering to applicable facility, local, state, federal, and reimbursement agencies. Documentation must effectively communicate the need and rationale for occupational therapy services. | Document occupational therapy services to ensure accountability of service provision and to meet standards for reimbursement of services, adhering to applicable facility and local, state, federal, and reimbursement agencies. Documentation must effectively communicate the need and rationale for occupational therapy services. |
| **In Summary** | |
| The occupational therapist initiates and directs the evaluation process. | The occupational therapy assistant contributes to the evaluation process by implementing delegated assessments and sharing the findings with the occupational therapist. |
| The occupational therapist interprets the data, including information provided by occupational therapy assistant, and develops the intervention plan. | |

Adapted from the Standards for an Accredited Master's-Level Educational Program for the Occupational Therapist and the Standards for an Accredited Educational Program for the Occupational Therapy Assistant (AOTA, 2006a, 2006b) and from the Reference Manual of the Official Documents of the American Occupational Therapy Association, Inc. (2004). Reprinted with permission from the American Occupational Therapy Association.

Other occupational therapy evaluation tools that measure occupational performance and capture the client's perspective regarding his or her performance include, but are not limited to, the Occupational Self-Assessment (Ay-Woan, Sarah, Lyinn, Tsyr-Jang, & Ping-Chuan, 2006; Baron, Kielhofner, Ienger, Goldhammer, & Wolenski, 2002; Kielhofner & Forsyth, 2001), the Child Occupational Self-Assessment (Keller, Kafkes, Basu, Federico, & Kielhofner, 2004; Keller & Kielhofner, 2005), and the Occupational Performance History Interview: Version 2.0 (Kielhofner et al., 1998).

The Occupational Self-Assessment (OSA), like the COPM, was developed to capture the client's perceptions of his or her own occupational competence. However, in addition to enabling the client to identify and prioritize his or her problems in occupational performance, it was also designed to assess the impact of the environment on the client's occupational adaptation. More specifically, the client is asked to respond to a series of statements about his or her occupational competence by labeling each as an area of strength, adequate functioning, or weakness, then indicate the level of importance of each item. Likewise, the client is asked to respond to a series of questions related to his or her environment by identifying components of the environment that either support or hinder occupational competence. Similarly, the client is asked to identify the level of importance of each item related to the environment. The last step in the OSA entails having the client identify specific items from both the occupational and environmental assessment forms that he or she would like to change/focus on in therapy. Comparable to the OSA, the Child Occupational Self-Assessment (COSA) was developed to provide an assessment tool in which a child can be actively involved in the occupational therapy evaluation and intervention process. Similar to the OSA, the COSA has the child identify and prioritize his or her problems in occupational performance on a child-friendly 4-point scale.

## Observation of Performance

After determining the person's occupational profile, the next essential step in the evaluation process, according to the framework, is to observe the client's occupational performance, ideally within the natural context, in order to determine what supports and hinders performance (AOTA, 2008). Observation of occupational performance is vital to the assessment process, especially since information from an interview alone may be inaccurate. For instance, a client may overestimate his or her functional abilities out of fear of being admitted to a nursing home. Or, perhaps the client may overestimate or underestimate his or her abilities because he or she has not even had the opportunity to perform his or her ADL or IADL since the onset of his or her accident, injury, or illness.

Since there are numerous standardized and nonstandardized methods available, the shrewd therapist will base his or her decision to use a particular ADL/IADL assessment tool on sound critical thinking skills. That is, the astute occupational therapist should ask him- or herself a series of questions before selecting an assessment tool. For example, the therapist should ask him- or herself the following:

1. Which specific ADL and/or IADL need to be evaluated for each individual client?
2. What are the advantages and disadvantages of the particular evaluation tools available to assess the explicit needs of each individual client?
3. Is the purpose of the evaluation to determine why the client is having difficulty performing his or her ADL and/or IADL, or is the purpose of the evaluation to determine if a client is able to perform his or her ADL and IADL safely and/or independently? Or, perhaps, is the purpose of the evaluation to demonstrate the extent of improvement or the effectiveness of intervention?
4. Is the selected method an efficient use of time?
5. Is there evidence to support the soundness of the selected evaluation tool?

Needless to say, the therapist who takes the time to ensure best practice in every step of the evaluation process is very different from the therapist who decides to use an evaluation tool just because "it's the tool that all of the therapists in the facility use" or because "I've always done it this way."

After completing the occupational profile, the occupational therapist should have a clear understanding of which specific ADL and/or IADL need to be observed for each individual. The specific ADL and/or IADL to be assessed should relate directly to the client's unique desires, choices, and needs. For example, the types of activities to be assessed for a client who lives alone, was previously independent in all ADL and IADL, does not have any support systems, plans on returning to his previous environment, and wants and needs to be independent in almost all ADL and IADL should be very different than the types of activities to be assessed for a client who lives with a spouse; participated in very few IADL previously; and has no desire or need to cook, clean, do the laundry, or pay the bills. Likewise, the types of ADL and IADL to be assessed throughout the lifespan (e.g., a very young child versus an adolescent versus a young adult versus an older adult) will differ as well.

Furthermore, since occupational performance involves a transaction between the individual, the task, and the environment (Law et al., 1996), it is essential that the therapist not only consider selecting a specific ADL and/or IADL assessment based on the type of activities it evaluates, but select a tool that provides the occupational therapy practitioner with critical information regarding the individual and the environment. Likewise, the framework (AOTA, 2008) asserted that the execution of a performance skill occurs when the performer, the context, and the demands of the activity unite in the performance of an activity. In other words, each factor (the individual, the task, and the environment) influences the execution of a skill and may support or hinder the performance skills and ultimately one's occupational performance. Thus, the most accurate means to assess one's ability to perform his or her ADL and/or IADL is to observe the client's performance within its natural context. Not only does the literature suggest that observation of occupational performance within the natural context is a more accurate means of assessment, but researchers have also indicated that it is a better predictor of safety and independence as well (Doble, Fisk, Fisher, Ritvo, & Murray, 1994; Linden, Boschian, Eker, Schalen, & Nordstrom, 2005; McNulty & Fisher, 2001; Park, Fisher, & Velozo, 1994). Lastly, observation of occupational performance in its natural context, as well as the identification of performance skill deficits, should provide the skilled therapist with the necessary information to determine the method of intervention (i.e., if the intervention will focus on remediation of performance skills, compensation, or a combination of remediation and compensation).

While there are a plethora of instruments to assess one's ability to perform his or her ADL and IADL, most standardized ADL and IADL assessments tools have the following characteristics:

- Are not designed to be flexible (i.e., meet the distinct needs of each individual client)
- Do not assess the individual's performance skills in the context of one's occupational performance
- Do not consider the impact of the environment on occupational performance
- Do not provide the therapist with information related to why the individual is having problems with his or her performance

These factors have probably led to the popularity of many "homegrown evaluation tools," which have little (if any) evidence to support their use.

As indicated above, the observation of ADL and IADL needs to consider the individual's skills underlying occupational performance. The performance skills are the goal-directed actions enacted in the context of occupational performance and consist of the individual's motor, process, and social/interaction skills (Fisher, 2005). To date, the Assessment of Motor and Process Skills (AMPS) (Fisher, 2005) is the only client-centered, performance-based, standardized occupational therapy ADL/IADL evaluation tool available to the occupational therapy practitioner. AMPS is unique for several reasons (Bernspang, 1999; Bernspang & Fisher, 1995; Dickerson & Fisher, 1995; Doble, Fisk, Lewis, & Rockwood, 1999; Ellison, Fisher, & Duran, 2001; Fisher, Liu, Velozo, Pan, 1992; Goldman & Fisher, 1997; Goto, Fisher, & Mayberry, 1996; Magalhães, Fisher, Bernspång, & Linacre, 1996; McNulty & Fisher, 2001; Sellers, Fisher, & Duran, 2001; Stauffer, Fisher, & Duran, 2000):

- The client is able to self-select which ADL and/or IADL he or she wants to perform.
- It contains over 10 standardized ADL tasks and over 75 standardized IADL tasks.
- It emphasizes the importance of the client performing each task in his or her usual manner.
- It measures the quality of a person's performance in terms of effort, efficiency, safety, and independence.
- It assesses the motor and process skills (not the person's underlying functions or capacities).
- It can be used with all persons above 3 years of age, regardless of the client's diagnosis/reason for his or her disability.
- It provides information to the occupational therapy practitioner that aids in the planning of effective interventions.
- It is a sensitive evaluation tool that can be used to document change and outcomes.
- There is strong evidence of its reliability and validity both internationally and cross-culturally.

Thus, in other words, AMPS is currently the only standardized assessment tool available to occupational therapists that evaluates the individual's performance skills during the performance of client-centered ADL and/or IADL occurring within its natural context.

Much like the AMPS evaluates performance skills during the natural context of ADL and IADL, the School AMPS evaluates performance skills during the natural context of schoolwork. When evaluating a child, adolescent, or young adult (if applicable), it is imperative that the occupational therapy practitioner assess that individual's ability to fulfill his or her role as a student. Since an individual is able to assume the role of student only to the extent that he or she can effectively perform those tasks integral to defining that role, it is vital that the occupational therapy practitioner observe and determine which of the student's activities support and/or hinder performance (Fisher et al., 2002). The School AMPS (Fisher et al., 2005) is a tool that enables a true top-down (Trombly, 1993), client-centered, and occupationally based approach to the assessment and intervention of the student's role performance within the classroom environment. However, the School AMPS addresses schoolwork performance only and not the ADL or IADL related to student role performance (e.g., getting on/off a bus, dressing for gym class, using communication devices).

On the other hand, the School Function Assessment (SFA) (Coster, Deeny, Haltiwanger, & Haley, 1998) is a criterion-referenced assessment that measures the student's ability to participate in most of the tasks expected of a student in the school setting. The SFA is a judgment-based questionnaire designed to measure the student's performance in a wide variety of functional tasks that support the student's participation in the academic and social aspects of elementary education. The SFA contains three scales. More specifically, the student's teacher or other knowledgeable professional within the school environment rates the following:

- Level of participation in a variety of school settings (e.g., in the classroom, on the playground or at recess, during lunch/snack time, during transportation, in the bathroom, and while moving from one location in the school to another)
- Type or amount of task support needed with a wide variety of physical and cognitive/behavioral tasks (e.g., using classroom materials, managing clothes and personal hygiene, ability to access the school environment)
- Performance on very specific physical and cognitive/behavioral tasks (e.g., using writing utensils, wiping or cleaning self after toileting, washing hands, opening and closing doors).

Thus, even though the SFA does assess the child's ability to perform a variety of ADL and IADL in the school setting and considers the environmental modifications and/or lack thereof, unfortunately it does not formally assess the student's performance skills as defined by the framework (AOTA, 2008). Furthermore, the SFA does not provide the therapist with any information regarding the student's opinion of his or her performance, the student's level of satisfaction, or which specific activities the student would prefer to address. Thus, if the SFA is administered, the occupational therapy practitioner will need to use his or her keen observational skills to determine why the client is unable to perform the various tasks in the school environment and, perhaps, may want to also consider using a client-centered assessment like the School Setting Interview (Hemmingsson, Egilson, Hoffman, & Kielhofner, 2005; Hemmingsson, Kottorp, & Bernspang, 2004) or the COPM (Law, Baptiste, et al., 2005) in order to gain a better appreciation of the student's opinion regarding his or her own level of satisfaction with his or her own performance in the school setting.

The Functional Independence Measure (FIM) (Uniform Data System for Medical Rehabilitation [UDSMR], 1999) and the WeeFIM (UDSMR, 2000) are two tools that are commonly used in rehabilitation settings and have a substantial amount of evidence to support their use as outcome measures (Cohen & Marino, 2000; Cottir, Burgio, Stevens, Roth, & Gitlin, 2002; Dickson & Köhler, 1995; Dodds, Martin, Stolov, & Deyo, 1993; Granger & Hamilton, 1992; Lundgren-Nilsson et al., 2005; Ottenbacher et al., 2000; Stineman, Ross, Fiedler, Granger, & Maislin, 2003). However, the therapist must keep in mind the purpose of these instruments and what type of information is gained through their administration. That is, the FIM and WeeFIM are part of the UDSMR and were developed to measure the effectiveness of medical rehabilitation services and programs. In other words, the FIM was not developed to specifically aid occupational therapists in their assessment and intervention process (i.e., it does not assess the person's performance skills and it does not provide the therapist with any information as to why the person is having difficulty with the observed tasks). However, since the FIM and WeeFIM are discipline-free assessments, they can be administered by any health care professional (e.g., nurse, physical therapist, speech therapist) and have the potential to create a common language that can be used across disciplines. In addition, the FIM and WeeFIM measure functional ability/degree of disability and were designed to detect change over time by rating the client's performance across three different domains (self-care, motor, and cognitive) on a 7-point scale (7 = complete independence and 1 = complete assistance).

# Summary

The purpose of this chapter was to introduce the occupational therapy practitioner to the general process of evaluating a person's ability to perform his or her ADL and IADL. As previously indicated, the first critical step in any occupational therapy evaluation is to obtain an understanding of the person's occupational profile (AOTA, 2008). After obtaining the occupational profile, it is vital that the occupational therapy practitioner observe the person's occupational performance in order to determine what supports and hinders performance (AOTA, 2008). Since occupational performance involves a transaction between the individual, the task, and the environment (Law et al., 1996), it is essential the therapist not only consider selecting a specific ADL and/or IADL assessment based on the type of activities it evaluates, but he or she should also consider selecting a tool that provides him or her with critical information regarding the individual and the environment. There are a plethora of ADL and IADL tools available to the occupational therapy practitioner. However, best practice entails selecting a specific evaluation tool based on sound critical thinking skills, as well as the evidence available to support its use. This chapter introduces the occupational therapy practitioner to a few of the ADL/IADL evaluation tools available (Table 11-2). Since there are an abundance of other tools available to the occupational therapy practitioner, it is imperative that he or she takes the time to go through the clinical reasoning process outlined in this chapter to ensure that whatever tool is chosen, it meets not only the needs of the therapist, but also the unique aspects of the client and his or her environment.

# Student Self-Assessment

1. Define the terms *occupation* and *activity*. Provide an example from your own life that demonstrates that you are able to differentiate the two terms.
2. Define the terms *activities of daily living* (ADL) and *instrumental activities of daily living* (IADL). Provide at least five examples of each term.

3. What is an occupational profile? Describe how an occupational therapy practitioner can best obtain information related to his or her client's occupational profile.
4. After obtaining the client's occupational profile, what is the next vital step in the evaluation process of one's ADL and IADL?
5. What is the ultimate purpose of observing the client's occupational performance?
6. Name at least two evaluation tools that capture the client's perception of his or her occupational performance and have the client identify the level of importance of each identified ADL and/or IADL.
7. What is the name of the client-centered, performance-based ADL/IADL evaluation tool that was designed to assist the occupational therapy practitioner in the intervention planning process?
8. Describe some of the principles that a therapist should consider before selecting which specific evaluation tool he or she should use to assess performance in ADL and IADL.
9. Become familiar with the assessment tools discussed in this chapter. Compare and contrast them. What do they assess? What are their strengths? Limitations?
10. Differentiate the role of the occupational therapist and the occupational therapy assistant.

# Electronic Resources

- The American Occupational Therapy Association: www.aota.org
- The Assessment of Motor and Process Skills (AMPS): http://ampsintl.com
- The Model of Human Occupation (MOHO) Clearinghouse: www.moho.uic.edu
- Occupational Therapy: Systematic Evaluation of Evidence: www.otseeker.com
- Evidence-Based Occupational Therapy: www.otevidence.info

**Table 11-2. Summary of Selected ADL and IADL Evaluation Tools**

| Name of Assessment | Areas of Assessment | Type of Client | Format of Assessment |
|---|---|---|---|
| Assessment of Motor and Process Skills (AMPS) | Quality of motor and process skills in the performance of 11 possible ADL and/or 73 possible IADL | 3 years and older<br><br>Any diagnosis or disability | Client self-selects one to three ADL/IADL items.<br>Therapist observes the client's motor and process skills concurrently with the observation of occupational performance and rates each motor and process skill item on a 4-point scale.<br>The calibrated AMPS rater is able to input data into computer scoring software.<br>Results of AMPS data can be used to answer: (1) Why is the client experiencing difficulty?, (2) What level of task challenge can the client manage?, (3) Is the client a candidate for restorative interventions via the use of therapeutic occupation or compensatory interventions via the use of adaptive occupations?, and (4) Has the client's ADL/IADL performance improved? |
| Canadian Occupational Performance Measure (COPM) | Client's self-perception of his or her performance in self-care, productivity, and leisure | Any age<br><br>Any diagnosis or disability | Semi-structured interview.<br>The client: (1) identifies concerns regarding his or her performance during self-care, productivity, and leisure activities; (2) evaluates his or her performance and satisfaction relative to the identified problematic occupational performance areas; and (3) prioritizes his or her problems in occupational performance.<br>The COPM is able to measure changes in the client's perception of his or her occupational performance over the course of occupational therapy intervention. |
| Child Occupational Self- Assessment (COSA) | The client's self-perception of sense of competence and level of importance in everyday activities in his or her home, school, and community. | Any child able to self-report | Self-report assessment comprised of 24 statements related to everyday activities in the client's home, school, and community.<br>Child rates each item in terms of personal competence and level of importance on a 4-point child-friendly scale.<br>There are two different formats to choose from: (1) card sort method; and (2) checklist format. |

| Table 11-2. Summary of Selected ADL & IADL Evaluation Tools (continued) | | | |
|---|---|---|---|
| **Name of Assessment** | **Areas of Assessment** | **Type of Client** | **Format of Assessment** |
| Functional Independence Measure (FIM) | Level of independence/disability on a total of 18 items related to: (a) self-care (eating, grooming, bathing, dressing, and toileting), (b) sphincter control (bowel and bladder management), (c) transfers (bed/chair/wheelchair, toilet, and tub/shower), (d) locomotion (walk/ wheelchair and stairs), (e) communication (comprehension and expression), and (f) social cognition (social interaction, problem solving, and memory). | Adults with various physical disabilities | Therapist observes client's performance and rates each item on a 7-point scale (7 = complete independence; 1 = total assistance).<br>Scores are intended to reflect the impact of the disability on the individual and on the human and economic resources in the community. |
| Occupational Self-Assessment (OSA) | Measures: (1) client's perceptions of his or her competence in occupational performance, using the Model of Human Occupation as a framework and (2) the impact of the environment on the client's occupational adaptation | All occupational therapy clients who can self-report | Self-rated occupational performance.<br>On a 4-point scale, the client labels: (1) each statement about his or her occupational performance as an area of strength, adequate functioning, or weakness; (2) components of the environment that either support or hinder occupational competence; (3) the level of importance of each item; and (4) specific items from both the occupational and environmental assessment forms that he or she would like to change/focus on in therapy. |
| Occupational Performance History Interview (OPHI-II) | Explores a client's life history in the areas of work, self-care, and play<br>Assesses the impact of disability on occupational performance<br>Identifies the direction in which the client would like to take in his or her life | Any client capable of responding to a life history interview | Semi-structured interview.<br>After the interview, the therapist fills out rating forms related to (1) occupational identity, (2) occupational competence, and (3) occupational settings. |
| Pediatric Evaluation of Disability (PEDI) | Describes a child's functional status as it relates to self-care, mobility, and social function<br>Monitors change in individuals or groups of children with functional disabilities<br>Can be used for program evaluation of inpatient, outpatient, or school-based programs | Children 6 months to 7½ years old (or older if their functional development is delayed) | Parents or professionals fill out a 3-part form related to: (1) functional skills, (2) caregiver assistance, and (3) modifications. Each of these three parts is further divided into a self-care domain, a mobility domain, and a social function domain. Items on Part I: Functional Skills are rated on a 2-point scale (able or unable to perform). Items on Part II: Caregiver Assistance are rated on a 6-point scale ranging from total assistance to independent. Items on Part III: Modification are rated on a 4-point scale ranging from extensive modifications to no modifications.<br>Scores can be put into a computer program or it can be scored manually.<br>Raw scores, normative standard scores, or scaled scores can be used. |
| School Function Assessment (SFA) | Measures and monitors a student's ability to participate in most of the tasks expected of a student in elementary school | Students in elementary school, grades kindergarten through 6th grade | A criterion-referenced assessment.<br>Teacher or other professional in the school setting fills out 3-part evaluation form.<br>Part I evaluates the student's level of participation in various school settings on a 6-point scale (1 = extremely limited participation; 6 = full participation).<br>Part II assesses the student's need for assistance or modifications on various physical and cognitive/behavioral tasks. Items are rated on a 4-point scale (1 = extensive assistance/modification; 4 = no assistance/modification).<br>Part III assesses the student's functional performance on specific activities in the school setting. Items are rated on a 4-point scale (1 = does not perform; 4 = consistent performance). |
| School Setting Interview | Allows the child/adolescent with a disability to describe the impact of the environment on his or her functioning in the school setting | Students 10 years old through high school with some type of motor dysfunction | A semi-structured interview containing 16 items regarding everyday school activities that provide the occupational therapy with information about the child's functioning and need for adjustments in the school setting. Each item is rated on a 4-point scale related to the student-environment fit (1 = unfit/needs new adjustments; 4 = perfect fit/no need for adjustments). |

| Evidence-Based Research Chart | |
|---|---|
| **Evaluation Tool** | **Evidence** |
| The Assessment of Motor and Process Skills (AMPS) | Bernspang, 1999; Bernspang & Fisher, 1995; Dickerson & Fisher, 1995; Doble et al., 1999; Ellison et al., 2001; Fisher et al., 1992; Goldman & Fisher, 1997; Goto et al., 1996; Magalhães et al., 1996; McNulty & Fisher, 2001; Sellers et al., 2001; Stauffer et al., 2000 |
| The School Assessment of Motor and Process Skills (School AMPS) | Atchison, Fisher, & Bryze, 1998; Fisher, Bryze, & Atchison, 2000; Fisher, Bryze, Hume, & Griswold, 2005 |
| The Barthel Index | Gauggel et al., 2004; Houlden, Edwards, McNeil, & Greenwood, 2006; Hsueh, Lin, Jeng, & Hsieh, 2006; Nicholl, Hobart, Dunwoody, Cramp, & Lowe-Strong, 2004; Sangha et al., 2005; van Exel, Scholte op Reimer, & Koopmanschap, 2004 |
| The Child Occupational Self-Assessment (COSA) | Keller et al., 2004; Keller, Kafkes, & Keilhofner, 2005; Keller & Kielhofner, 2005 |
| The Canadian Occupational Performance Measure (COPM) | Carswell et al., 2004; Dedding et al., 2004; Gilbertson & Langhorne, 2000; Harper et al., 2006; Kjeken et al., 2005; Pan et al., 2003; Persson et al., 2004; Verkerk et al., 2006; Wressel et al., 2003 |
| The Functional Independent Measure (FIM) and Wee FIM | Cohen & Marino, 2000; Cottir et al., 2002; Dickson & Köhler, 1995; Dodds et al., 1993; Granger & Hamilton, 1992; Lundgren-Nilsson et al., 2005; Ottenbacher et al., 2000; Stineman et al., 2003 |
| The Kohlman Evaluation of Living Skills (KELS) | Thomson, 1992; Pickens et al., 2007; Zimnavoda, Weinblatt, & Katz, 2002 |
| The Occupational Self-Assessment (OSA) | AyWoan et al., 2006; Baron et al., 2006; Kielhofner & Forsyth, 2001 |
| The Occupational Performance History Interview (OPHI-II) | Kielhofner, Dobria, Forsyth, & Basu, 2005; Kielhofner, Mallinson, Forsyth, & Lai, 2001; Mallinson, Mahaffey, & Kielhofner, 1998 |
| The Nottingham Extended Activities of Daily Living Scale | Green, Forster, & Young, 2001; Harwood & Ebrahim, 2002; Nicholl, Lincoln, & Playford, 2002 |
| The Pediatric Evaluation of Disability (PEDI) | Berg, Frøslie, & Hussain, 2003; Berg, Jahnsen, Frøslie, & Hussain, 2004; Haley, Coster, Ludlow, Haltiwanger, & Andrellos, 1992; Ho, Curtis, & Clarke, 2006; Iyer, Haley, Watkins, & Dumas, 2003; Kothari, Haley, Gill-Body, & Dumas, 2003; Vos-Vromans, Ketelaar, & Gorter, 2005; Wassenberg-Severijnen, Custers, Hox, Vermeer, & Helders, 2003 |
| The School Function Assessment (SFA) | Coster et al., 1998; Davies, Lee Soon, Young, & Clausen-Yamaki, 2004; Egilson & Costner, 2004; Hwang, Nochajski, Linn, & Wu, 2004 |
| The School Setting Interview | Hemmingsson et al., 2004; Hemmingsson et al., 2005 |

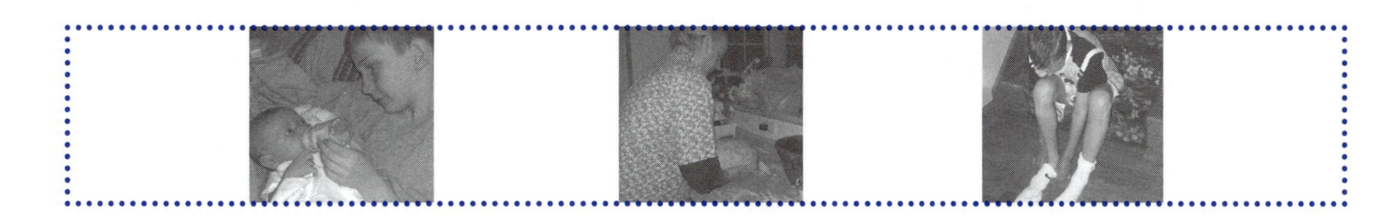

## References


American Occupational Therapy Association. (2004). *The reference manual of the official documents of the American Occupational Therapy Association* (10th ed.). Bethesda, MD: Author

American Occupational Therapy Association. (2006a). *Accreditation standards for a master's-degree level educational program for the occupational therapist*. Bethesda, MD: Author.

American Occupational Therapy Association. (2006b). *Accreditation standards for an educational program for the occupational therapy assistant*. Bethesda, MD: Author.

American Occupational Therapy Association. (2008). Occupational therapy practice framework: Domain and process, second edition. *American Journal of Occupational Therapy, 62*, 625-683.

Atchison, B. T., Fisher, A. G., & Bryze, K. (1998). Rater reliability and internal scale and person response validity of the School Assessment of Motor and Process Skills. *American Journal of Occupational Therapy, 52*, 843-850.

Ay-Woan, P., Sarah, C. P., Lyinn, C., Tsyr-Jang, C., & Ping-Chuan, H. (2006). Quality of life in depression: Predictive models. *Quality of Life Research, 15*(1), 39-48.

Baron, K., Kielhofner, G., Ienger, A., Goldhammer, V., & Wolenski, J. (2002). *Occupational self-assessment: Version 2.1*. Chicago, IL: Model of Human Occupation Clearinghouse.

Berg, M., Frøslie, K. F., & Hussain, A. (2003). Applicability of the pediatric evaluation of disability inventory in Norway. *Scandinavian Journal of Occupational Therapy, 10*(3), 118-126.

Berg, M., Jahnsen, R., Frøslie, K. F., & Hussain, A. (2004). Reliability of the pediatric evaluation of disability inventory (PEDI). *Physical & Occupational Therapy in Pediatrics, 24*(3), 61-77.

Bernspang, B. (1999). Rater calibration stability for the Assessment of Motor and Process Skills. *Scandinavian Journal of Occupational Therapy, 6*(3), 101-109.

Bernspang, B., & Fisher, A. G. (1995). Validation of the Assessment of Motor and Process Skills for use in Sweden. *Scandinavian Journal of Occupational Therapy, 2*(1), 3-9.

Carswell, A., McColl, M. A., Baptise, S., Law, M., Polatajko, H., & Pollock, N. (2004). The Canadian Occupational Performance Measure: A research and clinical literature review. *Canadian Journal of Occupational Therapy, 71*(4), 210-222.

Cohen, M. E., & Marino, R. J. (2000). The tools of disability outcomes research functional status measures. *Archives of Physical Medicine and Rehabilitation, 81*(12 suppl 2), S21-S29.

Coster, W. J., Deeny, T., Haltiwanger, J., & Haley, S. (1998). *School Function Assessment.* San Antonio, TX: The Psychological Corporation.

Cottir, E. M., Burgio, L. D., Stevens, A. B., Roth, D. L., & Gitlin, L. N. (2002). Correspondence of the Functional Independence Measure (FIM) self-care subscale with real-time observations of dementia patients' ADL performance in the home. *Clinical Rehabilitation, 16*(1), 36-45.

Davies, P. L., Soon, P. L., Young, M., & Clausen-Yamaki, A. (2004). Validity and reliability of the School Function Assessment in elementary school students with disabilities. *Physical and Occupational Therapy in Pediatrics, 24*(3), 23-43.

Dedding, C., Cardol, M., Eyssen, I. C., Dekker, J., & Beelen, A. (2004). Validity of the Canadian Occupational Performance Measure: A client-centered outcome measure. *Clinical Rehabilitation, 18*(6), 660-667.

Dickerson, A. E., & Fisher, A. G. (1995). Culture-relevant functional performance assessment of the Hispanic elderly. *Occupational Therapy Journal of Research, 15*(1), 50-68.

Dickson, H., & Köhler, F. (1995). Interrater reliability of the 7-Level Functional Independence Measure. *Scandinavian Journal of Rehabilitation Medicine, 27*(4), 253-256.

Doble, S. E., Fisk, J. D., Fisher, A. G., Ritvo, P. G., & Murray, T. J. (1994). Functional competence of community-dwelling persons with multiple sclerosis using the Assessment of Motor and Process Skills. *Archives of Physical Medicine and Rehabilitation, 75*(8), 843-851.

Doble, S. E., Fisk, J. D., Lewis, N., & Rockwood, K. (1999). Test-retest reliability of the Assessment of Motor and Process Skills in elderly adults. *Occupational Therapy Journal of Research, 19*(3), 203-215.

Dodds, T. A., Martin, D. P., Stolov, W. C., & Deyo, R. A. (1993). A validation of the Functional Independence Measurement and its performance among rehabilitation patients. *Archives of Physical Medicine and Rehabilitation, 74*(5), 531-536.

Egilson, S. T., & Coster, W. J. (2004). School Function Assessment: Performance of Icelandic students with special needs. *Scandinavian Journal of Occupational Therapy, 11*(4), 163-170.

Ellison, S., Fisher, A. G., & Duran, L. (2001). The alternate forms reliability of the new tasks added to the Assessment of Motor and Process Skills. *Journal of Applied Measurement, 2*(2), 121-134.

Fisher, A. (2005). *Assessment of Motor and Process Skills, Vol. 1: Development, Standardization, and Administration Manual* (6th ed.). Fort Collins, CO: Three Star Press.

Fisher, A. G., Bryze, K., & Atchison, B. T. (2000). Naturalistic Assessment of functional performance in school settings: Reliabilty and validity of the School AMPS. In R. M. Smith (Ed.), *Objective outcome measurement: Examples in physical medicine and rehabilitation* (Vol. 1). Chicago, IL: MESA Press.

Fisher, A. G., Bryze, K., & Hume, V. (2002). *School AMPS: School version of the Assessment of Motor and Process Skills.* Fort Collins, CO: Three Star Press.

Fisher, A. G., Bryze, K., Hume, V., & Griswold, L. A. (2005). *School AMPS: School version of the Assessment of Motor and Process Skills* (2nd ed.). Fort Collins, CO: Three Star Press.

Fisher, A. G., Liu, Y., Velozo, C. A., & Pan, A. W. (1992). Cross-cultural assessment of process skills. *American Journal of Occupational Therapy, 46*(10), 876-885.

Gauggel, S., Heinemann, A. W., Bocker, M., Lammler, G., Borchelt, M., & Steinhagen-Thiessen, E. (2004). Patient-staff agreement on Barthel Index scores at admission and discharge in a sample of elderly stroke patients. *Rehabilitation Psychology, 49*(1), 21-27.

Gilbertson, L., & Langhorne, P. (2000). Home-based occupational therapy: Stroke patients' satisfaction with occupational performance and service provision. *British Journal of Occupational Therapy, 63*(10), 464-468.

Goldman, S., & Fisher, A. G. (1997). Cross-cultural validation of the Assessment of Motor and Process Skills (AMPS). *British Journal of Occupational Therapy, 60,* 77-85.

Goto, S., Fisher, A. G., & Mayberry, W. L. (1996). The assessment of motor and process skills applied cross-culturally to the Japanese. *American Journal of Occupational Therapy, 50*(10), 798-806.

Granger, C. V., & Hamilton, B. B. (1992). UDS Report: The uniform data system for medical rehabilitation report of first admissions for 1990. *American Journal of Physical Medicine and Rehabilitation, 71*(2), 108-113.

Green, J., Forster, A., & Young, J. (2001). A test-retest reliability study of the Barthel Index, the Rivermead Mobility Index, the Nottingham extended Activities of Daily Living Scale and the Frenchay Activities Index in stroke patients. *Disability and Rehabilitation, 23*(15), 670-676.

Haley, S. M., Coster, W. J., Ludlow, L. H., Haltiwanger, J. T., & Andrellos, P. J. (1992). *Pediatric Evaluation of Disability Inventory: Development, standardization and administration manual, version 1.0.* Boston, MA: Trustees of Boston University, Health and Disability Institute.

Harper, K., Stalker, C. A., & Templeton, G. (2006). The use and validity of the Canadian Occupational Performance Measure in a posttraumatic stress program. *OTJR: Occupation, Participation and Health, 26*(2), 45-55.

Harwood, R. H., & Ebrahim, S. (2002). The validity, reliability and responsiveness of the Nottingham Extended Activities of Daily Living scale in patients undergoing total hip replacement. *Disability and Rehabilitation, 24*(7), 371-377.

Hemmingsson, H., Egilson, S., Hoffman, O., & Kielhofner, G. (2005). *A User's Manual for the School Setting Interview (SSI)* (Version 3.0). Chicago, IL: Model of Human Occupation Clearinghouse, University of Illinois at Chicago and Swedish Association of Occupational Therapists.

Hemmingsson, H., Kottorp, A., Bernspang, B. (2004). Validity of the School Setting Interview: An assessment of the student-environment fit. *Scandinavian Journal of Occupational Therapy, 11*(4), 171-178.

Ho, E. S., Curtis, C. G., & Clarke, H. M. (2006). Pediatric Evaluation of Disability Inventory: Its application to children with obstetric brachial plexus palsy. *Journal of Hand Surgery, 31*(2), 197-202.

Houlden, H., Edwards, M., McNeil, J., & Greenwood, R. (2006). Use of the Barthel Index and the Functional Independence Measure during early inpatient rehabilitation after single incident brain injury. *Clinical Rehabilitation, 20*(2), 153-159.

Hsueh, I. P., Lin, J. H., Jeng, J. S., & Hsieh, C. L. (2006). Comparison of the psychometric characteristics of the Functional Independence Measure, 5 Item Barthel Index, and 10 Item Barthel Index in patients with stroke. *Journal of Neurosurgery Psychiatry, 73*(2), 188-190.

Hwang, J. L., Nochajski, S. M., Linn, R. T., & Wu, Y. W. (2004). The development of the School Function Assessment-Chinese version for cross-cultural use in Taiwan. *Occupational Therapy International, 11*(1), 26-39.

Iyer, L. V., Haley, S. M., Watkins, M. P., & Dumas, H. M. (2003). Establishing minimal clinically important differences for scores on the Pediatric Evaluation of Disability Inventory for inpatient rehabilitation. *Physical Therapy, 83*(10), 888-898.

Keller, J., Kafkes, A., Basu, S., Federico, J., & Kielhofner, G. (2005). *Children's occupational self-assessment, version 2.1.* Chicago, IL: MOHO Clearinghouse.

Keller, J., Kafkes, A., & Kielhofner, G. (2005). Psychometric characteristics of the Child Occupational Self-Assessment (COSA), part one: An initial examination of psychometric properties. *Scandinavian Journal of Occupational Therapy, 12*(3), 118-127.

Keller, J., & Kielhofner, G. (2005). Psychometric characteristics of the Child Occupational Self-Assessment (COSA), part two: Refining the psychometric properties. *Scandinavian Journal of Occupational Therapy, 12*(4), 147-158.

Kielhofner, G., Dobria, L., Forsyth, K., & Basu, S. (2005). The construction of keyforms for obtaining instantaneous measures from the Occupational Performance History Interview rating scales. *OTRJ: Occupation, Participation & Health, 25*(1), 23-32.

Kielhofner, G., & Forsyth, K. (2001). Measurement properties of a client self-report for treatment planning and documenting therapy outcomes. *Scandinavian Journal of Occupational Therapy, 8*(3), 131-139.

Keilhofner, G., Mallinson, T., Forsyth, K., & Lai, JS. (2001) Psychometric properties of the second version of the Occupational Performance History Interview (OPHI-II). *American Journal of Occupational Therapy, 55*(3), 260-267.

Kielhofner, G., Mallinson, T., Crawford, C., Nowak, M., Rigby, M., Henry, A., et al. (1998). *The Occupational Performance History Interview (Version 2.0) OPHI–II.* Chicago, IL: Model of Human Occupation Clearinghouse.

Kjeken, I., Dagfinrud, H., Uhlig, T., Mowinckel, P., Kvien, T., & Finset, A. (2005). Reliability of the Canadian Occupational Performance Measure in patients with ankylosing spondylitis. *Journal of Rheumatology, 32*(8), 1503-1509.

Kothari, D. H., Haley, S. M., Gill-Body, K. M., & Dumas, H. M. (2003). Measuring functional change in children with acquired brain injury (ABI): Comparison of generic and ABI-specific scales using the Pediatric Evaluation of Disability Inventory (PEDI). *Physical Therapy, 83*(9), 776-785.

Law, M., Baptise, S., Carsweel, A., McColl, M., Polatajko, H., & Pollock, N. (2005). *Canadian occupational performance measure* (4th ed.). Ottawa, Ontario: CAOT Publications.

Law, M., Baum, C., & Dunn, W. (2005). *Measuring occupational performance: Supporting best practice in occupational therapy.* Thorofare, NJ: SLACK Incorporated.

Law, M., Cooper, B. A., Strong, S., Stewart, D., Rigby, P., & Letts, L. (1996). The person-environment-occupation model: A transactive approach to occupational performance. *Canadian Journal of Occupational Therapy, 63*(1), 9-23.

Linden, A., Boschian, K., Eker, C., Schalen, W., & Nordstrom, C. H. (2005). Assessment of Motor and Process Skills reflects brain-injured patients' ability to resume independent living better than neurological tests. *ACTA Neurologica Scandinavica, 111*(1), 48-53.

Lundgren-Nilsson, A., Grimby, G., Ring, H., Tesio, L., Lawton, G., Slade, A., et al. (2005). Cross-cultural validity of Functional Independence Measure items in stroke: A study using Rasch Analysis. *Journal of Rehabilitation Medicine, 37*(1), 23-31.

Magalhães, L., Fisher, A. G., Bernspang, B., & Linåcre, J. M. (1996). Cross-cultural assessment of functional mobility. *Occupational Therapy Journal of Research, 16,* 45-63.

Mallinson, T., Mahaffey, L., & Kielhofner, G. (1998). The Occupational Performance History Interview: Evidence for three underlying constructs of occupational adaptation. *Canadian Journal of Occupational Therapy, 65*(4), 219-228.

McNulty, M. C., & Fisher, A. G. (2001). Validity of using the Assessment of Motor and Process Skills to estimate overall home safety in person with psychiatric conditions. *American Journal of Occupational Therapy, 55*(6), 649-655.

Nicholl, C. R., Lincoln, N. B., & Playford, E. D. (2002). The reliability and validity of the Nottingham Extended Activities of Daily Living Scale in patients with multiple sclerosis. *Multiple Sclerosis, 8*(5), 372-376.

Nicholl, L., Hobart, J., Dunwoody, L., Cramp, F., & Lowe-Strong, A. (2004). Measuring disability in multiple sclerosis: Is the Community Dependency Index an improvement on the Barthel Index? *Multiple Sclerosis, 10*(4), 447-450.

Ottenbacher, K. J., Msall, M. E., Lyon, N., Duffy, L. C., Ziviani, J., Granger, C. V., et al. (2000). The WeeFIM Instrument: Its utility in detecting change in children with developmental disabilities. *Archives of Physical Medicine and Rehabilitation, 81*(10), 1317-1326.

Pan, A. W., Chung, L., & Hsin-Hwei, G. (2003). Reliability and validity of the Canadian Occupational Performance Measure for clients with psychiatric disorders in Taiwan. *Occupational Therapy International, 10*(4), 269-277.

Park, S., Fisher, A. G., & Velozo, C. A. (1994). Using the Assessment of Motor and Process Skills to compare occupational performance between clinic and home settings. *American Journal of Occupational Therapy, 48*(8), 697-709.

Persson, E., Rivano-Fischer, M., & Eklund, M. (2004). Evaluation of changes in occupational performance among patients in a pain management program. *Journal of Rehabilitation Medicine, 36*(2), 85-91.

Pickens, S., Naik, A. D., Burnett, J., Kelly, P. A., Gleason, M., & Dyer, C. B. (2007). The utility of the Kohlman Evaluation of Living Skills test is associated with substantiated cases of elder self-neglect. *Journal of the American Academy of Nurse Practitioners, 19*(3), 137-142.

Sangha, H., Lipson, D., Foley, N., Salter, K., Bhogal, S., Pohani, G., et al. (2005). A comparison of the Barthel Index and the Functional Independence Measure as outcome measures in stroke rehabilitation: Patterns of disability scale usage in clinical trials. *International Journal of Rehabilitation Research, 28*(2), 135-139.

Sellers, S. W., Fisher, A. G., & Duran, L. J. (2001). Validity of the Assessment of Motor and Process Skills with students who are visually impaired. *Journal of Visual Impairment and Blindness, 95*(3), 164-167.

Stauffer, L. M., Fisher, A. G., & Duran, L. (2000). ADL performance of Black Americans and White Americans on the Assessment of Motor and Process Skills. *American Journal of Occupational Therapy, 54*(6), 607-613.

Stineman, M. G., Ross, R. N., Fiedler, R., Granger, C. V., & Maislin, G. (2003). Functional Independence staging: Conceptual foundation, face validity, and empirical derivation. *Archives of Physical Medicine and Rehabilitation, 84*(1), 29-37.

Thomson, L. K. (1992). *The Kohlman Evaluation of Living Skills* (3rd ed.). Bethesda, MD: AOTA Press.

Trombly, C. (1993). Anticipating the future: Assessment of occupational function. *American Journal of Occupational Therapy, 47*(3), 253-257.

Uniform Data System for Medical Rehabilitation. (1999). *The Functional Independence Measure (FIM) user guide and self-guided training manual, version 5.20.* Buffalo, NY: Author.

Uniform Data System for Medical Rehabilitation. (2000). *The WeeFIM system clinical guide, version 5.01.* Buffalo, NY: Author.

van Exel, N. J., Scholte op Reimer, W. J., & Koopmanschap, M. A. (2004). Assessment of post-stroke quality of life in cost-effectiveness studies: The usefulness of the Barthel Index and the EuroQoL-5D. *Quality of Life Research, 13*(2), 427-433.

Verkerk, G. J., Wolf, M. J., Louwers, A. M., Meester-Delver, A., & Nollet, F. (2006). The reproducibility and validity of the Canadian Occupational Performance Measure in parents of children with disabilities. *Clinical Rehabilitation, 20*(11), 980-988.

Vos-Vromans, D. C., Ketelaar, M., & Gorter, J. W. (2005). Responsiveness of evaluation measures for children with cerebral palsy: The Gross Motor Function Measure and the Pediatric Evaluation of Disability Inventory. *Disability and Rehabilitation, 27*(20), 1245-1252.

Wassenberg-Severijnen, J. E., Custers, J. W., Hox, J. J., Vermeer, A., & Helders, P. J. (2003). Reliabilty of the Dutch Pediatric Evaluation of Disability Inventory (PEDI). *Clinical Rehabilitation, 17*(4), 457-462.

Wressle, E., Lindstrand, J., Neher, M., Marcusson, J., & Henricksson, C. (2003). The Canadian Occupation Performance Measure as an outcome measure and team tool in a day treatment programme. *Disability and Rehabilitation, 25*(10), 497-506.

Zimnavoda, T., Weinblatt, N., & Katz, N. (2002). Validity of the Kohlman Evaluation of Living Skills (KELS) with Israeli elderly individuals living in the community. *Occupational Therapy International, 9*(4), 312-325.

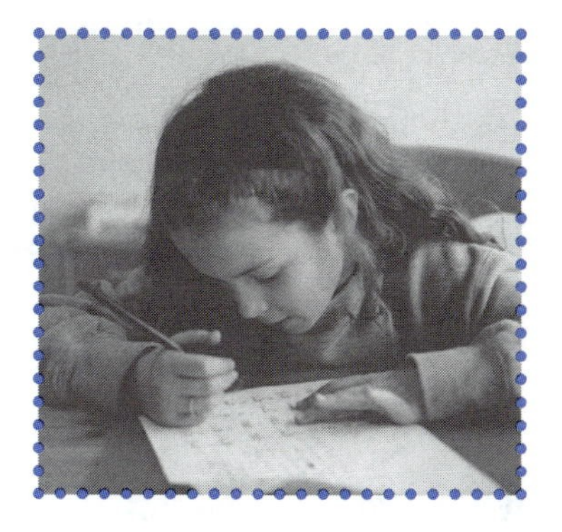

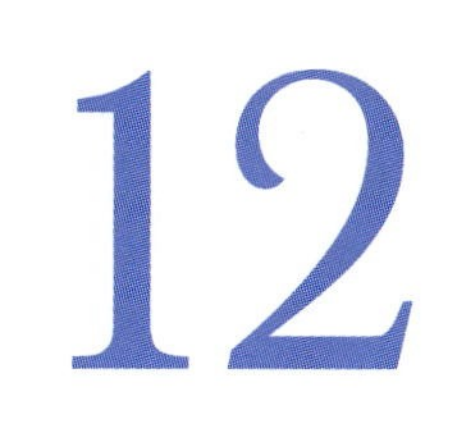

# 12 Evaluation of Education and Work

*Barbara Larson, MA, OTR/L, FAOTA*

**ACOTE Standard Explored in This Chapter**

B.4.4

**Key Terms**

| | |
|---|---|
| Client | Environment |
| Client-centered approach | Evaluation |
| Client factors | Work |
| Education | |

## Introduction

The focus of this chapter is the components and factors involved in the evaluation of education and work as occupational performance areas. The important task demands and performance factors that might need to be assessed in order to plan effective interventions will be discussed.

## Education

Education is both a primary therapeutic tool and a primary occupational performance area. When the educational experiences are being planned by the therapist, education is a primary therapeutic tool. For a child in a classroom or for a college student, education is a primary occupational performance area. In other cases, education might be a more casual experience, such as participating in a continuing education experience or otherwise learning a new skill. In each case, there are relevant barriers to learning.

Education has been described as the work of children (Larson, E., 2004). The barriers to a child being able to perform as a student may include sensory processing disorder, development delays, physical disabilities, psychosocial deficits such as autism, behavioral problems, and those things that interfere with the ability of a child to take advantage of a learning experience (Case-Smith, 2005). The occupational therapist must determine the most appropriate assessment for the identified problems. One example of a highly sophisticated assessment for limitations in sensory integration is the Sensory Integration and Praxis Tests (SIPT) (Bodison & Mailloux, 2006). Another assessment is the Sensory Profile, which measures sensory processing abilities in young children with autism (Watling, Deitz, & White, 2001).

Besides carefully selecting the accurate assessment, the occupational therapist must consider the environment and context in which the assessment takes place. The child's positioning, proximal distal stability (Smith-Zuzovsky & Exner, 2004), as well as the furniture he or she sits on related to the testing activity are important and could influence test performance and outcome (Naider-Steinhart & Katz-Leurer, 2007). In a study of children's work, the author's findings indicated that kindergarten, first, and second graders view handwriting as work, so the author cautions therapists to view this activity in a work context,



K. Sladyk, K. Jacobs, & N. MacRae (Eds.).
*Occupational Therapy Essentials for Clinical Competence* (pp. 127-134).

"promoting quiet and concentration, setting standards, and encouraging students to achieve them through persistent effort" (E. A. Larson, 2004, p. 377).

In like manner, there are numerous straightforward sensorimotor, cognitive, and psychosocial deficits (Law, Baum, & Dunn, 2005) that can interfere with the adult's occupational performance and, subsequently, the individual's ability to participate in educational experiences. Interviews, observations, a review of medical records, and client history information provide the necessary data to allow the therapist to gain an understanding of the individual's life activities. The therapist uses standardized or nonstandardized assessments to determine how the occupational performance in those life activities is affected (Law et al.).

Determining an individual's priorities during the assessment phase allows the occupational therapist to carefully and selectively design education programs that address the needs and wants of the adult. The importance of doing this is illustrated in a study involving the development of a health education program for an elderly population with macular degeneration (Dahlin Ivanoff, Sonn, & Svensson, 2002). The authors concluded that to maintain a sense of security in daily occupations, health education programs should be founded on the needs and problems of the elderly age group (Dahlin Ivanoff et al.).

In selecting assessment tools, the Canadian Occupational Performance Measure (COPM) can be used to identify client priorities and determine individual needs and wants. The COPM assesses self-perception of performance and satisfaction of daily occupations over time (McColl & Pollock, 2001). Problems in occupational performance areas are identified and weighted in terms of importance to the client. The therapist sets client-centered goals for the education program based on those identified priorities (Law et al., 2005).

Along with identifying problems carefully and selecting the appropriate assessment, the occupational therapist must interpret findings accurately and cautiously. It is important to understand the purpose and outcome of each assessment used in order to plan appropriate interventions. The contexts and activity demands must be taken into consideration when conducting assessments.

Changing behavior is an important outcome of client education. Whether looking at the occupation of children, the voluntary or educational occupations of adults, or the therapist using learning as a therapeutic approach, there are, as previously discussed, a host of barriers that can interfere with the educational process. These barriers must be evaluated in the context of relevant educational theories and models.

The Health Belief Model, which focuses on individual health behavior, supports that, in general, individuals will take action to ward off, screen for, or control ill-health under certain circumstances (Rosenstock & Strecher, 1997). For behavior change to succeed, people must feel threatened by their current situation and believe that change of a specific kind will be beneficial by resulting in a valued outcome at an acceptable cost (Rosenstock, 1990; Rosenstock & Strecher, 1997). People must also feel competent to implement that change. As clients move toward goal attainment, their successes should be reinforced verbally by the occupational therapy practitioner, while behavior problems should be treated as opportunities to analyze and control the factors that cause the problems.

## Value Expectancy Theory

Value expectancy theories, reasoned action, and multiattribute utility provide a method for operationally defining and systematically assessing the elements of a decision to perform a specific behavior. These theories do not attempt to describe how individuals make decisions.

The theory of reasoned action predicts an individual's intention to perform a given behavior in a specifically defined setting. This action is influenced by the individual's attitude toward the behavior and the influence of the social environment on the desired behavior (Carter, 1990).

Multiattribute utility theory predicts behavior directly from an individual's evaluation of the consequences or outcomes associated with the performance and nonperformance of the behavior in question. For both theories, the individuals who perform the behavior are the ones who identify the most important issues or barriers to behavioral performance (Carter, 1990). Designing any health education program requires a thorough understanding of the behavioral consequences or outcomes most important to the intended population (Carter, 1990).

## Attribution Theory

Lewis and Daltroy (1990) discussed attribution theory related to health behavior. They defined attributions as "the causes individuals generate to make sense of their world" (p. 92).

Determining how a person attributes causes to the state of his or her current health is often a first step in the development of a therapeutic relationship (Lewis & Daltroy, 1990). What is critical is that clients attribute potential effectiveness to their own behavior. Once this happens, clients can work through failures, initiate difficult tasks, and proceed in the face of obstacles (Lewis & Daltroy). Health-related skills will not be abandoned in the face of failure, difficult tasks will be initiated, and task persistence will occur even in the face of obstacles. The most potent attributions center around controllability and locus of causation of disease. Personal change needs to be reinforced to be sustained. Both environmental and personal change are important, and both should be addressed by health promotions efforts (Lewis & Daltroy).

## Social Learning Theory

Social learning theory addresses both the methods of promoting behavior change and the psychosocial dynamics underlying health behavior (Perry, Barnowski, & Parcel, 1990, 1997). From a cognitive view point, social learning theory emphasizes what people think. According to social learning theory, individuals with an internal locus of control are more likely to initiate change, whereas those who are externally controlled are more likely to be influenced by others. The literature provides evidence that giving people control over their lives improves their health outcomes (Perry et al., 1990).

Self-efficacy is the most important prerequisite for behavior change (Perry et al., 1990, 1997). Self-efficacy relates to the confidence a person feels about performing a given activity and affects the amount of effort invested in a given task and the levels of performance that are attained. Goal setting is important in self-efficacy (Perry et al., 1990, 1997). To make use of self-efficacy in promoting self-control of performance, goals should be set in increments similar to a given behavior, possible to achieve, and meaningful and relevant to the client.

Bandura (as cited in Perry et al., 1990) suggested that excessive emotional arousal inhibits learning and performance. Fearful thoughts produce emotional arousal and trigger defensive behaviors. When individuals experience heightened anxiety, it becomes difficult to attend to the health messages being sent by health professionals. Before health care professionals can help clients change their behavior, they must learn methods to aid people in their ability to minimize emotional arousal. If heightened anxiety cannot be minimized, education efforts should be postponed until anxiety has subsided. The health professional must plan interventions that will take into consideration the exploration of multiple relevant concepts.

The application of these models and theories supports clinical reasoning and helps the occupational therapist build therapeutic relationships with clients and caregivers, which are so vital to effecting behavior change.

Current theorists of client-provider relationships blend social and psychological perspectives and interpersonal influences to explain how the characteristics and behaviors of others affect a person's attitudes, feelings, and behavior. Joos and Hickam (1990) indicated that theories of cognition point to a number of factors that may interfere with clients' understanding and recall of information in the health care setting. Jargon and vocabulary that are too complex for the majority of clients are often present in verbal and written information, situational influences affect a client's ability to attend to and recall information, and the different backgrounds between provider and client often hamper their communication. Research on cognition and learning shows that providers can enhance the client's ability to understand written and verbal information by using shorter words and sentences, presenting and stressing the most important information first, using clear categories, giving specific rather than general instruction, and being aware of and checking for comprehension of major points (Joos & Hickam, 1990).

Clients have certain cultural expectations based on their social roles as group members and their behavior is influenced by the process of communication (Joos & Hickam, 1990). It is important for the health care provider to use culturally appropriate tools that match the client's educational and literacy levels (Pasick, 1997).

Rogers (as cited in Joos & Hickman, 1990) stated, "Empathy, genuineness, and acceptance of the client are the core conditions necessary for positive therapeutic change" (p. 221). A client-centered rather than provider-centered approach to care should be promoted.

Occupational behavior is influenced by the client's physiological, cognitive, and psychological conditions. These conditions also affect the client's ability to learn (Berkeland & Flinn, 2005). The occupational therapy practitioner needs to create a comfortable, safe environment in which the client can benefit from the educational experience.

Client education is important in the practice of occupational therapy. Written materials, while most commonly used in client education, need to reflect the reading level and comprehensibility of the reader to be effective (Griffin, McKenna, & Tooth, 2006). A survey of 147 Australian occupational therapists working with adults in physical disabilities found that 74% of therapists used client education often or most of the time (McEneany, McKenna, & Summerville, 2002).

Teaching and learning provide clients with a way to take action, explore possibilities, and engage in occupation, and they are fundamental to the occupational therapy process (Berkeland & Flinn, 2005). "In designing teaching and learning experiences, practitioners consider models or frameworks for client education, principles of adult learning and the mechanics of constructing education programs" (Berkeland & Flinn, 2005, p. 421). Client education is a vital link between the occupational therapy practitioner and those individuals under their care (Griffin et al., 2006).

## Work

Work is important socially and economically and it often defines our place in a community. In the evaluation of work, occupational therapists must consider the multiple context and activity demands that affect performance. According to Sandqvist and Henriksson (2004), work function assessment includes participation in work as it relates to society, work performance as it relates to the client, and the client's capacity as it relates to physical and psychological functioning. A client's deficits in the occupational performance area of work may be both physical and psychological. When work is interrupted, or when the individual is not able to continue working, the public recognition and identity as a worker is missing. The individual may lose the sense of being a productive member of society (Dickie, 2003). The order and expectations of work can provide the stability an individual needs to move forward with overall life activities.

Understanding the psychosocial aspects of disability is as important as having knowledge of those injuries and illnesses that affect the workers' abilities to perform essential job functions. Psychological events could be triggered by family or work stress. Sociocultural issues such as age discrimination could displace a worker (Rice & Luster, 2002). Neurological, sensory, or other changes related to aging could affect a worker's safety and productivity (B. Larson, 2001). The occupational therapist works with other professionals in addressing issues affecting an individual's ability to work. These individuals may include employers, human resource departments, safety personnel, or case managers. In the past, physical illnesses or injuries have been the primary focus of the employer. There is a definite need in the workplace for occupational therapists to address the performance deficits in those individuals who suffer the effects of mental illness. Competitive work has been shown to be valuable to integrating individuals with schizophrenia into the community. A study in Japan demonstrated how important competitive work, along with clinical support and occupational and vocational rehabilitation services, was in providing individuals with schizophrenia the motivation, income, and stability to move into the community (Oka et al., 2004).

Following a lack of acknowledgement, the recognition of anxiety and depressive disorders in the workplace and the employer costs associated with these illnesses are now being documented (Langlieb & Kahn, 2005). "Research, improved treatment options, and a gradual lessening of the stigma associated with mental illness have created an environment in which their importance to the employer community is more apparent" (Langlieb & Kahn, p. 1099).

In the evaluation of work, the ability to analyze job tasks is critical. Identifying the physical job requirements allows the occupational therapy practitioner to determine job adaptations or modifications or to assist an employer to make reasonable accommodations for a qualified individual with a disability (Americans with Disabilities Act [ADA], 1990). Knowing the physical job requirements is necessary to identify the potential for ergonomic changes, determine options for transitional work, write functional job descriptions, and design post-offer tests.

A comprehensive evaluation looks at the physical requirements of the work, the worker, and the workplace to gain an understanding of factors affecting participation in work. Consideration is given to the activity demands of the work, such as the forces, angles, weights, distances, and repetitions the job requires; the design or layout of the work area; organization of the work; and the tools and equipment used to perform the job. Knowledge of gender, age, skill level, and general health of an individual worker or worker population is an important factor in identifying both strengths and limitations in performance skills and patterns (Larson, Ellexson, & Commission on Practice, 2005).

The complexities involved in assessing work performance require observing and testing worker skills and abilities in the context of the job and workplace in which the worker intends to work. Environmental and psychosocial factors must also be considered (Sandqvist & Henriksson, 2004). After analyzing the assessment data, the occupational therapist draws conclusions on which to base clinical decisions that will guide workers toward engagement in meaningful, purposeful work activities.

Occupational therapy practitioners use education as a therapeutic tool, designing education programs for clients based on the needs and wants identified in the assessment. The programs could include injury prevention, stress management, safety, proper body mechanics, postural awareness, pain management strategies, joint protection, and symptom awareness (American Occupational Therapy Association [AOTA], 2008).

To be effective in the role of educator, the occupational therapy practitioner must create an environment for learning, becoming aware of the persons or populations being served, understanding the principles of how individuals learn, and selecting the most appropriate teaching approach. As stated earlier, it is important for occupational therapists to be aware of the reading level and comprehensibility of the education materials, as well as the individual client's or population's reading ability and comprehension level. Material should be written at a fifth to sixth grade reading level, have a clear purpose, and be meaningful and relevant to the audience (Griffin et al., 2006; Sharry, McKenna & Tooth, 2002).

A clinical example illustrates this point. A client arrived at an outpatient facility for a scheduled functional capacity assessment. Prior to beginning the test, the client was given medical forms to read and sign. He completed the required paperwork and the occupational therapist began the assessment. As the test progressed, the client followed directions but appeared frustrated and was not engaged in the process. The therapist decided to stop the test and talk with the client. The client confided that he was upset because of the paperwork he was given to fill out when he came into the clinic. He signed the forms but did not know what he was signing. He said he was a poor reader and embarrassed to ask for assistance. Once the therapist was made aware of the situation, she carefully and thoughtfully reviewed the forms to make sure he understood what he had signed. The client's attitude changed. He was now able to fully participate in the functional assessment.

This issue raised the following concerns. First, the client's uncooperative behavior was a result of his inability to read and understand the forms, not because he did not want to fully participate in the functional assessment. Second, the facility had not created an environment where the client felt comfortable to ask for assistance. The occupational therapist's ability to recognize and address the needs and wants of the client allowed him to fully participate in and benefit from the functional assessment. The results, in turn, will provide the occupational therapist vital information in intervention planning. With the engagement of the client in the process, the outcome is directed toward increasing the individual's health and well-being for participation in the occupational performance area of work (Law, 2002).

## Role of the Occupational Therapy Assistant

The occupational therapy assistant shares a collaborative role with the occupational therapist in the performance areas of work and education. The occupational therapist evaluates, while the occupational therapy assistant, working under the supervision of the occupational therapist, assists in the evaluation process by gathering and sharing data (Accreditation Council for Occupational Therapy Education [ACOTE], 2006).

The occupational therapist focuses on problem identification, problem analysis, and the planning required for problem solution. The occupational therapy assistant focuses on delivering direct services and documenting client response and progress (B. Larson, 2005). The occupational therapy assistant collects and reports selected information during the evaluation process. The occupational therapy assistant may be asked to participate in the interview process, assist in the development of an education program, or facilitate education and training sessions.

The occupational therapy assistant, having successfully completed an accredited occupational therapy assistant program, has the knowledge, skills, and abilities required to be part of a work rehabilitation team (Moyers, 1999). Assisting with job analysis, providing continuity in a work hardening or work conditioning program, and reporting client physical and behavior changes to the occupational therapist are important occupational therapy assistant roles. Specializing in work allows the occupational therapy assistant to gain a depth of skill and knowledge in this area (James & Kehrhahn, 2005). This valued experience enhances what the occupational therapy assistant brings to the team and benefits the therapeutic process for all occupational therapy practitioners.

## Summary

To facilitate meaningful participation in the evaluation of education or work, the occupational therapy practitioner needs to create an environment where clients can focus on and attend to tasks, have a sense of choice or control over the activity, and experience a sense of mastery (Law, 2002). In both the evaluation of the performance areas of work and education, identifying both the physical and psychosocial needs of the client is a crucial step in addressing problems manifested by those needs.

## Case Example

The client is a 54-year-old female who works in a light manufacturing industry that specializes in die cutting. Her job responsibilities include the production line and product inspection. The client has worked for the company for 15 years. She has been treated for thoracic outlet syndrome and continues to complain of left shoulder and neck pain. She has frequent doctor visits and has been on light duty for several years, stating she cannot do her regular job. The occupational therapist has been asked to evaluate the individual's current functional level related to her essential job functions. The human resources department at the company is working on case resolution and plans to use the functional assessment findings along with vocational data in the company's final placement decision.

| Worker Issues | Employer Issues |
|---|---|
| Bad body schema | Chronically absent from work |
| No responsibility for own health and well-being (i.e., poor shoes, footwear) | Employee did not rotate with the other employees; was permanently stationed on one part of the line |
| Multiple physical complaints | Employee was not performing the essential job functions on a fulltime basis |
| Poor work habits | Employee was frequently late, and needed reminders to keep on task |
| Various work restrictions | Employee had various work restrictions over the years that were never re-evaluated |
| Unhappy with job | Performance issues were never addressed |
| Personal issues outside of work affecting her job satisfaction | Employee had heavy use of workers' compensation, medical, and disability systems |
| Husband on disability | |

## Student Self-Assessment

1. Locate and review client education materials of your choice. Evaluate the clarity, reading level, and appropriateness for the intended population. Document positive findings as well as any changes you would make to improve the materials for the intended population.
2. Identify what contextual and environmental issues you need to consider when teaching handwriting skills to young children with sensory processing deficits.
3. Review the educational theories and models discussed in the chapter and identify the common themes.
4. Research the ADA Web site (www.ada.gov) to review cases involving rulings on mental health issues in the workplace.
5. List the 3 components of work function assessment described by Sandqvist and Henriksson.
6. Access the Job Accommodation Network (www.jan.wvu.edu) on the Internet and determine how it can be used to address the client's need for reasonable accommodations.
7. Explain why both physical and psychological issues must be considered when evaluating a client's deficits in the occupational performance area of work.
8. Describe how the principles from the educational theories and models discussed in the chapter are useful in establishing therapeutic relationships.
9. Working with a peer, identify the occupational therapy assistant's role in the evaluation of an individual with deficits affecting work performance.
10. Describe how education is both a primary therapeutic tool and a primary occupational performance area.

## Electronic Resources

- Job Accommodation Network (JAN): www.jan.wvu.edu
- Americans with Disabilities Act: www.ada.gov
- National Institute on Aging: www.nia.nih.gov
- National Institute for Occupational Safety and Health: www.cdc.gov/niosh

### Evidence-Based Research Chart

| Issue | Subject/Activity | Evidence |
|---|---|---|
| Educational theories and models | Behavior change; self-efficacy | Carter, 1990; Lewis & Daltroy, 1990; Perry et al., 1990, 1997; Rosenstock & Strecher, 1997 |
| Health education | Needs and problems | Dahlin Ivanoff et al., 2002 |
| | Comprehension, reading level; communication | Griffin et al., 2006; Joos & Hickam, 1990; McEneany et al., 2002 |
| Sensory deficits | Assessments | Bodison & Mailloux, 2006; Walting et al., 2001 |
| Handwriting | Positioning | Naider-Steinhart & Katz-Leurer, 2007 |
| Client centered | Self-perception | Joos & Hickam, 1990; Law, 2002; McColl & Pollock, 2001 |
| Work | Psychological issues | Dickie, 2003; Langlieb & Kahn, 2005; Oka et al., 2004; Rice & Luster, 2008; Sandqvist & Henriksson, 2004 |
| Children's work | Education; classroom | E. A. Larson, 2004 |
| Essential job functions | Reasonable accommodations | ADA, 1990 |

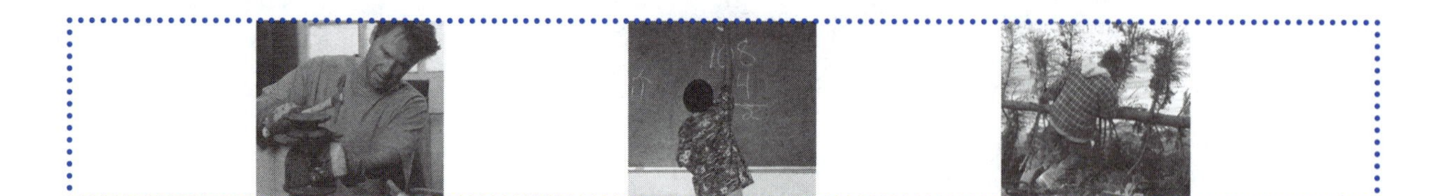

# References


Accreditation Council for Occupational Therapy Education. (2006). Standards for an accredited master's-level educational program for the occupational therapist. And Standards for an accredited educational program for the occupational therapy assistant. Retrieved February 10, 2006, from http://www.aota.org/Educate/Accredit/StandardsReview.aspx

Americans with Disabilities Act of 1990, Pub. L. No. 101-336, §2, 104 Stat. 328 (1991).

American Occupational Therapy Association. (2008). Occupational therapy practice framework: Domain and process, second edition. *American Journal of Occupational Therapy, 62*, 625-683.

Berkeland, R., & Flinn, N. (2005). Therapy as learning. In C. H. Christiansen, C. M. Baum, & J. Bass Haugen (Eds.), *Occupational therapy: Performance, participation, and well-being* (3rd ed., pp. 420-448.). Thorofare, NJ: SLACK Incorporated.

Bodison, S., & Mailloux, Z. (2006). The Sensory Integration and Praxis Tests: Illuminating struggles and strengths in participation at school. *OT Practice, 11*(17), CE1-CE8.

Carter, W. B. (1990). Health behavior as a rational process: Theory of reasoned action and multiattribute utility theory. In K. Glanz, F. M. Lewis, & B. K. Rimer (Eds.), *Health behavior and health education: Theory, research and practice* (pp. 39-62). San Francisco, CA: Jossey-Bass.

Case-Smith, J. (2005). *Occupational therapy for children* (5th ed.). St. Louis, MO: Mosby.

Dahlin Ivanoff, S., Sonn, U., & Svensson, E. (2002). A health education program for elderly persons with visual impairments and perceived security in the performance of daily occupations: A randomized study. *American Journal of Occupational Therapy, 56*(3), 322-330.

Dickie, V. A. (2003). Establishing worker identity: A study of people in craft work. *American Journal of Occupational Therapy, 57*(3), 250-261.

Griffin, J., McKenna, K., & Tooth, L. (2006). Discrepancy between older clients' ability to read and comprehend and the reading level of written educational materials used by occupational therapists. *American Journal of Occupational Therapy, 60*(1), 70-80.

James A. B., & Kehrhahn, M. T. (2005). Professional development. In S. Ryan & K. Sladyk (Eds.), *Ryan's occupational therapy assistant: Principles, practice issues, and techniques* (4th ed., pp. 560-570). Thorofare, NJ: SLACK Incorporated.

Joos, S. K., & Hickam, D. H. (1990). How health professionals influence health behavior: Patient-provider interaction and health outcomes. In K. Glanz, F. M. Lewis, & B. K. Rimer (Eds.), *Health behavior and health education: Theory, research and practice* (pp. 39-62.). San Francisco, CA: Jossey-Bass.

Langlieb, A. M., & Kahn, J. P. (2005). How much does quality mental health care profit employers? *Journal of Occupational and Environmental Medicine, 47*(10), 1099-1109.

Larson, B. (2001). The aging worker. *Work, 16*(1), 67-68.

Larson, B. (2005). Work injury activities. In S. Ryan & K. Sladyk (Eds.), *Ryan's occupational therapy assistant: Principles, practice issues, and techniques* (4th ed., pp. 462-469.). Thorofare, NJ: SLACK Incorporated.

Larson, B., Ellexson, M., & Commission on Practice. (2005). Occupational therapy services in facilitating work performance. *American Journal of Occupational Therapy, 59*(6), 676-679.

Larson, E. A. (2004). Children's work: The less-considered childhood occupation. *American Journal of Occupational Therapy, 58*(4), 369-379.

Law, M. (2002). Participation in the occupations of everyday life. *American Journal of Occupational Therapy, 56*(6), 640-649.

Law, M., Baum, C. M., & Dunn, W. (2005). Occupational performance assessment. In C. H. Christiansen, C. M. Baum, & J. Bass Haugen (Eds.), *Occupational therapy: Performance, participation, and well-being* (3rd ed., pp. 338-370.). Thorofare, NJ: SLACK Incorporated.

Lewis, F. M., & Daltroy, L. H. (1990). How causal explanations influence health behavior: Attribution theory. In K. Glanz, F. M. Lewis, & B. K. Rimer (Eds.), *Health behavior and health education: Theory, research and practice* (pp. 39-62.). San Francisco, CA: Jossey-Bass.

McColl, M. A., & Pollock, N. (2001). Measuring occupational performance using a client-centered approach. In M. Law, C. M. Baum, & W. Dunn (Eds.), *Measuring occupational performance: Supporting best practice in occupational therapy* (pp. 81-91.). Thorofare, NJ: SLACK Incorporated.

McEneany, J., McKenna, K., & Summerville, P. (2002). Australian occupational therapists working in adult physical dysfunction settings: What treatment media do they use? *Australian Occupational Therapy Journal, 49*(3), 115-127.

Moyers, P. A. (1999.) The guide to occupational therapy practice. American Occupational Therapy Association. *American Journal of Occupational Therapy, 53*(3), 247-322.

Naider-Steinhart, S., & Katz-Leurer, M. (2007). Analysis of proximal and distal muscle activity during handwriting tasks. *American Journal of Occupational Therapy, 61*(4), 392-398.

Oka, M., Otsuka, K., Yokoyama, N., Mintz, J., Hoshino, K., Niwa, S., et al. (2004). An evaluation of a hybrid occupational therapy and supported employment program in Japan for persons with schizophrenia. *American Journal of Occupational Therapy, 58*(4), 466-475.

Pasick, R. J. (1997). Socioeconomic and cultural factors in the development and use of theory. In K. Glanz, F. M. Lewis, & B. K. Rimer (Eds.), *Health behavior and health education: Theory and research* (pp. 425-440.). San Francisco, CA: Jossey-Bass.

Perry, C. L., Barnowski, T., & Parcel, S. (1990). How individuals, environments, and health behaviors interact: Social learning theory. In K. Glanz, F. M. Lewis, & B. K. Rimer (Eds.), *Health behavior and health education: Theory, research and practice* (pp. 162-186.). San Francisco, CA: Jossey-Bass.

Perry, C. L., Barnowski, T., & Parcel, S. (1997). How individuals, environments, and health behavior interact: Social cognitive theory. In K. Glanz, F. M. Lewis, & B. K. Rimer (Eds.), *Health behavior and health education: Theory, research, and practice* (2nd ed., pp. 153-178.). San Francisco, CA: Jossey-Bass.

Rice, V. J., & Luster, S. (2008). Restoring competence for the worker role. In C. A. Trombley & M. V. Radomski (Eds.), *Occupational therapy for physical dysfunction* (6th ed., pp. 875-908.). Baltimore, MD: Lippincott Williams & Wilkins.

Rosenstock, I. M. (1990). The health belief model: Explaining health behavior through expectancies. In K. Glanz, F. M. Lewis, & B. K. Rimer (Eds.), *Health behavior and health education: Theory, research and practice* (pp. 39-62.). San Francisco, CA: Jossey-Bass.

Rosenstock, I. M., & Strecher, R. J. (1997). The health belief model. n K. Glanz, F. M. Lewis, & B. K. Rimer (Eds.), *Health behavior and health education: Theory, research, and practice* (2nd ed., pp. 41-59.). San Francisco, CA: Jossey-Bass.

Sandqvist, J. L., & Henriksson, C. M. (2004). Work functioning: A conceptual framework. *Work, 23*(2), 147-157.

Sharry, R., McKenna, K., & Tooth, L. (2002). Occupational therapists' use and perceptions of written client educational materials. *American Journal of Occupational Therapy, 56*(5), 573-576.

Smith-Zuzovsky, N., & Exner, C. E. (2004). The effect of seated positioning quality on typical 6- and 7-year-old children's object manipulation skills. *American Journal of Occupational Therapy, 58*(4), 380-388.

Watling, R. L., Deitz, J., & White, O. (2001). Comparison of Sensory Profile scores of young children with and without autism spectrum disorders. *American Journal of Occupational Therapy, 55*(4), 416-423.

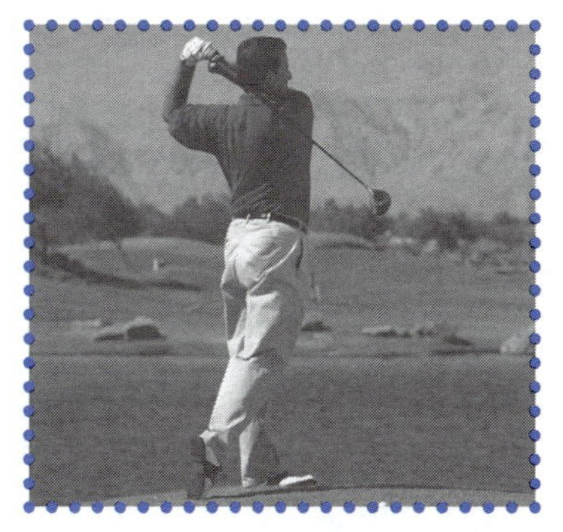

# 13

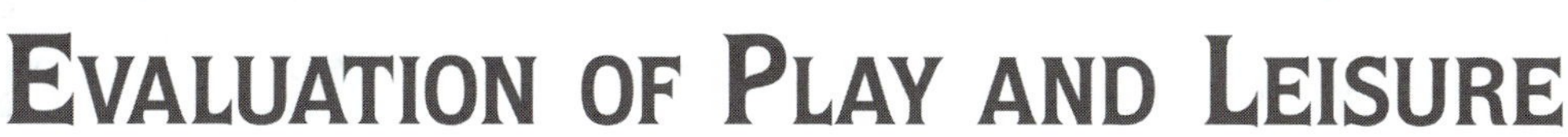

# Evaluation of Play and Leisure

*Lori Vaughn, OTD, OTR/L*

**ACOTE Standard Explored in This Chapter**

B.4.4

**Key Terms**

| | |
|---|---|
| Framing | Leisure activities |
| Freedom to suspend reality | Play activities |
| Internal control | Playfulness |
| Intrinsic motivation | |

## Introduction

### The Occupational Therapy Practitioner's Scope of Practice in Play and Leisure Assessment

The American Occupational Therapy Association (AOTA) *Scope of Practice* (LaVesser, Aird, & Lieberman, 2004), the core of occupational therapy practice, values the understanding and use of occupations. The domain of occupational therapy is the occupations people find purposeful and meaningful, enabling individuals to participate in everyday life activities and situations, desired roles, and contexts (LaVesser et al.). Play activities are defined as "spontaneous and organized activities that promote pleasure, amusement, and diversion" and leisure activities are described as "nonobligatory, discretionary, and intrinsically rewarding activities" (LaVesser et al., p. 674). In practice, occupational therapy practitioners must consider several factors, including the client's repertoire of occupations, performance skills and patterns utilized, the influence of contexts on participation, activity demands, and the structures and functions of the client's body (LaVesser et al.).

### The Role of the Occupational Therapist and Occupational Therapy Assistant in Play and Leisure Assessment

Evaluations are directed by occupational therapists and include the following:

- Determination of service need, problem identification, and definition
- Establishment of priorities, goals, and interventions
- Determination of additional assessment
- Interpretation of the data
- Integration of information

The occupational therapy assistant contributes to the process of evaluation by the implementation of assigned assessments if service competency has been established, provision of verbal and/or written reports based on observations and experience, and dissemination of other pertinent information necessary for the occupational therapist for interpretation and decision making (Brayman et al., 2004). Throughout the evaluation process, the



K. Sladyk, K. Jacobs, & N. MacRae (Eds.).
*Occupational Therapy Essentials for Clinical Competence* (pp. 135-150).

occupational therapist develops a client's occupational profile, assesses his or her ability to participate in everyday activities, and works with the client to determine areas of need and priorities for intervention to support engagements in meaningful occupations (LaVesser et al., 2004).

Evaluation includes several factors that can impact basic and instrumental activities of daily living (BADL, IADL), education, work, play, leisure, and social participation (LaVesser et al., 2004).

# Assessment of Play

*You can discover more about a person in an hour of play than in a year of conversation.*
—Plato, Greek philosopher (427 B.C. to 347 B.C.)

Play is a concept familiar to everyone. Just the mention of the word can evoke thoughts and emotions. However, the feelings induced are subjective to each individual. A child can be observed playing dress-up or chasing a friend on the playground. An adolescent can be engrossed in playing a video game, or a little leaguer can play baseball. Play is individual to the player and possesses meaning an outside observer can only assume. While the activities themselves can be labeled, a clear understanding remains elusive. Contributing to the difficulty with conceptualization are the divergent cultural and societal norms, beliefs, and values associated with play. While play is difficult to understand, it is an inherent part of who children are, how they learn and develop, and how they interact with people and objects in the environment. The first section of this chapter focuses on theories contributing to the concept of play and specific assessment tools used to evaluate play.

## What Is Play?

Despite an inherent personal concept of play subject to individual interpretations, theorists have long struggled to conceive of, develop, and concur on a definitive definition (Parham & Primeau, 1997; Takata, 1969). While observers might easily label the previous examples as play, the ability to determine what intrinsic value a task holds for the player and what elements of the task constitute a playful experience is much more complex. While lacking an operational definition may seem inconsequential, the inability to operationalize the term impacts the ability to develop appropriate assessment instruments (Parham & Primeau). Scholars have long attempted to form a consensus on a definition in an attempt to ensure that they were talking about the same thing (Garvey, 1990). Without the ability to find a common language, scholars are unable to adequately evaluate and research all of the intricacies of play (Parham & Primeau) and are unable to distinguish it from non-play (Bundy, 1993; Rubin, Fein, & Vandenberg, 1983). Labeling what constitutes play is much more challenging than determining what it is not (Takata), as it is easy to identify but difficult to define (Johnson, Christie, & Yawkey, 1987). One thing that scholars can agree on is that play is the primary occupation of children (Bundy, 1993; Heard, 1977; Knox, 1997; Muys, Rodger, & Bundy, 2006), and one in which people engage throughout their lifespan (Christiansen, 1991; Kielhofner, 1995; Primeau, Clark, & Pierce, 1989; Yerxa et al., 1989).

Some of the prevailing operational concepts are found within the constructs of occupational science (Clark et al., 1991), which focuses on the study of occupation (Parham & Primeau, 1997). Under this theory, in order to understand the occupation of play, scholars must study play rather than focus on the performance skills and client factors that can impact play (Parham & Primeau). In occupational science, play is open-ended, limitless, and a completely pleasurable experience (Burke, 1996). Yerxa et al. (1989) stressed the importance of understanding what the process of engagement means to the individual. Another view involves the belief that play is more than a method to achieve a therapeutic end but is an end in and of itself because of its intrinsic value and its ability to promote health. It is inappropriate to view play simply as a therapeutic tool but rather as an entity (Muys et al., 2006). It possesses the ability to promote the skills needed for present life while developing skills for the future (Bundy, 1993; Erikson, 1959; Ornstein & Sobel, 1989; Parham, 1996; Parham & Primeau, 1997; Reilly, 1974). Play is a process through which children learn how to interact within their environments; develop an understanding of the world; develop physical, cognitive, and social skills; enhance independence; and develop coping and problem-solving skills (Brown & Gottfried, 1985; Bruner, Jolly, & Sylva, 1976; Burke, 1996; Hess & Bundy, 2003; Hughes, 1999; Malone, 1999; Saunders, Sayer, & Goodale, 1999; Tanta, Deitz, White, & Billingsley, 2005). Play has also been linked to the development of creativity, curiosity, humor, imagination, and communication skills (F. Caplan & T. Caplan, 1973; McCune-Nicolich & Bruskin, 1982; Russ, 2003; Saltz & Brodie, 1982; Singer, D. & Singer J., 1992). While engaged in play, a child is at, or close to, his or her optimal level of development (Vygotsky, 1967, cited in Linder, 1993). It exists for the intrinsic pleasure of the player, and there is no correct or incorrect way to play (Olsen, 1999). It is also highly dependent upon the attitudes and beliefs of the player (Takata, 1974). For this reason, defining play is not the only challenge that is presented—evaluating play is equally difficult.

## Theories of Play

Occupational therapists have recognized the value of play as a role and as a method of health promotion. However, not until the work of Mary Reilly (1974) and her students did the profession contribute to the knowledge base of play. While there exists an extensive body of knowledge regarding play theories, much of that knowledge was acquired through other disciplines, especially education and psychology. Still, efforts to develop an occupational therapy theory of play have been limited (Parham & Primeau, 1997). Because much of the knowledge is derived from other disciplines, and because of the unique foci and perspectives of these other disciplines, the ability to develop a comprehensive occupational therapy taxonomy regarding the occupational components of play is challenging (Parham & Primeau). With the lack of an appropriate taxonomy, therapists often apply other models of practice to play, which may or may not appropriately address the deficits (Bryze, 1997). Despite the challenges, these disciplines provide a basis upon which occupational therapy can build. According to Reilly (1974), an interdisciplinary explanation is necessary because of the complexity of play.

# Historical Perspectives

History provides several play perspectives. In the research, these theories are typically labeled either classical or modern theories, with World War I as the marker between the two periods (Gillmore, 1971; Mellou, 1994). Classical theories attempted to identify why play existed and define its purpose. These theories were based on philosophical principles rather than scientific research (Ellis, 1973, cited in Parham & Primeau, 1997). Four classical theories were identified (Gillmore; Mellou) and are briefly described below:

1. *Surplus Energy Theory*: Hypothesized that every organism has a fixed quantity of energy available, which must be expended. When the energy is not required for self-preservation, it is manifested in non–goal-directed ways. Because children are typically cared for and do not expend a great deal of energy in these endeavors, they have excess energy, and play occurs as a result (Gilmore, 1971; Lieberman, 1977; Mellou, 1994; Parham & Primeau, 1997; Rubin, 1982; Stagnitti, 2004; Tsao, 2002).
2. *Recreation/Relaxation Theory*: Proposed that play was a result of a lack of energy and occurred to replenish depleted energy. Because children are always busy learning and acquiring new skills, a great deal of energy is utilized. Play is relaxing and rejuvenating because there are no cognitive demands (Gilmore, 1971; Lieberman, 1977; Mellou, 1994; Parham & Primeau, 1997; Stagnitti, 2004).
3. *Pre-Exercise Theory*: Hypothesized that play is instinctive and is preparatory for mature adult behavior in the future. As species become increasingly complex on the evolutionary scale, organisms are not born with the required skills to survive in adulthood. For this reason, periods of time during which adaptive skills are acquired are necessary, and play is a method of acquiring these skills. Play is utilized as rehearsal for adult roles and for the acquisition of skills necessary for survival and adaptation (Parham, 1996; Reilly, 1974; Saracho & Spodek, 1995; Stagnitti, 2004; Tsao, 2002).
4. *Recapitulation Theory*: Postulated that play is part of an evolutionary process. Human development follows an evolutionary path, and the development of play is no exception. For example, children swing and climb trees during an "animal" phase of development (Mellou, 1994; Rubin et al., 1983; Stagnitti, 2004).

Modern theories developed after World War I and were based on classical theories. These theorists were more interested in addressing play and how it relates to human development (Parham & Primeau, 1997). Parham and Primeau grouped modern theories into 4 categories—arousal modulation, psychodynamic, cognitive developmental, and sociocultural theories, which are briefly described below:

- *Arousal Modulation Theories*: Hypothesized that novelty and uncertainty increase arousal levels, and when aroused, organisms enter an exploratory state. When children are presented with a novel toy or are in a new environment, play is limited because they enter the discovery state, which is cognitively based and requires focused attention. Play is more relaxed as a child experiments with a familiar toy in a known environment (Mellou, 1994; Parham & Primeau, 1997).
- *Psychodynamic Theories*: Based on the works of Freud and Erikson, these theories hypothesized that children develop coping strategies through play. These strategies are "acted out" through play to rehearse for situations that might occur in reality later in life. This allows them to actively mediate stressful events rather than falling prey to anxiety and helplessness (Gilmore, 1971; Parham & Primeau, 1997; Rubin et al., 1983).
- *Cognitive Developmental Theories*: Postulated that play is volitional and contributes to the development of cognitive skills, symbolism, adaptation, flexibility, and a repertoire of skills necessary for later life (Bruner, 1972; Mellou, 1994; Parham & Primeau, 1997; Rubin et al., 1983; Sutton-Smith, 1967). These theories further postulate that creativity develops through play. Children also learn the consequences of their actions and self-expression (Gardner, 1982).
- *Sociocultural Theories*: Hypothesized that children learn social and cultural norms and behaviors through play, with both play and culture reciprocally influencing each other. Children also learn the rules of social conduct and concept of self-identity through playful activities. Empathy and the ability to function as a member of society are learned through game play and games with rules (Mead, 1934, cited in Parham & Primeau, 1997; Roopnarine & Johnson, 1994; Sutton-Smith, 1980).

While many of the classical and modern theories were based in philosophy, psychology, and education, the field of occupational therapy has also been interested in play throughout its history. The early founders stressed the importance of finding a balance between work, rest, play, and sleep (Parham & Primeau, 1997). Play developed as a primary tool when treating children and became synonymous with occupational therapy (Granoff, 1995 as cited in Parham and Primeau, 1997). Economic factors influenced the use of play as a therapeutic tool in the early 20th century. Individuals deemed able to work were placed in work programs, and those unable to work participated in recreational programs (Inch, 1936, cited in Parham & Primeau). The differentiation between work and play became less defined as practitioners learned that both could exist within a given activity (Parham & Primeau). Through Mary Reilly's work (1974), play was once again brought to the forefront of occupational therapy and utilized as a valuable therapeutic and research tool. Reilly recognized the complexity of play, which she described as a "cobweb" through which children learn mastery of their environment and gain the skills and competency required for adulthood. Many of Reilly's students continued her work and have added substantial information to the field and inspired a new generation of scholars and practitioners.

# Why Assess Play?

Researchers have stressed the importance of embracing play as a valid occupational therapy area of practice (Bundy, 1991; Couch, Deitz, & Kanny, 1998; Florey, 1981). While play is acknowledged as the primary occupation of children and one that lasts throughout the lifetime, it is rarely assessed (Bundy, 1997; Lawlor & Henderson, 1989). The reasons for this are varied but are likely related to the lack of assessment tools that truly evaluate play (Bundy, 1993; Bundy, Nelson, Metzger, & Bingaman, 2001; Morrison & Metzger, 2001; Sturgess, 1997). Because play and the components that comprise play are difficult to define, the ability to quantify and standardize these components can be even more challenging (Kalverboer, 1977). Other constraints diminishing the use of play as a therapeutic tool include negativity regarding play with an emphasis on non–play-based skill development, intervention based on site specific roles, and reimbursement issues (Couch et al.). Assessments exist, but they tend to focus more on play-related skills such as fine motor, gross motor, and cognitive abilities (Bundy, 1997). While these assessments assist in identifying a child's underlying capabilities and capacity to engage in play, they do not assess play as an occupation (Wallen & Walker, 1995).

Assessing the occupation of play provides the therapist with valuable information regarding his or her developmental levels across several domains, including socialization, preacademic, motor, communication, and self-awareness (Fewell & Glick, 1993; Florey, 1971; Michelman, 1974; Schaaf, 1990; Takata, 1974), and has been called the "window to development" (Stagnitti, Unsworth, & Rodger, 2000, p. 292). To effectively evaluate play, it is important to look at the entire occupation of play rather than simply evaluating the related client factors. Children who cannot play or who have difficulty engaging in play do not develop the skills necessary for typical development. This difficulty can precipitate lifelong difficulties, including decreased participation and satisfaction in occupational roles (Bledsoe & Shepherd, 1982; O'Brien & Shirley, 2001; Stagnitti & Unsworth, 2000).

Effective assessment of play serves multiple purposes. Play assessments can be used diagnostically to assess development across domains, as well as therapeutically for intervention planning and to determine the effectiveness of intervention (Kelly-Vance & Ryalls, 2005).

Lack of empirically researched assessment tools may also be related to the cultural value that has been placed on play as an occupation. Cultural and societal beliefs have impacted the prioritization of areas of focus within the profession, and play has historically been viewed as a volitional rather than compulsory activity such as self-care, work, and education (Bundy, 2005). This lack of tools often leads to the use of informal observation-based evaluation. While this can be a valuable and informative method of obtaining information, there are many factors that can impact the quality of such an evaluation, including the knowledge and experience of the practitioner and his or her ability to adequately interpret the information (Bundy, 2005).

Because play is central in the lives of children, and practitioners are ethically bound to utilize a client-centered approach with children and families, it is incumbent upon practitioners to evaluate it as an occupation when play is a concern. Evaluation of play should include the family and caregivers in the process, and whenever possible, it should occur within the child's natural settings of home, school, and community (Townsend, 1997, cited in Primeau, 2003). Using this top-down, collaborative approach to evaluation, the client and practitioner are able to identify the occupations that children want, need, and have to do and the factors that impact their ability to fully participate in these areas (Coster, 1998; Law et al., 1990; Trombly, 1993). According to Anita Bundy (1997), a comprehensive evaluation of play should include the following five factors:

1. What the player does
2. Why the player enjoys the chosen activity
3. How the player approaches play
4. The player's capacity to play
5. The relative supportiveness of the environment

## What the Player Does

Regardless of the words used to define play, theorists agree play is activity for its own sake and not one that is based on external factors (Parham & Primeau, 1997; Rubin et al., 1983). In play, it is the process of doing rather than the end product that is rewarding (Rubin et al.). There are three factors that researchers have identified that comprise play: intrinsic motivation, internal control, and freedom to suspend reality (Bundy, 2002; Morrison, Bundy, & Fisher, 1991; Neuman, 1971). Intrinsic motivation is what drives a child to participate in an activity for pleasure rather than for extrinsic reward (Bundy, 1993). However, it is difficult to assess, as children do not always demonstrate outward expressions of pleasure while engaged in play activities (Morrison et al.). With intrinsic motivation, children are actively engaged in the process of play and are able to continue participation despite barriers and obstacles experienced during the activity (Bundy, 1997; Primeau & Ferguson, 1999). Intrinsic motivation involves pleasure, which differentiates play from work (West, 1990). With internal control, the individual is the mechanism that drives the play. The player is in control of the materials, the play interactions, and some aspects of the outcome (Bundy, 1997; Connor, Williamson, & Siepp, 1978). The child is motivated, is able to modify his or her approach despite challenges, is willing to share materials and equipment, and seeks play opportunities with peers (Bundy, 1997). With the freedom to suspend reality, the child is able to defer the restrictions of realistic play and use his or her imagination to take on new roles and identities and to use objects in a creative way (Bundy, 1997; Rubin et al., 1983). With the ability to suspend reality, the child is able to be mischievous, playful, joking, teasing, and imaginative (Bundy, 1997). This is recognized as important for the acquisition and development of cognitive, social, and language skills (McCune-Nicholich & Fenson, 1984 cited in Rodger & Ziviani, 1999).

### Why the Player Enjoys the Chosen Activity

As an observer, it can be difficult to understand why an individual chooses a specific activity and what value participation holds for the individual. Theorists have struggled over this concept, attempting to deconstruct the value and purpose ascribed to one activity over another that appears equally enticing (Lawlor, 2003). According to Rubin et al. (1983), play involves self-imposed goals that are subject to change according to the wishes and desires of the player, making it spontaneous. Understanding why a person selects a particular activity and the intrinsic pleasure derived from it is difficult and equally challenging for the player to articulate. Intrinsic motivation is difficult to assess but important to understand if we are to consider play as an important occupation (Bundy, 1997). According to Bruner (1986), it is impossible to understand what an individual is experiencing while engaged in any activity. However, through observation, clues are emitted upon which inferences can be drawn. Although motivation is difficult to assess, information can be obtained through the observation of play patterns. Activities in which the child derives pleasure and engages in regularly can provide clues as to the player's motivation (Bundy, 1997). Pleasure is subjective, with each individual deriving something personal from any given activity. Evaluating personal meaning, while difficult, is important if intervention is aimed at building and improving an individual's repertoire of play skills and interests (Bundy, 2001).

### How the Player Approaches Play

It is important to consider not just what a player does, but also how the child approaches play (Bundy, 1993), which has been termed *playfulness* (Barnett, 1990; Bundy; Lieberman, 1977). Playfulness incorporates intrinsic motivation, internal control, and freedom to suspend reality, but it is not limited to play and may be seen in any activity (Bundy). In addition to the three factors that comprise play, Bateson (1972) described a fourth factor—framing—that he identified as essential for playfulness. He likened play to a frame through which the player offers cues about how he or she wants to be treated. For success, players must be able to give and receive these social cues (Bateson; Bundy, 1997). With playfulness, the outcome is not as important as the process. It is the individual who determines whether a task is playful, rather than the activity itself (Bryze, 1997; Bundy, 1997). Assessing playfulness may provide therapists with greater and more valuable information than assessing the play activities themselves (Bundy, 1997). Anita Bundy (1991) recognized the importance of incorporating several factors into the evaluation of play and developed a model of playfulness and a complementary assessment, the Test of Playfulness (ToP), which is described in the assessment section of this chapter.

### The Player's Capacity to Play

The player's capacity to play relates to active participation in a play activity (Rubin et al., 1983). Play assessments have historically focused on evaluating the skills necessary to participate in play activities (Bundy, 1997). Fine and gross motor, sensory, and neurological deficits may play a role in play deficits. While it is important to evaluate these skills to determine how skill performance impacts an individual's ability to play, it is not the only area that should be evaluated, and the best information will result from an evaluation of these skills within the context of play rather than in isolation (Bundy). Including a variety of recognizable toys in a familiar environment with minimal intrusion will aid in obtaining the most accurate information of play skills (Rubin et al.).

### Relative Supportiveness of the Environment

Play represents an interaction of the player and the environment in which he or she plays, and a complete evaluation of play must include how the environment supports participation (Bundy, 1997). This environmental assessment should include the caregivers and other individuals, objects, space, safety, comfort, and sensory input relative to their support of play (Bundy, 1997; Olsen, 1999; Parham & Primeau, 1997). A child's daily routines and interactions become incorporated into play experiences and are drawn upon for imagination (Harris, 2000). Children who are deemed "playful" exhibit a decrease in playfulness in a less supportive environment, and conversely, less playful children exhibit an increase in playfulness in a more supportive environment (Bronson & Bundy, 2001; Lieberman, 1977). If environmental factors impede an individual's ability to play, the development of required skills and behaviors may be inhibited (Bryze, 1997; Burke, 1993; Reilly, 1974). Theorists have espoused the benefits of a supportive environment and have advocated the benefits of the reciprocal person-environment interaction, with each influencing the other (Bronson & Bundy; Kielhofner, 1995; Wicker, 1987). Both physical and social aspects of the environment can influence the development of play skills. The "fit" between the environment and the person is considered positive when the environment is able to meet the individual's needs and when the individual's abilities match the demands imposed by the environment (Pervin, 1968 as cited in Bronson & Bundy; Rodger & Ziviani, 2006). Boredom or anxiety can exist if the demands of the environment are too low or too high relative to the abilities of the child (Bronson & Bundy). Play can occur when the child feels comfortable and safe within his or her environment (Hamm, 2006).

## Play Assessments

As indicated earlier in this chapter, play is complex. A thorough evaluation is necessary to determine which factors relate to deficits in this multifaceted occupation. A variety of assessment tools are available; however, they are not inclusive of all potential deficit areas. The selection of a play assessment should be carefully considered. Inclusion of the word *play* in the name of the tool does not necessarily mean that play is being assessed. Therefore, consideration of various tools and options is recommended for an accurate evaluation (Bundy, 1997). Play assessments generally consist of an observation of the child within the context of play to evaluate the child's abilities across all areas when compared to typically developing peers (Kelly-Vance & Ryalls, 2005). These assessments can provide a wealth of information related to a child's areas of strength and areas of need (Fewell, 1991; Kelly-Vance & Ryalls; Linder, 1993).

Neisworth and Bagnato (1988) outlined a continuum of assessment approaches that are typically utilized by multidisciplinary assessment teams. Norm-based assessments evaluate a child's developmental level to a similar cohort group. Curriculum-based assessments involve following an individual's achievement along a "developmentally sequenced curriculum" (Neisworth & Bagnato, p. 27). Adaptive-to-disability assessments allow for altered presentation and response modes and modified responses on test items by a child with sensory impairments to minimize incorrect or false failure on test items. Process assessments examine the changes in a child's reaction to changes in stimuli and can be indicative of a child's cognitive functioning. This includes changes in behavior and affects the response to the presentation of different stimuli. Judgment-based assessments quantify the impressions and observations of individuals familiar with the child, including parents, caregivers, teachers, and other professionals. This assessment approach is typically used for traits not easily evaluated through other means, including temperament, muscle tone, motivation, and impulse control (Linder, 1993). Ecological assessment examines the child's social, physical, and psychological contexts. Interactive assessment is considered a component of ecological assessment (Linder) and involves the examination of the social synchronicity of the infant and caregiver. Systematic observation occurs in a child's natural environment of home, school, or community. It may also occur through simulations and/or roleplaying and involves measurable, observed aspects of behavior, such as frequency, duration, and intensity (Neisworth & Bagnato). A brief description of play assessments is included in Appendix C to assist the practitioner in selecting the appropriate tool.

# Assessment of Leisure

*To be able to fill leisure intelligently is the last product of civilization, and at present, very few people have reached this level.*
—Bertrand Russell, British author and philosopher (1930)

According to Mary Reilly (1974), play possesses both social and biological components. Socially, a child learns to interact with both physical and nonphysical aspects of the environment and adapts his or her responses based upon those experiences. Biologically, living things engage in play, which lends itself to the assumption that as beings become increasingly complex, the activities in which they engage also become more physically and cognitively complex (Gilfoyle, Grady, & Moore, 1990). As individuals mature beyond childhood, play transforms to leisure, encompassing both social and solitary activities as they continue to refine their understanding of the world and the roles in which they participate (Gilfoyle et al.). While the theoretical beliefs related to leisure have changed throughout history, there is no disputing that, like play, it is an important occupation in which we engage.

## What Is Leisure?

Similar to play, theorists have long contemplated the characteristics and value of leisure. The definition of leisure has changed throughout history, adding new elements with each revision. Although each definition added a new dimension to leisure conceptualization, empirical research lagged behind (Esteve, San Martin, & Lopez, 1999). Research indicated that leisure participation, satisfaction, and attitude are positively correlated with satisfaction and quality of life (Hawkins, 1994; Hawkins, Ardovino, & Hsieh, 1998; Lloyd & Auld, 2002) and has been associated with contributing to promoting and maintaining mental and physical health (Caldwell & Smith, 1988; Coleman & Iso-Ahola, 1993; Passmore, 2003; Tinsley, H. & Tinsley, D., 1986). Some research also indicated that leisure impacts development by providing opportunities for skill acquisition (Evans & Poole,

1991), social competency, self-awareness, and self-control (Silbereisen, Noack, & Eyferth, 1986, cited in Passmore, 2003). There have been many terms that have become synonymous with leisure such as *relaxation, stress free, freedom from "necessaries,"* and *guilt free* (Sellar & Boshoff, 2006). Work is often considered obligatory, whereas leisure is the freedom from obligation (Kelly, 1987; Kleiber, 1999; Sellar & Boshoff). Historically, work has been more highly regarded than leisure, causing the work-leisure dichotomy to exist. Occupational choices were made out of financial necessity and responsibility, creating a barrier to leisure participation and a sense of guilt over what a person can do and what he or she should do (Sellar & Borshoff). By removing or minimizing the barriers of obligatory tasks, the meaning and experience of leisure is enhanced (Kelly; Sellar & Boshoff).

Like play in children, leisure has been linked to playfulness (Guitard, Ferland, & Dutil, 2005). The benefits of playfulness in everyday life have been linked to increased creativity, improved ability to heal, increased motivation, and enhanced affect and morale (Auerhahn & Laub, 1987; Etienne, 1982 as cited in Guitard et al., 2005; Lyons, 1987; Tegano, 1990). Despite the benefits, the components of playfulness are different in adults than in children, with adults expressing decreases in spontaneity and tolerance for joy and humor (Guitard et al.; Lieberman, 1977). Guitard et al. found that playfulness in adults is composed of five components: creativity, curiosity, sense of humor, pleasure, and spontaneity. They further found that playfulness, as defined by the aforementioned components, is helpful in enhancing an individual's occupational performance.

Leisure is also similar to play in that cultural values of leisure time vary. The meaning of "free time" holds different values and beliefs in different societies and cultures (Godbey & Jung, 1991). In English-speaking countries, leisure is equated with free time and can hold a negative value because of its contrast with the concept of work and the value therein (Goodale & Cooper, 1991). There are several factors that impact time use, including work beliefs and values, socioeconomic status, politics, gender roles, and weather (Godbey & Jung).

# Past and Present Theories of Leisure

Theories related to leisure and the use of discretionary time have been in a continuous state of evolution for centuries. It was first defined by Aristotle as being in a state in which an individual was free from the need to toil in laborious tasks and dedicated to more virtuous tasks of self-discovery, self-development, and the pursuit of pleasure (Dare, Welton, & Coe, 1987; Goodale & Cooper, 1991; Sellar & Boshoff, 2006; Veal & Lynch, 2001). These beliefs continued until the period of industrialization and the prevalence of the Protestant work ethic dichotomizing the concepts of work and leisure (Goodale & Cooper; Primeau, 1996; Sellar & Boshoff; Veal & Lynch). Leisure time became that which was left over after domestic and vocational tasks were completed (Veal & Lynch). It was viewed as a time for consumption, whereas work was a time for production (Goodale & Cooper). Focus on the concept of leisure as a component of residual time persisted until approximately 20 years ago, when a shift in thinking occurred. The focus became less of a concept of time and more a concept of the subjective experience of the individual (Primeau; Suto, 1998; Veal & Lynch). The perception of the individual became the prevailing determinant in the classification of an activity as leisurely, existing within the individual's consciousness (Kelly, 2000; McDowell, 1984).

# Why Assess Leisure?

Technological advancements, improved health care services, and increased awareness of wellness and prevention have led to an increased number of active, older adults (Stanley, 1995). This number is expected to continue to increase, highlighting the need to ensure that people are able to maintain healthy, active, satisfying existences throughout the lifespan (Stanley; Sellar & Boshoff, 2006). It is important for healthcare providers, including occupational therapy practitioners, to enhance their understanding of the meaning of roles and occupations. Leisure is an important area of practice and is related to improved quality of life (Lloyd & Auld, 2002; Sellar & Boshoff). As such, the necessity to incorporate the evaluation of leisure in occupational therapy is undeniable. However, until recently, the concept of including the subjective experience of the individual in the evaluation was minimal, with a greater focus on more objective factors, including the actual activity and time utilization. This led to the implication that the act of participation was more important than the meaning (Sellar & Boshoff; Suto, 1998). Understanding the meaning behind participation in certain activities can help therapists utilize leisure as a therapeutic activity and enhance the identification of specific barriers that preclude participation (Sellar & Boshoff; Suto). To do so effectively, it is important to explore common conceptual factors of leisure, including the temporal, activity, and experiential components. It is also important to consider the role of culture in leisure participation and the concept of leisure as a "flow" experience (Csikszentmihalyi & Kleiber, 1991).

## Leisure as Time

There are certain obligatory activities that everyone engages in to occupy their time. Once these activities are completed, certain discretionary time remains. This discretionary time has fluctuated throughout history depending upon the prevailing cultural and societal work demands (Csikszentmihalyi & Kleiber, 1991). Despite the existence of this discretionary time, family responsibilities, religious obligations, and personal ambition may drive a person to engage in externally driven projects rather than intrinsically motivating pursuits (Csikszentmihalyi & Kleiber). The distinction between work and nonwork time in defining leisure leads to identifying leisure not as what it is, but rather as what it is not (Henderson et al., 2001). Even when the workday ends, leftover time is not necessarily "free." Long drives are often associated with getting to and from work, and the end of one work day is often the beginning of a second shift of both paid and unpaid labor (Csikszentmihalyi & Kleiber). Time demands and time use vary from person to person, which is an important consideration in leisure assessment.

### Leisure as Activity

Leisure is identified as activity when engagement occurs for fun and enjoyment, and the activities are categorized according to similar characteristics, such as sports, games, outdoor and cultural activities, and socializing (Henderson et al., 2001). Despite the tendency to identify leisure by the activities in which people engage, it is difficult to identify the intrinsic pleasure derived by these activities (Csikszentmihalyi & Kleiber, 1991). This makes it unclear which activities constitute leisure to which individuals. When business executives play golf while discussing business, is this work or leisure? Do professional athletes who earn a living playing baseball or football actually work? Is gardening work or leisure to a retired person versus a farmer? It is difficult to determine which activities are considered work and which ones are considered leisure and by whom. Researchers tend to identify leisure as those activities that culture identifies as recreational and not engaged in for productive purposes (Csikszentmihalyi & Kleiber). Csikszentmihalyi (1981) argued that it is more than participation in an activity that constitutes leisure. A single meaningful leisure experience is more significant within a person's life than participation in mundane obligatory experiences over time. For example, a little league trophy may be a family centerpiece for years, with stories passed on to grandchildren. Frequency data on leisure participation are often used to establish local, state, and federal recreation programs (Henderson et al.). However, the frequency of participation in an activity does not determine importance, but perhaps it is the quality of the experience that determines relevance (Csikszentmihalyi & Kleiber). The activity is less important than the satisfaction derived from engagement (Brown, Frankel, & Fennell, 1991).

### Leisure as Experience

A trend has occurred over the past few decades to shift from the view of leisure as culturally defined, discretionary versus obligatory time, and the subjective experience of the individual (Csikszentmihalyi & Kleiber, 1991). Freedom and intrinsic motivation are essential features of the leisure experience—when an activity is freely selected and engaged in for intrinsic pleasure, it should be considered leisure (Csikszentmihalyi & Kleiber: Henderson et al., 2001; Neulinger, 1981; Parr & Lashua, 2004). It is a state of mind, and the value of the experience means different things to different people (Estes, 2003; Parr & Lashua, 2005). However, cultural norms and mores cannot be separated from this definition. Some delinquent and vandalistic acts can fall into that definition. Youth gang members who steal and vandalize do so out of free choice and some form of intrinsic pleasure (Csikszentmihalyi & Larson, 1978). Watching television can be considered leisure, but research indicated that it can lead to feelings of apathy and depression (Kubey & Csikszentmihalyi, 1990). To avoid the problem of defining leisure as experience based upon these dichotomous viewpoints, two rationalizations can be drawn. First is the admission that leisure can be depressing, tiresome, and even criminal. Second is the idea that an activity cannot be deemed leisure unless it leads to increased positive and culturally accepted experiences in addition to possessing intrinsic motivation and free choice (Csikszentmihalyi & Kleiber).

### Leisure as a Construct of Culture

Each society identifies certain activities as work and others as leisure (Henderson et al., 2001). How an individual experiences leisure is often dependent upon external factors, such as the societal value of work (Parker, 1971, cited in Henderson et al.). Leisure is encumbered by the influence of social norms, mores, beliefs, and values (Henderson et al.) and cannot occur without consideration of historically conditioned political, economic, and social contexts (Parr & Lashua, 2004). Social influences and peer pressure impact the meaning an individual places on both specific activities as well as the use of discretionary time. Preferences, behaviors, and expectations are dependent, at least in part, on the influence of cultural customs (Henderson et al.).

### Leisure and the Flow Experience

Because of the incongruence of theory related to leisure, the theory of leisure as a "flow experience" was developed and inspired by the work of Maslow (Csikszentmihalyi & Kleiber, 1991). The research on this theory indicated that when people enjoy what they are doing, the experiential states they report are similar across cultural, gender, and age boundaries (Csikszentmihalyi, 1990; Csikszentmihalyi & Kleiber). According to this theory, there is a change in the state of consciousness with the pleasure of the experience. The pleasurable state experienced envelopes the individual, creating a feeling likened to being engulfed in a current or flow. There is a melding of play and player into a single entity devoid of the "duality of consciousness" typically present in ordinary life—the player becomes the play, able to enjoy new experiences without repercussion (Csikszentmihalyi & Kleiber, p. 95).

## Leisure Assessments

A variety of leisure assessments are available to measure several domains of the leisure experience. Because leisure is subjective, many of the assessments are self-report or interviewer-guided questionnaires. Several assessments are described in Appendix C.

Theories of play and leisure have changed over time. However, both are valuable occupations in which people engage throughout the lifespan. Benefits have been linked to physical, social, and psychological well-being, as well as improved quality of life, self-esteem, and self-identity. As such, assessment of play and leisure through a variety of standardized and nonstandardized assessment tools, interviews, and observation in a variety of contexts is an essential component to developing a complete occupational profile and developing holistic, client-centered intervention.

# Summary

After our basic needs of food and shelter are addressed, play and leisure become a significant foundation for how we define ourselves as human beings. Play is so important in childhood because of its importance in early learning. Leisure provides adults with healthy outlets to the stresses of a fast-paced life. Even adults with strong and meaningful work relationships know the significance of play and leisure for forming important relationships in life. As play and leisure are so individualized, the occupational therapy practitioner must address the meaning of these activities to the client if the client is to return to a rich and full life.

# Student Self-Assessment

1. Observe a child at play. Take note of the following: What is the child playing with? Is the child intrinsically motivated? What evidence do you have to support your answer? Is the child demonstrating internal control? What evidence do you have to support your answer? Is the child free to suspend reality? What evidence do you have?
2. If possible, observe the child playing with a peer. Does he or she demonstrate the same level of intrinsic motivation, internal control, and freedom to suspend reality?
3. Attend a child or youth sporting event. Are all of the children demonstrating the same level of playfulness? Why or why not?
4. Interview people at different stages of life, such as a high school or college student, new parents, a baby boomer, and a recent retiree. What differences and similarities do they describe in their leisure pursuits? What about their leisure satisfaction? How does each describe his or her quality of life?
5. Make a play assessment kit. Pediatric therapists are often itinerant staff, traveling from site to site. This makes it necessary to travel with all of the items that you need for evaluation and intervention. Because you can only use what you can carry, develop a play assessment kit that you can carry in one bag. What toys/activities would you include? Why would you select these toys? Would you carry different items to assess a preschooler and a second grader?

**Evidence-Based Research Chart**

| Play Assessment | Evidence |
|---|---|
| Child Initiated Pretend Play Assessment (ChIPPA) | Stagnitti, 2002 as cited in Swindells & Stagnitti, 2006; Stagnitti & Unsworth, 2000, 2004; Stagnitti et al., 2000; Swindells & Stagnitti, 2006 |
| Children's Playfulness Scale | Barnett, 1990, 1991; Bundy & Clifton, 1998; Muys et al., 2006 |
| Knox Play Scale (now Preschool Play Scale or Revised Knox Preschool Play Scale) | Bundy, 1989; Clifford & Bundy, 1989; Harrison & Kielhofner, 1986; Knox, 1974, 1997; Rodger & Ziviani, 1999 |
| Play History | Behnke & Fetkovich, 1984; Rodger & Ziviani, 1999; Stagnitti et al., 2000; Takata, 1969 |
| Play in Early Childhood Evaluation System (PIECES) | Cherney, Kelly-Vance, Gill, Ruane, & Ryalls, 2003; Gill-Glover, McCaslin, Kelly-Vance, & Ryalls, 2001 as cited in Kelly-Vance & Ryalls, 2005; Kelly-Vance & Gill-Glover, 2002 as cited in Kelly-Vance & Ryalls, 2005; Kelly-Vance, Gill, Ruane, Cherney, & Ryalls, 1999 as cited in Kelly-Vance & Ryalls, 2005; Kelly-Vance, Needelman, Troia, & Ryalls, 1999; Kelly-Vance, Gill, Schoneboom, Cherney, Ryan, Cunningham, & Ryalls, 2000 as cited in Kelly-Vance & Ryalls, 2005; Kelly-Vance, Ryalls, & Glover, 2002; King, McCaslin, Kelly-Vance, & Ryalls, 2003 as cited in Kelly-Vance & Ryalls, 2005; McCaslin, King, Kelly-Vance, & Ryalls, 2003 as cited in Kelly-Vance & Ryalls, 2005; Ryalls, Gill, Ruane, Cherney, Schoneboom, Cunningham, & Ryan, 2000 as cited in Kelly-Vance & Ryalls, 2005; Kelly-Vance & Ryalls, 2005 |

| Evidence-Based Research Chart (continued) | |
|---|---|
| Preschool Play Scale | Bledsoe & Shepherd, 1982; Bundy, 1987 as cited in Bundy et al., 2001; Bundy, 1989; Clifford & Bundy, 1989; Couch, 1996; Harrison & Kielhofner, 1986; Kielhofner, Barris, Bauer, Shoestock, & Walker, 1983; Knox, 1974, 1997; O'Brien et al., 2000; Restall & Magill-Evans, 1994; Shepherd, Brollier, & Dandrow, 1994; Tanta et al., 2005; von Zuben, Crist, & Mayberry, 1991 |
| Symbolic Play Test | Casby, 1997; Cunningham, Glenn, Wilkinson, & Sloper, 1985; Gould, 1986; Lowe & Costello, 1988; Power & Radcliffe, 1989 |
| Test of Playfulness | Bundy, 1997, 2003; Bundy et al., 2001; Cameron et al., 2001; Gaik & Rigby, 1994 as cited in Cameron et al., 2001; Hamm, 2006; Harkness & Bundy, 2001; Hess & Bundy, 2003; Liepold & Bundy, 2000; Muys et al., 2006; O'Brien et al., 2000; O'Brien & Shirley, 2001; Okimoto, Bundy, & Hanzlik, 2000; Reed, Dunbar, & Bundy, 2000; Rodger & Ziviani, 1999 |
| Transdisciplinary Play-Based Assessment | Friedli, 1994; Kelly-Vance & Ryalls, 2005; Kelly-Vance et al., 1999; Myers, McBride, & Peterson, 1996; Rodger & Ziviani, 1999 |
| Penn Interactive Peer Play Scale (PIPPS) | Castro, Mendez, & Fantuzzo, 2002; Coolahan, Fantuzzo, Mendez, & McDermott, 2000; Fantuzzo, Coolahan, Mendez, McDermott, & Sutton-Smith, 1998; Fantuzzo, Mendez, & Tighe, 1998; Fantuzzo et al., 1995; Mendez, Fantuzzo, & Cicchetti, 2002; Mendez, McDermott, & Fantuzzo, 2002 |
| **Leisure Assessment** | **Evidence** |
| Activity Card Sort (ACS) | Katz, Karpin, Lak, Furman, & Hartman-Maeir, 2003; Sachs & Josman, 2003 |
| Children's Assessment of Participation and Enjoyment (CAPE) | King et al., 2003, 2007; Law et al., 2006 |
| Interest Checklist/Activity Checklist | Katz, 1988; Klyczek, Bauer-Yox, & Fiedler, 1997; Matsutsuyu, 1967, 1969; Rogers, Weinstein, & Figone, 1978 |
| Leisure Activity Profile (LAP) | Mann & Talty, 1991 |
| Leisure Assessment Inventory | Hawkins, 1993, 1994; Hawkins et al., 1998; Hawkins & Freeman, 1993 |
| Leisure Attitude Scale | Ragheb & Beard, 1982; Ragheb & Tate, 1993; Siegenthaler & O'Dell, 2000 |
| Leisure Boredom Scale | Gordon & Caltabiano, 1996; Iso-Ahola & Weissinger, 1990; Wegner, Flisher, Muller, & Lombard, 2002 |
| Leisure Competence Measure | Kloseck, Crilly, Ellis, & Lammers, 1996; Kloseck, Crilly, & Hutchinson-Troyer, 2001 |
| Leisure Diagnostic Battery [1] | Beard & Ragheb, 1983; Trottier, Brown, Hobson, & Miller, 2002 |
| Leisure Diagnostic Battery [2] | Chang & Card, 1994; Ellis & Witt, 1986; Peebles, McWilliams, Norris, & Park, 1999; Thomas, 1999; Witt & Ellis, 1984 |
| Leisure Satisfaction Scale | Beard & Ragheb, 1980; DiBona, 2000; Lysyk, Brown, Rodrigues, McNally, & Loo, 2002; Ragheb & Griffith, 1982; Ragheb & Tate, 1983; Raj, Manigandan, & Jacobs, 2006; Siegenthaler & O'Dell, 2000; Trottier et al., 2002 |
| Preferences for Activities of Children (PAC) | King et al., 2003, 2007 |

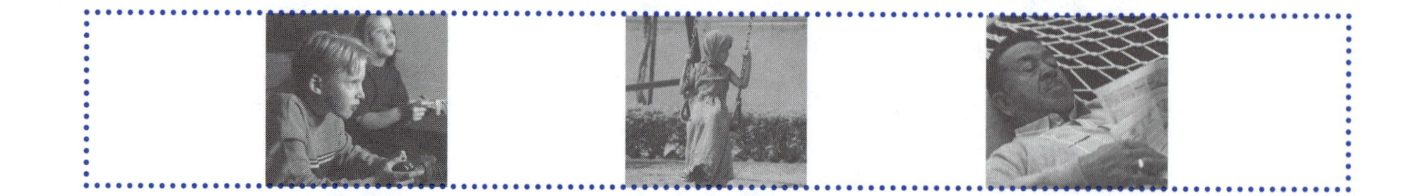

# References


Auerhahn, N., & Laub, D. (1987). Play and playfulness in Holocaust survivors. *Psychoanalytic Study of the Child, 42*, 45-58.

Barnett, L. A. (1990). Playfulness: Definition, design, and measurement. *Play and Culture, 3*(4), 319-336.

Barnett, L. A. (1991). The playful child: Measurement of a disposition to play. *Play and Culture, 4*(1), 51-74.

Bateson, G. (1972). Toward a theory of play and fantasy. In G. Bateson (Ed.), *Steps to an ecology of the mind* (pp. 14-20). New York, NY: Bantam.

Beard, J. G., & Ragheb, M. G. (1980). Measuring leisure satisfaction. *Journal of Leisure Research, 12*(1), 20-33.

Beard, J. G., & Ragheb, M. G. (1983). Measuring leisure motivation. *Journal of Leisure Research, 15*(3), 219-228.

Behnke, C. J., & Fetkovich, M. M. (1984). Examining the reliability and validity of the Play History. *American Journal of Occupational Therapy, 38*(2), 94-100.

Bledsoe, N. P., & Shepherd, J. T. (1982). A study of reliability and validity of a Preschool Play Scale. *American Journal of Occupational Therapy, 36*(12), 783-788.

Brayman, S. J., Clark, G. F., DeLany, J. V., Garza, E. R., Radomski, M. V., Ramsey, R., et al. (2004). Guidelines for supervision, roles, and responsibilities during the delivery of occupational therapy services. *American Journal of Occupational Therapy, 58*(6), 663-667.

Bronson, M. R., & Bundy, A. C. (2001). A correlational study of a Test of Playfulness and a Test of Environmental Supportiveness for play. *Occupational Therapy Journal of Research, 21*(4), 241-259.

Brown, B. A., Frankel, B. G., & Fennell, M. (1991). Happiness through leisure: The impact of type of leisure activity, age, gender, and leisure satisfaction on psychological well-being. *Journal of Applied Recreation Research, 16*(4), 368-392.

Brown, C. C., & Gottfried, A. W. (Eds.). (1985). *Play interactions: The role of toys and parental involvement in children's development.* Skillman, NJ: Johnson and Johnson.

Bruner, E. M. (1986). Experience and its expressions. In V. W. Turner & E. M. Bruner (Eds.), *The anthropology of experience* (pp. 3-30). Urbana, IL: University of Illinois.

Bruner, J. S. (1972). Nature and uses of immaturity. *American Psychologist, 27*(8), 687-708.

Bruner, J. S., Jolly, A., & Sylva, K. (Eds.). (1976). *Play: Its role in development and evolution.* New York, NY: Basic Books.

Bryze, K. (1997). Narrative contributions to the play history. In L. D. Parham & L. S. Fazio (Eds.), *Play in occupational therapy for children* (pp. 23-34). St. Louis, MO: Mosby.

Bundy, A. C. (1989). A comparison of the play skills of normal boys and boys with sensory integrative dysfunction. *Occupational Therapy Journal of Research, 9*, 84-100.

Bundy, A. C. (1991). Play theory and sensory integration. In A. G. Fisher, E. A. Murray, & A. C. Bundy (Eds.), *Sensory integration: Theory and practice* (pp. 46-68). Philadelphia, PA: F.A. Davis.

Bundy, A. C. (1993). Assessment of play and leisure: Delineation of the problem. *American Journal of Occupational Therapy, 47*(3), 217-222.

Bundy, A. C. (1997). Play and playfulness: What to look for. In L. D. Parham & L. S. Fazio (Eds.), *Play in occupational therapy for children* (pp. 52-66). St. Louis, MO: Mosby.

Bundy, A. C. (2001). Measuring play performance. In M. Law, C. Baum, & W. Dunn (Eds.), *Measuring occupational performance: Supporting best practice in occupational therapy* (pp. 89-102). Thorofare, NJ: SLACK Incorporated.

Bundy, A. C. (2002). Play theory and sensory integration. In A. C. Bundy, S. J. Lane, & E. A. Murray (Eds.), *Sensory integration: Theory and practice* (2nd ed.). Philadelphia, PA: F.A. Davis.

Bundy, A. C. (2003). *Test of Playfulness (ToP), version 4.* Sydney, Australia: School of Occupation and Leisure Sciences, The University of Sydney.

Bundy, A. C. (2005). Measuring play performance. In M. Law, C. M. Baum, & W. Dunn (Eds.), *Measuring occupational performance: Supporting best practice in occupational therapy* (2nd ed., pp. 128-149). Thorofare, NJ: SLACK Incorporated.

Bundy, A. C., & Clifton, J. (1998). Construct validity of the Children's Playfulness Scale. In M. C. Duncan, G. Chick, & A. Aycock, *Play & culture studies, volume 1: Diversions and divergences in fields of play* (pp. 37-47). New York, NY: Ablex Publishing.

Bundy, A. C., Nelson, L., Metzger, M., & Bingaman, K. (2001). Validity and reliability of a Test of Playfulness. *Occupational Therapy Journal of Research, 21*(4), 276-292.

Burke, J. P. (1993). Play: The life role of the infant and young child. In J. Case-Smith (Ed.), *Pediatric occupational therapy and early intervention* (pp. 198-224). Boston, MA: Andover Medical Publishers.

Burke, J. P. (1996). Variations in childhood occupations: Play in the presence of chronic disability. In R. Zemke & F. Clark (Eds.), *Occupational science: The evolving discipline* (pp. 413-418). Philadelphia, PA: F.A. Davis.

Caldwell, L. L., & Smith, E. A. (1988). Leisure: An overlooked component of health promotion. *Canadian Journal of Public Health, 79*(2), S44-S48.

Cameron, D., Leslie, M., Teplicky, R., Pollock, N., Steward, D., Toal, C., et al. (2001). The clinical utility of the Test of Playfulness. *Canadian Journal of Occupational Therapy, 68*(2), 104-111.

Caplan, F., & Caplan, T. (1973). *The power of play.* New York, NY: Doubleday.

Casby, M. W. (1997). Symbolic play of children with language impairments: A critical review. *Journal of Speech, Language, and Hearing Research, 40*(3), 468-479.

Castro, M., Mendez, J. L., & Fantuzzo, J. (2002). A validation study of the Penn Interactive Peer Play Scale with urban Hispanic and African American preschool children. *School Psychology Quarterly, 17*(2), 109-127.

Chang, Y. S., & Card, J. A. (1994). The reliability of the Leisure Diagnostic Battery Short Form Version B in assessing healthy, older individuals: A preliminary study. *Therapeutic Recreation Journal, 28*(3), 163-167.

Cherney, I. C., Kelly-Vance, L., Gill, K., Ruane, A., & Ryalls, B. O. (2003). The effects of stereotyped toys and gender on play-based assessment in children aged 18-47 months. *Educational Psychology, 22*(5), 95-106.

Christiansen, C. H. (1991). Occupational therapy: Intervention for life performance. In C. H. Christiansen & C. M. Baum (Eds.), *Occupational therapy: Overcoming human performance deficits* (pp. 4-43). Thorofare, NJ: SLACK Incorporated.

Clark, F. A., Parham, D., Carlson, M. E., Frank, G., Jackson, J., Pierce, D., et al. (1991). Occupational science: Academic innovation in the service of occupational therapy's future. *American Journal of Occupational Therapy, 45*(4), 300-310.

Clifford, J. M., & Bundy, A. C. (1989). Play preference and play performance in normal boys and boys with sensory integrative dysfunction. *Occupational Therapy Journal of Research, 9*(4), 202-217.

Coleman, D., & Iso-Ahola, S. E. (1993). Leisure and health: The role of social support and self-determination. *Journal of Leisure Research, 25*(2), 111-128.

Connor, F. P., Williamson, G. G., & Siepp, J. M. (Eds.). (1978). *Program guide for infants and toddlers with neuromotor and other developmental disabilities.* New York, NY: Teachers College Press.

Coolahan, K., Fantuzzo, J., Mendez, J., & McDermott, P. (2000). Preschool peer interactions and readiness to learn: Relationships between classroom peer play and learning behaviors and conduct. *Journal of Educational Psychology, 92*(3), 458-465.

Coster, W. (1998). Occupation-centered assessment of children. *American Journal of Occupational Therapy, 52*(5), 337-344.

Couch, K. J. (1996). The use of the Preschool Play Scale in published research. *Physical and Occupational Therapy in Pediatrics, 16*(4), 77-84.

Couch, K. J., Deitz, J. C., & Kanny, E. M. (1998). The role of play in pediatric occupational therapy. *American Journal of Occupational Therapy, 52*(2), 111-117.

Csikszentmihalyi, M. (1981). Some paradoxes in the definition of play. In A. T. Cheska (Ed.), *Play as context* (pp. 14-26). West Point, NY: Leisure Press.

Csikszentmihalyi, M. (1990). *Beyond boredom and anxiety: The experience of play in work and games.* San Francisco, CA: Josey-Bass.

Csikszetmihalyi, M., & Kleiber, D. A. (1991). Leisure as self actualization. In P. J. Brown, B. L. Driver, & G. L. Peterson (Eds.), *Benefits of leisure* (pp. 91-102). State College, PA: Venture Publishing.

Csikszentmihalyi, M., & Larson, R. (1978). Intrinsic rewards in school crime. *Crime and Delinquency, 24*(3), 322-335.

Cunningham, C. C., Glenn, S. M., Wilkinson, P., & Sloper, P. (1985). Mental ability, symbolic play and receptive and expressive language of young children with Down's Syndrome. *Journal of Child Psychology and Psychiatry and Allied Disciplines, 26*(2), 255-265.

Dare, B., Welton, G., & Coe, W. (1987). *Concepts of leisure in western thought: A critical and historical analysis.* Dubuque, IA: Kendall/Hunt.

DiBona, L. (2000). What are the benefits of leisure? An exploration using the Leisure Satisfaction Scale. *British Journal of Occupational Therapy, 63*(2), 50-58.

Ellis, G. D., & Witt, P. A. (1986). The Leisure Diagnostic Battery: Past, present, and future. *Therapeutic Recreation Journal, 20*(4), 31-47.

Erikson, E. H. (1959). Identity and the life cycle. *Psychology Issues, 1*(Monograph 1). New York, NY: International Universities Press.

Estes, C. (2003). Knowing something about leisure: Building a bridge between leisure philosophy and recreation practice. *Schole, 18,* 51-66.

Esteve, R., San Martin, J., & Lopez, A. E. (1999). Grasping the meaning of leisure: Developing a self-report measurement tool. *Leisure Studies, 18*(2), 79-91.

Evans, G., & Poole, M. E. (1991). *Young adults: Self perceptions and life contexts.* London, England: Falmer Press.

Fantuzzo, J., Coolahan, K., Mendez, J., McDermott, P., & Sutton-Smith, B. (1998). Contextually relevant validation of peer play constructs with African-American Head Start children: Penn Interactive Peer Play Scale. *Early Childhood Research Quarterly, 13*(3), 411-431.

Fantuzzo, J., Mendez, J., & Tighe, E. (1998). Parental assessment of peer play: Development and validation of the parent version of the Penn Interactive Peer Play Scale. *Early Childhood Research Quarterly, 13*(4), 659-676.

Fantuzzo, J., Sutton-Smith, B., Coolahan, K. C., Manz, P. H., Canning, S., & Debnam, D. (1995). Assessment of preschool play interaction behaviors in young low-income children: Penn Interactive Peer Play Scale. *Early Childhood Research Quarterly, 10*(1), 105-120.

Fewell, R. R. (1991). Trends in the assessment of infants and toddlers with disabilities. *Exceptional Children, 58*(2), 166-173.

Fewell, R. R., & Glick, M. P. (1993). Observing play: An appropriate process for learning and assessment. *Infants and Young Children, 5*(4), 35-43.

Florey, L. L. (1971). An approach to play and play development. *American Journal of Occupational Therapy, 25*(6), 275-280.

Florey, L. L. (1981). Studies of play: Implications for growth, development, and for clinical practice. *American Journal of Occupational Therapy, 35*(8), 519-524.

Friedli, C. (1994). Transdisciplinary play-based assessment: A study of reliability and validity. Unpublished doctoral dissertation, University of Colorado at Boulder.

Gardner, H. (1982). *Art, mind, and brain: A cognitive approach to creativity.* New York, NY: Basic Books.

Garvey, C. (1990). *Play.* Cambridge, MA: Harvard University Press.

Gilfoyle, E. M., Grady, A. P., & Moore, J. C. (1990). *Children adapt: A theory of sensorimotor-sensory development* (2nd ed.). Thorofare, NJ: SLACK Incorporated.

Gilmore, J. B. (1971). Play: A special behavior. In R. E. Herron & B. Sutton-Smith (Eds.), *Child's play* (pp. 311-325). New York, NY: John Wiley and Sons.

Godbey, G. C., & Jung, B. (1991). Relations between the development of culture and philosophies of leisure. In B. L. Driver, P. J. Brown, & G. L. Peterson (Eds.), *Benefits of leisure* (pp. 37-45). State College, PA: Venture Publishing.

Goodale, T. L., & Cooper, W. (1991). Philosophical perspectives on leisure in English-speaking countries. In B. L. Driver, P. J. Brown, & G. L. Peterson (Eds.), *Benefits of leisure* (pp. 25-35). State College, PA: Venture Publishing.

Gordon, W. R., & Caltabiano, M. L. (1996). Urban-rural differences in adolescent self-esteem, leisure boredom, and sensation-seeking as predictors of leisure-time usage and satisfaction. *Adolescence, 31*(124), 883-901.

Gould, J. (1986). The Lowe and Costello Symbolic Play Test in socially impaired children. *Journal of Autism and Developmental Disorders, 16*(2), 199-213.

Guitard, P., Ferland, F., & Dutil, E. (2005). Toward a better understanding of playfulness in adults. *OTJR: Occupation, Participation and Health, 25*(1), 9-22.

Hamm, E. M. (2006). Playfulness and the environmental support of play in children with and without developmental disabilities. *OTJR: Occupation, Participation and Health, 26*(3), 88-96.

Harkness, L., & Bundy, A. C. (2001). The Test of Playfulness and children with physical disabilities. *OTJR: Occupation, Participation and Health, 21*(2), 73-89.

Harris, P. L. (2000). *The work of the imagination.* Oxford, England: Wiley-Blackwell.

Harrison, H., & Kielhofner, G. (1986). Examining reliability and validity of the Preschool Play Scale with handicapped children. *American Journal of Occupational Therapy, 40*(3), 167-173.

Hawkins, B. A. (1993). An exploratory analysis of leisure and life satisfaction of aging adults with mental retardation. *Therapeutic Recreation Journal, 27*(2), 98-109.

Hawkins, B. A. (1994). Leisure as an adaptive skill area. *AAMR News & Notes, 7*(1), 5-6.

Hawkins, B. A., Ardovino, P., & Hsieh, C. M. (1998). Validity and reliability of the Leisure Assessment Inventory. *Mental Retardation, 36*(4), 303-313.

Hawkins, B. A., & Freeman, P. A. (1993). Correlates of self-reported leisure among adults with mental retardation. *Leisure Sciences, 15,* 131-147.

Heard, C. (1977). Occupational role acquisition: A perspective on the chronically disabled. *American Journal of Occupational Therapy, 31,* 243-247.

Henderson, K. A., Bialeschki, M. D., Hemingway, J. L., Hodges, J. S., Kivel, B. D., & Sessoms, H. D. (2001). *Introduction to recreation and leisure services* (8th ed.). State College, PA: Venture Publishing.

Hess, L. M., & Bundy, A. C. (2003). The association between playfulness and coping in adolescents. *Physical and Occupational Therapy in Pediatrics, 23*(2), 5-17.

Hughes, F. P. (1999). *Children, play, and development* (3rd ed.). Boston, MA: Allyn & Bacon.

Iso-Ahola, S. E., & Weissinger, E. (1990). Perceptions of boredom in leisure: Conceptualization, reliability, and validity of the Leisure Boredom Scale. *Journal of Leisure Research, 22*(1), 1-17.

Johnson, J. E., Christie, J. F., & Yawkey, T. D. (1987). *Play and early childhood development.* Glenview, IL: Scott Foresman.

Kalverboer, A. F. (1977). Measurement of play: Clinical application. In B. Tizard & D. Harvey (Eds.), *Biology of play* (pp. 100-122). Philadelphia, PA: Lippincott.

Katz, N. (1988). Interest checklist: A factor analytical study. *Occupational Therapy in Mental Health, 8*(1), 45-55.

Katz, N., Karpin, H., Lak, A., Furman, T., & Hartman-Maeir, A. (2003). Participation in occupational performance: Reliability and validity of the Activity Card Sort. *OTJR: Occupation, Participation and Health, 23*(1), 10-17.

Kelly, J. R. (1987). *Freedom to be: A new sociology of leisure.* New York, NY: Macmillan.

Kelly, J. R. (2000). Leisure, play, and recreation. In J. R. Kelly & V. J. Freysinger (Eds.), *21st century leisure: Current issues* (pp. 14-24). San Francisco, CA: Benjamin-Cummings Publishing Company.

Kelly-Vance, L., Needelman, H., Troia, K., & Ryalls, B. O. (1999). Early childhood assessment: A comparison of the Bayley Scales of Infant Development and a play-based assessment in two-year-old at-risk children. *Developmental Disabilities Bulletin, 27*(1), 1-15.

Kelly-Vance, L., & Ryalls, B. O. (2005). A systematic, reliable approach to play assessment in preschoolers. *School Psychology International, 26*(4), 398-412.

Kelly-Vance, L., Ryalls, B. O., & Glover, K. G. (2002). The use of play assessment to evaluate the cognitive skills of two- and three-year-old children. *School Psychology International, 23*(2), 169-185.

Kielhofner, G. (1995). Environmental influences on occupational behavior. In G. Kielhofner, *A model of human occupation: Theory and application* (pp. 91-111). Baltimore, MD: Lippincott Williams & Wilkins.

Kielhofner, G., Barris, R., Bauer, D., Shoestock, B., & Walker, L. (1983). A comparison of play behavior in nonhospitalized and hospitalized children. *American Journal of Occupational Therapy, 37*(5), 305-312.

King, G. A., Law, M., King, S., Hurley, P., Hanna, S., Kertoy, M, et al. (2007). Measuring children's participation in recreation and leisure activities: Construct validation of the CAPE and PAC. *Child: Care, Health and Development, 33*(1), 28-39.

King, G., Law, M., King, S., Rosenbaum, P., Kertoy, M. K., & Young, N. L. (2003). A conceptual model of the factors affecting the recreation and leisure participation of children with disabilities. *Physical and Occupational Therapy in Pediatrics, 23*(1), 63-90.

Kleiber, D. A. (1999). *Leisure experience and human development: A dialectical interpretation.* New York, NY: Basic Books.

Kloseck, M., Crilly, R. G., Ellis, G. D., & Lammers, E. (1996). Leisure Competence Measure: Development and reliability testing of a scale to measure functional outcomes in therapeutic recreation. *Therapeutic Recreation Journal, 30*(1), 13-26.

Kloseck, M., Crilly, R. G., & Hutchinson-Troyer, L. (2001). Measuring therapeutic recreation outcomes in rehabilitation: Further testing of the Leisure Competence Measure. *Therapeutic Recreation Journal, 35*(1), 31-42.

Klyczek, J. P., Bauer-Yox, N., & Fiedler, R. C. (1997). The Interest Checklist: A factor analysis. *American Journal of Occupational Therapy, 51*(10), 815-823.

Knox, S. (1974). A play scale. In M. Reilly (Ed.), *Play as exploratory learning: Studies of curiosity behavior* (pp. 247-266). Thousand Oaks, CA: Sage Publications.

Knox, S. (1997). Development and current use of the Knox Preschool Play Scale. In L. D. Parham & L. S. Fazio (Eds.), *Play in occupational therapy for children* (pp. 35-51). St. Louis, MO: Mosby.

Kubey, R., & Csikszentmihalyi, M. (1990). *Leisure and the benefits of television.* New Brunswick, NJ: L. Erlbaum.

LaVesser, P. D., Aird, L., & Lieberman, D. (2004). Scope of practice. *American Journal of Occupational Therapy, 58*(6), 673-677.

Law, M., Baptiste, S., McColl, M., Opzoomer, A., Polatajko, H., & Pollock, N. (1990). The Canadian Occupational Performance Measure: An outcome measure for occupational therapy. *Canadian Journal of Occupational Therapy, 57*(2), 82-87.

Law, M., King, G., King, S., Kertoy, M., Hurley, P., Rosenbaum, P., et al. (2006). Patterns of participation in recreational and leisure activities among children with complex physical disabilities. *Developmental Medicine and Child Neurology, 48*(5), 337-342.

Lawlor, M. C. (2003). The significance of being occupied: The social construction of childhood occupations. *American Journal of Occupational Therapy, 57*(4), 424-434.

Lawlor, M. C., & Henderson, A. (1989). A descriptive study of the clinical practice patterns of occupational therapists working with infants and young children. *American Journal of Occupational Therapy, 43*(11), 755-764.

Lieberman, J. N. (1977). *Playfulness: Its relationship to imagination and creativity.* New York, NY: Academic Press.

Liepold, E. E., & Bundy, A. C. (2000). Playfulness in children with attention deficit hyperactivity disorder. *OTJR: Occupation, Participation, and Health, 20*(1), 61-82.

Linder, T. W. (1993). *Transdisciplinary Play-Based Assessment: A functional approach to working with young children* (2nd ed.). Baltimore, MD: Paul H. Brookes.

Lloyd, K. M., & Auld, C. J. (2002). The role of leisure in determining quality of life: Issues of content and measurement. *Social Indicators Research, 57*(1), 43-71.

Lowe, M., & Costello, A. J. (1988). *Symbolic Play Test* (2nd ed.). Windsor, Berkshire, England: NFER-Nelson.

Lyons, M. (1987). A taxonomy of playfulness for use in occupational therapy. *Australian Journal of Occupational Therapy, 34*(4), 152-156.

Lysyk, M., Brown, G. T., Rodrigues, E., McNally, J., & Loo, K. (2002). Translation of the Leisure Satisfaction Scale into French: A validation study. *Occupational Therapy International, 9*(1), 76-89.

Malone, D. M. (1999). Contextual factors informing play-based program planning. *International Journal of Disability, Development and Education, 46*(3), 307-324.

Mann, W. C., & Talty, P. (1991). Leisure Activity Profile: Measuring use of leisure time by persons with alcoholism. *Occupational Therapy in Mental Health, 10*(4), 31-41.

Matsutsuyu, J. S. (1967). The Interest Checklist. *American Journal of Occupational Therapy, 11*, 179-181.

Matsutsuyu, J. S. (1969). The Interest Checklist. *American Journal of Occupational Therapy, 23*(4), 323-328.

McCune-Nicholich, L., & Bruskin, C. (1982). Combinatorial competency in symbolic play and language. In D. J. Pepler & K. H. Rubin (Eds.), *The play of children: Current theory and research* (Vol. 6, pp. 30-45). New York, NY: Karger.

McDowell, C. F. (1984). An evolving theory of leisure consciousness. *Society and Leisure, 7*, 53-87.

Mellou, E. (1994). Play theories: A contemporary review. *Early Child Development and Care, 102*, 91-100.

Mendez, J. L., Fantuzzo, J., & Cicchetti, D. (2002). Profiles of social competence among low-income African American preschool children. *Child Development, 73*(4), 1085-1100.

Mendez, J. L., McDermott, P., & Fantuzzo, J. (2002). Identifying and promoting social competence with African American preschool children: Developmental and contextual considerations. *Psychology in the Schools, 39*(1), 111-123.

Michelman, S. (1974). Play and the deficit child. In M. Reilly (Ed.), *Play as exploratory learning* (pp. 157-207). Thousand Oaks, CA: Sage Publications.

Morrison, C. D., Bundy, A. C., & Fisher, A. G. (1991). The contribution of motor skills and playfulness to the play performance of preschoolers. *American Journal of Occupational Therapy, 45*(8), 687-694.

Morrison, C., & Metzger, P. (2001). Play. In J. Case-Smith, A. S. Allen, & P. N. Pratt (Eds.), *Occupational therapy for children* (pp. 528-544). St. Louis, MO: Mosby.

Muys, V., Rodger, S., & Bundy, A. C. (2006). Assessment of playfulness in children with autistic disorder: A comparison of the Children's Playfulness Scale and the Test of Playfulness. *OTJR: Occupation, participation and Health, 26*(4), 159-170.

Myers, C. L., McBride, S. L., & Peterson, C. (1996). Transdisciplinary, play-based assessment in early childhood special education: An examination of social validity. *Topics in Early Childhood Special Education, 16*, 102-127.

Neisworth, J. T., & Bagnato, S. J. (1988). Assessment in early childhood special education: A typology for independent measures. In S. L. Odom & M. B. Karnes (Eds.), *Early intervention for infants and children with handicaps: An empirical base* (pp. 23-49). Baltimore, MD: Paul H. Brookes Publishing Co.

Neulinger, J. (1981). *To leisure: An introduction*. Boston, MA: Allyn & Bacon.

Neuman, E. A. (1971). *The elements of play*. New York, NY: MSS Information Corp.

O'Brien, J., Coker, P., Lynn, R., Suppinger, R., Pearigen, T., Rabon, S., et al. (2000). The impact of occupational therapy on a child's playfulness. *Occupational Therapy in Health Care, 12*(2), 39-51.

O'Brien, J. C., & Shirley, R. J. (2001). Does playfulness change over time? A preliminary look using the Test of Playfulness. *Occupational Therapy Journal of Research, 21*(2), 132-139.

Okimoto, A. M., Bundy, A., & Hanzlik, J. (2000). Playfulness in children with and without disability: Measurement and intervention. *American Journal of Occupational Therapy, 54*(1), 73-82.

Olsen, L. J. (1999). Psychosocial frame of reference. In P. Kramer & J. Hinojosa (Eds.), *Frames of reference for pediatric occupational therapy* (2nd ed., pp. 323-375). Baltimore, MD: Lippincott Williams & Wilkins.

Ornstein, R., & Sobel, D. (1989). *Healthy pleasures*. Reading, MA: Addison-Wesley.

Parham, L. D. (1996). Perspectives on play. In R. Zemke & F. Clark (Eds.), *Occupational science: The evolving discipline* (pp. 71-80). Philadelphia, PA: F.A. Davis.

Parham, L. D., & Primeau, L. A. (1997). Play and occupational therapy. In L. D. Parham & L. S. Fazio (Eds.), *Play in occupational therapy for children* (pp. 2-21). St. Louis, MO: Mosby.

Parr, M. G., & Lashua, B. D. (2004). What is leisure? The perceptions of recreation practitioners and others. *Leisure Sciences, 26*(1), 1-17.

Parr, M. G., & Lashua, B. D. (2005). Students' perceptions of leisure, leisure professionals and the professional body of knowledge. *Journal of Hospitality, Leisure, Sport, and Tourism Education, 4*(2), 16-26.

Passmore, A. (2003). The occupation of leisure: Three typologies and their influence on mental health in adolescence. *OTJR: Occupation, Participation and Health, 23*(2), 76-83.

Peebles, J., McWilliams, L., Norris, L. H., & Park, K. (1999). Population-specific norms and reliability of the Leisure Diagnostic Battery in a sample of patients with chronic pain. *Therapeutic Recreation Journal, 33*(3), 135-141.

Power, T. J., & Radcliffe, J. (1989). The relationship of play behavior to cognitive ability in developmentally disabled preschoolers. *Journal of Autism and Developmental Disorders,19*(1), 97-107.

Primeau, L. A. (1996). Work and leisure: Transcending the dichotomy. *American Journal of Occupational Therapy, 50*(7), 569-577.

Primeau, L. (2003). Play and leisure. In E. B. Crepeau, E. S. Cohn, & B. A. Boyt Schell (Eds.), *Willard & Spackman's occupational therapy* (10th ed., pp. 354-363). New York, NY: Lippincott Williams & Wilkins.

Primeau, L. A., & Ferguson, J. F. (1999). Occupational frame of reference. In P. Kramer & J. Hinojosa (Eds.), *Frames of reference for pediatric occupational therapy* (2nd ed., pp. 469-516). Philadelphia, PA: Lippincott Williams, & Wilkins.

Primeau, L. A., Clark, F., & Pierce, D. (1989). Occupational therapy alone has looked upon occupation: Future applications of occupational science to pediatric occupational therapy. *Occupational Therapy in Health Care, 6*, 19-32.

Ragheb, M. G., & Beard, J. G. (1982). Measuring leisure attitude. *Journal of Leisure Research, 14*(2), 155-167.

Ragheb, M. G., & Griffith, C. A. (1982). The contribution of leisure participation and leisure satisfaction to life satisfaction of older persons. *Journal of Leisure Research, 14*(4), 295-306.

Ragheb, M. G., & Tate, R. L. (1993). A behavioral model of leisure participation, based on leisure attitude, motivation and satisfaction. *Leisure Studies, 12*(1), 61-70.

Raj, J. T., Manigandan, C., & Jacob, K. S. (2006). Leisure satisfaction and psychiatric morbidity among informal carers of people with spinal cord injury. *Spinal Cord, 44*(11), 676-679.

Reed, C. N., Dunbar, S. B., & Bundy, A. C. (2000). The effects of an inclusive preschool experience on the playfulness of children with and without autism. *Physical & Occupational Therapy in Pediatrics, 19*(3), 73-89.

Reilly, M. (1974). *Play as exploratory learning*. Thousand Oaks, CA: Sage Publications.

Restall, G., & Magill-Evans, J. (1994). Play and preschool children with autism. *American Journal of Occupational Therapy, 48*(2), 113-120.

Rodger, S., & Ziviani, J. (1999). Play-based occupational therapy. *International Journal of Disability, Development and Education, 46*(3), 337-365.

Rodger, S., & Ziviani, J. (Eds.). (2006). *Occupational therapy with children: Understanding children's occupations and enabling participation*. Malden, MA: Wiley-Blackwell.

Rogers, J. C., Weinstein, J. M., & Figone, J. J. (1978). The interest check list: An empirical assessment. *American Journal of Occupational Therapy, 32*(10), 628-630.

Roopnarine, J. L., & Johnson, J. E. (1994). The need to look at play in diverse cultural settings. In J. L. Roopnarine, J. E. Johnson, & F. H. Hooper (Eds.), *Children's play in diverse cultures* (pp. 1-8). Albany, NY: State University of New York Press.

Rubin, K. H. (1982). Early play theories revisited: Contributions to contemporary research and theory. In D. J. Pepler & K. H. Rubin (Eds.), *Play of children: Current theory and research* (Vol. 6, pp. 4-14). New York, NY: Karger.

Rubin, K. H., Fein, G. G., & Vandenberg, B. (1983). Play. In P. Mussen & E. M. Hetherington (Eds.), *Handbook of child psychology, socialization, personality and social development* (Vol. 4, 4th ed., pp. 693-774). New York, NY: Wiley.

Russ, S. W. (2003). Play and creativity: Developmental issues. *Scandinavian Journal of Educational Research, 47*(3), 291-303.

Sachs, D., & Josman, N. (2003). The Activity Card Sort: A factor analysis. *OTJR: Occupation, Participation and Health, 23*(4), 165-174.

Saltz, E., & Brodie, J. (1982). Pretend play training in childhood: A review and critique. In D. J. Pepler & K. H. Rubin (Eds.), *Play of children: Current theory and research* (Vol. 6, pp. 97-113). New York, NY: Karger.

Saracho, O. N., & Spodek, B. (1995). Children's play and early childhood education: Insights from history and theory. *Journal of Education, 177*(3), 129-148.

Saunders, I., Sayer, M., & Goodale, A. (1999). The relationship between playfulness and coping in preschool children: A pilot study. *American Journal of Occupational Therapy, 53*(2), 221-226.

Schaaf, R. C. (1990). Play behavior and occupational therapy. *American Journal of Occupational Therapy, 44*(1), 68-75.

Sellar, B., & Boshoff, K. (2006). Subjective leisure experiences of older Australians. *Australian Occupational Therapy Journal, 53*(3), 211-219.

Shepherd, J., Brollier, C., & Dandrow, R. (1994). Play skills of preschool children with speech and language delays. *Physical and Occupational Therapy in Pediatrics, 14*(2), 1-20.

Siegenthaler, K. L., & O'Dell, I. (2000). Leisure attitude, leisure satisfaction, and perceived freedom in leisure within family dyads. *Leisure Sciences, 22*(4), 281-296.

Singer, D. G., & Singer, J. L. (1992). *The house of make-believe: Children's play and the developing imagination*. Cambridge, MA: Harvard University Press.

Stagnitti, K. (2004). Understanding play: The implications for play assessment. *Australian Occupational Therapy Journal, 51*(1), 3-12.

Stagnitti, K., & Unsworth, C. (2000). The importance of pretend play in child development: An occupational therapy perspective. *British Journal of Occupational Therapy, 63*(3), 121-127.

Stagnitti, K., & Unsworth, C. (2004). The test-retest reliability of the Child-Initiated Pretend Play Assessment. *American Journal of Occupational Therapy, 58*(1), 93-99.

Stagnitti, K., Unsworth, C., & Rodger, S. (2000). Development of an assessment to identify play behaviors that discriminate between the play of typical preschoolers and preschoolers with pre-academic problems. *Canadian Journal of Occupational Therapy, 67*(5), 291-303.

Stanley, M. (1995). An investigation into the relationship between engagement in valued occupations and life satisfaction for elderly South Australians. *Journal of Occupational Science, 2*(3), 100-114.

Sturgess, J. L. (1997). Current trend in assessing children's play. *British Journal of Occupational Therapy, 60*(9), 410-414.

Suto, M. (1998). Leisure in occupational therapy. *Canadian Journal of Occupational Therapy, 65*(5), 271-278.

Sutton-Smith, B. (1967). The role of play in cognitive development. *Young Children, 22*, 361-370.

Sutton-Smith, B. (1980). A sportive theory of play. In H. B. Schwartzman (Ed.), *Play and culture* (pp. 10-19). West Point, NY: Leisure Press.

Swindells, D., & Stagnitti, K. (2006). Pretend play and parents' view of social competence: The construct validity of the Child-Initiated Pretend Play Assessment. *Australian Occupational Therapy Journal, 53*(4), 314-324.

Takata, N. (1969). The play history. *American Journal of Occupational Therapy, 23*(4), 314-318.

Takata, N. (1974). Play as prescription. In M. Reilly (Ed.), *Play as exploratory learning* (pp. 209-246). Thousand Oaks, CA: Sage Publications.

Tanta, K. J., Deitz, J. C., White, O., & Billingsley, F. (2005). The effects of peer-play level on initiations and responses of preschool children with delayed play skills. *American Journal of Occupational Therapy, 59*(4), 437-445.

Tegano, D. W. (1990). Relationship of tolerance ambiguity and playfulness to creativity. *Psychological Reports, 66*, 1047-1056.

Thomas, D. W. (1999). Evaluating the relationship between premorbid leisure preferences and wandering among patients with dementia. *Activities, Adapting and Aging, 23*(4), 33-48.

Tinsley, H. A., & Tinsley, D. J. (1986). A theory of attributes, benefits, and causes of the leisure experience. *Leisure Sciences, 8*, 1-45.

Trombly, C. (1993). Anticipating the future: Assessment of occupational function. *American Journal of Occupational Therapy, 47*(3), 253-257.

Trottier, A. N., Brown, G. T., Hobson, S. J., & Miller, W. (2002). Reliability and validity of the Leisure Satisfaction Scale (LSS—short form) and the Adolescent Leisure Interest Profile (ALIP). *Occupational Therapy International, 9*(2), 131-144.

Tsao, L. (2002). How much do we know about the importance of play in child development? Review of research. *Childhood Education, 78*(4), 230-234.

Veal, A. J., & Lynch, R. (2001). *Australian leisure* (2nd ed.). Frenchs Forest, New South Wales, Australia: Longman.

von Zuben, M. V., Crist, P. A., & Mayberry, W. (1991). A pilot study of differences in play behavior between children of low and middle socioeconomic status. *American Journal of Occupational Therapy, 45*(2), 113-118.

Wallen, M., & Walker, R. (1995). Occupational therapy practice with children with perceptual motor dysfunction: Findings of a literature review and survey. *Australian Occupational Therapy Journal, 42*, 15-25.

Wegner, L., Flisher, A. J., Muller, M., & Lombard, C. (2002). Reliability of the Leisure Boredom Scale for use with high school learners in Cape Town, South Africa. *Journal of Leisure Research, 34*(3), 340-351.

West, J. (1990). Play, work, and play therapy: Distinctions and definitions. *Adoption and Fostering, 14*(4), 31-37.

Wicker, A. W. (1987). Behavior settings reconsidered: Temporal stages, resources, internal dynamics, context. In D. Stokols & I. Altman (Eds.), *Handbook of environmental psychology* (pp. 613-653). New York, NY: Wiley.

Witt, P. A., & Ellis, G. D. (1984). The Leisure Diagnostic Battery: Measuring perceived freedom in leisure. *Society and Leisure, 7*(1), 109-124.

Yerxa, E. J., Clark, F., Jackson, J., Parham, D., Pierce, D., Stein, C., et al. (1989). An introduction to occupational science, a foundation for occupational therapy in the 21st century. *Occupational Therapy in Health Care, 6*(4), 1-17.

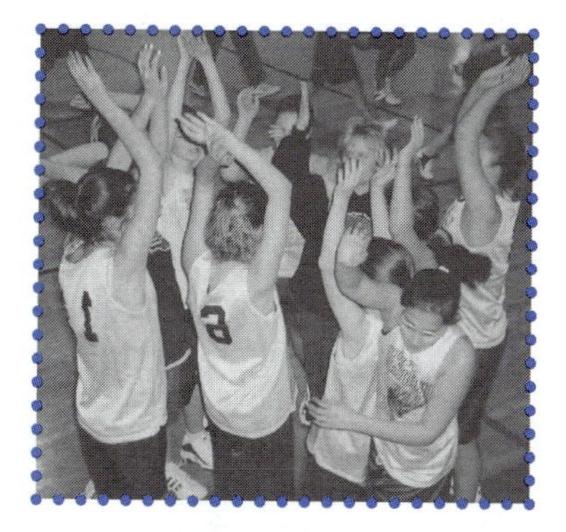

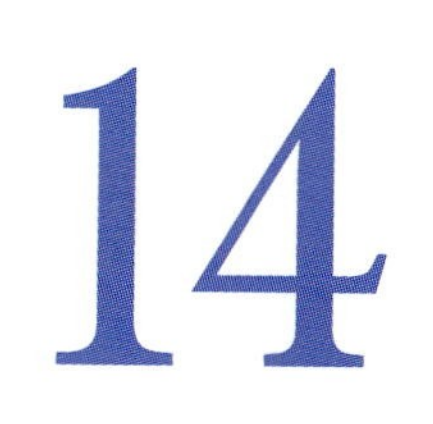

# 14

# Evaluation of Social Participation

*Mary V. Donohue, PhD, OTL, FAOTA*

**ACOTE Standard Explored in This Chapter**

B.4.4

**Key Terms**

Associative level participation
Basic cooperative level participation
Mature level participation
Parallel level participation
Social participation
Supportive cooperative level participation

## Introduction

Several of the basic tenets of occupational therapy relate closely to the principles of interpersonal interactions and relationships emphasized by the *International Classification of Functioning, Disability, and Health* (ICF) of the World Health Organization (WHO) in its section on Activities and Participation (2001). The role of the occupational therapist is delineated as one who understands the "effects of health, disability, disease processes, and traumatic injury to the individual within the context of family and society" (ACOTE, B.2.7, 1998).

In particular, ICF guidelines point out the importance of every level of relationship from how to relate appropriately to strangers as well as in formal and informal, family, and intimate relationships (WHO, 2001) that can apply to occupational therapy and practitioners' intervention focus in social performance.

The Accreditation Council for Occupational Therapy Education (ACOTE) tenets also expect clinicians to understand how vital the balance of performance areas are to health, wellness, and quality of life. These tenets echo the ICF expectations of becoming a part of organized social life outside the family by developing community and civic relationships (WHO, 2001). Perceptions developed in evaluating the social participation of individuals are preparation for designing interventions for both individual and group interactions. The therapeutic use of self, a social approach to intervention, has been designated as a means of achieving therapeutic goals. These same perceptions developed in observing individuals and groups and in designing interventions prepare the practitioner to consider social aspects of the larger community for an understanding of contextual factors in the management of service delivery.

## Social Skill Tools in Occupational Therapy

Several occupational therapy tools partially addressing social issues are reviewed here. They include the Bay Area Functional Performance Evaluation (BaFPE), the Assessment and Communication of Interaction Skills (ACIS), the Role Activity Performance Scale (RAPS), and the Model of Human Occupation Screening Tool (MOHOST).



K. Sladyk, K. Jacobs, & N. MacRae (Eds.).
*Occupational Therapy Essentials for Clinical Competence* (pp. 151-160).

The BaFPE (Bloomer & Williams, 1979) was developed as a comprehensive tool with Part B called the Social Interaction Scale. This assessment examines people through interviews, at mealtime, and in unstructured and structured oral and activity groups. It examines their verbal communications, psychomotor behaviors, social appropriateness, response to authority, independence, ability to work with others, and participation in groups and programs. The BaFPE evaluates individuals but not a group as a whole. See Table 14-1 for research carried out to provide evidence of the BaFPE's usefulness. For further research on the BaFPE, refer to Hemphill-Pearson's book on mental health assessment tools (1999).

The ACIS (Forsyth, Salamy, Simon, & Kielhofner, 1998) also focuses on individuals and the skills they use to accomplish occupations of daily living. The behavioral categories of the ACIS include an examination of physicality, information exchange, and relations with others. Specifically, as examples, it looks at gestures, focus of attention, and respect for others as items of assessment. Table 14-1 provides citations of studies used to provide evidence of the value of the ACIS.

The RAPS (Good-Ellis, 1987) includes a social role component as 1 of 12 sections. Likewise, the Occupational Performance History Inventory (OPHI) (Kielhofner et al., 2005) includes social roles from the individual's present and past in a semi-structured interview.

In 2006, MOHOST was developed (Kielhofner et al., 2009; G. Kielhofner, personal communication, November 3, 2006). It includes a section on communication and interaction skills, assessing behavioral categories of nonverbal cues, conversation, vocal expression, and relationships. Studies using the Rasch model, factor analysis, and analysis of variance (ANOVA) are in the process of developing this tool. To track this process, there is online access to the University of Illinois at Chicago Department of Occupational Therapy MOHO Clearinghouse. This tool also studies individuals (see Table 14-1).

For further references to assessment tools used in occupational therapy, see *Occupational Therapy Assessment Tools: An Annotated Index*, a comprehensive volume that includes tools from psychology (Asher, 2007).

In summary, all of these tools described previously examining the dimensions of social participation focus on detailed interaction skills by individuals, which is valuable. However, most treatment of social skills in occupational therapy is carried out in activity groups. In order to assess the larger issues of levels of interaction in groups and of individuals in groups, a theoretical construct with dimensions of social skill developmental stages was selected to design a social profile as criteria for evaluation. A later section will provide the background of designing such a profile.

## Social Participation Studies

Several occupational therapy studies in 2004 focused on evaluating social participation. Bedell and Dumas (2004) carried out research examining social participation of

**Table 14-1. Tools Used in Occupational Therapy Evaluating Social Participation in Individuals and in Groups**

| Tool Focus | Behavioral Categories | Research |
|---|---|---|
| Bay Area Functional Performance Evaluation (BaFPE) (1979): Individuals<br>Part B: Social Interaction Scale (SIS) during: Interview of individual, mealtime, unstructured group situation, structured activity group, structured oral group | 1. Verbal communications<br>2. Psychomotor behaviors<br>3. Socially appropriate<br>4. Response to authority<br>5. Independence/dependence<br>6. Ability to work with others<br>7. Participation in group and program activities | Klyczek, Bloomer, & Fiedler, 1999; Klyczek & Mann, 1990; Mann & Klyczek, 1991 |
| Assessment and Communication of Interaction Skills (ACIS) (1998): Individuals<br>Used to accomplish occupations of daily living—gesturing, respecting others, focusing | 1. Physicality<br>2. Information exchange<br>3. Relations with others | Forsyth, Lai, & Kielhofner, 1999; Helfrich & Aviles, 2001; Keller & Forsyth, 2004 |
| Model of Human Occupation Screening Tool (MOHOST) (2006): Individuals<br>Section on communication and interaction skills | 1. Nonverbal cues<br>2. Conversation<br>3. Vocal expression<br>4. Relationships | Parkinson, Forsyth, & Kielhofner, 2006.; G. Kielhofner, personal communication, November 3, 2006 |
| Social Profile (Unpublished): Groups or individuals<br>Parallel level, associative level, basic cooperative level, supportive cooperative | 1. Activity participation<br>2. Social interaction<br>3. Group membership and roles | Donohue, 2003, 2005, 2007, 2009 |

children and youth with acquired brain injuries who had been treated in inpatient rehabilitation. They found children to be most restricted in peer social play and structured community activity in contrast to activities carried out at home.

Coster and Haltiwanger (2004) used Part III, Activity Performance, of the School Function Assessment (Coster, Deeney, Haltiwanger, & Haley, 1998) to measure social behavior skills of elementary children with physical disabilities who were included in general education classrooms. On 6 of the 7 scales, more than 40% of students with physical disabilities performed below the expected grade level for social skills.

Bedell, Coster, and Law are continuing to develop measures of activity participation and environment through sponsorship by the U. S. Department of Education (2007-2010). They are standardizing these instruments through psychometric testing.

## Integration of Evaluation With Concepts of Social Participation

On the one hand, many people perceive the evaluation of social participation as abstract, complex, and subjective in nature. On the other hand, a recent study (Roney, Hanson, Durante, & Maestripieri, 2006) indicated that people in general size up social cues in potential mates whom they perceive will like children and are kind to others. The challenge here is how practitioners can evaluate, as accurately as possible, within a range of social levels of function because the assessment of social cues is not a hard science.

In this chapter, there is a need to distinguish between the conceptual parts of the term *social activity participation*. Throughout occupational therapy intervention, activity participation is planned for and incorporated as its basis. In group settings of intervention, the type of participation designed and expected is social activity participation. This distinction is necessary because many mechanical or physical types of intervention may employ activity participation for individuals but not social activity participation (Isaksson, Lexell, & Skär, 2007). Social participation can be defined as consisting of verbal and interpersonal activity interactions among people.

In 1932, Parten designed a study to evaluate activity group participation of preschool children using the concepts of parallel, associative, and cooperative play. Parten's theoretical base was developmental across children's ages, with the expectation that children would function at higher levels of participation as they advanced in age. She observed 30 children—six children in each of five preschool ages. Collecting 360 data points, Parten reported an association between ages and the three developmental group concept levels. Parten defined the concepts of participation as follows:

- *Parallel participation*: Play, activity, or work side-by-side without interaction. Examples include children playing side-by-side in a sandbox without talking, and seniors doing movement to music (Figure 14-1).
- *Associative participation*: Approaching others briefly in verbal or nonverbal interactions. Examples include the games of "Simon Says" and "Musical Chairs" with brief interactions, and adults using a parachute and calling each other's names to run underneath the parachute and change places (Figure 14-2).
- *Basic cooperative participation*: Selecting longer activity or tasks for mutual self-interest. Examples include dressing up in costumes to role play and adults choosing to play charades where two teams of people compete against each other (Figure 14-3).

Over the years, many child psychologists have evaluated children's groups using Parten's concepts. More recently, Parten's schema or construct of group participation has been used to evaluate outdoor play, symbolic play, block play, cooperative play, day care center, and free play programs (Aureli & Colecchia, 1996; Fantuzzo et al, 1996;

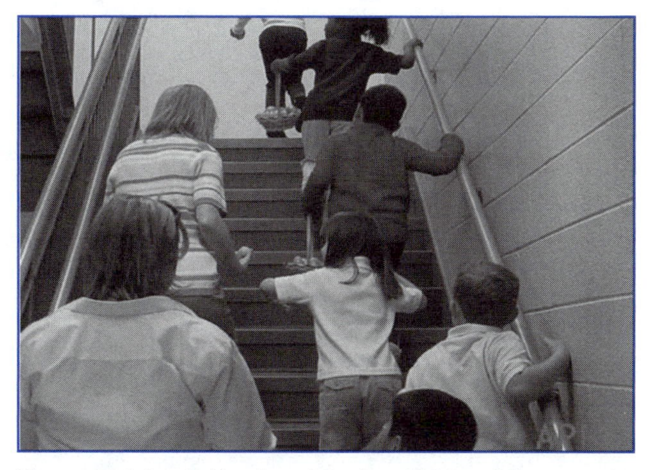

**Figure 14-1.** Parallel level participation: Children follow upstairs without interaction one by one, behind each other.

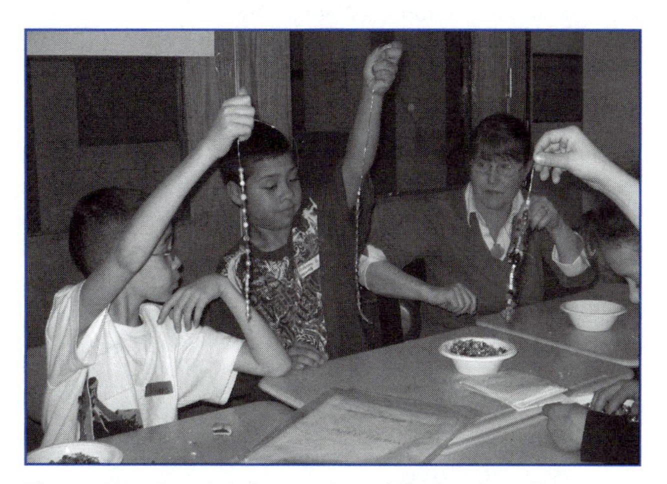

**Figure 14-2.** Boys briefly associate while showing off creativity in a group activity of beading.

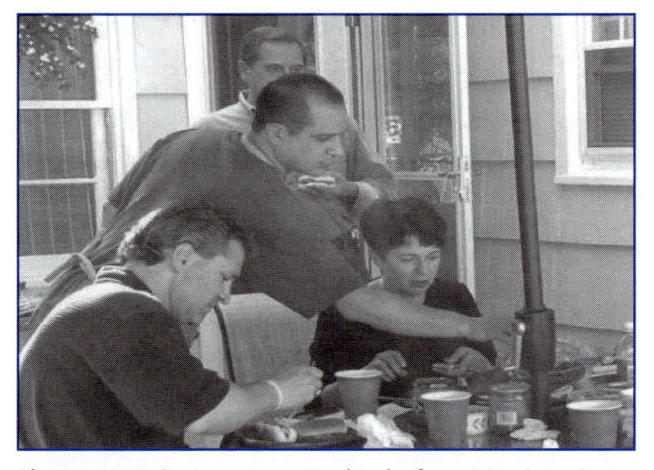

**Figure 14-3.** Basic cooperative level of participation: Group members coordinate a longer, structured task of picnic preparation and eating together.

Field, 1984; Garnier & Latour, 1994; Guralnick, 1990; Howes, 1988; Petrakos & Howe, 1996; Saracho, 1993). All but one study confirmed the association of the children's ages with their level of participation delineated by Parten's three concepts (see the Evidence-Based Research Chart at the end of the chapter).

In Mosey's developmental frame of reference (1968, 1986), she incorporated the concepts of Parten and added participation levels of performance for adolescents and adults. She separated the cooperative level into two parts—an Egocentric Cooperative level and a Cooperative level—and added a Mature level. While Mosey's interaction skills appeared to have clinical face validity, they were not tested empirically until recently. However, the concepts of Mosey's five levels of social interactive skills have appealed to many occupational therapy practitioners who continue to publish them in recent textbooks (Borg & Bruce, 1991; Cole, 2005; Howe & Schwartzberg, 2001; Posthuma, 2002) and use them in activity group process therapy. These five level concepts have formatted the perceptual observations and interventions of occupational therapy practitioners working in mental health, pediatric, rehabilitation medicine, and geriatric settings.

# The Social Profile

In order to empirically evaluate the concepts of social participation as valid and reliable and then evaluate the level of performance of individuals and group members, a tool of a developmental nature was designed and named the Social Profile (Donohue, 2009). For the Social Profile, *supportive cooperative* and *mature participation* are defined as follows:

- Supportive cooperative participation consists of interactions that express feelings and emotions designed to foster social cohesion.
- Mature participation combines basic and supportive cooperative participation fostering task completion and social interaction.

The five levels of social participation concepts (Parallel, Associative, Basic Cooperative, Supportive Cooperative, and Mature) were assembled in an ordinal manner and rated using a Likert scale of 0 to 5. Forty items spread across the five levels were arranged under three topics of activity participation, social interaction, and group membership/roles. These three topics provide an analysis of group participation skill levels designed for practitioners to understand the meaning and dynamics of evaluation of interactive occupation in an appropriate context. Activity participation items evaluate social performance contexts of interaction fostered by the activity. Social interaction items evaluate performance components of a psychosocial nature. Finally, group membership/roles items evaluate performance areas of application to the family and society.

In defining the additional levels of social participation for adolescents and adults, the conceptual terms have been modified, as indicated previously in defining basic cooperative participation, by changing the label from egocentric cooperative. This new label was considered because in situations where people might self-evaluate using the social profile, they would not wish to designate themselves as egocentric. The upper two developmental concepts of participation have been defined as follows:

1. *Supportive cooperative participation*: Enjoys homogeneous membership and fulfills emotional needs. For example, teens decorating a gym for a dance, enjoying each other's company, listening to music, and expressing their feelings about the words of songs (Figure 14-4).
2. *Mature participation*: Mutual leadership balances activity goals and emotional needs. For example, members of a writers' critique group giving feedback about each other's writings and providing suggestions for edits and changes (Figure 14-5).

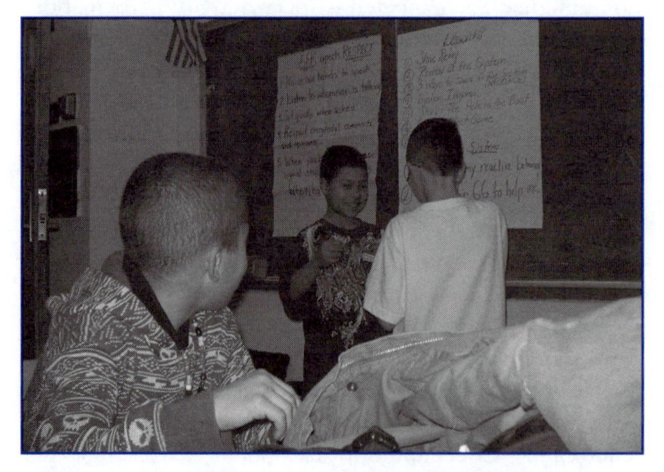

**Figure 14-4.** In a Supportive Cooperative manner, two boys express emotion in role playing scenarios in class.

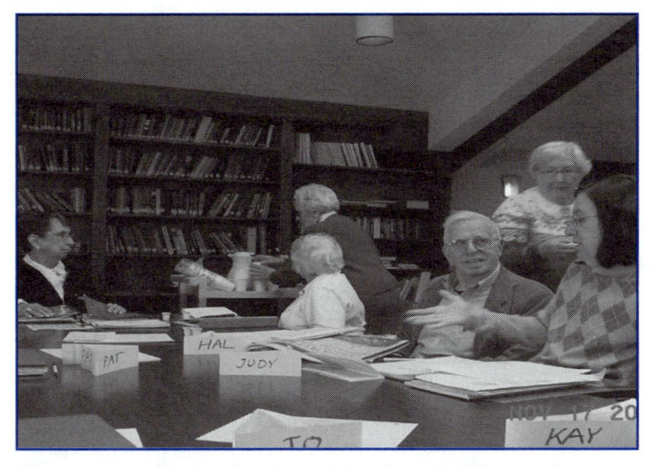


**Figure 14-5.** Mature level participation: Members take turns leading the group, a book discussion club, combining Basic and Supportive participation, so that the task is as important as the group interaction and emotions.

The items for the profile were drawn from a large universe of possible behaviors in social situations in clinical practice and group processes literature (Borg & Bruce, 1991; Cole, 2005; Howe & Schwartzberg, 2001; Johnson, D. & Johnson, F., 2000; Lisina, 1985; Mosey, 1986; Parten, 1932). They were narrowed to a practical number of items through the assistance of 11 expert occupational therapy master practitioners who served as judges.

Groups and individuals in groups can perform at several levels of participation even within one session depending on the activities and the individual's social skills, thus his or her participation is summarized and recorded on a profile graph. Groups and individuals in groups can also participate at levels across the developmental group interaction range, even levels below their prime or highest level, if the activity calls for participation at an earlier level. An example would be a group of seniors who are capable of interacting in a mature group preparing food packets for needy neighbors, but for an exercise group, they appropriately participate at a parallel level of performance.

# Expertise in Observation for Evaluation of Social Participation

Some people are "naturals" at keen observation of other's social participation. Many have acquired expertise through experience with working with individuals and groups of people. Others need guidance or structure to learn what to discern. For some practitioners, an assessment tool can provide structure, which will develop observation skills. In whichever of these categories practitioners find themselves, professional development demands that the prospective observer review the available guidelines, manual, or training opportunities before beginning to use a tool. Some of the methods employed to prepare students and therapists to use the social profile are training workshops, in-service presentations, seminars, individual coaching, videotapes, worksheets, and discussion. Of these methods, discussion with others and with someone familiar with the developmental model of social participation or this tool is most helpful (Smith, 1986). If an observer is at the beginning of the process of developing observation skills, the use of a general observation worksheet during 30 minutes in groups is recommended. Factors such as cooperation, goals, roles, activity involvement, power, attraction, norms, and interaction are valuable to begin with as a focus of interpersonal aspects of function (Borg & Bruce, 1991; Cole, 2005; Howe & Schwartzberg, 2001; Johnson, D. & Johnson, F., 2000; Posthuma, 2002). Familiarity with these general components of activity group process before undertaking observations with the social profile or other tool for measurement of social participation adds to the validity and reliability of the results.

While assessment in the field of occupational therapy is the prerogative of the registered therapist, certified occupational therapy assistants may report and discuss behavioral observations from groups with their occupational therapist supervisor.

# Tests of Validity and Reliability of the Social Profile

## Design of the Studies

Tests of content, construct, and criterion validity were carried out, along with an exploratory factor analysis to study the validity of the social profile. Item analysis internal consistency and interrater reliability statistical analyses were also undertaken (Donohue, 2003, 2005, 2007).

## Participants

For the validity and item analysis research, a study of 21 groups of preschool children ($n$ = 242) ranging from 2 to 5 years of age, with a minimum of 53 children in each age group was designed. These were typically developing children of a variety of socioeconomic and ethnic backgrounds. Observations were made of groups as a unit engaged in free play in an effort to study the children engaged in activities that they selected (Donohue, 2003).

## Construct Validity

Using age groups as a developmental guide or construct, the relationship between age and social participation skills of the Social Profile was examined. Results yielded correlations in the expected range for 2 and 3 year olds with parallel behaviors ($r$ = .8805), for 3 and 4 year olds with associative behaviors ($r$ = .7139), and for 4- and 5-year-old groups with basic cooperative behaviors ($r = .8309$). All correlations' probability was $p = .0003$ or less. The age groups were clustered in overlapping ranges since, as observed in social participation, social behaviors are developed gradually across a sliding, overlaying scale or continuum (Donohue, 2003).

## Criterion Validity

Using Parten's (1932) research results as a criteria, this type of validity study was designed to compare the social profile's data on the three basic levels of parallel, associative, and basic cooperative levels in an overall correlation. The Spearman correlation coefficient of Parten's age associated that concept results compared to those of the Social Profile was $r = .85$ at the $p = .01$ level of confidence (Donohue, 2003).

## Interrater Reliability

Several populations—children, seniors, and psychiatric and drug-abusing adults—were observed by pairs of students and clinician and student pairs using the social profile. The groups were located in inpatient psychiatric services, schools, and senior centers. An intraclass correlation coefficient (ICC) statistic was .8359, or .84 for interrater reliability (Donohue, 2007). Certified occupational therapy assistants on these units assisted in the research by approaching prospective participants to invite them into the study.

# Further Evaluation of Social Participation in the Social Profile

A factor analysis and test of internal consistency reliability were carried out in early stages of development of the social profile and can be examined in earlier literature (Donohue, 2003, 2005, 2007).

An expanded study is underway in a hospital on several units: in adult drug rehabilitation groups and psychiatric and geriatric inpatient groups. In addition, a training video of community adult groups is being prepared by one occupational therapy academic program for training practitioners and students in the use of the social profile.

# Summary

While several published and unpublished occupational therapy tools include items and sections examining the area of social participation, the social profile is broadly devoted to the measurement of social participation around activities and roles that group members assume during group interaction for clinical, educational, and well populations. ACOTE (2006) reminds occupational therapy students and practitioners of the importance of social and behavioral foundations of intervention across the life span. The social profile incorporates levels of social function for children, adolescents, adults, and senior groups.

In emphasizing the need for standardized and nonstandardized screening and assessment tools, *ACOTE Standards* (2006) provide opportunity for both occupational therapy clinicians and assistants to begin with their informal observations of human social behavior in social settings. Occupational therapy assistants can report and discuss their observations of social participation during therapy groups with their occupational therapy supervisors and other team professionals. The occupational therapists may then validate and record these social participation behaviors on occupational therapy assessment tools such as have been described in this chapter in order to determine therapeutic levels of intervention for the individuals and groups whom they and the occupational therapy assistants treat.

# Student Self-Assessment

1. Are my observation skills adequate to use the social profile?
2. Do I need training or practice to strengthen my skills of observation of group interaction?
3. Is my knowledge of the statistical aspects of evaluation of social participation mentioned in this chapter current? Do I need to review my statistics and research books and notes?
4. Would I like to study some aspect of social participation in a research study during my student program in occupational therapy?
5. Should internet sites, exchanges, or chat room interaction be considered social participation?

# Electronic Resources

- National Alliance of the Mentally Ill: www.nami.org
- Suicide Prevention: www.save.org
- AOTA Special Interest Section—Mental Health: www.aota.org
- National Organization on Disability: www.nod.org
- American Speech-Language-Hearing Association: http://asha.org (See study on "The Role of Social Participation Intervention.")

## Communicative Participation: Construct and Scale Development

Brian J. Dudgeon and Jean C. Deitz

Participation has emerged as an important construct relative to the disability experience and appraisal of rehabilitation outcomes. Multiple dimensions of participation are evident and key skills of individuals used in participation can involve mobility, manipulation, or handling of objects, communication, and cognition. The presence of disability has been found to lead to participation that is often less diverse, restricted to a residential setting, involves fewer social relationships, and includes less active recreation (Law, 2002). Because of the central role participation occupies in understanding disabling conditions, participation is becoming an important outcome measure in the field of rehabilitation (Dijkers, Whiteneck, & El-Jaroudi, 2000). Communication skills are inherent in many aspects of participation, yet traditional measures of speech and language skills do not often address participation (Worral, McCooey, Davidson, Larkins, & Hickson, 2002).

Communicative participation can be defined as taking part in life situations where knowledge, information, ideas, or feelings are exchanged (Eadie et al., 2006). It may take the form of speaking, listening, reading, writing, or nonverbal means of communication. Since many life situations involve communication, it is logical to assume that communication is an important aspect of participation across a wide variety of domains, including personal or household management, work or education, leisure, relationships, and community involvement. These contexts of life situations served as the basis for the design of specific questions relative to communicative participation. Scale development regarding this construct is developing using a mixed method approach around specific tasks, activities, and situations related to life situations. Thus far, 150 or more items have been written and are starting to be qualitatively and quantitatively trialed with various populations who have communication disorders due to neurological or other voice disorders. A pared down version of the scale will then be ready for use in client-specific or disability-population measures of communication participation.

An important theme of judging participation is that self-report about one's participation and satisfaction is important. Self-report measures are advocated for on the basis that the judgment of the individual with disability is the ultimate determinant of whether his or her participation is adequate (Cardol et al., 1999; Hemmingsson & Jonsson, 2005; Whiteneck, 1994). "What is valued is not community participation in terms of a standard set of activities but community participation as defined by the person" (Johnston, Goverover, & Dijkers, 2005).

How one self-reports about one's communicative participation is important and can also be determined by asking persons with disability directly. Yorkston et al. (2007) discussed important aspects of communicative participation with persons with disability and determined that comfort, ease, and confidence were important dimensions, along with the success or function achieved and the connections made through communication. Participation can have personal meaning and asking about it may be best done by directly probing for satisfaction and what dimensions of communication are important to change.

Abstracted from a presentation by the authors and researchers at the 2006 Conference of the American Occupational Therapy Association, Charlotte, NC. Reproduced with permission.

### Evidence-Based Research Chart

| Population of Program | Intervention Activities | Evidence |
|---|---|---|
| Pediatrics; Preschool groups | Free play | Aureli & Colecchia, 1996; Field, 1984; Henniger, 1994; Petrakos & Howe, 1996; Saracho, 1993; Tanta, Deitz, White, & Billingsly, 2005 |
| | Peer interaction | Bedell & Dumas, 2004; Coster & Haltiwanger, 2004; Fantuzzo et al., 1996; Garnier & Latour, 1994; Guralnick & Groom, 1987, 1988; Parten, 1932 |
| Adult psychiatric | Social activity groups | DeCarlo & Mann, 1985; Duncombe & Howe, 1995; Salo-Chydenius, 1996; Schwartzberg, Howe, & McDermott, 1983 |
| Well elderly | Individual occupational therapy program | Clark et al., 1997; Jackson, Carlson, Mandel, Zemke, & Clark, 1998 |

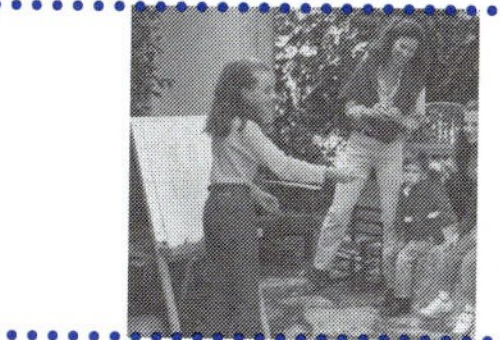

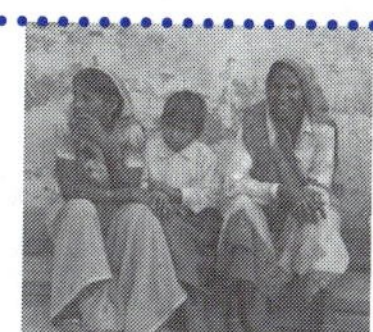

# References


Accreditation Council for Occupational Therapy Education. (2006). *ACOTE Standards*. Bethesda, MD: AOTA Press.

Asher, I. E. (Ed.). (2007). *Occupational therapy assessment tools. An annotated index* (3rd ed.). Bethesda, MD: AOTA Press.

Aureli, T., & Colecchia, N. (1996). Day care experience and free play behavior in preschool children. *Journal of Applied Developmental Psychology, 17*(1), 1-17.

Bedell, G. M., Coster, W., & Law, M. (2007-2010). Development of measures of participation and environment for children with disabilities. U.S. Department of Education National Institute for Disability and Rehabilitation Research Grant #H133G070140. Boston University.

Bedell, G. M., & Dumas, H. M. (2004). Social participation of children and youth with acquired brain injuries discharged from inpatient rehabilitation: A follow-up study. *Brain Injury, 18*(1), 65-82.

Bloomer, J., & Williams, S. (1979). *The Bay Area Functional Performance Evaluation (BaFPE)*. Palo Alto, CA: Consulting Psychologists Press.

Borg, B., & Bruce, M. A. G. (1991). *The group system: The therapeutic activity group in occupational therapy*. Thorofare, NJ: SLACK Incorporated.

Cardol, M., Brandsma, J. W., de Groot, I. J., van den Bos, G. A., de Haan, R. J., & de Jong, B. A. (1999). Handicap questionnaires: What do they assess? *Disability & Rehabilitation, 21*(3), 97-105.

Clark, F., Azen, S. P., Zemke, R., Jackson, J., Carlson, M., Mandel, D., et al. (1997). Occupational therapy for independent-living older adults. A randomized controlled trial. *Journal of the American Medical Association, 278*(16), 1321-1326.

Cole, M. B. (2005). *Group dynamics in occupational therapy: The theoretical basis and practice application of group treatment* (3rd ed.). Thorofare, NJ: SLACK Incorporated.

Coster, W. J., Deeny, T., Haltiwanger, J., & Haley, S. (1998). *School Function Assessment*. San Antonio, TX: The Psychological Corporation.

Coster, W. J., & Haltiwanger, J. T. (2004). Social-behavioral skills of elementary students with physical disabilities included in general education classrooms. *Remedial and Special Education, 25*(2), 95-103.

DeCarlo, J. J., & Mann, W. C. (1985). The effectiveness of verbal versus activity groups in improving self-perceptions of interpersonal communication skills. *American Journal of Occupational Therapy, 39*(1), 20-27.

Dijkers, M. P., Whiteneck, G., & El-Jaroudi, R. (2000). Measures of social outcomes in disability research. *Archives of Physical Medicine and Rehabilitation, 81*(12 suppl 2), S63-S80.

Donohue, M. V. (2003). Group Profile Studies with children: Validity measures and item analysis. *Occupational Therapy in Mental Health, 19*(1), 1-23.

Donohue, M. V. (2005). Social Profile: Assessment of validity and reliability with preschool children. *Canadian Journal of Occupational Therapy, 72*(3), 164-175.

Donohue, M. V. (2007). Interrater reliability of the Social Profile: Assessment of community and psychiatric group participation. *Australian Occupational Therapy Journal, 54*(1), 49-58.

Donohue, M. V. (2009). Social Profile. Unpublished assessment tool. Retrieved July 28, 2009, from http://www.Social-Profile.com

Duncombe, L. W., & Howe, M. C. (1995). Group treatment: Goals, tasks, and economic implications. *American Journal of Occupational Therapy, 49*(3), 199-206.

Eadie, T. L., Yorkston, K. M., Klasner, E. R., Dudgeon, B. J., Deitz, J. C., Baylor, C. R., et al. (2006). Measuring communicative participation: A review of self-report instruments in speech-language pathology. *American Journal of Speech-Language Pathology, 15*(4), 307-320.

Fantuzzo, J., Sutton-Smith, B., Atkins, M., Meyers, R., Stevenson, H., Coolahan, K., et al. (1996). Community-based resilient peer treatment of withdrawn maltreated preschool children. *Journal of Consulting and Clinical Psychology, 64*(6), 1377-1386.

Field, T. (1984). Play behaviors of handicapped children who have friends. In T. Field, J. L. Roopnarine, & M. Segal (Eds.), *Friendships in normal and handicapped children*. Santa Barbara, CA: Greenwood Publishing Group.

Forsyth, K., Lai, J., & Kielhofner, G. (1999). The assessment of communication and interaction skills (ACIS): Measurement properties. *British Journal of Occupational Therapy, 62*(2), 69-74.

Forsyth, K., Salamy, M., Simon, S., & Kielhofner, G. (1998). *The Assessment of Communciation and Interaction Skill (ACIS), version 4.0*. Chicago, IL: MOHO Clearinghouse.

Garnier, C., & Latour, A. (1994). Analysis of group process: Cooperation of preschool children. *Canadian Journal of Behavioural Science, 26*(3), 365-384.

Good-Ellis, M. A. (1999). The Role Activity Performance Scale. In B. J. Hemphill-Pearson (Ed.), *Assessments in occupational therapy in mental health: An integrated approach*. Thorofare, NJ: SLACK Incorporated.

Guralnick, M. J. (1990). Peer interactions and the development of handicapped children's social and communicative competence. In H. C. Foot, M. J. Morgan, & R. H. Shute (Eds.), *Children helping children*. London, England: Wiley.

Guralnick, M. J., & Groom, J. M. (1987). The peer relations of mildly delayed and nonhandicapped preschool children in mainstreamed playgroups. *Child Development, 58*(6), 1556-1572.

Guralnick, M. J., & Groom, J. M. (1988). Friendships of preschool children in mainstreamed playgroups. *Developmental Psychology, 24*(4), 595-604.

Helfrich, C., & Aviles, A. (2001). Occupational therapy's role with victims of domestic violence: Assessment and intervention. *Occupational Therapy in Mental Health, 16*(3/4), 53-70.

Hemmingsson, H., & Jonsson, H. (2005). An occupational perspective on the concept of participation in the international classification of functioning, disability and health—Some critical remarks. *American Journal of Occupational Therapy, 59*(5), 569-576.

Hemphill-Pearson, B. J. (Ed.). (1999). *Assessments in occupational therapy mental health. An integrative approach*. Thorofare, NJ: SLACK Incorporated.

Henniger, M. L. (1994). Planning for outdoor play. *Young Children, 49*(4), 10-15.

Howe, M. C., & Schwartzberg, S. L. (2001). *A functional approach to group work in occupational therapy* (3rd ed.). Philadelphia, PA: Lippincott Williams & Wilkins.

Howes, C. (1988). Peer interaction of young children. *Monographs of the Society for Research in Child Development, 53*(1), 1-88.

Isaksson, G., Lexell, J., & Skär, L. (2007). Social support provides motivation and ability to participate in occupation. *OTJR: Occupation, Participation and Health, 27*(1), 23-30.

Jackson, J., Carlson, M., Mandel, D., Zemke, R., & Clark, F. (1998). Occupations in lifestyle redesign: The Well Elderly Study occupational therapy program. *American Journal of Occupational Therapy, 52*(5), 326-336.

Johnson, D. W., & Johnson, F. P. (2000). *Joining together: Group theory and group skills* (7th ed.). Upper Saddle River, NJ: Prentice Hall.

Johnston, M. V., Goverover, Y., & Dijkers, M. (2005). Community activities and individuals' satisfaction with them: Quality of life in the first year after traumatic brain injury. *Archives of Physical Medicine & Rehabilitation, 86*(4), 735-745.

Keller, J., & Forsyth, K. (2004). The model of human occupation in practice. *Israel Journal of Occupational Therapy, 13*, E99-E106.

Kielhofner, G., Fogg, L., Braveman, B., Forsyth, K., Kramer, J., & Duncan, E. (2009). A factor analytic study of the Model of Human Occupation Screening Tool of hypothesized variables. *Occupational Therapy in Mental Health, 25*, 127-137.

Kielhofner G., Mallinson, T., Crawford, C., Nowak, M., Rigby, M., Henry, A., et al. (2005). *Occupational performance history inventory. (OPHI-II, Version 2.1)*. Chicago, IL: Model of Human Occupation Clearinghouse.

Klyczek, J. P., & Mann, W. C. (1990). Concurrent validity of the Task-Oriented Assessment component of the Bay Area Functional Performance Evaluation with the American Association on Mental Deficiency Adaptive Behavior Scale. *American Journal of Occupational Therapy, 44*(10), 907-912.

Klyczek, J., Bloomer, J., & Fiedler, R. (1999). *Analysis of a shortened BaFPE: Task oriented assessment*. Buffalo, NY: D'Youville College.

Law, M. (2002). Participation in the occupations of everyday life. *American Journal of Occupational Therapy, 56*(6), 640-649.

Lisina, M. I. (1985). *Child-adults-peers: Patterns of communication*. Moscow, Russia: Progress Publishers.

Mann, W. C., & Klyczek, J. P. (1991). Standard scores for the Bay Area Functional Performance Evaluation Task Oriented Assessment. *Occupational Therapy in Mental Health, 11*(1), 13-24.

Mosey, A. C. (1968). Recapitulation of ontogenesis: A theory for practice of occupational therapy. *American Journal of Occupational Therapy, 22*(5), 426-438.

Mosey, A. C. (1986). *Psychosocial components of occupational therapy*. New York, NY: Raven Press.

Parkinson, S., Forsyth, K., & Kielhofner, G. (2006). *The Model of Human Occupation Screening Tool (MOHOST), version 2.0*. Chicago, IL: MOHO Clearinghouse.

Parten, M. B. (1932). Social participation among pre-school children. *Journal of Abnormal and Social Psychology, 27*, 243-269.

Petrakos, H., & Howe, N. (1996). The influence of the physical design of the dramatic play center on children's play. *Early Childhood Research Quarterly, 11*(1), 63-77.

Posthuma, B. W. (2002). *Small groups in counseling and therapy: Process and leadership* (4th ed.). Columbus, OH: Allyn & Bacon.

Roney, J. R., Hanson, K. N., Durante, K. M., & Maestripieri, D. (2006). Reading men's faces: Women's mate attractiveness judgments track men's testosterone and interest in infants. *Proceedings: Biological Sciences, 273*(1598), 2169-2175.

Salo-Chydenius, S. (1996). Changing helplessness to coping: An exploratory study of social skills training with individuals with long-term mental illness. *Occupational Therapy International, 3*, 174-189.

Saracho, O. N. (1993). A factor analysis of young children's play. *Early Childhood Development and Care, 84*(1), 91-102.

Schwartzberg, S. L., Howe, M. C., & McDermott, A. (1983). A comparison of three treatment group formats for facilitating social interaction. *Occupational Therapy in Mental Health, 2*(4), 1-16.

Smith, D. E. (1986). Training programs for performance appraisal: A review. *Academy of Management Review, 11*(1), 22-40.

Tanta, K. J., Deitz, J. C., White, O., & Billingsly, F. (2005). The effects of peer-play level on initiations and responses of preschool children with delayed play skills. *American Journal of Occupational Therapy, 59*(4), 437-445.

Whiteneck, G. G. (1994). The 44th annual John Stanley Coulter Lecture. Measuring what matters: Key rehabilitation outcomes. *Archives of Physical Medicine & Rehabilitation, 75*(10), 1073-1076.

World Health Organization. (2001). *International classification of functioning, disability, and health (ICF)*. Geneva, Switzerland: Author.

Worral, L., McCooey, R., Davidson, B., Larkins, B., & Hickson, L. (2002). The validity of functional assessments of communication and the Activity/Participation components of the ICIHD-2: Do they reflect what really happens in real-life? *Journal of Communication Disorders, 35*(2), 107-137.

Yorkston, K. M., Baylor, C. R., Klasner, E. R., Deitz, J., Dudgeon, B. J., Eadie, T., et al. (2007). Satisfaction with communicative participation as defined by adults with multiple sclerosis: A qualitative study. *Journal of Communication Disorders, 40*(6), 433-451.

# Suggested Reading

Bernard, H. R. (2000). *Social research methods: Qualitative and quantitative approaches*. Thousand Oaks, CA: Sage Publications.

Burns, N., & Grove, S. K. (1993). *The practice of nursing research: Conduct, critique, and utilization* (2nd ed.). Philadelphia, PA: W.B. Saunders Company.

Campanelli, L. C. (1996). Theories of aging. In C. B. Lewis (Ed.), *Aging: The health care challenge* (3rd ed.). Philadelphia, PA: F.A. Davis.

Cohen, R. J., Swerdlik, M. E., & Smith, D. K. (1992). *Psychological testing and assessment: An introduction to tests and measurement* (2nd ed.). Mountainview, CA: Mayfield.

Crepeau, E. B., Cohn, E. S., & Schell, B. A. B. (2003). *Willard & Spackman's occupational therapy* (10th ed.). New York, NY: Lippincott Williams & Wilkins.

Davis, C. M. (1996). Psychosocial aspects of aging. In C. B. Lewis (Ed.), *Aging: The health care challenge* (3rd ed.). Philadelphia, PA: F.A. Davis.

Donohue, M. V. (1999). Theoretical bases of Mosey's group interactions skills. *Occupational Therapy International, 6*(1), 35-51.

Erdfelder, E., Faul, F., & Buchner, A. (1996.). G Power: A general power analysis program. *Behavior Research Methods, Instruments and Computers, 28*, 1-11.

Erikson, E. H. (1968). *Identity: Youth and crisis*. New York, NY: W. W. Norton & Company.

Gliner, J. A., & Morgan, G. A. (2000). *Research methods in applied settings: An integrated approach to design and analysis*. Mahwah, NJ: Lawrence Erlbaum.

Guralnick, M. J., Neville, B., Hammond, M. A., & Connor, R. T. (2007). The friendships of young children with developmental delays: A longitudinal analysis. *Journal of Applied Developmental Psychology, 28*(1), 64-79.

Hinojosa, J., & Kramer, P. (1998). *Evaluation: Obtaining and interpreting data*. Bethesda, MD: AOTA Press.

Kaplan, K. L. (1988). *Directive group therapy. Innovative mental health treatment*. Thorofare, NJ: SLACK Incorporated.

Kielhofner, G. (2002). *Model of Human Occupation: Theory and application* (3rd ed.). Baltimore, MD: Lippincott Williams and Wilkins.

Lengua, L. J., Honorado, E., & Bush, N. R. (2007). Contextual risk and parenting as predictors of effortful control and social competence in preschool children. *Journal of Applied Developmental Psychology, 28*(1), 40-55.

McIntire, S. A., & Miller, L. A. (2000). *Foundations of psychological testing*. Boston, MA: McGraw-Hill.

Nachmias, D., & Nachmias, C. (1987). *Research methods in the social sciences* (3rd ed.). New York, NY: St. Martin's Press.

Polit, D. F. (1995). *Nursing research principles and methods*. Philadelphia, PA: Lippincott Williams & Wilkins.

Reinertsen, L. D. (2006). Adults with dementia in social adult day care: Changes in cognitive status, sleep and activity behaviors and caregiver stress. Unpublished doctoral dissertation, New York University.

Ross, M. (1997). *Integrative group therapy: Mobilizing coping abilities with the five stage group*. Bethesda, MD: AOTA Association.

Shrout, P. E., & Fleiss, J. L. (1979). Intraclass correlations: Uses in assessing rater reliability. *Psychological Bulletin, 86*(2), 420-428.

Stein, F., & Cutler, S. K. (2000). *Clinical research in occupational therapy* (4th ed.). San Diego, CA: Singular.

Weinberg, S. L., & Goldberg, K. P. (1990). *Statistics for the behavioral sciences*. New York, NY: Cambridge University Press.

Williams, S., & Bloomer, J. (1987). *Bay Area Functional Performance Evaluation* (2nd ed.). Palo Alto, CA: Consulting Psychologists Press.

Yaffee, R. A. (1998). Enhancement of reliability analysis: Application of intraclass correlations with SPSS/Windows v.8. Retrieved February 12, 2002, from http://www.nyu.edu/its/socsci/Docs/intracls.html

Yalom, I. D. (1985). *The theory and practice of group psychotherapy* (3rd ed.). New York, NY: Basic Books.

# Section V

## Intervention Plan: Formulation and Implemention

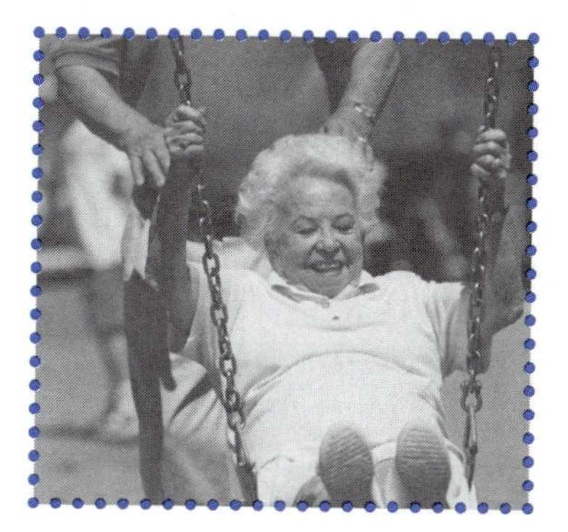

# 15

# The Interpretation, Development, and Use of Evidence, Safety, and Grading in Intervention Planning

*Jane O'Brien, PhD, OTR/L*

**ACOTE Standards Explored in This Chapter**

B.5.1-5.3, 5.19, 5.21

**Key Terms**

| | |
|---|---|
| Adapting | Grading |
| Context | Models of practice |
| Frames of reference | Occupation-based |

## Introduction

Occupational therapy practitioners work with a variety of clients who have a wide range of abilities and disabilities. Therefore, a crucial skill in the development of effective intervention planning is the ability to interpret, develop, and use evidence to support practice. Furthermore, occupational therapy practitioners must be able to analyze activity so that they may grade or adapt intervention according to a client's needs. Finally, clinicians must be aware of safety issues throughout the process and ensure that clients are safe once discharged from services. Occupational therapy practitioners use activity to help clients return to engagement in those things they find meaningful. This chapter provides an overview of the intervention process by examining the use of activities in intervention by describing how Models of Practice and Frames of Reference guide practitioners in their decision making. A description of the role of the occupational therapist and occupational therapy assistant in intervention is provided. A discussion of how to develop occupational-based intervention plans reflective of the client's needs is followed by suggestions in how to select and provide occupational therapy intervention. Finally, this chapter provides guidelines on how to grade and adapt activities to meet the client's needs.

## Overview of the Intervention Process

Intervention plans provide a map for the occupational therapy process. The plan requires that the occupational therapy practitioner problem solve, reason, and decide based upon knowledge, past experiences, and the setting in which the intervention takes place. Intervention planning requires creativity, knowledge of available resources,



K. Sladyk, K. Jacobs, & N. MacRae (Eds.).
*Occupational Therapy Essentials for Clinical Competence* (pp. 163-174).

and practice. The plan includes the goals of the intervention, who will perform the intervention, and where, when, how often, and how long the intervention will take place. The plan includes a rationale for the type of intervention with desired outcomes. Intervention plans clarify the role of the occupational therapy practitioner and specify the team members (see Appendix D for an outline of an intervention plan). Occupational therapy students and novice practitioners learn from carefully describing each part of the intervention plan with a well-developed rationale. As practitioners gain experience, the rationale may not necessarily be written in the plan. However, experienced practitioners should always be able to articulate the rationale for intervention.

The occupational therapist is ultimately responsible for the intervention plan, yet receives input from the occupational therapy assistant. The occupational therapy assistant assists in the plan by providing data, updates, and information about the client. Once the plan is developed, the occupational therapy assistant and occupational therapist work toward the selected goals (AOTA, 1990; 1994; 2008). The occupational therapist provides supervision to the occupational therapy assistant as needed depending on the occupational therapy assistant's experience. Both the occupational therapy assistant and occupational therapist design activities to meet the plan. The occupational therapy practitioner must be able to adapt and grade activities as needed.

## Models of Practice and Frames of Reference

Occupational therapy is based upon the premise that engagement in activity (that is meaningful to the client) is beneficial to clients and will help them recover, relearn, or re-engage in life's activities (AOTA, 2008). A model of practice provides an overview of how to look at the client and, as such, models of practice help clinicians organize their thinking (MacRae, 2001). Occupational therapy models of practice include occupation and describe how, in a holistic manner, factors influence an individual's engagement in occupation. Occupational therapy models of practice include: Model of Human Occupation (Kielhofner, 1985, 2002), Person-Environment-Occupation model (Law et al., 1996), Canadian Occupational Performance Model (Townsend, Brintnell, & Staisey, 1990), and Occupational Adaptation (Schkade & Schultz, 1992). Table 15-1 provides a description of the above-mentioned occupational therapy models of practice. Readers are encouraged to explore these models to choose the one that will be of greatest help to the client.

Occupational therapy practitioners use the model of practice to organize their thinking of clients and their abilities (see Chapter 10 for more information on evaluation). The frame of reference helps the occupational therapy practitioner develop an intervention plan and provides

**Table 15-1. Models of Practice**

| Model | Author(s) | Components | Premises |
|---|---|---|---|
| Model of Human Occupation (MOHO) | Kielhofner, 1985 | • Volition<br>• Habituation<br>• Performance<br>• Environment | The human is an open system. Volition drives the system. The clinician's role is to understand the client in terms of these systems (and subsystems) and intervene to facilitate engagement in occupation. |
| Canadian Occupational Performance Model (COPM) | Canadian Occupational Therapy Association (Townsend et al., 1990) | • Spirituality<br>• Occupation<br>• Context (institutional included) | The worth of the individual is central to this model. Spirituality is the core of a person. Thus, occupational therapy practitioners must understand the client's spirituality to facilitate engagement in occupations. Performance of occupations takes place within social, physical, and cultural environments. |
| Occupational Adaptation (OA) | Schkade & Schultz, 1992 | • Occupations<br>• Physical and emotional strengths and weaknesses<br>• Examination of available support systems (physical and emotional) | Help people participate in their desired occupations by adapting or modifying the occupation or using other methods to perform the occupation. |
| Person Environment Occupation (PEO) | Law et al., 1996; Christiansen & Baum, 1997 | • Person<br>• Environment<br>• Occupation | Occupations are the everyday things people do. PEO looks at the person in terms of physical, social, and emotional factors. The environment (context) influences the person and occupations. The environment includes culture and political institutions. |

Adapted with permission from O'Brien, J. C., & Solomon, J. W. (2006). Scope of practice. In J. W. Solomon & J. C. O'Brien (Eds.), *Pediatric Skills for Occupational Therapy Assistants* (2nd ed.). St. Louis, MO: Mosby. Copyright Elsevier Mosby, 2006.

specific intervention techniques. It should be noted that some models (e.g., the Model of Human Occupation and Canadian Occupational Performance Model) are both models of practice and frames of reference. Frames of reference include a description of the theory, principles surrounding the intervention, description of function and dysfunction, the role of the clinicians, the intervention process, and techniques (Mosey, 1981). Frames of reference also include assessment and measurement tools. Commonly used occupational therapy frames of reference include Model of Human Occupation, sensory integration, biomechanical, motor control, neurodevelopmental treatment, cognitive disabilities, and developmental. See Table 15-2 for a description of the frames of reference used in pediatric occupational therapy practice.

Students and occupational therapy practitioners commonly ask, "Why do we need to use a frame of reference or theory?" While expert practitioners may rely on experience and prior knowledge to determine what to do with certain clients, novice practitioners and students rely on the research of others to determine the most effective intervention techniques. The model of practice frames the evaluation and intervention session as it provides parameters for viewing the client. The frame of reference provides a systematic manner to conduct intervention. Together, the model of practice and frame of reference help the occupational therapy practitioner define and observe factors influencing function. Occupational therapy practitioners who do not use a model of practice or frame of reference may waste time and energy organizing intervention.

Those who say they do not use a frame of reference or theory may, in fact, not be able to articulate the frame of reference or theory ("It is just what we do"). For example, when practitioners perform range of motion, they are using the biomechanical frame of reference and the principles of stretching. Neurodevelopmental (NDT) approaches are based upon the theories of brain plasticity. A neurodevelopmental approach relies on repeating activities so that the client learns them and is more able to perform the activity due to improved brain plasticity.

Since frames of reference change as new research becomes available, occupational therapy practitioners must become consumers of research if they want to provide the best care to their clients. For example, changes have been made in the NDT approaches with the realization that children learn motorically through mistakes and that children with cerebral palsy may need to make some motor mistakes to be functional (Howle, 2005; Nichols, 2005; Schoen & Anderson, 1999). Therefore, the best compromise might be to allow the child to perform the movement and help him or her perform it in the best way for him or her. The goal does not have to be a perfect movement pattern as was previously implied by this frame of reference. The newest models for NDT include functional movement throughout the therapy session.

Clinicians evaluate whether the intervention strategies associated with the frame of reference are working. If the client is not making the desired progress, a closer review of the techniques, principles, and assessment tools described in the frame of reference may provide an alternative plan. A closer inspection of the research or protocols associated with the frame of reference may promote success. Alternatively, the occupational therapy practitioner may decide to try another frame of reference altogether. Informed practitioners benefit from the knowledge of many frames of reference in that they are able to treat diverse client issues. Once practitioners understand the principles and theory guiding the frame of reference, they are better able to adapt techniques for clients for whom the frame of reference was not originally intended. Occupational therapy practitioners evaluate many factors when choosing a model of practice or frame of reference. See Table 15-3 for guiding questions to consider when selecting a model of practice or frame of reference.

## Occupational-Based Intervention Plans

Once the occupational therapist has evaluated the client and determined the client's needs through interpretation of the data, the occupational therapist develops the intervention plan. After establishing service competency [ensuring that two practitioners will obtain the same results (AOTA, 1990)] in administering standardized tests, the occupational therapy assistant may assist by providing information and administering standardized tests as requested by the occupational therapist. The occupational therapy assistant is not responsible for interpreting the data. The first step in developing the intervention plan is to collaborate with the client on the goals for the intervention.

The goals are based on helping clients re-engage in their occupations, the everyday things we do that provide us with meaning (AOTA, 2008). Occupations vary from person to person. The occupational therapy practitioner collaborates with the client, family, and team members to develop appropriate goals that reflect the client's occupations. Intervention is based upon these occupationally-based goals developed with the client and family. Therapy goals are designed to create/promote, establish/restore, maintain, modify, and prevent, according to the framework (AOTA, 2008).

## Collaboration with Clients

Collaborating with clients and family members on developing goals for occupational therapy services helps occupational therapists gain trust from clients. Clients who collaborate in goal setting are motivated to participate in therapy and home programs, and make better gains (Maurer, Smith, & Armetta, 1989; Melchert-McKearnan, Dietz, Engel, & White, 2000; Steinbeck, 1986).

| Table 15-2. Pediatric Frames of Reference | | | | |
|---|---|---|---|---|
| **Frame of Reference** | **Author(s)** | **Principles** | **Sample Populations** | **Treatment Modalities** |
| Developmental | Llorens, 1976 | Development occurs over time and between skills (e.g., gross and fine motor). Some children experience a "gap" in their development due to physical, emotional, or social trauma. Occupational therapist's role is to "fill in the gap." | • Down Syndrome<br>• Mental retardation<br>• Failure to thrive<br>• Cerebral palsy<br>• Pervasive Developmental Disorder<br>*principles are used in conjunction with other frames of reference | Identify current level of functioning. Work on the next step to achieve the skill. Intervention includes practice, repetition, education, modeling of skills. |
| Biomechanical | Pedretti & Paszuinielli, 1990 | Improve strength, endurance, range of motion | • Children with cardiac concerns<br>• Brachial plexus<br>• Cerebral palsy<br>• Juvenile Rheumatoid Arthritis<br>• Down Syndrome | Strength: Increase weight of toys or repetitive use of objects.<br>Endurance: Increase time engaged in occupation.<br>Range of motion: Repetitively provide slow sustained stretch to increase end range. |
| Sensory Integration | Ayres, 1979 | Children with sensory integration dysfunction have difficulty processing sensory information (vestibular, proprioceptive, tactile). Improvements in sensory processing lead to improved engagement in occupations. | • Sensory integrative dysfunction<br>• Developmental Coordination Disorder<br>• Sensory Modulation disorder<br>• Pervasive Developmental Disorder | Provide controlled sensory input to improve the child's ability to process sensory stimuli. Use of suspended equipment and the "just-right challenge." Activities are child-directed. |
| Motor Control | Shumway-Cooke & Woollacott, 2007 | Acquisition of motor skills is based upon dynamical systems theory. (All systems work on each other for movement to occur, including sensory, motor, and cognitive). | • Cerebral palsy<br>• Developmental Coordination Disorder<br>• Down Syndrome | Task-oriented approach—Children learn motor skills best by repeating the occupations in the most natural setting, varying the requirements. Children learn from their motor mistakes. |
| Neurodevelopmental | Bobath, 1975<br>Schoen & Anderson, 1993 | Children learn motor patterns when they "feel" normal movement patterns. | • Cerebral palsy<br>• Traumatic brain injury | Clinician uses handling techniques and key points of control to inhibit abnormal muscle tone and facilitate normal movement patterns. Children learn through "feeling" normal patterns and thus, should not make motor mistakes. |
| Sensorimotor | Trombly, 1994 | Sensory input to change the muscle tone or promote a muscle contraction. | • Cerebral palsy<br>• Traumatic brain injury | Icing techniques, neutral warmth, slow stroking, vibration are all techniques used in this approach. |

Adapted with permission from O'Brien, J. C., & Solomon, J. W. (2006). Scope of practice. In J. W. Solomon & J. C. O'Brien (Eds.), *Pediatric Skills for Occupational Therapy Assistants* (2nd ed.). St. Louis, MO: Mosby. Copyright Elsevier Mosby, 2006.

**Table 15-3. Considerations When Deciding Upon a Model of Practice or Frame of Reference**

| | |
|---|---|
| **Setting** | Does this model of practice or frame of reference fit within the setting? |
| **Population** | Does this model of practice or frame of reference address the needs of the population being treated? |
| **Basic principles** | What is the theory of this model of practice or frame of reference and does it make sense for the population being treated? Is this model of practice or frame of reference congruent with occupational therapy practice? Is there adequate research to support the theory and principles? |
| **Evidence** | Has the research supported the use of this model of practice or frame of reference and, if so, with which population? Does this model of practice or frame of reference support cost-effective intervention? Are the assessment tools associated with this model of practice or frame of reference well designed and clinically relevant? Is there documentation that this model of practice or frame of reference can improve the occupations of clients? |
| **Assessment/ Evaluation** | What assessments or tests are compatible with the model of practice or frame of reference? Are the assessments standardized, reliable, and valid? |
| **Practical considerations** | Does the clinic or site have the equipment necessary to competently use this model of practice or frame of reference? |
| **Clinical expertise** | Is the practitioner adequately trained to use the associated techniques or assessment tools? How much training is necessary? |

Therapists use their awareness of the client's strengths and weaknesses, occupational desires, and contextual support to develop goals. Collaborating with clients on goal setting requires skill in interviewing and, until a client is ready, the therapist may need to look for nonverbal clues, work with family, and investigate possible alternative goals. However, the time taken to really understand clients and develop an intervention plan that meets their needs makes for a more successful session (AOTA, 2008; Kielhofner, 2008; Law et al., 1996).

**Possible Questions to Ask When Collaborating on Goal Setting:**

- What would you like to do?
- What is causing you trouble?
- When you leave, what would you like to be doing?
- What is your favorite thing to do?
- Describe a typical day.

The mechanics of goal writing are described in Chapter 32. Occupational therapists developing occupational-based goals may be successful by using the documentation guidelines. Goals must be meaningful and relevant to the person, measurable, achievable, and written clearly. As a general rule, successful practitioners write goals that clients hope to achieve. The short-term goals are steps toward the long-term goals. The steps are not so challenging as to discourage the client. Furthermore, goals must be written so that all who read them can determine how they will be met. People are more likely to achieve those things that they can see and understand.

Intervention plans and strategies are dependent upon the context in which the goal must be achieved. The framework (AOTA, 2008) lists contexts or environments as including cultural, physical, social, personal, temporal, and virtual (see the sidebar on the next page for a description of each). The following examples describe important issues showing how contexts may impact the intervention plan.

## Cultural

Culture is reflected in everyday events such as feeding, dressing, grooming, and hygiene. The goal of occupational therapy is to help the person regain function within his or her culture. Thus, practitioners must be sensitive to how the person and/or culture views the occupation. Goals and subsequent intervention plans are designed around the cultural expectations and beliefs for the occupation.

Since occupational therapy practitioners work with clients who have experienced some form of disability, an awareness of the client's cultural view of disability may prove insightful. In fact, an awareness of the culture of disability is beneficial. For example, it may not be the wish of every disabled client to "fit in." In fact, disability scholars argue that the disability is part of the person's identity and rehabilitation professionals may reinforce the idea that the client is "abnormal" (Giangreco, 1995 as cited in Kielhofner, 2005). Kielhofner and colleagues propose that occupational therapy practitioners rethink how they view disability (Kielhofner, 2005; McColl, 2005; Neville-Jan, 2005; Taylor, 2005; Thibodaux, 2005).

Black and Wells (2007) proposed that occupational therapy practitioners become first aware of their own culture and be open to other cultures through experience and discussion (see Chapter 2).

**Contexts**

- *Cultural*: Customs, beliefs, activity patterns, behavior standards, and expectations accepted by the society of which the individual is a member. Includes ethnicity and values as well as political aspects, such as law that affect access to resources and affirm personal rights. Also includes opportunities for education, employment, and economic support.
- *Physical*: Natural, nonhuman, and built and the objects in them. Includes the accessibility to and performance within environments having natural terrain, plants, animals, buildings, furniture, objects, tools, or devices.
- *Social*: Is constructed by presence, relationships, and expectations of persons, organizations, populations. Availability and expectations of significant individuals, such as spouse, friends, and caregivers. Also includes relationships with individual groups or organizations and systems.
- *Personal*: Features of the individual that are not part of the health conditions or health status (WHO, 2001, p. 17). Personal context includes age, gender, socioeconomic status, and educational status.
- *Temporal*: Location of occupational performance in time (Neistadt & Crepeau, 1998, p. 292).
- *Virtual*: Environment in which communication occurs by means of airways or computers and an absence of physical contact.



# Physical

Occupations are performed in many different physical settings. Occupational therapy practitioners consider all of the physical factors required for success. For example, while a client may be successful cooking in the occupational therapy clinic with all materials readily available, the same client may not be able to maneuver around his or her own kitchen. Intervention may need to include making the kitchen accessible to the client.

In another case, a child with Juvenile Rheumatoid Arthritis was provided with an electronic wheelchair. This worked well at school, and the teachers, parents, and child were happy. The chair fit well. However, the mom complained of a sore back, and upon further discussion, revealed that she had to lift the wheelchair up the stairs into the house. In this situation, the child was successful in the school, but not at home. These examples show the importance of understanding all of the physical contexts in which the occupations occur.

# Social

Social demands change the interpersonal and sometimes physical demands of occupations. Therefore, occupational therapy practitioners planning intervention consider the social expectations and demands of a given occupation. For example, going to lunch with your sister requires very different social skills than attending a large formal dinner party. Occupational therapy practitioners provide interventions aimed to help clients function in both of these situations as well as many different scenarios. For clients to successfully engage in occupations, they must be prepared for the social expectations. This may require education to those in the support system (e.g., teachers sometimes ask children to discuss differences within a supportive environment with their classmates). Caregivers may not understand the social differences observed in their loved one. Occupational therapy practitioners can play an important role in helping others understand so that they may support intervention plans.

# Personal

Occupational therapy practitioners develop activities and intervention plans based upon a person's age, gender, socioeconomic status, and educational status. For example, elderly clients typically do not wish to engage in the same type of activities as adolescents or young children. Age-related and gender differences are easily identified. However, practitioners must also be open to differences in terms of other cultures and individual preferences (see Chapter 2). For example, many elderly people engage in activities that may be considered limited to young people (e.g., snowboarding, lifting weights, surfing).

# Temporal

People participate in different activities at certain stages of life. The temporal aspects of occupations also include time of day, time of year, and duration of the activity. For example, some activities are dependent upon the season (e.g., snowboarding, skiing). Some activities are part of a morning routine (e.g., breakfast, dressing, grooming) while others may be more suitable for afternoon (e.g., lunch). For some clients, performing activities in their natural temporal context allows them to be more successful.

# Virtual

Many driving simulator programs use virtual context to help retrain individuals to drive. The virtual context of this activity may help prepare the individual for driving. Occupational therapy practitioners analyze the virtual nature of activities and may address how a person accesses the virtual environment.

# Activity Analysis

The importance of finding activities that are motivating and purposeful to clients is a key assumption of occupational therapy practice. Occupational therapy practitioners examine individual motivations and desires as essential to the intervention process. Once the goals and objectives have been established for clients, practitioners design intervention activities to reach these goals. Prior to performing the actual occupation, clients may have to engage in preparatory activities. Preparatory activities may include exercise, stretching, range of motion, postural preparation, and positioning (Fisher, 1998). These activities are designed to provide the person with the necessary prerequisite skills. For example, runners stretch prior to running long distances. In this case, stretching is considered a preparatory activity. Children may participate in hand warm-up exercises prior to completing handwriting in school (Figure 15-1).

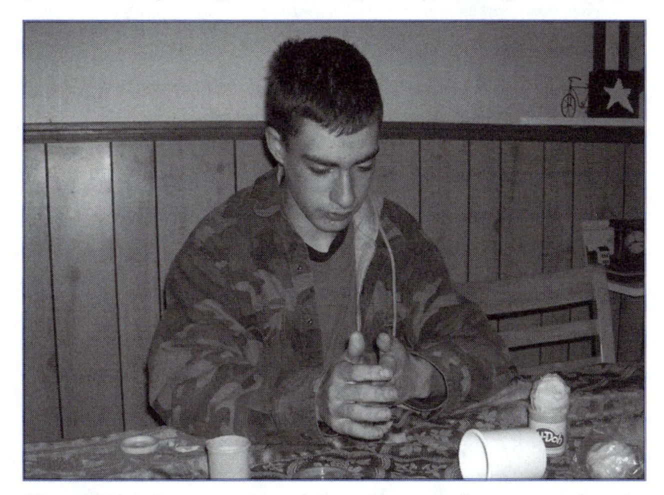

**Figure 15-1.** Preparatory activity—Scott performs some hand exercises to get ready for writing. Photo by Scott O'Brien.

Once preparatory work is completed, the occupational therapy practitioner may engage the client in some purposeful activities. Purposeful activities are those activities that are meaningful to the person or may help the client reach his or her goals (Fisher, 1998). Purposeful activities are chosen by the client, have an end goal, and involve many separate skills and abilities. In the case of running, purposeful activities may include doing some speed work to get faster. In this case, the activity relates to the occupation, but is not performed in the same context as the actual occupation. In the case of the child, purposeful activity may include practicing letter formation or painting (Figure 15-2).

The goal of occupational therapy intervention is that the client engages in the chosen occupation. Occupation-based activity involves doing the actual occupation, which provides meaning and is part of one's identity (Fisher, 1998). Using occupation-based activity requires the person use the actual materials and context in which the activity is performed. For example, running along the road for the distance runner, or the child writing a story in school (Figure

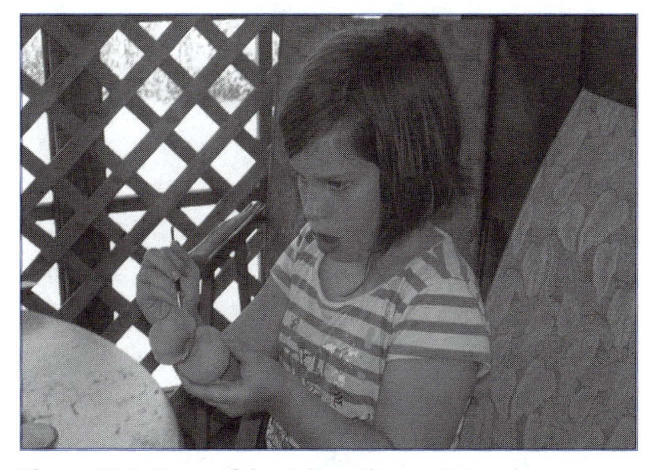

**Figure 15-2.** Purposeful activity—Alison paints a clay vase as a way to improve her hand skills for writing. Photo by Scott O'Brien.

15-3). Occupations are personal and thus will depend upon the client. A skilled occupational therapist takes the time to find out what occupations are most vital to the person's identity and targets intervention on those. A person who enjoys gardening may identify him- or herself as a gardener. This may provide him or her with pleasure, a sense of being, and accomplishment. For this person, returning to gardening is important and a part of his or her identity (AOTA, 2008). For others, gardening may be a task they accomplish every year because it makes the home look better, and for them, being a homemaker is important. In this case, gardening is an activity associated with taking care of the home. Still other people may find gardening a chore that comes along with owning a home, but it is not enjoyable and not important to their identity.

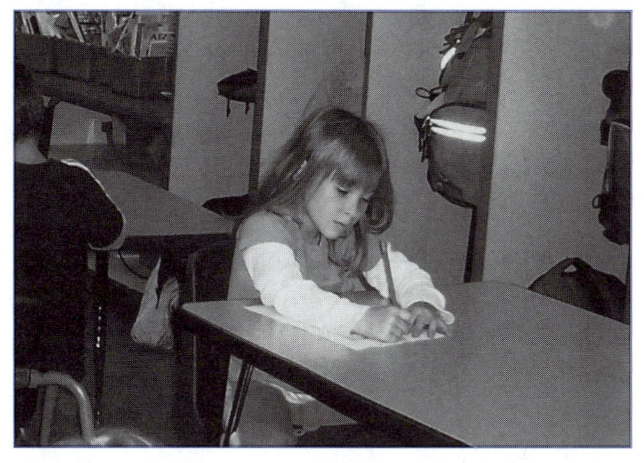

**Figure 15-3.** Occupation-based activity—Molly writes a story about her dog during writing time at school. Photo by Scott O'Brien.

Occupational therapy practitioners use all types of activity in practice. However, intervention should be made up mostly of occupation-based activity (AOTA, 2008; Fisher, 1998). Occupational therapy practitioners believe that engaging in occupations is therapeutic and will lead to larger gains. Furthermore, participating in the actual occupation in the actual context promotes adaptation, generalization, and transfer of learning.

## Safety

Throughout the intervention process, the occupational therapy practitioner considers safety issues and addresses the ability of the client to return to occupations in a safe manner. The occupational therapy practitioner carefully watches clients as they perform occupations to determine if judgment, cognition, and physical abilities allow them to be safe. Frequently, the occupational therapist will perform a home evaluation prior to discharge to assure the client and team that the environment is safe. It may be the occupational therapy practitioner's role to adapt and modify equipment so the client is able to use safety devices (e.g., phone, grab bars). Prevention of accidents may be achieved with analysis of the environment (e.g., get rid of throw rugs). Creating a safe environment by teaching safety skills (e.g., lock doors) may be the occupational therapist's role.

## Grading and Adapting

The ability to analyze activities is learned early in occupational therapy curricula with activity analysis coursework. These skills are refined and enhanced, leading to improved observational skills. Entry-level occupational therapy practitioners are successful at analyzing activities and using activities to improve function.

Grading refers to making an activity easier or harder for the client. Providing clients with the "just-right challenge" (a challenge that is neither too hard nor too easy), is motivating and therapeutic. If the activity is too difficult or too easy, clients become discouraged or bored and do not want to continue. Thus, occupational therapy practitioners work to challenge clients toward their goals without overwhelming or boring them. Activities may be graded by:

- Adding or subtracting steps
- Providing more or less direction
  - Verbal
    - 1 step
    - 2 step
  - Demonstrative
  - Written
- Providing more or less physical assistance
- Increasing or decreasing the time
- Adding or subtracting the environmental demands
- Adding or subtracting choices
- Adding or subtracting cognitive or psychological demands
- Adding or subtracting physical demands

Adapting activities involves changing the actual task to make it easier or harder for the client. Adapting may involve the use of assistive technology. For example, providing clients with a built-up handled spoon makes gripping easier. Other adaptations may include teaching a person to dress using one-hand techniques. Adaptations may include:

- Technology to change tasks (e.g., cooking food using a microwave instead of an oven)
- Eliminating steps or performing activities differently (e.g., buying fruit already cut up)
- Providing adaptive equipment (e.g., picking things up using a "reacher")
- Changing the physical demands of the task (e.g., sitting while dressing).

All activities can be graded and adapted to meet the needs of the client. Occupational therapy practitioners may change activities by examining the client factors required to perform or by changing the contextual aspects of the tasks. Suggestions to change the contextual aspects of the task include:

- *Cultural*: Increase or decrease the cultural nature of the activity. Discuss the cultural aspects.
- *Physical*: Increase the distance required for walking; change the terrain. Conduct the activity in a familiar or unfamiliar setting. Make the materials larger or smaller. Change the lighting of the room. Increase or decrease the size of the space.
- *Social*: Increase or decrease the number of people in the activity. Involve familiar or unfamiliar people. Require the client to organize an event or attend only. Vary the time of the interactions or the intensity of the exchanges. Provide varying degrees of structure to the interactions.
- *Personal*: Consider gender and age when selecting activities.
- *Spiritual*: Change the intensity, focus, and meaning of activity. Ask the individual to discuss the meaning of the activity or reflect on the event.
- *Temporal*: Perform the activity at the same time. Vary length of time for the activity or change time expectations.
- *Virtual*: Require the client to use more or less familiar or unfamiliar technology.

## Environmental Modifications and Adaptations

Occupational therapists analyze context (cultural, physical, social, personal, spiritual, temporal, and virtual) and the client factors required for success to determine the activity demands on the person. The goal of therapy is for the client to engage in the occupation in its most natural context.

Thus, if the person comes from a large social and talkative family, the therapist's job is to help him or her return to this social context. Intervention aimed at having the person return to this environment differs from that in which the client may be returning home with minimal visitors.

## Tools

The tools used in occupational therapy intervention include therapeutic use of self (see Chapter 22), therapeutic use of occupations or activities, consultation (see Chapter 31), and education (see Chapter 20). The tools used when conducting therapeutic use of occupations and activities include:

- Materials (e.g., arts and crafts, self-care, work, leisure, communication)
- Social (e.g., role playing, acting, dance, sports)
- Animal-assisted (e.g., dogs, pet care, hippotherapy)
- Specialized setting (e.g., aquatic therapy, vocational rehabilitation)
- Personal reflections (e.g., writing, singing, meditation, artwork)

## Materials

The materials used in occupational therapy intervention include any materials used for self-care, work, education, leisure, and social participation. In the clinic setting, occupational therapists may use craft activities, computer-based cognitive activities, or simulators to ensure that clients are ready for the actual occupation. The occupational therapist must analyze the materials used and help the client be successful through adapting the materials. Table 15-4 provides a description of some of the activities that may be used in practice.

# Case Example Intervention Plan Using Model of Practice

Evidence exists to support the use of the Model of Human Occupation (Kielhofner, 2008) in practice (Forsyth, Mann, & Kielhofner, 2005; Keller & Forsyth, 2004; Lee, Taylor, Kielhofner, & Fisher, 2008). MOHO provides occupational therapy practitioners with a framework for viewing occupational performance. The following case example provides an overview of how one might use this model for intervention planning.

Mabel is a 75-year-old woman who experiences health issues of diabetes, heart disease, and arthritis. Recently, Mabel fell and fractured her hip. Mabel has difficulty walking up stairs and is unable to lift heavy objects. She has recently lost her husband and lives on her own in the country. Her daughter lives 1 hour away from her; she is concerned about her mother's ability to live on her own. The occupational therapy practitioner working in acute care received a referral to evaluate and treat Mabel.

*Volition*: Mabel loves to cook. She enjoys watching soap operas and talking to family and friends. Mabel has 2 dogs. She used to love to do puzzles with her husband. She will not do puzzles now.

**Table 15-4. Suggested Activities**

| Activity | Description | Goals | Comments |
|---|---|---|---|
| Treasure hunt | Ask child to follow the written steps to find a "treasure." Reinforce the concept of the list. Ask the child to write steps down for an activity to reinforce organization skills. | • Increase organization for school | Children will do better if they come up with the system for organizing their work. Be sure to include them in the process and be flexible with the outcome. |
| Lunch group | Have a regular lunch group requiring each client to prepare a part of the meal depending upon his or her ability. Once clients are able, require one client to make the entire lunch for the group. Praise the success and have the clients enjoy a lunch break. | • Increase ability to prepare meals<br>• Increase ability to play with others (e.g., share playthings) | Asking family members, friends, or even other staff members to lunch may help the person feel special and proud of his or her accomplishments. |
| Picture frame | Glue beads on a wooden or cardboard picture frame to decorate it. Place a picture inside the frame upon completion. | • Increase hand function | Providing a variety of beads, stickers, and paint changes the complexity of the project. |

*Habituation*: Mabel reported that recently, she has no desire to watch television or talk to friends. Mabel stated she gets up "whenever," sort of eats, and takes a shower. Mabel stated she spent her day "hanging out at home." She has a few friends who come to visit. Her daughter visits at least once a week.

*Performance*: Mabel moved slowly and made little contact with the therapist. She followed simple verbal directions and answered questions in complete sentences. Mabel had difficulty moving from her bed to the chair. She has a R hip fracture.

*Environment*: Mabel lives in the country in a cold climate. She has a few friends nearby who visit her (weekly). Her daughter visits her weekly. Mabel lives in a two-story house. She does not drive and there is no bus available.

*Intervention Plan*: The occupational therapy practitioner considers Mabel's volition, habituation, performance, and environment when selecting activities and designing the intervention plan. The practitioner decides (with Mabel's input) that they will work to help her revisit her joy of cooking. Since the practitioner is working in an acute care setting, the goal of the intervention is to provide Mabel with R hip precautions for healing. Thus, the practitioner is able to determine if Mabel is capable of safe living at home while evaluating her kitchen skills. Furthermore, the practitioner considers Mabel's environment and works with the physical therapists to be sure that Mabel is mobile in her home. Since winter is approaching, the practitioner meets with the daughter and Mabel to develop strategies for home safety concerning snow shoveling and emergency preparedness in case of power outages. Intervention also includes goals to improve Mabel's habits and routines so that she can re-engage in occupations such as cooking, visiting with friends, watching television, and making puzzles.

# Case Sample Intervention Plan Using Frame of Reference

The developmental frame of reference (Llorens, 1976) is frequently used to facilitate learning and development in children. This frame of reference relies on identifying the child's level of ability and providing activity to promote the next step. Thus, a developmental approach uses practice in a variety of activities. The central principle underlying the developmental approach is that through practice, improved neural synapses occur resulting in improved performance and improved motor patterns. The following example illustrates the use of the developmental frame of reference to structure intervention.

Trevor is a 2-year-old boy diagnosed with global developmental delays. Trevor lives at home with his mother, father, and 4-year-old brother in the city. The occupational therapy practitioner begins intervention planning by conducting a developmental assessment to determine the level at which Trevor is functioning in terms of feeding, dressing, bathing, and play. After completing the Hawaii Early Learning Profile (HELP), a developmental checklist, the practitioner determines a level of functioning for Trevor for gross motor, fine motor, social participation, feeding, dressing, and play. Once age levels for these systems are established, the practitioner is able to design intervention to address the next logical step in development. For example, Trevor will pick up a variety of foods and feed himself (9 to 12 months skill), but he will not bring a spoon to his mouth (12 to 15 months skill) or hold a cup handle (12 to 15.5 months skill). The practitioner works on a variety of developmental skills through play each session and provides parents with a home program to reinforce the concepts. This approach relies on practice to teach the child.

# Summary

Planning intervention involves determining occupational-based goals, adapting and grading activities, and being mindful of the impact the context has upon the success of the activity. Intervention planning requires a clear evaluation of the clients' strengths and weaknesses and collaboration on occupational-based goals. The occupational therapy practitioner bases intervention on a well-developed frame of reference. The materials, activities, and techniques used vary with clients and goals. Practice and experience with reflection make the process of activity analysis creative and meaningful, which benefits clients.

# Student Self-Assessment

1. Develop an activity. Decide on the age, client population, goals, and purpose of the activity. Describe how the activity can be adapted or modified to meet various clients' needs.
2. Examine an activity using Appendix D as your guide. Describe the contextual aspects of the activity, the client factors involved, and the performance habits required. Present the activity to the class as a teaching-learning experience.
3. Conduct an activity with classmates role-playing different client issues. Discuss how to intervene and change the activity so that all are successful.

4. Cultural considerations—Interview a person from a culture different from your own. Discuss occupations of importance to them and the activities involved. Present the activity to the class, discussing the importance of this to the culture. Provide directions for each class member.
5. Compile a notebook of activities that you may use in clinical settings. Include website references and handouts that may be helpful. Organize the activities so that you can readily find an appropriate one for a client.
6. Examine an occupation prevalent in your area (e.g., lobsterman, basket weaver). What are the skills, client factors, habits, and contextual aspects of this activity? How could you adapt or grade the activity?
7. Find a local resource that may help a client (e.g., senior citizens' center, therapeutic horseback riding clinic). Find out the cost, benefits, times, and services provided. Share these with your classmates.

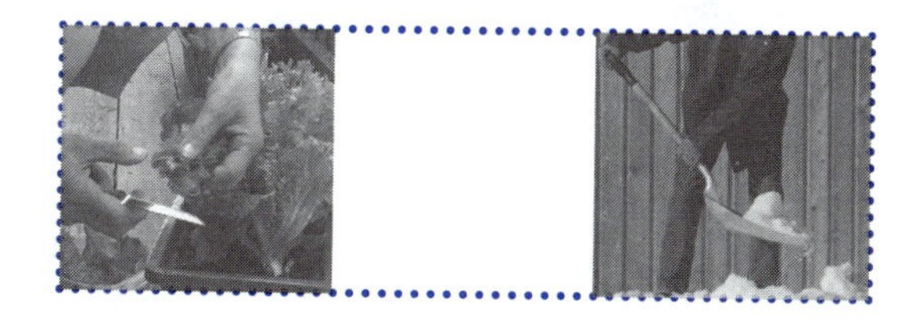

# References


American Occupational Therapy Association. (1990). Entry-level role delineation for registered occupational therapists (OTRs) and certified occupational therapy assistants (COTAs). *American Journal of Occupational Therapy, 44*(12), 1091-1102.

American Occupational Therapy Association. (1994). Guide for supervision of occupational therapy personnel. *American Journal of Occupation Therapy, 48*(11), 1045-1046.

American Occupational Therapy Association. (2008). Occupational therapy practice framework: Domain and process, second edition. *American Journal of Occupational Therapy, 62*, 625-683.

Ayres, A. J. (1979). *Sensory integration and the child.* Los Angeles, CA: Western Psychological Services.

Black, R. M., & Wells, S. A. (2007). *Culture and occupation: A model of empowerment in occupational therapy.* Baltimore, MD: AOTA Press.

Bobath, B. (1975). Sensorimotor development. *NDT Newsletter, 7*, 1.

Christiansen, C., & Baum, C. M. (1997). Person-environment occupational performance: A conceptual model for practice. In C. Christiansen & C Baum (Eds.), *Occupational therapy: Enabling function & well-being* (2nd ed.). Thorofare, NJ: SLACK Incorporated.

Fisher, A. G. (1998). Uniting practice and theory in an occupational framework. 1998 Eleanor Clarke Slagle Lecture. *American Journal of Occupational Therapy, 52*(7), 509-521.

Forsyth, K., Mann, L. S., & Kielhofner, G. (2005). Scholarship of practice: Making occupation-focused, theory-driven, evidence-based practice a reality. *British Journal of Occupational Therapy, 68*(6), 260-268.

Keller, J., & Forsyth, K.(2004). The model of human occupation in practice. *Israel Journal of Occupational Therapy, 13*(3), E99-E106.

Kielhofner, G. (1985). *A model of human occupation: Theory and application* (2nd ed.), Philadelphia, PA: Lippincott Williams & Wilkins.

Kielhofner, G. (2002). Dimensions of doing. In G. Kielhofner (Ed.), *A model of human occupation: Theory and application* (3rd ed.). Philadelphia, PA: Lippincott Williams & Wilkins.

Kielhofner, G. (2005). Rethinking disability and what to do about it: Disability studies and its implications for occupational therapy. *American Journal of Occupational Therapy, 59*(5), 487-496.

Kielhofner, G. (2008). *A model of human occupation: Theory and application* (4th ed.). Baltimore, MD: Lippincott Williams & Wilkins.

Howle, J. (2005). Neuro-developmental treatment approach: Theoretical foundations and principles of clinical practice. In J. Case-Smith. *Occupational therapy for children* (5th ed., p. 296). St. Louis, MO: Mosby.

Law, M., Cooper, B. A., Strong, S., Stewart, D., Rigby, P., & Letts, L. (1996). The person-environment-occupation model: A transactive approach to occupational performance. *Canadian Journal of Occupational Therapy, 63*(1), 9-23.

Lee, S. W., Taylor, R., Kielhofner, G., & Fisher, G. (2008). Theory use in practice: A national survey of therapists who use the Model of Human Occupation. *American Journal of Occupational Therapy, 62*(1), 106-117.

Llorens, L. A. (1976). *Application of a developmental theory for health and rehabilitation.* Rockville, MD: AOTA Press.

MacRae, N. (2001). Unpublished lecture notes: OT 301 foundations of occupational therapy. Biddeford, ME: University of New England.

Maurer, T., Smith, D., & Armetta, C. (1989). Purposeful activity as exercise. *Occupational Therapy in Mental Health, 9*, 9-20.

McColl, M. A. (2005). Disability studies at the population level: Issues of health service utilization. *American Journal of Occupational Therapy, 59*(5), 516-526.

Melchert-McKearnan, K., Dietz, J., Engel, J. M., & White, O. (2000). Children with burn injuries: Purposeful activity versus rote exercise. *American Journal of Occupational Therapy, 54*(4), 381-390.

Mosey, A. C. (1981). *Occupational therapy: Configuration of a profession.* New York, NY: Raven Press.

Neistadt, M., & Crepeau, E. B. (1998). *Willard & Spackman's occupational therapy* (9th ed.). Philadelphia, PA: Lippincott Williams & Wilkins.

Neville-Jan, A. (2005). The problem with prevention: The case of spina bifida. *American Journal of Occupational Therapy, 59*(5), 527-539.

Nichols, D. (2005). Development of postural control. In J. Case-Smith. *Occupational therapy for children* (5th ed.). St. Louis, MO: Mosby.

Pedretti, L. W. & Paszuinielli, S. (1990). A frame of reference for occupational therapy in physical dysfunction. In L. W. Pedretti & B. Zoltan (Eds.), *Occupational therapy: Practice skills for physical dysfunction* (3rd ed., pp. 1-17) St. Louis, MO: Mosby.

Schkade, J. K., & Schultz, S. (1992). Occupational adaptation: Toward a holistic approach in contemporary practice, Part I. *American Journal of Occupational Therapy, 46*(9), 829-837.

Schoen S., & Anderson, J. (1993). Neurodevelopmental treatment frame of reference. In P. Kramer & J. Hinojosa. *Frames of reference for pediatric occupational therapy.* Baltimore, MD: Lippincott Williams & Wilkins.

Schoen, S., & Anderson, J. (1999). Neurodevelopmental treatment frame of reference. In P. Kramer & J. Hinojosa. *Frames of reference for pediatric occupational therapy* (2nd ed.). Philadelphia, PA: Lippincott Williams & Wilkins.

Shumway-Cook, A., & Woollacott, M. (2007). *Motor control: Theory and practical applications.* Philadelphia, PA: Lippincott Williams & Wilkins.

Solomon, J. W., & O'Brien, J. C. (2006). Scope of practice. In J. W. Solomon & J. C. O'Brien (Eds.), *Pediatric skills of the occupational therapy assistant* (2nd ed.). St. Louis, MO: Mosby.

Steinbeck, T. M. (1986). Purposeful activity and performance. *American Journal of Occupational Therapy, 40*(8), 529-534.

Taylor, R. R. (2005). Can the social model explain all of disability experience? Perspectives of persons with chronic fatigue syndrome. *American Journal of Occupational Therapy, 59*(5), 497-506.

Thibodaux, L. R. (2005). Habitus and the embodiment of disability through lifestyle. *American Journal of Occupational Therapy, 59*(5), 507-515.

Townsend, E., Brintnell, S., & Staisey, N. (1990). Developing guidelines for client-centered occupational therapy practice. *Canadian Journal of Occupational Therapy, 57*(2), 69-76.

Trombly, C. A. (1994). Rood approach. In C. Trombly (Ed.), *Occupational therapy for physical dysfunction* (4th ed.). Baltimore, MD: Williams & Wilkins.

World Health Organization. (2001). *International classification of functioning, disability, and health (ICF)*. Geneva, Switzerland: Author.

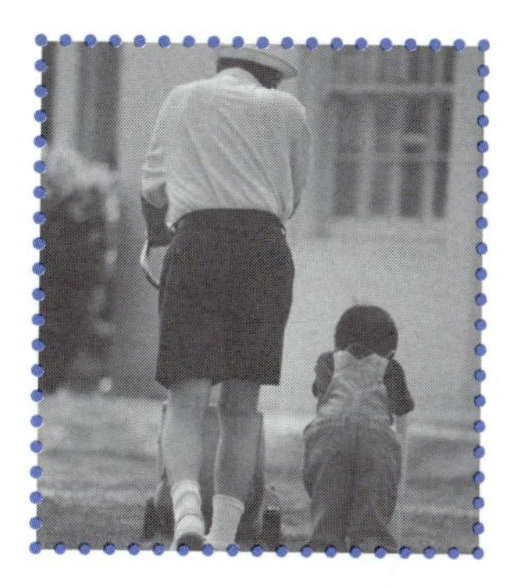

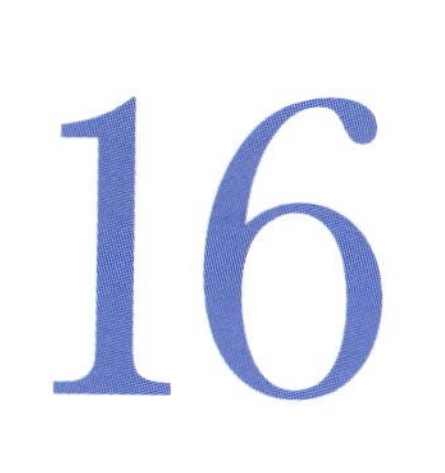

# 16

# Interventions of Activities of Daily Living and Instrumental Activities of Daily Living

*Michael E. Roberts, MS, OTR/L*

**ACOTE Standards Explored in This Chapter**

B.5.1-5.6, 5.19-5.21

**Key Terms**

Activities of daily living (ADL)
Adaptation
Instrumental activities of daily living (IADL)
Maintenance
Performance context

## Introduction

Occupational performance in activities of daily living (ADL) and instrumental activities of daily living (IADL) serve as the foundation for the expression of meaning and identity for clients of occupational therapy practitioners (American Occupational Therapy Association [AOTA], 2008; Christiansen, 1999). It follows logically and, therefore, the evaluation, intervention, and outcomes related to these areas of occupation are of critical importance to effective service delivery. Indeed, this focus on effective self-management of these areas of occupation has served as the defining core of the profession since its earliest days (Meyer, 1922).

## Assessment of ADL and IADL Performance

An evaluation of ADL and IADL performance is comprised of an initial occupational profile and a more focused performance analysis, frequently involving direct observation and standardized assessments (AOTA, 2008). During this first phase of developing and implementing the intervention plan, the frame of reference or model of practice most appropriate for the client is selected, client priorities and perspective are evaluated and incorporated, and the influence of the context of performance are assessed. This process must be ultimately directed by the needs of the



K. Sladyk, K. Jacobs, & N. MacRae (Eds.).
*Occupational Therapy Essentials for Clinical Competence* (pp. 175-186).

client and their input. The frame of reference or model of practice must be selected exclusively by an assessment of the client's needs and capacities, not practitioner preference. An evaluation of client priorities drives intervention selection and goal setting. Accurate assessments of client perspective and context are critical to ensuring the durability and applicability of goals and intervention plans throughout the continuum of care.

The occupational profile frequently includes questions like, "Tell me about your typical day," or "What activities or roles are most important to you?" or "How has your life changed because of your disease/trauma/life change?" These questions allow for the client to identify the most typical patterns of performance, habits, or roles that comprise their occupational existence. Follow-up questions or active listening techniques can elicit important information about client priorities, perceived obstacles to effective performance, or adaptive/maladaptive strategies for improving performance. Also, occupational history, influence of caregivers or other contextual issues, and client goals may be understood more effectively through effective strategic use of initial interviews with clients. It is important to remember that effective use of the occupational profile and initial interview period must result in specific, occupation-focused priorities in order to result in an effective intervention plan (Neistadt, 1995). This occupation-directed outcome is important for defining our profession for our clients, and continues as a challenge for practitioners in current practice (McAndrew, McDermott, Vitzakovitch, Warunek, & Holm, 2000).

The next step in the evaluation of ADL and IADL performance is to determine more specifically how to focus the practitioners' efforts through analysis of occupational performance (AOTA, 2008). Informed by the occupational profile, evidence-based practice strategies, and the frame of reference or model of practice most effective for the client, performance is directly observed in the most appropriate context, using standardized assessments where possible (AOTA, 2008). Ideally, tasks such as meal preparation, laundry management, bathing, or dressing are observed and performance is assessed in the environment most commonly used by the client. In certain clinical settings, or due to particular medical issues, this is not always possible. In these instances, the alternative context must be specifically documented in order to provide the most complete picture of ADL/IADL performance. Also, observation of performance in a clinical context or a client's usual or home context is preferable to relying exclusively on self-report of function. Research comparing standardized assessments with self-reported IADL status suggested greater accuracy is obtained through performance-based measures (Hilton, Fricke, & Unsworth, 2001), as practitioners may expect.

The order or priority given to the assessment of specific performance skills, performance patterns, or client factors depends on the needs and priorities of the client. Utilization of an occupation-focused or "top-down" approach may be effective for certain clients, while a "bottom-up" or component-based approach may be best for other clients (Trombly, 1993, p. 253), and still others receive the most effective intervention through an assessment of the client's context and its impact (Weinstock-Zlotnich & Hinojosa, 2004). For example, in a client who presents with diabetic peripheral polyneuropathy, an assessment from a "top-down" approach may identify decreased client satisfaction with her role as an independent grandparent who cooks brunch for her family every Sunday morning. Based on the occupational profile, her occupational therapist may perform a more focused assessment of safety with sharp objects in the kitchen, foot care as part of her morning self-care routine, and functional mobility assessments in the kitchen during meal preparation to directly identify the roles or occupational priorities most important to this client.

A "bottom-up" approach may also be determined to be the best for this client, including standardized assessments of balance, peripheral sensation, safety awareness, or other foundational skills that, when addressed in the intervention plan, are expected to result in the resolution of the larger occupational performance issues. The client may benefit most from a contextual assessment first, evaluating the effectiveness of resource utilization, impact of caregivers, and influence of the physical, social, cultural, or temporal environments on the client's performance of her Sunday morning brunch routine.

The most effective approach is the one that is most effective for meeting the needs of the client, not the approach with which the practitioner is most comfortable or the one that is routinely used in the setting where assessment occurs. Rather, effectiveness in evaluation depends upon the "fit" of the approach to the client (Weinstock-Zlotnich & Hinojosa, 2004), while maintaining the focus on occupation inherent in occupational therapy practice.

Non-standardized assessments of ADL and IADL performance can provide valuable information for intervention plan development, but the selection of a frame of reference or model of practice, or an intention of adherence to evidence-based practice often necessitate the incorporation of standardized assessments of the performance of basic and instrumental ADL. It is important to note that standardized assessments need not be full self-care assessments in order to inform intervention planning. Standardized assessments of client factors may prove to be predictive of self-care performance, such as deficits in categorization and deductive reasoning logically proving effective predictors of IADL performance (Goverover & Hinojosa, 2002).

The following is a selection of standardized assessments of ADL and IADL performance in current use in occupational therapy clinical practice and mentioned in this chapter:

- *Arnadottir Occupational Therapy ADL Neurobehavioral Evaluation (A-ONE)*: Two-part observational assessment focusing on ADL (Arnadottir, 1990).

- *Assessment of Living Skills and Resources (ALSAR)*: Interview-based assessment for IADL that incorporates available resource utilization in determining the true relevance and prioritization of IADL dysfunction (Williams et al., 1991).
- *Assessment of Motor and Process Skills (AMPS)*: Fifty-six tasks typical to IADL routines of children, adolescents, or adults to allow standardized ratings on specific motor and process skills (Fisher, 1999).
- *Canadian Occupational Performance Measure (COPM)*: This semi-structured interview is used to identify the client's perception of his or her occupational performance in self-care, productive, and leisure tasks (Law et al., 2005).
- *Functional Independence Measure (FIM)*: A widely used multidisciplinary assessment of functional performance in physical dysfunction settings, and adapted for use with children as the WeeFIM. The FIM uses a 7-point scale to describe the amount of assistance required for the subject to perform 18 tasks relating to self-care, cognition, and communication (Uniform Data System for Medical Rehabilitation, 2000).
- *Klein-Bell Activities of Daily Living Scale (Klein-Bell)*: One hundred seventy subtasks of dressing, elimination, mobility, hygiene and bathing, emergency communication, and eating are rated and weighted according to relative importance and difficulty. This assessment may be used in children and adults (Klein & Bell, 1979).
- *Kohlman Evaluation of Living Skills (KELS)*: Interview and observation utilized primarily to determine the likelihood of safe, independent function in the community for clients with psychiatric diagnoses and/or cognitive dysfunction (McGourty, 1979).
- *Minimum Data Set (MDS)*: Used in long-term care and covering a large and comprehensive view of the client's health and function, occupational therapy practitioners contribute to section G, which relates to mobility and ADL/IADL performance (Nelson & Glass, 1999). The performance of these components must be observed, and scores must represent the resident's performance at his or her status of greatest need across all hours within the previous 7 days (Centers for Medicare and Medicaid Services, 2005).
- *Occupational Self Assessment (OSA)*: The OSA is a Model of Human Occupation self-report assessment that measures clients' satisfaction with their performance of tasks and activities, as well as their perceived mastery of their environment (Kielhofner & Forsyth, 2001).
- *Outcome and Assessment Information Set (OASIS)*: Sixteen ADL/IADL performance subtests are included in this comprehensive home-care assessment. Questions on this assessment are used to determine reimbursement based on acuity, functional assistance required, complexity, and other factors (Center for Health Services and Policy Research, 1998).
- *Performance Assessment of Self-Care Skills (PASS)*: Used with adults to evaluate performance in functional mobility, home management, and basic ADL, with differing protocols depending upon whether assessment occurs at the client's home or in the clinic of the assessing occupational therapy clinician (Rogers & Holm, 1994).
- *Routine Task Inventory (RTI)*: For clinicians operating within Allen's cognitive disability model, this assessment relates observed and reported self-care performance to Allen's cognitive levels (Allen, Earhart, & Blue, 1992).
- *Safe At Home*: Specific to safety and safety awareness of adult clients in the home environment, Safe At Home involves 12 test items related to typical environmental hazards in the home (Robnett, Hopkins, & Kimball, 2002).
- *Satisfaction with Performance Scaled Questionnaire (SPSQ)*: Subjects for this assessment report the percentage of time in the last 6 months that they were satisfied by their performance in 46 ADL/IADL tasks (Yerxa, Burnett-Beaulieu, Stocking, & Azen, 1988).

## Contextual Issues With Assessment

In the current practice environment, there are a number of factors that can impact or influence assessments and outcomes, which must be considered in the anticipation of developing an intervention plan. A necessary consideration in contemporary practice is reimbursement (see Chapter 34). Whether discussing the Prospective Payment System (PPS), Resource Utilization Groups (RUGs), Individualized Education Plans (IEPs), Health Maintenance Organizations (HMOs), Managed Care Organizations (MCOs), Preferred Provider Options (PPOs), or any other configuration of reimbursement for occupational therapy services, practitioners must strive for effective outcomes and optimal intervention planning regardless of payer source (AOTA, 2000).

Despite expected adherence to the AOTA Code of Ethics, some discrepancies have surfaced (see Chapter 40 on knowledge of AOTA's Code of Ethics, Core Values, and Standards of Practice). One typical example is research describing functional outcomes for clients with a cerebral vascular accident (CVA) who receive rehabilitation services. Those who utilized a Medicare HMO instead of the traditional fee-for-service plans for their intervention received fewer therapy and medical specialist visits and more home care visits, made less progress in functional performance, and were more likely to be living in a nursing home 1 year after their stroke (Kramer et al., 2000). Ideally, practitioners are developing intervention plans as if they were "blind" to reimbursement issues, but incorporating an appreciation of expected utilization limits may help ensure an equality of outcomes across payer sources.

Practitioners must also be aware of how they are perceived by their clients and their clients' perceptions of their own function, as these may impact the data collected in assessments and thereby impact intervention planning. Mothers who are engaged in the IADL of child rearing report that practitioners who present with a more relaxed and friendly demeanor are perceived as having better insight into the daily routine of child rearing and having a greater capacity to "tailor" services to the specific needs of the family (Thompson, 1998). This fact encourages practitioners to be aware of their interactive styles from the development of the intervention plan and to reassess the effectiveness of their therapeutic use of self through the intervention process.

Practitioners may also be affected by their own prejudices regarding settings, populations, and ADL/IADL function. Misguided generalizations may negatively impact the capacity of an intervention plan to most directly and efficiently enhance the functional independence and quality of life for our clients. Research has identified that residents in long-term care facilities perceived themselves to present with significantly higher levels of function than that documented by clinicians (Atwood, Holm, & James, 1994). Dunford, Missiuna, Street, and Sibert (2005) reported that children with a developmental coordination disorder described concerns regarding limitations in performance of self-care and leisure activities, while these deficits were largely not identified by parents or teachers for these children. Self-awareness regarding pre-conceptions in the assessment of clients becomes a matter of ensuring a professional level of intervention, and this information must be incorporated into the assessment and intervention planning processes.

The environment utilized for assessment and intervention may also affect results of assessment and intervention. As described earlier, assessment in the client's most commonly used performance context is ideal, while an observation of performance, regardless of setting, is still preferable to relying solely on self-report of status. Some inpatient facilities invest significant resources into replicating, as closely as possible, contextually-appropriate environments for their clients, with the expectation that contextually-appropriate settings lead to contextually-appropriate carryover. This theory, however, has not been borne out. Richardson, Law, Wishart, and Guyatt (2000) demonstrated that no significant functional performance difference was achieved with the use of contextually-appropriate intervention settings. Davis, Hoppes, and Chesbro (2005) reported that there is no substitute for assessment in the clients' home (their most personally-relevant context), wherein clients with dementia and IADL dysfunction were found to be largely similar in functional profile, except that clients exhibited higher levels of motor skills in their homes.

# Intervention

Once evaluation data is obtained, an intervention plan can be developed, including objectives, expected time frame for goal completion, roles for practitioners, and an evidence-based intervention approach within the chosen model of practice or frame of reference (AOTA, 2008). Throughout implementation of the intervention plan, a constant intervention outcome "feedback loop" informs an evaluation of the plan's efficacy, including not only functional progress with ADLs and IADLs, but also the effectiveness of changes to the available resources, performance context, or therapeutic use of self strategies.

Once the evaluation data has been compiled and the objectives have been determined in collaboration with the client and other members of the client's health care team, the most appropriate intervention approach must be selected. The framework (AOTA, 2008) describes five approaches: create or promote, establish or restore, maintain, modify, and prevent. Each of these approaches is used in combination with some or all of the others with each client depending upon the client's needs.

- *Create or promote*: The create or promote approach, also described as health promotion, involves interventions that facilitate the enhancement of health and function in natural contexts of life (AOTA, 2008). This approach may involve utilization of universal design strategies for living spaces, or offering cooking classes to enhance nutrition, socialization, and mobility practice in an assisted living facility.
- *Establish or restore*: The establish or restore or remediation approach seeks to ensure acquisition and mastery of skills that are absent, lost, or impaired (AOTA, 2008). This approach may include establishing a well-balanced and effective morning ADL routine for a client with a chronic disease, enhancement of activity tolerance in standing for meal preparation or cleanup, or addressing limitations of fine motor control and hand strength to allow a return to independence with grooming and oral care after carpal tunnel release surgery.
- *Maintain*: The maintenance approach, while frowned upon in documentation for rehabilitation settings, is also important for ensuring maximal ADL/IADL performance (AOTA, 2008). For example, practitioners using this approach may use magnifiers and templates to allow clients with low vision to complete budgeting, check writing, or developing grocery lists. Practitioners may teach the use of timers and

pill boxes with clients with chronic mental illness to ensure effective medication management once they are discharged from an inpatient clinical setting. This approach may also be used to train clients with amyotrophic lateral sclerosis (ALS) in energy conservation and work simplification to delay the outpacing of ADL demands with declining activity tolerance.

- *Modify*: The modify or adaptation approach (AOTA, 2008) is used quite frequently in rehabilitation settings. In this setting, practitioners use adaptation to decrease the demands of the environment and task to meet the client's expected skill level after remediation. This approach is evident when practitioners teach the use of a sock aid after a client's hip replacement surgery, modify workspaces to maximize ergonomic fit of the client and task, or train clients with chronic obstructive pulmonary disease in the use of tub seats, hand-held showers, and long-handled sponges to decrease trunk flexion and conserve energy during bathing. Given this information, it is important to use adaptive equipment and adaptations judiciously, as too many changes to the home environment, too many new strategies at once, or too great an expenditure of resources to ensure success with adaptations may defeat the initial purpose. The social, developmental, and cultural impact of adaptations and adaptive equipment must be taken into consideration before time and effort are carved out of the intervention plan for their training and use.
- *Prevent*: Prevention is also utilized as an intervention approach in clients and populations determined to be at-risk. Teaching communication skills to school-age children to reduce school violence, teaching proper body mechanics during home maintenance and laundry tasks for clients with chronic low back pain, or incorporating effective foot care into the ADL routines of clients with diabetes are all examples of preventative approaches with at-risk clients.

As described earlier, these approaches are not necessarily mutually exclusive, and most effective intervention plans incorporate all of the approaches. For instance, a client with rheumatoid arthritis who presents with pain in both hands with grooming tasks, difficulties with lower body ADL due to limited joint range of motion and low back pain, difficulty with food preparation, opening pill bottles, and writing checks due to hand deformities may require all of the approaches in order to achieve ADL/IADL independence and improved quality of life. This client may require joint protection retraining to prevent any future deterioration of joint function. The client may use an occupational therapy selected or fabricated upper extremity splint to prevent further deterioration of joints in his or her hands, as well as maintain range and alignment in the hands at this point. The demands of the client's environment may be modified by introducing adaptive equipment that decreases the demands of tasks to meet the client's current status, such as an adapted built-up toothbrush to decrease the pain and coordination demands of oral care tasks or a dressing stick to reduce the trunk range and low back pain demands of lower body dressing. The practitioner may also assist the client in establishing a new daily routine of ADL and IADL to enhance joint protection and energy conservation strategies for daily living tasks that must be completed by the client. Finally, the creation of adaptive equipment or strategies within the client's home environment may reduce dysfunction and pain and may promote greater participation and engagement in occupations that enhance functional independence, such as money management, medication management, laundry and clothing management, or other potentially difficult IADL tasks.

In the previously described example, a number of different "instruments" are utilized by the practitioner in conjunction with the client. These instruments have classifications depending upon their complexity and intention. Preparatory activities are interventions that help a client prepare for functional performance. These may include splinting, modalities, or joint mobilization. In the arthritis example, a practitioner may don or doff a splint for the client, apply moist heat or paraffin to their hands, or perform manual joint distraction to enhance joint range of motion and reduce pain. These are not specifically occupation-based activities. However, if they are completed in advance of meal preparation retraining or grooming retraining and the results of the preparatory activities enhance and improve performance, they have been used effectively and appropriately by the practitioner.

Some activities used in occupational therapy are described as purposeful activities, which achieve movement along therapeutic continua through engagement in goal-directed activities (AOTA, 2008). Practice with durable medical equipment (DME) for bathroom mobility, such as grab bars, tub seats, or commodes, would qualify as purposeful activities. These practice sessions addressing components of ADL/IADL are intended to enhance functional performance, yet they have the added benefit of additional focus on the most troublesome components leading to dysfunction, or breaking down occupational performance into manageable "pieces" without losing a focus on ultimate functional independence for the client or their caregivers.

Occupation-based activities involve participation in the specific occupations identified by the clients and practitioners as priorities to ensure independence and quality of life. Making a meal in the client's kitchen, training in donning and doffing the client's prosthesis, or practicing wheelchair-level toileting in the client's home bathroom are all examples of occupation-based activities used therapeutically. As expected, progression up the hierarchy of activities to occupation-based activities is often the goal of the intervention plan and an effective strategy for ADL/IADL retraining (Richards et al., 2005).

These different types of activities are then directed appropriately to address each of the components of the domain of occupational therapy. Client factors are addressed by adaptive equipment use, upper extremity (UE) orthosis construction and use, or preparatory methods like joint distraction or modalities. Performance patterns are addressed by joint protection and energy conservation training. Contextual issues are addressed when making environmental changes, using adaptive devices, or addressing temporal issues in training with ADL and IADL routines. The use of upper extremity orthoses, adaptive equipment for lower body dressing, or enhancing body mechanics training may all change activity demands. Teaching joint protection strategies, practicing them, and providing informed feedback to the client would impact and improve performance skills. In this way, all components of the domain of occupational therapy may be addressed (AOTA, 2008). In fact, comprehensive interventions of this type, and of joint protection retraining specifically, have been reported to be effective occupational therapy interventions with clients with rheumatoid arthritis (RA) (Steultjens et al., 2004).

It is important to remember that these interventions may address several approaches or aspects of occupational therapy's domain at once, and that the goals of effectively selected occupational tasks address as many components of independence and quality of life as possible. For instance, in the previously described example, an occupational therapist or occupational therapy assistant may address the client's difficulty with check writing through the use of an adapted writing implement and more ergonomically correct writing environment. Addressing this relatively small area of the client's occupational performance may accomplish many objectives at once. Joint degradation may be reduced, pain may be reduced, the client's satisfaction with maintaining financial independence may enhance quality of life and mood, and confidence in the occupational therapy team may improve, therefore enhancing the likelihood of carryover and success of other components of the intervention plan. In this way, an elegantly simple "melody" may enhance the overall effect of the occupational therapy intervention "symphony."

The previous example provides a description of ADL/IADL interventions with a client with a chronic disease. The domain remains the same for acute trauma and disease as well. For example, a client diagnosed with a left hemiparesis and left neglect after a stroke will require a number of different interventions from his or her occupational therapy team members. Given that all of the aspects of the occupational therapy domain will be affected in this clinical situation, a wide variety of interventions are possible. Evidence must be utilized to determine which of the interventions will most likely be of benefit to the client and his or her family. Expected ADL and IADL dysfunctions for a client with left hemiparesis are many. Limited motor function will make bilateral self-care tasks (donning socks, tying shoes) very difficult. Clothing management during toileting, meal preparation, grooming, medication management, kitchen and bathroom mobility, transfers in the home environment, sexuality, safety with sharp objects in the kitchen and temperatures in the bathroom, learning use of adaptive equipment or strategies, attention to the left side for functional tasks, balance during functional transfers, and health maintenance of the left side of the body are all components of occupational performance that may be negatively affected by the onset of the stroke. All of these may have different and changing priorities for the client, and they all may have dozens of different activities that are appropriate for use in intervention by practitioners with this client.

The ADL/IADL retraining process for more acute cases is the same as for chronic cases. The activity selection process depends upon the evidence available, the frame of reference or model of practice, the resources available to the client, the client's priorities, and the impact of other contextual issues, such as service delivery issues or family concerns. For this population in particular, recent research describes the following components critical to successful occupational therapy intervention (Trombly & Ma, 2002):

- Use of specific client-identified activities
- Use of and training with appropriate adaptations
- Maximizing the familiarity of the context
- Providing feedback to improve performance
- Providing ample practice with the activities

To illustrate, a number of client characteristics may impact independence in bathing, an important and foundational ADL. The client may highly value the activity and prioritize it for intervention. The client's left hemiparesis, left neglect, and impaired sensation on the left side may negatively affect task completion, safety, and bathroom mobility. Family members may express specific concerns about their ability to use the resources available to them to assist in ensuring the client's independence with this activity. The client may be concerned about the expertise of the occupational therapy team, the efficacy of the bathing retraining plan, or the possibility of institutionalization, all lending expanded meaning to bathing as an occupation-based activity.

The inherent complexity of meaning of the activity within occupational performance for this client in this situation must be seen as an opportunity and not an obstacle by the practitioners with whom this client works. One effective option for the occupational therapy team would be to incorporate the family members in the bathing retraining therapy sessions in as familiar a context as possible given the clinical situation. If, for instance, the practitioner demonstrates the use of adaptations like tub benches, hand-held showers, long-handled sponges, long mirrors, or grab bars to the client and family during a bathing retraining session, a number of objectives are addressed. Primarily, the client's functional performance improves. This activity may also reinforce transfer retraining, skin inspection or other health management strategies, enhancement of activity tolerance, sitting balance, attention to the affected side, problem-solving and scanning retraining, or energy conservation strategies. Demonstrated success with occupational therapy retraining may also enhance self-esteem, build confidence in the occupational therapy team and intervention plan, reduce family concerns about functional outcomes, and enhance carryover of other components of the intervention plan. Utilizing self-care retraining to enhance functional performance directly is also borne out as the most effective strategy for enhancing ADL performance (Walker et al., 2004).

Both of these clinical examples demonstrate the richness of ADL and IADL tasks as modalities within the intervention plan, or as "melodies" within the occupational therapy intervention "symphony." Because so many of these tasks are profoundly meaningful, defining, and personal for the clients, even the simplest of ADL or IADL tasks wield significant power to affect many or all aspects of occupational therapy's domain, and therefore are invaluable "instruments" within the occupational therapy "orchestra" of potential interventions and strategies.

## Therapeutic Outcomes

There are a number of different areas for intervention by practitioners in collaboration with their clients. Practitioners can incorporate movement along an adaptation-gradation continuum to match the demands of the retraining activity to the client's performance level and expected goals. An understanding of the performance skills that are intact may be used to enhance the skills that are lacking. Contexts must be understood and incorporated into intervention planning, especially available resources, influence of caregivers, expected disease or recovery process, and other therapies active with the client. Performance patterns, habits, routines, and roles of the client also may be affected and therefore prioritized for intervention planning (AOTA, 2008). Communication skills, client insight, client goals/priorities, socio-cultural and socio-economic influences, setting, acuity, and developmental level are also important potentially impactful issues to be addressed and utilized in enhancing or focusing the collaboration between clinician and client to maximize the effectiveness of the intervention plan.

Each of these potential intervention-maximizing components has an influence on the effectiveness of the practitioner's efforts to improve their client's quality of life and move with the client toward functional independence. Not all of the components need to be in effect or be actively addressed at all times in all situations, but it stands to reason that in order to "treat the whole person," clinicians should be utilizing or manipulating many of these components at once with each intervention.

One way to envision this strategy is to picture each of the potential intervention components or influences as a musical instrument. Just as there are different kinds of music appropriate for different situations in life, different combinations of these components of ADL/IADL function are addressed in whole or in part depending upon the client and their context. For instance, a relatively uncomplicated case such as an otherwise well client status post an elective orthopedic procedure may require a simpler "melody" or fewer "instruments" (e.g., 1950s-style rock-and-roll). The instruments still need to work together in rhythm, tempo, and key, and be adaptable to the demands of the situation, but can match the complexity of the case more directly.

More complex clinical cases, such as a client who is socio-economically disadvantaged, diagnosed with a chronic disease, and serves as caregiver to a spouse with a progressive neurological syndrome, will require more intricate interweaving of "instruments." A highly-skilled clinician "conductor" must ensure that all of the interventions are of one purpose, directing the production of one elegant symphonic masterpiece where the varied, unique, and inherently complex components construct a whole greater than the sum of the parts—more Mozart than Buddy Holly. Regardless of situation or complexity, recruiting and effectively utilizing as many of the "instruments" as possible for each client will enhance the holistic, life-changing potential of each intervention plan and thereby ensure the most effective collaboration with clients in their efforts to achieve success in ADL and IADL performance.

## Current Service Delivery Environment

The value of functional independence in self-care is appreciated not only by practitioners and their clients, but also by regulators and purchasers of health care services. More outcome measures related to the efficacy of therapy and health care services in general are focused on function and quality of life, which are traditional practice domains of practitioners. For example, Minimum Data Set (MDS) data is collected on all residents of long-term care facilities that receive Medicare or Medicaid funding. Ninety percent of occupational therapists responding to a survey reported they were involved in the MDS data collection in the long-term care facilities where they worked, mostly with subsections related to self-care and changes in ADL function (Nelson & Glass, 1999). Given the need for practitioners with this expertise, it is not surprising, therefore, that the change in Medicare reimbursement from a cost-based system to a client-specific resource utilization system has been associated with a greater likelihood of receiving occupational therapy services for non-elderly institutional long-term care residents (Wodchis, Fries, & Pollack, 2004).

The value associated with self-care and quality of life is also increasingly appreciated by other clinical professionals with whom practitioners frequently collaborate. Lysaght &

Wright (2005) suggested that in work-related practice settings, physical therapy approaches and interventions closely resembled those of occupational therapy practitioners. A psychiatric pilot study described the efficacy of a combined nursing case management and health management skills training program intended to enhance functional independence, independent living, and social functioning, which utilized case workers and nurses, not practitioners (Bartels et al., 2004). In other research, non-occupational therapy psychosocial programs focusing on promoting functional independence and utilizing ADL retraining, client-centered practice, "skill elicitation," and group therapies were lauded as "innovations" in the care of residents with dementia in nursing homes (Haitsma & Ruckdeschel, 2001). Perhaps the most direct example is a description of a one-week retreat for persons with multiple sclerosis staffed by physical therapists who assessed participants on self-esteem, quality of life, and ADL self-care (Beatus, O'Neill, Townsend, & Robrecht, 2002). The results of their retreat were described as a significant increase in quality of life related to mental components, but there was a lack of significant differences in self-esteem, physical components of quality of life, or functional independence.

These examples are important in that they describe an increased appreciation of professionals with whom practitioners collaborate for the traditional goals of occupational therapy's practice domain. Some are even attempting to expand their own practice domains to include these traditional occupational therapy goals. Two such examples are physical therapists attempting to expand their scope of practice to include "functional training in self-care and in home, community, or work integration" (American Physical Therapy Association [APTA], 2003) and athletic trainers claiming knowledge about implementation of return-to-work programs (Smith, 2006).

This increased appreciation for functional training in other professions is not a substitute, however, for the unique history, tradition, and skill set of occupational therapy practitioners honed over generations, informed by evidence-based practice, and tempered through a client-centered approach. Current occupational therapy practice has been shown to uniquely enhance occupational functioning in recent research (Alexander, Bugge, & Hagen, 2001; Hagsten, Svensson & Gardulf, 2004; Hastings, Gowans, & Watson, 2004; Walker et al., 2004). It should be noted, therefore, that appreciation for enhancing quality of life and functional independence among non-occupational therapy clinicians is not a substitute for occupational therapy practitioners' unequalled expertise in addressing ADL and IADL performance.

# Summary

Perhaps the most emblematic interventions utilized by occupational therapy practitioners are those involving basic and instrumental activities of daily living. Effective evaluation and intervention of deficits in these occupational performance areas are critical to a client-centered approach, particularly because of their potential for expression of uniquely personal meaning for clients. Successful assessment and interventions related to these areas include standardized evaluations, clinical reasoning within an appropriate model of practice or frame of reference, effective use of proper strategies and approaches, and judicious application of an appreciation for the impact of contextual issues on occupational performance.

# Student Self-Assessment

## IADL Group Discussion

Each of these questions can be asked of students in groups, then compiled answers can be presented to the rest of the class and discussed. Discussion can focus on identifying personal stereotypes or assumptions that may impair intervention planning, enhancing understanding of the client perspective, expression of personal values or identity through occupational performance, or the impact of resources on occupational performance, including contextual and caregiver issues.

1. Which IADL tasks are most important to you?
2. Do you believe that there are particular client populations less focused on certain components of self-care?
3. When you are busy or not feeling well, with which ADL and IADL tasks does your performance slip first, either by necessity or choice?
4. If you were working with a client with advanced Parkinson's disease in home care, how would your ADL retraining differ between your work with the client, their spouse, and the home health aide?

## Non-Traditional Case Study

This activity encourages thinking about function and personal values as opposed to rigid diagnosis-based reasoning. Additional information may be added to match recent course content, or role playing may be used to enhance incorporation of a client-centered approach into intervention planning.

Veronica, a 42-year-old married mother of two teenage daughters, had suffered from intractable right hip joint pain for many months. She had worked in a state government office for about 8 years but was increasingly unable to work because of the pain. Doctors suspected osteoarthritis despite its solitary presentation in her hip. She agreed to an elective total hip replacement and went in for surgery reluctantly.

When the surgeons opened up her hip joint for the arthroplasty, they found not arthritic changes, but a stage III osteosarcoma within the joint capsule. She was brought out of the anesthesia and told she instead needed a hemipelvectomy. She underwent the procedure and was admitted to inpatient rehabilitation. She was very tearful and withdrawn for the first 2 weeks of intervention. Later weeks of functional mobility and self-care intervention were hampered by her significant anxiety. She had been assured that it would be very unlikely that the cancer would recur as it was well encapsulated and later scans showed no evidence of recurrence anywhere else in her body.

Consider the following questions:

1. What are her priorities for effective functioning at home?
2. Which model of practice and which assessments would you use in intervention planning?
3. What impact will her family have on her recovery?
4. What potential areas of psychosocial dysfunction could limit her function?
5. What would your intervention plan include?
6. Which of Veronica's strengths will you utilize to improve her function?

# Group Activities

### Non-Traditional Occupations

This activity can engender discussions about cultural sensitivity, unique challenges to client education or teaching, communication issues, or enhancing the scope of available occupational performance components for use in intervention planning.

- Have students gain an appreciation for ADL or IADL retraining from the client's perspective by teaching others how to perform tasks not common to their cultural experience, such as learning to roll sushi, wrap a sari, tie a bowtie, or other tasks with or without simulated impairments/disabilities.

### Stump Your Classmates

This activity is a lower complexity activity that can be fun as well as educational. Teams of students can either ask other groups to guess the function of a device, or present three potential uses for the device and have competing groups guess which potential use is actually correct.

- Have students dig through catalogs of DME and medical suppliers to find obscure adaptive equipment, and attempt to "stump" each other in groups as to the purpose and application of the devices.

### Desert Island

This can be completed in groups with each group's results discussed and critiqued by their classmates.

- Each group is given a "desert island" scenario where they are assigned a disability, impairment, or limitation and an occupational performance context. They are then asked to select the three most important ADL/IADL in which to be independent and three most important resources or assistive equipment to have to enhance function and safety. For example: a married client with total hip replacement precautions in a two-story house, a client with low vision in elderly housing, a married mother of three with hemiplegia, and perceptual difficulties in an urban apartment.

# Electronic Resources

- AliMed—Medical and Ergonomic Products for Healthcare, Business, and Home: www.alimed.com
- Sammons Preston: www.sammonspreston.com
- Invacare: www.invacare.com

# References


Alexander, H., Bugge, C., & Hagen, S. (2001). What is the association between the different components of stroke rehabilitation and health outcomes? *Clinical Rehabilitation, 15*(2), 207-215.

Allen, C. K., Earhart, C., & Blue, T. (1992). *Occupational therapy treatment goals for the physically and cognitively challenged.* Rockville, MD: AOTA Press.

American Occupational Therapy Association. (2000). Occupational therapy code of ethics. *American Journal of Occupational Therapy, 54*, 614-616.

American Occupational Therapy Association. (2008). Occupational therapy practice framework: Domain and process, second edition. *American Journal of Occupational Therapy, 62*, 625-683.

American Physical Therapy Association. (2003). *Guide to physical therapist practice* (Revised 2nd ed.). Alexandria, VA: Author.

Arnadottir, G. (1990). *The brain and behavior: Assessing cortical dysfunction through tasks of daily living.* St. Louis, MO: Mosby.

Atwood, S. M., Holm, M. B., & James, A. (1994). Activities of daily living capabilities and values of long-term-care facility residents. *American Journal of Occupational Therapy, 48*(8), 710-716.

Bartels, S. J., Forester, B., Mueser, K. T., Miles, K. M., Dums, A. R., Pratt, S. I., et al. (2004). Enhanced skills training and health care management for older persons with severe mental illness. *Community Mental Health Journal, 40*(1), 75-90.

Beatus, J., O'Neill, J., Townsend, T., & Robrecht, K. (2002). The effect of a one-week retreat on self-esteem, quality of life, and functional ability for persons with multiple sclerosis. *Neurology Report, 26*(3), 154-159.

Bendstrup, K. E., Ingemann Jensen, J., Holm, S., & Bengtsson, B. (1997). Out-patient rehabilitation improves activities of daily living, quality of life and exercise tolerance in chronic obstructive pulmonary disease. *European Respiratory Journal, 10*(12), 2801-2806.

Center for Health Services and Policy Research. (1998). *Outcome and Assessment Information Set (OASIS-BI).* Denver, CO: Author.

| Evidence-Based Research Chart | | |
|---|---|---|
| **Population** | **Evidence** | **References** |
| CVA | Client-specific interventions, particularly ADL-specific retraining enhances independence of function | Kwan & Sandercock, 2006; Richards et al., 2005; Trombly & Ma, 2002; Walker, Gladman, Lincoln, Siemonsma, & Whiteley, 1999; Walker et al., 2004 |
| COPD | ADL performance and quality of life improved with simple program | Bendstrup, Ingemann Jensen, Holm, & Bengtsson, 1997 |
| Alzheimer's Disease | ADL retraining can improve client quality of life and decrease sense of burden for caregivers | Dooley & Hinojosa, 2004 |
| SCI | Client-centered intervention planning requires a focus on self-care and mobility | Donnelly et al., 2004 |
| TBI | Behavioral observation, task analysis, consistent practice, cue fading, acclimation to electronic aids to daily living are key to success with ADL/IADL | Erikson, Karlsson, Söderström, & Tham, 2004; Giles, Ridley, Dill, & Frye, 1997 |
| MS/Ataxia | Combination of contextual changes, adaptations, and orthoses increase ADL function | Gillen, 2000 |
| PTSD, homeless | Role identified for occupational therapy in addressing IADL, especially financial management | Davis & Kutter, 1998 |
| Intellectual disabilities | ADL performance hierarchy of difficulty for clients with mild and moderate intellectual disability identified, ADL performance can be improved, even in absence of change in insight | Hällgren & Kottorp, 2005; Kottorp, Bernspång, & Fisher, 2003 |
| RA | Impact of comprehensive occupational therapy, instruction in joint protection, and splints on functional ability | Steultjens et al., 2004 |
| Orthopaedics/Hip fracture | Individualized occupational therapy training enhances ADL function, likelihood of independent living, and reduces need for care at home | Hagsten et al., 2004 |
| Pediatrics/Teens/Young adults | Occupational therapy contributes to increased function, cognition, mobility in inpatient setting, increases peer connection, environmental adaptation, independence in 20-day summer program | Chen, Heinemann, Bode, Granger, & Mallinson, 2004; Healy & Rigby, 1999 |
| Cancer/Brain Tumors | Quality of life improvements may occur later than functional improvements, functional assessments may not sufficiently represent changes in clients | Huang, Wartella, & Kreutzer, 2001; Perez de Heredia, Cuadrado, Rodriguez, Lopez & Miangolarray, 2001 |
| Medical/Surgical: Organ transplantation, emergency medicine | Direct correlations between contact with occupational therapy and greater independence with ADL | Hastings et al., 2004; Patterson & Williams, 2005 |

CVA = Cerebral vascular accident
COPD = Chronic obstructive pulmonary disease
SCI = Spinal cord injury
TBI = Traumatic brain injury
MS = Multiple Sclerosis
PTSD = Posttraumatic Stress Disorder
RA = rheumatoid arthritis

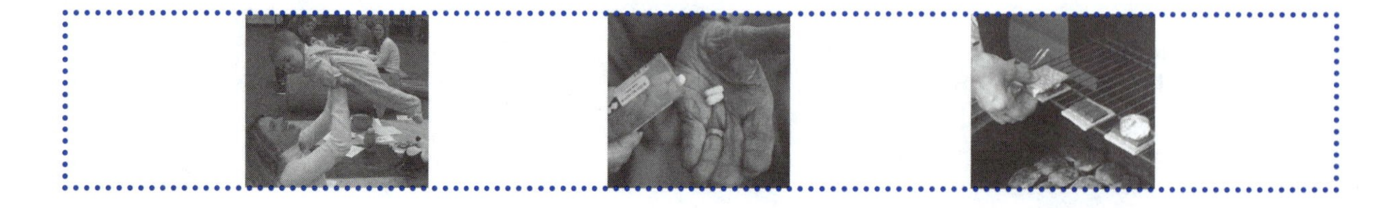

Centers for Medicare and Medicaid Services. (2005). *Minimum Data Set, 2.0*. Washington, DC: U.S. Government Printing Office.

Chen, C. C., Heinemann, A. W., Bode, R. K., Granger, C. V., & Maillinson, T. (2004). Impact of pediatric rehabilitation services on children's functional outcomes. *American Journal of Occupational Therapy, 58*(1), 44-53.

Christiansen, C. H. (1999). The 1999 Eleanor Clarke Slagle Lecture. Defining lives: Occupation as identity: An essay on competence, coherence, and the creation of meaning. *American Journal of Occupational Therapy, 53*(6), 547-558.

Davis, J., & Kutter, C. J. (1998). Independent living skills and posttraumatic stress disorder in women who are homeless: Implications for future practice. *American Journal of Occupational Therapy, 52*(1), 39-44.

Davis, L. A., Hoppes, S., & Chesbro, S. B. (2005). Cognitive-communicative and independent living skills assessment in individuals with dementia: A pilot study of environmental impact. *Topics in Geriatric Rehabilitation, 21*(2), 136-143.

Donnelly, C., Eng, J. J., Hall, J., Alford, L., Giachino, R., Norton, K., et al. (2004). Client-centred assessment and the identification of meaningful treatment goals for individuals with a spinal cord injury. *Spinal Cord, 42*(5), 302-307.

Dooley, N. R., & Hinojosa, J. (2004). Improving quality of life for persons with Alzheimer's disease and their family caregivers: Brief occupational therapy intervention. *American Journal of Occupational Therapy, 58*(5), 561-569.

Dunford, C., Missiuna, C., Street, E., & Sibert, J. (2005). Childrens' perceptions of the impact of developmental coordination disorder on activities of daily living. *British Journal of Occupational Therapy, 68*(5), 207-214.

Erikson, A., Karlsson, G., Söderström, M., & Tham, K. (2004). A training apartment with electronic aids to daily living: Lived experiences of persons with brain damage. *American Journal of Occupational Therapy, 58*(3), 261-271.

Fisher, A. G. (1999). *Assessment of motor and process skills* (3rd ed.). Fort Collins, CO: Three Star Press.

Giles, G. M., Ridley, J. E., Dill, A., & Frye, S. (1997). A consecutive series of adults with brain injury treated with a washing and dressing retraining program. *American Journal of Occupational Therapy, 51*(4), 256-266.

Gillen, G. (2000). Improving activities of daily living performance in an adult with ataxia. *American Journal of Occupational Therapy, 54*(1), 89-96.

Goverover, Y., & Hinojosa, J. (2002). Categorization and deductive reasoning: Predictors of instrumental activities of daily living performance in adults with brain injury. *American Journal of Occupational Therapy, 56*(5), 509-516.

Hagsten, B., Svensson, O., & Gardulf, A. (2004). Early individualized postoperative occupational therapy training in 100 patients improves ADL after hip fracture: A randomized trial. *Acta Orthopaedica Scandinavica, 75*(2), 177-183.

Haitsma, K. V., & Ruckdeschel, K. (2001). Special care for dementia in nursing homes: Overview of innovations in programs and activities. *Alzheimer's Care Quarterly, 2*(3), 49-56.

Hällgren, M., & Kottorp, A. (2005). Effects of occupational therapy intervention on activities of daily living and awareness of disability in persons with intellectual disabilities. *Australian Occupational Therapy Journal, 52*(4), 350-359.

Hastings, J., Gowans, S., & Watson, D. E. (2004). Effectiveness of occupational therapy following organ transplantation. *Canadian Journal of Occupational Therapy, 71*(4), 238-242.

Healy, H., & Rigby, P. (1999). Promoting independence for teens and young adults with physical disabilities. *Canadian Journal of Occupational Therapy, 66*(5), 240-249.

Hilton, K., Fricke, J., & Unsworth, C. (2001). A comparison of self-report versus observation of performance using the Assessment of Living Skills and Resources (ALSAR) with an older population. *British Journal of Occupational Therapy, 64*(3), 135-143.

Huang, M. E., Wartella, J. E., & Kreutzer, J. S. (2001). Functional outcomes and quality of life in patients with brain tumors: A preliminary report. *Archives of Physical Medicine and Rehabilitation, 82*(11), 1540-1546.

Kielhofner, G., & Forsyth, K. (2001). Measurement properties of a client self-report for treatment planning and documenting therapy outcomes. *Scandinavian Journal of Occupational Therapy, 8*(3), 131-139.

Klein, R. M., & Bell, B. (1979). *The Klein-Bell ADL Scale manual*. Seattle, WA: Educational Resources, University of Washington.

Kottorp, A, Bernspång, B., & Fisher, A. (2003). Activities of daily living in persons with intellectual disability: Strengths and limitations in specific motor and process skills. *Australian Occupational Therapy Journal, 50*, 195-204.

Kramer, A. M., Kowalsky, J. C., Lin, M., Grigsby, J., Hughes, R., & Steiner, J. F. (2000). Outcome and utilization differences for older persons with stroke in HMO and fee-for-service systems. *Journal of the American Geriatrics Society, 48*(7), 726-734.

Kwan, J., & Sandercock, P. (2006). In-hospital care pathways for stroke. *Cochrane Database of Systematic Reviews, 18*(4), CD002924.

Law, M., Baptiste, S., Carswell, A., McColl, M. A., Polatajko, H., & Pollack, N. (2005). *Canadian Occupational Performance Measure* (4th ed.). Ottawa, Ontario: CAOT Publications.

Lysaght, R., & Wright, J. (2005). Professional strategies in work-related practice: An exploration of occupational and physical therapy roles and approaches. *American Journal of Occupational Therapy, 59*(2), 209-217.

McAndrew, E., McDermott, S., Vitzakovitch, S., Warunek, M., & Holm, M. B. (2000). Therapist and patient perceptions of the occupational therapy goal-setting process: A pilot study. *Physical & Occupational Therapy in Geriatrics, 17*(1), 55-63.

McGourty, L. K. (1979). *Kohlman evaluation of living skills*. Seattle, WA: KELS Research.

Meyer, A. (1922). The philosophy of occupational therapy. *Archives of Occupational Therapy, 1*, 11-17.

Neistadt, M. E. (1995). Methods of assessing clients' priorities: A survey of adult physical dysfunction settings. *American Journal of Occupational Therapy, 49*(5), 428-436.

Nelson, D. L., & Glass, L. M. (1999). Occupational therapists' involvement with the Minimum Data Set in skilled nursing and intermediate care facilities. *American Journal of Occupational Therapy, 53*, 348-352.

Patterson, S., & Williams, M., Townsville Hospital Occupational Therapy Department. (2005). An occupational therapy consultation provided to older adults presenting to accident and emergency improves ADL functioning and reduces falls and hospital stays. Retrieved June 30, 2006, from http://www.otcats.com/topics/CAT-OT&ADLTownsville12Jan2006.html

Perez de Heredia, M., Cuadrado, M. L., Rodriguez, G., Lopez, S., & Miangolarray, J. C. (2001). Eficacia de la Terapia Ocupacional en adolescentes con neoplasias intracraneales: Estudio piloto [Efficacy of occupational therapy in adolescents with intracranial neoplasia: Pilot study]. *Rehabilitacion, 35*(3), 140-145.

Richards, L. G., Latham, N. K., Jette, D. U., Rosenberg, L., Smout, R. J., & DeJong, G. (2005). Characterizing occupational therapy practice in stroke rehabilitation. *Archives of Physical Medicine and Rehabilitation, 86*(12, suppl 2), S51-S60.

Richardson, J., Law, M., Wishart, L., & Guyatt, G. (2000). The use of a simulated environment (Easy Street) to retrain independent living skills in elderly persons: A randomized controlled trial. *Journal of Gerontology, 55*(10), M578-M584.

Robnett, R. H., Hopkins, V., & Kimball, J. G. (2002). The SAFE AT HOME: A quick home safety assessment. *Physical & Occupational Therapy in Geriatrics, 20*(3/4), 77-102.

Rogers, J. C., & Holm, M. B. (1994). Performance Assessment of Self-Care Skills (PASS) (version 3.1). Unpublished manuscript. Pittsburgh, PA: University of Pittsburgh.

Smith, K. (2006). Athletic trainers aim to expand scope. [Electronic Version]. *OT Practice, 11*(5), 6.

Steultjens, E. M., Dekker, J., Bouter, L. M., van Schaardenburg, D., van Kuyk, M. A., & van den Ende, C. H. (2004). Occupational therapy for rheumatoid arthritis. *Cochrane Database of Systematic Reviews, 1*, CD003114.

Thompson, K. M. (1998). Early intervention services in daily family life: Mothers' perceptions of 'ideal' versus 'actual' service provision. *Occupational Therapy International, 5*, 206-221.

Trombly, C. (1993). Anticipating the future: Assessment of occupational function. *American Journal of Occupational Therapy, 47*(3), 253-257.

Trombly, C. A., & Ma, H. I. (2002). A synthesis of the effects of occupational therapy for persons with stroke, part 1: Restoration of roles, tasks, and activities. *American Journal of Occupational Therapy, 56*(3), 250-259.

Uniform Data System for Medial Rehabilitation [UDSMR]. (2000). *Guide for the Uniform Data Set for Medical Rehabilitation (including the FIM instrument (Version 5.1)*. Buffalo, NY: State University of New York.

Walker, M. F., Gladman, J. R., Lincoln, N. B., Siemonsma, P., & Whiteley, T. (1999). Occupational therapy for stroke patients not admitted to hospital: A randomized controlled trial. *Lancet, 354*(9175), 278-280.

Walker, M. F., Leonardi-Bee, J., Bath, P., Langhorne, P., Dewey, M., Corr, S., et al. (2004). Individual patient data meta-analysis of randomized controlled trials of community occupational therapy for stroke patients. *Stroke, 35*(9), 2226-2232.

Weinstock-Zlotnick, G., & Hinojosa, J. (2004). Bottom-up or top-down evaluation: Is one better than the other? *American Journal of Occupational Therapy, 58*(5), 594-599.

Williams, J. H., Drinka, T. J., Greenburg, J. R., Farrell-Holtan, J., Euhardy, R., & Schram, M. (1991). Development and testing of the Assessment of Living Skills and Resources (ALSAR) in elderly community-dwelling veterans. *Gerontologist, 31*(1), 84-91.

Wodchis, W. P., Fries, B. E., & Pollack, H. (2004). Payer incentives and physical rehabilitation therapy for nonelderly institutional long-term care residents: Evidence from Michigan and Ontario. *Archives of Physical Medicine and Rehabilitation, 85*(2), 210-217.

Yerxa, E. J., Burnett-Beaulieu, S., Stocking, S., & Azen, S. P. (1988). Development of the Satisfaction With Scaled Performance Questionnaire (SPSQ). *American Journal of Occupational Therapy, 42*(4), 215-221.

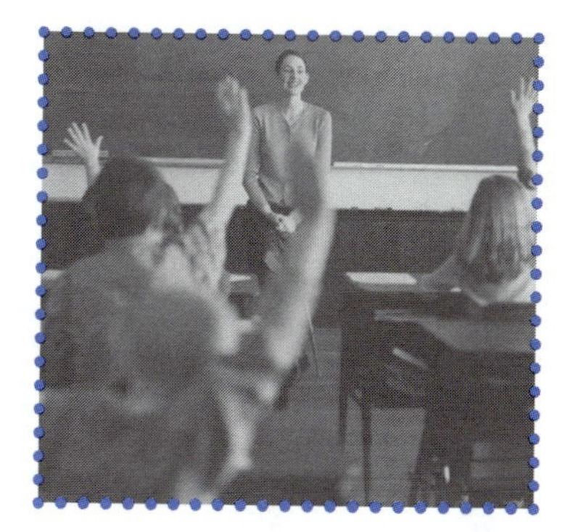

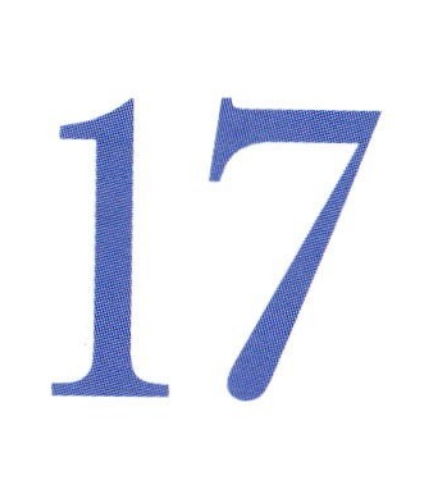

# 17

# Interventions in School and Work

Barbara J. Steva, MS, OTR/L

**ACOTE Standards Explored in This Chapter**

B.5.1-5.6, 5.19-5.21

**Key Terms**

| | |
|---|---|
| Consultation | Individual education plan (IEP) |
| Educational activities | Least restrictive environment (LRE) |
| Exceptional educational need (EEN) | Objective |
| Goal | Related service |
| Inclusion | |

## Introduction

This chapter addresses client identification, evaluation, and intervention within the educational setting and during the process of transition into the work force or post-secondary education. Models of practice are reviewed and discussed as to how they impact practice. Federal laws and regulations are outlined with the outcome of each on occupational therapy practice. The role of the occupational therapy practitioner is discussed throughout the chapter.

## Medical and Educational Models of Service Delivery

Occupational therapy practitioners must have a clear understanding of the medical and educational service delivery models guiding practice in these areas. Within the medical model, occupational therapy is a primary service provider. Services promote wellness and independence within the individual's daily occupations. In contrast, occupational therapy within the educational model is a related service. Services supplement the educational program, are provided within the educational setting, and are related to the student's success in that environment. The occupational therapy practitioner chooses between medical necessity and educational needs before implementing services within the educational setting. Although services may be helpful to the overall function of the student, the therapist evaluates whether the disability or disease impacts the student's ability to access and benefit from the academic instruction before recommending and implementing services. Practitioners adhere to federal and state mandates by selecting evaluation tools, goals, and objectives, and interventions that will address identified education goals. Mandates within the Individuals with Disabilities Education Act (IDEA) (U.S. Department of Education, n.d.) require that services be provided within the least restrictive environment (LRE) and support access to the general education or special education curriculum. A student should therefore



K. Sladyk, K. Jacobs, & N. MacRae (Eds.).
*Occupational Therapy Essentials for Clinical Competence* (pp. 187-198).

receive occupational therapy services within the classroom environment whenever possible, with goals and objectives that reflect these needs.

# Occupational Therapy in the Educational Setting

Occupational therapy services employed within the public education setting are provided under federal mandates as outlined in Table 17-1. The Education of Handicapped Children Act (Cengage Learning, n.d.), ensures a free public education without discrimination based on disability. This act was amended to become IDEA in 1990 with further amendments made in 1994 and 2004. The Rehabilitation Act was enacted in 1973 (U.S. Department of Education, 2004). This act requires services for all eligible students, enabling them to participate in their regular or special education program.

## The Individual Education Program Team

Practitioners collaborate with the educational staff and support personnel to ensure that services are available in a timely and appropriate manner. An individual education program team (IEP team) is formed when a student is not benefiting from academic instruction. The team consists of the parent or guardian, the student (when appropriate), at least one regular education teacher, at least one special education teacher, a school administrator, and all appropriate support service representatives such as occupational therapy, physical therapy, and social work. Practitioners are related service providers and are included when the team makes a referral stating that the student would benefit from an occupational therapy evaluation.

## Evaluation of the Student

Evaluation in the school setting looks at the primary areas of function and uses a problem-solving approach to identify issues impacting the student's academic progress. Table 17-2 lists the skills assessed and their functional implications. For example, evaluation addresses sensorimotor skills that limit access to the physical environment, self-care, or participation in daily tasks expected within the academic setting. Fine motor skills are addressed to ensure adequate ability in tasks requiring manipulation of objects or use of writing utensils. Visual motor skills are assessed with a focus on spatial organization, directionality, and the ability to control the writing tool for legible writing and organization of work on the page. Visual perception, inclusive of discrimination, figure ground, form constancy, spatial relationships, part or whole concepts, and memory for one or more forms are important aspects of the evaluation. These areas can impact reading ability, multi-step task completion, part or whole concepts, and spatial concepts used in telling time, mathematical operations, and science concepts. Challenges in the area of perceptual skills can also suggest a nonverbal learning disability or assist in excluding this as an identifier if strong perceptual skills are present. Finally, functional self-care skills such as toileting, feeding, grooming, and hygiene are assessed as they relate to the student's ability to participate in the school day.

## IEP Development

The team reviews the evaluation/assessment material collected by all disciplines to determine whether the student meets state eligibility requirements for special education. Eligibility is based upon exceptional educational need (EEN). The team determines whether the information from the evaluations indicate a specific disabling or handicapping condition that prevents the student from participating in and benefiting from academic instruction.

Suchomel (2000) lists the following considerations when determining eligibility of occupational therapy service within the school:

- Does the student have an EEN that qualifies him or her for special education services, or does he or she qualify for services under Section 504 of the Rehabilitation Act?

**Table 17-1. Public School Laws**

| Law | Provisions |
|---|---|
| The Education of Handicapped Children<br>Public Law 94-142<br>http://college.cengage.com/education/resources/res_prof/students/spec_ed/legislation/pl_94-142.html | • All children, age 3 to 21, are entitled to a free and appropriate education.<br>• Parent and student rights and legal recourses are outlined in the event this right is denied. |
| Individuals with Disabilities Education Act (IDEA)<br>Public Law 108-446<br>http://idea.ed.gov | • Services are to be provided to assist the student with a disability to benefit from special education. |
| Section 504 of the Rehabilitation Act<br>Public Law 93-112<br>www.ed.gov/policy/speced/reg/narrative.html | • Services are to be provided without discrimination of disability.<br>• Ensures free and appropriate accommodations and services for eligible students and entitles students with chronic diseases or disabling conditions to modifications that will allow them to participate within the regular or special education program. |

**Table 17-2. Performance Areas and Functional Implications Assessed in the Educational Setting**

| Skill Assessed | Functional Implication |
|---|---|
| Visual perception, Discrimination | Ability to read and identify safety signs, letters, shapes, or pictures for communication |
| Memory | Ability to recall letters, shapes, numbers, and mathematical operations |
| Sequential memory | Ability to remember a series of letters or numbers for tasks such as spelling, copying text, remembering phone numbers, and sequencing visual cues within the environment for vocational activities |
| Form constancy | Ability to mentally manipulate visual information when some attributes (i.e., size or orientation) have been changed; recognize letters or forms in different contexts such as print to cursive; impacts ability to use mental pictures for tasks such as sequencing the alphabet, using the calendar, telling time, reading maps, and applying mathematical concepts; important skill for sewing and construction |
| Figure ground | Ability to locate salient information within a busy background such as words, numbers, or mathematical operations on worksheets, text, desk, drawer, bookshelf, or grocery store shelf |
| Visual closure/Part or whole relationships | Ability to recognize forms or objects partially hidden or incomplete letters or words; also related to part-whole integration and the ability to see the overall picture of a situation; impacts ability to tell time, perform mathematical skills, and perform mechanical or constructional tasks |
| Spatial relationships | Ability to recognize the directionality of letters and numbers (i.e., "b" and "d"); spatial organization of work within lines or on the page; also impacts the ability to use mental pictures to perform tasks such as sequencing the alphabet, using the calendar, telling time, reading maps, and applying mathematical concepts |
| Visual motor Spatial organization | Ability to organize work on a page, space letters and words, set up mathematical operations, complete artwork or projects, conceptualize parts as they relate to the whole |
| Directionality | Ability to correctly orient letters, numbers, and shapes; follow instructions of "up, down, right, left" |

- Does the evaluation indicate a need for occupational therapy service by demonstrating a significant delay in one or more areas of occupational performance that is impacting the ability to participate in academic tasks?
- Will occupational therapy assist the student in accessing and benefiting from academic instruction?
- Does the student require the skilled service of an occupational therapist or occupational therapy assistant or can the tasks and interventions be carried out by other personnel?

## Role of the Practitioners in the Evaluation and Development of IEP

The occupational therapist establishes the areas and methods that will be used in the evaluation of the student. The occupational therapy assistant collaborates with the occupational therapist by providing observations, collecting data, and administering/scoring assessments within their level of competency. The occupational therapist interprets and reports the information from the assessments. The practitioners collaborate in the development of goals and objectives for intervention. The occupational therapy assistant is a member of the individualized education program (IEP) team and can attend the IEP meeting under the direction and supervision of the occupational therapist to report the findings and review the goals and objectives (Solomon, 2000).

The occupational therapist provides supervision to the occupational therapy assistant by overseeing service delivery and assisting in his or her professional growth and competence. Frequency of supervision may vary depending upon the knowledge and experience of the occupational therapy assistant and his or her ability to ensure safe, effective intervention. The practitioners collaborate to decide upon an appropriate amount and method of supervision. Factors to consider include the practice setting, complexity of client needs, requirements of the practice setting, and skills of both the practitioners. Regulations set forth by state and federal agencies must be followed with completion of clear and appropriate documentation of the supervision.

## Goals and Objectives

Together, the team determines the student's strength and need areas in order to develop goals and objectives for the IEP. Occupational therapy goals and objectives are specific to the student, address educational needs, and are measurable. The goal is overarching and less specific than the objectives. The objectives break the goal down into specific tasks or skills required to successfully achieve the goal. Each objective defines the conditions in which you expect to see the student perform well, along with the behavior you wish the student to exhibit, how you are going to measure the behavior, and why you are intervening in this area. The goals and objectives must be directly linked to educational development. Table 17-3 shows a sample goal and objectives (Figure 17-1).

Table 17-3. Representative Goal and Objectives

| Condition | Behavior | Measurement | Outcome |
|---|---|---|---|
| Under what circumstances you expect the student to perform | What you are expecting the student to do | How you will measure success | Why this area of performance is being addressed |
| "Given..." | "Joey will..." | "...trials, over a 2 week period" "...% of the time during 3 consecutive intervention sessions" | "for use in..." |

**Goal**

Joey will demonstrate improved strength, endurance, and control in the trunk and upper extremity required for fine motor, visual motor, and academic occupations by December 2009.

**Objectives**

Given therapeutic activities, Joey will demonstrate improved trunk strength and control as seen by the ability to maintain an upright sitting position in a chair or on the floor without external support for 5 minutes (1st trimester), 10 minutes (2nd trimester), and 15 minutes (3rd trimester), 3 times per day on 4 of 5 consecutive school days, for use in daily occupations.

Given therapeutic activities, Joey will demonstrate the ability to use bilateral upper extremities at midline for writing, cutting, and playing while in an unsupported sitting position for 3 minutes (1st trimester), 5 minutes (2nd trimester) and 10 minutes (3rd trimester), 3 times per day on 4 of 5 consecutive school days, for use in daily occupations.

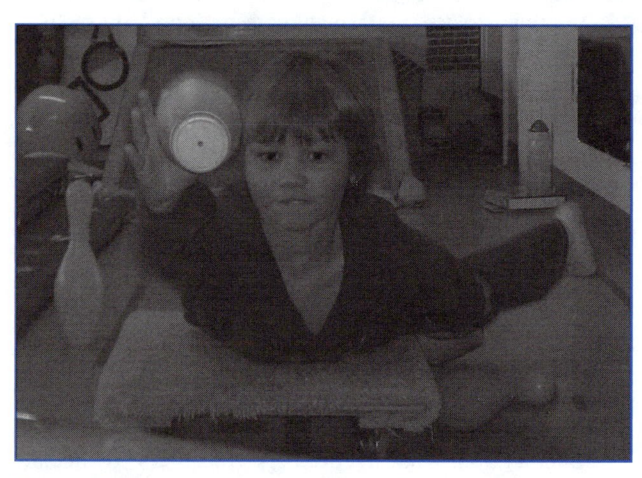

**Figure 17-1.** Joey performing activities for postural strength.

# Service Delivery Models

The type of practice model the therapist chooses to employ depends upon the educational setting and student needs. Current federal mandates call for instruction to take place in the least restrictive environment (LRE). This challenges the practitioner to develop an intervention program that can be incorporated into the classroom whenever possible. The model of practice must be determined by carefully examining the classroom environment, the student's needs, and the ability to accomplish the prescribed goals and objectives.

# Direct Service

Direct service occurs individually or in a small group setting. The therapist decides whether this should take place in a setting outside of the classroom, often referred to as "pullout," or in an inclusive setting within the classroom environment. Pullout services involve removal of the student from the classroom for the duration of the therapy session. Inclusive therapy involves the practitioner providing therapy within the classroom environment in a nonintrusive manner. The inclusive model allows the therapist to gain knowledge regarding skills the student needs to be successful within the classroom and allows the teacher to observe the therapeutic approach, preparing him or her to assist the student during activities when the practitioner is not present. Services are typically provided on a weekly basis for an amount of time discussed and decided upon by the IEP team. Inclusion therapy ensures that the intervention supports the educational process and increases the likelihood of generalization of therapeutic techniques throughout the school day. Direct pullout services require ongoing consultation with educational staff outside of the therapy session to ensure carryover of learned tasks. This service delivery is most effective when a student is working on a skill that is significantly below that of peers and intervention within the classroom would be a distraction to other students.

# Consultation

The consultation, or collaboration, model involves the practitioner providing service through direct contact with the teacher or other educational staff working with the student. This can be the primary method of service delivery and should always be pursued in addition to the provision of direct services. When providing consultation, the practitioner must have good communication skills and insight to recognize when the tasks being asked of the teaching staff cannot be successfully implemented in their classroom. Teachers provide motivating instruction while implementing modifications and accommodations to students with varying learning styles and speeds. A common mistake of therapists is to overwhelm a teacher with activities, equipment, and specialized programs for one or two children within their classroom. As a result, teachers can become resentful and less receptive to the practitioner's ideas. It is important for the practitioner to be a part of the classroom to which he or she is consulting by observing the environment on an ongoing basis to better understand the inner workings and expectations of the environment and to tailor recommendations to the flow of the classroom schedule.

Dunn (1990) conducted a study of direct service and consultation and the effect of each practice model on student outcomes and adult attitudes. Fourteen preschool- and kindergarten-aged children were randomly assigned to either a direct service or a consultation model. Children in both groups achieved nearly 75% of all IEP goals. Teachers in the consultation group, however, reported a 24% greater occupational therapy contribution to goal attainment than the direct service group. Palisano (1989) researched the use of therapist-directed groups and consultation groups. Results revealed statistically higher scores between pre-test and post-test scores for the consultation group in the area of motor skills, while the therapist-directed group showed clinically higher scores in the area of visual perception. There was no difference in visual motor scores. These findings suggest the need for care in determining the service delivery model to implement and to assess its effectiveness on a regular basis.

### Termination of Services

A recommendation to discontinue services is made by the occupational therapist when the established goals and objectives have been achieved. The IEP team is reconvened to review progress and discuss discontinuation of services. The student's disabilities are not necessarily "cured" but are functioning within the academic setting with supports and strategies acquired through occupational therapy intervention. With effective collaboration with the student's teacher, the practitioner can identify and address concerns regarding the dismissal. There can be a safety net put in place in the event of regression by developing a measurable goal outlining expected performance. The occupational therapist can step back in to provide more consultation or support to the teacher and student if the goal is not being met. The occupational therapist can help the teacher intervene immediately and support the student when challenged. The therapist does not want to promote a situation in which the student and teacher are unable to function without ongoing intervention by the occupational therapist. The practitioner may slowly withdraw from the immediate environment.

## Alternative Education Settings

Recommendations for an alternative education setting are often made for students at risk for dropping out of school or failing in the public school. Risk factors include:

- Truancy
- Low-motivation
- Inability to maintain attention
- Low self-esteem
- Behavioral difficulties

These settings incorporate the student's social, emotional, intellectual, physical, spiritual, and moral development with their education. Classroom size, teaching styles, and methods are commonly different from those seen in public or traditional school settings. Using questionnaires distributed to educational staff, Dirette and Kolak (2004) studied the needs of students within alternative educational settings. The top three areas of student concern included:

1. Difficulty with time management
2. Lack of participation in healthy play and leisure activities
3. Maintenance of healthy lifestyle behaviors

Other areas of concern included:

- Cognitive deficits such as multitasking or the ability to follow multi-step instructions
- Higher level thinking skills such as problem solve and retain/recall information
- Coping skills
- Anger management
- Poor self-concept

Occupational therapy services are provided within this setting as in a public school setting. These settings are often privately funded and are not obligated by the federal and state mandates guiding special education services. The student's public school district is responsible for evaluating, developing, and implementing an IEP for the student.

## Transition Planning

Legislation guiding the transition from school to the work place is defined in section 602(30) of IDEA (U.S. Department of Education, n.d.), which describes "transition services" for students with disabilities beginning at age 14. By age 16, the IEP should contain a statement regarding services to be provided and designate responsibilities for the student's successful transition into the workplace and/or community. Specifically, the mandate is designed as an outcome-oriented process, promoting transition of the student from school to post-school activities. Post-school activities may include post-secondary education, vocational training, supported or unsupported employment, adult services, independent living, or community participation. The transition plan is based upon the student's strengths, preferences, and interests. Transition services should include instruction, related services, community experiences, development of employment, post-school adult living objectives, acquisition of daily living skills (as appropriate), and vocational evaluation (U.S. Department of Education, n.d.). The Americans with Disabilities Act (ADA) (U.S. Equal Employment Opportunity Commission [EEOC], n.d.) provides individuals with disabilities an opportunity to fulfill typical roles in the community. The act requires reasonable accommodations for the qualified individual with a disability, including accessibility, job restructuring, modifications to equipment and training materials, and provision of qualified readers or interpreters. The intention of the School to Work Opportunities Act (Fessler State Board of Education Site, n.d.), jointly managed by the Department of Education and the Department of Labor, is to build partnerships between schools and communities and provide school to work programs. This mandate serves to provide opportunities for students to engage in performance-based education and training to prepare them for competitive employment, participation in post-secondary education, and navigation of the workplace.

The National Organization on Disability (Louis Harris and Associates, 1998) reported that only 32% of individuals with disabilities within the working age of 18 to 64 were employed full- or part-time compared to 81% of same-age peers without disabilities. The findings of the President's Commission on Excellence in Special Education of the United States Department of Education (2002) are consistent with this, showing a stable 70% unemployment rate of individuals with disabilities over the previous 12 years. The Commission reported that students with disabilities who chose a nonacademic path following high school were not prepared for or supported in achieving employment goals.

Practitioners contribute to the transition from school to work by offering skills in the assessment, training, and reinforcement of work skills and behavior. Despite the knowledge and expertise practitioners have to offer in this area, few are providing the services. In a study conducted by Spencer, Emery, and Schneck (2003), special education directors within the Kentucky Department of Education were surveyed regarding the use of occupational therapy practitioners in the delivery of transition services to secondary education students. Findings revealed that special education teachers and job coaches provided the majority of transition services for work components. Occupational therapy practitioners provided job placement, exploration, and community-based transition services 5% or less of the time. Asher (2003) described factors that potentially impact successful transition from school to community and areas where practitioners can provide meaningful intervention. These are outlined in Table 17-4.

## Work

Thomas (1999) wrote:

> On the one hand, work has, since time immemorial, been seen as a curse, a result of the Fall and punishment for sin. It was something that, it was assumed; everyone would naturally try to avoid... The ideal society was a land of Cockaigne, where all things came by nature and the need to work had vanished.
>
> On the other hand, work was widely admired as a divine activity, practiced by God during the creation of the world and by Adam and Eve in Eden. It was a sacred duty and the source of all human comforts, creating wealth and making civilization possible. It was a cure for boredom and melancholy, and a remedy for vice. It was the only sure route to human happiness, bringing health, contentment, and personal fulfillment. It structured the day, gave opportunities for sociability and companionship, fostered pride in individual creativity, and created a sense of personal identity. Idleness could never make people happy; and the ideal society was one in which there was satisfying work available for everybody (p.xvii).

**Table 17-4. Factors For Successful School/Work Transition**

| Factor | Evaluation/Assessment Area | Intervention |
|---|---|---|
| Accessibility of the work area | Is adaptive equipment required for positioning or accessibility? | Training in appropriate use of the equipment |
| Student | Sensory, motor, and cognitive-perceptual skills | Development and training in the use of adaptations |
| Task | Analysis of job requirements and components | Pre-teach the sequence or specific job tasks that may be problematic. Develop supports to assist with successful completion of the tasks |
| Skill development | Assessment of job requirements (i.e., standing, finger dexterity) | Develop and implement a program into the school day to work on needed skills |
| Personal care | Independence in self-care | Develop and implement a program involving personal hygiene (i.e., grooming, toileting, eating) into the school day |
| Communication | Evaluate the need for assistive technology | Develop and implement assistive technology in conjunction with the speech and language clinician as appropriate to enhance communication |
| Job carving | Assessment of the job site to discern any other job possibilities not previously considered | Training in areas required to fulfill other responsibilities within the site |

Work is one of the primary roles in life essential for health and wellness. However, there have been several incomplete definitions. Work has been defined as what people do to earn a living (Brief & Nord, 1990); as an activity done in a specific place and time, on a regular basis (Hearnshaw, 1954); and as employment perceived by individuals as their main occupation, by which they are known, and from which they derive their societal role (Shimmin, 1966). Work may mean different things to different individuals. One may see it as obligatory while another may find it enjoyable whether there is a monetary value attached to it or not. Young individuals participate in work as a means of supporting themselves and their families financially. After retirement from this role, senior citizens and the elderly often continue to contribute to the work force through volunteering. This provides a fulfilling experience to individuals who have spent most of their lives in the worker role and may have difficulty transitioning to retirement. The terms *work* and *occupation* have evolved to be used synonymously, creating confusion. The Merriam Webster dictionary defines work as the labor, task, or duty that is one's accustomed means of livelihood, and occupation as an activity in which one engages or the principal business of one's life. Regardless of the reason, an individual participates in work-related activities, financial reimbursement, or enjoyment. The role of the worker often encompasses the majority of the individual's time each day, making work a primary occupation for him or her.

Before providing any type of intervention within the work environment, a comprehensive evaluation of the work site and the worker must be completed. A conceptual framework, proposed by Sandqvist and Henriksson (2004), identifies three dimensions for the assessment of work function. These are work participation, work performance, and individual capacity. Work participation refers to the ability of the individual to gain and maintain employment within society. Factors such as public support and the demands upon the individual are considered. Work performance refers to the individual's ability to perform the tasks associated with the work activity. Finally, individual capacity refers to the individual's ability to physically and psychologically complete the work activities.

## Intervention

Intervention is required for those individuals with physical, cognitive, and developmental disabilities such as Down Syndrome or cerebral palsy, as well as those who become injured as a result of work-related stress or other activities such as carpal tunnel injury, chronic back pain, or brain injury. Interventions may include direct service in the form of job training, training to perform a specific task, muscle strengthening, implementation of task modifications, and accommodations, such as ergonomic supports, to assist with back pain or repetitive use injuries. Occupational therapists may be used as consultants to the employer to ensure that hiring procedures and job descriptions are nondiscriminatory and the workplace is ergonomically safe for workers and meets ADA regulations (AOTA, 2000). Regardless of the reason for initial referral to occupational therapy, a thorough evaluation of the client's needs and abilities, as well as an analysis of the work task, are required before developing an intervention plan. Goals and objectives are developed and written in conjunction with the client and caregiver when appropriate. These are objective, task-oriented, and measurable to assist in planning for dismissal from occupational therapy services. Knowledge of universal design, construction guidelines, specialized products, and government guidelines are essential in providing guidance to the employer and solutions for the worker within the work place.

Pohlman, Poosawtsee, Gerndt, and Lindstrom-Hazel (2001) surveyed workers' compensation carriers to assess how occupational therapy programs can best meet the needs of the carriers. Results showed that carriers consider a rehabilitation program successful if the worker is able to return to any job position. The carriers reported that occupational therapy programs are beneficial for return to work, although it was stated that most carriers did not understand what occupational therapy was or how they can assist in returning an individual to the work force. This study suggests the need for educating insurance carriers as to the role of the practitioner with the worker with an injury or disability (Table 17-5).

A model of practice is used to guide the practitioner's thinking and subsequent intervention plan and activities. The following section summarizes five models of practice used in school and work intervention. Practitioners may use several different models within their practice. Some practitioners choose one model to guide their philosophy and interventions with all students/clients, while others may choose to use several different models based on the presentation of the client. It is important to focus on the student's/client's occupation and desired outcome when choosing a model of practice.

# Models of Practice

## Neurodevelopmental Model

The original theory and practice of neurodevelopmental treatment (NDT) was developed from the work of Karel and Berta Bobath's intervention of individuals with brain injury. NDT is a sensori-motor approach focusing on motor and postural aspects that translate to independence in active tasks (Dunn, 1990). The theory has a strong foundation in normal development and the interpretation of motor responses. These include motor control developing from head to foot, midline to the limbs, and large to small movements. The theory progresses through the developmental sequence, integrating primitive reflexes and achieving developmental milestones. Mobility is built on stability and progresses outward as the child begins

| Table 17-5. Workplace Laws Guiding Services for Individuals With Disabilities | |
|---|---|
| Americans with Disabilities Act (ADA) of 1990<br>Public Law 101-336<br>www.eeoc.gov/ada | • "To provide a clear and comprehensive prohibition of discrimination on the basis of disability" (sec2.b.1) |
| The Rehabilitation Act<br>www.ed.gov/policy/speced/reg/narrative.html | • Authorizes the formula grant programs of vocational rehabilitation, supported employment, independent living, and client assistance<br>• Authorizes a variety of training and service discretionary grants administered by the Rehabilitation Services Administration |
| Ticket to Work and Work Incentive Improvement Act of 1999<br>Public law 106-170<br>www.wid.org/publications/the-ticket-to-work-and-work-incentives-improvement-act-of-1999-federal-fact-sheet-on-public-law-106-170 | • Aims to improve the ability to choose and obtain vocational services for the individual with disabilities<br>• Removes the need for the individual with disabilities to choose between work and health benefits<br>• Decreases the individual's dependence on public benefits by improving participation in work |

to explore the environment. The trunk is typically where intervention is initiated, progressing to more advanced movements performed away from the trunk. Because NDT focuses on abnormal movement patterns and attempts to extinguish these in favor of more appropriate or typical motor patterns, this theory may not always be effective in treating children with changes in muscle tone, such as cerebral palsy. These children build motor patterns that are successful for them. By changing their motor pattern, they may become dependent in areas or tasks in which they were previously independent.

## Biomechanical Model

The biomechanical model is based in a physical science such as kinesiology and physics. A balance between stability and mobility is a primary focus of this model, which takes into consideration muscle tone and skeletal alignment (Dunn, 2000). Muscle tone is the amount of tension in a muscle or muscle group at any given time. Muscle tone is not an exact science and exists along a continuum. Many individuals with high or low muscle tone, relative to "typical," lead functional and productive lives with no detriment to themselves or their lifestyle. An individual with a disorder of the central nervous system may have more severe challenges in regulating the amount of tension present in the muscles during activity or rest. An individual with cerebral palsy may have "high" or "increased" muscle tone resulting from excess tension in the muscles. This leaves the individual at risk for shortened muscle length or contractures due to poor stretch and relaxation. Function is impacted due to the decreased ability to relax and tense the muscle as needed for mobility. An individual exhibiting "low" or "decreased" muscle tone results from an excessive relaxation of the muscles. This leaves the individual at risk for subluxation of joints due to laxity and poor tension in the muscles. Function is impacted by a lack of stability. The underlying goal of the biomechanical practice model is improved skeletal alignment by developing postural control for use in functional occupations (Dunn, 2000). This can be done through strengthening exercises and activities or the use of positioning devices. Indicators of poor postural control are a decreased ability to maintain an upright position without external support. This is often seen when the individual leans on a table or desk for support or slouches in a chair. These are often seen in school and work settings and can impact an individual's ability to work effectively and efficiently. The biomechanical approach is most commonly used when assessing and providing wheelchairs or splints to improve positioning and function.

## Motor Learning

The motor learning theory focuses on the process of learning rather than a specific task. Approaches of feedback, feed-forward, and event are described in the literature (Breslin, 1996). The feedback approach relies on information from the environment to provide feedback regarding movement. Arguments to this approach include the closed loop system, which does not allow for variability in the routine (Gliner, 1985). The feed-forward approach suggests that a motor plan is created prior to carrying out the motor task and is adapted during future use based on feedback from the environment. This is felt to promote variability, although Croce and DePaepe (1989) argued that a separate motor plan for every motor task would be very complex. Gliner (1989) pointed out that these approaches focus on the learner as the primary component with the environment being a secondary factor. The event approach brings both the learner and the environment together and brings purposeful activity to the forefront. This approach describes the learner as subconsciously choosing the motor plan for a purposeful task from a learned repertoire. The environment provides the learner with feedback regarding the success of the plan, and movements are adjusted at that time or stored for future use. The therapist provides intervention through the use of feedback regarding the success or failure of a movement, structuring the environment or task while the individual engages in a purposeful movement activity (Breslin, 1996). This model is commonly used within the academic and work settings to address fine motor skill development and skills needed to engage in physical education or playground activities.

## Sensory Integration

A. Jean Ayres developed sensory integration theory in the early 1970s as she attempted to apply neuro-scientific knowledge to her practice with children diagnosed with "minimal brain dysfunction," today known as attention deficit hyperactivity disorder (ADHD). The theory emphasizes the individual's ability to interact with the environment by receiving and organizing sensory information. This information is used to produce an adaptive response and adjust to changes within the environment. Sensory input impacts aspects of physical, cognitive, and emotional responses. An individual exhibiting an extreme response to an otherwise benign input such as a gentle tap on the shoulder by a friend would be displaying over-responsivity. Over-responsivity describes the nervous system's state of hyper arousal or fright, fight, or flight where all input is interpreted as a threat. An individual displaying under-responsivity requires excessive input to register sensory stimulation. This may be the case with the child who loves to spin and purposely crashes to the floor or doesn't cry when injured. Sensory integration theory attempts to normalize sensory input to produce an adaptive response that fits the situation at hand.

Sensory integration theory can be implemented in several ways within the educational or work environment. Many schools and most work places do not have the equipment or space to apply optimal intervention using this theory. This approach can be effectively used to develop and implement a sensory diet of activities or strategies to provide individuals with an optimal level of arousal to participate in their academic or work occupations. Table 17-6 reviews the sensory systems and the type of stimulation used to facilitate a calming or alerting response in an individual. These strategies can be used throughout the day to maintain an optimal level of arousal for productive work.

## Model of Human Occupation

The Model of Human Occupation (MOHO) as described by Kielhofner (1995) identifies four factors influencing work behavior. Volition describes the manner in which the individual chooses, experiences, anticipates, and interprets the occupational behaviors. Personal causation, interest, and value components all contribute to volition. Habituation describes internal roles and habits that convey a pattern and regularity in daily life. Performance, or the individual's innate abilities, are the foundation for adept function. Finally, the environment always results from the interaction of the previous three factors. In applying this model to practice, the occupational therapist takes the individual and setting into consideration, looking at the four subsystems. The occupational therapist must also attend to how the individual's injury or disability is affecting his or her relationship to the setting (Kielhofner et al., 1999).

The choice of a practice model depends upon the practice setting and client's needs. One approach may work with a client in one setting while a different model is most effective in another practice setting. Examples of these are work hardening and ergonomics (see Chapter 24, Environmental Adaptation and Ergonomics). However, these specialized areas of practice require further training, and the occupational therapy practitioner must be open to all approaches and use the one or pieces of several that provide the best care for the client.

# Summary

The implementation of occupational therapy services within the education and work models requires teamwork and ongoing collaboration with the members of the IEP team or the employers to ensure the individual is capable of interacting and participating in the tasks being asked of them. The practitioner assists with the transition from secondary education into the workforce, independent/supported living, or post-secondary education.

# Student Self-Assessment

Sam is a 7-year-old boy with cerebral palsy. He is in a regular first-grade classroom with educational support from an educational technician 100% of the day. Sam is independent with ambulation using a rear walker. His upper extremity strength and control is poor with ataxic movements impacting precision with fine motor tasks. He uses raking finger movements and a lateral pinch to retrieve objects. Release is not always volitional and he drops many items. Sam is independent with toileting with the exception of clothing management. At this time, there is a private bathroom within the classroom where Sam's educational technician can assist him as needed. Sam's difficulty in this area has been an ongoing area of need described by his parents at the IEP meeting. The team agrees that this is an area of need, particularly as he gets older and needs to use one of the public restrooms while at school.

1. Write at least one goal and two objectives to address Sam's independence in self-care while in school.
2. Describe the theoretical model, intervention activities, and potential accommodations or modifications the occupational therapy practitioner may use in Sam's intervention.

| Table 17-6. Factors Impacting Sensory Regulation | | |
|---|---|---|
| **Type of Input** | **Relaxing/Calming** | **Alerting** |
| Vestibular movement of the head through space | • Slow<br>• Rhythmic<br>• Linear—one plane<br>• Movement while on stable ground | • Fast<br>• Jerky<br>• Frequent changes of direction<br>• Angular movement<br>• Suspended equipment |
| Proprioception—compression or stretch of a joint | • Joint compression<br>• Slow stretch<br>• Heavy and sustained resistance | • Quick/unexpected changes<br>• Jarring/jerking<br>• Abrupt stop and starts |
| Tactile—any kind of touch | • Firm/deep pressure<br>• Swaddling<br>• Firm stroking over large areas<br>• Smooth texture<br>• Familiar and predictable<br>• Warmth | • Light touch<br>• Poking<br>• Touch on the face<br>• Rough texture<br>• Unexpected touch<br>• Cold |
| Visual | • Rhythmic<br>• Constant<br>• Blue and green shades<br>• Dim or dark<br>• Familiar and predictable | • Unexpected<br>• Bright colors or lights<br>• Red/yellow shades<br>• Black on white<br>• Changing or moving stimuli |
| Auditory | • Expected<br>• Familiar<br>• Quiet gentle rhythm<br>• Melodic | • Unexpected<br>• Loud<br>• Complex |
| Olfactory | • Familiar—associated with comforting experiences | • All odors |

Susan, a receptionist, is referred to occupational therapy due to chronic back and shoulder pain resulting from work-related stress. During your evaluation, you find that her computer desk is above elbow level when she is sitting. The computer is set to her right, at an angle to the keyboard, causing Susan to rotate her upper body while working. She schedules appointments and is frequently using the telephone and computer simultaneously, needing to hold the telephone between her ear and shoulder. Susan enjoys her job and does not want to leave in pursuit of other opportunities.

3. Describe the model of intervention most beneficial in the intervention of Susan's pain.
4. Write a Care Plan for Susan including outcome potential, at least one goal, and two objectives.
5. How can the occupational therapy practitioner work with Susan's employer to provide accommodations to assist her in working pain-free? What are those accommodations?

# Electronic Resources

- Sensory Integration and Special Needs Resources: www.comeunity.com
- Sensory Processing Disorder Resources: www.spd-foundation.net
- Sensory Integration Resources: www.fhsensory.com
- Work and School Intervention/Practice Resources: www.aota.org
- Education Mandates, Regulations, And Resources: www.ed.gov/index.jhtml
- Model of Human Occupation Clearinghouse: www.moho.uic.edu

| Evidence-Based Research Chart | | |
|---|---|---|
| **Topic** | **Area Addressed** | **Evidence** |
| Sensory Integration | Effectiveness | Humphries, Wright, McDougall, & Vertes, 1990; Soper & Thorley, 1996; Urwin & Ballinger, 2005; Wilson, Kaplan, Fellowes, Gruchy, and Faris, 1992 |
| Neurodevelopmental Intervention | Effectiveness | Brown & Burns, 2001; DeGangi, 1994a, 1994b; Jonsdottir, Fetters, & Kluzik, 1997; Kluzik, Fetters, & Coryell, 1990; Lilly & Powell, 199; Miles Breslin, 1996; Tsorlakis, Evaggelinou, Grouios, & Tsorbatzoudis, 2004 |
| Motor Learning | Effectiveness | Baron & Littleton, 1999; Miles Breslin, 1996 |
| Model of Human Occupation | Effectiveness | Basu, Jacobson, & Keller, 2004; Parrott, 2001 |
| Intervention | Alternative education settings | Dirette & Kolak, 2004 |
| | Transition planning | Spencer et al., 2003 |
| | Fine motor development | Case-Smith, 1996 |
| | Handwriting remediation | Lockhart & Law, 1994 |
| Sensory Diet Strategies | Effectiveness: Wilbarger brushing and joint compression protocol | Moore & Henry, 2002 |
| | Oral motor activity | Scheerer, 1992 |
| | Weighted vest | Fertel-Daly, Bedell, & Hinojosa, 2001; VandenBerg, 2001 |

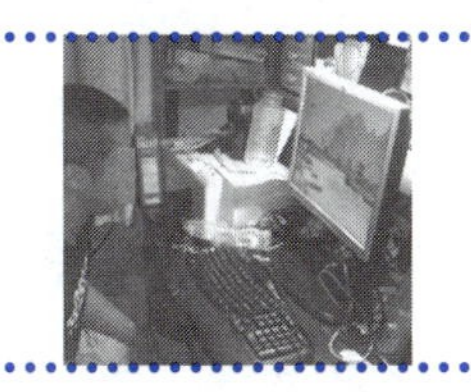
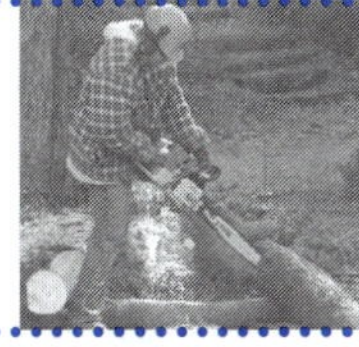
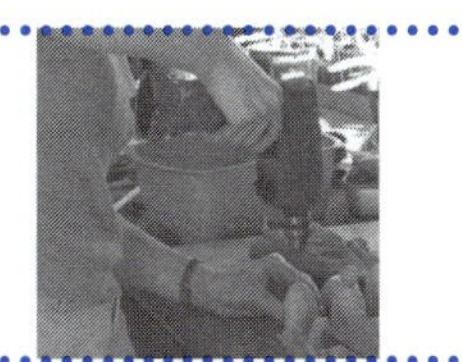

# References


American Occupational Therapy Association. (2000). Occupational therapy and the Americans with Disabilities Act (ADA). *American Journal of Occupational Therapy, 54*(6), 622-625.

Asher, A. (2003). From student to employee: Helping students with disabilities make the transition. *Developmental Disabilities Special Interest Section Quarterly, 26*(4), 1-4.

Baron, K. B., & Littleton, M. J. (1999). The model of human occupation: A return to work case study. *Work, 12*(1), 3-12.

Basu, S., Jacobson, L., & Keller, J. (2004). Child-centered tools: Using the model of human occupation framework. *School System Special Interest Section Quarterly, 11*(2), 1-3.

Breslin, D. (1996). Motor learning theory and the neurodevelopmental treatment approach: A comparative analysis. *Occupational Therapy in Health Care, 10*(1), 25-40.

Brief, A. P., & Nord, W. R. (1990). *The meanings of occupational work: A collection of essays*. Lanham, MD: Lexington Books.

Brown, G. T., & Burns, S. A. (2001). The efficacy of neurodevelopmental treatment in paediatrics: A systematic review. *British Journal of Occupational Therapy, 64*(5), 235-244.

Case-Smith, J. (1996). Fine motor outcomes in preschool children who receive occupational therapy services. *American Journal of Occupational Therapy, 50*(1), 52-61.

Cengage Learning. (n.d.). The Education For All Handicapped Children Act (PL 94-142) 1975. Retrieved July 31, 2009, from http://college.cengage.com/education/resources/res_prof/students/spec_ed/legislation/pl_94-142.html

Croce, R., & DePaepe, J. (1989). A critique of therapeutic intervention programming with reference to an alternative approach based on motor learning theory. *Physical & Occupational Therapy in Pediatrics, 9*(3), 5-33.

DeGangi, G. A. (1994a). Examining the efficacy of short-term NDT intervention using a case-study design: Part 1. *Physical & Occupational Therapy in Pediatrics, 14*(1), 71-88.

DeGangi, G. A. (1994b). Examining the efficacy of short-term NDT intervention using a case-study design: Part 2. *Physical & Occupational Therapy in Pediatrics, 14*(2), 21-61.

Dirette, D., & Kolak, L. (2004). Occupational performance needs of adolescents in alternative education programs. *American Journal of Occupational Therapy, 58*(3), 337-341.

Dunn, W. (1990). A comparison of service provision models in school-based occupational therapy services: A pilot study. *Occupational Therapy Journal of Research, 10*(5), 300-320.

Dunn, W. (2000). *Best practice occupational therapy: In community service with children and families*. Thorofare, NJ: SLACK Incorporated.

Fertel-Daly, D., Bedell, G., & Hinojosa, J. (2001). Effects of a weighted vest on attention to task and self-stimulatory behaviors in preschoolers with pervasive developmental disorders. *American Journal of Occupational Therapy, 55*(6), 629-640.

Fessler State Board of Education Site. (n.d.) School-to-Work Opportunities Act of 1994. Retrieved August 26, 2009, from http://www.fessler.com/SBE/act.htm

Gliner, J. A. (1985). Purposeful activity in motor learning: An event approach to motor skill acquisition. *American Journal of Occupational Therapy, 39*(1), 28-34.

Hearnshaw, L. S. (1954). Attitudes of work. *Occupational Psychology, 28*, 129-139.

Humphries, T., Wright, M., McDougall, B., & Vertes, J. (1990). The efficacy of sensory integration therapy for children with learning disability. *Physical and Occupational Therapy in Pediatrics, 10*(3), 1-17.

Jonsdottir, J., Fetters, L., & Kluzik, J. (1997). Effects of physical therapy on postural control in children with cerebral palsy. *Pediatric Physical Therapy, 9*(2), 68-75.

Kielhofner, G. (1995). *A model of human occupation: Theory and application*. Baltimore, MD: Williams and Wilkins.

Kielhofner, G., Braveman, B., Baron, K., Fisher, G., Hammel, J., & Littleton, M. (1999). The model of human occupation: Understanding the worker who is injured or disabled. *Work, 12*(1), 37-45.

Kluzik, J., Fetters, L., & Coryell, J. (1990). Quantification of control: A preliminary study of effects of neurodevelopmental treatment on reaching in children with spastic cerebral palsy. *Physical Therapy, 70*(2), 65-76.

Lilly, L. A., & Powell, N. J. (1990). Measuring the effects of neurodevelopmental treatment on the daily living skills of 2 children with cerebral palsy. *American Journal of Occupational Therapy, 44*(2), 139-415.

Lockhart, J., & Law M. (1994). The effectiveness of a multi-sensory writing programme for improving cursive writing in children with sensorimotor difficulties. *Canadian Journal of Occupational Therapy, 61*(4), 206-214.

Louis Harris and Associates. (1998). *The N.O.D./Harris Survey Program on Participation and Attitudes: Survey of Americans with disabilities*. New York, NY: Author.

Miles Breslin, D. M. (1996). Motor-learning theory and the neurodevelopmental treatment approach: A comparative analysis. *Occupational Therapy in Health Care, 10*(1), 25-40.

Moore, K. M., & Henry, A. D. (2002). Treatment of adult psychiatric patients using the Wilbarger protocol. *Occupational Therapy in Mental Health, 18*(1), 43-63.

Palisano, R. J. (1989). Comparison of two methods of service delivery for students with learning disabilities. *Physical & Occupational Therapy in Pediatrics, 9*(3), 79-100.

Parrott, M. (2001). Further research into specific models of practice. *British Journal of Occupational Therapy, 64*(10), 519.

Pohlman, J., Poosawtsee, C., Gerndt, K., & Lindstrom-Hazel, D. (2001). Improving work programs' delivery of information and service to workers' compensation carriers. *Work, 16*(2), 91-100.

Sandqvist, J. L., & Henriksson, C. M. (2004). Work functioning: A conceptual framework. *Work, 23*(2), 147-157.

Scheerer, C. R. (1992). Perspectives on an oral motor activity: The use of rubber tubing as a "chewy." *American Journal of Occupational Therapy, 46*(4), 344-352.

Shimmin, S. (1966). Concepts of work. *Occupational Psychology, 40*, 195-201.

Soper, G., & Thorley, C. R. (1996). Effectiveness of an occupational therapy program based on sensory integration theory for adults with severe learning disabilities. *British Journal of Occupational Therapy, 59*(10), 475-482.

Solomon, J. W. (2000). *Pediatric skills for occupational therapy assistants*. St. Louis, MO: Mosby.

Spencer, J. E., Emery, L. J., & Schneck, C. M. (2003). Occupational therapy in transitioning adolescents to post-secondary activities. *American Journal of Occupational Therapy, 57*(4), 435-441.

Suchomel, S. K. (2000). Educational system. In J. W. Solomon (Ed.), *Pediatric skills for occupational therapy assistants*. St. Louis, MO: Mosby.

Thomas, K. (1999). *The Oxford Book of Work*. New York, NY: Oxford University Press.

Tsorlakis, N., Evaggelinou, C., Grouios, G., & Tsorbatzoudis, C. (2004). Effect of intensive neurodevelopmental treatment in gross motor function of children with cerebral palsy. *Developmental Medicine and Child Neurology, 46*(11), 740-745.

Urwin, R., & Ballinger, C. (2005). The effectiveness of sensory integration therapy to improve functional behaviour in adults with learning disabilities: Five single-case experimental designs. *British Journal of Occupational Therapy, 68*(2), 56-66.

U.S. Departmenr of Education. (2004). The Rehabilitation Act. Retrieved July 31, 2009, from http://www.ed.gov/policy/speced/reg/narrative.html

U.S. Department of Education. (n.d.). Building the lagacy: IDEA 2004. Retrieved July 31, 2009, from http://idea.ed.gov

U.S. Equal Employment Opportunity Commission. (n.d.). American with Disabilities Act (ADA): 1990–2002. Retrieved July 31, 2009, from http://www.eeoc.gov/ada

President's Commission on Excellence in Special Education. (2002). *A new era: Revitalizing special education for children and their families*. Washington, DC: Author. Retrieved July 13, 2009, from http://www.ed.gov/inits/commissionsboards/whspecialeducation/reports/index.html

VandenBerg, N. L. (2001). The use of a weighted vest to increase on-task behavior in children with attention difficulties. *American Journal of Occupational Therapy, 55*(6), 621-628.

Wilson, B. N., Kaplan, B. J., Fellowes, S., Gruchy, C., & Faris, P. (1992). The efficacy of sensory integration treatment compared to tutoring. *Physical & Occupational Therapy in Pediatrics, 12*(1), 1-36.

World Institute on Disability. (n.d.). The Ticket to Work and Work Incentives Improvement Act of 1999: Federal fact sheet on Public Law 106-170. Retrieved July 31, 2009, from http://www.wid.org/publications/the-ticket-to-work-and-work-incentives-improvement-act-of-1999-federal-fact-sheet-on-public-law-106-170

# Suggested Reading

Baker, N. A., & Jacobs, K. (2003). The nature of working in the United States: An occupational therapy perspective. *Work, 20*(1), 53-61.

Barris, R., & Kielhofner G. (1985). Generating and using knowledge in occupational therapy: Implications for professional education. *Occupational Therapy Journal of Research, 5*(2), 113-124.

Berry, J., & Ryan, S. (2002). Frames of reference: Their use in pediatric occupational therapy. *British Journal of Occupational Therapy, 65*(9), 420-427.

Brayman, S. J., Clark, G. F., DeLany, J. V., Garza, E. R., Radomski, M. V., Ramsey, R., et al. (2004). Guidelines for supervision, roles and responsibilities during the delivery of occupational therapy services. *American Journal of Occupational Therapy, 58*(6), 663-667.

Fetters, L., & Kluzik, J. (1996). The effects of neurodevelopmental treatment versus practice on the reaching of children with spastic cerebral palsy. *Physical Therapy, 76*(4), 346-358.

Kemmis, B. L., & Dunn, W. (1996). Collaborative consultation: The efficacy of remedial and compensatory interventions in school contexts. *American Journal of Occupational Therapy, 50*(9), 709-717.

King, G. A., McDougall, J., Tucker, M. A., Gritzan, J., Malloy-Miller, T., Alambets, P., et al. (1999). An evaluation of functional, school-based therapy services for children with special needs. *Physical & Occupational Therapy in Pediatrics, 19*(2), 5-29.

Shamberg, S. (2005). Occupational therapy practitioner role in the implementation of worksite accommodations. *Work, 24*(2), 185-194.

Storch, B. A., & Eskow, K. G. (1996). Theory application by school-based occupational therapists. *American Journal of Occupational Therapy, 50*(8), 662-668.

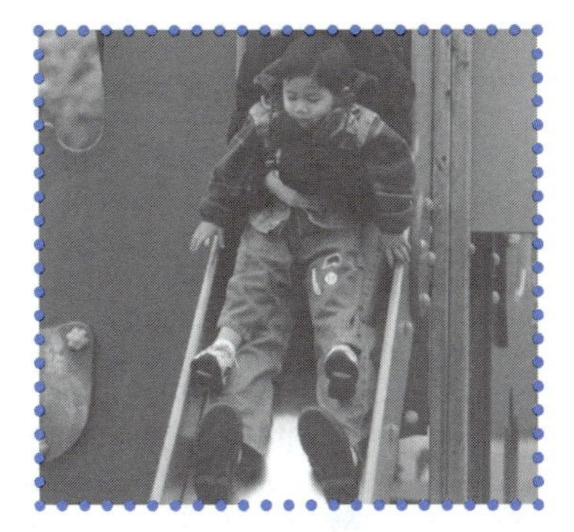

# 18

# Interventions of Play and Leisure

*Kathryn M. Loukas, MS, OTR/L, FAOTA and Bevin J. Journey, MS, OTR/L*

**ACOTE Standard Explored in This Chapter**

B.5.3

**Key Terms**

| | |
|---|---|
| Freedom to suspend reality | Leisure |
| Fun | Play |
| Internal control | Playfulness |
| Intrinsic motivation | Recreation |

## Introduction

Play and leisure activities are one part of the important triad of balance in occupational performance areas: work, play, and self-care across the lifespan (American Occupational Therapy Association [AOTA], 2008; Christiansen, 1991; Kielhofner, 2008). Occupational therapy practitioners should employ the use of play and leisure in the process and product of occupations in evaluation, intervention planning, intervention implementation, consultation, and discharge planning. Holistic intervention in occupational therapy is enhanced through the use of conceptual models. Models of practice guide holistic critical thinking in occupational therapy, and theory provides a foundation and rationale for practice (Scaffa, 2001). Recent scholars agree that occupation should be the central construct in our practice (Christiansen, Baum, & Bass-Haugen, 2004; Kielhofner, 2004; Wood, 1998; Yerxa, 1992). Occupation-centered interventions focus beyond impairment reduction, toward meaningful participation in life (Lee, Taylor, Kielhofner, & Fisher, 2008). Play and leisure pursuits can be highly meaningful, adding much to the health, well-being, and social participation of human beings. In occupational practice, we often neglect this important part of occupation, perhaps because present society seems to favor work and self-care. This chapter focuses on interventions specific to play and leisure across the lifespan. It is based on goal-directed preparatory activities, purposeful activities, and occupational performance (Figure 18-1).

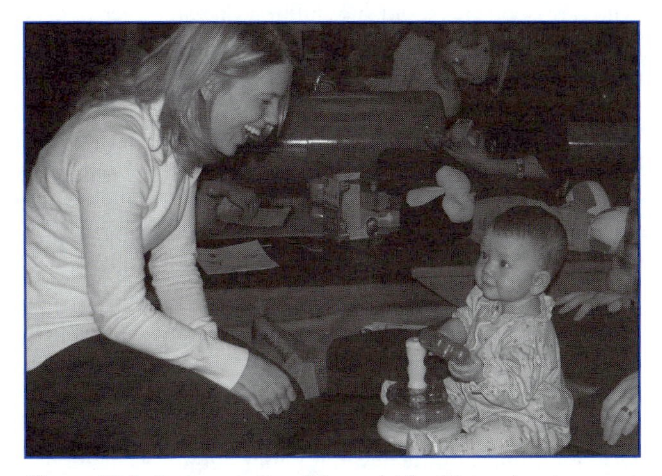

**Figure 18-1.** An occupational therapist facilitates development through play.



K. Sladyk, K. Jacobs, & N. MacRae (Eds.).
*Occupational Therapy Essentials for Clinical Competence* (pp. 199-206).

Play is the primary activity, and playfulness is the primary process in which occupational therapy practitioners address young children and infants (Bundy, 1997). Playfulness, according to Bundy, has three elements: intrinsic motivation, internal control, and the freedom to suspend reality. Suspending reality, or pretend or symbolic play, incorporates an imaginative element that can facilitate a child to develop the skills for real life (Bundy, 1993). Therefore, an occupational therapy practitioner working with young children should try to create a safe environment, make activities fun, make routines part of a game or song, and engage the family or friends in the playful process. Creating contexts that enhance development is also an important aspect of the occupational therapy process as the child and the environment are interdependent in a transactional relationship (Humphry & Wakeford, 2006). Play facilitates dynamic development in physical, cognitive, social, and emotional skills, and is the underlying mechanism of learning during the developmental years. During play, a child should feel comfortable, safe, and engaged. The process should be enjoyable for both the client and the therapist. In western culture, play is often considered to be the occupational role of children (Rodger & Ziviani, 1999). However, in some cultures, both play and leisure are often incorporated into work and self-care activities (S. Bazyk, Stalnaker, Llerena, Ekelman, & J. Bazyk, 2003; Primeau, 1995). For this reason, it is important for the occupational therapy practitioner to understand the role of play or leisure in the culture of the client and/or family.

Play activities throughout infancy and childhood can lead to decisions about which leisure activities to participate in later in life. Leisure activities are those that we fill our free time with as we take on adult roles and are important to leading a balanced life. Leisure activities have individual meaning to the persons participating in them. Adults have both coordinated leisure activities, which are work-related, such as playing on the company softball team or attending holiday parties at work; or complementary leisure, which is role-related, such as a mother who coaches soccer, a father who works on the set of his children's theater, or partners who accompany an elderly family member on a trip to their homeland (Glantz & Richman, 2001).

When intervention incorporates play or leisure activities, it is vital for the occupational therapist to consider the meaning a certain activity has to the client. Also, it is important to note that although occupational therapy practitioners promote play and leisure occupations, not all play and leisure occupations are healthy or positive. Children and adults can have negative occupations such as self-destructive behavior; addictions such as gambling, substance abuse, or compulsions; or aggressive, illegal, or unsafe behaviors during their free time (Moyers, 1999). They may also have impoverished habits such as watching television and eating fatty foods most of the day. It is important for occupational therapy practitioners to promote healthy occupations and prevent or decrease unhealthy ones. Having strong and meaningful leisure occupations can prevent the development or recurrence of negative occupations.

# Play and Leisure Across the Lifespan

## Infancy

In infancy, play focuses around exploration of surroundings and is sensorimotor-based. Infants and young children discover cause and effect relationships to develop a purpose to their actions. Play occurs as an interaction between infant and caregiver, and later evolves to include siblings or other children (Knox, 1998).

## Preschool Age

During the preschool years, play becomes more constructive, and symbolic play is refined. Children start to use play to explore social roles. Play often incorporates fine motor activity, refining this skill as well. Play at this stage often occurs at home with parents or siblings.

## School Age

School-aged play frequently revolves around rule-governed games, with emphasis on turn-taking (Knox, 1998). Play is part of life for school-aged children on the playground at recess, in afterschool activities, and during free time. School-aged children also have free leisure time that they need to find positive ways of fulfilling. Middle childhood is a time of engagement with peers in real and important ways. It is a time of making decisions about what occupations are fulfilling and meaningful to them, which can lead to decisions about what leisure activities to pursue in coming years.

## Adolescence

As children approach adolescence, they begin to engage in more organized or "structured" play and leisure activities, such as arts, sports, and other specific individual interests (Figure 18-2). The main focus of most play and leisure activities in adolescence is socialization. For this age group, it has been found that participation in structured activities can lead to decreased antisocial behavior (Mahoney & Stattin, 2000), and even higher academic grades (Fletcher, Nickerson, & Wright, 2003).

## Adulthood

Time spent pursuing leisure activities widely varies depending on contexts during adulthood. A single man or woman's leisure activities differ greatly from those of new parents, which differ from those of parents of adolescents or a business man or woman, which are again different from those of a retired couple. For parents, leisure activities might center around their children's activities. As adults age and

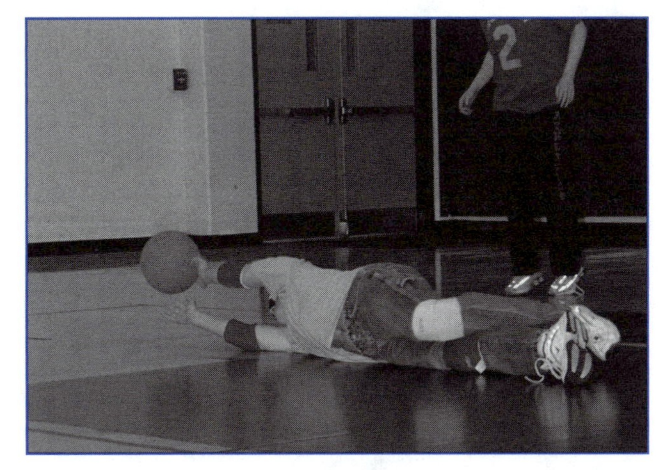


**Figure 18-2.** An athlete plays "Goalball," a sport designed for people who are blind or visually impaired.

children leave the house, more free time emerges for leisure activities such as reading, sewing, ballroom dancing, kayaking, or hiking. Social clubs or religious organizations might become important. Older adults and elders may engage in card groups, restaurant nights, and gardening as an empty nest, retirement, or disability opens up more leisure time.

# Intervention Plan

The intervention plan should progress in the following manner according to the framework (AOTA, 2008):

- The client's goals (or those of the family), values, and beliefs should be taken into consideration in the plan. For instance, a family who feels that an infant or child is too fragile for play but would enjoy motor activities could be educated to follow precautions while given specific ideas for interactive play with a medically fragile child.
- The health and well-being of the client should always be the primary focus of the occupational therapist. Knowing and following precautions may enable a client to feel safe and engaged in a therapeutic play or leisure setting.
- Performance skills: Physical performance skills include posture, mobility, coordination, strength, effort, and energy. Goals can often target specific areas of performance through interventions that are play- or leisure-based, creating a fun and engaging therapeutic activity.
- The context: The dynamic and complex nature of context, environment, and circumstances should be considered, utilized, and adapted for optimal therapeutic outcomes. Often play and recreational contexts are outdoors or in the community; this can have a very positive therapeutic influence on intervention outcomes. Because the natural environment is less controlled and predictable, safety considerations specific to each client, his or her age, and ability levels should always be in place for any therapeutic context. (See Chapter 29).

For more specific components of the occupational therapy intervention plan, see Chapter 15.

The occupational therapy intervention plan utilizing play or leisure activities is geared toward four common approaches (Moyers, 1999):

1. *Remediation/restoration*: Here, the play or leisure activity is geared toward client factors that are interfering with overall function. The occupational therapist creatively selects a play or leisure activity that will improve the targeted areas of function through play or leisure activities.
2. *Compensation/adaptation*: This is an approach to help clients participate in the occupations of their lives by adapting the environment, using adaptive devices, or implementing a compensatory strategy. Adapting toys or games for children with physical disabilities or enlarging text for people with visual impairment in order to read are examples of this. Training family members to include their loved one using adaptations is also under this area of intervention.
3. *Disability prevention*: This area may entail helping people with disabilities engage in activities that require movement safely and effectively. Wearing a helmet when using the adaptive bicycle, using a reacher to pick up the golf balls, or assuring that a person with cognitive impairment understands not to swim alone are examples of this. People with chronic problems such as back injuries, chronic pain, or mental illness may need an occupational therapist to assist them with a play or leisure program that is healthy and will not exacerbate their disability.
4. *Health promotion*: Play or leisure programs that target a specific population are examples of occupational therapy intervention that promote healthy lifestyles. An afterschool play and fitness program to promote physical activity and prevent obesity is an example. A Tai Chi program for older adults to improve balance, prevent falls, and promote relaxation and circulation is another example (Figure 18-3). Occupational therapists are finding more and more ways to promote health in their communities or work places. Many of these programs are play- or leisure-based.

# Goals Using Play or Leisure for Occupational Performance Intervention

Play and leisure are often used in two ways in occupational therapy practice: play/leisure as a means, or play/leisure as an end. Play/leisure as a means is described as using these activities as a tool for other goal-oriented outcomes.

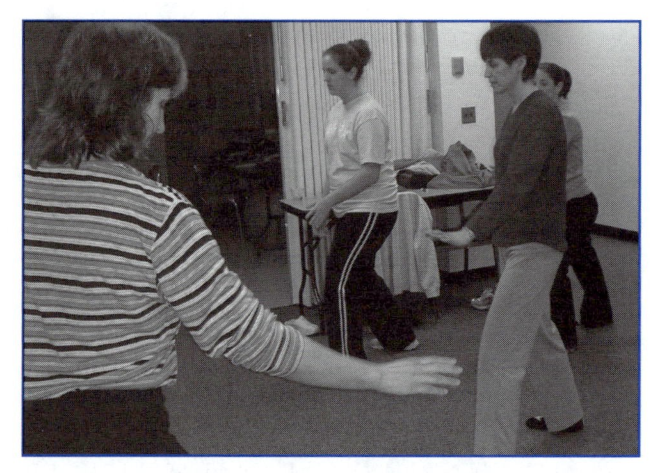

**Figure 18-3.** Occupational therapy practitioners learn Tai Chi as a leisure-based intervention activity.

This can be an important part of occupational therapy intervention and can be used to address many different client factors, as clients are more likely to engage and cooperate in a fun activity (O'Brien, 2006). Play/leisure as a goal or "end" is used when the occupational therapy practitioner is focused on helping the client gain skills and utilize daily routines in engagement in play or leisure activities (O'Brien, 2006).

Occupational therapy goals should be objective, measurable, and client-centered to individual clients. The goals presented here are broad in scope and meant to give goal-based ideas for intervention planning:

1. Play or leisure to improve targeted motor skills or development:
   - Johnny will improve gross and fine motor skills through play with objects and toys in his environment in a variety of developmental positions as measured by improvement to an 18-month developmental level as measured by the Peabody Developmental Motor Scales.

     *Activity ideas*: Creating a supportive context of developmental play incorporating the interdependent contexts of family, play, and childcare in the natural environment. Explorative play in positions such as supportive sitting, prone on elbows, or supported standing and interaction with age-appropriate sensorimotor toys should be facilitated.
   - Through play-based motor activities, Christine will improve trunk control, sitting balance, and upper body control as measured by clinical observations data.

     *Activity ideas*: horseback riding, swimming, or playing on a playground.
   - William will engage in selected leisure activities 30 minutes per day in order to improve overall energy, bilateral arm use, and social participation as measured by self-reported journal entries.

     *Activity ideas*: Involvement in afterschool programming of choice, shooting baskets, playing catch with a friend, swimming with a group, playing waffle ball, or playing volleyball.
2. Goals to improve playfulness:
   - Jessie will engage in make-believe play with her sister with activity set-up as measured by sustaining pretend play activity for three interactions.

     *Activity ideas*: Family training and facilitation of make-believe play such as puppet theater, dress-up, or bath-time play.
3. Goals to improve psychosocial and behavioral skills:
   - Annie will improve emotional control and social interactions when engaging in peer group activities as measured by successful interactions without behavioral outburst three out of four times.

     *Activity ideas*: The occupational therapist can consult with the staff to create contexts that support this goal. Other ideas include board games with one or more peers, "New Games," or initiative and cooperative games (possibly done in the physical education class).
   - Mrs. Cooper will actively engage in a leisure activity with her husband without outburst for 30 minutes daily as measured by husband report.

     *Activity ideas*: Consultation with the family and caregivers to create a context of support, safety, and recreation. Simple card games, walking around the block, reading a book to their grandchild, or baking cookies together are ideas that could be incorporated into the intervention plan.
4. Goals to improve social interactions/community participation:
   - Dustin will interact with peers during recess to negotiate and share equipment 3 out of 4 times as measured by Educational Technician recordkeeping.

     *Activity ideas*: Facilitating play with a group of children along with the client. Modeling and scripting communication to share the swings, helping a child wait and then try the slides, or engaging a group of children in a 4-square game alternating participants are some examples.
   - Susan will successfully join the fitness center, interacting with staff as needed as measured by therapist observation one time per month.
5. Goals to add structure and leisure occupations to the daily routine:
   - Isabelle will engage in three leisure activities that she will perform independently during free time as measured by Group Home recordkeeping.

     *Activity ideas*: Explore and engage in leisure activities to add to her list.
   - James will engage in three meaningful leisure-based heavy work activities to effectively transition from home to school daily as measured by sensory diet report card.

*Activity ideas*: Pogo stick, medicine ball, mini-trampoline, book deliveries.

6. Goals with play or leisure occupations as the outcome:
   - As part of the group home program, members will plan and engage in two community recreation activities per month as measured by recordkeeping and client report.

     *Activity ideas*: Choosing and going to a movie or theater event, going to the mall, walking on the high school track, or going to an outdoor concert.
   - The Samson family will develop at least five play or leisure activities they can engage in as a family and do one family activity per week as measured by family reporting.
7. Goals that use adaptation/compensation for play/leisure involvement:
   - Simon will use adaptation in the community, such as his adapted bicycle, for safe and effective play participation with his siblings as measured by family report.
   - Given adaptations for visual deficits including enlarging the targets, creating tactile boundaries, and adding noise to sports equipment, Lynn will fully participate in sports at recreation camp as measured by staff reports, photos, and anecdotal data.
   - Given adaptations such as a card-holder, Emma will effectively play with her friends on Cards Night for 30 minutes using her hemiplegic left arm as a functional assist as measured by therapist observation and recordkeeping.
8. Goals to prevent disability:
   - Amanda will learn and participate in three safe activities to engage in on the playground without injury as measured by inclusive playground therapy recordkeeping by the occupational therapist.
   - Markus will learn and utilize safe body mechanics while playing outdoor games such as bocci ball with his friends without pain behaviors as measured by client pain journal data.
9. Goals to promote health:
   - The group of people recovering from substance abuse will show increased insight about their addictions and less recidivism following the outdoor adventure program as measured by a 6-week follow-up study.
   - The elders in assisted living will show improved balance following the ballroom dance session as measured by improved performance on the Berg Balance Scale.
10. Goals to develop positive occupational leisure choices:
    - Isabelle will learn three positive leisure activities for physical input that she will engage in instead of reverting to self-abusive behaviors (such as cutting) as measured by staff recordkeeping.
    - John will engage in recreation of his choice three times a week and refrain from online gambling as measured by reflection journal and anecdotal records.
11. Goals to improve self-esteem:
    - Kayla will improve self-confidence and self-esteem through success in community programs such as Special Olympics and choir as measured by an increase of 10% on scores of the self-esteem checklist.

# Summary

Occupational therapy practitioners promote and facilitate play with a purpose. Play and leisure are an important part of the triad of balance in occupational performance skills involved in life and occupational therapy practice. Using models and frames of reference as a guide, play and leisure activities in occupational therapy intervention should be carefully selected and performed with cultural sensitivity and individualized plans. Taking client factors into consideration such as developmental level, physical and cognitive ability levels, psychosocial skills, and cultural considerations, a wide range of activities can be used in play and leisure interventions. The natural environment of intervention should also be considered and modified to facilitate participation of play, leisure, and recreation in context. The outcomes of play and leisure intervention are as dynamic and broad as the occupational therapy spectrum, but they are all successful when they are performed with safety, fun, and enjoyment.

# Student Self-Assessment

## Occupations of Children

The instructor brings in a variety of toys and games for a wide spectrum of developmental levels and interests. Every student goes to a toy, game, or creative childhood item.

Answer the following questions:

1. What thoughts or memories does this item bring back for you?
2. What ages and gender would most likely use this toy/game?
3. What skills are necessary to use this toy/game?
4. What areas of motor development does this toy/game facilitate?
5. What levels of visual/perceptual/cognitive development does this toy/game facilitate?

6. How could this toy/game develop social interaction with other people?
7. How could this toy/game be modified for a person with physical special needs? For cognitive special needs?
8. Is this something that an occupational therapist might use during an intervention? Describe how and with what client and client factors, and include age, diagnosis, and environment.

## Service Learning Project

Students are to find a child with special needs through fieldwork or other means and design a piece of play equipment, toy, game, or sport specifically for that individual child or family. The student will then give the child/family the project. Cost limitation: $20.00. Lab time can be provided for this project (See Figure 18-4 for examples).

Criteria:

- Level of sophistication: Complexity of project
- Individualization, client-centered
- Safety
- Functionality: How well does it work?
- Fun factor
- Family friendly
- Presentation in class
- Aesthetics
- Level of learning for the student
- Creativity

## Leisure and Recreation

The instructor should bring in a variety of arts and crafts, games, and sports equipment such as croquet, bocci ball, checkers, Connect Four, Twister, a deck of cards, Kings in the Corner, a playground ball, table tennis, art activities such a scrapbooking, etc.

Students are divided into groups. Each group has 5 to 10 minutes to plan, and 5 minutes to present/demonstrate one activity. Groups will choose a scenario below and an activity to adapt for a successful occupational leisure activity:

1. You are working with a middle school child who is significantly visually impaired in a recreational after-school program with typical peers.
2. You need to plan an activity evening for young adult clients with mental retardation and mild obesity who generally like to sit and watch TV and are resistant to physical activity.
3. You are working with a client with chronic low back pain and over-medication who is sedentary and depressed. Occupational therapy goals are to promote pain-free movement.
4. You are working with a 60-year-old man with significant tremors and balance deficits from Parkinson's Disease who wants to participate in activities with his wife.
5. You are working with a young man with Schizophrenia in a mental health group of 4 people who have significant difficulties with social interaction.

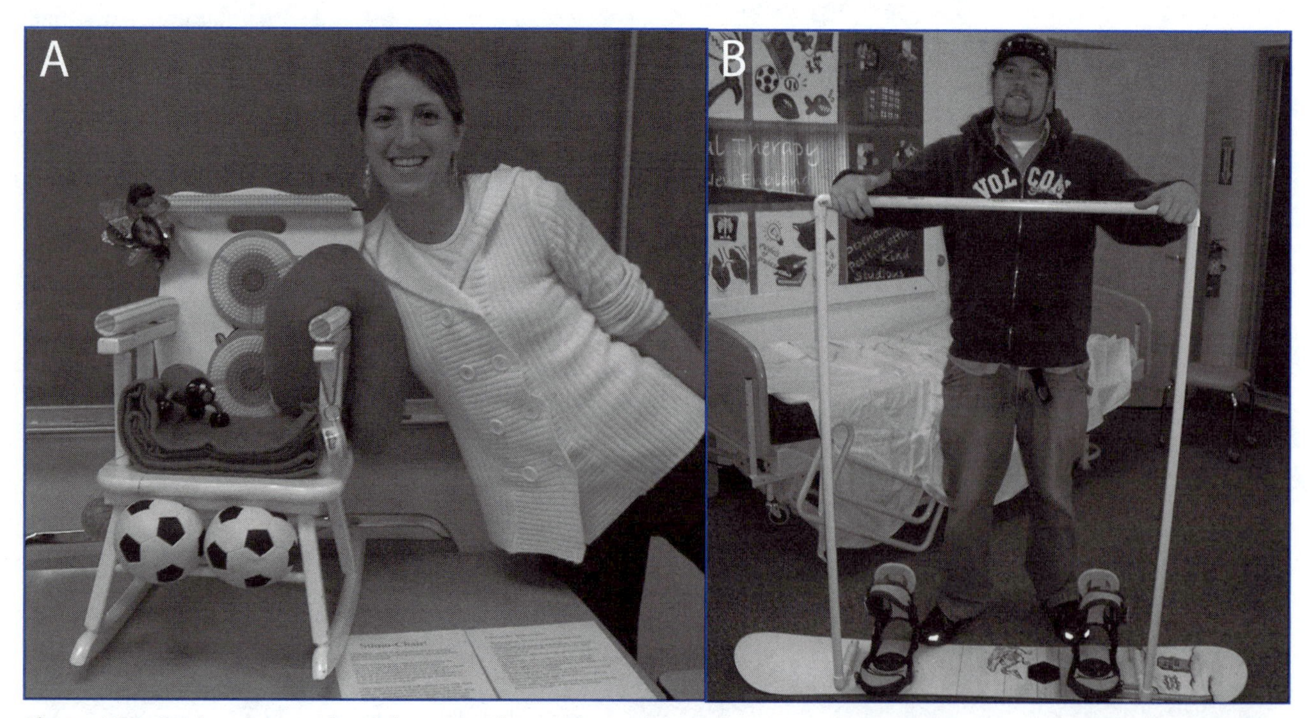


**Figure 18-4.** Sarah, an occupational therapy student, with an adapted chair (A), and Duncan, another occupational therapy student, with a ski board (B).

## Experiential Learning

Students who have been involved with work or volunteer work with people in adapted play, leisure, or recreational programming gain valuable insight into the importance and skills involved in adaptive activities. Consider the following experiential activities for students through volunteer experiences, work, or Level 1 Fieldwork:

- Therapeutic horseback riding
- Adaptive aquatics
- Camps for children with special needs (Easter Seals)
- Martial arts for people with physical challenges
- Special Olympics
- Ski programs for people with physical challenges
- School-based summer recreational programs with inclusion
- Sensory integrative camps
- Developmental preschools

### Evidence-Based Research Chart

| Program/ Content | Intervention | Evidence |
|---|---|---|
| Playfulness | Occupational therapy intervention targeted at improving playfulness in 4- to 6-year-old children with autism spectrum disorder | Improvements indicated in playfulness and recommendations made (O'Brien et al., 2000) |
| | Play behaviors of random preschool children were studied | Positive correlation found between playfulness and coping skills (Saunders, Sayer, & Goodale, 1998) |
| Play as occupation | Purposeful "play" activity versus rote exercise was studied on children with burn injuries | Study of two children found purposeful activity results to favor rote exercise (Melchert-McKearnan, Deitz, Engle, & White, 2000) |
| | The parasympathetic and sympathetic nervous system are influenced during the important developmental play activities of children | There is a relationship with the neuro-occupation of play in development of children's occupations. The role of internal and external processes should be equally considered (Way, 1999) |
| Play to improve sensorimotor skills/development | Preschool-aged children with fine motor delays engaged in occupational therapy-based play | Occupational therapy focus on play can improve fine motor and visual motor performance (Case-Smith, 2000) |
| | Mastery of play was one area targeted through sensory integrative intervention for preschool children with autism. | Children increased goal-directed play through occupational therapy intervention (Case-Smith & Bryan, 1999) |
| | Positioning equipment for children with physical disabilities | Positive impact on play skills as measured by parent survey (O'Brien et al., 1998) |
| Peer play | Initiation and response in free-play dyads of children with delayed play skills | Children demonstrated more initiation and response when engaged with higher level peers (Tanta, Deitz, White, & Billingsly, 2005) |
| Cultural influences | Play is incorporated into work activities with Mayan children | Qualitative study of Mayan families (Bazyk et al., 2003) |
| | Sociocultural comparison of Nigerian and American children's games | Diversity of styles, values, and approach to play in different cultures (Nwokah & Ikekeonwu, 1998) |
| Leisure activity involvement | Reading, playing board games, playing music, and dancing | Associated with reduced risk of dementia (Verghese et al., 2003) |
| | Leisure benefits for persons with congenital disabilities by involvement in leisure activities | Reported improvement of mental and physical health, enjoyment, increased self-concept, and enhanced social relationships (Specht, King, Brown, & Foris, 2002) |
| Structured leisure activity | Structured leisure activities (clubs, sports, classes) | Linked to lower levels of antisocial behavior in adolescents (Fletcher et al., 2003; Mahoney & Stattin, 2000) |
| Occupational identity | Older, retired persons involved in creative occupations such as woodworking, painting, knitting, etc. | Improvement of occupational identity measured by occupational narratives (Howie, Coulter, & Feldman, 2004) |
| Leisure assessment | Study looked at how frequently occupational therapists assess leisure as part of evaluation and how much value is placed on leisure in occupational therapy | Survey of occupational therapy practitioners indicated few use formal leisure assessments, but most use informal assessment. Leisure is valued by practitioners, more research is needed (Turner, Chapman, McSherry, Krishnagiri, & Watts, 2000) |

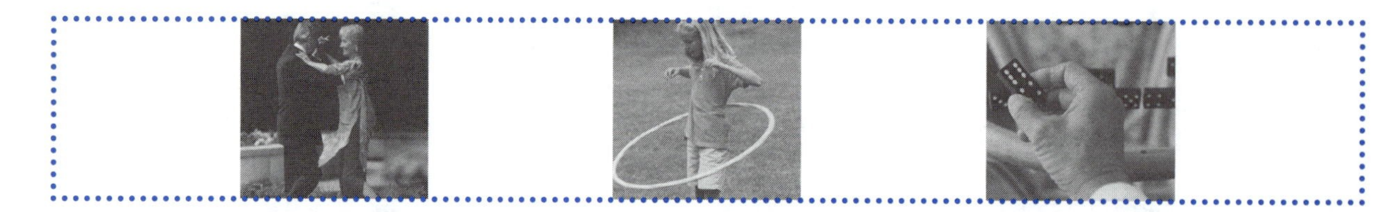

# References


American Occupational Therapy Association. (2008). Occupational therapy practice framework: Domain and process, second edition. *American Journal of Occupational Therapy, 62*, 625-683.

Bazyk, S., Stalnaker, D., Llerena, M., Ekelman, B., & Bazyk, J. (2003). Play in Mayan children. *American Journal of Occupational Therapy, 57*(3), 273-283.

Bundy, A. C. (1993). Assessment of play and leisure: Delineation of the problem. *American Journal of Occupational Therapy, 47*(3), 217-222.

Bundy, A. C. (1997). Play and playfulness: What to look for. In L. D. Parham & L. S. Fazio (Eds.), *Play in occupational therapy for children* (pp. 52-66). St. Louis, MO: Mosby.

Case-Smith, J. (2000). Effects of occupational therapy services on fine motor and functional performance in preschool children. *American Journal of Occupational Therapy, 54*(4), 372-380.

Case-Smith, J., & Bryan, T. (1999). The effects of occupational therapy with sensory integration emphasis on preschool-age children with autism. *American Journal of Occupational Therapy, 53*(5), 489-497.

Christiansen, C. H. (1991). Occupational therapy: Intervention for life performance. In C. H. Christiansen & C. M. Baum (Eds.), *Occupational therapy: Overcoming human performance deficits*. Thorofare, NJ: SLACK Incorporated.

Christiansen, C. H., Baum, C. M., & Bass-Haugen, J. (Eds.). (2004). *Occupational therapy: Performance, participation, and well-being* (3rd ed.). Thorofare, NJ: SLACK Incorporated.

Fletcher, A. C., Nickerson, P., & Wright, K. L. (2003). Structured leisure activities in middle childhood: Links to well-being. *Journal of Community Psychology, 31*(6), 641-659.

Glantz, C. H., & Richman, N. (2001). Leisure activities. In L. W. Pedretti & M. B. Early (Eds.), *Occupational therapy practice skills for physical dysfunction* (5th ed., pp. 249-256). St Louis, MO: Mosby.

Howie, L., Coulter, M., & Feldman, S. (2004). Crafting the self: Older persons' narratives of occupational identity. *American Journal of Occupational Therapy, 58*(4), 446-454.

Humphry, R., & Wakeford, L. (2006). An occupation-centered discussion of development and implications for practice. *American Journal of Occupational Therapy, 60*(3), 258-267.

Kielhofner, G. (2004). *Conceptual foundations of occupational therapy* (3rd ed.). Philadelphia, PA: F.A. Davis.

Kielhofner, G. (2008). *Model of human occupation: Theory and Application* (4th ed.). Baltimore, MD: Lippincott Williams & Wilkins.

Knox, S. H. (1998). Treatment through play and leisure. In M. E. Neistadt & E. B. Crepeau (Eds.), *Willard & Spackman's occupational therapy* (9th ed., pp 382-390). New York, NY: Lippincott Williams and Wilkins.

Lee, S. W., Taylor, R., Kielhofner, G., & Fisher, G. (2008). Theory use in practice: A national survey of therapists who use the Model of Human Occupation. *American Journal of Occupational Therapy, 62*(1), 106-117.

Mahoney, J. L., & Stattin, H. (2000). Leisure activities and adolescent antisocial behavior: The role of structure and social context. *Journal of Adolescence, 23*(2), 113-127.

Melchert-McKearnan, K., Deitz, J., Engel, J. M., & White, O. (2000). Children with burn injuries: Purposeful activity versus rote exercise. *American Journal of Occupational Therapy, 54*(4), 381-390.

Moyers, P. (1999). The guide to occupational therapy practice. *American Journal of Occupational Therapy, 53*(3), 246-322.

Nwokah, E. E., & Ikekeonwu, C. (1998). A sociocultural comparison of Nigerian and American children's games. In M. C. Duncan, G. Chick, & A. Aycock (Eds.), *Play and culture studies, volume 1: Diversions and divergences in fields of play*. London, England: Ablex Publishing.

O'Brien, J. C. (2006). Play and playfulness. In J. W. Solomon & J. C. O'Brien (Eds.), *Pediatric skills for occupational therapy assistants* (2nd ed., pp. 321-342). St Louis, MO: Mosby.

O'Brien, J., Boatwright, T., Chaplin, J., Geckler, C., Gosnell, D., Holcombe, J., et al. (1998). The impact of positioning equipment on play skills of physically impaired children. *Play and culture studies, volume 1*. London, England: Ablex Publishing Corporation.

O'Brien, J., Coker, P., Lynn, R., Suppinger, R., Pearigen, T., Rabon, S., et al. (2000). The impact of occupational therapy on a child's playfulness. *Occupational Therapy in Health Care, 12*(2/3), 39-51.

Primeau, L. A. (1996). Work and leisure: Transcending the dichotomy. *American Journal of Occupational Therapy, 50*(7), 569-577.

Rodger, S., and Ziviani, J. (1999). Play-based occupational therapy. *International Journal of Disability, Development and Education, 46*(3), 337-365.

Saunders, I., Sayer, M., & Goodale, A. (1999). The relationship between playfulness and coping in preschool children: A pilot study. *American Journal of Occupational Therapy, 53*(2), 221-226.

Scaffa, M. E. (2001). *Occupational therapy in community-based practice settings*. Philadelphia, PA: F.A. Davis.

Specht, J., King, G., Brown, E., & Foris, C. (2002). The importance of leisure in the lives of persons with congenital physical disabilities. *American Journal of Occupational Therapy, 56*(4), 436-445.

Tanta, K. J., Deitz, J. C., White, O., & Billingsley, F. (2005). The effects of peer-play level on initiations and responses of preschool children with delayed play skills. *American Journal of Occupational Therapy, 59*(4), 437-445.

Turner, H., Chapman, S., McSherry, A., Krishnagiri, S., & Watts, J. (2000). Leisure assessment in occupational therapy: An exploratory study. *Occupational Therapy in Health Care, 12*(2/3), 73-85.

Verghese, J., Lipton, R. B., Katz, M. J., Hall, C. B., Derby, C. A., Kuslansky, G., et al. (2003). Leisure activities and the risk of dementia in the elderly. *New England Journal of Medicine, 348*(25), 2508-2516.

Way, M. (1999). Parasympathetic and sympathetic influences in neuro-occupation pertaining to play. *Occupational Therapy in Health Care, 12*(1), 71-86.

Wood, W. (1998). It is jump time for occupational therapy. *American Journal of Occupational Therapy, 52*(6), 403-411.

Yerxa, E. J. (1992). Some implications of occupational therapy's history for its epistemology, values, and relation to medicine. *American Journal of Occupational Therapy, 46*(1), 79-83.

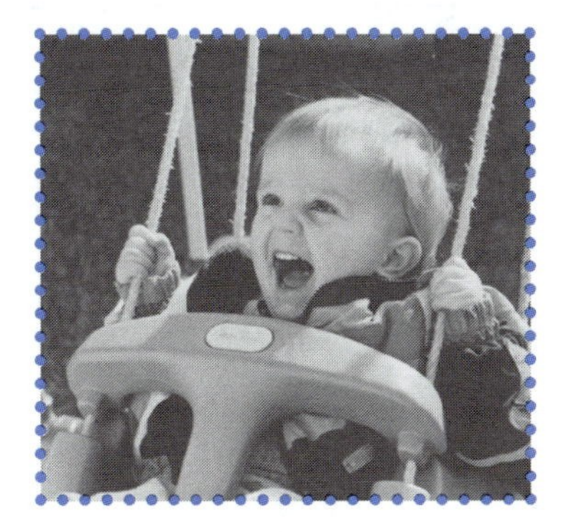

# Interventions of Social Participation

*Jane O'Brien, PhD, OTR/L*

**ACOTE Standards Explored in This Chapter**

B.5.4-5.6, 5.19-5.21

**Key Terms**

Compensation
Occupation-based activity
Practice skills
Preparatory activity
Remediation

## Introduction

This chapter will introduce readers to therapeutic use of occupations and activities for helping clients increase social participation, as well as self-management and community and work integration. Techniques to provide development, remediation, and compensation for social behaviors will be introduced. Examples of how to grade and adapt the environment, tools, materials, occupations, and interventions to reflect the client's social participation needs will be provided. Finally, a description of compensatory strategies that may be helpful in terms of social participation will be included. The role of the occupational therapist and occupational therapy assistant in intervention of social participation will be differentiated throughout the chapter.

## Social Participation

Social participation is an area of occupation targeted in intervention by occupational therapy practitioners. Social participation includes activities associated with organized patterns of behavior that are characteristic and expected of an individual or an individual interacting with others within a given social system (American Occupational Therapy Association [AOTA], 2008, adapted from Mosey, 1996, p. 340). As such, social participation includes activities that occur with the community, family, peer, or friend.

The first step in planning intervention to improve engagement in social participation is to understand the client's needs. This involves collaboration with clients, family members, and significant others. Therefore, the occupational therapist designs intervention based on "the client's goals, values, and beliefs as well as the health and well-being of the client" (AOTA, 2008, p. 655). While the occupational therapist is ultimately responsible for the intervention plan, the occupational therapist assistant may provide input and data to the process and may be responsible for designing the activities based upon the established plan (AOTA, 1990, 1994).

In addition to collaborating with clients, the occupational therapy practitioner analyzes the performance skills required for successful social participation. Performance skills are observable elements of action (AOTA, 2008; Fisher & Kielhofner, 1995) and include motor, processing, and communication/interactions skills (Table 19-1).



K. Sladyk, K. Jacobs, & N. MacRae (Eds.).
*Occupational Therapy Essentials for Clinical Competence* (pp. 207-216).

**Table 19-1. Communication/Interaction Skills**

| | |
|---|---|
| Physicality—Pertains to using the physical body when communicating within an occupation. | • Contacts: Makes physical contact with others<br>• Gazes: Uses eyes to communicate and interact with others<br>• Gestures: Uses movements of the body to indicate, demonstrate, or add emphasis<br>• Maneuvers: Moves one's own body in relation to others<br>• Orients: Directs one's body in relation to others and/or occupational forms<br>• Postures: Assumes physical positions |
| Information Exchange—Refers to giving and receiving information within an occupation. | • Articulates: Produces clear, understandable speech<br>• Asserts: Directly expresses desires, refusals, and requests<br>• Asks: Requests factual or personal information<br>• Engages: Initiates interactions<br>• Expresses: Displays affect/attitude<br>• Modulates: Uses volume and inflection in speech<br>• Shares: Gives out factual or personal information<br>• Speaks: Makes oneself understood through the use of words, phrases, and sentences<br>• Sustains: Keeps up speech for appropriate duration |
| Relations—Relates to maintaining appropriate relationships within an occupation. | • Collaborates: Coordinates action with others toward a common goal<br>• Conforms: Follows implicit and explicit social norms<br>• Focuses: Directs conversation and behavior to ongoing social action<br>• Relates: Assumes a manner of acting that tries to establish a rapport with others<br>• Respects: Accommodates to other people's reactions and requests |

Reprinted with permission from American Occupational Therapy Association. (2002). Occupational therapy practice framework: Domain & process. *American Journal of Occupational Therapy, 56*, 622.

The occupational therapist evaluates performance skills required for social interactions by observing, interviewing, and conducting evaluations. This process is outlined in the following case example.

> Mabel is a 75-year-old woman who had a stroke resulting in right-sided weakness. She lives alone and has limited social contact. The occupational therapist observes Mabel interacting with other senior citizens as they wait for rehabilitation services. Mabel seems to "light up" and become more verbal around other people her age. She enjoys talking about television programs and listens well to others. Mabel is liked by her peers in the rehabilitation program. The occupational therapy practitioner is concerned that Mabel will have limited social contact upon discharge.
>
> During the interview, the occupational therapist learns that Mabel has no transportation or opportunities for social activities. She speaks slowly and has trouble expressing herself since the stroke. Mabel's strengths include the ability to listen, make appropriate eye contact, and that she is viewed as personable and approachable. Mabel works slowly but is capable of completing tasks.
>
> The occupational therapy practitioner works with the social worker to arrange for weekly transportation to the local senior citizens' center upon discharge, and to a weekly support group for those with stroke. Mabel is pleased with this arrangement.

Prior to discharge, the occupational therapist further evaluates the motor skills required to interact at the senior citizens' center and in the support group. Mabel needs to develop adequate sitting and standing posture, walk to and from the center entrance, sit for extended periods of time at the center and in the car, get up out of the car and chair, use fine motor skills for activities, and eat a light meal. The processing skills required include choosing and using words, inquiring, and sequencing conversation. Mabel speaks slowly but is able to make conversation. She has difficulty with word finding and articulation, but she will have support in the senior citizens' group and support group.

Communication/interaction skills are a large component of engagement in social participation (See Table 19-1). The framework (AOTA, 2008) provides guidelines to direct observation. From these guidelines, the practitioner observes that Mabel is good at making physical contact and eye contact; she is neither too forward nor too shy and easily "connects" with others. She shows some difficulty maneuvering around others (due to motor difficulties associated with the stroke). In terms of information exchange, Mabel asks, engages in interactions, and shares easily. However, she has articulation difficulties and speaks slowly. While Mabel has facial weakness, she is able to convey affect/attitude through her eyes and body posture. Mabel shows strength in the area of relations. She works with others toward a common goal. In the rehabilitation setting, Mabel establishes a rapport easily with others. This case illustrates the many factors associated with social participation.

While performance skills are important, the pattern of engagement in social activities provides direction for occupational therapy intervention. The practitioner determines whether the social activity is part of the client's established routine or role. Activities performed on a regular basis may become routine and part of the client's identity. Generally, clients wish to return to engaging in routines as they are conducted as part of one's role. Roles are "a set of behaviors that have some socially agreed upon function for which there is an accepted code of norms" [i.e., mother, father, student, and worker] (Christiansen & Baum, 1997, p. 603).

To distinguish between roles and routines, consider Gordon, a 78-year-old grandfather who enjoys walking. As part of his routine, he walks to the store for the paper each morning, converses with others, and returns home to report. This routine has become part of his social role within the community. Gordon would be distressed if he could not partake in this routine. Furthermore, as part of his grandfather role, Gordon frequently brings back "treats" for his grandchildren.

Clients may possess performance patterns that foster engagement in social participation (useful habits) or patterns of performance considered limitations (impoverished habits). Self-stimulating behaviors (e.g., head banging, hand biting) are considered dominating habits that interfere with social participation.

Habits and patterns may interfere with social participation as observed with Kenny, a 58-year-old client with traumatic brain injury, who hopes to return to "hanging out" with a group of work friends, but has trouble remembering to bathe or groom himself. His habits around hygiene are impoverished as he has no routine or pattern of performance. While Kenny has many useful habits (e.g., he takes public transportation), his impoverished pattern interferes with successful participation.

Once the practitioner has an understanding of the client's performance skills and patterns, further evaluation of the context in which the social interaction takes place is considered. The framework lists cultural, physical, social, temporal, personal, and virtual contexts as important to consider when developing occupation-based intervention. A description of how each context may be considered in terms of social participation is presented.

## Cultural

Cultures hold different expectations for social participation. The occupational therapy practitioner evaluates expectations for such things as proximity, eye contact, and physical contact (e.g., touch). Since the expectations of participation in social events vary among cultures and impact the goals for occupational therapy, it is the occupational therapy practitioner's responsibility to be aware of cultural complexities.

Occupational therapy practitioners must be aware that cultural differences are also observed within families. For example, Tonya expressed concern that her 3-year-old son with autism could not play with his cousin at family gatherings every Sunday. The occupational therapy practitioner realized the cultural value of this to the family and worked on play skills with the child, encouraging the mom to bring in his cousin on occasion. Being sensitive to the family's values enabled the practitioner to design client-centered intervention that made a difference to the child and family.

## Physical

The physical space in which the social interaction occurs becomes important when examining the activity demands on the client. Physical space includes the building, location, surroundings, objects, and setup of the event. Small intimate gatherings require different social skills than large public events. Activities that occur outside on uneven or hilly terrain may not be accessible to some clients. Background noise or certain smells may even be bothersome to some clients, especially elderly or children with olfactory sensitivity.

## Social

Everyone makes social mistakes varying from wearing the wrong clothes to saying the wrong thing. Social situations require different behaviors and may become the source of occupational therapy intervention. Social manners may need to be addressed to help clients engage in social events. Helping clients address others properly, make conversation, and participate in events with others are all part of occupational therapy intervention.

Other peoples' expectations affect the skills necessary to participate in social events. For example, the training and standards for success differ between formal and informal events and between familiar persons and strangers. Clients are expected to behave differently with peers or loved ones than in public settings. Social activities differ in the type and amount of personal disclosure required.

Therefore, occupational therapy practitioners analyze the social requirements to prepare clients for social outings, as in the case of Max, a 20-year-old with muscular dystrophy who freely (and inappropriately) discusses personal issues. Prior to the actual outing, the occupational therapy practitioner reviewed social expectations for attending the art museum and led clients in a role play activity to illustrate social behaviors appropriate for the art museum. Max and the occupational therapy practitioner developed a system to remind him when his behavior was not appropriate. After the outing, they discussed Max's performance to reinforce what he did well and to change what he did not.

## Personal

Social participation requirements may vary depending upon one's age, gender, or educational or socioeconomic status. Although the occupational therapy practitioner is not able to change personal context, this must be considered when designing intervention. Examples along the developmental continuum are offered to illuminate this aspect of social participation.

As commonly understood, adults interact and express differently than children. For example, occupational therapy practitioners working with clients with mental retardation may need to design "age-appropriate" activities. Thus, the occupational therapy practitioner does not give a rattle to a 12-year-old girl who still mouths objects as this is not considered socially appropriate. Developing social activities commensurate with educational level requires the practitioner consider the client's reading level. Socioeconomic status may include considering cost as a factor to certain social activities.

## Spiritual

The social nature of a spiritual event may influence the activity requirements. For example, persons must be reflective, quiet, and respectful when attending a spiritual event. Some spiritual events allow individuals to be festive and boisterous, but still reflective and respectful of others. Furthermore, many events hold meaning and may be deemed spiritual by the client, thereby changing the activity demands. The occupational therapy practitioner must be respectful of the meaning and spiritual aspects of activities.

## Virtual

Communication via computers may provide a social outlet for some clients, but they may require help navigating Internet sources. Occupational therapy practitioners may help clients understand the social expectations and guidelines to protect themselves while using Internet sources or communicating with unknown people.

## Temporal

The demands for social participation vary over the lifespan. Early social experiences with children involve their parents. As children gain experience and develop social and cognitive skills, parallel play develops, followed by cooperative play and games with rules. Children learn to negotiate and read others' cues early in their development (Bundy, 1997). Expectations for social behavior increase as school-aged children are expected to behave in socially appropriate manners.

Frequently, young children receiving occupational therapy services have difficulty playing with others. They may experience difficulty reading nonverbal cues or "framing" play situations (Bundy, 1997). Occupational therapy intervention may be designed to increase the child's ability through role playing, practice, and verbalization.

Children may exhibit other problems with social participation. For example, children may hug strangers and exhibit self-stimulating behaviors. Occupational therapy intervention may include techniques to eliminate these behaviors.

Social groups are important to adolescents who are beginning to develop their personal identity. Adolescent peer groups pressure the adolescent to conform to certain rules and expectations. For example, adolescents dress alike, use certain slang phrases, and collectively take up similar mannerisms. Adolescents may be working and, thus, have to show social skills for work. Adolescents need to learn to get along in groups, be heard, negotiate, stand up for themselves, and resist negative peer influences.

Occupational therapy practitioners work with adolescents who have experienced disease, trauma, or an event that has changed or interrupted their development (Llorens, 1976). In terms of social participation, adolescents may exhibit a host of difficulties including inappropriate affect, difficulty initiating or sustaining conversation, and difficulty with boundaries, articulation, or poor judgment. The occupational therapist's role is to close the gap (Llorens) and work on foundational social skills such as making eye contact, greeting people, and social manners. Activities may be structured to help the adolescent understand social rules prior to spending time in social settings. The occupational therapy practitioner may decide to include peers in activities.

Social participation related to work and relationships becomes important to adolescents and adults. Work relationships require different skills than intimate relationships. Adults are expected to take the lead and participate in community and family activities, each requiring social skills. Raising a family introduces situations that require the adult to model behaviors for children.

Finally, older adults often experience loss as they retire and lose work relationships. As the social activities provided through work decline, they may need to establish new social avenues. Some elders may experience a loss of a spouse or loved one, changing the social support to which they are accustomed.

Once the occupational therapist evaluates and develops the goals with clients and family members, the occupational therapist and occupational therapy assistant together design an intervention plan in collaboration with the client and family. The occupational therapist is responsible for the intervention plan, but the occupational therapy assistant may design the actual activities used and communicates with the occupational therapist as needed (AOTA, 1990, 1994). Both the occupational therapist and occupational therapy assistant are skilled at adapting and grading activities so that intervention involves the "just-right" challenge. The "just-right" challenge refers to activities that are not so difficult as to cause frustration nor so easy as to cause boredom and consequently are not therapeutic (Ayres, 1979). The occupational therapy practitioner regularly monitors the level of difficulty of the activity in relationship to the client's skills and abilities and makes adjustments as needed.

# Family, Community, Peer, or Friend

Social participation occurs with family, community, or peer/friends (Figures 19-1 through 19-3). The relationships of those involved in the social interactions change the activity demands. For example, clients are expected to behave differently in community settings (e.g., a public fair) than with family (e.g., at home). Clients exhibit closer displays of affection with significant others than with co-workers. Many social rules exist to describe the relationship boundaries and associated interactions. Thus, social training differs for community versus family activities. For example, family activities generally evoke deeper emotional responses and closer physical contact.

Socialization is an aspect of work settings and, thus, helping clients return to work may require remediation of social participation skills. Role playing, practice, and cognitive awareness of social behaviors appropriate for work may help a client return to work successfully.

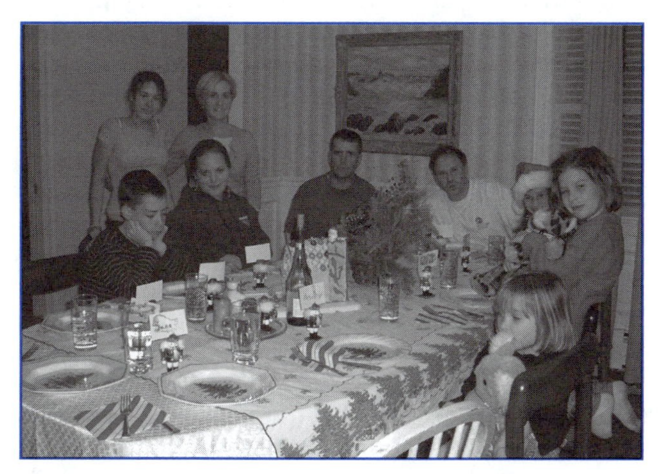

**Figure 19-1.** The O'Brien and Cohn families celebrate the holiday together.

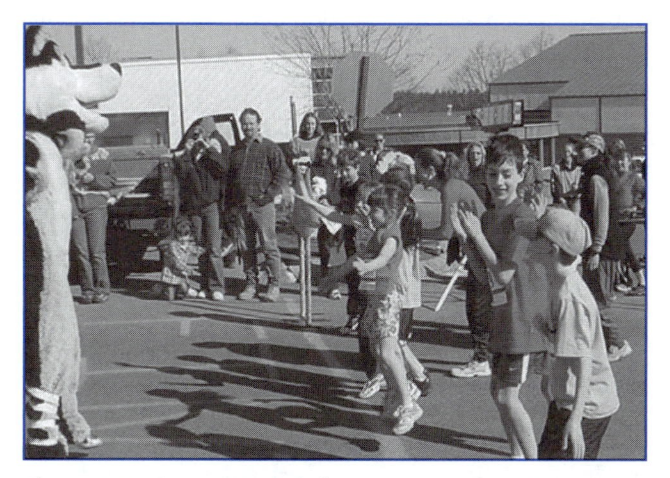

**Figure 19-2.** Scott gets ready for a community Fun Run.

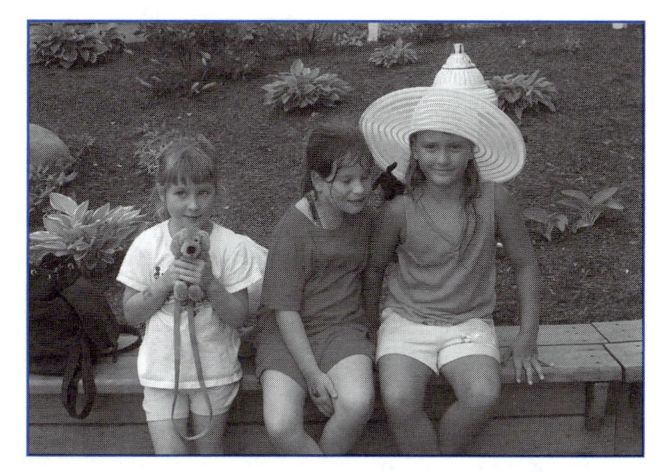

**Figure 19-3.** Molly, Alison, and Shelby enjoy a day trip to StoryLand.

# Development of Social Participation

## Preparatory

Clients may experience stress or discomfort prior to engaging in a social activity. Preparatory activities help clients get ready for the interaction and may include relaxation techniques, sensory-based activities, role-playing, or discussion. Breathing techniques, mental rehearsal, or reviewing the schedule of the events have been found to be helpful preparatory activities. For example, some children or adults may experience tactile defensiveness and dislike crowds, being touched, or even noises. The occupational therapy practitioner may work with the client on preparatory activities aimed at preparing the nervous system for the interaction. These preparatory activities may be used by the client on a regular basis after therapy to "calm" the system so that the client is not fearful.

## Purposeful Activity

When working on social participation, occupational therapy practitioners may help clients learn specific skills through engagement in purposeful activity. Purposeful activity is a goal-directed activity with an end product (Fisher, 1998). Typically, purposeful activity is used in intervention to target given client factors. See Table 19-1 for a description of client factors that may interfere with interactions. For example, the client may show poor interaction skills by sharing inappropriate personal information with strangers. Using purposeful activity, the occupational therapy practitioner may address this skill level through education, role playing, or discussion prior to actually having the client perform the social activity. Another example may be sharing craft supplies as one way to increase the ability to ask and communicate with others. Working on group projects may be purposeful and work on selected areas of social participation. Cooperating with others and playing a sport together are examples of how an occupational therapy practitioner may help clients improve their social participation skills. Clients may work in small groups on expressing frustration appropriately in hopes that this will transfer to the actual occupation in which the person engages. The client may work on eye contact, appropriate conversations, body language, and relating to others during many different group events. Frequently, the occupational therapy practitioner sets up scenarios for clients to role play so that they may practice the skills prior to the actual event.

## Occupation-Based Activity

Performing social activities in their actual context is the goal of occupational therapy. For example, helping children get along with others on the playground at the school or daycare they attend is the preferred activity. Working with siblings so they may play and socialize together at home is an occupation-based activity. In this scenario, the occupational therapy practitioner may encourage children to play games and facilitate socialization when the client is showing signs of stress or decreased ability. Taking clients to a public event such as the swimming pool and encouraging them to use socially appropriate behaviors is an occupation-based activity. The occupational therapy practitioner may deal with difficulties the client exhibits during the occupation through many techniques depending on the client and the frame of reference (refer to Chapter 15). For example, practitioners using a behavioral frame of reference reward clients for positive social behaviors (e.g., verbal cue, token, or smile). Clinicians using a cognitive-behavioral approach may help the client identify the behaviors that were positive during the occupation so that the client helps determine the solution.

# Consultation

Consulting requires clear communication and negotiation skills. Consulting is most frequently conducted by an occupational therapist. The occupational therapist may decide to serve as a consultant to improve social participation. In this case, the role of the occupational therapist is to help the client identify the problem, try some solutions, and alter them as necessary (AOTA, 2008). The occupational therapist does not do the activity with the client, but instead recommends activities to enhance the client's functioning. For example, the occupational therapist may suggest that an adolescent join Special Olympics. The child may require consultation from the occupational therapist to be successful in the desired sport. This consultation may require the occupational therapist visit the site and make suggestions to the coach, client, or family member.

Consultation for social participation may include identifying social groups that the client would enjoy and making specific recommendations to the client or family. The occupational therapist may serve as a consultant on an as-needed basis to help the client problem solve situations as they arise. When consulting, the occupational therapist is not directly responsible for the outcome (AOTA, 2008).

Consultation may occur to increase social behaviors of clients in group homes, schools, etc. The occupational therapist provides information on the client's abilities and disabilities along with suggestions to help the client be successful. Implementation is overseen by others and responsibilities for outcomes lie with the client.

# Education

Occupational therapy practitioners frequently educate others about occupations and the impact a disorder, disease, or trauma may have upon the client's functioning. Imparting knowledge or educating others about the occupation is part of the intervention process (AOTA, 2008). The occupational therapy practitioner may educate family members or caregivers on social expectations consistent with a client's diagnosis. Family members may need education on how to best approach and communicate with clients who do not use traditional methods (e.g., computer systems, communication boards). Family members, caregivers, or significant others may need education on the prognosis of the client to help develop realistic expectations (not to be confused with giving up hope). Frequently, occupational therapy practitioners teach others what to expect developmentally from the client, how to grade and adapt activities so the client is successful, how to make social situations successful for clients with all abilities and disabilities, the legal rights that will help the clients be more successful in their occupations (e.g., access, billing), and the possibilities for engagement in occupations.

Occupational therapy practitioners are resources to those with disabilities since they frequently know which programs adapt to clients with special needs. Other resources available to clients allow them to engage in social activities, such as transportation systems, adapted sailing programs, hippotherapy programs, or aquatic programs.

# Designing Intervention Using Frames of Reference

Understanding the theory and rationale for a specific frame of reference helps practitioners design intervention. Occupational therapy practitioners evaluate clients based upon the frame of reference and design goals that the frame of reference can address. For example, when providing intervention to improve the play skills of a child with developmental delays, occupational therapy practitioners frequently use the developmental frame of reference (Llorens, 1976). This frame of reference postulates that practice will improve the child's abilty (by improving neural synapses). Thus, the practitioner determines the level of play in which the child currently functions and addresses therapy at that level with the intent to grade the challenge slightly so the child can succeed and move to the next level. Using the intervention approaches (as outlined in the framework; AOTA, 2008) provides practitioners with strategies to address.

## Occupational Therapy Intervention Approaches

Overall occupational therapy intervention aimed to increase social participation has been reported to have positive results (Carter, et al., 2004; Gol & Jarus, 2005; Steultjens, Dekker, Bouter, Leemrijse, & van den Ende, 2005). However, more research is required to substantiate this claim using randomized controlled trials with larger samples and specific populations. See Table 19-2 for a review of studies specifically examining social participation in occupational therapy.

According to the framework, occupational therapy intervention consists of five approaches: create, establish, maintain, modify, prevent (AOTA, 2008). The following describes each approach and how occupational therapy practitioners apply the approach to enhance social participation:

- *Create, promote* (health promotion): This approach develops experiences for everyone, not just those with disability. Occupational therapy practitioners use this approach to create social experiences for all persons and promote healthy social activities. Examples are as varied as clients but include developing afterschool programs for children or creating social opportunities, such as a tea party or dance, appropriate to clients. An occupational therapy practitioner using this type of approach sets up the scenario under the premise that the clients have the abilities but need the opportunity. A practitioner working to improve play skills in a young child might add novelty to the play area (e.g., large boxes, new toys) or add play groups.
- *Establish, restore* (remediation, restoration): This intervention approach works on establishing abilities that have not developed or restoring those that may have been lost (AOTA, 2008). Developing a client's social skills through role playing and coaching techniques is one way to establish abilities. This approach requires restoring the underlying factors interfering with the occupation. Helping a client who has had a stroke interact with loved ones is an example of attempting to restore social skills. Many of the behavioral frames of reference work on establishing appropriate social skills through reinforcement methods. Clients are rewarded when their behavior meets the appropriate social standards. Motor control or biomechanical approaches work to increase physical skills that may be interfering with social participation. The developmental frame of reference postulates that practice helps children establish abilities.

**Table 19-2. Studies on Occupational Therapy Intervention and Social Participation**

| Author/year | Population | Measurement | Intervention | Results |
|---|---|---|---|---|
| Carter et al., 2004 | Children with Asperger Syndrome ages 8 to 15 (*n* = 12) | Lifestyle Performance Profile Interview | An afterschool program for children | Positive results per report from children and parents |
| Dumont, Gervais, Fougeyrollas, & Bertrand, 2005 | 53 adults with traumatic brain injury | Self-efficacy and social participation questionnaire | | Perceived self-efficacy explained 40% variance of social participation |
| Gol & Jarus, 2005 | Children with ADHD (*n* = 27) and without ADHD (*n* = 24) | Assessment of Motor Processing (AMPS) | Social skills training through meaningful occupations (e.g., art, games, cooking) in groups | AMPS for children with ADHD improved from first to second evaluation (*p* = .008). |
| Paul-Ward, Kielhofner, Braveman, & Levin, 2005 | Staff members (*n* = 21) and clients with AIDS (*n* = 16) | Focus groups | | Staff identified systematic and personal barriers; clients identified only systemic barriers as impacting participation |
| Steultjens et al., 2005 | 14 systematic reviews (4 reviewed stroke) | Systematic search for evidence | Comprehensive occupational therapy | Occupational therapy intervention improved social participation in clients with stroke |
| Thibodaux, 2005 | 2 years post spinal cord injury (*n* = 976) | Craig Handicap Assessment | | 83.6% reported involvement in recreation |

- *Maintain*: Occupational therapy practitioners may help clients keep the skills and abilities they currently possess so they do not decline in function. This type of approach may be readily used with deteriorating conditions in which maintaining function is difficult. In this case, the client is expected to keep the appropriate skills they have without losing function. Thus, the practitioner helps the client keep the social skills they currently have and develops strategies so the client may participate in social activities. For example, the occupational therapist may work with the client to continue attending a weekly yoga class. The occupational therapist may work to help the client communicate with others despite decreased functioning. Maintaining social networks may require educating others involved or helping the client overcome fears. The developmental frame of reference postulates that once a child gains a skill, he or she will not lose that skill. Therefore, the goal of the developmental approach is that the child maintain all established skills and build upon them.
- *Modify* (compensation, adaptation): This intervention approach requires the occupational therapy practitioner to make changes to the activity or the way in which the client performs the activity. In this case, the expectation is not that the client makes improvements in his or her abilities, but rather learns to perform the activity differently. Compensation is used to help clients engage in occupations without trying to change the degree of disability. Clients may need to compensate in social activities for poor verbal skills by using assistive technology. More subtle but equally important compensations may be required when a client experiences psychological difficulties interfering with social participation. For example, clients anxious in new social systems may be encouraged to seek out a familiar person with whom to attend social activities. The compensation strategy may be that the client only attends those functions for short periods of time, or the client is encouraged to participate in activities with a few familiar peers. For example, using the developmental frame of reference, the occupational therapy practitioner may have to change an activity to help a child be successful.
- *Prevent* (disability prevention): Some occupational therapy practitioners develop programs to help those who may be at risk for disability, such as programs targeting backpack awareness, healthy computing, childhood obesity, well elderly, work simplification, or fall prevention. The goal of this type of intervention is to prevent future impairments. Social participation programs such as Big Brother Big Sister, peer mentoring groups, day intervention, and adult recreational leagues are designed to increase socialization, friendships, and a sense of belonging. Structured groups provide resources to individuals. These groups may prevent anti-social behaviors or psychosocial disorders (e.g., depression and loneliness) caused by lack of social interactions. The occupational therapy practitioner may develop a specific group around preventing disability, or help a client participate in an existing group. Clients may be involved in book clubs, dance classes, school programs, craft classes, parenting classes, and exercise groups. Clients may form support groups with persons with similar diagnoses. These support groups provide resources and are a source of social participation. Therefore, they help the client meet his or her social needs and identify with others.

# Grading and Adapting Social Participation

Grading and adapting social participation first involves a thorough analysis of the social behaviors and expectations required of the activity. Table 19-3 provides a description of questions to ask when grading or adapting social participation activities. These areas can be modified to make the activity more or less challenging for the client. For example, the rules and expectations of the social activity may be formal or informal, flexible or inflexible, explicit or implicit. The social activity may be new versus old or active versus passive. Occupational therapy practitioners also consider the number of people involved in the activity and the relationships of group members. The diversity of group members and the content of the activity change the degree of difficulty.

The difficulty level may be changed by altering the group structures. For example, the task group requires members to complete a given activity. Clients work on individual goals toward the end product. This group requires interactions, but the occupational therapy practitioner is able to grade those interactions as needed. In a task group, the degree of sharing and negotiation required is more difficult when supplies are limited. Cooperative groups require clients interact closely toward a collective end goal. Therefore, cooperative groups require a great deal of interaction, communication, and negotiation.

Adapting and grading activities requires that the practitioner consider the client's strengths and weaknesses when deciding on the type of social activity and how to change the activity so the client will be successful. Generally, small task-oriented groups are the least stressful socially. Pairing clients with others who have similar issues may be helpful. Working one-to-one with the client to establish a rapport prior to a social event may prove useful. Discussing the social rules, boundaries, and consequences prior to the activity promotes success. Setting firm limits and helping clients work through and socially adapt to different situations is necessary prior to performing the actual occupation.

| Table 19-3. Factors to Consider When Grading and Adapting Social Participation Activities | |
|---|---|
| Size of group | |
| Location | • Familiar versus unfamiliar |
| Physical space | • Outdoors versus indoors<br>• Small versus large<br>• Quiet versus noisy<br>• Public versus private<br>• Formal versus informal |
| Purpose of the interactions | • Project<br>• Goals of group |
| Structure | • Expectations of others<br>• Roles<br>• Degree of investment required<br>• Time commitment |
| Behavioral expectations | • Eye contact<br>• Speaking requirements<br>• Dress<br>• Participation requirements |
| Novelty of experience | |
| Transportation | |
| Frequency of activity | |
| Client's goal for activity | |

# Summary

Humans are social beings and, as such, social participation is an important occupation for clients of all ages and abilities. Occupational therapy practitioners evaluate the social skills required, considering the contexts of the activity including the setting in which the activity occurs. Occupational therapy practitioners help prepare clients for the social interactions by providing them with many opportunities to practice the pre-requisite skills, consulting with them and team members, and educating clients on appropriate social behaviors. In this way, the goal of improved social participation can be reached.

# Student Self-Assessment

1. Describe the social behaviors required to participate in one social activity. Describe the context in which this activity takes place.
2. Change the context of the above-mentioned activity. Compare and contrast the differences.
3. Describe the social aspects of an activity using Table 19-3.
4. Make a list of social activities in which you participate. Describe the motor, processing, and communication/interaction factors involved in three of them.
5. Develop a notebook of social activities and resources for children, adolescents, adults, and elderly persons.
6. Summarize three research articles describing social participation in a given population.

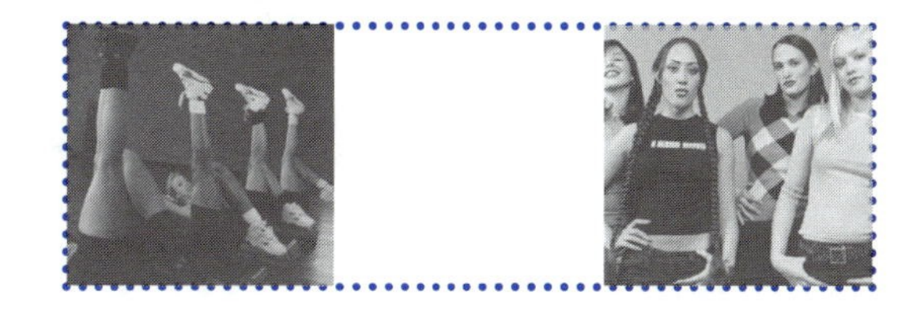

# References


American Occupational Therapy Association. (1990). Entry-level role delineation for registered occupational therapists (OTRs) and certified occupational therapy assistants (COTAs). *American Journal of Occupational Therapy, 44*(12), 1091-1102.

American Occupational Therapy Association. (1994). Guide for supervision of occupational therapy personnel. *American Journal of Occupation Therapy, 48*, 1045-1046.

American Occupational Therapy Association. (2008). Occupational therapy practice framework: Domain and process, second edition. *American Journal of Occupational Therapy, 62*, 625-683.

Ayres, A. J. (1979). *Sensory integration and the child.* Los Angeles, CA: Western Psychological Services.

Bundy, A. C. (1997). Play and playfulness: what to look for. In L. S. Parham & L. S. Fazio (Eds.), *Play in occupational therapy for children.* St. Louis, MO: Mosby.

Carter, C., Meckes, L., Pritchard, L., Swensen, S., Wittman, P. P., & Velde, B. (2004). The Friendship Club: An after-school program for children with Asperger syndrome. *Family and Community Health, 27*(2), 143-150.

Christiansen C., & Baum, C. (1997). Person-environment occupational performance: A conceptual model for practice. In C. Christiansen & C. Baum (Eds.), *Occupational therapy: Enabling function and well-being.* Thorfare, NJ: SLACK Incorporated.

Dumont, C., Gervais, M., Fougeyrollas, P., & Bertrand, R. (2005). Perceived self-efficacy is associated with social participation in adults with traumatic brain injury. *Canadian Journal of Occupational Therapy, 72*(4), 222-233.

Fisher, A. G. (1998). Uniting practice and theory in an occupational framework. 1998 Eleanor Clarke Slagle Lecture. *American Journal of Occupational Therapy, 52*(7), 509-521.

Fisher, A. G., & Kielhofner, G. (1995). Skill in occupational performance. In G. Kielhofner (Ed.), *A model of human occupation: Theory and application* (2nd ed., pp. 113-128). Philadelphia, PA: Lippincott Williams & Wilkins.

Gol, D., & Jarus, T. (2005). Effect of a social skills training group on everyday activities of children with attention-deficit-hyperactivity disorder. *Developmental Medicine & Child Neurology, 47*(8), 539-545.

Llorens, L. A. (1976). *Application of a developmental theory for health and rehabilitation.* Rockville, MD: AOTA Press.

Mosey, A. C. (1996). *Psychosocial components of occupational therapy.* Philadelphia, PA: Lippincott Williams & Wilkins.

Paul-Ward, A., Kielhofner, G., Braveman, B., & Levin, M. (2005). Resident and staff perceptions of barriers to independence and employment in supportive living settings for persons with AIDS. *American Journal of Occupational Therapy, 59*(5), 540-545.

Steultjens, E. M., Dekker, J., Bouter, L. M., Leemrijse, C. J., & van den Ende, C. H. (2005). Evidence of the efficacy of occupational therapy in different conditions: An overview of systematic reviews. *Clinical Rehabilitation, 19*(3), 247-254.

Thibodaux, L. R. (2005). Habitus and the embodiment of disability through lifestyle. *American Journal of Occupational Therapy, 59*(5), 507-515.

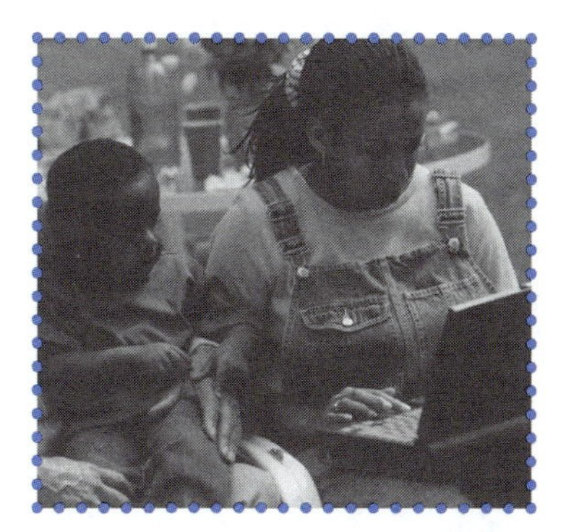

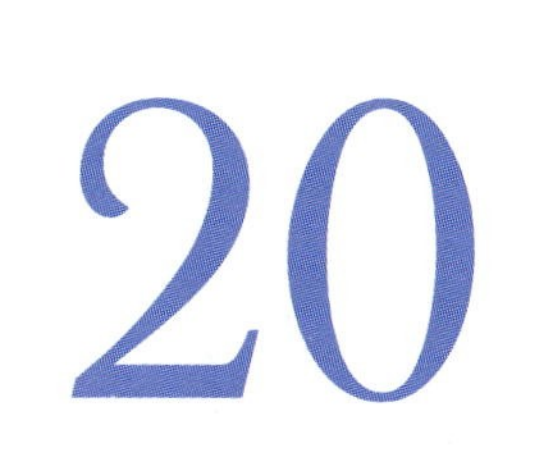

# 20

# TRAINING, EDUCATION, TEACHING, AND LEARNING

*Nancy MacRae, MS, OTR/L, FAOTA*

**ACOTE Standards Explored in This Chapter**

B.5.4, 5.16-5.17

**Key Terms**

| | |
|---|---|
| Backward chaining | Modeling |
| "Just right" challenge | Scaffolding |

## Introduction

Since occupational therapy's inception, teaching and learning have been crucial aspects of the profession. Education helps students at the occupational therapist or occupational therapy assistant level gain the necessary knowledge, skills, and ethics to become practitioners, and it keeps practicing clinicians current with new developments. Education also provides clients and their families with the knowledge they need to improve the quality of their lives. Consequently, it behooves the profession to know which components of teaching are required for an optimal learning experience to occur. This means knowing the principles of learning (particularly adult learning), relevant teaching and learning theories, varied learning styles, transfer of learning or training concepts, developmental stages of learning, how best to assess what has been learned, and how to imbue good techniques for learning and teaching in our varied encounters with students and clients. All of these will be addressed in this chapter with the intent of designing effective educational experiences for the client, family, significant others, colleagues, other health providers, and the public.

## Occupational Therapy Research on Teaching and Learning

Research articles providing evidence on teaching and learning are sparse, with most describing the use of evidence-based information and student-centered or experiential learning in the education or continuing education of occupational therapy practitioners (Bondoc, 2005; Stern, 2005; Tickle-Degnen, 2002). An evidence-based research chart can be found at the end of this chapter and includes relevant articles pertaining to topics covered. The use of evidence-based research coupled with the judicious decisions based on clinical experience and the individual being treated is touted as best practice. Although, the dearth of evidence-based articles specifically examining the teaching and learning process makes this a wish rather than a reality. Clearly this is a sign that the profession needs to generate more research on those components of our practice that are critical to our success and progress.



K. Sladyk, K. Jacobs, & N. MacRae (Eds.).
*Occupational Therapy Essentials for Clinical Competence* (pp. 217-228).

# Principles of Learning

To learn is to acquire information and understanding through experience or study. Learning is essential for all humans. Neuro and cognitive scientists declare that learning changes the physical structure of the brain, organizing and reorganizing the brain. There are different readiness levels in different parts of the brain (National Research Council, 2000). Knowing changes occur as a result of learning and learning depends on neurological readiness levels, it becomes especially important for learning exercises to be personally meaningful and functional and to be a concept that applies to students, clients, and their families.

## Readiness to Learn

First of all, a readiness for learning must be present. The student or client must see a need to learn what is being taught. Personal investment in the learning process will allow the best outcomes. The individual's systems, especially sensory systems, need to be functioning at an appropriate level so that information can be both received and processed (Ayres, 1973). The same applies to emotional or psychological readiness. If the client is still reeling from loss and the grieving process is strong, optimal learning may not be possible. If psychotropic drugs to diminish an individual's psychosis have not yet modulated that person's behavior, little learning is likely to occur. Areas of disability, such as memory and physical abilities, also need to be given careful scrutiny.

## Motivation to Learn

Motivation to learn additionally helps with grasping concepts. If the new learning is utilitarian, helps with the solving of a current problem, or contributes to helping others, it is more meaningful to the learner. Material needs to provide the "just right" challenge to the learner—it cannot be too difficult or it will be discouraging, and if it is too easy, it will be boring. When this "just right" challenge has been provided in therapy, it becomes apparent quickly and is one of the "a-ha!" gratifying moments for that person.

## Developmental Levels

Identifying the developmental level at which a student/client functions will help the teacher/therapist decide what to present and how to present it. This refers to both developmental progression in the case of children and developmental regression in the cases of adults with injuries to the brain or dementia. In education, it refers to both the life, including work experience, and the prior educational experiences of the individual. Clinically, this means the practitioner plans a session based on the developmental level of the client (i.e., for a child, the next step would be in the development of grasp; for the adult who has regressed due to nervous system insult, it would be a relearning of the skill, like using adaptive techniques to successfully accomplish the task).

## Context

The context in which such experiences occur also becomes important, as context can help or hinder the ability to transfer or extend what has been learned into a new context. The framework (American Occupational Therapy Association [AOTA], 2008) lists a number of contexts: cultural, physical, social, personal, spiritual, temporal, and virtual. Since transfer of knowledge provides the foundation upon which a professional develops or a client is made more likely to be safe at home, we need to understand what increases the likelihood of it occurring. Careful thought needs to go into the designing of a learning environment. A consideration of contexts helps with the appropriate design for a client or student. Learning environments need to be pleasant, comfortable surroundings. They need to be as authentic as possible, as posited by The Situated Learning Theory (Lave & Wagner, 1991). The environment or context can be stationary or dynamic; it can be rich in resources for a student, or it can be a quiet and structured surrounding for a person with attention difficulties. Determining which type of environment to strive for can impact the learning possibilities for the involved person.

## Focus of Learning

The focus of the learning can be learner centered, concentrating on the specific needs of the learner at that time or within the near future; it can be knowledge centered, highlighting what information students or clients need to know; or it can be assessment centered, providing opportunities for feedback, practice, and revision. Social and cultural components of a learning environment also need to be carefully considered. The amount and quality of learning can be helped or hindered by social support, depending on the individual's perception of the social factors. Cultural context can also support or negate learning. Environments can also be community centered, where connections to others (in a clinic during fieldwork, a classroom, or an actual community) are stressed (National Research Council, 2000). Collaborative goals and the freedom to safely err may be among the norms of such an environment and therefore foster learning in a safe place.

A fieldwork student will likely be exposed to all of these environments at different times during clinical experiences. Fieldwork provides students with the ability to practice and the freedom to safely make a mistake (Figure 20-1). Mistakes can be wonderful learning experiences, providing teachable moments if handled sensitively by supervisors, teachers, and therapists.

The focus of learning in environments include the following (National Research Council, 2000):

- Learner centered focuses on needs of learner
- Knowledge centered focuses on what learner needs to know

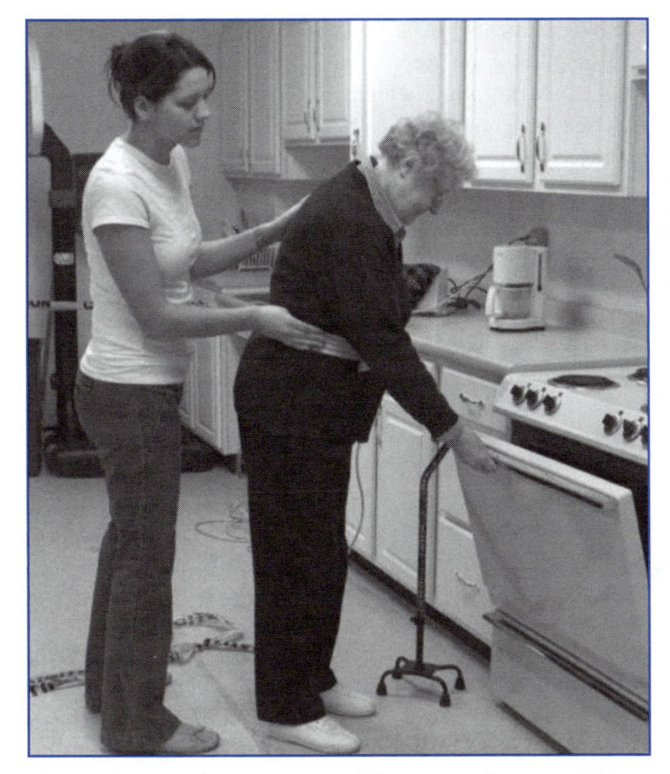

**Figure 20-1.** Erin, an occupational therapy student, provides assistance in the kitchen.

- Assessment centered focuses on provision of opportunities to practice, receive feedback, make revisions
- Community centered focuses on connections to others

## Dimensions of a Task

The dimensions of the task to be learned are also important considerations when designing a learning environment. A simple to complex direction needs to be taken into account, matching the level of readiness of a client with the difficulty of the task being presented. Whether the task is a novel one to be learned or an acquired task that needs to be relearned or refined is an important consideration. Dimensions that need to be considered include weight of an object, posture, distance from the object, repetitions, time it takes to perform and the usual time the task is done during the day or evening (temporal context considerations), softness or hardness, etc. Examples are progressing from grasping a larger but lighter object to a smaller but heavier one, or having a child use a marker, then progress to using a smaller-in-diameter pencil (Figure 20-2). How the task is presented and the preference of the individual's learning style must also be taken into account in devising an optimal learning situation.

Occupational therapists use scaffolding (Vygotsky, 1978) as a tool when teaching the breakdown of occupations and activities into hierarchical component parts (occupational

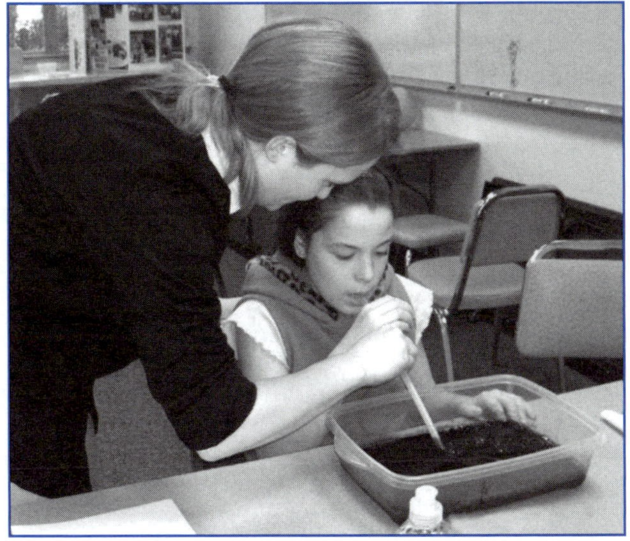

**Figure 20-2.** Another occupational therapy student helps with a fine motor activity.

analysis is an example), thus devising an organized and sequential way to teach. Each component builds on the foundation or platform of the earlier-learned component.

An example is that when students are learning medical terminology, memorization is necessary at first in the learning process. Once memorization is completed, the true test is being able to apply the learning to understand the use of the medical terminology in print. The final step would be being able to use that terminology in a documentation format. Thus, the scaffolding is the entire process, beginning with memorization and then ending with various forms of application (Figure 20-3).

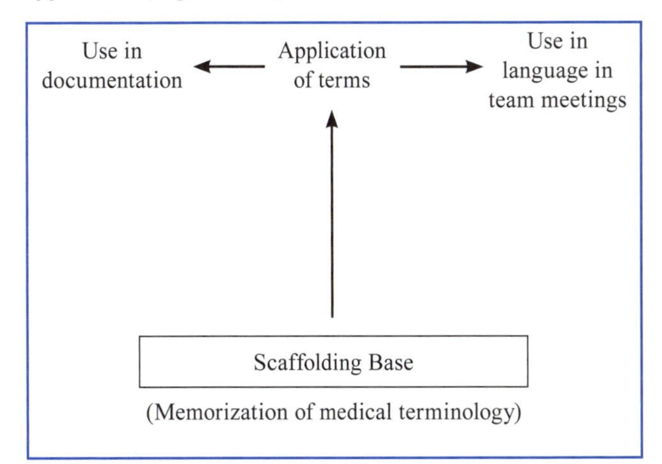


**Figure 20-3.** Table for scaffolding.

The use of this analysis can then be employed in a method such as backward chaining (Nannay, 1976), where one step—the final step—is taught first. With practice, the step that precedes the final step will be taught, and so on until the whole sequence is learned. Teaching a client with developmental disabilities how to independently wash hands is a clinical example, with the process beginning with the client hanging the towel used to dry his or her hands back up on the rack. The necessary steps for completing this task would look like the following:

- Hanging towel back up on rack
- Using towel to dry both sides of both hands
- Reaching for towel
- Turning off faucets
- Rinsing hands under water
- Soaping hands
- Grasping soap
- Reaching for soap
- Adjusting temperatures of water
- Turning on faucets
- Reaching for faucets

This process can ensure success and is vital for clients or students who are uncertain about their abilities.

# Transfer of Learning

Learning builds on previous knowledge. Some key characteristics of learning and transfer are as follows (National Research Council, 2000):

- Learning must have occurred to support transfer
- Abstract representations of knowledge can assist transfer
- Transfer is an active, dynamic process
- "All new learning involves transfer based on previous learning" (p. 53)

For learning to be effective, it must be accompanied with understanding, the learning must be accessible, and the learner needs metacognition or the ability to think about thinking skills (Lauder, Sharkey, & Booth, 2004). The social dimension also has an impact on transfer. A "community of practice" (Lauder et al.) is where groups and/or teams can become learning units, with the culture of the group having an influence on both learning and knowledge transfer. Cultural values, structure of groups and/or teams, and cooperation within them all interplay in a learning experience. Examples for students include learning within a problem-based learning group or learning specific techniques in class, being evaluated on performance of techniques in practical experience, and then completing the transfer to an actual client in a clinical setting. For a client, transfer of learning would occur when dressing strategies could be successfully implemented at home upon discharge. Using reflection on performance, a client thinking back about the quality of performance of a task can assist in focusing the client's attention on the next performance and, hopefully, improve the quality of the performance.

Requiring students to think about problems at a higher level of abstraction will again help, ensuring they understand the basic concepts inherent in what they are learning. Helping students become aware of their learning processes and to think about their thinking assists with their ability to actively monitor themselves and determine when more practice or knowledge is necessary. This holds true for clients and is part of the Motor Control Theory (Shumway-Cook & Woollacott, 2001) for motor learning since a client needs to know when actions are performed correctly or when they need adjustments to enhance motor learning.

# Importance of Time

Time must be allotted to allow learning to occur with complex material or a large amount of material, or when a client is learning something for the first time or relearning skills. This is especially true for those who are older (over 65 years of age). The necessary amount of time and pace of learning vary with each individual and are dependent on many of the topics that will be considered in this chapter, such as level of cognition, social support, environments, motivation to learn, and readiness to learn. Encouraging a generation of underlying concepts such as human development follows a proximal to distal progression and connections with what is being learned will cement the learning and facilitate transfer, but it takes time and practice.

Practicing new skills is required with the similarity of tasks in different environments necessary for successful transfer to occur. Generalization is a closely related skill and has to do with being able to transfer what has been learned to a similar task. Varying the situations and the tasks routinely can improve the abilities to both transfer and generalize.

# Practice Considerations

Practice reinforces learning. Practicing in a number of different contexts or ways will reinforce the learning and help with the transfer of knowledge. According to Williams (Solomon & O'Brien, 2006), there are a number of types of practice. Practice can occur with short intervals between sessions (massed), it can occur with longer rest intervals (distributed), or it can be presented with variability in both tasks and environmental contexts. Practice can also be done by engaging in the whole task (best when the task is simple) or by engaging in part of the task (best when the task is complex). Finally, there can be mental practice, where cognitive or mental rehearsal occurs prior to task completion. Mental practice (Solomon & O'Brien) helps prepare for performance and is frequently used by top-notch athletes to enhance their performances.

Types of practice include the following (Williams, 2006):

- *Massed*: When short intervals occur between practice sessions
- *Distributed*: When longer intervals occur between practice sessions

- *Variable*: When variety exists in both task and environment
- *Mental*: When cognitive rehearsal occurs prior to task completion

Practice can be enhanced with modeling and demonstration. It is best used in the early stages of learning (Figure 20-4) and can be given throughout practice as often as necessary.

Verbal instruction and cueing can also be used to help with learning. The verbal instruction can be simple words or more complex directions that provide critical cues, depending on the client and student needs (Williams, 2006). Physical prompting is another technique that may help a client initiate a task performance (e.g., touching a client's elbow to encourage the initiation of a motor task). Feedback regarding one's performance also enhances learning. Feedback can be formative or summative. Formative feedback or assessment occurs during the activity being learned and allows for change and correction to be made. Examples are feedback on performance given to a client periodically during a session or to a student on multiple drafts of a paper. Summative feedback occurs after the task is completed and gives a final judgment of the learning experience. An example would be a final grade for a course or the decision to discharge a client home.

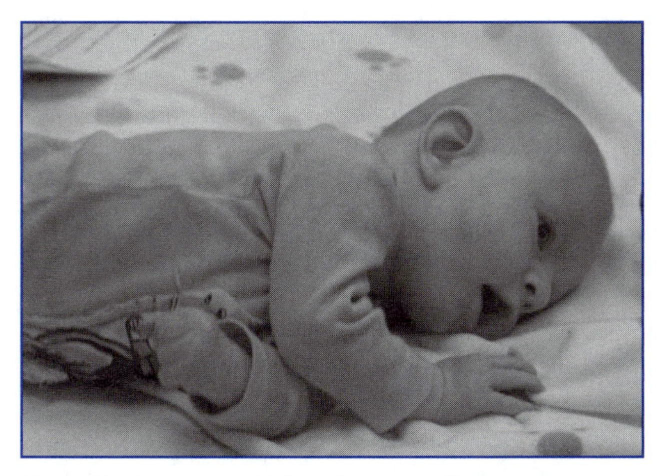

**Figure 20-4.** A young child turning over, with prompting.

## Adult Learning Principles

An awareness of adult learning principles factors into learning and teaching. Hallmarks of this approach are that adult learners have a need to know and are self-directed. They exhibit a readiness to learn, want to be involved in their learning, and are thus strongly internally motivated. They also want to immediately apply what they have learned, often to solve a problem that spawned their interest in learning. Adult learners bring a host of experiences with them, one of which is a unique orientation or a problem-centered approach to learning. They desire choices as to how they will learn and often what they will learn, and they assume responsibility for their learning. They want to voice what they already know based on their life experience and build on that. They value the experience of others, are willing to take risks, and are committed to lifelong learning (Cross, 1984; Knowles, 1980). These concepts also apply to adult clients who are the experts on their lives and who often know what they want but need help strategizing how to get there.

## Teaching

A teacher is one who instructs by imparting knowledge to a learner. As such, a teacher decides what is to be learned and when it is to be learned, and designs an appropriate environment in which the learning can occur. This is considered a pedagogical (the teaching of children) approach to teaching. Another viewpoint, andragogy (the teaching of adults), is that of a teacher being a facilitator and assisting as a guide with learning. In this format, the learner assumes more responsibility for the learning, often choosing what is to be learned. Adults, as nontraditional students, often flourish with this type of approach. The teacher and the student are both joint learners, each learning from and with one another. Another concept of an andragogical teacher is one who challenges the learner to progress to higher levels of personal development (Cross, 1984). The typical role of a therapist is to facilitate learning by clarifying the goal, designing appropriate learning environments, teaching strategies for acquiring learning, providing feedback, and structuring practice opportunities to enhance transfer (Trombly, 1995). In the provision of occupational therapy services, the practitioner may need to make use of both approaches and their varied concepts, depending on the client and the progress in therapy. A clinical example is structuring the environment at the beginning of therapy and, with progress, having the client choose which task to work on and self-structure the environment.

## Educational Theories

Education has a number of teaching and learning theories and embedded frames of reference that need to be understood to design the environment that will best meet the needs of the client or student. Block and Chandler (2005) identified three frames of reference often used in schools:

1. *Behaviorism*: Teachers/therapists design classroom structure and/or goals for students/clients
2. *Cognitivism*: Teachers/therapists encourage discovery within the classroom/clinic
3. *Constructionism*: Teachers/therapists facilitate with students/clients constructing their own meaning

Behaviorism grew out of stimulus-response, classical, and operant conditioning theories and promotes the teacher/therapist to design the structure of the classroom/clinic and the goals for students/clients. Cognitivists encourage discovery within a less-structured environment, while constructivists believe that learners construct their own meaning and thus create their own learning. A behaviorist approach may be used with clients who have problems controlling their behavior, such as clients recovering from brain injury or children with emotional problems. Students may need more of this approach as they begin to learn about the traits of a professional, with a lessening structure occurring as they progress in their learning. Graduate-level occupational therapy education, particularly after clinical experience, would encourage a constructionist approach, providing choices for focused learning goals and the opportunity to reflect upon and integrate the resultant learning. A clinical example would be that during the last stages of community re-integration, a client could be encouraged to choose on which area to focus and expected to recount areas of success or problems with implementation.

# Learning Styles

Learning styles differ for each individual and need to be considered when planning a learning experience. Individual preferences can be based on feeling, thinking, doing, or intuiting ways of learning. Kolb (1976) has labeled people with those preferred styles of learning as accommodators, divergers, convergers, and assimilators. Each style moves along a continuum from active experimentation to reflective observation. Accommodators prefer active experimentation or doing, while divergers prefer to learn via concrete examples. Convergers, on the other hand, prefer a combination of abstract conceptualization and active experimentation, while assimilators prefer reflective observation and abstract conceptualization for their learning. Beyond this distinction, some individuals may learn best through a visual mode, an auditory mode, or via kinesthetic techniques. An example of a visual mode is reinforcing learning by providing clients with visual cues (list of items found within cupboards) or students with paper copies that depict or summarize necessary information. Others may be stimulated with imaginative musings, such as poems, while others may use a reflection of an observed situation to gain learning. Many need to be actively involved in doing in order to learn. Learners typically proceed from a concrete to abstract learning in the course of their professional education (Katz & Heimann, 1991) with a master learner comfortable and successful in any learning environment (Sandmire & Boyce, 2003). Adapting a learning experience to accommodate to learning styles and preferences increases the likelihood of learning.

# Other Relevant Teaching/Learning Models

Other teaching/learning models used with adults include the following:

- Health belief model
- Attributions model
- Social cognitive theory
- Theory of reasoned action
- Situated learning theory
- Transtheoretical theory

Understanding these approaches helps the therapist/teacher discern at which level the client/student is in his or her thinking. These models used in combination have the greatest likelihood for success (Christiansen & Baum, 2005). A combination allows for such factors as motivation, attitude, self-efficacy, and social support to be addressed.

## Health Belief Model

The health belief model describes the client reacting to a perceived health threat, determining the benefits and barriers to making a change in the health behavior, and believing in self-efficacy (belief in ability to be successful with a task) to make the needed change. For example, receiving a diagnosis of diabetes faces the client with choices as to how to maintain and/or improve his or her health status. A belief in the ability to be successful with instituting healthy behaviors will allow for a more successful outcome.

## Attributions Model

The attributions model defines an attribution as a particular cause or source of a problem (Weiner, 1974). Attributions help a person make sense of the world. Since attributions are not always realistic, correcting them may be necessary to alter a person's focus and allow self-efficacy to develop. For example, a client may believe that success cannot be obtained in recovering from an addiction. Providing correct information about taking one day at a time (a new attribution) will strengthen the client's potential for small victories and ultimately, long-term success.

## Social Cognitive Theory

Social cognitive theory (Bandura, 1977) supports a belief in the interdependent relationship of behavior, person, and environment that is critical to our understanding of the person and the meaning of occupation in individuals' lives. It posits that learning occurs via observation of others' behavior, and perceptions of self-efficacy influence learning. For example, a student watching the behavior of a professional (occupational therapist) with clients and other colleagues influences how that student will behave in similar settings.

### Theory of Reasoned Action

The theory of reasoned action (Ajzen, 2002) links motivation and attitude with promoting health behavior, specifically when a change in behavior is linked to the attitudes of those admired by the person, as well as to the person's willingness to change. For example, a parent who successfully diets and exercises to reduce cholesterol levels may provoke similar changes in his or her children.

### Situated Learning Theory

The situated learning theory (Lave & Wagner, 1991) underscores the social dimension of learning and advocates for an authentic context to promote learning. For example, this type of learning would occur in clinical fieldwork at either Level I or Level II.

### Transtheoretical Theory

The transtheoretical theory (Prochaska et al., 1994) is about the readiness to change. It is a complex model of change that proffers five stages (precontemplation, contemplation, preparation, action, and maintenance) of change and encourages the educator to match the readiness stage of the client to what is being taught/learned. An example of this would be a person considering cessation of smoking.

## Perry's Work

Perry's (1968) work on the developmental levels of thinking, or the ability to make your own meaning, can also provide insight into learning. He classified making meaning into four different and developmental levels: dualism, multiplicity, contextual relativism, and commitment within relativism. A dualistic thinker views knowledge from a black/white perspective and wants to learn the correct answers and perform the task accurately. In other words, a dualistic thinker wants a recipe card. This type of thinker is challenged by ambiguity and uncertainty and wants and needs structure and concrete examples. The learner at the mutiplicity level is learning to think with support from evidence, sees peers as legitimate sources of knowledge, and values independent thought. The student desires evidence to support opinions and may balk at structure, while the client may ask for justification or proof that the approach being used is a valid one. Those within the contextual relativism level find all knowledge to be contextual, use metacognition, seek out many opinions, and look for connections. They insist upon choice and commitment and may seek help from an authority figure. Clinically, this is the client who may combine traditional therapy with complementary approaches. The commitment within relativism stage would be represented by the expert clinician who has made professional commitments. Clinically, it would be represented by a client who has committed to providing education and support to those clients with similar diagnoses (Table 20-1). Knowing at which Perry level students or clients are performing provides some of the information needed to design an appropriate learning environment. The new Level II fieldwork student will likely need the structure a dualistic thinker wants. At the end of the clinical experience, fieldwork educators hope that the student is thinking independently, functioning autonomously, and pursuing evidence prior to making a decision. With the start of a second Level II fieldwork experience, the student can be expected to regress (hopefully for only a short period of time) to a dualistic level, progressing more rapidly due to prior experience and transfer of learning to the next level or levels. Client expectations would be similar (i.e., the need for concrete, real examples and practice within a structured environment to support learning and transfer).

## Dynamic Process

Information processing emphasizes change as a continuing and dynamic process of learning. Input, throughput, and output affected by a feedback loop influence new learning. A dynamic system theory advances that changes occur over time, with the central nervous system being only one component of the cooperation of underlying systems necessary for motor learning to occur. Motor learning theory proposes that practice can lead to permanent change when trying to produce a skilled action (Shumway-Cook & Woollacott, 2001). Motor learning involves a process (perception-cognition-action) that experience and practice reinforce, is inferred from behavior, and results in permanent change in behavior. Clients are encouraged to have a "knowledge of performance" as they are doing a task, as well as a "knowledge of results" after they have completed the task. Knowledge of performance allows detection of errors and a performance change based on it, while knowledge of results encourages a reflection on the entire performance. Both types of knowledge equate with formative and summative feedback. Knowledge of results, or metacognitive thinking, can help them to achieve the desired results of skill. For example, metacognitive thinking uses thinking about or reflecting on what has happened to gain insight about performance. This can assist in improving future results.

## Therapeutic Relationship

Establishing a therapeutic relationship with a client is an integral part of the occupational therapy philosophy. Having a student or client feel respected and valued by a teacher/therapist facilitates an open environment in which genuine goals can be discussed and collaboratively formulated and where feedback can be meaningful. Formulation of goals and the ability to change one's performance are necessary for learning that is practical and able to be applied to occur.

| Table 20-1. Learning Characteristics Implied by Perry's Schema | | | | | | |
|---|---|---|---|---|---|---|
| **Student** | | | | **Client** | | |
| **Dualistic** | **Multiplicity** | **Contextual Relativism** | | **Dualistic** | **Multiplicity** | **Contextual Relativism** |
| Black/white; right/wrong | Explorer uncertain | Knowledge contextual | **Role of Knowledge** | Black/white; right/wrong | Explorer uncertain | Specific recommendations for unique situation (expert on own life) |
| Source of knowledge | Metacognition begins; questions authority | One source of expertise; mutual learning experience | **Teacher/ Therapist Role** | Seen as expert | Questions authority | Valued as one source of information |
| Do right | Support thinking with evidence | Metacognition used in various contexts | **Role of Student/ Client** | Performs correctly | Wants justification for therapy activities | Applies what he or she knows to various contexts (transfers) |
| No legitimacy | Legitimate source of knowledge | Process varied opinions | **Role of Peers/Family** | Not interested yet, too overwhelmed with own situation | Support groups prove helpful; talking with others with same diagnosis | Takes opinions of others and applies to specific situations |
| Uncertainty and ambiguity | Evidence | Choice, commitment | **Source of Challenge** | Future uncertainties | Number of possibilities, accepting responsibility | Making decisions regarding own situation |
| Hands-on structure; concrete examples | Balks at structure; looking for diversity | Intellectual mastery | **Source of support** | Structured learning environment with practice | Number of choices | Peers, therapist can be sought out for more specific information |

Adapted from MacRae, N. (1999). Supervision. In K. Jacobs & M. K. Logigian (Eds.), *Functions of a manager in occupational therapy* (3rd ed., pp. 63-79.). Thorofare, NJ: SLACK Incorporated.

# Novice/Expert Distinction

The mission of occupational therapy education is to educate entry-level practitioners. Understanding what differentiates an expert therapist from a novice (Mattingly & Fleming, 1994) helps discern the characteristics that set apart the expert's way of thinking. Experts have developed meaningful patterns of information they can rapidly and flexibly access. These patterns are based on a deep understanding of content material, which they can apply to various contexts—they know when, where, and why to use information. Experts' organization of extensive material, based on their broad experience, aids them in clinically reasoning with a speed and efficiency the novice does not possess. This ability to interpret and transfer meaningful knowledge or organized conceptual structures or schemas to novel situations is a wonderful aid in effective client intervention and outcomes. Experts recognize "big ideas" (National Research Council, 2000) and establish meaningful relationships around what they have learned, allowing for a quicker discovery of the problem and ignoring what is tangential and the applicability of the knowledge they have so efficiently stored. Finally, experts use metacognition to assess their knowledge and its areas of deficiency, and then teach themselves what they need to know. What becomes critical to improving the profession is the ability of these experts to transmit their knowledge to novices in both the classroom and clinical arenas. However, being an expert practitioner does not guarantee one can teach well.

# Designing a Learning Environment: Review of Considerations

Designing learning or training situations involves the consideration of a tremendous amount of information. A solid knowledge of educational theories, occupational therapy models of practice, and frames of reference provide the framework for the learning or training session. To be effective with helping a client or student learn, a practitioner/teacher needs to consider the characteristics that affect learning. These include the traits and learning style of the individual, the dimensions of learning required, the components of the task, and a careful consideration of the evidence-based content related to what you will be teaching and how you will be presenting the material. Critical to devising a plan is the involvement of the individual: what is it that the client/student wishes to learn, what are the specific goals of the session(s), and what are the learner's responsibilities? According to Bloom's taxonomy (1956), the type of knowledge to be pursued also needs to be considered. Is it cognitive, psychomotor, affective, or a combination of all three? Bloom's taxonomy places descriptive words in acquiring knowledge in a hierarchical structure to assist educators in designing learning environments that can be developmentally appropriate and then made more complex as learning deepens. An example is recognizing a concept such as spasticity. Recognition is at a lower level than understanding. Being able to demonstrate an understanding of that concept in intervention is a higher level of learning.

The "just right" challenge needs to be planned, with a quick ability to adapt it, as needed. Varied practice opportunities in a real or closely simulated environment also need to be of concern to assist with learning and the transfer of that learning. Feedback that will be meaningful to the client or student needs to be provided at optimal times to promote self-care, home management, and community and work integration. A clinical example would be providing specific feedback after the third practice session on adhering to safety precautions while making a hot lunch. Simultaneous self-evaluation of performance needs to be encouraged to aid the learner to detect problems as well as success.

## Flexibility

A plan is important, but just as important is the ability to be flexible and change "on the spot" to meet the dynamic needs of the situation. Careful planning with a number of available schemes help with flexibility. The ability to "reflect-in-action" (Schon, 1987) (to think about what you are doing at the time of doing) enhances the prospect for a successful learning experience and occurs more frequently with experience and practice. Table 20-2 is a checklist of such considerations.

## Assessment of Session

As important as good planning and implementation of a teaching and learning session is an assessment of the teaching and learning that occurred in the session. Such assessment is best done by both sides (i.e., the therapist and the client or the educator and the student). Questions that need to be addressed are: Were goals met? What was the quality of performance? How much more practice and variability are needed to guarantee transfer of learning? Gaining the client's perception of the session provides valuable information for future sessions and encourages self-reflection by the client. Pre- and post-test assessments such as degrees of flexion obtained or a tool such as the Canadian Occupational Performance Measure (Law et al., 1998), which has clients identify prioritized occupational performance goals and then rate their satisfaction in meeting better performance outcomes at the end of their therapy, also provide valuable information. When working with families

### Table 20-2. Checklist for Considerations for Learning

- ❐ Readiness to learn
- ❐ Motivation to learn
- ❐ Developmental level
    - ❐ Age
    - ❐ Regression
    - ❐ Perry's levels of thinking
- ❐ Abilities and disabilities
- ❐ "Just right" challenge
- ❐ Occupational analysis and task dimensions
- ❐ Focus of learning
    - ❐ Learner centered
    - ❐ Knowledge centered
    - ❐ Assessment centered
    - ❐ Community centered
- ❐ Context—include consideration of all listed in the framework
- ❐ Other relevant teaching/learning models
    - ❐ Social cognitive theory
    - ❐ Theory of reasoned action
    - ❐ Situated learning theory
    - ❐ Transtheoretical theory
    - ❐ Health belief model
    - ❐ Attributions model
- ❐ Learning styles
- ❐ Adult education principles
- ❐ Practice opportunities
    - ❐ Massed
    - ❐ Distributed
    - ❐ Variable
    - ❐ Mental
    - ❐ Modelling
    - ❐ Demonstration
    - ❐ Verbal and physical cueing
- ❐ Transfer of learning
- ❐ Educational theories
    - ❐ Behaviorism
    - ❐ Cognitivism
    - ❐ Constructionism
- ❐ Therapeutic relationship
- ❐ Novice/expert distinction
- ❐ Designing a learning environment
- ❐ Assessment and feedback

or significant others, time to absorb the material presented and time for questions become critical for carry-over at home. The same is true for students. They need to be able to consider carefully what has been discussed and pose any queries they may have. Taking such time can facilitate clients and their families and students grasping the critical concepts presented to improve the likelihood of appropriate application. The success of therapy and education hinges on a meaningful understanding of what is being taught and the ability to transfer that knowledge to situations when it is needed.

## Summary

This chapter has presented an overview of some of the important issues involved in teaching and learning. Occupational therapy practitioners need to be aware of these issues, understand them, and incorporate them into their clinical and educational interventions for clients, families, and students. Doing this allows for the development of optimal learning environments that foster successful learning and growth and are cornerstones for enhanced independence and understanding.

## Student Self-Assessment

1. Using the Checklist for Considerations for Learning (see Table 20-2), apply as many of the components as necessary to devise an appropriate learning environment for Sam. Justify your choice of learning components.

> Sam is a 25-year-old male who has sustained a C6 complete injury resulting from a diving accident in an unfamiliar lake. He is married with no children, and his relationship with his wife was strained premorbidly. He is a self-employed carpenter. He presents as a depressed man concerned about his ability to fulfill the roles of husband and provider and to stay alone in his home while his wife works.

2. Devise an optimal learning environment and teaching plan for a group of beginning occupational therapy students who need to understand how to prepare for their first interview with assigned elderly residents in a nursing home.
3. Describe how to best facilitate the transfer of learning for a cerebrovascular accident (CVA) client who has been working on making a light lunch in the clinic's kitchen.
4. Think of a client with whom you have worked. Based on this client's attributes, devise an intervention plan that incorporates appropriate practice and feedback techniques to facilitate the client's progress. Describe the techniques you will use and why you will use them.

## Electronic Resources

- What Works Clearinghouse—U.S. Department of Education: www.whatworks.ed.gov
- The Cochrane Collaboration: www.cochrane.org
- American Occupational Therapy Association: www.aota.org

**Evidence-Based Research Chart**

| Topic | Evidence |
|---|---|
| Continuing education for practitioners | Coldham, 2003; Grimshaw et al., 2001; Rappolt & Tassone, 2002 |
| Education of caregivers | Jarvis & Worth, 2005; Smith, Forster, & Young, 2004; Wilken & Isaacson, 2005 |
| Education of practitioners | Diekelmann, 2005; Gaudine, 2001; McCartney & Morin, 2005 |
| Evidence-based education | S. Bennett & J. Bennett, 2000; Bondoc, 2005; Covell, 2006; Ferguson & Day, 2005; Ross & Anderson, 2004; Slavin, 2004; Stern, 2005; Tickle-Degnen, 2000 |
| Evidence-based practice | Abreu & Chang, 2002; Chiu & Tickle-Degnen, 2002; Johnson, 2005; Tickle-Degnen, 2002 |
| Transfer of learning | Lauder et al., 2004 |

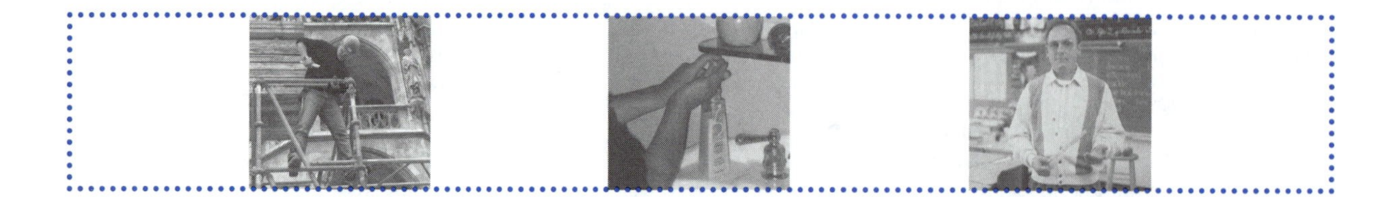

# References


Abreu, B. C., & Chang, P. F. (2002). Getting started in evidence-based practice. *OT Practice, 7*(18), CE1-CE8.

Ajzen, I. (2002). Perceived behavioral control, self-efficacy, locus of control, and the theory of planned behavior. *Journal of Applied Social Psychology, 32*(4), 665-683.

American Occupational Therapy Association. (2008). Occupational therapy practice framework: Domain and process, second edition. *American Journal of Occupational Therapy, 62*, 625-684.

Ayres, A. J. (1973). *Sensory integration and learning disorders*. Los Angeles, CA: Western Psychological Services.

Bandura, A. (1977). Self-efficacy: Toward a unifying theory of behavioral change. *Psychological Review, 84*, 191-215.

Bennett, S., & Bennett, J. W. (2000). The process of evidence-based practice in occupational therapy: Informing clinical decisions. *Australian Occupational Therapy Journal, 47*(4), 171-180.

Block, M., & Chandler, B. E. (2005). Understanding the challenge: Occupational therapy and our schools. *OT Practice, 10*(1), CI1-CE8.

Bloom, B. S. (1956). *Taxonomy of educational objectives in the classification of educational goals: Cognitive domain (handbook 1)*. New York, NY: McKay

Bondoc, S. (2005). Occupational therapy and evidence-based education. *Education Special Interest Section Quarterly, 15*(4), 1-4.

Chiu, T., & Tickle-Degnen, L. (2002). Learning from evidence: Service outcomes and client satisfaction with occupational therapy home-based services. *American Journal of Occupational Therapy, 56*(2), 217-220.

Christiansen, C. H., & Baum, C. M. (2005). *Occupational therapy: Performance, participation and well-being*. Thorofare, NJ: SLACK Incorporated.

Coldham, S. (2003). Educating the reflective practitioner: Graduates in practice. *Journal of Alternative and Complementary Medicine, 9*(5), 795-798.

Covell, C. L. (2006). BCLS certification of the nursing staff: An evidence-based approach. *Journal of Nursing Care Quality, 21*(1), 63-69.

Cross, P. K. (1984). *Adult learners: Increasing participation and facilitating learning*. San Francisco, CA: Jossey-Bass Publishers

Diekelmann, N. (2005). Keeping current: On persistently questioning our teaching practice. *Journal of Nursing Education, 44*(11), 485-488.

Ferguson, L., & Day, R. A. (2005). Evidence-based nursing education: Myth or reality. *Journal of Nursing Education, 44*(3), 107-115.

Gaudine, A. P. (2001). Demonstrating theory in practice: Examples of the McGill model of nursing. *Journal of Continuing Education in Nursing, 32*(2), 77-85.

Grimshaw, J. M., Shirran, L., Thomas, R., Mowatt, G., Fraser, C., Bero, L., et al. (2001). Changing provider behavior: An overview of systemic reviews of interventions. *Medical Care, 39*(8 suppl 2), II2- II45.

Jarvis, A., & Worth, A. (2005). Meeting carers' information needs. *Community Practitioner, 78*(9), 322-326.

Johnson, L. S. (2005). From knowledge transfer to knowledge translation: Applying research to practice. *OT Now*, 11-14.

Katz, N., & Herman, N. (1991). Learning styles of students and practitioners in five health professions. *Occupational Therapy Journal of Research, 11*, 238-244

Knowles, M. (1980). *The modern practice of adult education*. Chicago, IL: Follett Publishing.

Kolb, D. A. (1976). *Learning style inventory*. Boston, MA: McBer.

Lauder, W., Sharkey, S., & Booth, S. (2004). A case study of transfer of learning in a family health nursing course for students in remote and rural areas. *Nurse Education in Practice, 4*(1), 39-44.

Lave, J., & Wagner, E. (1991). *Situated learning: Legitimate peripheral participation*. Cambridge UK: Cambridge University Press.

Law, M., Baptiste, S., Carswell, A, McColl, M. A., Polatajko, H., & Pollock, N. (1998). *Canadian occupational performance measure* (3rd ed.). Thorofare, NJ: SLACK Incorporated.

MacRae, N. (1999). Supervision. In K. Jacobs & M. K. Logigian (Eds.), *Functions of a manager in occupational therapy* (3rd ed., pp. 63-79). Thorofare, NJ: SLACK Incorporated.

Mattingly, C., & Fleming, M. H. (1994). *Clinical reasoning: Forms of inquiry in a therapeutic practice*. Philadelphia, PA: F.A. Davis.

McCartney, P. R., & Morin, K. H. (2005). Where is the evidence for teaching methods used in nursing education? *MCN: American Journal of Maternal Child Nursing, 30*(6), 406-412.

Nannay, R. W. (1976) A comparison of forward chaining to backward chaining as an approach to teaching manipulative activities in industrial education. *Journal of Industrial Teacher Education, 13*(3), 56-62.

National Research Council. (2000). *How people learn: Brain, mind, experience and school, expanded edition*. Washington, DC: National Academy Press.

Perry, W. G. (1968). *Forms of intellectual and ethical development in the college years: A scheme*. New York, NY: Holt, Rinehart and Winston

Prochaska, J. O., Velicer, W. F., Rossi, J. S., Goldstein, M. G., Marcus, B. H., Rakowski, W., et al, (1994). Stages of change and decisional balance for 12 problem behaviors. *Health Psychology, 13*(1), 39-46.

Rappolt, S., & Tassone, M. (2002). How rehabilitation therapists gather, evaluate, and implement new knowledge. *Journal of Continuing Education in the Health Professions, 22*(3), 170-180.

Ross, E. C., & Anderson, E. Z. (2004). The evolution of a physical therapy research curriculum: Integrating evidence-based practice and clinical decision-making. *Journal of Physical Therapy Education, 18*(3), 52-57.

Sandmire, D. A., & Boyce, P. F. (2003). Pairing of opposite learning styles among allied health students: Effects on collaborative performance. *Journal of Allied Health, 33*(2), 156-163.

Schon, D. A. (1987). *Educating the reflective practitioner*. San Francisco, CA: Jossey-Bass.

Shumway-Cook, A., & Woollacott, M. J. (2001). *Motor control: Theory and practical applications* (2nd ed.). Philadelphia, PA: Lippincott Williams & Wilkins.

Slavin, M. D. (2004). Teaching evidence-based practice in physical therapy: Critical competencies and necessary conditions. *Journal of Physical Therapy Education, 18*(3), 4-11.

Smith, J., Forster, A., & Young, J. (2004). A randomized trial to evaluate an education programme for patients and carers after strokes. *Clinical Rehabilitation, 18*(7), 726-736.

Solomon, J. W., & O'Brien, J. C. (Eds.). (2005). *Pediatric skills for occupational therapy assistants* (2nd ed.). St. Louis, MO: Mosby Elsevier.

Stern, P. (2005). A holistic approach to teaching evidence-based practice. *American Journal of Occupational Therapy, 59*(2), 157-164.

Tickle-Degnen, L. (2000). Teaching evidence-based practice. *American Journal of Occupational Therapy, 54*(5), 559-560.

Tickle-Degnen, L. (2002). Client-centered practice, therapeutic relationship, and the use of research evidence. *American Journal of Occupational Therapy, 56*(4), 470-474.

Trombley, C. A. (1995). *Occupational therapy for physical dysfunction* (4th ed.). Baltimore, MD: Williams & Wilkins.

Vygotsky, L. S. (1978). *Mind in society*. Cambridge, MA: Harvard University Press.

Weiner, B. (1974). *Achievement motivation and attribution theory*. Morristown, NJ: General Learning Press.

Wilken, C. S., & Isaacson, M. (2005). Educating caregivers of geriatric rehabilitation consumers. *Topics in Geriatric Rehabilitation, 21*(4), 263-274.

Williams, H. G. (2005). Motor control: Fine motor skills. In J. W. Solomon & J. C. O'Brien (Eds.), *Pediatric skills for occupational therapy assistants* (2nd ed., pp. 461-480). St. Louis, MO: Mosby Elsevier.

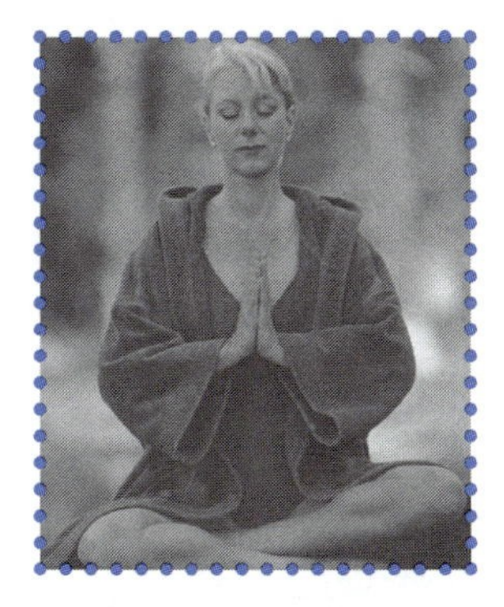

# 21

# Occupational Therapy Intervention in the Realms of Cognitive, Physical, and Sensory Functioning

*Regula H. Robnett, PhD, OTR/L*

**ACOTE Standard Explored in This Chapter**

B.5.5

**Key Terms**

| | |
|---|---|
| Executive skills | Kinesthesia |
| Ideational apraxia | Proprioception |
| Ideomotor apraxia | |

## Introduction

Occupational therapy practitioners work with people who have a variety of impairments. While these impairments are rarely seen in isolation, this chapter divides some of the major categories of impairments into separate sections to more clearly and succinctly explain each one at a fundamental level. However, in occupational therapy intervention, combinations of techniques are usually used simultaneously in addressing a number of occupational performance problem areas. This chapter gives an overview of occupational therapy interventions that focus on remediating or developing physical, cognitive, perceptual, sensory, neuromuscular, and behavioral skills or compensating for the absence or loss of skills in these realms. Each section provides a definition or overview of the specific area and then reviews some of the more common occupational therapy interventions currently in use. Evidence-based practice is included when it is available.

## Certified Occupational Therapy Assistants

Throughout this chapter, clinicians involved in the intervention process have been referred to as occupational therapy practitioners. This was done intentionally because the Accreditation Council for Occupational Therapy Education (ACOTE) standard upon which this chapter was based is exactly the same for both the registered occupational therapist and the certified occupational therapy assistant. Both carry out interventions using clinical reasoning, evidence-based practice (to the extent available), and occupational therapy principles. However, the title *occupational therapist* is used when referring to the practitioner with a professional role as an evaluator.



K. Sladyk, K. Jacobs, & N. MacRae (Eds.).
*Occupational Therapy Essentials for Clinical Competence* (pp. 229-244).

# Intervention Within the Occupational Therapy Practice Framework

The occupational therapy process, as described in the framework (American Occupational Therapy Association [AOTA], 2008), involves intervention planning, implementation, and follow-up review. Although intervention is the crux of the occupational therapy process, in order to be effective, it is imperative that the intervention phase be based on a comprehensive occupational therapy evaluation appropriate for the setting and the client. The process of intervention planning needs to incorporate a solid theoretical basis and relevant research to the extent these are available. The process, involving the practitioner working with one or more clients, includes the following types of intervention: creating or promoting, establishing or restoring, maintaining, modifying or preventing, establishing, remediating or developing, and compensating. The ultimate goal of occupational therapy intervention is "engagement in occupation" or successful participation in those areas of occupation that have personal meaning. Intervention techniques can follow a more functional and real-life, top-down approach, which includes engagement in occupational tasks as primary elements of each intervention session, or a bottom-up approach, in which therapeutic sessions focus more on the underlying client performance skills or factors. Performance skills include motor skills and process skills, whereas client factors include mental functions, sensory functions, neuromuscular and movement-related functions, and bodily functions (AOTA).

# Intervention Related to Cognitive Skills

In this chapter, cognition is considered foremost because occupational performance relies on at least a minimal level of cognition. Cognition includes all "mental activities associated with thinking, learning, and memory" (*Stedman's*, 1997, p. 174). All purposeful activity is regulated or supervised by one's brain. Therefore, cognition is the backdrop for all of the skill areas. In other words, adequate cognitive functioning is an essential, but not necessarily an adequate, underpinning for successful occupational performance. For example, even if a person has the cognitive skills to understand the motions and rules of a specific sport, he or she still may not have the physical performance capabilities to carry through these skilled motions in order to be a successful player.

Occupational therapy practitioners assess cognition in the realm of functional performance in clients of all ages and play a role in promoting optimal cognitive performance in the clients' chosen occupations. Assessment and client-centered goal setting are the keys to meaningful intervention, whether the intervention is based on enhancing or maintaining performance in those who are already doing well or whether intervention is for those who have impairments currently interfering with optimal performance. Based broadly on a statement put forth by the Commission on Practice (AOTA, 1999), occupational therapy services in the realm of cognition fall into the following broad categories:

- Remediation or development of cognitive skills and training in specific tasks
- Maintaining cognitive skills for those who are at risk of losing skills
- Compensating for decreased cognitive skills
- Education on cognitive performance in relation to safety, independent living, and/or life quality for the client and the family

The development of cognitive skills most often takes place in younger clients who have not attempted the task before, whereas remediation implies that the client was once able to do the task but now cannot due to impairments in brain functioning. Diagnoses and conditions related to cognitive dysfunction are extremely varied and may cause slight, moderate, or severe impairments.

Even the highest performing individuals cannot be expected to perform at an optimal cognitive level at all times. An important consideration for all populations is how cognitive performance can be enhanced by providing conditions and environments that promote optimal learning. Factors to consider include ensuring comfort level, body positioning for attention to task, an optimal amount of environmental stimulation, and physical condition (e.g., nutrition, level of fatigue, pain). The Quadraphonic Approach (Abreu, 1997) is a holistic cognitive rehabilitation approach that considers the client from both the macro and micro levels, and strongly emphasizes the contextual dimensions of intervention in order to ensure all of the influential factors on learning are included. The approach, which involves both retraining programs such as practice drills and compensatory programs such as memory aids, was designed specifically for those who exhibit cognitive dysfunction.

## Orientation

Remediation of cognitive performance generally focuses on improving one or more global or specific mental functions such as orientation, attention, memory, and visuospatial perception. Orientation training involves the repetition of basic orienting information answering pertinent questions about the client's life situation such as who, where, what, when, and how. Being able to improve orientation skills is based on the theoretical notion that repetition or practice will help the information stick, especially for those who are expected to make improvements, such as those who had a brain injury and are now in the midst of the healing process. Orientation is related to memory in that it involves remembering key information about aspects of one's life. In a study by Arkin (2000) using 30 biographical items, even those with Alzheimer's disease (AD) could improve in basic orientation skills when compared to a control group who had a similar amount of contact but no commensurate orientation training.

## Attention

Attention, in its various forms, is mediated by the reticular activating system in the brain. Attention is an important aspect of memory in that it is believed that one must be attending to environmental stimulation in order to remember the information. As might be expected, adequate attention is needed to complete many daily tasks, with more difficult tasks such as driving in an unfamiliar city requiring more focused attention, and automatic tasks such as teeth brushing requiring less. Attention process training (APT) is a common aspect of the cognitive neurorehabilitation techniques developed by Sohlberg and Mateer (2001) and is sometimes undertaken by occupational therapy practitioners. The system is based on practicing bottom-up cognitive exercises in order to hone in on improving one particular aspect of attention at a time. A number of studies have found APT to be effective in improving attention (e.g., all cited in Sohlberg & Mateer, 2001, p. 134). A Cochrane Database of Systematic Reviews, in an overview of two trials with 56 participants, found attention training following a stroke was generally effective (Lincoln, Majid, & Weyman, 2000). However, these studies did not find a correlation between improved attention on retraining exercises and improved functional performance in daily life tasks.

## Memory

Memory has many different facets, including remembering language, common knowledge, and events; how to do tasks; and to actually do set tasks at a specific time in the future. Not all aspects of memory are amenable to improvement and not all people are candidates for memory training. However, in some countries such as Switzerland, memory training is offered to adults of all ages through widespread continuing education courses. The courses focus on improving visual memory, using mnemonics effectively, teaching the method of loci, and increasing the level of attention to environmental stimulation (Scweizerische Verband der Gedaechtnistrainerinnen und-trainer, www.gedaechtnistraining.ch). Strong empirical evidence supporting the improvement of memory ability after memory practice drills is still lacking, and Sohlberg and Mateer (2001) suggested that if improvement does occur, it is more likely due to improvements in the foundational skill of attention.

## Executive Skills

Levy and Burns (2005) described cognition as based on a hierarchy in which the base is attention and the tip is executive functioning. Executive skills are defined as high-level cognitive skills that involve planning, problem solving, cognitive flexibility, and judgment/insight. Monitoring one's own behavior and adapting one's behavior to fit the current situation are also part of executive skills. These high-level skills develop during adolescence and are easily damaged in common brain injuries involving the frontal and prefrontal lobes. Also with brain diseases such as AD, the loss of ability in executive skills happens early in the disease process, while more basic skills are lost later (often in a reverse ontogenetic sequence) (Levy & Burns, 2005). A number of approaches for the management of executive dysfunction are detailed in Sohlberg and Mateer (2001). All involve repeated engagement in cognitive activities that challenge the person's level of thinking. Improvement is only expected to occur after rigorous and recurring practice.

## Metacognition

Another aspect of executive functioning is self-awareness, which AOTA (1999) refers to as metacognition. The awareness of one's self, including self-monitoring and being able to assess one's own strengths and weaknesses, is necessary for successful "functioning in any occupation" (p. 602). Metacognitive training is listed as a recommended occupational therapy intervention in the realm of cognition (AOTA). Fleming, Lucas, and Lightbody (2006) recently conducted a pilot study on four adult males with acquired brain injury (ABI) who demonstrated decreased self-awareness. They determined that an occupation-based program to improve awareness was effective in all four cases, but increased self-awareness was accompanied by increased anxiety across the board. This result highlights the necessity of considering psychosocial aspects of intervention along with the cognitive (and the physical) at all times.

## Evidence-Based Practice Findings

Carney et al. (1999) and Cicerone et al. (2000) completed detailed overviews of evidence-based practice in cognitive rehabilitation with follow-up recommendations for general clinical practice standards (strongly supported by empirical research), practice guidelines (a fair amount of support), or practice options (unclear level of support). Attention training attained the recommendation of practice guideline, although specific techniques for attention improvement were not outlined. Compensatory memory training was recommended as a practice standard for those with mild memory deficits. The study group also found the remediation of mild memory impairments to be effective but did not support the use of remediation techniques for those with severe memory impairments. Training in problem solving and executive functioning related to everyday tasks was recommended as a practice guideline. While both study groups (Cicerone et al.; Carney et al.) found strong evidence for the overall effectiveness of cognitive rehabilitation, Carney et al. mentioned the ethical dilemma that surfaces because those with impairments cannot be randomly assigned to a "no intervention" group. Therefore, studies usually compare one type of intervention to another, which can pose difficulties in determining true effects (versus the effect of general stimulation). Carney et al. also mentioned the common problem encountered in evidence-based research that more highly significant effects tend to be found in single case studies or in studies not as rigorously carried out (i.e., "as the strength of the evidence decreased, the effect increased" [p. 302]).

Cicerone, Mott, Azulay, and Friel (2004) concluded through a nonrandomized controlled intervention study that intensive, holistic cognitive rehabilitation was an effective form of rehabilitation, especially for community re-entry for those with traumatic brain injury, and an additional positive effect resulted when clients felt satisfied with their level of cognitive functioning. Cicerone et al. (2000) strongly recommended "comprehensive-holistic" (p. 1608) cognitive rehabilitation to be undertaken by a team of experts in the field. Occupational therapy practitioners certainly can be key players in this team of cognitive rehabilitation experts, especially with their level of expertise in wholly functional and individualized client-centered intervention.

## Maintaining Cognitive Performance

Maintaining cognitive performance can also be a goal of occupational therapy rehabilitation, especially for those with neurological conditions expected to worsen over the course of time. Diagnoses such as AD, Parkinson's disease, and Huntington's chorea are associated with cognitive decline. Therefore, maintaining cognitive performance could be the best hoped-for outcome for short-term intervention. Maintaining cognitive skills can involve all of the aforementioned intervention techniques, with the goal being the absence of decline rather than improvement in function. Yet even maintaining function can pose significant challenges. Nussbaum (2003) encouraged those who want to improve or maintain brain health into old age to actively engage the brain through lifestyle choices that encourage new learning. In his list of 10 behaviors to foster optimal brain health, he included healthy eating, not smoking, adequate physical activity, socializing, learning to relax, building strong ties to others, engaging in new and novel learning experiences, and finally, the occupational therapy practitioner's favorite: maintaining a role or purpose in life.

## Compensation for Decreased Cognition

When neither improvement nor maintenance of cognitive functioning is the anticipated outcome, therapeutic intervention adjusts its focus to the safe engagement in occupation in spite of persistent cognitive impairments. Compensation for decreased cognition puts the emphasis on changing the actions of others and the context rather than expecting a change in the self. For example, if one has decreased safety awareness, then supervision and/or a more constricted environment may be necessary. Certain complex cognitive activities such as driving are simply no longer appropriate, so other arrangements need to be made. Environments often may need to be more structured and simplified. Establishing routines to capitalize on the use of basic overlearned tasks can help those with significant cognitive deficits maintain activities of daily living (ADL) skills. Studies by Graff, Vernooij-Dassen, Hoefnagels, Dekker, and de Witte (2003) and, more recently, Hällgren and Kottorp (2005) have demonstrated the effectiveness of occupational therapy in improving ADL skills for those with cognitive impairments. Occupational therapy practitioners, through their keen observation skills, their use of functional cognitive assessments and activity analyses, and their ability to adapt the environment, are often instrumental in maintaining a person in the least restrictive living environment possible. For example, the simple act of disconnecting the stove or putting a safety bar in a strategic location may be what it takes to keep the home safe for the client.

## Cognitive Disabilities Model

A common occupational therapy approach used for those with cognitive impairments is the Cognitive Disabilities Model, which is based on Allen's early work (1985). In this approach, the expectation is not that occupational therapy will improve cognition, but rather that intervention will optimize current cognitive functioning through the use of environmental cues and adaptations. First, the practitioner must identify the level of functioning, possibly based on the Allen Cognitive Level Screening. The determined cognitive level (1 to 6, with specific modes) guides intervention so that the occupational therapy practitioner can capitalize on the person's cognitive strengths (Levy & Burns, 2005). For example, someone functioning at a level 4 can pay attention to visual cues and may need set-up and reminders to successfully complete daily tasks. People functioning at this level pose a safety risk because if a hazard is out of sight, they are not likely to attend to it. The occupational therapy practitioner can educate others about the needs of people functioning at different cognitive levels and can structure the environment for optimal task engagement.

# Intervention Related to Behavioral Skills

Behavioral impairments are not entirely different from cognitive impairments because neurological or cognitive deficits have behavioral manifestations. Behavioral intervention in the framework (AOTA, 2008) is extremely broad and focuses on changing behavior that is inadequate to support successful occupational engagement. Starting at one end of the age spectrum, an example might be a premature infant who has difficulty regulating environmental stimulation and thereby flails, cries, and becomes easily agitated. On the other end of the age spectrum, an elderly person with AD may have the same difficulty with similar behavioral manifestations. The elder with dementia might lash out and yell instead of cry, but in both cases, the person is not able to respond to the environment appropriately. In these examples, and in myriad other cases involving behavioral dysfunction, occupational therapy intervention can help regulate one's response to the environment.

## Sensory Integration

Occupational therapists rely on their knowledge of the evaluation of human performance and activity analysis to develop interventions that will assist people who need to make changes in their behavior. A common behavioral intervention in the field of pediatric occupational therapy is the use of sensory integration (SI) originated by the late Jean Ayres (1979). SI is based on the principle that children with sensory defensiveness cannot process sensory input from the environment adequately so they tend to respond in maladaptive ways. An occupational therapist using SI intervention principles designs individualized intervention programs based on the results of a thorough evaluation. One goal of intervention is to teach children with sensory defensiveness to regulate their own behavioral responses. The SI program may include a variety of means of self-regulated or self-determined sensory inputs such as suspension devices to provide vestibular input, an open environment in which children can easily move and jump around, and deep pressure to make it possible for children to focus their attention. Each child with SI dysfunction will need an individualized plan. The theory base is that by learning to manage one's own sensory environment, children with this disorder are then able to manage and respond appropriately to everyday sensory stimulation. In successful cases, their behavior no longer interferes with their occupational performance. In their 2003 statement, the Commission on Practice authors (Roley, Clark, Bissell, and Brayman) recognized SI as a frame of reference used in occupational therapy. While a great deal has been written about the theory of SI (e.g., Bundy, Lane, & Murray, 2002; Dunn, 2001; Kimball, 1993; all cited in Roley, Clark, Bissell, Brayman, & Commission on Practice) and the psychometric properties of the Sensory Integration and Praxis Tests (e.g., Mulligan, 1998, 2000, cited in Roley et al.), little empirical research has been conducted on the use of SI in children. Nonetheless, improved function in the realm of occupational performance is noted as a goal for SI intervention in the school system.

## Behavioral Management Strategies

Behavioral management strategies are often used for children with disruptive behaviors such as aggression, screaming, or self-injurious behaviors that may accompany autism, attention deficit disorder (with or without hyperactivity), as well as SI dysfunction. Once again, the empirical evidence demonstrating successful outcomes is scant, but anecdotal evidence and single-case studies are more abundant. Rosen and Scott (2003) described the behavioral management techniques that can be used with children with autism who appear to be less aware of others in the environment and more focused on their own needs. The occupational therapy practitioner can use the analysis and interpretation of ongoing behavior to formulate a plan. The goal is successful occupational engagement in learning activities and at home. Primary techniques include the consistent use of rewards for positive behaviors, redirection or natural consequences for negative behaviors, and environmental restructuring. Watling and Schwartz (2004) described the use of applied behavior analysis on children with developmental disabilities, specifically positive reinforcement, based on decades of research. Rosen and Scott wrote about the use of positive reinforcement, natural consequences, and redirection techniques with "Patty," a 9 year old with severe self-destructive tendencies. The behavior management strategies allowed "Patty" to have some choice in selecting tasks, which were introduced slowly with the initial expectation being that she would engage in the task only briefly. The occupational therapy practitioner used edible reinforcements and picture symbol communication since "Patty" was initially unable to clearly verbalize her needs. Through a rearrangement of the environment to decrease the level of compulsory stimulation to which "Patty" was exposed and by providing deep sensory input (e.g., joint compression, bear hugs, and deep massage), occupational therapy intervention was able to help "Patty" relate to her environment more effectively and to tolerate being in a classroom setting without resorting to maladaptive behaviors.

Making behavioral changes in life is a goal of many adults as well. Often, these changes are focused on habits that no longer are, or never were, productive or healthy. For example, a few of the common behavioral changes sought by people relate to improving diet, exercising, and giving up unhealthy habits such as smoking or substance abuse. Occupational therapy practitioners can be helpful in moving people through the stages of change, by helping people determine reasonable goals, and by breaking down these goals into more distinct and achievable steps or objectives. Based on the Transtheoretical Model of Behavior Change (Prochaska & Velicer, 1997) there are five phases of behavioral change:

1. Precontemplation
2. Contemplation
3. Preparation
4. Action
5. Maintenance

The role of the occupational therapy practitioner is to move the person from one stage to the next, always closer to the ultimate goal of an improved and healthier lifestyle. For example, in the precontemplation phase when the person is not yet thinking about making a change in lifestyle, the occupational therapy practitioner can assist the person in making a list of the benefits and drawbacks of a new behavior, such as adopting a diabetic diet for someone with diabetes. Just by acknowledging there are pros and cons of making a change, the person is beginning to move into the contemplation phase in which the person acknowledges that the current diet or any dissatisfactory situation is not promoting optimal health.

# Intervention Related to Physical Performance

Typical physical performance, which cannot free itself of the supervisory control exerted by the brain, relies on intact neurological connections within the brain that control the movement in question and proceed to the body part under consideration. The brain provides the control center for motor performance, but the person also needs intact musculature in order to move and to complete manipulation tasks. The aspects of physical performance of primary concern in occupational therapy intervention at the impairment level are range of motion (ROM), strength, balance, coordination, and functional mobility. Occupational tasks generally require at least minimal levels of ability in these client factors. A task analysis, completed by an occupational therapy practitioner, can determine the specific physical demands of any task under consideration. Ideally, the practitioner can then assist the person by adapting the task or the environment if the task currently exceeds the capabilities of the client. The physical factors mentioned are applicable for all age groups, but not all people need to be equally capable in all areas to be successful and to feel fulfilled occupationally. For example, lumberjacks need to have excellent strength and gross motor coordination in order to be successful at their chosen job. On the other hand, a computer programmer is likely to need less upper body ROM and strength, though intact fine motor coordination is a prerequisite for using a computer the way it is normally used. Fortunately, technology has advanced to the point that much of the programmer's job can be done without the stated prerequisites if necessary (e.g., through voice activation or head pointing devices).

The occupational therapy process for those with physical disabilities is much like the process for those with cognitive disabilities. An evaluation is followed by mutual goal setting, and intervention then takes place to move the client toward the agreed-upon meaningful occupational goals. The process may involve remediation to improve physical performance in one or more of the areas listed, compensation, or a combination of both, always depending on the needs of the client. A crucial element of any intervention plan also involves client and/or family education related to safe and effective occupational performance. Although this section focuses on the physical aspects of intervention, it should be noted that simple physical outcome goals such as improved strength, ROM, and balance are never sufficient; occupational therapy must always include functional aspects of goals following upon the heels of improved physical performance. For example, in occupational therapy, a client may work on improving ROM, but the ultimate goal is improved ability in ADL or home management skills.

Occupational therapy is often involved in providing physical performance interventions in both individual and group settings. These interventions may be component- or client factor-based such as an upper extremity exercise group, balance training, or motor control practice, or sessions may use more purposeful activity such as engagement in meaningful daily tasks. The preferred method is to strive toward occupation. However, since the areas of occupation that include physical aspects are covered in other chapters, intervention at the physical client-factor level is addressed briefly here.

## Range of Motion

As learned through the study of kinesiology, every joint in the human body has a normal or usual ROM. If the joint is compromised in some way through injury, disease, or disuse and performance on life tasks is compromised, then ROM needs to be addressed as a part of therapeutic intervention. Depending on the cause of the decrease, it may be appropriate to attempt to improve joint mobility through ROM exercises, joint mobilization, and stretching. When exercises are used in occupational therapy, the use of active ROM is preferred to passive ROM whenever possible, but if the client is in a coma, for example, active ROM on command is obviously not an option. However, engaging the client in a ROM program is still necessary to avoid contractures of the joints due to immobilization as well as to provide the person with some degree of normal proprioceptive input, which may enhance personal awareness of the body and the environment. After a stroke, if clients cannot actively move their hemiparetic side, they may benefit from learning how to complete a self-ROM exercise program. Pain must always be a consideration in treating ROM deficits, especially when completing passive- or active-assisted ROM for the client. Assisting clients in ROM can be beneficial to promote normal movement patterns as well as to increase available ROM. When ROM is less than full due to weakness (rather than joint obstruction), then the occupational therapy practitioner may work on increasing ROM through the use of gravity-assisted or gravity-neutral positions, which require a lower level of limb strength. Stretching can increase ROM at a joint beyond the current level, but it must be undertaken with caution. It is contraindicated for inflamed joints as well as in those with recent fractures or surgery (Brody, 2005). A low-resistance stretch of longer duration is preferred to repeated quick, bouncing stretches (Breines, 2006). Relaxation techniques may enhance the person's ability to stretch beyond existing ROM (Brody, 2005).

## Strength

Strength is integrally linked to ROM. When ROM is compromised, strength is generally impaired as well. Strength is the "degree of muscle power when movement is resisted as with objects or gravity" (*Stedman's*, 1997, p. 832) and "is the result of complex interactions of neurologic, biomechanical, and cognitive systems" (Hall & Brody, 2005, p. 58). The human body has over 430 voluntary muscles. For these to be considered "normal," people need to be able to move their limbs through full ROM and be able to withstand the application of a maximal amount of resistance. Before being able to lift additional weight beyond the weight of the limb or before being able to resist outside pressure, the limb must be able to move through full ROM (unless ROM is compromised by a joint obstruction). Decreased strength, like decreased ROM, can be caused by disuse, injury, or disease. While average muscle strength does tend to decline with age, an active, well elder who works diligently at strength training easily may be able to outperform a sedentary teen or young adult.

When the muscles are too weak to move the limb properly, the person may "substitute" other muscles to try and get the job done. This is not the optimal way to move unless it is necessary due to permanent deficits following a complete spinal cord injury, for instance. To increase the strength of a muscle, it needs to repeatedly contract at near maximal capacity. Different types of contractions are used in an exercise program, including isotonic, which takes place when a muscle contracts or shortens "against a constant load" such as when a weight is lifted against gravity (*Stedman's*, 1997, p. 457), and isometric, which involves holding a muscle contraction at an increased tension point in the muscle. An example of isometric contraction would be trying to push a car out of a mud or snow bank if the car is stuck and does not budge. Exercise groups or individual exercise sessions in occupational therapy often use repeated isotonic contractions with weights and resistance bands. While muscles do need to fatigue to gain strength, overfatiguing muscles can cause more harm than good. Using common sense is usually the best overall plan.

Once again, to promote symmetrical and effective movement, the practitioner should continually monitor the level of pain and proper body mechanics. Also, if people can build muscle strength through engagement in activities they find especially interesting such as sports, hobbies, or games, they will certainly enjoy the process more than involvement in a rote exercise program. This contention is supported by research such as the Nelson et al. study (1999), which found that the group involved in an occupationally based exercise program significantly outperformed a rote exercise group in a randomized control trial of 26 clients who had had a stroke. In an interesting aside to usual exercise training, one study compared a program of exercises including a virtual reality bicycle exercise with a control program just involving the physical exercises. Grealy, Johnson, and Rushton (1999) found the addition of virtual reality exercise was associated not only with more significantly improved strength but also with enhanced reaction times and cognitive performance. This finding highlights, once again, the interconnectedness of the physical and the cognitive client factors.

Strength training has been shown to decrease heart rate, normalize blood pressure, increase cardiac output, and it may lower bad cholesterol levels (Hall & Brody, 2005). Proper diaphragmatic breathing techniques should be incorporated into all strength and ROM exercise programs. Not breathing deeply enough or holding one's breath can even be dangerous, especially for those with compromised cardiac systems. Resistance training for healthy adults is recommended by the American Heart Association, the American College of Sports Medicine, and the Surgeon General's 1996 report (as cited in Feigenbaum, 2001). The exercise program should be rhythmical, performed at a slow-to-moderate rate of speed, completed at minimum level 2 or 3 days per week, and include 8 to 10 exercises with 1 to 2 sets of 8 to 15 repetitions. Although discomfort can be acceptable if tolerated, a high level of pain should be avoided, especially if the movement causes the level of pain to escalate.

The sources mentioned above also recommended strength training for populations who have physical impairments, although the program would be expected to start at a lower intensity level and the progression would be expected to be slower (Figure 21-1). Feigenbaum recommended a slow and temperate start in order to avoid an over-ambitious beginning with a subsequent high dropout rate. Progression to a higher level of resistance should occur every 1 to 2 weeks if possible when the person can lift the current weight comfortably a dozen times but still perceives the intensity to be hard. These guidelines apply to all adult age groups. Sedentary elders, however, may need to start with weights of 1 kilo or even less, take more care in stabilizing at the hip, and may do better on machines not requiring the exerciser to have normal postural control (Feigenbaum). Few guidelines for specific client populations are available, highlighting once again the need for further empirical research. Interesting, creative, and occupationally based research projects would involve comparing rote ROM and strength training to the use of repetitive functional tasks such as sports, hobbies, or home management skills.

## Endurance

Endurance as a physical component of occupational therapy intervention is included here only as an adjunct to the other physical aspects of intervention. Decreased endurance manifests itself as an inability to carry through repetitive motions or sustained resistance over time. It results in a decreased ability to complete daily tasks because the person lacks energy. Clients are not likely to be referred to occupational therapy intervention for impaired endurance alone. However, decreased strength is often coupled with lowered endurance. Each muscle contraction of a weakened

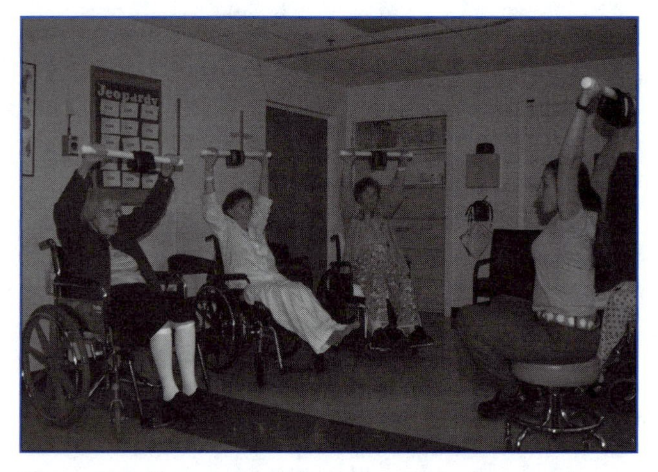

**Figure 21-1.** Those in rehabiliation hospitals often partake in upper extremity exercise group to help regain strength. Coutesy of New England Rehabilitaion Hopital Portland.

muscle uses a larger proportion of the overall performance capacity, resulting in the muscle fatiguing more quickly. When aiming to build muscle strength, a high-load regimen with a lower number of repetitions is preferred, but when the focus is on building endurance, a lower amount of resistance or weight over a greater number of repetitions has been determined to be more effective (Breines, 2006).

## Balance/Postural Control

Intact balance or postural control is a prerequisite for safe, ambulatory, functional mobility. Since many of our daily occupations involve ambulating or moving from one place to another, postural control is an important consideration for the occupational therapy practitioner. This is especially true for practitioners working with those who have sustained strokes, head injuries, or diagnoses associated with impaired balance such as multiple sclerosis or cerebral palsy. According to Peterson and Clemson (2008), occupational therapy practitioners are well suited to working with elders on fall prevention and rehabilitation due to our in-depth understanding of physical functioning and the contextual and intrinsic factors impacting balance, as well as our ability to implement multifactorial, evidence-based interventions.

Falls are common among the elderly, with about 1 out of 3 community living elders falling annually (Gillespie et al., 2003). One direct cause of falls is decreased postural control. Balance training can occur in groups, on an individual basis by providing balance exercises and education, or through occupational therapy-related interventions such as virtual reality or Tai Chi courses. Gillespie et al., in their systematic review, concluded that fall prevention interventions are often effective. A number of studies have now been completed on Tai Chi as an intervention to improve balance and strength with overall positive results (e.g., Han et al., 2004; Li et al., 2005; Taylor-Piliae, Haskell, Stotts, & Froehlicher, 2006). Hsieh, Nelson, Smith, and Peterson (1996), in an occupation-based study, found that small groups of stroke survivors who participated in real or simulated functional activities in addition to rote exercise had better outcomes related to dynamic standing balance.

A more general community-based course intended to improve balance is "Stepping On," a 7-week program offered for people 70 and over in Australia. Clemson et al. (2004) reported that the "Stepping On" program resulted in a 31% reduction in falls ($p = 0.025$), and that the program was particularly effective for men. A "Matter of Balance," designed by rehabilitation scientists at Boston University, is a similar 8-week program that uses volunteer instructors with occupational therapy and physical therapy consultants or visiting instructors.

In a systematic review of 19 randomized control trials of interventions to decrease fear of falling, Zijlstra et al. (2007) found overwhelming support for the effectiveness of interventions (including Tai Chi, "Matter of Balance," "Stepping On," and other multifactorial balance programs). Along with a decreased fear of falling, Zijlstra and colleagues also recommended looking at functional outcomes for balance programs (e.g., decreased incidence of falling and increased safe engagement in meaningful activities).

Besides remediating balance through the interventions mentioned, occupational therapy practitioners play a significant role in ensuring safety by helping the client to compensate when balance is impaired. Compensatory safety measures can involve removing clutter from the home and improving organization in the living space. Adaptive equipment such as safety bars, bath seats, and long-handled dustpans can facilitate successful occupational performance in the client's customary daily tasks. Education on fall prevention is a crucial component of occupational therapy in this realm as well. For example, if elders understand the factors impacting balance and the ways to make the environment safer, they are more likely to feel a higher degree of efficacy related to balance and to complete mobility tasks with more awareness of proper body mechanics.

# Intervention Related to Neuromuscular Disorders

Neuromuscular disorders are a combination of cognitive and physical impairments, often with accompanying sensory dysfunction. This discussion will focus on motor control, which encompasses coordination and movement in general. According to Shumway-Cook and Woollacott (2001), motor control is "the ability to regulate or direct the mechanisms essential to movement" (p. 1). Movement is the result of neuromuscular interactions involving sensory input to the brain. The central nervous system organizes and interprets this input then directs subsequent physical actions. When functioning at an adequate level, motor control allows the person to complete essential and optional daily tasks. Intact perceptual and cognitive processes are necessary for the enactment of purposeful and efficient movement. For example, tossing and catching a ball, feeding one's self, and writing numbers and letters all represent skills that require a high degree of coordination or motor control. An interested reader should be aware that there are several theories of motor control (systems, motor programming, hierarchical, dynamical action, and ecological) and that entire textbooks have been written about this subject. Shumway-Cook and Woollacott provide a comprehensive resource for those seeking more detail.

## Motor Control

Although motor control covers the entire life span, the focus for occupational therapy practitioners using motor control models of intervention is on initial motor learning in the young and in relearning movement patterns in adults, specifically those with a diagnosis or condition that impairs normal movement. Cerebral palsy and developmental coordination disorder are two common diagnoses causing movement impairments in children, whereas cerebrovascular accident (CVA or stroke), multiple sclerosis, and Parkinson's disease are common diagnoses interfering with normal movement in those who are older. The ultimate goal of the intervention is to improve occupational performance through the use of the most effective movement patterns possible. While evidence-based practice exists within this realm, it is lacking in its scope. Much has been written in occupational therapy and physical therapy literature about different aspects of motor control intervention, including assessment of motor control, types of learning, types of practice, practice schedules, instructions, and the parameters surrounding feedback. In guiding intervention, O'Brien and Savoyski (2006) contend that optimal motor learning is best achieved through occupational therapy intervention that is both individualized and allows for active experimentation, as well as being occupation-based in the client's natural environment.

More research has been conducted on assessing motor control performance than on occupational therapy intervention for motor control impairments. A few research-based articles specifically address the effectiveness of techniques designed to promote the development or relearning of motor skills. They generally compare one type of motor control intervention to another. The following research projects are worth noting, especially for those wishing to expand their knowledge in this realm. DeGangi, Wietlisbach, Goodin, & Scheiner (1993) compared two methods of motor control intervention in 12 preschoolers with sensorimotor deficits and found no order effect of the structured sensorimotor versus child-centered approaches, with all of the children in the project gaining in motor skills. The structured sensorimotor approach promoted gross motor skills better, while the child-centered approach promoted the more rapid development of fine motor coordination. Miyahara and Wafer (2004) also found general support for the motor control approaches of a skill theme program and a movement concepts program in a group of seven children with developmental coordination disorder, with the former focusing more on targeted skills training and the latter focusing more on self-esteem building and creativity. Similarly, Thorpe and Valvano (2002) examined three different practice protocols in a group of 13 children with cerebral palsy. They found that the majority of children improved no matter what strategy was used, but they did conclude that some children especially benefited from using cognitive strategies to augment practice in motor tasks. In a physiotherapy review that focused on intervention of postural control for those who have had a stroke, Pollock, Baer, Pomeroy, and Langhorne (2007) compared orthopedic, neurophysiologic, and motor learning approaches. They determined one approach was not significantly more effective than the others in improving balance. Since occupational therapy practitioners also work in the realm of postural control, this finding, imprecise as it is, still has meaning for the profession and highlights once again the need for more occupation-based research projects in this intervention area and beyond.

## Intervention Involving Functional Activities

While specific types of motor control intervention approaches may not be overwhelmingly better than others based on the research available thus far, a few studies did come to a conclusion that does greatly impact the practice of occupational therapy. Neistadt (1994) demonstrated that the 45 adult males with brain injuries in her study performed significantly better in fine motor coordination tasks when the intervention involved functional activities such as meal preparation as compared to when the intervention involved the contrived remedial task of parquetry puzzle construction. In quite a different study with yet a similar outcome, Wu, Trombly, Lin, and Tickle-Degnen (2000) found the condition of using real-life objects elicited better kinematic reaching performance than having the person simulate reaching for objects without the objects being present. To occupational therapy practitioners, the conclusion that occupation-based rather than contrived intervention activity promotes better functioning is self-evident. Yet the need for additional empirical research to substantiate this claim using various daily living tasks that involve motor control remains paramount.

# Intervention Related to Sensory Dysfunction

Occupational therapy intervention in the realm of sensory dysfunction is often compensatory and concerns primarily the sensory system of vision since the majority of sensory input to the brain comes through this modality (at least for those with normally functioning visual systems). Other sensory systems can sometimes be the focus of occupational therapy intervention, and these will be considered first.

## Smell and Taste

Olfaction and gustation are closely related sensory systems. Olfaction has the distinct characteristic of being the only sensory system that does not digress through the thalamus before progressing to the specific sensory processing area in the cortex. Because of the direct linkage of the sense of smell to sensory processing, using scents might be most effective in eliciting a response when stimulating a person in a coma. Olfaction can sometimes be impacted by disease processes such as sinus infections and traumatic brain injuries, but it tends to be more significantly impacted by the aging process, often without awareness of its decline. Nordin, Monsch, and Murphy (1995) found that the majority of elderly subjects had a decreased sense of olfaction, yet most of these respondents reported that their sense of smell was intact. Since the decline of olfaction sense with age appears to be insidious, the occupational therapy practitioner has a responsibility to educate elders about this potentiality. Problems secondary to anosmia (loss of smell sensation) beyond being disconcerting or annoying (e.g., not being able to notice if one is wearing too much cologne) can also impair one's ability to live independently. Someone with a normal sense of smell can readily detect spoiled food in the refrigerator, burning food in the oven, or a natural gas leak. Utility companies may have "scratch and sniff" cards available for easy detection of olfaction sensory loss. Occupational therapy intervention following smell loss can involve labeling food in the refrigerator with dates and teaching the client and family about the need for additional caution during cooking tasks. Unawareness and an inability to learn compensatory techniques would require having someone check on the person regularly.

Since the sense of smell is a backdrop for the sense of taste, similar issues arise with deceased gustation. Heckmann et al. (2005) reported that taste dysfunction following stroke is common. Gustatory sense losses were exhibited by 30% of their 102 clients, while others had distortions in their sense of taste. The person with decreased gustation, whether the impairment is caused by stroke or the aging process, also may not follow a healthy diet. In addition to perhaps ingesting spoiled food, they may eat foods that are too salty and consume too many sweets. As people age, their sense of salty and bitter naturally decreases, while sensation for sweet and sour is maintained (Hayflick, 1994). Besides making sure a client can either prepare or attain proper meals, a dietary consultation might be in order.

## Touch, Proprioception, and Kinesthesia

Touch, proprioception, and kinesthesia are sensory systems people rarely consciously think about until there is a problem. Perhaps the most common robber of sensation in these realms is the diagnosis of stroke, which often impacts sensory functioning on the contralateral (opposite) side of the body to where the lesion occurred. Diabetes is another common diagnosis impacting distal sensation in the form of diabetic peripheral neuropathy. Loss of sensation can result in significant safety concerns in nearly every daily task. Even if movement is normal, the person must take extra care in doing everything in order to make sure the limb is maintained in a safe position and is protected from excess pressure. Whereas sharp items could puncture the skin without the person being aware, sustained pressure brought about by not moving enough or by something pressing against the skin can also cause skin damage. In the worst case scenario, the sustained pressure can cause decubitus ulcers, which are very serious single to multi-layered skin lesions that heal extremely slowly and only with the utmost of care. Skin breakdown can occur within hours (of sustained pressure) and may eventually penetrate to the level of bone. With proper initial positioning, frequent repositioning, and other protective measures, decubitus ulcers should never or only rarely occur. Compensatory measures for decreased touch sense and proprioception/kinesthesia include using vision to carefully watch what one is doing, the removal of sharp items in the environment, as well as client and family education to ensure safety.

Since stroke often leads to sensory losses or distortions, occupational therapy practitioners may be involved in retraining sensory discrimination if sensation is present but not accurate in the affected limb(s). In a quasi-experimental research project using graded sensory discrimination tasks, sensory exploratory tasks without the use of vision, and specific feedback, Carey, Matyas, and Oke (1993) found long-term clinically significant improvements in the ability to distinguish sensory stimuli in a small group of stroke survivors in Australia.

## Hearing

Although the sense of hearing is not an area for which occupational therapy practitioners are primarily responsible, nonetheless the consideration of one's ability to hear is still a crucial element in promoting successful occupational performance. If one cannot hear, then compensatory measures need to be taken for safety. For example, using a vibrating alarm to alert one to wake up or a light to signal the doorbell just rang could be ways to adapt the home environment. Hearing is a sensory modality that also decreases with age, so impairments in this realm are encountered frequently in the field of rehabilitation. An occupational therapy practitioner may be called upon to work with the client on the ADL of hearing aid care and insertion after the loss of these skills (i.e., due to a stroke or injury). When working with clients who have a decreased sense of hearing, optimal intervention depends on appropriate communication techniques. Therapeutic use of self includes an awareness of and ability to modify verbal interactions, perhaps by enunciating words more clearly, speaking more slowly, lowering pitch, and eliminating background noise whenever possible (Robnett, 1999).

## Vision

Vision is often a focus of occupational therapy intervention either as a primary or secondary diagnosis. An estimated one of every two clients in a rehabilitation hospital has visual impairments that impact functioning, and an estimated one out of every four children has visual impairments. Specialists in the field of vision, including rehabilitation teachers and orientation and mobility specialists, work on a full-time basis with those who have visual losses. While occupational therapy practitioners and physical therapists undertake similar jobs in this realm, the previously mentioned two types of professionals have much more specialized education and training in the field of vision exclusively. The visual system is a complex sensory system involving many different pathways and components. Deficits can therefore be extremely varied. Warren (1993) describes the visual system as a hierarchy. The basic skills of visual acuity, oculomotor control, visual fields, and visual attention are foundational skills providing the backdrop for the more complex visual and perceptual skills such as scanning, pattern recognition, visual memory, and visuocognition. Interested readers are directed to two comprehensive occupational therapy textbooks on the topic of intervention for those with decreased vision: *Functional Visual Behavior in Adults, Second Edition* (Gentile, 2005) and *Vision, Perception, and Cognition, Fourth Edition* (Zoltan, 2007).

Occupational therapy intervention in the area of vision often involves starting with a functional visual assessment and following with compensation for decreased visual skills. Occasionally, however, development or remediation of visual skills occurs in occupational therapy. For example, after an acquired brain injury, intervention may involve training and functional tasks to promote better scanning and attention, especially to the side that tends to get neglected (Figure 21-2). Occupational therapy practitioners may sometimes work with behavioral optometrists in helping clients follow through with eye exercises for the purpose of restoring visual functioning in the realm of scanning, attention, and binocular visual skills. Occupational therapy practitioners may also be involved in teaching eccentric viewing, a special viewing technique for those who have macular degeneration. In addition, occupational therapy was shown to be effective, along with other disciplines, in assisting those with low vision to attain their functional goals, as demonstrated by the results of an experimental visual rehabilitation program for older adults in the mid-west (Pankow, Luchins, Studebaker, & Chettleburgh, 2004).

As people age, visual skills tend to decrease, which already starts in the third decade of life. Common diagnoses more prevalent in older clients include age-related macular degeneration, glaucoma, diabetic retinopathy, cataracts, and visual losses secondary to stroke. Completing a full evaluation to determine the client's needs in the realm of vision is paramount to improving the environment to promote optimal visual functioning. Besides corrective lenses, some

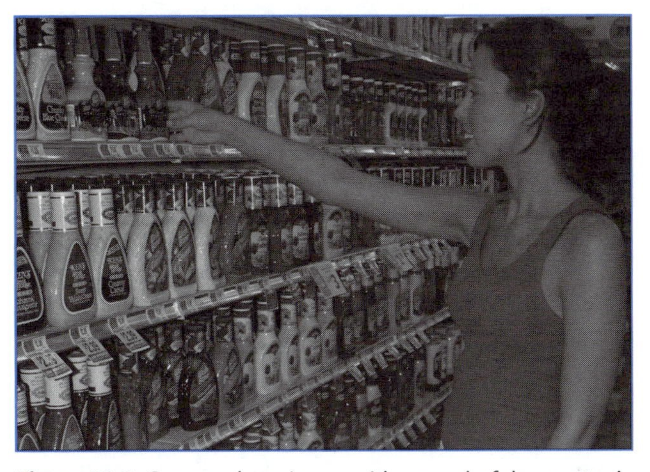

**Figure 21-2.** Grocery shopping provides wonderful opportunities to work on various cognitive and visual skills. Here a client is scanning for a certain item.

of the more common compensatory and adaptive measures include the following:

- Increasing the size of the object under scrutiny (e.g., printed material, images, signs)
- Using magnifying glasses or closed circuit television when actual object enlargement is not possible
- Protective lenses to reduce glare and shield out bright sunlight
- Increasing the contrast of items to one another (e.g., plate and placement, black print on white paper, safety strips on the edges of stairs)
- Improved lighting (e.g., effective spot lighting for work area, nightlights, shielding glare from bright light bulbs)
- Avoiding tasks that can no longer be completed safely due to decreased vision (e.g., driving at night)
- Making sure the home environment is as safe as possible (e.g., well-organized, clutter-free, removal of loose rugs)

## Visual Perception

Perceptual skills are higher level, top-of-the-pyramid visual skills that require not only intact visual pathways but also an accurate interpretation of the visual information in the occipital and parietal lobes of the brain. Perception also involves the processing and analysis of other types of sensory information in the brain. Due to their complexity, perceptual deficits are some of the most fascinating and difficult problems to treat. They are rarely seen in isolation and are often combined with more general cognitive impairments. Visual perceptual disorders include the inability to recognize common objects (e.g., agnosia), the inability to understand spatial relationships (e.g., figure-ground, right-left, and depth perception impairments), the inability to recognize subtle differences in similar objects and people (e.g., form constancy disorder), the inability to distinguish objects by touch (e.g., astereognosis), and a distortion of body scheme. Included in the realm of perceptual disorders are both ideomotor and ideational apraxias. These are defined as an inability to carry out common motor tasks due to perceptual impairments rather than because of decreased sensation or motor skills. Ideomotor apraxia is less severe because the person can do the task automatically but cannot simulate the task or do it on command. Ideational apraxia is a complete loss of the ability to do the task and, therefore, is much more difficult to remediate.

Remediation of perceptual deficits involves repetitive engagement in tasks requiring perceptual skills, starting at the client's level and working up to more complicated tasks as the person is able (Figure 21-3). In a pivotal study involving occupational therapy, Neistadt (1992) compared 45 men who had perceptual deficits due to brain injuries in two intervention groups. One group completed remedial parquetry block assembly and the other worked on functional meal preparation. The results showed that the functional approach was preferable to the remedial approach, although both groups did show improvements in the realm of perception. Compensation for decreased perceptual skills can involve simplifying the environment, establishing basic daily routines, and making sure the environment is safe for someone who has decreased awareness of their surroundings, supervision, and cueing.

Frequently, the research completed on the intervention of perceptual disorders has focused on unilateral neglect, which more often accompanies right-sided lesions of the brain. A Cochrane Review of cognitive rehabilitation for spatial neglect following stroke (Bowen, Lincoln, & Dewey, 2006) found that cognitive rehabilitation clearly did result in decreased visual neglect at the impairment level as measured by neuropsychological assessments, but additional research endeavors in this area were recommended to ensure these improvements actually transfer to enhanced functioning in day-to-day tasks. Cicerone et al. (2000) recommended "relatively intense (i.e., daily)" (p. 1601) visuospatial training, which includes scanning to decrease the level of visual neglect as a practice standard based on robust evidence of its effectiveness. However, this research group did not recommend the use of isolated computerized exercises as intervention. Warren (1993), who described the hierarchical model of visual functioning, recommended that occupational therapy practitioners focus on restoring basic visual functioning (visual acuity, visual fields, and oculomotor control) because in doing so, a natural consequence may be the spontaneous recovery of higher level skills.

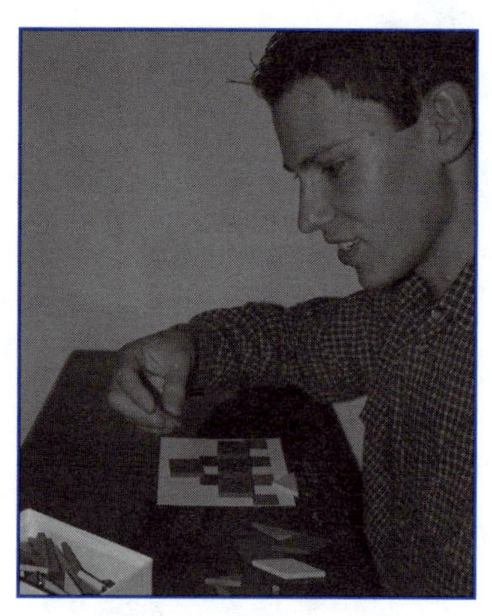

**Figure 21-3.** Parquetry puzzles are sometimes used to help clients regain skills in perceptual functioning.

## Summary

All of the interventions described in this chapter have been condensed for the sake of parsimony in an introductory text. As stated initially, the impairments—though described individually—are nonetheless rarely seen in isolation. In addition, although the primary impairment may be cognitive, sensory, or physical, these typically have accompanying psychosocial implications. Losses in the realm of client factors and/or performance skills can be traumatic and can result in deep emotional responses in the clients and in their significant others. These feelings definitely impact the rehabilitation process and should not be ignored. Effective occupational therapy intervention is based on a thorough review of the biopsychosocial factors pertinent to the individual case, as well as a strong dose of clinical reasoning to ensure that the intervention plan is both client-centered and based on the best and most accurate empirical knowledge currently available. In this chapter, further references are often cited and should be consulted prior to working with clients in the areas described. Striving for excellence in occupational therapy and doing our utmost best to help "build the skills for the job of living" is, after all, our ultimate goal as professionals within this exhilarating and challenging field.

## Student Self-Assessment

1. Many people have a rather superficial level of understanding of disabilities. We can define them, but we do not truly comprehend what it is like to have impairments. Therefore, a valuable learning tool is to simulate life with a disability. This activity can lend insight into the difficulties encountered in everyday life. The activity can be completed in a classroom or lab setting or in the community (although care should be taken not to offend people with disabilities in the community). All of these exercises should be undertaken only under supervision. The following list is just a few examples of how this exercise can work:
   - Simulating paralysis of the legs, use a wheelchair to get around. Be sure to go around several buildings and roll on graded surfaces.
   - Wearing heavy gloves, try to make a peanut butter and crackers snack (or another snack requiring opening containers and using utensils).

- Using just one arm, put on a shirt and shoes, including tying them. You are not allowed to move your "affected" arm.
- Smear lotion on some old sunglasses and put them on. Then try doing a puzzle or playing a game.
- Wearing ear plugs and earmuffs, try to write down the words to a song you are listening to on the radio (if there is static on the radio, that's even better).
- Try cleaning a kitchen area or dusting while blindfolded.

2. In small groups of two to four, brainstorm intervention ideas for the impairments listed. Be sure to think of ideas that incorporate remediation and ideas that incorporate compensation or adaptation whenever possible. For example, for decreased sense of smell, although remediation is probably not possible, compensation might involve labeling leftovers with dates, getting a second opinion about perfume (or not wearing any), and making sure areas are well-ventilated when working with any harmful airborne substances. Remember that the broad list you devise will not be client centered, but it will stimulate your individualized intervention planning when working with people who have the following impairments:
   - Decreased vision
   - Unilateral neglect
   - Ideational/ideomotor apraxia
   - Figure ground deficit
   - Orientation deficit
   - Decreased attention
   - Decreased short-term memory
   - Decreased endurance
   - Decreased strength
   - Impaired self-awareness

## Evidence-Based Research Chart

| Area | Intervention | Evidence |
|---|---|---|
| Cognitive | General cognitive rehabilitation | Carney et al., 1999; Cicerone et al., 2000, 2004; AOTA, 1999 |
| | Attention training | Lincoln et al., 2006; Sohlberg & Mateer, 2001 |
| | Memory training | Cicerone et al., 2000 |
| | Self-awareness | Fleming et al., 2006; Ownsworth, Fleming, Desbois, Strong, & Kuipers, 2006 |
| Behavioral | Sensory dysfunction (SI) | Case-Smith & Bryan, 1999; Roley et al., 2003; Smith, Press, Koenig, & Kinnealey, 2005 |
| | Behavior—children | Rosen & Scott, 2003; Watling & Schwartz, 2004 |
| | Behavioral change—adults | Clark, Nigg, Greene, Riebe, & Saunders, 2002; Glasgow, Bull, Gillette, Klesges, & Dzewaltowski, 2002 |
| Physical | Range of motion | Bemben, Bemben, Fields, & Walker, 1996 |
| | Strength | Andrews & Bohannon, 2003; Grealy et al., 1999; Kauranen, Siira, & Vanharanta, 1998; Latham, Anderson, Bennett, & Stretton, 2003; Nelson et al., 1999; Teixeira-Salmela et al., 1999; Weiss, Suzuki, Bean, & Fielding, 2000 |
| | Endurance | McMurdo & Burnett, 1992 |
| | Balance/postural control | Clemson et al., 2004; Davison, Bond, Dawson, Steen, & Kenny, 2005; Gillespie et al., 2003; Han et al., 2004; Hsieh et al., 1996; Li et al., 2005; Taylor-Piliae et al., 2006; Zijlstra et al., 2007 |
| Neuro-muscular | Motor control | DeGangi et al., 1993; Miyahara & Wafer, 2004; Neistadt, 1994; Pollock et al., 2007; Stevens & Stoykov, 2004; Thorpe & Valvano, 2002; Ward & Rodger, 2004; Whitall, McCombe Waller, Silver, & Macko, 2000; Wu et al., 2000 |
| Sensory | Olfactory and gustatory | Zasler, McNeny, & Heywood, 1992 |
| | Touch, proprioception, and kinesthesia | Carey, Matyas, & Oke, 1993; Dannenbaum & Jones, 1993 |
| | Hearing | Andersson, Green, & Melin, 1997 |
| | Vision | Pankow et al., 2004 |
| | Visual perception | Aki & Kayihan, 2003; Bowen et al., 2006; Cicerone et al., 2000; Lin, Cermak, Kinsbourne, & Trombly, 1996; Neistadt, 1992 |
| | Sensory stimulation—coma | Mitchell, Bradley, Welch, & Britton, 1990; Oh & Seo, 2003 |

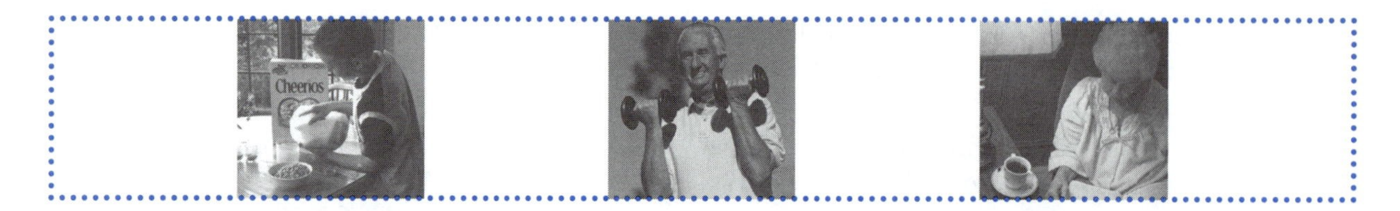


# References


Abreu, B. C. (1997). *The quadraphonic approach*. Galveston, TX: Unpublished course manual.

Aki, E., & Kayihan, H. (2003). The effect of visual perceptual training on reading, writing, and daily living activities in children with low vision. *Fizyoterapi Rehabilitasyon, 14*(3), 95-99.

Allen, C. K. (1985). *Occupational therapy for psychiatric diseases: Measurement and management of cognitive disabilities*. Boston, MA: Little, Brown, and Company.

American Occupational Therapy Association. (1999). Management of occupational therapy services for persons with cognitive impairments (statement). *American Journal of Occupational Therapy, 53*(6), 601-607.

American Occupational Therapy Association. (2008). Occupational therapy practice framework: Domain and process, second edition. *American Journal of Occupational Therapy, 62*, 625-683.

Andersson, G., Green, M., & Melin, L. (1997). Behavioural hearing tactics: A controlled trial of a short treatment programme. *Behaviour Research and Therapy, 35*(6), 523-530.

Andrews, A. W., & Bohannon, R. W. (2003). Short-term recovery of limb muscle strength after acute stroke. *Archives of Physical Medicine and Rehabilitation, 84*(1), 125-130.

Arkin, S. M. (2000). Alzheimer memory training: Students replicate learning successes. *American Journal of Alzheimer's Disease and Other Dementias, 15*(3), 152-162.

Ayres, A. J. (1979). *Sensory integration and the child.* Los Angeles, CA: Western Psychological Services.

Bemben, M. G., Bemben, D. A., Fields, D. A., & Walker, L. S. (1996). The effects of 16 weeks of resistance training on strength and flexibility in elderly women. *Issues on Aging, 19*(2), 10-14.

Bowen, A., Lincoln, N. B., & Dewey, M. (2007). Cognitive rehabilitation for spatial neglect following stroke. *Cochrane Database for Systemic Reviews, 2*, CD003586.

Breines, E. B. (2006). Therapeutic occupations and modalities. In H. M. Pendleton & W. Schultz-Krohn (Eds.), *Pedretti's occupational therapy: Practice skills for physical dysfunction* (6th ed.). St. Louis, MO: Mosby Elsevier.

Brody, L. T. (2005). Impaired joint mobility and range of motion. In C. M. Hall & L. T. Brody (Eds.), *Therapeutic exercise: Moving toward function* (2nd ed.). Philadelphia, PA: Lippencott, Williams & Wilkins.

Carey, L. M., Matyas, T. A., & Oke, L. E. (1993). Sensory loss in stroke patients: Effective training of tactile and proprioceptive discrimination. *Archives of Physical Medicine and Rehabilitation, 74*(6), 602-611.

Carney, N., Chestnut, R. M., Maynard, H., Mann, N. C., Patterson, P., & Helfand, M. (1999). Effect of cognitive rehabilitation on outcomes for persons with traumatic brain injury: A systematic review. *Journal of Head Trauma Rehabilitation, 14*(3), 277-307.

Case-Smith, J., & Bryan, T. (1999). The effects of occupational therapy with sensory integration emphasis on preschool-age children with autism. *American Journal of Occupational Therapy, 53*(5), 489-497.

Cicerone, K. D., Dahlberg, C., Kalmar, K., Langenbahn, D. M., Malec, J. F., Bergquist, T. F., et al. (2000). Evidence based cognitive rehabilitation: Recommendations for clinical practice. *Archives of Physical Medicine and Rehabilitation, 81*(12), 1596-1615.

Cicerone, K. D., Mott, T., Azulay, J., & Friel, J. C. (2004). Community integration and satisfaction with functioning after intensive cognitive rehabilitation for traumatic brain injury. *Archives of Physical Medicine and Rehabilitation, 85*(6), 943-950.

Clark, P. G., Nigg, C. R., Greene, G., Riebe, D., & Saunders, S. D. (2002). The study of exercise and nutrition in older Rhode Islanders (SENIOR): Translating theory into research. *Health Education Research, 17*(5), 552-561.

Clemson, L., Cumming, R. G., Kendig, H., Swann, M., Heard, R., & Taylor, K. (2004). The effectiveness of a community-based program for reducing the incidence of falls in the elderly: A randomized trial. *Journal of the American Geriatrics Society, 52*(9), 1487-1494.

Dannenbaum, R. M., & Jones, L. A. (1993). The assessment and treatment of patients who have sensory loss following cortical lesions. *Journal of Hand Therapy, 6*(2), 130-138.

Davison, J., Bond, J., Dawson, P., Steen, I. N., & Kenny, R. A. (2005). Patients with recurrent falls attending Accident & Emergency benefit from multifactorial intervention—A randomized controlled trial. *Age and Ageing, 34*(2), 162-168.

DeGangi, G. A., Wietlisbach, S., Goodin, M., & Scheiner, N. (1993). A comparison of structured sensorimotor therapy and child-centered activity in the treatment of preschool children with sensorimotor problems. *American Journal of Occupational Therapy, 47*(9), 777-786.

Feigenbaum, M. S. (2001). Rational and review of current guidelines. In J. E. Graves & B. A. Franklin (Eds.), *Resistance training for health and rehabilitation*. Leeds, UK: Human Kinetics Publishers.

Fleming, J. M., Lucas, S. E., & Lightbody, S. (2006). Using occupation to facilitate self-awareness in people who have acquired brain injury: A pilot study. *Canadian Journal of Occupational Therapy, 73*(1), 44-55.

Gentile, M. (2005). *Functional visual behavior in adults: An occupational therapy guide to evaluation and treatment options* (2nd ed.). Bethesda, MD: AOTA Press.

Gillespie, L. D., Gillespie, W. J., Robertson, M. C., Lamb, S. E., Cumming, R. G., & Rowe, B. H. (2003). Interventions for preventing falls in elderly people. *Cochrane Database for Systematic Reviews, 4*, CD000340.

Glasgow, R. E., Bull, S. S., Gillette, C., Klesges, L. M., & Dzewaltowski, D. A. (2002). Behavior change intervention research in healthcare settings: A review of recent reports with emphasis on external validity. *American Journal of Preventive Medicine, 23*(1), 62-69.

Graff, M. J. L., Vernooij-Dassen, M. J. F. J., Hoefnagels, W. H. L., Dekker, J., & de Witte, L. P. (2003). Occupational therapy at home for older individuals with mild to moderate cognitive impairments and their primary caregivers: A pilot study. *OTJR: Occupation, Participation and Health, 23*(4), 155-164.

Grealy, M. A., Johnson, D. A., & Rushton, S. K. (1999). Improving cognitive function after brain injury: The use of exercise and virtual reality. *Archives of Physical Medicine and Rehabilitation, 80*(6), 661-667.

Hall, C. M., & Brody, L. T. (2005). Impairment in Muscle Performance. In C. M. Hall & L. T. Brody (Eds.), *Therapeutic exercise: Moving toward function* (2nd ed.). Philadelphia, PA: Lippincott Williams & Wilkins.

Hällgren, M., & Kottorp, A. (2005). Effects of occupational therapy intervention on activities of daily living and awareness of disability in persons with intellectual disabilities. *Australian Occupational Therapy Journal, 52*(4), 350-359.

Han, A., Robinson, V., Judd, M., Taixiang, W., Wells, G., & Tugwell, P. (2004). Tai Chi for treating rheumatoid arthritis. *Cochrane Database for Systemic Reviews, 3*, CD004849.

Hayflick, L. (1994). *How and why we age.* New York, NY: Ballantine Books.

Heckmann, J. G., Stössel, C., Lang, C. J. G., Neundörfer, B., Tomandl, B., & Hummel, T. (2005). Taste disorders in acute stroke: A prospective observational study on taste disorders in 102 stroke patients. *Stroke, 36*(8), 1690-1694.

Hsieh, C. L., Nelson, D. L., Smith, D. A., & Peterson, C. Q. (1996). A comparison of performance in added-purpose occupations and rote exercise for dynamic standing balance in persons with hemiplegia. *American Journal of Occupational Therapy, 50*(1), 10-16.

Kauranen, K. J., Siira, P. T., & Vanharanta, H. V. (1998). A 10-week strength training program: Effect on the motor performance of an unimpaired upper extremity. *Archives of Physical Medicine and Rehabilitation, 79*(8), 925-930.

Latham, N., Anderson, C., Bennett, D., & Stretton, C. (2003). Progressive resistence strength training for physical disability in older people. *Cochrane Database of Systematic Reviews, 2*, CD002759.

Levy, L. L., & Burns, T. (2005). Cognitive disabilities reconsidered. In N. Katz (Ed.), *Cognition and occupation across the lifespan* (2nd ed.). Bethesda, MD: AOTA Press.

Li, F., Harmer, P., Fisher, K. J., McAuley, E., Chaumeton, N., Eckstrom, E., et al. (2005). Tai Chi and fall reductions in older adults: A randomized controlled trial. *Journals of Gerontology Series A, Biological Sciences and Medical Sciences, 60*(2), 187-194.

Lin, K. C., Cermak, S. A., Kinsbourne, M., & Trombly, C. A. (1996). Effects of left-sided movements on line bisection in unilateral neglect. *Journal of the International Neuropsychological Society, 2*(5), 404-411.

Lincoln, N. B., Majid, M. J., & Weyman, N. (2000). Cognitive rehabilitation for attention deficits following stroke. *Cochrane Database of Systematic Reviews, 4*, CD002842.

McMurdo, M. E. T., & Burnett, L. (1992). Randomized controlled trial of exercise in the elderly. *Gerontology, 38*, 292-298.

Mitchell, S., Bradley, V. A., Welch, J. L., & Britton, P. G. (1990). Coma arousal procedures: A therapeutic intervention in the treatment of head injury. *Brain Injury, 4*(3), 273-279.

Miyahara, M., & Wafer, A. (2004). Clinical intervention for children with developmental coordination disorder: A multiple case study. *Adapted Physical Activity Quarterly, 21*(3), 281-300.

Neistadt, M. E. (1994). The effects of different treatment activities on functional fine motor coordination in adults with brain injury. *American Journal of Occupational Therapy, 48*(10), 877-882.

Neistadt, M. E. (1992). Occupational therapy treatments for constructional deficits. *American Journal of Occupational Therapy, 46*(2), 141-148.

Nelson, D. L., Konosky, K., Fleharty, K., Webb, R., Newer, K., Hazboun, V. P., et al. (1999). The effects of an occupationally embedded exercise on bilaterally assisted supination in persons with hemiplegia. *American Journal of Occupational Therapy, 50*(8), 639-646.

Nordin, S., Monsch, A. U., & Murphy, C. (1995). Unawareness of smell loss in normal aging and Alzheimer's Disease: Discrepancy between self-reported and diagnosed smell sensitivity. *Journals of Gerontology Series B. Psychological Sciences and Social Sciences, 50*(4), P187-P192.

Nussbaum, P. (2003). *Brain health and wellness.* Tarentum, PA: Word Association Publishers.

O'Brien, J., & Savoyski, J. (2006). *Application of motor control and motor learning concepts in pediatric occupational therapy practice.* Charlotte, NC: American Occupational Therapy Association National Conference.

Oh, H., & Seo, W. (2003). Sensory stimulation programme to improve recovery in comatose patients. *Journal of Clinical Nursing, 12*(3), 394-404.

Ownsworth, T., Fleming, J., Desbois, J., Strong, J., & Kuipers, P. (2006). A metacognitive contextual intervention to enhance error awareness and functional outcome following traumatic brain injury: A single case experimental design. *Journal of the International Neuropsychological Society, 12*(1), 54-63.

Pankow, L., Luchins, D., Studebaker, J., & Chettleburgh, D. (2004). Evaluation of a vision rehabilitation program for older adults with visual impairment. *Topics in Geriatric Rehabilitation, 20*(3), 223-232.

Peterson, E. W., & Clemson, L. (2008). Understanding the role of occupational therapy in fall prevention for community-dwelling older adults. *OT Practice, 13*(3), CE1-CE8.

Pollock, A., Baer, G., Pomeroy, V., & Langhorne, P. (2007). Physiotherapy treatment approaches for the recovery of postural control and lower limb function following stroke. *Cochrane Database of Systemic Reviews, 1*, CD001920.

Prochaska, J. O., & Velicer, W. F. (1997). The transtheoretical model of health behavioral change. *American Journal of Health Promotion, 12*(1), 38-48.

Robnett, R. H. (1999). The psychological, behavioral, and cognitive aspects of aging. In W. C. Chop & R. H. Robnett (Eds.), *Gerontology for the Health Care Professional.* Philadelphia, PA: F.A. Davis.

Roley, S. S., Clark, G. F., Bissell, J., Brayman, S. J., & Commission on Practice. (2003). Applying sensory integration framework in educationally related occupational therapy practice. *American Journal of Occupational Therapy, 57*(6), 652-659.

Rosen, S., & Scott, J. B. (2003). Behavior management strategies for students with Autism. *OT Practice, 8*(11), 16-20.

Shumway-Cook, A., & Woollacott, M. H. (2001). *Motor control: Theory and practical applications* (2nd ed.). Philadelphia, PA: Lippincott Williams & Wilkins.

Smith, S. A., Press, B., Koenig, K. P., & Kinnealey, M. (2005). Effect of sensory integration intervention on self-stimulating and self-injurious behaviors. *American Journal of Occupational Therapy, 59*(4), 418-425.

Sohlberg, M. M., & Mateer, C. A. (2001). *Cognitive rehabilitation: An integrative neuropsychological approach.* New York, NY: Guilford Press.

*Stedman's concise medical dictionary for the health professions* (3rd ed.). (1997). Baltimore, MD: Lippincott Williams & Wilkins.

Stevens, J. A., & Stoykov, M. E. (2004). Simulation of bilateral movement training through mirror reflection: A case report demonstrating occupational therapy for hemiparesis. *Topics in Stroke Rehabilitation, 11*(1), 59-66.

Taylor-Piliae, R. E., Haskell, W. L., Stotts, N. A., & Froehlicher, E. S. (2006). Improvement in balance, strength, and flexibility after 12 weeks of Tai Chi exercise in ethnic Chinese adults with cardiovascular disease risk factors. *Alternative Therapies in Health & Medicine, 12*(2), 50-58.

Teixeira-Salmela, L. F., Olney, S. J., Nadeau, S., & Brouwer, B. (1999). Muscle strengthening and physical conditioning to reduce impairment and disability in chronic stroke survivors. *Archives of Physical Medicine, 80*(10), 1211-1218.

Thorpe, D. E., & Valvano, J. (2002). The effects of knowledge of performance and cognitive strategies on motor skill learning in children with cerebral palsy. *Pediatric Physical Therapy, 14*(1), 2-15.

Ward, A., & Rodger, S. A. (2004). The application of cognitive orientation to daily occupational performance (CO-OP) with children 5-7 years with developmental coordination disorder. *British Journal of Occupational Therapy, 67*(6), 256-264.

Warren, M. (1993). A hierarchical model for evaluation and treatment of visual perception dysfunction in adult acquired brain injury, part 1. *American Journal of Occupational Therapy, 47*(1), 42-54.

Watling, R., & Schwartz, I. S. (2004). Understanding and implementing positive reinforcement as an intervention strategy for children with disabilities. *American Journal of Occupational Therapy, 58*(1), 113-116.

Weiss, A., Suzuki, T., Bean, J., & Fielding, R. A. (2000). High intensity strength training improves strength and functional performance after stroke. *Archives of Physical Medicine and Rehabilitation, 79*(4), 369-376.

Whitall, J., McCombe Waller, S., Silver, K. H., & Macko, R. F. (2000). Repetitive bilateral arm training with rhythmic auditory cueing improves motor function in chronic hemiparetic stroke. *Stroke, 31*(10), 2390-2395.

Wu, C. Y., Trombly, C. A., Lin. K. C., & Tickle-Degnen, L. (2000). A kinematic study of contextual effects on reaching performance in persons with and without stroke: Influences of object availability. *Archives of Physical Medicine and Rehabilitation, 81*(1), 95-101.

Zasler, N. D., McNeny, R., & Heywood, P. G. (1992). Rehabilitation management of olfactory and gustatory dysfunction following brain injury. *Journal of Head Trauma Rehabilitation, 7*(1), 66-75.

Zijlstra, G. A., van Haastregt, J. C., van Rossum, E., van Eijk, J. T., Yardley, L., & Kempen, G. I. (2007). Interventions to reduce the fear of falling in community-living older people: A systematic review. *Journal of the American Geriatrics Society, 55*(4), 603-615.

Zoltan, B. (2007). *Vision, perception, and cognition: A manual for the evaluation and treatment of the adult with acquired brain injury* (4th ed.). Thorofare, NJ: SLACK Incorporated.

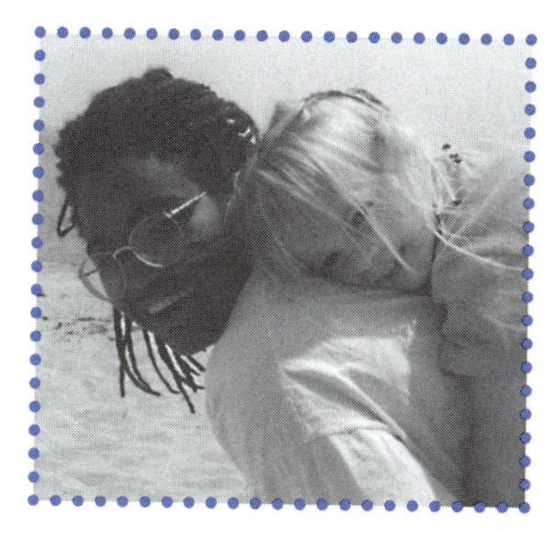

# 22

# Therapeutic Use of Self

*Jan Froehlich, MS, OTR/L*

**ACOTE Standard Explored in This Chapter**

B.5.6

**Key Terms**

| | |
|---|---|
| Caring | Effective communication |
| Client-centered practice | Empathy |
| Counter-transference | Transference |

## Introduction

Jody, the occupational therapist, has tried many strategies with Annabelle, but none have motivated her to get out of bed. Exasperated, Jody says, "How about if I wear my wedding dress to work tomorrow, will you get out of bed for me then?" Jody wears her wedding dress to the nursing home the next day, and sure enough, Annabelle chuckles as she gets out of bed and engages in occupational therapy interventions related to her self-care.

## Caring

One of the most rewarding aspects of being an occupational therapy practitioner is that we get to care about our clients. Every time we show our caring toward our clients, we are using ourselves as a therapeutic tool. Sometimes, therapeutic use of self is the most profound aspect of the therapy process. Conversely, if we have not achieved therapeutic use of self with a given client, the most expert techniques may be ineffective. Jody was able to inspire Annabelle to engage in occupational therapy because she was creative enough and cared enough about her to try something as outlandish as wearing her wedding dress to work to get Annabelle out of bed.

Allowing ourselves to care for our clients comes naturally to many occupational therapy practitioners. We chose occupational therapy as our profession because we wanted to make a difference in the lives of clients in need of our services. We show our caring for our clients in a variety of ways. On a most basic level, occupational therapy practitioners are required to care for clients by providing technically competent occupational therapy services that are based on sound judgment. Beyond providing technically competent care, some practitioners show their care by spending time creating adaptive equipment for their clients or engaging in research on a particular occupational therapy intervention or assessment instrument. Others, like Jody, have a talent for bringing humor to the occupational therapy relationship. Still others deepen the therapeutic relationship by allowing themselves to cry right alongside their clients as tragedies and losses are expressed and faced. Many offer deep hope to clients who find little meaning and hope in their lives.



K. Sladyk, K. Jacobs, & N. MacRae (Eds.).
*Occupational Therapy Essentials for Clinical Competence* (pp. 245-254).

Obviously, there are a multitude of different ways that occupational therapists show their caring for their clients, and the way we show our caring is in part related to our personality. There is no "right" way to care for our clients. Often, caring occurs right from the start in a therapy relationship, and many times, it deepens over the course of the therapy relationship. Other times, we initially may find ourselves not being able to notice we like or care for a particular client, yet we offer our care just the same. Paradoxically, we can care about people even if we do not feel we like them.

To elucidate the nature and importance of caring in occupational therapy, the 60th American Occupational Therapy Association (AOTA) conference theme was on caring. At that conference, Gilfoyle (1980) identified the importance of knowledge, skill, and attitudes in caring. She emphasized how important it is to truly know our client—what a person's strengths, limitations, and needs are and what will enable them to grow and change. In addition, she felt that knowledge must include the ability to know how to respond to another person's needs and to know your own abilities and limitations as a practitioner. Flexibility was identified as a key skill in caring as we continually assess and reassess our effectiveness. Patience, honesty, trust, humility, hope, and courage were identified as the attitudes we bring to caring.

King (1980) challenged therapists to provide both effective and creative caring in occupational therapy. Like Gilfoyle, she also emphasized the importance of knowledge in caring, yet she highlighted the importance of the practitioner's engagement in independent thinking and examination of the broad issues related to therapy. Generating creative alternatives in occupational therapy was stressed as a deep form of caring.

A few years later, Devereaux (1984) described occupational therapy practitioners as specialists in making caring and connection happen. She highlighted seven elements of the caring, therapeutic relationship:

1. Belief in the dignity and worth of the individual—respect
2. Belief in our clients' innate potential for change and growth
3. Effective communication: Listening and empathy and client-centered therapy and empowerment
4. Humor
5. Values
6. Touch
7. Competence

Other scholars have applied their own fresh thinking to therapeutic use of self and caring in occupational therapy. Peloquin (2002, 2003) emphasized empathy in therapeutic relationships. Many therapists have contributed to the development of client-centered practice in occupational therapy (Law & Mills, 1998). Wells and Black (2000) inspired occupational therapy practitioners to develop cultural competence. Schwartzberg (2002) articulated the nature of interactive reasoning in occupational therapy. Tickle-Degnen (2002) interwove the principles of client-centered practice and therapeutic use of self with the use of evidence-based research. Black (2005) drew an intersection of caring between client-centered practice, culturally competent care, and the feminist ethic of caring. Taylor (2008) developed an intentional relationship model for occupational therapists.

From the author's experience, Devereaux's (1984) seven elements of a caring therapeutic relationship are still important today, yet they can be expanded upon by the rich contributions of many other scholars from within and outside of occupational therapy. Each element will now be explored and expanded upon from the perspective of multiple scholars. This will be done in the context of occupational therapy clinical examples drawn from the author's own clinical experience and that of her occupational therapy colleagues in northern New England so the readers can gain an increasing appreciation and understanding of therapeutic use of self in occupational therapy.

## Belief in the Dignity and Worth of the Individual–Respect

The first client I worked with on an inpatient psychiatric unit was Kenny, a 15 year old who had stabbed his mother to death. He was psychotic at the time and believed his mother was poisoning him. As a new therapist, I found it a little challenging to notice that I did not like this client, but I could offer my care and respect. As his life story unfolded before me, I never doubted that when the entire situation was taken into account, he had done his best. I grew to like this client over time, yet right from the beginning, I cared about his well-being. Occupational therapy sessions aimed at boosting his self-confidence regarding his ability to master a variety of age-appropriate social, leisure, and prevocational activities were effective.

The most effective occupational therapy practitioners approach their clients with an attitude of deep respect and belief in the dignity and worth of every individual. Respect can be offered even when we do not feel like we like somebody. This respect generally acknowledges that the client we are assisting has probably been through many ups and downs in his or her life and has done his or her best with the cards he or she has been dealt. Jackins (1993) expresses this well in the following quote: "Every single human being, when the entire situation is taken into account, has always, at every moment, done the very best that he or she could do, and so deserves neither blame nor reproach from anyone, including self" (p. 3).

A caring attitude that communicates respect is one that separates people from their problems, behaviors, and distresses. In my work with Kenny, not only did I offer respect, but in my mind, I made a sharp distinction between who he was and what his problems and distresses were at that time. I held a mental picture of him as a smart, caring boy who had had many hard experiences in his lifetime. Yet at the same time, I did not forget that in a distressed and psychotic state, he had killed his mother. I did not respect his distress.

Not confusing our clients with their distresses or problems is a crucial element in maintaining respect for a client and for enhancing the therapeutic use of self. I worked with a young woman, Martha, who, after experiencing whiplash from a car accident, had bilateral wrist and foot drop that was a conversion disorder. In other words, her physical disability was in her mind. Her paralysis followed no neurological pattern. She was dependent on others for all of her self-care needs, including toileting. My gut response to this situation was judgmental. However, I quickly checked that response at the door and replaced it with an attitude of respect for her as a human, not for her distresses. I assumed that when the entire situation was taken into account, this woman was doing her best. Therapy proceeded well because I could separate Martha as a human being from her problems or distresses. Using a physical rehabilitation approach and a caring attitude, Martha regained complete independence with her self-care and decided it was time to begin exploring childhood trauma in psychotherapy.

## Belief in Our Clients' Innate Potential for Change and Growth

I worked with Alice for several months on an inpatient psychiatric unit. She was lethally suicidal (attempted to hang herself) as she recalled the trauma of sexual abuse in her early life. The team and I worked with her and were able to separate Alice from her distresses and problems. She was a very intelligent, witty, attractive young woman, yet she battled with irrational thoughts in her mind that she was no good and should die. We communicated our belief in Alice that she could face the trauma of her past and move on to a brighter future. With plenty of psychotherapy, occupational therapy, expressive therapy, and assistance from a social worker, Alice was able to reconstruct a new life. After discharge from a long hospitalization, she completed a bachelor's and a master's degree and worked as a victim's advocate for years before marrying and becoming a mother of two children.

Belief in our client's ability to recover is also an important attitude we bring to a caring relationship. Psychiatric rehabilitation literature, particularly the work of Anthony (1993), provides us with a compelling picture of the power of believing in our clients' with psychiatric challenges ability to recover. The recovery perspective, which assumes psychiatric clients can find new meaning and hope in their lives, can be used in physical rehabilitation as well.

It appears that many occupational therapy practitioners intuitively offer hope to their clients, even those with the most disabling conditions. The simple statement that we frequently use in occupational therapy, "You can," is a strong contradiction to the despair that many people with disabilities feel about their ability to regain function, occupation, meaning, and purpose in their lives. We may need to follow this statement with a reminder that it may take a great deal of work to achieve particular goals a client has identified. When we notice we are not feeling hopeful about a particular client with whom we are working, it is useful for us to seek supervision so we can explore any personal roadblocks to being hopeful about particular clients.

## Effective Communication

### Listening and Empathy

Claire worked on a general medical acute, inpatient unit. She introduced herself to her client, Robert, to let him know she would work with him in the afternoon. Robert perceived Claire's kind attention and began right then to talk about his situation. He was a chiropractor who had a son who had been in a car accident and needed extensive rehabilitation. Unable to find life worth living with his disability, his son committed suicide. Robert felt betrayed by his son and shameful that this could have happened to him, a man so knowledgeable about disability. He had never told anyone his son had killed himself prior to this moment with Claire. He cried heavily with Claire and she gently touched his shoulder and let him cry for a while. She thanked him for sharing his difficult story and said she would be back later. As she was leaving, a nurse came in and Robert said, "That is the best damn occupational therapist I have ever met."

Claire was able to listen not only to Robert's story but also to all of the emotions that accompanied it. She was able to know Robert in ways he had never shared with anyone before. Caring is a feeling and an attitude, yet it is also expressed through listening. One of the most profound actions that a practitioner may offer his or her clients is the gift of listening and paying attention so we can reach for the true knowing that Gilfoyle (1980) described.

As Schwartzberg (2002) suggested, the therapist's job is to facilitate the flow of communication and to validate the person as the meaning and the content come forth. If we return to Alice, my client who was lethally suicidal, over time, more and more of her traumatic experiences were shared with members of the intervention team who could listen to what she endured and to all of the emotions that accompanied those experiences, while validating her for surviving her childhood. As Isham (2006) stated, "Listening is an attitude of the heart, a genuine desire to be with another which both attracts and heals."

Empathy is closely linked to caring and is an important part of the listening process (Davis, 2006). Peloquin (2002, 2003) described empathy as a process of reaching for both the hands and the heart of our client. In doing so, we enter the experience of our clients through a communication partnership that is often deeply moving and inspiring. This partnership changes both the client and the therapist.

Claire will never forget her time with Robert, nor will I forget my time with Alice. Alice expressed deep grief, fear, and anger as her life story unfolded. I was able to listen to her well by allowing myself to enter her experience and shed a few tears of my own, as well as voice my own indignation at what had occurred while laughing with relief that it was all in the past. This level of empathy deepened the effectiveness of the occupational therapy process. Yet, as much as I allowed myself to enter Alice's experience as I listened to her, I was also able to remind both of us that the abuse was in the past and she had survived. Chapter 30, Effective Communication, provides the reader with a process for becoming an effective listener.

### Client-Centered Therapy and Empowerment

Janey, a 4-year-old girl at a center for children with disabilities, had hypoglossia-hypodactylia, which presented with the absence of hands and feet. She was a brilliant and determined little girl who was eager to participate in the world by using all kinds of utensils and craft tools. Bilateral activities were extra challenging for Janey, but 6 months into therapy, she expressed with vehemence that she really wanted to use scissors. With some trial and error, her occupational therapist, Marie, created a custom scissor block, with mounted spring-loaded scissors angled so gravity assisted in cutting. This scissor block enabled Janey to use one residual limb to stabilize the paper and the other to actively cut. When she saw the scissor block and tried it for the first time, Marie said, "She lit up like a Christmas tree." Despite being a shy girl, she proclaimed to everyone in her class, "Look at me, look at what I can do!" She wanted to cut paper grass for spring baskets for all eight of her peers.

Client-centered occupational therapy has been defined as "an approach to service that embraces a philosophy of respect for, and partnership with, people receiving services" (Law, Baptiste, & Mills, 1995, p. 253). Canadian occupational therapists have developed and disseminated seminal thinking about the nature of client-centered practice in occupational therapy. The key concepts of client-centered practice include the following (Law & Mills, 1998):

- Respect for clients
- Clients have the ultimate responsibility for decisions about occupations and occupational therapy
- Person-centered communication with an emphasis on provision of information
- Physical comfort and emotional support
- Facilitation of client participation in all aspects of occupational therapy
- Flexible and individualized occupational therapy service delivery
- Enabling clients to solve occupational performance issues
- A focus on the person-environment-occupation relationship

It would appear obvious that Marie engaged in client-centered occupational therapy that empowered Janey to achieve her goals. Tickle-Degnen (2002) described the client-centered relationship as involving the formation of two types of relationship bonding: a working alliance and rapport building. The working alliance is formed when clients and therapist collaborate with one another to develop common goals, and they develop a sense of shared responsibility for working on tasks that are involved in achieving those goals. In order for a practitioner to ascertain what a client's true concerns are and therefore be client centered, he or she must be able to first build rapport and then listen well enough to accurately know what these concerns are. Marie quickly bonded with Janey as they instantly took a great liking to one another. They saw each other 5 days a week for 2 years. The working alliance between them was strong because Marie was deeply respectful and listened well to Janey's wishes and goals, which besides using scissors included working with markers, feeding herself with a spoon, and learning to hang onto a swing independently.

As Jackins (1993) stated, "Happiness is the overcoming of obstacles on the way to a goal of one's own choosing" (p. 34). The more occupational therapy practitioners can truly listen to their clients to find out what their real goals and concerns are, the more they will be able to engage in client-centered occupational therapy that is satisfying to their clients. Not surprisingly, a number of studies have reported that client satisfaction does increase when therapists truly use a client-centered approach (Calnan et al., 1994; Henbest & Fehrsen, 1992; Wasserman, Inui, Barriatua, Carter, & Lippincott, 1984). However, as Maitra and Erway (2006) demonstrated, there is still a gap between occupational therapists' perception of their use of client-centered therapy and clients' perceptions of how involved they were in decisions about occupational therapy. As occupational therapy practitioners continue to refine their communication skills, client-centered therapy will be more readily achieved.

## Humor

Florence was attempting to get her client, Carla, who had mild mental retardation and depression, to increase her engagement in self-care and social activities in her residence. Carla was so unmotivated one day that she opened the door to allow Florence into her apartment, and then began walking back to her bedroom stating that she wasn't going to cook today, she was just going to lie down. Florence ran ahead of her and got in her bed before Carla could lie down. Carla laughed and said, "OK, what are we cooking today?"

Like Jody, Florence was able to convey her caring to Carla by using humor to break Carla's depressed state. Physician and clown Patch Adams stated that the greatest success in health care involves caring for others, and that fun is as important as love (Adams & Mylander, 1993). He found that humor contributes to the success of many professional and social relationships because we deepen connections when we laugh together. The therapeutic value of humor and laughter has been noted by many health professionals. Laughter increases the secretion of catecholamines and endorphins, natural chemicals in the brain that make people feel good. Laughter also enhances immune function by decreasing cortisol secretion. Although when we initially laugh our heart rate and blood pressure rise, as our arteries relax, both of these lower, resulting in a general relaxation response. After a hearty laugh, this therapeutic response can last up to 45 minutes (Adams & Mylander).

Adams and Mylander (1993) suggested that we all learn to cultivate our sense of humor by paying closer attention to what makes ourselves and those around us laugh. Workshops on humor and health care are well worth attending so we can learn to bring laughter to even the most trying and difficult situations we encounter as occupational therapists. Ultimately, we will enhance and deepen our relationships in occupational therapy by cultivating our own sense of humor.

## Values

At his mother's insistence, John, a young adult man with schizoaffective disorder, was receiving home health occupational therapy to increase his participation in daily routines and to work on becoming more independent. An initial interview using the Canadian Occupational Performance Measure revealed that the most important goal for John was going to the gym to increase his strength and endurance. His second most important goal was learning some social skills so he could make friends. Goals important to his mother, but less important to John, were learning to cook, managing his money, and finding an apartment. The second week into therapy, Florence, his occupational therapist, successfully assisted John in establishing a routine of working out at one of the local gyms three times a week. Other goals were eventually achieved as they became important to John.

Altruism, equality, freedom, justice, dignity, truth, and prudence are the core values of occupational therapy (AOTA, 1993), and they provide the foundation for a caring therapeutic relationship. In the case of John, Florence valued John's own freedom of choice regarding his engagement in occupation, and because of this, she was successful with him and client-centered therapy was achieved. Each core value of occupational therapy has significant implications for how we relate to our clients. The reader is referred to Chapter 40, Ethics and Its Application, for a review of the meaning of each of these values and is reminded of the commitment we make to upholding these values as occupational therapists.

### Touch

Marie works with children with severe developmental disabilities. One of the greatest aspects of her job is that she gets to be physically close with young people day in and day out while helping them become active participants in the world. They rely on her physical presence and caring touch for external support in order to explore textures, to activate switches connected to toys, to experience movement by bouncing on a ball or riding a horse, to be in water, or to use a paint brush or spoon. They experience great joy and exuberance with many of these occupations. Marie finds that there is a touch that is custodial such as wiping a mouth or nose, and then there is a whole other kind of touch that is affectionate, is playful, and facilitates experiencing the world. There is also touch that is comforting and consoling, and it is often more acceptable to give this kind of touch to young children.

As humans, we all need close physical contact. Young people instinctively seek out large amounts of physical closeness and touch. Infants often protest loudly when they are not held. It is only as we mature through childhood that we become resigned to less and less physical contact and loving touch. In adolescence, human closeness becomes less available and in many societies, it becomes sexualized. In the United States, the sexualization of closeness has resulted in increased homophobia or fear of closeness with someone of the same gender. The net result has been less physical closeness and touch for many people (D'Arc, 2003).

Despite some of the societal taboos on closeness, health care workers often have opportunities to use touch in thoughtful and caring ways as Marie described. Purtilo and Haddad (1996) speak of touching privileges that are granted to health professionals. Comforting touch, such as Claire touching Robert's shoulder, has particular legitimacy and may speak more loudly than the kindest words. Yet on the other hand, some health care professionals may provide only functional touching because of concerns about a client's misinterpretation of their touch. Guided by our ethics as a practitioner and paying close attention to the nonverbal and verbal communication of our clients, occupational therapists can determine what is appropriate therapeutic touch.

### Competence

Dom worked in a rehabilitation hospital with an elderly gentleman, William, who was recovering from a stroke. William was despondent and shut down. Doctors and therapists could not engage him in therapy routines. Aware of how withdrawn William was, Dom went into his room and got down on his knees near his bed and said, "I can hardly imagine how hard this is for you. I know it has been hard for you to want to participate in therapy. What did you enjoy doing in the past?" The gentleman mentioned that he used to enjoy reading and writing and that some of his poetry had been published. As Dom listened to William, he decided that he was going to the library to check-out his book. He brought it into work with him the next day and read to William one of his own poems about living life well.

Dom read the first few sentences and William recited the rest from memory. He closed the book with gratitude and said, "Thank you for reminding me that I want to live." He got up and began to engage in occupational therapy.

Many of the chapters in this text address the development of theoretical, technical, and practical competence in the delivery of occupational therapy services. As Devereaux (1984) pointed out, this is one of the most fundamental aspects of the occupational therapy relationship. Every client deserves an occupational therapy practitioner who is technically competent. In addition, every client also deserves a therapist who is competent in developing a therapeutic relationship. Dom's work with William beautifully demonstrates such competence.

Taylor (2008) developed an intentional relationship model to assist practitioners in refining their interpersonal competence with clients. She proposed that therapists tend to adopt a preferred mode of relating to and caring for their clients. These modes include advocating, collaborating, empathizing, encouraging, instructing, and problem solving. Although practitioners tend to have a preference for a particular mode, the most effective ones are able to shift modes in their practice. Nonpreferred modes can be developed and enhanced. In the example above, Dom exemplifies an encouraging mode with William. By reading some of William's own poetry about the value of life, Dom has encouraged William to move forward in his own life and in therapy. A full text on this model is in print and serves as an invaluable source to occupational therapists in refining and expanding their therapeutic use of self.

Cultural competence is also a critical ingredient in competent therapeutic use of self. Black (2005) found that much of the literature on cultural competence agrees that a culturally competent individual exhibits cultural self-awareness, knowledge of diverse groups, and skill in relating to diverse groups of people. Obviously, cultural competence is an ongoing process as health care providers continually learn new information about different cultures, so an open mind and willingness to learn is also essential. Chapter 2, Culture and Meaningful Occupations, more fully addresses cultural competence, and Chapter 30, Effective Communication, will guide the reader through a process of becoming a culturally sensitive communicator.

# Therapeutic Use of Self in Group Work

The most technically, culturally, and interpersonally competent occupational therapy practitioner—one who believes in the dignity and worth of the individual; believes in an innate potential for change and growth; who effectively communicates with caring, empathy, and good listening skills; who is client-centered; who is committed to the core values of occupational therapy; and who uses touch and humor therapeutically—may or may not be effective as a group leader. Although development of all of the aforementioned attitudes and skills will enhance therapeutic use of self as a group leader, some additional information needs to be imparted and a few more important skills need to be addressed, including the following:

- Understanding of group development
- Fostering mutual support
- Handling challenging group and individual behaviors

## Understanding Group Development

Groups often take on a life of their own, and group dynamics can be complex. A number of theorists have described group development, yet perhaps Tuckman's (1965) ideas are most well known. He identified four stages to group development, including forming, storming, norming, and performing. In the forming stage, group members are often somewhat anxious as they become acquainted with one another and become more clear about the nature and purpose of the group. They are often very dependent on the group leader. In the storming stage, conflict occurs as group members challenge the rules, expectations, tasks, and leadership of the group. During the norming stage, these conflicts are resolved and relationships deepen as the group learns to work together. The performing stage occurs when group members work together on mutually agreed-upon goals in a manner that is supportive and growth promoting.

Based on her work in leading groups primarily composed of women, Schiller (2003) constructed a relational model of group development that is somewhat different. The relational model has a stronger emphasis on the development of relationships within groups, and consequently, the stage of conflict is replaced by one of challenge and change. It includes the following stages:

- Pre-affiliation
- Establishing a relational base
- Mutuality and interpersonal empathy
- Challenge and change
- Separation

Similar to Tuckman's forming stage, in the pre-affiliation stage, group members are somewhat anxious and determining with who they can relate and be close. During the stage of establishing a relational base, group members seek out friendship and support and begin to share openly about themselves. During the phase of mutuality and interpersonal empathy, trust is deepened and group members take greater risks in sharing their experiences. Commonalities are noted and empathy for each other is experienced. The challenge and change stage occurs when group members feel safe enough with each other to challenge each other, yet at the same time, they maintain connections and relationships. The separation stage is identified as an important part of the overall group, and time is spent on reviewing both positive and challenging experiences in the group and saying goodbye. Schiller finds her model of group development occurs not only in groups that are all female but in groups that have both men and women in them when the leader adopts a relational perspective. The relational perspective intentionally fosters caring and connection between group members.

## Fostering Mutual Support

Occupational therapy practitioners may find some of the groups that they lead follow the relational model of group development and others follow Tuckman's model. This may have to do with the practitioner's leadership style, the focus of the group, or it may have to do with the membership of a particular group. Regardless, practitioners will be effective group leaders with many different kinds of groups when they can foster mutual support within their groups. In order to do this, the group leader or facilitator will need to model therapeutic use of self with each client in a group and, at the same time, support group members in relating to each other therapeutically as well. This will enable group members to play a profound role in empowering each other.

In order for clients in a group to play an empowerment role with each other, it is useful to establish group norms at the beginning of a group regarding confidentiality and respect. In addition, group members can be taught the importance of truly listening to each other without interrupting. A useful guideline for groups is that no one person is permitted to speak twice unless each person in the group has had a chance to speak once. It is the group leader's job to insure every voice is heard in a group. It is generally tedious for all group members when one group member tends to dominate with his or her ideas or experiences. A simple way to intervene in this situation is to simply thank the group member who is dominating for speaking and then asking what other group members think about a given subject. Giving each group member a particular amount of time to speak on a particular topic or experience can assist group members in truly getting to know each other and therefore develop empathy and support.

Supporting the leadership development of group members by giving them specific tasks and responsibilities will enhance group member empowerment as well. Group member tasks and responsibilities may include leading an opening circle or an icebreaker, sharing thoughts on a reading, or organizing clean-up or refreshments.

## Handling Challenging Group and Individual Behaviors

From time to time, challenging individual behaviors will develop in therapeutic interactions. This is typically transference and counter-transference. Transference is when one person (usually the client) places a role on another (usually the therapist). Counter-transference is when one person (usually the therapist) accepts the role that has been placed on him or her. Both are handled by reflection on the part of the therapist and limit setting when appropriate with the client (Schwartzberg, 2002).

There is much to learn about how to handle challenging group behaviors such as criticism or attacks toward the group leader or facilitator, group member conflict, the silent nonparticipating group member, the hostile group member, and other forms of disruptive behavior. Based on many years of leading a variety of groups, the following are good general guidelines for leading groups so that conflict is productive and empowerment of group members occurs:

- Whenever possible, involve the group in determining group norms
- Listen, listen, and listen to find out where people are coming from
- Be respectful of people but not of any negative patterns of behavior
- When a group member is very challenging, you can always ask the group to take a break or discuss a particular topic in pairs while you discuss with that person what you need from him or her in order for him or her to stay in your group
- When workable, use humor to assist in conflict resolution
- Do not assume that someone who appears not to be participating is not gaining things from your group
- Use work or discussion in pairs to foster new interconnections
- Allow a range of behaviors that are not disruptive or distracting
- Always remember as a group leader that you have the right to ask someone to leave your group if he or she is making it impossible for you to lead

The reader is referred to Cole's (2005) text, *Group Dynamics in Occupational Therapy*, and Howe and Schwartzberg's (1995) text, *A Functional Approach to Group Work in Occupational Therapy*, for an understanding of the theoretical underpinnings of group work in occupational therapy.

# Summary

Ultimately, in caring therapeutic relationships, we bring together our minds and our hearts. Every time we think about how to offer our assistance to our clients so their lives go better, we are caring for that individual. Much can be learned about how to enhance therapeutic use of self in occupational therapy by continually refining our technical, cultural, and interpersonal competence. In doing so, we need to recommit to the core values of occupational therapy and hold firm to our belief in the dignity and worth of the individual and to our belief in an innate potential for change and growth. We need to continually refine our use of empathy, touch, humor, and listening as important aspects of client-centered practice. The novice and experienced occupational therapy practitioner alike can expect to experience many successes and to make mistakes as they attempt to build rapport and a working alliance with their clients. As Gilfoyle (1980) suggested, skill in caring is achieved by continually assessing and reassessing our practice. Having opportunities to reflect on these experiences with supportive peers and/or a supervisor will prove invaluable in refining therapeutic use of self in occupational therapy.

# Student Self-Assessment

Use the following questions to either guide a discussion with a peer or to guide your thoughts in a journal regarding therapeutic use of self in occupational therapy.

1. Describe what caring means to you and how you will use caring in occupational therapy.
2. Can you respect someone even if you do not like him or her? What do you think of the Jackins (1993) quote, "Every single human being, when the entire situation is taken into account, has always, at every moment, done the very best that he or she could do, and so, deserves neither blame nor reproach from anyone, including self" (p. 3).
3. What will it be like to offer hope to your future occupational therapy clients? Are there some people you will find it difficult to be hopeful about? Has it been helpful to you when someone offered you his or her hope? If so, discuss this time.
4. Describe a time you noticed you felt empathy for someone or that someone felt empathy for you.
5. Have you ever been assisted in pursuing a goal of your own choosing? Describe what was and was not effective in this situation.
6. Pay attention to what makes you laugh and what makes other people laugh, and journal about this on a daily basis for 1 week. Do you have any new insights about humor from this exercise? How confident are you about using humor as an occupational therapist?
7. What is your own comfort level with touch? Describe how this varies in different situations.
8. In friendships, do you tend to be an encourager, empathizer, instructor, problem solver, advocate, or collaborator? Describe a situation when you functioned in one of these interpersonal modes.
9. Describe a time when you have interacted with someone from a different cultural group. Did you gain any new insights from this interaction? Once you know what your future clinical site will be, find out about the different ethnic populations served by your site and do some research to become better informed about those groups.
10. Describe how a group that you have participated in followed either Tuckman's or Schiller's model of group development.

**Evidence-Based Research Chart**

| Elements | Key Concepts | Evidence |
|---|---|---|
| Caring | Knowledge, skills, and attitude | Devereaux, 1984; Gilfoyle, 1980; King, 1980 |
| Respect | Belief in the dignity and worth of our clients | Devereaux, 1984 |
| Hope | Belief in the client's ability to change and grow | Anthony, 1993 |
| Effective communication | Empathy | Davis, 2006; Peloquin, 2002 |
| | Listening | Jackins, 1993; Schwartzberg, 2002; Taylor, 2008 |
| | Client-centered practice and empowerment | Calnan et al., 1994; Henbest & Fehrsen, 1992; Law, 1998; Law et al., 1995; Maitra & Erway, 2006; Tickle-Degnen, 2002; Wasserman et al., 1984 |
| Values | Altruism, equality, freedom, justice, dignity, truth, and prudence | AOTA, 1993 |
| Touch | Comforting and functional | Purtilo & Haddad, 1996 |
| Humor | Therapeutic effects | Adams & Mylander, 1993 |
| Competence | Cultural | Black, 2005; Wells & Black, 2000 |
| | Interpersonal | Taylor, 2008 |
| Group work | Group development | Cole, 2005; Howe & Schwarzberg, 1995; Schiller, 2003; Tuckman, 1965 |

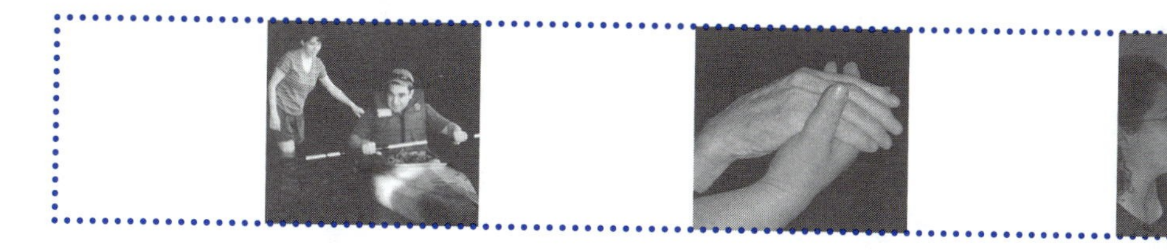

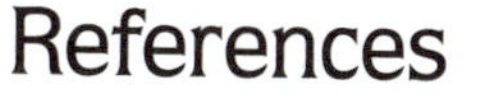

# References


Adams, P., & Mylander, M. (1993). *Gesundheit!: Bringing good health to you, the medical system, and society through physician service, complementary therapies, humor, and joy.* Rochester, VT: Healing Arts Press.

American Occupational Therapy Association. (1993). Core values and attitudes of occupational therapy practice. *American Journal of Occupational Therapy, 47,* 1085-1086.

Anthony, W. A. (1993). Recovery from mental illness: The guiding vision of the mental health service system in the 1990s. *Psychosocial Rehabilitation Journal, 16*(4), 11-23.

Black, R. M. (2005). Intersections of care: An analysis of culturally competent care, client-centered care, and the feminist ethic of care. *Work, 24*(4), 409-422.

Calnan, M., Katsouyiannopoulos, V., Ovcharov, V. K., Prokhorskas, R., Ramic, H., & Williams, S. (1994). Major determinants of consumer satisfaction with primary care in different health systems. *Family Practice, 11*(4), 468-478.

Cole, M. B. (2005). *Group dynamics in occupational therapy: The theoretical basis and practice application of group intervention* (3rd ed.). Thorofare, NJ: SLACK Incorporated.

Davis, C. M. (2006). *Patient practitioner interaction: An experiential manual for developing the art of health care* (4th ed.). Thorofare, NJ: SLACK Incorporated.

D'Arc J. (2003). *Allies to Gay/Lesbian/Bisexual/Transgendered Workshop.* A Re-evaluation Counseling workshop at China Lake, ME.

Devereaux, E. B. (1984). Occupational therapy's challenge: The caring relationship. *American Journal of Occupational Therapy, 38*(12), 791-798.

Gilfoyle, E. (1980). Caring: A philosophy for practice. *American Journal of Occupational Therapy, 34*(8), 517-521.

Henbest, R. J., & Fehrsen, G. S. (1992). Patient-centeredness: Is it applicable outside the West? Its measurement and effect on outcomes. *Family Practice, 9,* 311-317.

Howe, M. C., & Schwartzberg, S. L. (1995). *A functional approach to group work in occupational therapy* (3rd sub ed.). Philadelphia, PA: JP Lippincott.

Jackins, H. (1993). *Quotes* (2nd ed.). Seattle, WA: Rational Island Publishers.

Isham, J. (2006). Quotes of the heart. Retrieved August 3, 2006, from http://www.heartquotes.net/Listening.html

King, L. J. (1980). Creative caring. *American journal of Occupational Therapy, 34*(8), 522-528.

Law, M., Baptiste, S., & Mills, J. (1995). Client-centered practice: What does it mean and does it make a difference? *Canadian Journal of Occupational Therapy, 62*(5), 250-257.

Law, M. & Mills, J. (1998). Client-centered occupational therapy. In M. Law (Ed.), *Client-centered occupational therapy* (pp. 1-18). Thorofare, NJ: SLACK Incorporated.

Maitra, K. K., & Erway, F. (2006). Perception of client-centered practice in occupational therapists and their clients. *American Journal of Occupational Therapy, 60*(3), 298-310.

Peloquin, S. M. (2002). Reclaiming the vision of reaching for heart as well as hands. *American Journal of Occupational Therapy, 56*(5), 517-526.

Peloquin, S. M. (2003). The therapeutic relationship: Manifestations and challenges in occupational therapy. In E. B. Crepeau, E. S. Cohn, & B.A. Boyt Schell (Eds.), *Willard & Spackman's occupational therapy* (10 ed., pp. 157-170). Philadelphia, PA: Lippincott Williams & Wilkins.

Purtilo, R. B., & Haddad, A. M. (1996). *Health professional and patient interaction* (5th ed.). Philadelphia, PA: W.B. Saunders Co.

Schiller, L. Y. (2003). Women's group development from a relational model and a new look at facilitator influence on the group. In M. B. Cohen & A. Mullender (Eds.), *Gender and groupwork* (pp. 16-40). London, England: Routledge.

Schwartzberg, S. L. (2002). *Interactive reasoning in the practice of occupational therapy.* Upper Saddle River, NJ: Prentice Hall.

Taylor, R. R. (2008). *The intentional relationship: Occupational therapy and use of self.* Philadelphia, PA: F.A. Davis.

Tickle-Degnen, L. (2002). Evidence-based practice forum: Client-centered practice, therapeutic relationship, and the use of research evidence. *American Journal of Occupational Therapy, 56,* 470-474.

Tuckman, B. W. (1965). Developmental sequence in small groups. *Psychological Bulletin, 63*(6), 384-399.

Wasserman, R. C., Inui, T. S., Barriatua, R. D., Carter, W. B., & Lippincott, P. (1984). Pediatric clinician's support for parents makes a difference: An outcome-based analysis of clinician-parent interaction. *Pediatrics, 74*(6), 1047-1053.

Wells, S. A., & Black, R. M. (2000). *Cultural competency for health professionals.* Bethesda, MD: AOTA Press.

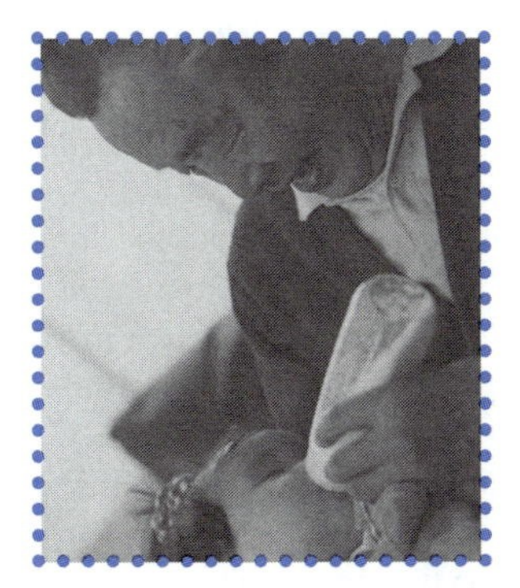

# Case Management and Coordination

*Diane P. Bergey, MOT, OTR/L and Erica A. Flagg, OT*

**ACOTE Standard Explored in This Chapter**

B.5.7

**Key Terms**

| | |
|---|---|
| Care coordination | Managed care |
| Case management | Transition services |
| Clinical pathway | |

## Introduction

The role of the occupational therapist in care coordination, case management, and transition services is not only an area of emerging practice but is already a role occupational therapists are filling in traditional practice environments. With our education, we are prepared to fill case management roles, utilizing our skills well and meeting the demands of society and our clients effectively. In order to be marketable in an environment highly influenced by managed care, it is important to realize case management as a career option.

## What Is Case Management?

The Case Management Society of America (CMSA) defines case management as:

> A collaborative process that assesses, plans, implements, coordinates, monitors, and evaluates the options and services required to meet the client's health and human services needs. It is characterized by advocacy, communication, and resource management, and promotes quality and cost-effective interventions and outcomes (Blass & Reed, 2003, p. 81).

Case management being a practice area and not a profession allows practitioners from a variety of disciplines and work settings to enter the field. For decades, health care organizations have used case managers to manage resources and reduce costs. This trend in managed care has only increased in recent years. Van Deusen (1995) stated that managed care is here to stay; as such, the issue is how occupational therapists can function effectively within this system. Case managers are utilized in numerous settings, including traditional health care settings as well as educational programming and community health services. Lohman (1999) proposed that occupational therapy be "proactive" in the current health care environment and take on nontraditional roles, such as case manager.

The term *case manager* is a title; *care coordination* is the function. Care coordination entails looking at the big picture, assessing needs and goals, identifying resources, and efficiently coordinating services to best meet the client's needs. The case manager's support and coordination facilitates and sustains movement through the health care system toward optimal health. An individual's health



K. Sladyk, K. Jacobs, & N. MacRae (Eds.).
*Occupational Therapy Essentials for Clinical Competence* (pp. 255-262).

care needs often change based on a variety of factors, including nature of condition, age, availability of services, environmental factors, and individual choices. As the single point of entry, the case manager will coordinate care and facilitate transitions. Transition services are an integral part of case management. For instance, per the Individuals With Disabilities Education Act (IDEA) 2004, a student with an identified disability will receive services through the school system until graduation. This individual will then require transition services that are vocational, residential, and life-skill based. Additionally, a person with a hip replacement will first require acute services in a hospital for stabilization, possible transfer to a skilled facility, and home health services. Each example benefits from the skills of a case manager to assure a smooth transition.

## How Is Managed Care Affecting Case Management?

"The purpose of managed care is to provide affordable, quality health care with functional outcomes in a reasonable time frame. Access, quality, cost, and satisfaction are the usual goals that exist in health care" (Pope, 1995, p. 110). Case management and managed care are not synonymous. Trends in health care reflect the need for continued and creative resource management, which is driven by managed care. Case managers provide a vehicle to reach these goals. The demand for case management services is likely to increase given limited financial and human resources. We are living in a society that is aging, clients are returning home after shorter acute in-client stays, people are living longer with chronic conditions (Markle, 2004), and more children are being identified with persistent medical conditions. With these demands on our system, limited resources are available, necessitating cost efficiency and streamlining of services. Even though insurers use case management to obtain timely cost-effective outcomes, we need to stress the importance of doing this in a positive way to meet the client's needs (Fricke, 2006). Most importantly, we are there to improve quality of life for the client and family by continued assessment and evaluation. To summarize, managed care is creating a need for case managers, but there is a shortage of nurses who often act as case managers. This should encourage more allied health professionals to enter the practice area of case management (Baldwin, 2005).

## Why Is Case Management an Appropriate Role for Occupational Therapists?

Occupational therapy is the only discipline with the sole focus of understanding function. We evaluate occupational performance, routines, and volition as these factors interact with the client's environment. Our training provides us with strong human interaction skills, knowledge of occupational performance, and the ability to see the "big picture." Occupational therapists are a "tremendous untapped talent in terms of case management" (Hettinger, 1996).

There are clear parallels between the criteria for case management and the *Standards of Practice for Occupational Therapy*. Thurkettle & Noji (2003) described case management as a process consisting of assessing, planning, implementing, coordinating, monitoring, and evaluating. These six functions are dependent upon effective communication skills. The case manager must communicate with a number of people, including the client, family members, service providers, vendors, insurance companies, and employers.

As illustrated in Table 23-1, educational standards prepare entry-level occupational therapists to take on case management roles.

**Table 23-1. Comparison of Case Manager Functions and Standards of Practice**

| **Case Manager Functions** (Thurkettle & Noji, 2003) | **Standards of Practice for Occupational Therapy** (American Occupational Therapy Association [AOTA], 2005) |
|---|---|
| *Assessment*: Gathers, compares, and evaluates information from various sources to determine client needs. | *Standard II—Screening, Evaluation, Re-evaluation*: Occupational therapists collaborate with the client and support providers to assess ability to participate in daily occupations in their context. |
| *Planning*: Develops plan based on assessment and case management needs. | *Standard III—Intervention*: Develops intervention based on evaluation goals, evidence, and clinical reasoning. |
| *Implementation*: Provides client with options to make intervention choices. | *Standard II—Intervention*: Implements plan based on client goals and current best evidence. |
| *Coordination*: Organizing and supporting services to meet goals and monitor progress. | *Standard III—Intervention*: Networking with appropriate others to establish progress toward goals, including safety, benefits, and risks. |
| *Monitoring*: Assessment of client adherence, achievement of goals, and progress. | *Standard IV—Outcomes*: Monitoring expected or achieved outcomes. |
| *Evaluation*: Evaluates desired outcomes and cost effectiveness. | *Standard IV—Outcomes*: Determine and document changes in performance, capacities and need to discontinue services, achieved goals and reached maximum benefit, and client motivation. |

The specific qualities that have supported excellence in occupational therapy will also foster competency as a case manager. The occupational therapy perspective considers meaning in context of the client's condition and environment. The client's medical, spiritual, and psychosocial needs are holistically considered. Consideration of all contexts and participants is essential, both in occupational therapy and case management. All factors, including family interaction, environment, and response to illness and intervention measures, are critical when determining a person's ability to engage in meaningful occupations.

Occupational therapists often consider factors missed by other disciplines. "In the case management role, occupational therapists can help to facilitate a continuum of care from the acute setting to the community by developing clinical pathways that include the whole episode of care that emphasize functional status" (Lohman, 1999, p. 112). Additionally, other professionals may focus more on symptomatic relief and less on functional outcomes. For example, a particular individual with a lower limb amputation may be more functional utilizing a wheelchair rather than being fitted for a prosthetic. In the school system, the push to focus on proper grip and handwriting is not appropriate for all. Some students are better served by technology, meeting needs with the use of a keyboard, saving energy, and achieving success in the academic environment.

Clinical pathways are an essential function of care coordination. Occupational therapists acting as case managers can incorporate their knowledge about work, play, daily activities, disability, and environment into realistic clinical pathways. Accurate assessment is critical in the application of reasonable clinical pathways. Our assessment tools are geared toward understanding occupational impact and will possibly lead to better intervention planning.

Any case manager coordinating the care of a client is concerned with the functional level of the person in these areas (activities of daily living, ADL). The skills that case managers need are an understanding of the injury or illness, ability to act as lifespan coordinator (i.e., being able to project future care and responsibilities of the person who is ill or injured), knowledge of costs for specific health care procedures and intervention, and understanding of clinical pathways (Fisher, 1996). Consequently, better quality of care emerges.

The basic tenets of occupational therapy have long focused on person-centered planning and care. It is the occupational therapist's intention to assure each individual is able to meet personally chosen goals. "The client/patient is an active partner in care, sharing risk for the impact of choices on quality of life, functional ability, and subsequent income generation" (Thurkettle & Noji, 2003, p. 90). At times, goals are set without input of the individual and are based on assumptions of need. Occupational therapy embraces education as a vital step in including the client in the decision-making process. Clients are provided with information that allows decisions reflective of possible consequences and risks. In order to remain person centered, it is important to empower the client, educating them about their disease process and giving them a larger voice in their care delivery and more personalized attention to their needs (Mullahy, 1998).

Occupational therapy's holistic nature allows us to get a broader picture and supports person-centered planning. Our view of the environment does not focus solely on the physical environment. It also considers the sensory environment, recognizing the fact that we all must function within larger systems. There are a number of factors that must be considered in care coordination. Awareness of cultural differences; medical, spiritual, and psychosocial needs; unique gender and role beliefs; and generational norms are essential to person-centered planning. Our holistic view recognizes that we affect change by addressing individual factors as well as the broader system. For instance, when working within the school system, it may be necessary to educate direct care staff, educational technicians, special staff, teachers, and administrators in order to achieve good outcomes. In order to support the student, all team members must be working toward a common goal. The holistic focus of occupational therapy allows for case management to occur in the most supportive environment. Although specific clinical pathways are prescribed, it is always necessary to take into consideration the unique characteristics of the individual case that may influence the norm and the success of the plan. Fricke (2006) asserted that the client still remains the priority in an environment of resource management. Within the current system, which demands cost effectiveness, the client's needs must be considered foremost.

# Barriers to Case Management

The realm of case management is an exciting area of potential growth for occupational therapists. However, breaking into a new niche can have its challenges. To be best prepared to meet challenges, it is important for occupational therapists to be aware of the potential barriers that may be encountered.

Occupational therapy programs are currently providing a good base of education to prepare new therapists for the specialty practice area of case management. However, therapists are likely to find that there will be skills that need to be developed in order for therapists to be proficient as case managers. As an occupational therapist enters the realm of case management, weaker skills will become more apparent. Once need areas are determined, further education, networking, or exploration can occur. The need areas will be highly dependent on the setting, client base, community resources, etc. Lohman (1999) noted that in her experience as a "participant observer of case management" in an acute care setting, she found she did not have all of the medical background necessary to be an effective case manager in that particular context. However, through networking with other professionals and reading current journals and textbooks, she was able to gain a better understanding of pertinent issues. She noted that it was important to understand the medical chart using a functional perspective. This observation is likely to be consistent across many settings. She also noted that advanced training or continuing education addressing the specifics of case management such as the development of multidisciplinary clinical pathways and economic aspects of interventions would be beneficial (Lohman).

Also significant is the current shortage of resources for case managers. For example, there are more nonprofessionals involved in the carry-through of care for our consumers (i.e., personal care assistants, nursing technicians, and other paraprofessionals) (Boling & Hoffman, 2001). Paraprofessionals and family members are commonly used now in order to control costs. However, with this trend, more oversight is necessary to assure good care for our clients. "...case managers must become an even stronger link along the care continuum to oversee the efficient implementation of intervention plans and, at the same time, become instrumental in developing innovative solutions to fill those care gaps already emerging" (Boling & Hoffman, p. 54). Family support and community programming are essential to good outcomes.

Case management positions have traditionally been held by social workers and nurses. At this time, there is a shortage of nurses, which will inevitably affect the provision of case management services. If occupational therapists choose to fill these roles effectively, they are likely to have to prove themselves. As outsiders, the challenge is to demonstrate the ability to fill these roles well. Tensions regarding boundaries can be overcome with good interdisciplinary communication. Communication can be enhanced with an understanding of each profession's educational background, values, roles, norms, and thinking differences (Lohman, 1999). An effective interdisciplinary team requires solid communication skills, the ability to resolve conflict, and respect for each team member's role. Occupational therapists as case managers must be willing to collaborate with those better equipped to address their client's particular needs. Seeking the assistance of other professionals will lead to better care, as well as increased respect from one's peers. Through effective case management, turf barriers should eventually dissolve. "Effective case managers understand the organization's informal political system. They have good communication skills, show a willingness to do a fair workload, respect differences, and have good conflict resolution and negotiating skills" (Lohman, p. 112).

Barriers to effective care coordination include the following (American Academy of Pediatrics, 2005; Boling & Hoffman, 2001):

- Lack of knowledge: chronic conditions, resources, or the coordination process
- Lack of effective communication
- Poor team building
- Lack of clearly defined roles
- Insufficient acknowledgment for amount of time/work spent
- Inadequate reimbursement
- Lack of an organized system
- Language/cultural barriers
- Decreased client education
- Increased percentage of clinical complications
- Increased nursing/medical error rates
- Decreased client satisfaction
- Decreased clinical outcomes

## How to Become a Certified Case Manager

Case management is a practice area, not a profession. Presently, there are no accredited degree programs specifically for case management. In fact, a comprehensive literature review completed by Baldwin (2005) determined that there are no official guidelines regarding educational standards or training. More often, case managers receive on-the-job training through employee training, supervision, and team meetings. Since its inception, case management has evolved as a multidisciplinary specialty practice with the case manager position filled by those trained in a variety of health care disciplines, including nursing, social work, and rehabilitation counseling. "The Case Management Society of America (CMSA), through the development of its core curriculum for case managers, recently established the first national, standardized, basic knowledge and skill set for case managers" (Boling & Hoffman, 2001, p. 54). The opportunity for certification should allow qualified health care professionals from a variety of disciplines to enter the field.

In the absence of a degree program in case management, one can now become a certified case manager (CCM). The CCM designation is offered through the Commission for Case Manager Certification (1996). Certification is a voluntary process. The credentialing process is described below. One must do the following:

- Be registered as an occupational therapist in good standing with the National Board for Certification in Occupational Therapy (NBCOT) and one's state licensure board. License or certification must be based on a post-secondary program in a field that promotes the physical, psychosocial, or vocational well-being of the persons being served.
- Show documented employment experience as a case manager or as a supervisor of case management services. There are three categories of acceptable employment based on time frames for employment

and amount of supervision provided by either a CCM or noncertified case manager:

- *Category 1*: 12 months of full-time employment under the supervision of a CCM
- *Category 2*: 24 months of employment as a case manager, with no requirements for supervision
- *Category 3*: A minimum of 12 months directing case management services

- Use the six essential case management activities of assessment, planning, implementation, coordination, monitoring, and evaluation to five core practice components, as documented in one's job description.
- Pass a certification examination that covers the five core practice components of coordination and service delivery, physical and psychological factors, benefit systems and cost benefit analysis, case-management concepts, and community resources.
- Display good moral character and reputation.
- Be independently licensed and able to practice without the supervision of another licensed professional, performing the six functions of a case manager as indicated above.

Once one becomes a case manager, either certified or noncertified, it is important to remain current. CMSA hosts professional conferences that provide case managers the opportunity to maintain professional licensure and credentials through continuing education. Training that pertains to a case manager's specific client population is also available to remain current.

# Applications

Case manager skills parallel those used by therapists in all settings. Occupational therapists use the skills of case management for best practice in daily decision making, therapeutic intervention, collaboration, and transition planning. Currently, occupational therapists fill essential roles as team members, providing direct service as need presents. They provide information on baseline functioning, work collaboratively with the team, and support the care plan with the ultimate goal of discharge from service. Insurance companies, including workman's compensation and return-to-work programs, depend on occupational therapy to provide the information for planning and coverage.

> Occupational therapy practitioners understand productive living. They understand job analysis, job accommodations, and many of the issues facing injured workers. Because of this knowledge and their background in the psychosocial sciences, occupational therapists are a natural possibility as case managers for the worker's compensation population...understanding a variety of occupations and skills necessary to do certain jobs is an advantage to case management in this area as is understanding specific task modifications and job accommodations (Fisher, 1996, p. 453).

Less traditionally, occupational therapists can act as case managers, making valuable contributions in high-risk communities, community-based health centers located in schools, churches, day care centers, or other population centers (Thurkettle & Noji, 2003). Occupational therapists are also qualified to work directly with these companies as case managers.

Occupational therapists have a unique perspective on functioning, viewing the whole system and the person within their context. They are a valuable asset to case management because of their understanding of all of the vital components. Occupational therapists are unique because their education includes the intensive study of all of the vital components of human functioning, recognizing how the interrelationships of the components affect well-being and quality of life (Hafez & Brockman, 1998).

Occupational therapists' education addresses physical and lifestyle factors and their application in the complex task of helping a client continue to live a meaningful and purposeful life. Occupational therapists are likely to be the only professionals analyzing all factors influencing a client to determine how to build supports that are truly compatible. Good case management is achieved through a team process. The cornerstone of a healthy team process must be consumer driven and all parts must be well matched. For instance, a vocational rehabilitation counselor might select a job coach based on availability and not compatibility. If the client required motor-based modeling and demonstration to learn tasks but was paired with a coach who used an extensive verbal cueing system, success would be diminished. It is the ability of an occupational therapist to analyze each component of support that increases the potential for success.

One way occupational therapists coordinate services can be exemplified by the community-based practice of Linda Learnard in rural Maine. Occupational Therapy Consultation and Rehabilitation Services (OTCRS) coordinates care through consultation. Although not labeled case management, the services provided directly impact the intervention plan, thus driving care coordination. The functional occupational therapy assessment completed by OTCRS provides recommendations for the client based on the client's occupational capabilities and areas of needs. Clear identification of strengths and weaknesses in the areas of sensory processing, perceptual abilities, and cognitive learning style allows the team to use the dynamic process in a truly client-centered approach. The functional assessment includes recommendations for the system, for the environment, and for individual skill building. This format reflects an all-inclusive view of a person's functioning. The following illustrates how this process unfolds.

An occupational therapist would be called in when an individual was not functioning effectively in his or her environment. For instance, a resident with unhealthy eating habits, aggression, and poor hygiene is at risk of losing placement. The first step in working with this individual would be to complete a functional assessment. Next, feedback involving the individual and the team would be provided. Through this feedback and the process of collaboration, an intervention plan is developed. This intervention plan needs to address how the system will assist this person, what skill building needs to occur, and how the environment can be set up to facilitate individual growth and functioning. After the completion of a thorough functional evaluation, a number of strategies to address the resident's clinical needs can be determined. For instance, the individual may require more joint compression to calm the nervous system and minimize aggression. It would be important to work with the direct care providers to find appropriate activities to increase deep pressure, weight bearing, and heavy muscle work. The case manager may want to make a referral to vocational rehabilitation services to match this person with an appropriate job with physical components. This would be in addition to helping the individual develop and use strategies to reduce arousal level and minimize aggressive outbursts. In this example, the occupational therapist did not assume the role of case manager but as a consultant helped to direct the provision of services.

Another example of case management's effectiveness can be seen in coordinating transition services for a young person "aging out" of high school or foster care. This is an appropriate role for an occupational therapist whose expertise in human development facilitates the client's transition from childhood/adolescence occupational roles to those of a young adult.

Ms. Learnard also acts as a clinical consultant as part of her practice. For example, on a regular basis, a review of intervention plans is conducted for individuals with mental illness and/or mental retardation who attend a community-based day program. Her care plan, created from information supplied by direct support providers, is used to guide intervention until her next visit, at which time adjustments are made to the plan to address new or different needs. This plan provides specific guidelines that drive the direct support for provider's interventions. The plan also provides a means for documentation and a crisis intervention plan. Team collaboration may reveal the need to bring in additional professionals to address goals and support function.

The goal of case management is to manage limited resources. A means of reaching this goal is to provide comprehensive training to address functional needs. If we provide functionally based training with the intent of teaching direct care providers how to better support their clients, we will be supporting more efficient use of resources. For example, a referral for a behaviorally disregulated client would require functional assessment. Assessment may determine that, in order to support the least restrictive living environment, additional one-on-one staffing was needed. By providing a structured routine full of motor-based activities, the client was able to remain calm and organized. For this routine and interventions to truly be supportive, proper training would need to be provided to direct service providers. This training would identify the needs of persons with sensory defensiveness, detail his learning style, and describe sensory interventions and how to structure the environment. With effective services, the individual no longer required emergency room visits, no longer was being incarcerated, and no longer was eloping and putting himself and others at risk.

Occupational therapists are able to look at the big picture using a systems approach to drive services in an effective manner. The examples above detailed how case management can be applied in both traditional settings and in emerging practice areas. Although these are only a few examples, many opportunities exist in our practice. Three important differences between a traditional case manager and an occupational therapist as a case manager are as follows:

1. Our ability to understand functional abilities needed to match the person to the task.
2. Our occupational analysis skills, which allow us to adapt and be creative with support systems and solutions.
3. Our ability to guide support providers to facilitate effective interventions.

## Summary

Understanding the clear connections between the skills of a case manager and the skills of an occupational therapist magnifies the many opportunities that exist. Occupational therapists can use these skills in roles specifically designated as "case manager." There are also alternative applications that may not carry the title but have the same end result. Occupational therapists can be part of care coordination, transition services, management of resources, and good outcomes in any role that they fill. Good case management demands excellent communication with the client and the interdisciplinary team. It requires comprehensive knowledge of available human, financial, and community-based resources and an ability to use these in the most cost-effective manner. Flexibility and ability to adjust the plan based on the client's functional level and changing goals is vital. Occupational therapists only add to these general principles, bringing a truly holistic view of the client and their context.

## Student Self Assessment

1. Using a local newspaper, find a position that requires case management services. Determine the needs of the target population and, using the unique skills of occupational therapy, demonstrate how our solutions to any problems would differ from those offered by a different profession, such as social work.

| Evidence-Based Research Chart | |
|---|---|
| **Issue** | **Evidence** |
| Impact of managed care on case management | Baldwin, 2005; Fricke, 2006; Markle, 2004; Pope, 1995 |
| Occupational therapy attributes that are a match for case management | Fisher, 1996; Hettinger, 1996; Lohman, 1999; Mullahy, 1998; Thurkettle & Noji, 2003 |
| Understanding barriers to case management | Boling & Hoffman, 2001; Lohman, 1999 |
| Case management outcomes | Allison, 2004; Blass & Reed, 2003; Lohman, 1999; Van Deusen, 1995 |

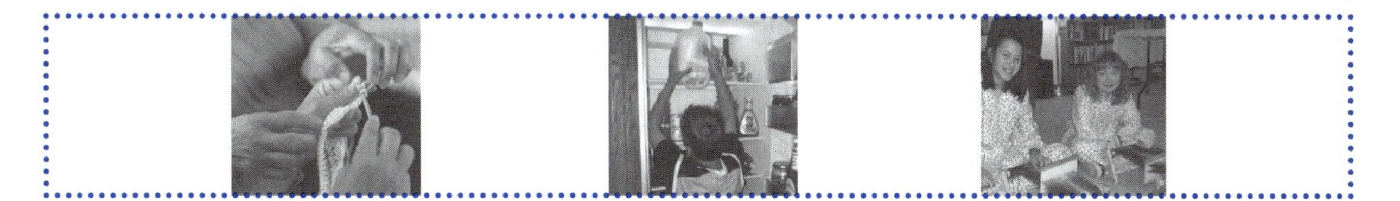

2. List three non-traditional populations who might benefit from case management services provided by an occupational therapist. What other title might an occupational therapist function under to influence the plan of care?
3. In your own words, explain what occupational therapy can bring to case management that other professions cannot.

# Electronic Resource

- Case Management Society of America: www.cmsa.org

# References


Allison, L. (2004). Evidence-based practice as tool for case management. *The Case Manager, 15*(5), 62-65.

American Academy of Pediatrics. (2005). Policy statement: Care coordination in the medical home: Integrating health and related systems of care for children with special health care needs. *Pediatrics, 116*(5), 1238-1244.

American Occupational Therapy Association. (2005). Standards of practice for occupational therapy. *American Journal of Occupational Therapy, 59*(6), 663-665.

Baldwin, T. M. (2005). Case management: Entry level practice for occupational therapists? *The Case Manager, 16*(4), 47-51.

Blass, T. C., & Reed, T. L. (2003). Consider case management. *Nursing Management, 34*(10), 81-83.

Boling, J., & Hoffman, L. (2001). The nursing shortage and its implications for case management. *The Case Manager, 12*(6), 53-57.

Commission for Case Management Certification. (1996). *CMM certification guide*. Rolling Meadow, IL: Author.

Fisher, T. (1996). Roles and functions of a case manager. *American Journal of Occupational Therapy, 50*(6), 452-454.

Fricke, K. (2006). Client centered case management in today's health care. *Lippincott's Case Management, 11*(12), 112-114.

Hafez, A., & Brockman, S. (1998). Occupational therapists: Essential team members as service providers and case managers. *Journal of Care Management, 4*(2), 10-20.

Hettinger, J. (1996). Case management: Do OTs have what it takes? Yes! *OT Week, 10*, 12-14.

Lohman, H. (1999). What will it take for more occupational therapists to become case manager? Implications for education, practice and policy. *American Journal of Occupational Therapy, 53*(1), 111-113.

Markle, A. (2004). The economic impact of case management. *The Case Manager, 15*(4), 54-58.

Mullahy, C. (1998). *The case manager's handbook* (2nd ed.). Gaithersburg, MD: Aspen.

Pope, T. (1995). Case managers help define managed care. *Case Manager, 6*(4), 109-114.

Thurkettle, M., & Noji, A. (2003). Case management: A source of support and stability for the client and the health care system. *Lippincott's Case Management, 8*(2), 88-94.

Van Deusen, J. (1995). What is the role of the occupational therapist in managed care? *American Journal of Occupational Therapy, 49*(8), 833-834.

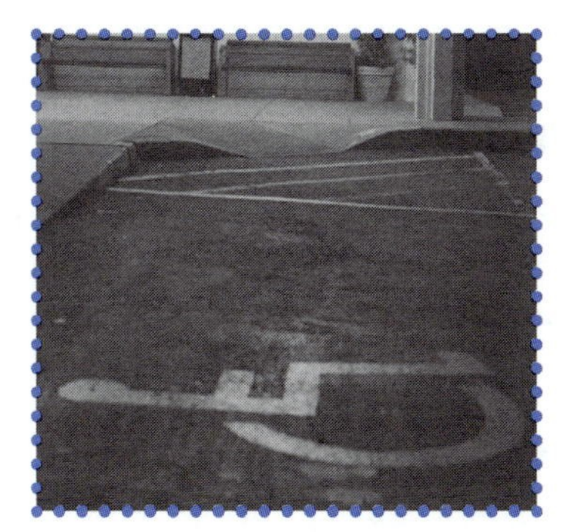

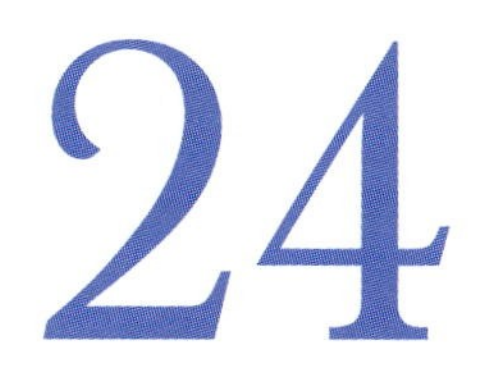

# 24

# ENVIRONMENTAL ADAPTATION AND ERGONOMICS

*William R. Croninger, MA, OTR/L; John E. Lane, Jr., OTR/L; and Betsy DeBrakeleer, COTA/L, ROH*

**ACOTE Standards Explored in This Chapter**

B.5.8, 5.20

**Key Terms**

Americans With Disabilities Act (ADA)
AbleData
Ergonomics
Human factors engineering
Universal design

## Introduction

The role of the occupational therapy practitioner is to consider the client's occupational performance in the environment in which is it performed. Environmental adaptation has as its goal the modification of the client's environment to maximize participation in his or her occupational roles. It is an attempt, then, to modify the environment to match the abilities of the client rather than expecting an individual to meet the demands of the environment. In assessing an environment, regardless of whether it is home, work, school, or community, it is desirable to organize around the following tasks:

- Movement to a site (e.g., public or private transportation)
- Access to the structures or areas (e.g., parking, entering and exiting a building)
- Movement within common areas (e.g., foyers, halls, cafeteria/kitchen, bathroom)
- Tasks specific to each activity area (e.g., dressing, bathing, word processing, fabrication, note taking, shopping)

An additional point to remember is that the environment may be appropriate, but the activities, processes, or procedures within task areas may lead to injury secondary to repetition or strain.

## Transportation

### Public Transportation

The Americans With Disabilities Act (ADA) of 1990 prohibits discrimination against individuals with disabilities in the area of public transportation. As with all elements of the Act, this section continues to be upgraded and modified. The ultimate goal, however, remains the provision of access to "basic mobility" for all individuals with disabilities.



K. Sladyk, K. Jacobs, & N. MacRae (Eds.).
*Occupational Therapy Essentials for Clinical Competence* (pp. 263-270).

## Private Transportation

Private transportation is access to and the independent operation of motor vehicles. Public transportation assumes an individual with a disability needs only to access a conveyance. Private transportation can place greater demands on your client if he or she is expected to also be the vehicle operator. The client must then be able to enter and exit the vehicle unassisted, store and access necessary mobility devices, and safely operate the vehicle.

A standard-sized automobile may well be sufficient in situations where the client can transfer to and from the vehicle unassisted. Vehicles with sufficient room behind the front seat can be appropriate when a client has the strength and balance to stow a wheelchair or other devices there independently. When the weight of the mobility aid becomes prohibitive or an individual does not have the strength to load a wheelchair, car-top mounted power lifts are available.

In situations where independent transfers are impossible or not inappropriate, a van can become the best solution. Vans may be modified to allow entrance and exit via power lift or ramp.

Independent operation of the vehicle requires the ability to access controls such as the ignition and accelerator, to control the direction of travel, and to be able to stop. Modifications may entail mechanical assists to lessen the force needed to use traditional controls such as steering wheel, accelerator, or brake. However, adaptations using nontraditional controls, such as hand accelerators, also exist.

## Site Accessibility

Once the client arrives at a destination, access to the structure or area becomes the next potential challenge. If arriving in a personal vehicle, the initial challenge will be parking and egress, followed by movement through common areas, and finally, passage through doorways or openings.

- *Parking places*: The ADA specifies the number of parking places that must be accessible. Additionally, there are regulations that specify the number of these spaces that must be larger to accommodate van access.
- *Walkways*: The ADA requires at least one "accessible route" be provided that allows an individual access to and between all accessible areas.
- *Entry doors*: The following section provides guidance on the ADA regulations as they apply to the width, handle type, and force required in constructing doors in accessible structures.

### Ramps

One common means of providing access to a private or public structure is via ramps. A ramp for a public structure will have to meet state and local codes. Ramps for a private residence may or may not be covered by a local code. Quite often, family, friends, or a civic organization may want to assist the client with construction.

The most common specification encountered for determining how long to make a ramp is the ratio 1:12, which translates to 12 inches in length for every 1 inch the ramp must rise. Note that this ratio is the maximum angle allowed. When possible, it will be desirable to make the ramp longer to place less stress on the person propelling the chair, whether it is a client or a caregiver.

Wheelchair ramps are commonly built over concrete posts, which must be constructed so they extend lower than the normal frost line found in the area. This procedure, although necessary when using concrete posts to support the ramp's uprights, greatly increases the cost and difficulty of construction.

Information on a clever alternative method of supporting uprights can be found at:

Minnesota Center for Independent Living (MCIL)
600 University Ave, St. Paul, MN 55104-3825

The Handyman's Club of America published the original article on the ramp in Figure 24-1. In this method, the uprights sit on 12" x 12" plates. The plates are standard treated 3/4" thick plywood. The entire deck "floats" with the thawing and freezing of the underlying ground.

The method utilized in the ramp in Figure 24-2 has the added advantage of being modular—it can be fabricated off site and later assembled at the residence. It can also be taken apart and reused in the future.

## Common Area Access

Common areas can be thought of as areas within a structure that a client will need to navigate or utilize. This might include hallways, a cafeteria, bathrooms, as well as utilization of devices such as a drinking fountain. Guidance for the acceptable dimensions and location can be found under Electronic Resources.

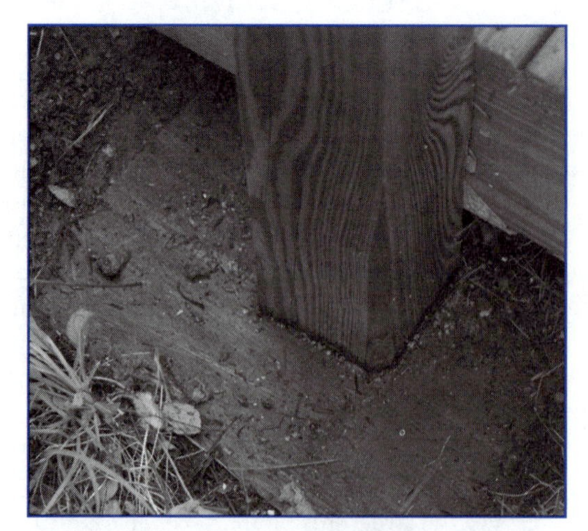

**Figure 24-1.** Detail of "floating base." For the original article, visit http://www.wheelchairramp.org/rampman/articles/handyman/handyman.htm. Photo courtesy of William R. Croninger.

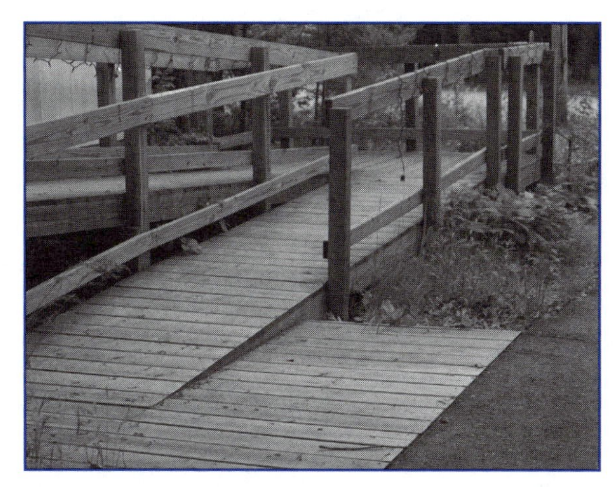

**Figure 24-2.** A 42-foot ramp constructed by an occupational therapist for his wheelchair-bound neighbor. Photo courtesy of Wiliam R. Croninger.

# Task Areas

Task areas may be thought of as the sites where primary occupations take place. Examples include the following:

- *Home*: Kitchen and bathroom
- *School*: Classroom and gym
- *Work*: Storeroom and office
- *Community*: Stores, restaurants, and theaters

Task areas offer the occupational therapist the opportunity to utilize the unique training received in activity analysis.

The following case example provides an overview for assessing any environment in which a client will function (home, school, work, community).

Shortly after the death of her husband, Grace's family began to notice changes in her behavior. She began calling her adult children numerous times on the same day, each time asking the same question. It became apparent that she was opening cards and letters repeatedly prior to mailing them to see whom she had written them to or if she had included the letter. Most alarming was that her friends began calling to report she was becoming increasingly forgetful. An assessment by a neuropsychologist returned a diagnosis of mild dementia.

An occupational therapist assisted the family by utilizing the framework (American Occupational Therapy Association [AOTA], 2008) to define Grace's goals and the requirements of her environment and to determine her ability to meet those requirements.

With the assistance of the therapist, the family helped their mother identify her goals related to living independently, her continued operation of a motor vehicle, and her desire to continue to participate in social activities. In the areas of independent living and motor vehicle operation, Grace and her children were able to define "threshold events" that would require her to give up her driver's license or move to residential living facility.

Utilizing the Context and Activity Demands portions of the framework, the therapist identified the performance skills and client factors needed to be successful in the context and activity demands of Grace's environment. The therapist then requested the family use a common activities of daily living (ADL) checklist to identify both performance skills and performance patterns they had observed in their mother. The therapist stressed that it was important to look at change over time, always considering her performance in these areas at her "best" rather than focusing only on current issues.

Finally, using the assessment reports provided by the neuropsychologist, Grace, her children, and the therapist were able to develop a plan, that included environmental adaptations and weekly visits by a caregiver.

Adaptations:

- Decrease clutter throughout the house
- Create "workstations" where Grace could place bills and other important mail for later pickup by a friend who paid her bills
- Place a whiteboard over the phone and have Grace write answers to her questions on the "first" call

She was able to live successfully in her home for 2 additional years, relinquishing her driver's license during this period when the threshold event occurred.

# The Process

Using Context and Activity portions of the framework, define the demands of the environment and activities within the following:

- *Educational setting*: Watson and Wilson (2003) stressed the importance of "participation and engagement" by modifying the classroom and its demands to allow all students to participate more fully. Participation in learning activities is argued to be more effective than simply providing a piece of assistive technology, which makes it possible to participate. Thus, it is imperative for the school-based therapist to work with the classroom teacher and caregivers to fully understand the contexts of the classroom as well as performance skills and activity demands prior to suggesting alterations in the space or activities.

- *Work setting*: Prior to performing an ergonomic or job task analysis at the workplace, the therapist should contact the employer to determine what safety equipment is required, such as steel-toed shoes, safety glasses, or hearing protection. Although most employers have hearing and eye protection available for visitors, presenting with your own equipment will impress upon them the professionalism and experience you possess. Generally speaking, open-toed footwear should never be worn to the workplace, as you may not know when you are going on the production floor. If the production areas are for medical or food processing, be prepared to don a hairnet, beard net, shoe covers, and smocks. You may also be required to wear company uniforms when job shadowing an employee who interacts with the public, such as package car drivers for United Parcel Service (UPS). If the area you are evaluating is particularly noisy, interview the employer prior to going out on the production floor. Obtain an understanding of product flow and materials, and use the terminology of the employer versus the medical community.
- *Computer workstation setting*: Computers are no longer limited to the accounting office or administrative areas of work. From tracking orders to making paper, the employee interfaces with a computer as a regular part of his or her occupation. When looking at a computer workstation, the Occupational Safety and Health Administration (OSHA) Web site (www.osha.gov/SLTC/etools/computerworkstations) can be used as a reference. When making recommendations for equipment or a change in the work process, review these recommendations with the employer before committing them to the report or discussing with the employee. You do not want to make demands on the employer that cannot be immediately honored due to costs or production restraints. However, instruction to the employee regarding tool positioning, body mechanics, and other basic safety practices can be recommended at the time of the evaluation.
- *Community setting*: Interview the client to determine goals and pre-existing performance patterns. Performance skills and client factors can be assessed using standardized or nonstandardized means to understand observed or potential issues related to the client's ability to successfully and safely function in the environment.

# Overview of Ergonomics and Human Factors Engineering

In the preceding pages of this chapter, a process for assessing an environment prior to determining what modifications might be desirable has been detailed. Ergonomics provides a very useful body of knowledge that will assist practitioners in understanding the activity demands of task areas (AOTA, 2008), particularly those found in work settings.

Jacobs (1999) traced the understanding of the importance of ergonomics back to the earliest tools created by humanoids as they shaped stone implements to fit their own hands and abilities. An Internet search for the term will yield a wide range of definitions. However, the recurring theme is that the practice of ergonomics seeks to match the demands of work with the abilities of the worker. In this way, worker safety, comfort, and productivity are maximized. A term closely related to ergonomics and often used interchangeably is *human factors engineering* (HFE). Both involve knowledge of human physiology and psychology and the ability to process information (U.S. Army Human Engineering Laboratory, 1984).

The pilots of some World War II era aircraft frequently displayed puzzling behavior after landing. While taxing back to parking areas, the pilots would retract their landing gear, dropping the aircraft to the ground and causing considerable damage to the aircraft. The surprised and embarrassed pilot would later relate that he thought he was retracting the flaps, a necessary practice following landing. Investigators discovered this error was not common across all types of aircraft. Rather, it was most frequently seen in specific models of fighters and bombers.

In looking deeper, it was noted that the "problem" models had flap and gear levers or switches side by side. In fact, on many aircrafts, the controls were of identical shape. Pilots of aircrafts that had the levers separated or those that used a different sequence for each action did not commonly embarrass themselves by retracting their plane's landing gear while on the ground.

It was wartime, so one could not simply recall all of the aircrafts and move the controls. However, when human factors engineering was applied to the problem, a quick and easily applied solution was readily found. The fix? Small rubber tires were added to the ends of the landing gear levers, while the flap lever was modified so it ended in a same wedge shape as the actual flaps.

Pilots of World War II aircrafts were too busy to look away from the runway, landing at high speed, with limited control, and with the likelihood of battle damage. However, having levers that resembled the action intended could easily be interpreted through their flying gloves, and incidences of wheels up after landing decreased significantly (Roscoe, 1997).

Ergonomics requires knowledge in a wide range of topics. Table 24-1 provides an overview (Headquarters Department of the Army, 1983).

The field of ergonomics then holds considerable promise for the occupational therapist. It allows for a thorough understanding of the contexts and performance skills required by a task and its environment. Further, it can help the practitioner understand the interrelationship of these skills and better plan for an environment that will promote client independence. It can also assist a practitioner in analyzing an environment or process to better understand the sources of injury and in devising the means to prevent it.

# Universal Design

Closely aligned with ergonomics is the concept of universal design. This term is attributed to architect Ronald Mace and describes that tools and spaces should be designed to be at the same time aesthetically pleasing as well as usable by all individuals, regardless of their abilities (About the Center: Ronald L Mace, 2008). Universal design, at its core, has seven principles. They are as follows (Copyright © 1997 NC State University, The Center for Universal Design):

1. Equitable use
2. Flexibility in use
3. Simple and intuitive use
4. Perceptible information
5. Tolerance for error
6. Low physical effort
7. Size and space for approach and use

Universal design could be thought of as an attempt to "get it right from the start." Rather than adapting the environment as a user's abilities change, universal design seeks to anticipate these changes by building "tolerance" for different abilities and processes.

In the following case example, note how the practitioner analyzed the activity demands of the task. Using HFE principles, he recognized potential sources of hazards for the workers. His suggested fix demonstrates a low-tech, cost-effective strategy for greatly reducing worker risk.

A contract-manufacturing firm was required to modify their standard operating procedure to accommodate the demands of a customer. Specifically, they were required to retool from bottling a single flavor to bottling three flavors. Initially, the pails of product would be palletized by each flavor, then repalletized so three flavors were on each pallet, increasing the handling of each pail 3-fold and exposing the worker to increased risk of injury.

The onsite occupational therapist performed a job task analysis and recommended the pails be stacked by flavor, one flavor per row as they came off the production line, reducing the pail handling to once per pail.

**Table 24-1. Fields Contributing to Knowledge of Ergonomics**

| Subject | Operational Definition | Example |
|---|---|---|
| Physiology | Sensory information: visual, auditory, olfactory, touch, taste | What color would make a shut-off switch most visible in an emergency situation? |
| Skills | What is the skill set required to operate a piece of equipment? | What is the longest password that the average person can remember? |
| Performance | What are the factors that influence an operator's ability to perform an operation? | How long can a long-distance truck driver safely operate his or her vehicle on the highway? |
| Anthropometrics | Study of human body dimensions; examines both averages and extremes | How far can the average person reach into a refrigerator? |
| Biomedical factors | Effects of environment on workers: sound levels, temperature, vibration, altitude, humidity, odor, etc. | What effect does temperature have on a worker's ability to perform fine adjustments on a piece of equipment? |
| Safety factors | What could go wrong? What are the consequences of making a wrong choice? | What are the consequences of a distracted vehicle operator shifting the transmission into "park" while moving? |
| Training | How long should a training program be? | What is the minimal amount of time a driver education program needs to significantly reduce the accident rate among new drivers? |
| Manning implications | What is the minimum number of workers we need? | How many craftspeople should be on a team that manufacturers custom-made stairways onsite? |

Adapted from Headquarters Department of the Army. (1983). *Man-material systems: Human factors engineering program.* AR 602-1, Washington, DC: Author.

To decrease the potential for shoulder injuries, an adaptive piece of equipment was designed by the occupational therapist and fabricated by the employer's maintenance department. Now, instead of reaching at arm's length with a pail weighing 40 pounds, the employee places the pail on top of the first row and slides it into place (Figures 24-3 and 24-4).

By John E. Lane, Jr., OTR/L

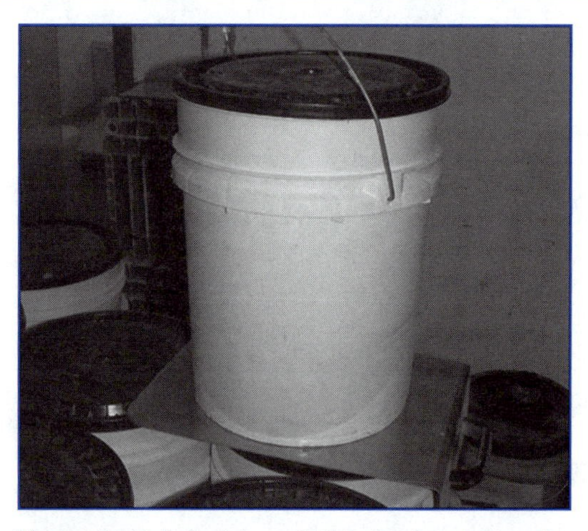

**Figure 24-3.** Palletizing of 40 lb. buckets by hand requires frequent lifting and unsupported forward reaching at or above shoulder height. Photo courtesy of John E. Lane, Jr.

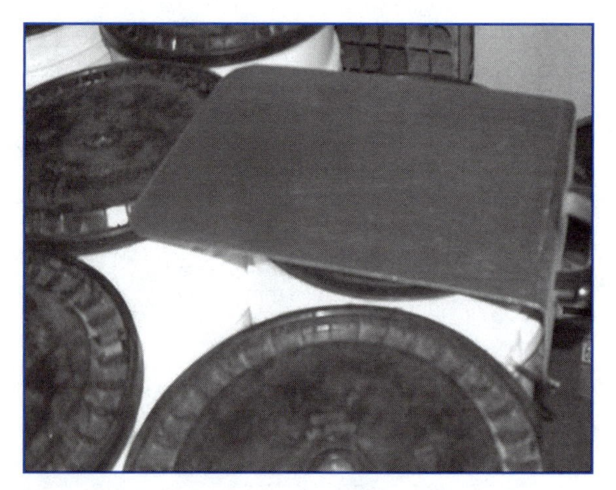

**Figure 24-4.** An example of a simple Engineering Control to reduce shoulder strain. Stainless steel "slide board" made by employer's in-house maintenance department per recommendation of on-site occupational therapist. Photo courtesy of John E. Lane, Jr.

# Overview of Ergonomics and Process Modification

Job modifications to decrease risk of injury fall under three categories (Cohen, Gjessing, Fine, Bernard, & McGlothing, 1997):

1. *Engineering controls*: Design of the job, the workstation, the tools, and work process are created from the beginning to accommodate the capability and capacities of the workers. It is independent of the worker's capabilities or techniques.
2. *Administrative controls*: The policies or work practices used to prevent or control exposure to ergonomic risks (e.g., frequent rest breaks to offset fatigue, limiting overtime or rotating between tasks, broadening job responsibilities to decrease repetition or awkward postures, slowing of production rates).
3. *Personal protective equipment*: Provides a barrier between the worker and the hazard source. This is the least-preferred intervention and should only be implemented when engineering and administrative controls have not been effective.

The practitioner chose to address the task by altering the work process and workstation, found under engineering controls. It was also necessary for him to convince the administration that work practices needed to be modified (administrative controls). For the practitioner practicing in worksite assessments, the "toolbox" items include (J. Lane, personal communication, June 26, 2006):

- Appropriate foot and headwear for the site
- Clipboard
- Tape measure
- Push-pull force gauge
- Bathroom scales
- Digital photo or video equipment (determine photo policy of employer prior to bringing equipment in)

# Occupational Therapist/ Occupational Therapy Assistant Teams in Environmental Adaptation

The occupational therapy assistant may work with an occupational therapist in the provision of services in environmental adaptation. The standard, however, makes it clear that the occupational therapy assistant may also work independently to modify, adapt, and teach once service competency has been demonstrated.

# Summary

Environmental adaptation and ergonomics present the occupational therapist with an important professional challenge. To be effective, the practitioner must be familiar with the client, environment, and tasks involved. In this chapter, a process for addressing each of these has been presented.

## Student Self-Assessment

1. Specify a ramp for the residence you live in or one nearby. Your work should be specific enough that a contractor could fabricate it without additional questions. You should include length of ramp, width, height of handrails, and wheelchair rails. If you need "switchback," you should also state the dimensions for the platform that ties the sections together. Use any of the Web sites listed to assist you.
2. Assess your computer workstation or that of a friend or member of your faculty. Create a detailed report that specifies how the workstation should be altered to meet Occupational Safety and Health Administration (OSHA) guidelines.
3. Using a diagnosis provided by your faculty, perform a home evaluation on your residence, your parents', or a relative's. How should the site be modified to allow the "client" to remain in the home at a maximal level of independence?
4. Write a job description for one of your faculty members. How would the environment need to be changed to allow that person to continue to teach were he or she to lose his or her sight, hearing, or mobility?
5. Conduct an informal assessment of a supermarket aisle. How might this aisle be confusing for a client following a head injury? How would you suggest modifying the environment to make it less problematic for this client?

## Electronic Resources

- Accessibility-Equal Access to Transportation (deals with air carriers): www.dot.gov/citizen_services/disability/disability.html
- U.S. Architectural and Transportation Barriers Compliance Board Americans with Disabilities Act (transportation in general): www.access-board.gov/publications/ADAFactSheet/a13.html
- National Council on Disability (limited information on bus access): www.ncd.gov/newsroom/publications/2005/quickreference.htm
- U.S. government site for the law: www.ada.gov
- AbleData: www.abledata.com
- Adapting Vehicles for People with Disabilities: www.nhtsa.dot.gov/cars/rules/adaptive/brochure/brochure.html
- Department of Justice, ADA Standards for Accessible Design: www.ada.gov/adastd94.pdf
- Seven Principles of Universal Design and their guidelines: www.design.ncsu.edu/cud/pubs_p/docs/poster.pdf
- Center for an Accessible Society: www.accessiblesociety.org/topics/universaldesign

### Evidence-Based Research Chart

| Intervention | Keywords | Evidence |
|---|---|---|
| ADA | Mixed results in workplace; limited to negative results in employment; per student expenditures; preliminary findings suggested improvements in transportation, and accessibility of public buildings | Bell & Heitmueller, 2005; Frieden, 2005; Gius, 2005; Wells, 2001 |
| Ergonomics, HFE | Return to work; cost effectiveness of ergonomics improvements; parents rank RSI injury low on concerns for children using computers at home, interventions; aircraft cockpit design and HFE | Anema et al., 2004; Helander & Burri, 1995; Kimmerly & Odell, 2009; Schmelzer, n.d. |
| Universal Design | Designing instructional materials for all learners; designing computer interface (email) for seniors; potential role for physiological anthropologists in improving independence of elders; downloadable booklet: principles, history, case studies in universal design | Crews & Zovotka, 2006; Hawthorn, 2003; Pisha & Coyne, 2001; Story, Mueller & Mace, 1998 |
| Environmental adaptation | Positive and negative aspects of adapting homes for children with disabilities; poor housing related to poor health; justifying occupational therapy at home; effectiveness of home adaptation decreases as client limitations increase in eldery | Donald, 2009; Mathieson, Kronenfeld, & Keith, 2002; Richards, 2003; Roy, Rousseau, Allard, Feldman, & Majnemer, 2008 |

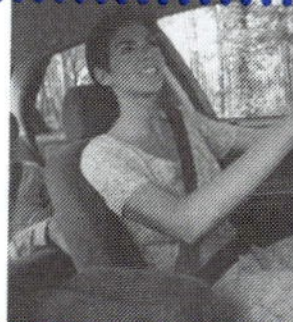

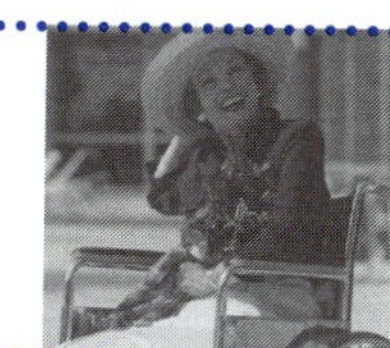

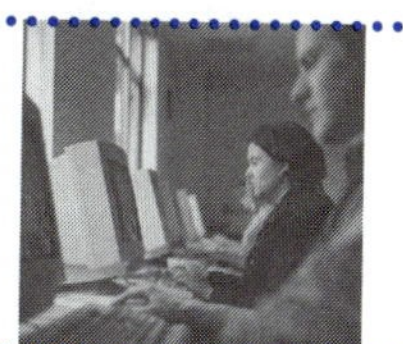

# References


About the Center: Ronald L. Mace. Retrieved June 2, 2008, from http://www.design.ncsu.edu/cud/about_us/usronmace.htm

American Occupational Therapy Association. (2008). Occupational therapy practice framework: Domain and process, second edition. *American Journal of Occupational Therapy, 62*, 625-683.

Anema, J., Cuelenaere, B., van der Beek, A, Knol, D., de Vet, H., & van Mechelen, W. (2004). The effectiveness of ergonomic interventions on return-to-work after low back pain; a prospectice two year cohort study in six countries on low back pain patients sick-listed for 3-4 months. *Occupational and Environmental Medicine, 61*, 289-294. Retrieved July 31, 2009, from http://oem.bmj.com/cgi/content/abstract/61/4/289

Bell, D., & Heitmueller, A. (2008). The Disability Discrimination Act in the UK: Helping or hindering employment among the disabled? Retrieved July 30, 2009, from http://www.ncbi.nlm.nih.gov/pubmed/19091434?ordinalpos=9&itool=EntrezSystem2.PEntrez.Pubmed.Pubmed_ResultsPanel.Pubmed_DefaultReportPanel.Pubmed_RVDocSum

The Center for Universal Design. (1997). *The principles of universal design, version 2.0*. Raleigh, NC: North Carolina State University.

Cohen, A., Gjessing, C., Fine, L., Bernard, B., & McGlothing, D. (1997). Elements of ergonomic programs. *NIOSH Pub., 97-117*, 31-37.

Crews, D., & Zavotka, S. (2006). Aging, disability, and frailty: Implications for universal design. *Journal of Physiological Anthropology, 25*, 113-118. Retrieved August 2, 2009, from http://www.jstage.jst.go.jp/article/jpa2/25/1/113/_pdf

Donald, I. (2009). Housing and health care for older people. *Age and Ageing, 38*(4), 364–367.

Frieden, L. (2005). NCD and the Americans With Disabilities Act: 15 years of progress. Retrieved July 28, 2009, from http://www.ncd.gov/newsroom/publications/2005/15yearprogress.htm

Hawthorn, D. (2003). How universal is good design for older users? Presented to the Proceedings of the 2003 Conference on Universal Usability.

Headquarters Department of the Army. (1983). *Man-material systems: Human factors engineering program*. AR 602-1, Washington, DC: Author.

Helander, M., & Burri, G. (1995). Cost effectiveness of ergonomics and quality improvements in electronics manufacturing. *Journal of Industrial Ergonomics, 15*(2), 137-151. Retrieved July 31, 2009, from http://md1.csa.com/partners/viewrecord.php?requester=gs&collection=ENV&recid=3705219&q=author%3A%22Helander%22+intitle%3A%22Cost+effectiveness+of+ergonomics+and+quality+...%22+&uid=788134953&setcookie=yes

Jacobs, K. (Ed.). (1999). *Ergonomics for therapists* (2nd ed.). Newton, MA: Butterworth Heinemann.

Kimmerly, L., & Odell, D. (2009). Children and computer use in the home: Workstations, behaviors and parental attitudes. *Work, 32*(3), 299-310.

Gius, M. (2005). The effect of the American With Disabilities Act on public education expenditures, *Journal of Social Sciences, 1*(3), 162-165. Retrieved July 31, 2009, from http://www.scipub.org/fulltext/jss/jss13162-165.pdf

Mathieson, K., Kronenfeld, J., & Keith, V. (2002). Maintaining functional independence in elderly adults: The roles of health status and financial resources in predicting home modifications and use of mobility equipment. *The Gerontoligist, 42*(1), 24-31. Retrieved August 2, 2009, from http://intl-gerontologist.gerontologyjournals.org/cgi/reprint/42/1/24.pdf

Pisha, B. & Coyne, P. (2001). Smart from the start: The promise of universal design for learning. *Remedial and Special Education, 22*(4), 197-203. Retrieved August 2, 2009, from http://rse.sagepub.com/cgi/reprint/22/4/197

Richards, S. (2003). People leave hospital stable, but not necessarily able: We must help them. Retrieved August 2, 2009, from http://0-proquest.umi.com.lilac.une.edu:80/pqdweb?did=351348661-&sid=14&Fmt=3&clientId=8421&RQT=309&VName=PQD

Roscoe, S. (1997). The adolescence of engineering psychology. Retrieved June 14, 2006, from http://www.hfes.org//PublicationMaintenance/FeaturedDocuments/27/adolescencehtml.html

Roy, L., Rousseau, J., Allard, H., Feldman, D., & Majnemer, A. (2008). Parental experience of home adaptation for children with motor disabilities. *Physical & Occupational Therapy in Pediatrics, 28*(4), 353-368.

Schmelzer, R. (n.d.). Human interaction with aircraft cockpit displays. Retrieved August 2, 2009, from http://www.eas.asu.edu/~humanfac/ringo.html

Story, M., Mueller, J. & Mace, R. (1998). The universal design file: Designing for people of all ages and abilities. Retrieved August 2, 2009, from http://eric.ed.gov:80/ERICDocs/data/ericdocs2sql/content_storage_01/0000019b/80/19/ac/11.pdf

U.S. Army Human Engineering Laboratory. (1984). *Human factors engineering: Supplement for HEO 101-108*. Aberdeen Proving Ground, MD: The Army Institute for Professional Development, Army Correspondence Course Program.

Watson, D., & Wilson, S. (2003). *Task analysis: An individual and population approach*. Baltimore, MD: AOTA Press.

Wells, S. (2001). Is the ADA working-Americans With Disabilities Act. Retrieved July 30, 2009, from http://findarticles.com/p/articles/mi_m3495/is_4_46/ai_73848278

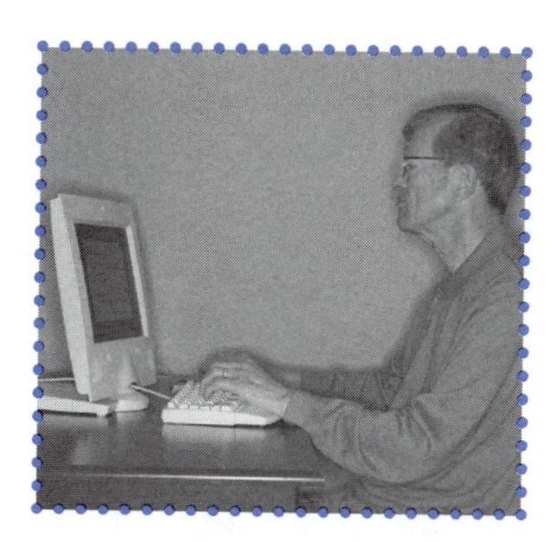

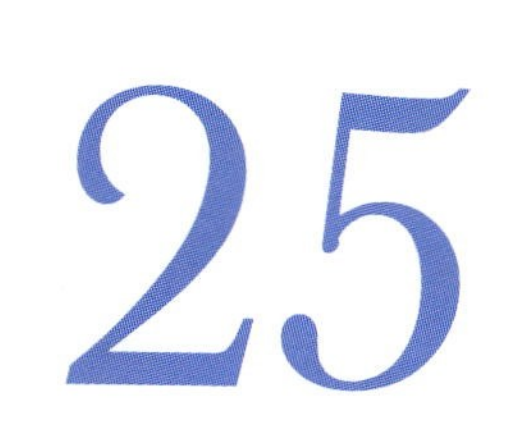

# 25

# Assistive Technology

William R. Croninger, MA, OTR/L and Betsy DeBrakeleer, COTA/L, ROH

**ACOTE Standards Explored in This Chapter**

B.5.9-5.10, 5.20

**Key Terms**

AbleData
Assistive technology
Hi-tech
Low-tech

## Introduction

It is altogether too easy to think of assistive technology as being appropriate only for individuals with a deficit of some type. We may believe our clients "need" assistive technology because they are unable to do something. In fact, the definition of assistive technologies would seem to promote the disability label. "Assistive technology can be defined as any item, piece of equipment, or product system, whether acquired commercially off the shelf, modified, or customized, that is used to increase, maintain, or improve the functional capabilities of individuals with disabilities" (Office of the Federal Register, 2000).

Mann and Lane (1991) offered a different paradigm when they stated, "Tools augment existing human functions or add new functions" (p. 6.). If we look at assistive technology as a collection of tools that augment or add to the functions possible for our clients, we de-emphasize the disability label. All humans and many animals use tools. A length of pipe added to a wrench is often used to increase the force generated when trying to free a stubborn bolt. Chimpanzees have been observed in the wild using sticks to gather food and otters are regularly observed to use rocks to open sea urchins. In this chapter, assistive technologies will be explored as tools that extend and augment our client's ability to function in a variety of settings and roles.

Assistive technologies have traditionally been divided into two types:

1. *Low-tech devices*: Characterized as being "inexpensive and easy to obtain" (Cook & Hussey, 1995, p. 7). Examples would include built-up handles on utensils, adapted doorknobs, dressing sticks, and sock aids.
2. *High-tech devices*: Thought of as more expensive, more difficult to obtain, and often requiring training to operate. They are usually electrical or electronic. Falling into this classification would be robotic assistants, augmented speaking devices, and prosthetic limbs.

Although common, there are difficulties with this classification system. Technologies continue to move from "high" to "low" in terms of their cost and availability. In 1995, computers were considered high-tech devices (Cook & Hussey, 1995). Today, they would hardly be thought of as such under this classification system. Another example would be the cellular phone. The first call was placed on one in 1973 (Bellis, n.d.) and until recently, they would have been considered high technology devices. Now they are nearly ubiquitous and affordable for many of the world's



K. Sladyk, K. Jacobs, & N. MacRae (Eds.).
*Occupational Therapy Essentials for Clinical Competence* (pp. 271-280).

population. Possibly the best method of conceptualizing assistive technologies is that they exist in a continuum with technologies that were once considered high-tech, gradually moving to low-tech as new tools come into existence.

# Evaluation

Assessment should start with a thorough analysis of the demands of the task, which under the framework (American Occupational Therapy Association [AOTA], 2008) fall under the category of activity demands and performance skills. Common tasks such as those found in activities of daily living (ADL) will likely be familiar to the practitioner. Tasks that are unfamiliar, such as those found in school, work, or leisure, will require additional consultation. In work settings, a job description will be helpful, while team members, co-workers, and supervisors may also be able to deepen the practitioner's understanding of demands and skills necessary. Co-workers or peers who might be affected by the device also need to be considered. To be successful, the practitioner needs a firm grasp of all of the task components.

Simultaneously, the practitioner should interview the client relative to his or her impressions of the roles, demands, and skills required. At this time, it is also appropriate to work with the client to understand performance patterns. What are the habits and routines historically used by the client? Were they successful in the past? What parts of the routine or habit does the client value and seek to maintain? Finally, what limitations does the client place on the nature of any intervention or tool?

The final set of assessments fall into the areas of performance skills and client factors (AOTA, 2008). At this point, the practitioner has assessed the skills required by the task. How do the performance skills and contextual factors of the task match with the performance skills and client factors? When mismatches are noted that cannot be addressed solely by environmental and/or process changes, assistive technology devices may be appropriate.

We met Maryanne when she was in her mid-seventies. Despite severe arthritis, she had continued to live independently in her own home after the death of her husband. Maryanne had been referred for occupational therapy following replacement of the metacarpophalangeal joint of her left hand. During therapy, she related that she was experiencing significant issues centered on ADL and home management. Permission for a home evaluation was obtained from her attending physician.

Maryanne escorted us through her home, pointing out problem areas and detailing strategies she had used with various degrees of success. In coming up with a set of possible interventions, we paid attention to her impressions of the task demands, the contexts in which the tasks took place, as well as her habits and routines. We tried each task to get a feel of the performance skills required. Our understanding of her "space" was then compared to the formal assessments we had on her range of motion, strength, endurance, and information from the physician relative to the expected progress of both her therapy and the disease.

We then met again with Maryanne to present our list of solutions and to get her feedback on her willingness to accept changes to habit and routine. Financial considerations related to the final choice of assistive devices were also discussed.

One major issue was that her limited range of motion made opening doors with traditional knobs almost impossible. We selected a commercially available device that clamps over the doorknob and featured a lever she could easily utilize.

A second issue related to controlling the faucets in her kitchen. Replacing the controls was not a financial option. However, she was able to use the controls when we attached wooden clothespins to them. These adaptations allowed her to use her closed fist to turn the water on and off. The pins initially slid off the controls quickly, but this was rectified by a small bolt with a nut running through the open portion of the pin.

A final problem of great aggravation to her was her inability to open the windows in her living area on hot days. She was able to close windows with her fists but could not grasp the window hardware to open it. Maryanne had shown us, with great pride, how she used a back scratcher to remove her winter coat. Since she always left her windows open a small amount, we devised a plan where we attached small blocks to each of the windowsills. We then fabricated a slightly stronger "scratcher" that allowed her to use the block as a fulcrum to lever the windows up on warm days. She now had a combination scratcher-lever. A few weeks later, she demonstrated, with great pride, how she could also use the device to open her refrigerator by inserting it into the door handle and pushing against it with her chest.

All tools were decidedly "low-tech" interventions, and only the door handles entailed any cost for Maryanne. She took a considerable amount of pride in helping "her" therapists. One unintended consequence was that she also became one of the strongest advocates in our community for occupational therapy.

# Assistive Devices

There are a variety of methods for classifying assistive technologies. Angelo (1997) looked at mobility, methods of access, switch types, and the level of technology. Mann and Lane (1991) presented a system that sorts devices by disability: physical, sensory, speech, and cognition. Cook and Hussey (1995) ordered their work by activity area: communication, mobility, sensation, manipulation, and control. All of these ordering systems would seem to be appropriate. A look at assistive technology using a combination of the preceding classification systems follows.

## Occupational Therapy's Role in Assistive Technology Provision

Mann and Lane (1991) noted that the occupational therapist may work independently in some situations, as when training a client to use a "sock aid" following a total hip arthroplasty. When the complexity of the task(s) requires a team approach, they argued that the occupational therapist is the individual best prepared to act as its leader.

Angelo (1997) stated that the occupational therapist frequently serves as the "interface specialist" (p. 8). In this role, the responsibility of the occupational therapist is to assess the client's performance skills and client factors to determine the body part or motion over which the client demonstrates the greatest and most consistent control. Working with other team members, the specific method of access, the switch, and its mounting location can then be selected.

All authors are in agreement that one primary role for the occupational therapist and other team members is in positioning and seating. Effective, consistent control will not be possible until the client is positioned correctly.

# Augmenting or Adding Mobility

Problems with mobility have a wide variety of potential causes, which may include problems with balance, muscle strength, joint range, control, or sensation. Finally, a limb may not be present in whole or part.

- *Low-tech examples*: Canes, walkers, crutches, lower extremity orthosis, manual wheelchair. Low-tech mobility devices such as canes, walkers, and crutches are commonly prescribed by the physical therapist who will perform the initial selection, set-up, and training. Thereafter, all team members frequently work to improve a client's functional mobility as during ADL.
  - *Lower extremity orthosis*: Lower extremity orthoses can take many forms and can impact the body at the ankle, knee, hip, or any combination of these. They are frequently used to stabilize the lower extremity, to correct deformity, or to slow the progression of deformity. In addition to stability functions, they are used to assist in mobility by correcting problems in gait. They are generally fabricated and fitted by an orthotist.
  - *Manual wheelchairs*: Generally co-prescribed by the attending physical and occupational therapists.
- *High-tech examples*: Power wheelchairs, personal mobility devises, lower extremity prosthesis, and robotic walker.
  - *Powered wheelchairs*: These items change dramatically every year. The therapist should know the products and have good working relationships with the equipment vendors in order to assure that the client receives the most appropriate equipment.
  - *Personal mobility devices*: A wide range of devices fall into this category, from the three-wheeled scooters to electric carts to the high-tech two wheel devices such as the Segway personal transportation device (Figures 25-1 and 25-2).

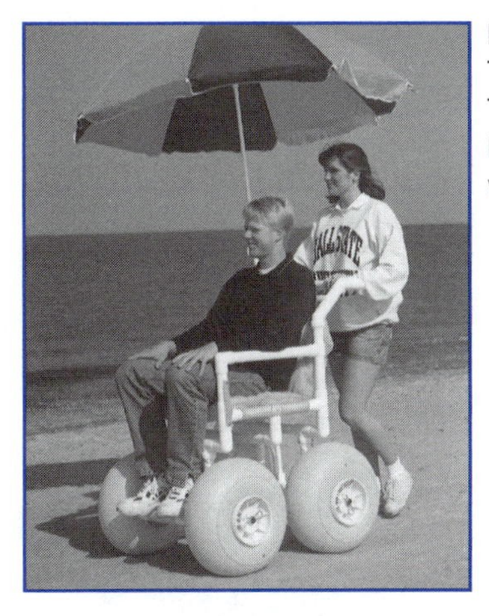

**Figure 25-1.** All Terrain Chair (Assistive Technology, Inc, New Buffalo, MI). Reproduced with permission.

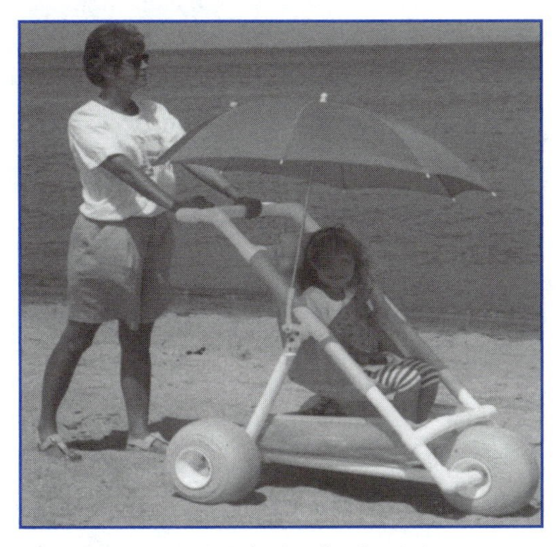

**Figure 25-2.** Beach Baby Stroller (Assistive Technology, Inc, New Buffalo, MI). Reproduced with permission.

- *Lower extremity prosthesis*: While a lower extremity orthosis is utilized to augment an existing body part, the prosthesis functions to replace a missing body part (Bodeau, 2002). Assessment and prescription require the team to look at a diverse set of criteria that includes cognitive status, function, environment in which the device will be used, client goals, client financial situation, as well as the level of amputation.
- *Robotic walker*: The robotic walker is a hybrid system under development that adds global positioning, obstacle avoidance, and speech recognition to a rolling walker. Researchers envision this device as a means to allow individuals with cognitive and balance deficits to ambulate more safely.
- *Exoskeleton walker*: Although still in the realm of science fiction, considerable research is being conducted in this area. Unlike the robot walker, the exoskeleton attaches to or is donned by the user. Current devices are aimed at augmenting or enhancing an individual's ability to walk or carry heavy loads over a variety of terrain types.

## Assistive Technology for Upper Extremity Augmentation

The upper extremities are frequently impacted by a number of conditions, both congenital and acquired. This classification will look at assistive technology for situations requiring the augmentation or extension of gross motor upper extremity functions: range of motion, strength, sensation, and control.

- *Low-tech devices*: Dressing sticks, reachers, long-handled shoe horn, long-handled bath sponge, sock aids, button hooks, nosey cups, lipped plates, plate guards, built-up utensils, card holders, mouth sticks, pointing devices, and static splints (Figures 25-3 to 25-6).
- *High-tech devices*: Environmental controls, upper extremity prosthetic, robotics, and dynamic splints.

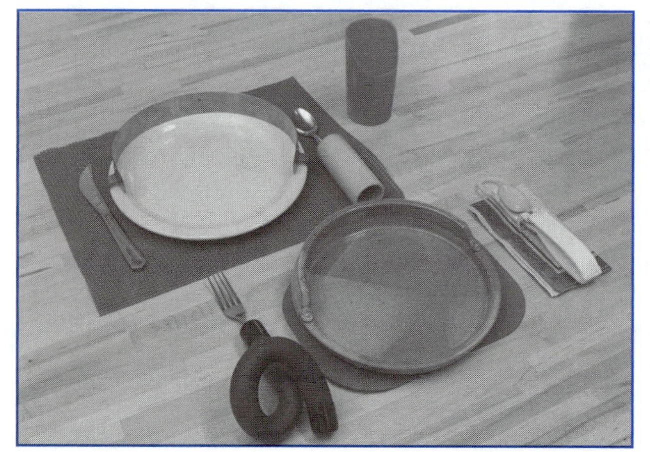

**Figure 25-3.** Low-tech assists for eating. Photo courtesy of William R. Croninger.

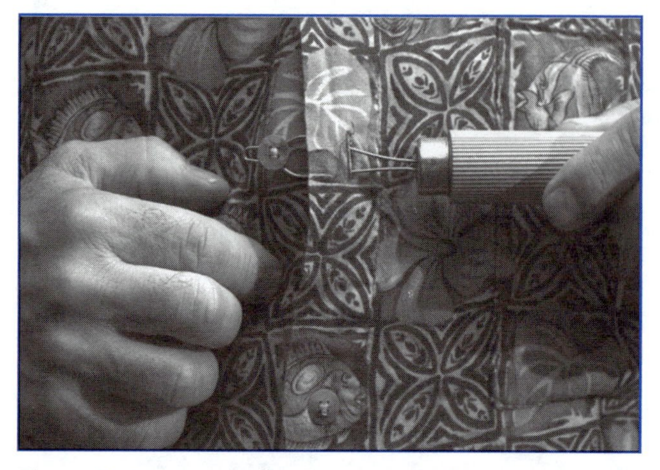

**Figure 25-4.** Low-tech assist for buttoning. Photo courtesy of R. Robnett.

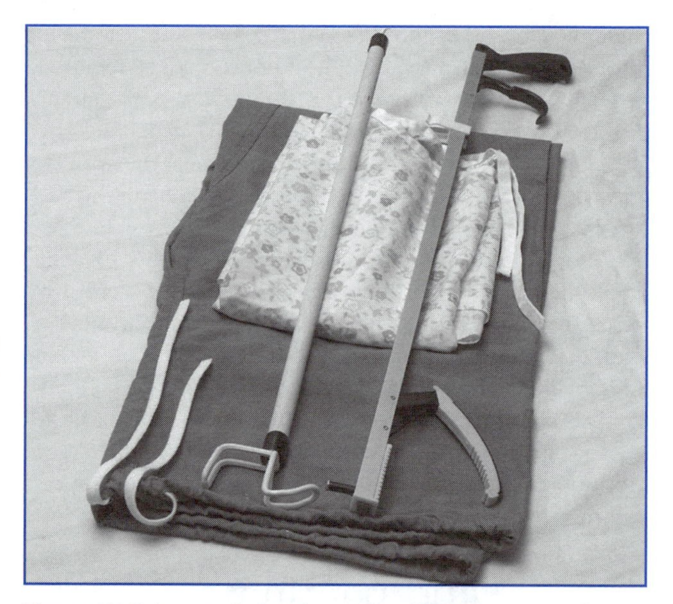

**Figure 25-5.** Low-tech dressing assists. Photo courtesy of William R. Croninger.

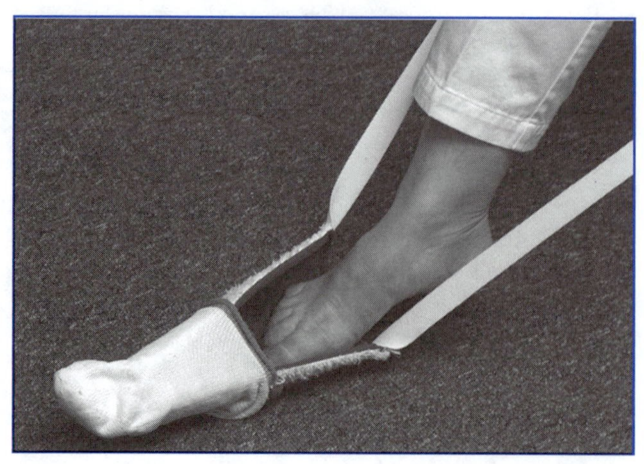

**Figure 25-6.** Low-tech assist for sock donning. Photo courtesy of William R. Croninger.

# Assistive Technology for Fine Motor Augmentation

Most of the devices discussed in this chapter allow a user to approach or participate in a task. The fine motor assistive technology is commonly some type of switch. It is critically important as it is the point of interface between user and device. AbleData is again an excellent point to begin to understand the large variety and types of switches available.

Most critical is that the switch be accessible and appropriate for the client. Since it is the most heavily used portion of the intervention, it is also the most common point of failure. Therapists should always consider the impact of switch failure, both on the client's ability to access the device and on the impact to client safety if a switch fails while the device is being used. There are two types of switches:

- *Latched*: Latched switches turn a device on or off. Once activated the device stays in that mode until the switch is activated again. Examples include light switches, on/off knobs on appliances, and tools that require two-handed operation (Figures 25-7 and 25-8).

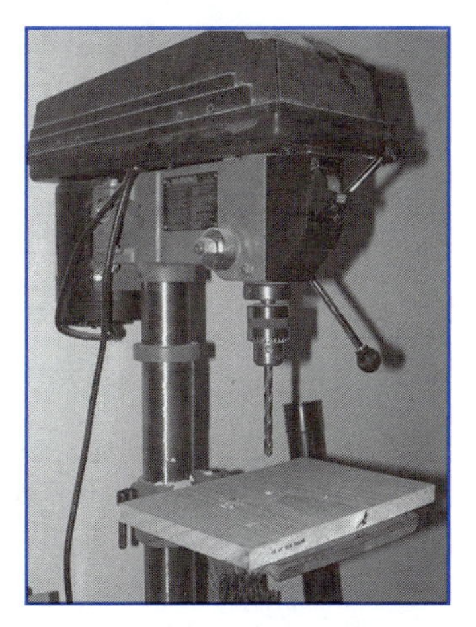

**Figure 25-7.** Example of tool with latching switch. Photo courtesy of William R. Croninger.

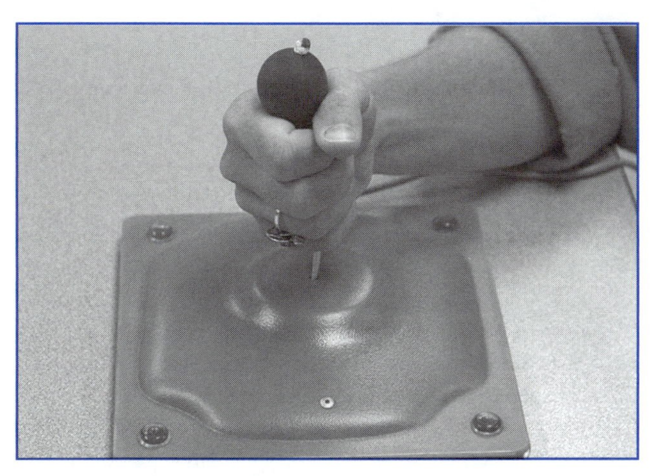

**Figure 25-8.** Example of latched switch. Photo courtesy of William R. Croninger.

- *Momentary*: Momentary switches require constant input or attention to operate. Examples include automobile accelerators and the "triggers" on tools that require fine adjustments while operating (Figures 25-9 and 25-10).

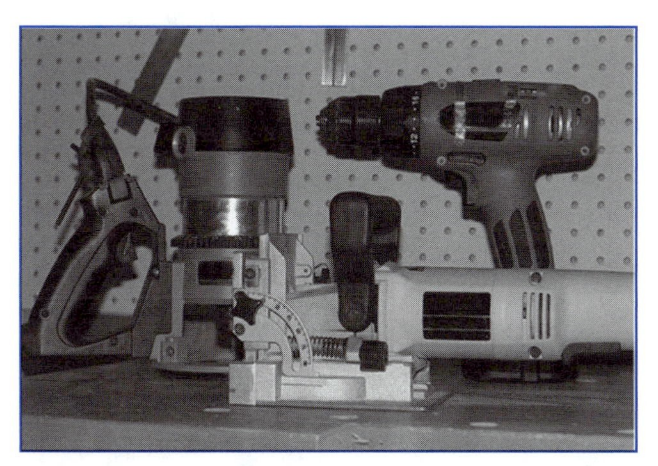

**Figure 25-9.** Tools with momentary switches. Photo courtesy of William R. Croninger.

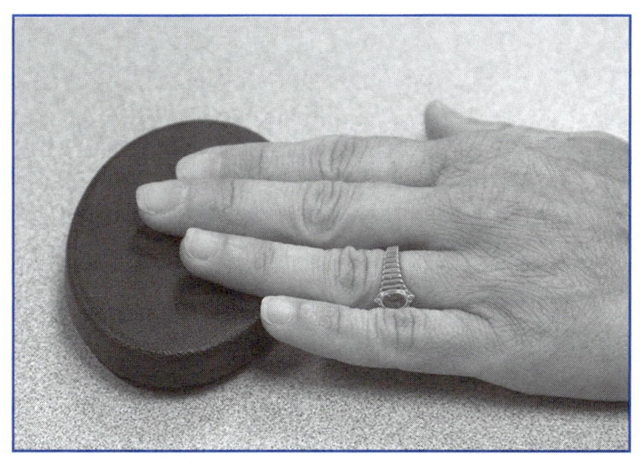

**Figure 25-10.** Example of momentary switch. Photo courtesy of William R. Croninger.

# Assistive Technology for Sensory Augmentation

This assistive technology area is generally thought of as including deficits in vision and hearing. To this, however, should be added technology for those individuals who experience altered sensation, whether it be epicritic or protopathic (informational versus safety) pathways.

## Hearing

- *Environmental adaptations*: Includes modifications to environment to reduce background noise and "auditory clutter."

- *Low-tech*: This could include sound deadening materials, amplification, or choice/positioning of furniture. This also includes modifications speakers make, which may include not standing in front of bright light sources and trimming of mustaches/beards to allow a listener who lip-reads a clear view of the speaker's lips.
- *High-tech*: In some situations, selective amplification, as in assisted listening devices, is more appropriate. The assisted listening devices involve a microphone (speaker), transmitter, receiver, and earphone (listener) system that allows an individual with diminished hearing to adjust the sound levels produced at the earphones. In this way, an audience can be made up of those who do and do not need amplification.

- *Hearing aids* (generally all high-tech): Falling into this category are devices that alert and/or augment hearing. Buzzers, strobes, flashing lights, or vibratory devices can signal an individual that he or she needs to attend to some event or situation. Hearing aids are classified by the National Institute of Health (National Institute on Deafness and Other Communications Disorders, 2002) using a number of categories:
  - *By style*: In the ear fits into the outer ear; behind the ear is located behind the ear, while the earpiece is within the canal; canal aids fit completely within the ear canal; body aids are large devices carried external to the ear and located on the wearer's clothing.
  - *By circuitry*: Analog/adjustable is built for a specific client to augment a specific level of hearing loss; analog/programmable is fabricated to an individual's specific needs—the users can often select a variety of settings depending upon the environment they are in; digital/programmable contain a microchip, which increases the ability of the device to adjust to the acoustics of varying environments.
- *Cochlear implants*: This assistive technology involves implantation of a device implanted behind the ear. The device bypasses damaged or nonfunctioning parts of the user's ear, sending information directly to the brain.

## Vision

- *Low tech*: Glasses, magnifying glass, large print, large fonts, alterations to light levels, contrast enhancement, reduction of glare, books/signage in Braille, walking cane (Figure 25-11).
- *High tech*: Scanning/large display device, character enhancement via computer, Braille talkers/typers (Figure 25-12).
  - Scanning/large display: A large number of devices allow a user to scan print on a page and display it on a screen in real time.

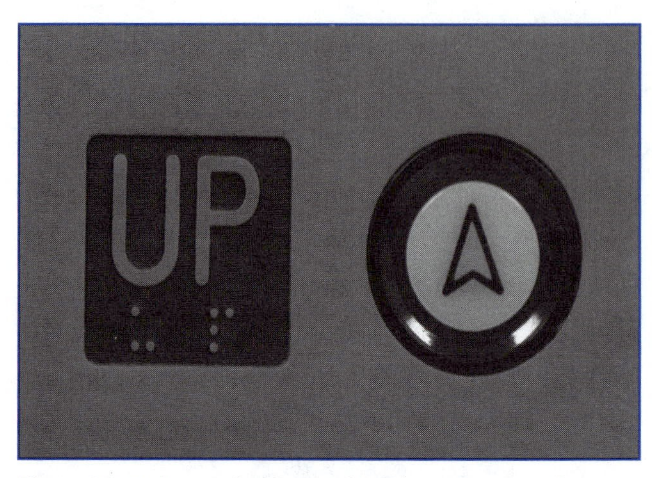


**Figure 25-11.** Low tech vision assists. Photo courtesy of William R. Croninger.

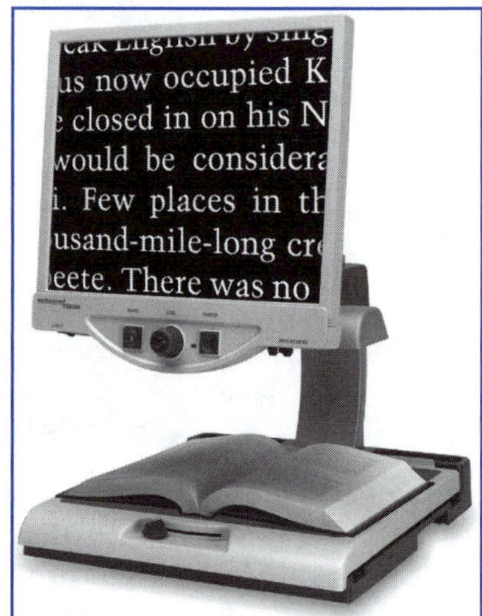


**Figure 25-12.** Merlin: LCD (Enhanced Vision, Huntingdon Beach, CA). Reproduced with permission.

  - Character enhancement: Adds a computer that can enlarge fonts and/or "speak" words on a page.
  - Braille typers: Braille typers utilize a scanner, which is moved over a printed page. The device converts the text input to Braille and raises the correct pins under the reader's fingers. Another strategy again uses a scanner to convert text to Braille but the output is in Braille via a specialized printer.

## Touch

Altered sensation, particularly tactile and pain, has the potential to impose a significant impact on a client's life and well-being. Since the hands are the most common means in which we interact with our environment, loss of tactile sensation will make it more difficult to choose effective assistive technology for other existing conditions. Therapists should remember switches need not always be activated by hand. The key is that the switch be positioned where motor ability allows consistent and accurate access (Figure 25-13).

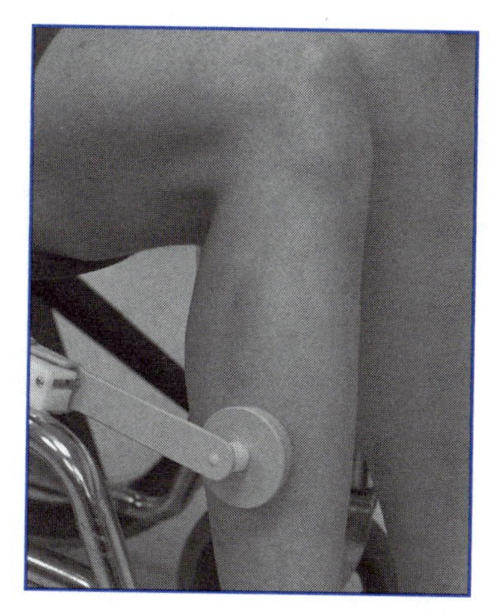

**Figure 25-13.** Locate switch where user has greatest amount of control. Photo courtesy of William R. Croninger.

Loss of sensation in the protopathic pathways (sharp/dull and hot/cold) brings a safety issue into the equation. Clients may not recognize they have come into contact with an object that is sharp or sufficiently cold or hot enough to cause tissue damage. Individuals with decreased peripheral sensation, such as found after trauma or with diabetes, may not recognize that fingers, toes, or a complete limb is too cold or hot.

The first strategy could be deemed to be "no-tech" in that clients should be trained to attend visually to affected body parts. When the body part cannot be readily visualized, it can often be viewed using a hand-mirror or mirror fitted with a universal cuff. Clients should always use thermometers in situations where extremes of temperature may be encountered.

# Assistive Technology for Communications Augmentation

A wide variety of conditions can lead to a decreased ability to communicate. Problems may be congenital as in a child with dysarthria acquired following a cerebral vascular accident (CVA) or progressive as seen in amyotrophic lateral sclerosis (ALS). Strategies involve a wide range of low- and high-tech interventions.

- *No-tech*: Gestures, grimaces, "mouthing," eye gaze
- *Low tech*: Paper and pencil, picture boards, symbol boards, touch talkers, and speech recognition software. Speech recognition and touch talkers were originally considered high-tech interventions. However, both have now become much more commonly available to the general public.
- *High tech*: Dedicated software/computer systems that use variable strategies for word selection and/or prediction. Mann and Lane (1991) grouped electronic communication devices into three types by method of access, each with its own advantages and drawbacks.
    1. *Direct*: Here, the user touches or uses a form of fine motor augmentation to select the response from among a group. The fine motor augmentation could be a mouth stick or one of the many head-mounted electronic pointers that use lasers, infrared, or radio waves.
    2. *Scanning*: In this strategy, the device moves through the available choices in a pre-arranged pattern at a pre-set pace. When the desired choice is available, often signaled by light emitting diode (LED) near the choice, the user responds. This method requires less user action but is slower than direct selection.
    3. *Encoding*: Symbols, numbers, colors, or letters for the desired words or phrases. It requires the least action on the part of the client in exchange for the client learning a new system of symbolizing.

**Morse Code**

Morse code is an example of an encoding strategy. In this system, combinations of short and long tones stand for letters, numbers, and abbreviations.

With modern equipment, very small hand movements are needed to generate the tonal sequences, which could then be displayed on a computer screen as letters. The computer would add the ability to have a short letter combination, such as "az" stand for an entire phrase just as in when a word processor is used to create a "macro" (Figure 25-14).

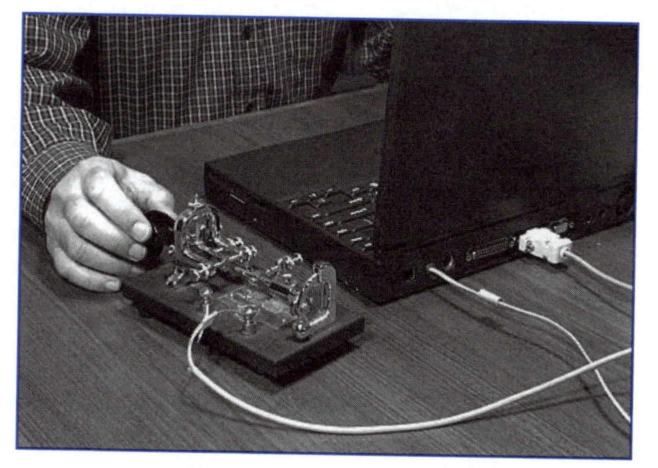

**Figure 25-14.** Example of morse code keyer (N7RZ). Photo courtesy of Less Kerr.

# Occupational Therapy Assistant in Assistive Technology

The occupational therapy assistant may work with an occupational therapist in the provision of services in assistive technology provision. The Accreditation Council for Occupational Therapy Education (ACOTE) standard, however, makes it clear that the occupational therapy assistant may also work independently to modify, adapt, and teach once service competency has been demonstrated.

## Summary

Assistive technology, whether it be a low-tech reacher or high-tech communication device, has the potential to greatly enhance the ability of occupational therapy clients to engage in occupations. Careful use of the framework (AOTA, 2008) greatly enhances the potential interventions that using these technologies will be successful. The practitioner, however, should pay particular attention to the sources cited in the following chart on evidence-based practice, which document why and when assistive technology interventions have failed. It is not enough to provide assistive technologies for our clients. Practitioners must be certain that what is provided is the proper tool, the client is adequately trained, and ongoing support and post-discontinuation of services is provided.

## Student Self-Assessment

1. Write a definition of assistive technology you could use to explain an assistive technology intervention to the partner of a client.
2. Review Maryanne's story. What other assistive technologies could have been used to assist her in her dressing, cooking, and home management activities?
3. Pick one of your instructors and imagine he or she has lost the use of his or her right upper-extremity. Analyze the tasks required by his or her environment and roles. What assistive technology interventions might assist him or her in maintaining his or her occupations?
4. How would you assist him or her with assistive technology if the problem were decreased memory? Decreased mobility?

## Electronic Resources

- AbleData, sponsored by the U.S. Department of Education: www.abledata.com
- Job Accomodation Network: www.jan.wvu.edu
- Rehabilitation Engineering & Assistive Technology Society of North America: www.resna.org
- Hearing Loss Association of America: www.shhh.org/learn/hat.asp
- Gallaudet University: www.gallaudet.edu
- American Speech-Language-Hearing Association—Assistive technology: www.asha.org/public/hearing/treatment/assist_tech.htm
- National Institute on Deafness and Other Communication Disorders (NIDCD)—Cochlear implants: www.nidcd.nih.gov/health/hearing/coch.asp
- National Institute on Deafness and Other Communication Disorders (NIDCD)—Hearing aids: www.nidcd.nih.gov/health/hearing/hearingaid.asp
- American Foundation for the Blind: www.afb.org/Section.asp?SectionID=3&TopicID=135&DocumentID=2424
- American Speech-Language-Hearing Association: http://www.asha.org/members/divs/div_12.htm
- International Society for Augmentative and Alternate Communication: www.isaac-online.org/select_language.html

**Evidence-Based Research Chart**

| Intervention | Keywords | Evidence |
|---|---|---|
| Pediatric | Improve writing, verbal communication | Lancioni et al., 2007; Lau & O'Leary, 1993; Mihailidis, Tam, McLean, & Lee, 2005 |
| | Caregiver reasons for use versus non-use (mobility, augmentative communications) | Benedict, Lee, Marrujo, & Farel, 1999 |
| Cognitive | Memory loss, conversation skills | Bourgeois & Mason, 1996; Van Hulle & Hux, 2006 |
| Functional mobility, communication, ADL | Improved independence | Dahlin Ivanoff & Sonn, 2005; Eriksrud & Bohannon, 2005; Hoenig, Taylor, & Sloan, 2003; Nordenskiöld, 1997; Uustal & Minkel, 2004 |
| | Reasons for use versus non-use | Agree & Freedman, 2003; Sonn, 1996 |

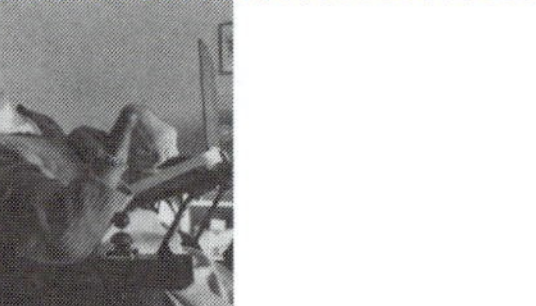
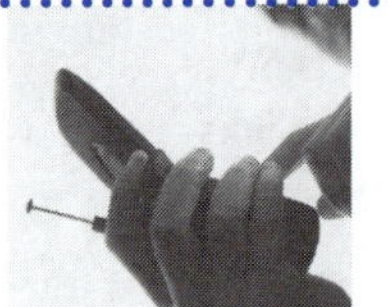
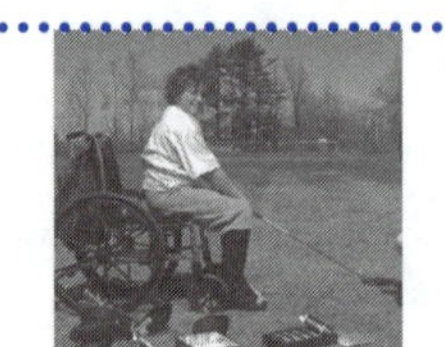

# References

Agree, E., & Freedman, V. (2003). A comparison of assistive technology and personal care in alleviating disability and unmet need. *The Gerontologist, 43*(3), 142-151.

American Occupational Therapy Association. (2008). Occupational therapy practice framework: Domain and process, second edition. *American Journal of Occupational Therapy, 62*, 625-683.

Angelo, J. (1997). *Assistive technology for rehabilitation therapies.* Philadelphia, PA: F.A. Davis.

Bellis, M. (n.d.). Martin Cooper—History of cell phone: Martin Cooper talks about the first cell phone call. Retrieved June 6, 2006, from http://inventors.about.com/cs/inventorsalphabet/a/martin_cooper.htm

Benedict, R. E., Lee, J. P., Marrujo, S. K., & Farel, A. M. (1999). Assistive devices as an early childhood intervention: Evaluating outcomes. *Technology and Disability, 11*(1/2), 79-90.

Bodeau, V. (2002). Lower limb prosthetics. In EMedicine from WebMD. Retrieved June 6, 2006, from http://www.emedicine.com/pmr/topic175.htm

Bourgeois, M., & Mason, L. A. (1996). Memory wallet intervention in an adult day-care setting. *Behavioral Interventions: Theory and Practice in Residential and Community-based Clinical Programs, 11*(1), 3-18.

Cook, A. M., & Hussey, S. (1995). *Assistive technologies: Principles and practice.* St. Louis, MO: Mosby.

Dahlin Ivanoff, S., & Sonn, U. (2005). Assistive devices in activities of daily living used by persons with age-related macular degeneration: A population study of 85-year-olds living at home. *Scandinavian Journal of Occupational Therapy, 12*(1), 10-17.

Eriksrud, O., & Bohannon, R. (2005). Effectiveness of the easy-up handle in acute rehabilitation. *Clinical Rehabilitation, 19*(4), 381-386.

Hoenig, H., Taylor, D. H., Jr., & Sloan, F. A. (2003). Does assistive technology substitute for personal assistance among the disabled elderly? *American Journal of Public Health, 93*(2), 330-337.

Lancioni, G. E., Singh, N. N., O'Reilly, M. F., Sigafoos, J., Olivia, D., & Baccani, S. (2007). Enabling students with multiple disabilities to request and choose among environmental stimuli through microswitch and computer technology. *Research in Developmental Disabilities: A Multidisciplinary Journal, 28*(1), 50-58.

Lau, C., & O'Leary, S. (1993). Comparison of computer interface devices for persons with severe physical disabilities. *American Journal of Occupational Therapy. 47*(11), 1022-1030.

Mann, W. C., & Lane, J. P. (1991). *Assistive technology for persons with disabilities: The role of occupational therapy.* Bethesda, MD: AOTA Press.

Mihailidis, A., Tam, T., McLean, M. & Lee, T. (2005). An intelligent health monitoring and emergency response system. In S. Giroux & H. Pigot (Eds.), *From smart homes to smart care* (pp. 272-281.). Amsterdam, The Netherlands: IOSPress.

National Institute on Deafness and Other Communications Disorders. (2002). Hearing aids. Retrieved June 6, 2006, from http://www.nidcd.nih.gov/health/hearing/hearingaid.asp

Nordenskiöld, U. (1997). Daily activities in women with rheumatoid arthritis. Aspects of patient education, assistive devices and methods for disability and impairment assessment. *Scandinavian Journal of Rehabililitation Medicine Supplement, 37*, 1-72.

Office of the Federal Register, National Archives and Records Service, General Services Administration. (2000). Electronic and information technology accessibility standards. *The Federal Register, 65*(246), 80499-80528.

Sonn, U. (1996). Longitudinal studies of dependence in daily life activities among elderly persons. *Scandinavian Journal of Rehabililitation Medicine Supplement, 34*, 1-35.

Uustal, H., & Minkel, J. (2004). Study of the Idependence IBOT 3000 Mobility System: An innovative power mobility device, during use in community environments. *Archives of Physical Medicine and Rehabilitation, 85*(12), 2002-2010.

Van Hulle, A., & Hux, K. (2006). Improvement patterns among survivors of brain injury: Three case examples documenting the effectiveness of memory compensation strategies. *Brain Injury, 20*(1), 101-109.

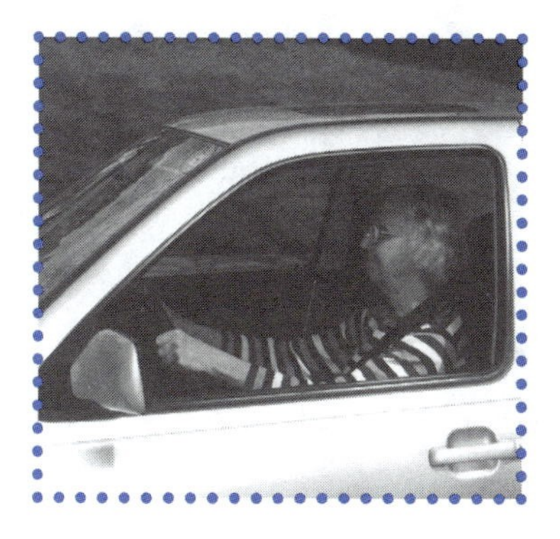

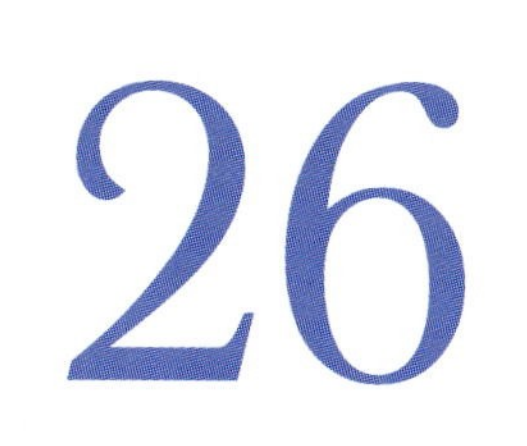

# 26

# Occupation-Centered Mobility

*Kathryn M. Loukas, MS, OTR/L, FAOTA*

**ACOTE Standard Explored in This Chapter**

B.5.11

**Key Terms**

| | |
|---|---|
| Bed mobility | Functional mobility |
| Body mechanics | Physical transfers |
| Community mobility | Seating systems |
| Driver rehabilitation | Wheelchair management |

## Introduction

Occupational engagement and participation in activities of life require people to move about their environment. Social participation is greatly enhanced when people can freely move about their homes, communities, and gathering places that hold purpose. *Functional mobility intervention* is the term occupational therapy practitioners most often use to describe the therapeutic tenets of bringing a client from bed mobility through transfers, and finally to community mobility and driving. Safe and effective participation in occupations is the goal of such intervention. It is usually an interdisciplinary intervention as the occupational therapy practitioner must work closely with the physical therapist, who addresses gait training and functional ambulation, as well as physicians and durable medical equipment vendors involved in wheeled mobility. The occupational therapy practitioner must be fully informed of important factors involved in functional mobility through evaluation of overall important client factors, including strength, range of motion, balance, coordination, cognitive processing, perceptual understanding, and visual skills (Creel, Adler, Tipton-Burton, & Lillie, 2001).

Pierce (2002) proposed a basic hierarchy of mobility to address the order in which these skills should be addressed. This adapted pyramid forms the stability, positioning, and mobility necessary to begin meaningful occupations and goes from the foundation or base and moves to the top (Figure 26-1).

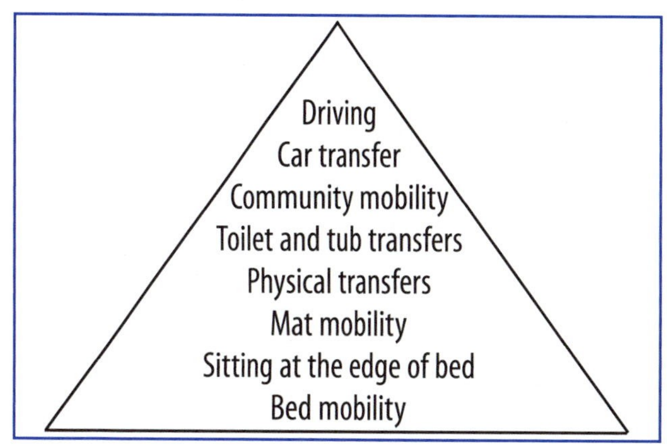


**Figure 26-1.** The occupation-based mobility pyramid. Adapted from Pierce, S. (2002). Restoring competence in mobility. In C. A. Trombly & M. V. Radomski (Eds.), *Occupational therapy for physical dysfunction* (5th ed., p. 667). Philadelphia, PA: Lippincott Williams & Wilkins.



K. Sladyk, K. Jacobs, & N. MacRae (Eds.).
*Occupational Therapy Essentials for Clinical Competence* (pp. 281-294).

The occupational therapy practitioner must keep in mind that every client is unique in his or her abilities and approach to mobility in occupation. Prerequisites to functional mobility training include critical thinking of the occupational therapy practitioner regarding client factors and performance patterns, including primary and secondary medical conditions, age, medications, family unit, and lifestyle, and how these factors might affect the client's functioning now and in the future (AOTA, 2008). Context and environmental opportunities and obstacles are also important to incorportate and adapt if necessary. It is imperative that occupational therapy practitioners learn and utilize proper body mechanics in order to safely move, position, and transfer clients.

## Basic Principles of Body Mechanics

Use of proper body mechanics is key for the safety of both the occupational therapy practitioner and the client. Alnaser (2007) found in a literature review that patient handling was the most common occupational factor involved in work-based injuries. In addition, the occupational therapy practitioner may teach caretakers or instruct the client to facilitate the proper body mechanics of handling and lifting in the home or community.

The basic principles include the following:

- Keep a stable center of gravity. Keep a square orientation to the client with a straight or neutral spine and back. Bend at the hips and knees.
- Maintain a wide base of support while handling or lifting.
- Maintain proper body alignment and do not twist.

Techniques to utilize during handling or lifting include the following (Brookside Associates, 2007; Creel et al., 2001):

- Make sure that you are strong enough to handle the situation; seek assistance if necessary.
- Communicate with the person you are handling or lifting and seek their assistance in any way possible.
- Use the larger, stronger muscles such as the legs for lifting.
- Bend at the knees or hips while keeping the back straight.
- Lift in one smooth motion.
- Stay as close to the person you are lifting or handling as possible.
- Avoid twisting or over-stretching.

# Bed Positioning and Mobility

Movement in the bed is often the first physical task involved in the recovery of occupational performance. The occupational therapy practitioner is often involved with the interdisciplinary team in assisting the client to position or move in the bed. It is important that the team collaborate and communicate the best positioning movement techniques for each individual client. All team members should facilitate the positioning and movement of the client in the same manner in order to help the client move in an independent or interdependent manner.

## Goals of Bed Positioning

- Provision of support, comfort, and pain relief
- Normalization of muscle tone
- Promotion of symmetrical positioning
- Improved awareness of affected side and safety of limbs
- Prevention of positions of deformity and decubitus ulcers
- Facilitation of occupational mobility and meaningful activities
- Optimization of occupational performance (Wilson, Lange, & Mandac, 2006)

## Precautions

The occupational therapy practitioner should be aware of her or his own physical capabilities as well as the medical and psychosocial needs and attributes of the client when preparing for occupational mobility. Common client precautions include the following (Bolding, Adler, Tipton-Burton, & Lillie, 2006):

- Absent or impaired sensation
- Pressure points and length of positioning
- Awareness of skin integrity as friction during movement may cause shearing, particularly over boney prominences
- Deep vein thrombosis (DVT) from lack of circulation in the legs
- Abnormal muscle tone (hypertonia or hypotonia) with impaired sensation
- Head of bed position (keep client up in bed to prevent foot entrapment)
- Orthostatic hypotension caused by a sudden drop in blood pressure when moving from supine to upright positions following long periods of bed rest resulting in dizziness, nausea, or possible loss of consciousness
- Cognitive challenges

# Bed Mobility Skills

The occupational therapist can facilitate the basic movements needed in the occupational performance task of bed mobility. Breaking these tasks into manageable steps can be an effective way to facilitate bed mobility. The occupational therapy practitioner should work with the interdisciplinary team to develop an approach to bed mobility based on the evaluation of individual client factors, performance patterns, and contexts. Practicing skills can help the client gain skills and confidence to begin to combine movements for occupational performance. The occupational therapy practitioner should then facilitate the use of these skills in independent or interdependent performance patterns and daily routines. The following skills are needed for effective bed mobility:

- Rolling (to either side) (Figure 26-2)
- Bridging (pulling the hips up in supine while supporting the pelvis from the legs)
- Scooting up in bed (necessary to reposition one's self in bed)
- Supine to side lying to sit (Figures 26-3 and 26-4)
- Moving to either side of the bed
- Sitting on the edge of the bed (Figure 26-5)

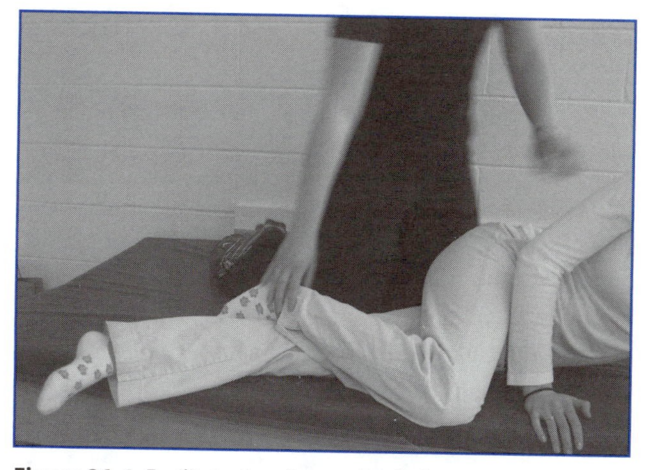

**Figure 26-4.** Facilitate the client to hook the stronger leg over a weaker one and push legs off the end of the bed while spotting carefully for safety.

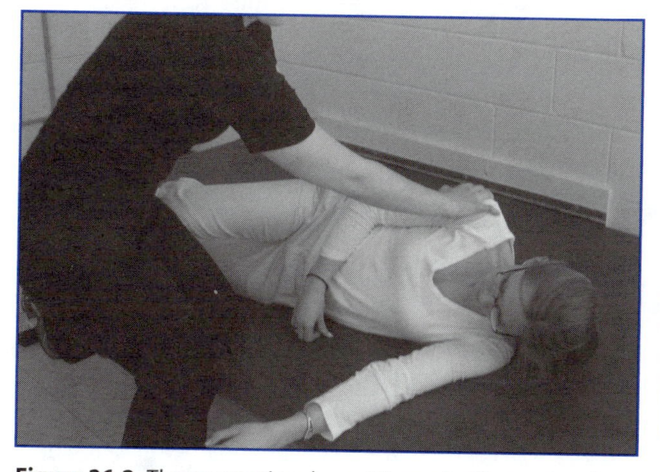

**Figure 26-2.** The occupational practitioner facilitates the client to roll to her side.

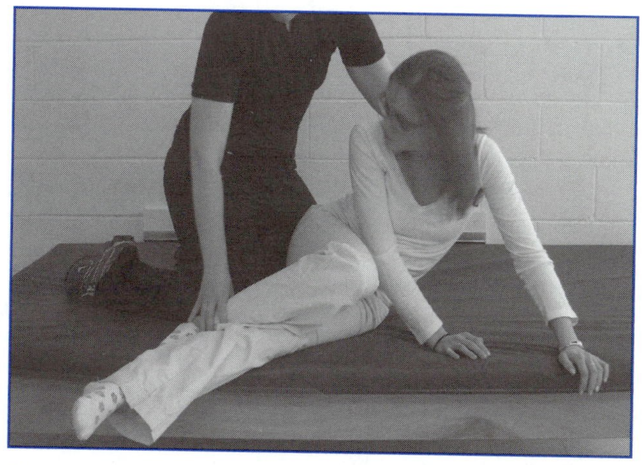

**Figure 26-5.** The client should come to sitting slowly.

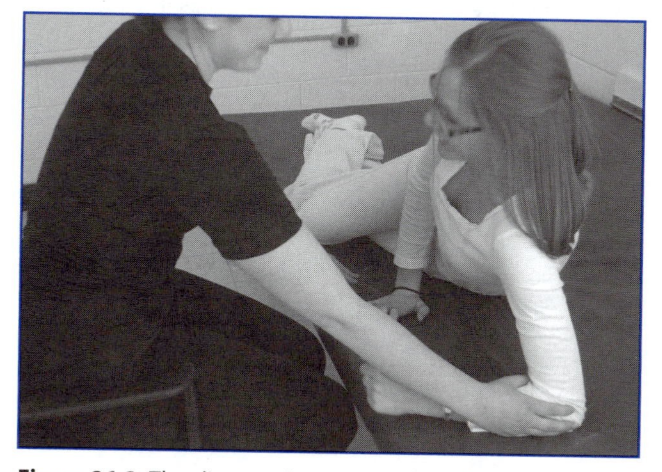

**Figure 26-3.** The client pushes up onto one elbow.

## Therapeutic Bed Mobility

Bed mobility can be used as the occupational product of therapy, such as when a client is given adaptations for independence, and/or as occupational process, such as when the therapist is facilitating movement, cognitive processing, or perceptual awareness through the occupation of bed mobility. Some examples of physically based occupational process skills that can be incorporated into bed mobility include the following:

- Awareness of affected side (hemiparesis) or affected extremities (spinal cord injury [SCI])
- Upper extremity movement, including scapular mobility
- Weight shift and weight bearing
- Trunk stability and postural control
- Management of affected extremities
- Safe movement and cognitive awareness

## Adaptive Devices for Bed Mobility

Adaptive equipment may assist a client to move effectively in bed. The occupational therapist should work with the interdisciplinary team to facilitate independent or interdependent bed mobility individualized to each client. Devices that can facilitate bed mobility in the medical setting or home include:

- Bed ladder pull-up (Figure 26-6)
- Leg lifter
- Overhead trapeze bar
- Bed rail assist (Figure 26-7)
- Transfer pole
- A draw sheet or positioning sheet can be placed perpendicular to the client under the trunk and hips for dependent bed mobility with two people on either side of the bed (Pierce, 2002).

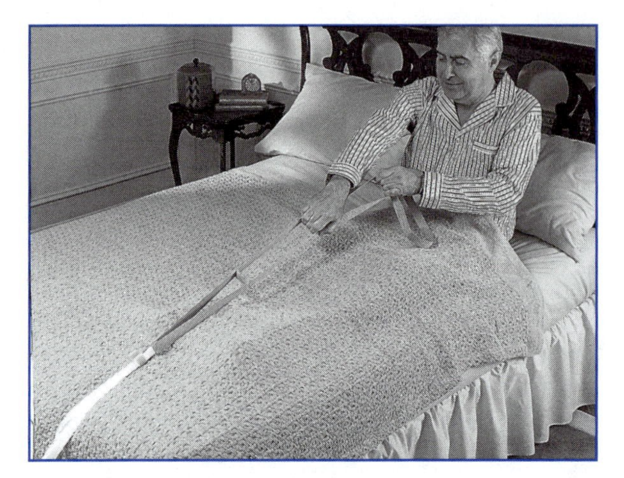

**Figure 26-6.** Bed Pull-up, product #C5130. Reproduced with permission from Sammons Preston, a Patterson Medical Company (2006).

# Transfers

The next step in functional mobility is teaching your client who uses a wheelchair to move from one surface to another. This is called transferring.

Some facilities and occupational therapy departments require use of a transfer belt for safety when transferring clients. Occupational therapy practitioners should be aware of the protocol of their facility/department regarding use of a transfer belt or any protocol.

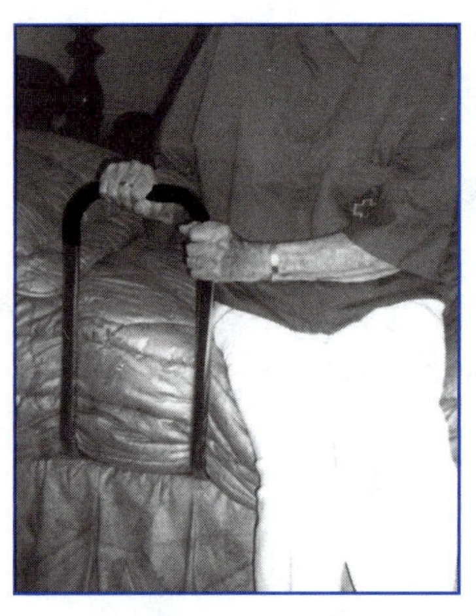

**Figure 26-7.** Freedom Grip, product #C552888. Reproduced with permission from Sammons Preston, a Patterson Medical Company (2006).

# Wheelchair Safety/Etiquette

The occupational therapy practitioner should have respect for the physical and psychosocial difficulties a client may have with use of the wheelchair. The wheelchair is a wonderful tool to facilitate occupational mobility. However, it also carries with it stigma regarding disability and loss of ambulation, whether that be temporary or permanent. The occupational therapy practitioner, who is skilled in both physical and psychosocial aspects of human life, should be attuned to the client as they begin to be mobilized by a wheelchair. Language is key to acceptance of mobility using a wheelchair. The occupational therapy practitioner should refer to the client as "using" or "mobilized" by a wheelchair. Care should be taken that clients are not referred to as "confined" to a wheelchair (Loukas, 2008).

### Tips for Wheelchair Etiquette

- Talk to clients at wheelchair height when you can, do not stand over them to talk.
- Teach the client, caretakers, and interdisciplinary team to always lock brakes for all transfers.
- The client should be wearing shoes with a nonslip sole.
- The client should never stand on the footrests; the practitioner should not lean on the chair.
- In most transfers, you should swing the footrests aside for ease of movement.
- Transfers are most efficient when the surfaces are the same height.
- A client with hemiparesis or other one-sided impairment will most easily transfer toward his or her stronger side.

## As You Prepare for the Transfer

- Be aware of the client's assets and limitations.
- Recognize the dynamic nature of your own physical abilities and limitations.
- Use optimal body mechanics.

## Therapeutic Principles Incorporated in the Transfer

Therapeutic approaches and client factor remediation can be incorporated into the occupation of transferring. The following can be related to the occupational therapy intervention plan, model, or frame of reference:

- Anterior pelvic tilt
- Trunk alignment
- Weight bearing and weight shifting
- Use of manual cues (neurodevelopmental treatment [NDT])(Runyan, 2006)
- Lower extremity positioning
- Upper extremity positioning and functional use
- Cognitive, perceptual, and/or visual awareness
- Facilitating independence by encouraging the client to do as much of the process him- or herself as possible. The occupational therapy practitioner should provide the minimal amount of physical assistance for safe transfer.
- In the case of the client who is interdependent with a caregiver, teach the client how to teach others, including family, caregivers, and paid attendants.

## Preparation for the Transfer to the Wheelchair

1. Communicate with the client about the procedure and provide rapport and meaning to this mobility occupation.
2. The client should wear and secure a transfer belt (Figure 26-8).
3. Position the wheelchair at a 30-degree angle to the surface to which you are transferring and remove the armrest closest to the transfer site if necessary (Figure 26-9).
4. Be certain that the brakes are locked. Facilitate the client's awareness of safety. Check the brakes again (Figure 26-10).
5. The client should scoot forward (Figure 26-11).
6. The client should lean forward (nose over toes) (Figures 26-12 through 26-14).
7. Stabilize the lower extremities or the hemiplegic leg if necessary and support any upper extremity limbs with abnormal tone.
8. Help the client squat down to the wheelchair (Figure 26-15).

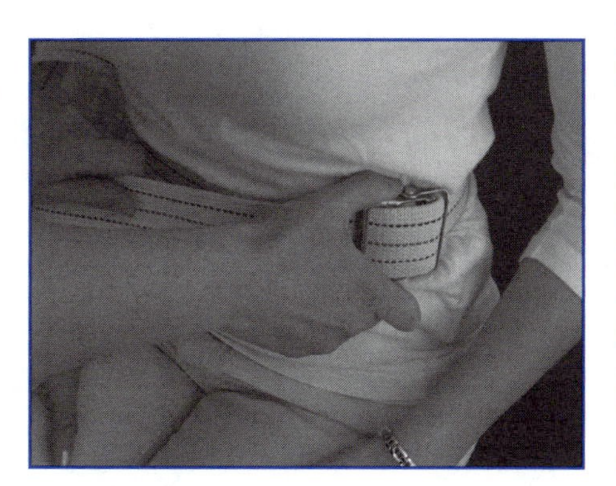

**Figure 26-8.** Secure transfer (gait) belt for safety.

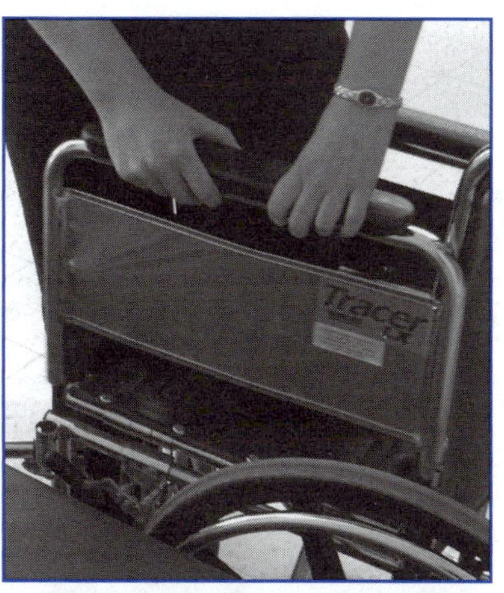


**Figure 26-9.** Position wheelchair, remove armrest closest to the client for some transfers.

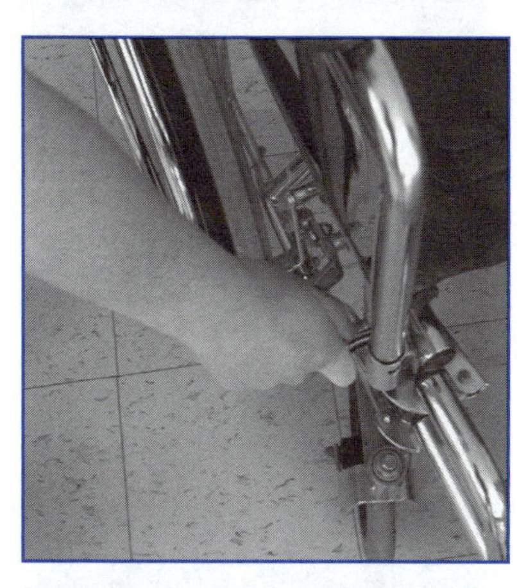

**Figure 26-10.** Be certain that the wheelchair brakes are locked!

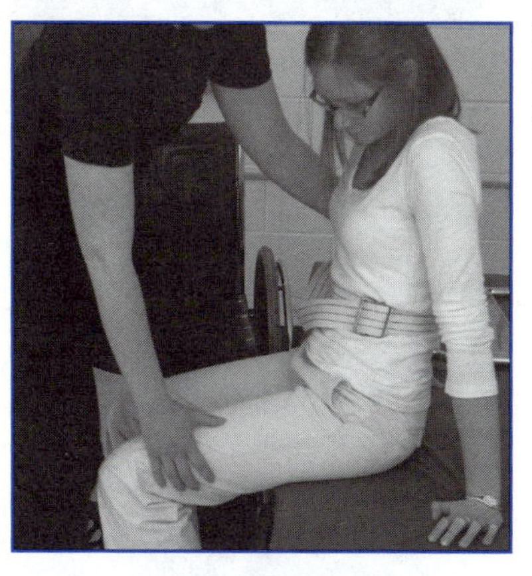

**Figure 26-11.** Facilitate the client to safely scoot forward.

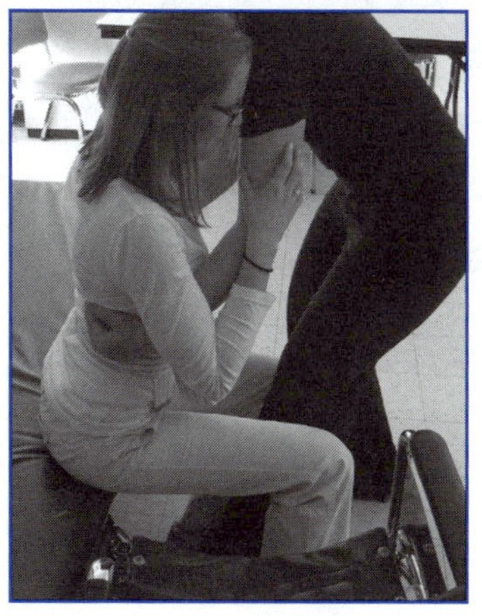

**Figure 26-12.** Facilitate the client into the "nose over toes" position; block the knee or knees if there is weakness there.

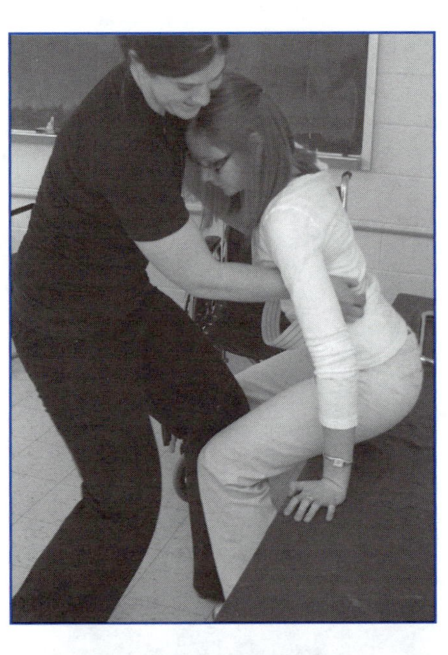

**Figure 26-13.** Client pushes off of the mat. Note the proper body mechanics of the occupational therapy practitioner and facilitation of client participation in the process.

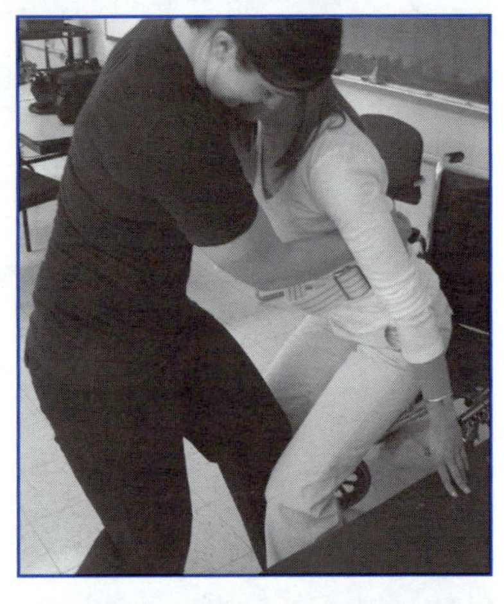

**Figure 26-14.** The client reaches back and leans forward as she is seated in the wheelchair.

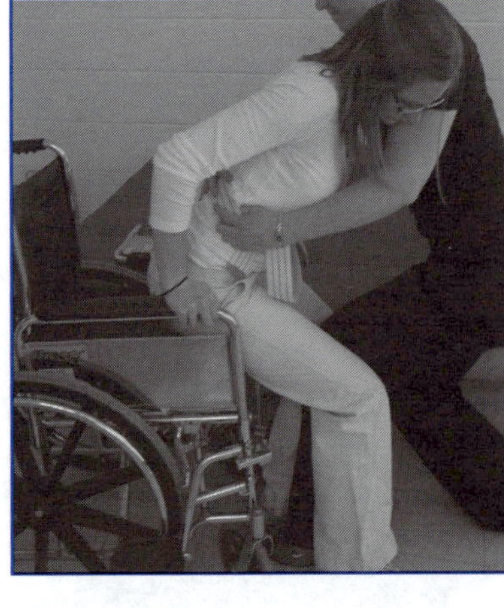

**Figure 26-15.** Transfer: In a squat-pivot transfer, the practitioner pivots while the client maintains hip flexion and the "nose over toes" position.

# Types of Transfers

These first three types of transfers can be performed as an intervention progression and are often used for clients with hemiparesis or other central nervous system impairments:

- Squat or bent pivot
- Stand pivot
- Stand step

The following are equipment used for transfers:

- *Sliding board*: Commonly used for people who have a spinal cord injury, overall weakness, and above-knee or double amputation.
- *Dependent transfers*: Use of mechanical device such as a hoyer lift (Figure 26-16).
- *Cueing systems*: Clients with cognitive impairments may be physically able but need verbal, tactile, or visual cues to break down the steps of the task for safety.

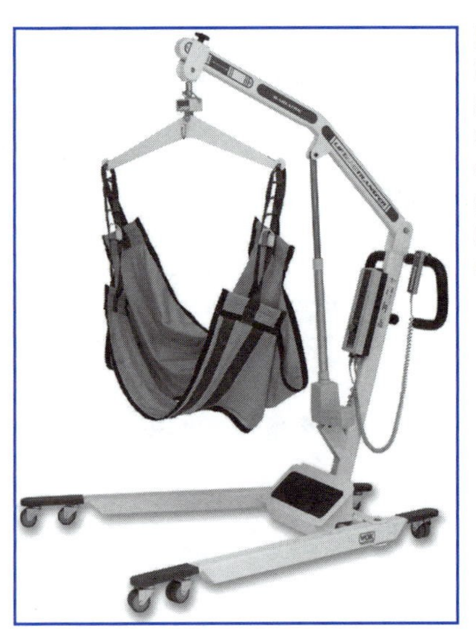

**Figure 26-16.** BCW Lift and Transfer System, product #563436. Reproduced with permission from Sammons Preston, a Patterson Medical Company (2006).

## Levels of Assistance in Transfer

- One or two people assist with device, if needed
- Two or more assistants (Maximum Assist x 2)
- Verbal cues needed (tactile, visual cues)
- Dependent: 75% to 100% assistance
- Maximum assist: 50% to 74% assistance
- Moderate assist: 25% to 49% assistance
- Minimum assist: up to 24% assistance
- Contact guard (CG): Practitioner has his or her hand on the client at all times
- Supervision: No hands-on assistance
- Set up
- Independent (means completely independent) (Matthews & Jabri, 2001)

## Physical Transfer Procedures

### Bent (Squat) Pivot

- Remove armrest
- Scoot forward and lean forward (nose over toes)

- Position affected arm
- Support affected leg
- Transfer, keeping the client in a bent forward position

Stand Pivot

- Same as above, although you do not need to remove armrests
- Bring client to a standing position, gain equilibrium, do not rush
- Client pivots on unaffected leg, or both
- Reach back for the chair
- Lean the client forward as you descend as well

Stand Step

- Same as stand pivot, with weight shift of the lower extremities
- Should need less physical assistance

Sliding Board Transfers

- Set up wheelchair as described previously
- Shift weight to the opposite side of the transfer and maneuver the sliding board under the leg and buttock closest to the wheelchair (when there are sensation losses, male clients need to be careful of the positioning of their genitalia) (Figure 26-17)
- Block the client's knees with your own knees (the practitioner may be seated during the transfer)
- The client should make sure the board is in a good position to travel into the chair
- Instruct the client to lean forward and put his or her hands on the board (clients with a SCI that are preserving the tenodesis grasp should keep their hands fisted as to not overstretch the wrist and hand extensors)
- The client should slowly and carefully scoot or move toward the wheelchair with the practitioner directly in front of him or her (the transfer should become more independent as the client's skill progresses) (Figures 26-18 and 16-19)

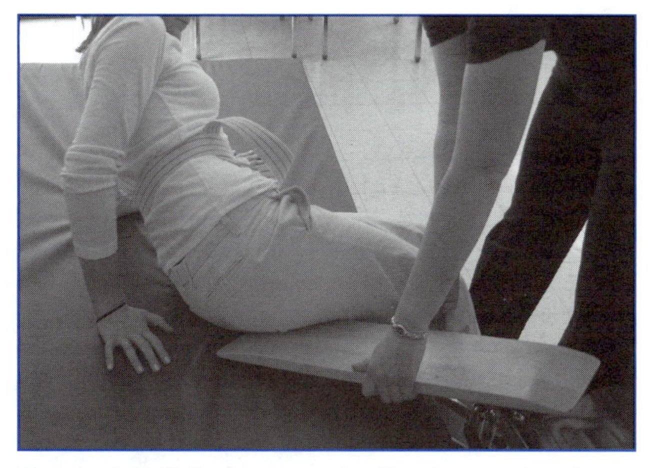

**Figure 26-17.** Sliding board transfer: The client supports herself in a tripod arm position while un-weighting the hip closest to the wheelchair.

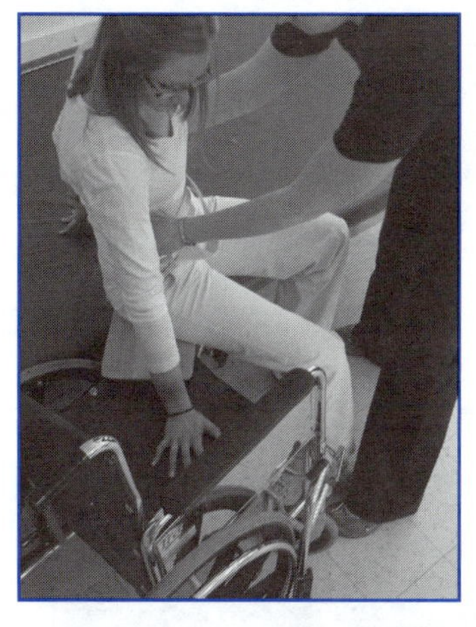

**Figure 26-18.** The client uses a slow un-weighting procedure as the practitioner provides manual cues and safety.

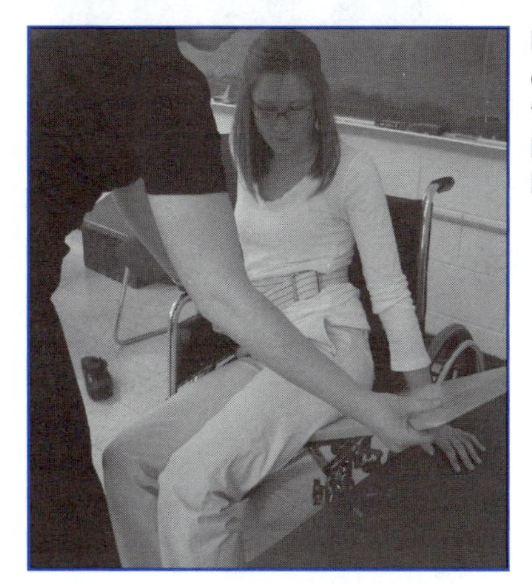

**Figure 26-19.** The client un-weights or "slides" into the chair, hips should be as far back as possible.

## Dependent Transfers

Many clients with significant client factors will be dependent in their transfers. It is important for occupational therapy practitioners to know their own limitations and protect their own bodies when attempting dependent transfers for clients. Dependent transfers can be accomplished by use of a team approach. However, if a client needs to transfer dependently long-term, the best solution is a client lift system. If a client is very heavy, there are bariatric lift systems available to lift up to 600 pounds. The role of the occupational therapy practitioner then becomes selection and training of the family or caregiver to use the device. The occupational therapy practitioner can work with more involved clients to assure that they have the skills to do their own transfer training over the lifespan as caregivers may come and go. An example of this is a client with quadriplegic cerebral palsy making a CD of a caregiver performing a model transfer in order to train others.

# Occupation-Based Mobility for Larger, Heavier Clients

Occupational therapy practitioners are often called upon to meet the needs of the larger, heavy (obese) client. In the areas of beds, mats, transfer aids, adaptive equipment, and lift systems; specialized equipment is often needed to meet the needs of large clients. It is important to use equipment that can handle the weight for maximal safety and comfort of our larger clients. Occupational therapy practitioners should work with their durable equipment vendors and manufacturing representatives in order to keep current with the evolving adaptive equipment and assistive technology available to meet client needs (Figure 26-20).

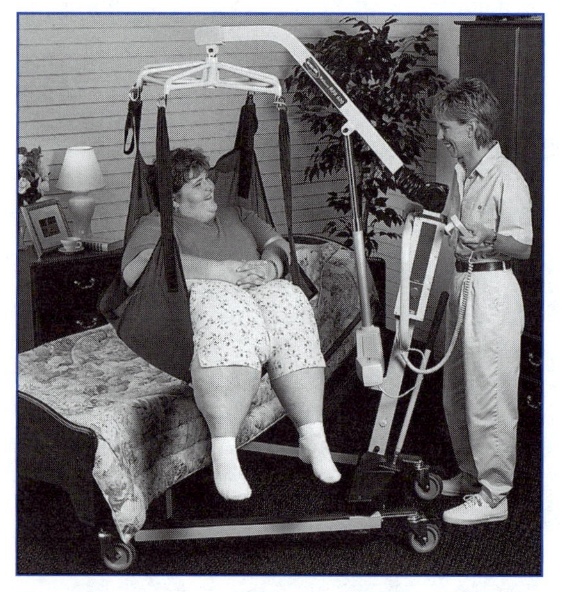

**Figure 26-20.** Invacare Bariatric Lift, product #926766. Reproduced with permission from Sammons Preston, a Patterson Medical Company (2009).

# Wheelchair Management

The wheelchair is the primary mobility device for many people who live with mobility impairment. Because of the cost and importance of the wheelchair, there are often multiple disciplines involved in ordering the wheelchair. This includes the client and his or her family/caregiver, a physician, a physical therapist, a wheelchair vendor, and an occupational therapist. Other specialists such as a respiratory therapist may also be involved, as well as speech and language pathologists when the client uses an electronic communication device. In this circumstance, the positioning and attachment of the device becomes essential to functional use of the communication system (Wilson et al., 2006).

## Wheelchair Seating and Positioning

Sling seats in a wheelchair are for very short-term, occasional use. Any individual who spends time sitting in a wheelchair should be fitted with a foam-, gel-, or air-based seating system. Pressure mapping is important for individuals who are at high risk for skin breakdown. Specialized, customized seating is recommended for consumers with significant postural deformities.

Goals for proper wheelchair seating and positioning include the following (Bolding et al., 2006, p. 212):

- To facilitate postural control and head stability
- To provide symmetry and prevent deformity
- To normalize muscle tone and facilitate postural control
- To maintain skin integrity and pressure management
- To promote occupational performance and function to maximize sitting endurance and stamina for activity
- To optimize respiratory function

The client must have adequate strength and control to mobilize the wheelchair. For clients who will propel their wheelchairs manually, techniques include giving clients protective gloves or lacing the wheelchair with rubber tubing to improve grip. Other techniques, such as using wheeled mobility or electric devices, can conserve energy and improve occupational functioning and community participation for many clients. For clients with high-level paralysis, a breath-controlled or head-controlled electronic system can be used to operate the wheelchair, thus providing important independence and mobility. For children with mobility impairments, there are myriad pediatric mobility devices. These include push-chairs, positioning chairs, and adaptable level chairs for school-based occupations (Figures 26-21 and 26-22).

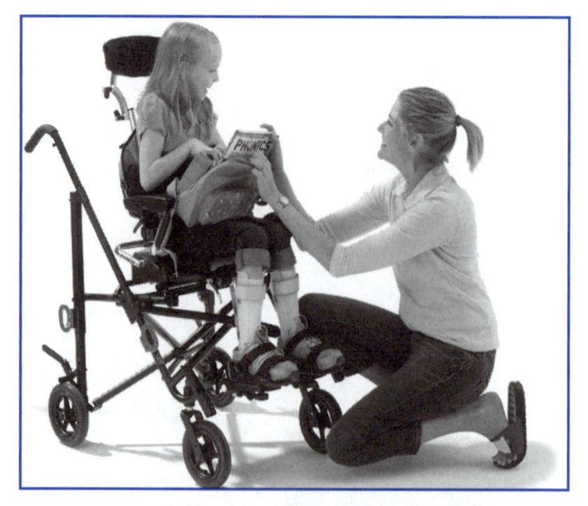


**Figure 26-21.** Convaid EZ Rider Mobility Base, product #081433572. Reproduced with permission from Sammons Preston, a Patterson Medical Company (2009).

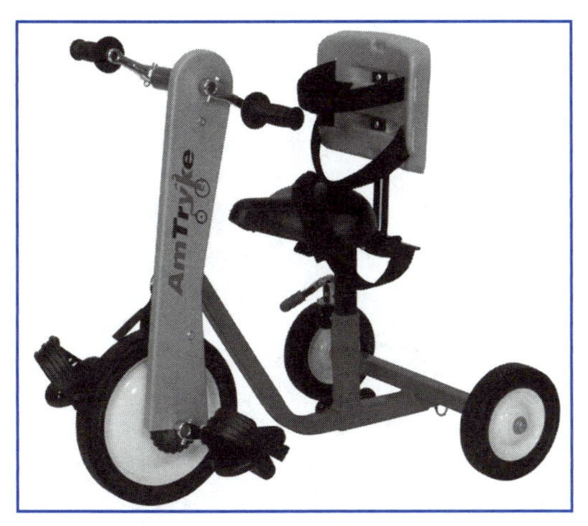


**Figure 26-22.** Am Tryke, product #45232. Reproduced with permission from Sammons Preston, a Patterson Medical Company (2009).

## Leisure-Based Mobility Devices

There are also a number of bicycles and recreation-based, fun mobility devices for children and adults. These can be adapted in a number of ways to provide more support or stability.

## Wheelchair Selection and Measurement

When determining the wheelchair needs of a person, the occupational therapy practitioner should be sure to consider the client's context (home, school, work) accessibility, outdoor terrain, and climate. It is important to help consumers understand their needs and make the best selection. Some good questions for a consumer to ask are as follows (Wheelchair Net, 2006):

- Where will I use my wheelchair most?
- What will be occasional needs I will have for wheelchair mobility?
- What kinds of activities do I intend to do? What are my occupational needs?
- How will I transport my wheelchair?
- How much time will I be spending in the wheelchair?
- How will I transfer from the wheelchair into different surfaces?
- If I am dependent or interdependent with my wheelchair, what features might be helpful to my aide or caregiver?
- How will I mobilize my chair in my neighborhood or yard? Are there other surfaces that I might frequently encounter?

An occupational therapy practitioner should always work with the client and an inter-disciplinary team that includes a physician and durable equipment vendor to make determinations regarding the use, payment, and type of wheelchair and accessories to meet the mobility needs of individual clients. The occupational therapy practitioner should use critical thinking to assure that the mobility device facilitates the client's occupational performance, enabling the client to participate as fully as possible in occupations in the home, worksite, and community (Figures 26-23 through 26-26).

## Community Mobility

Community participation is a very important aspect to a full life and occupational functioning. The Americans With Disabilities Act (ADA) of 1990 has provided important

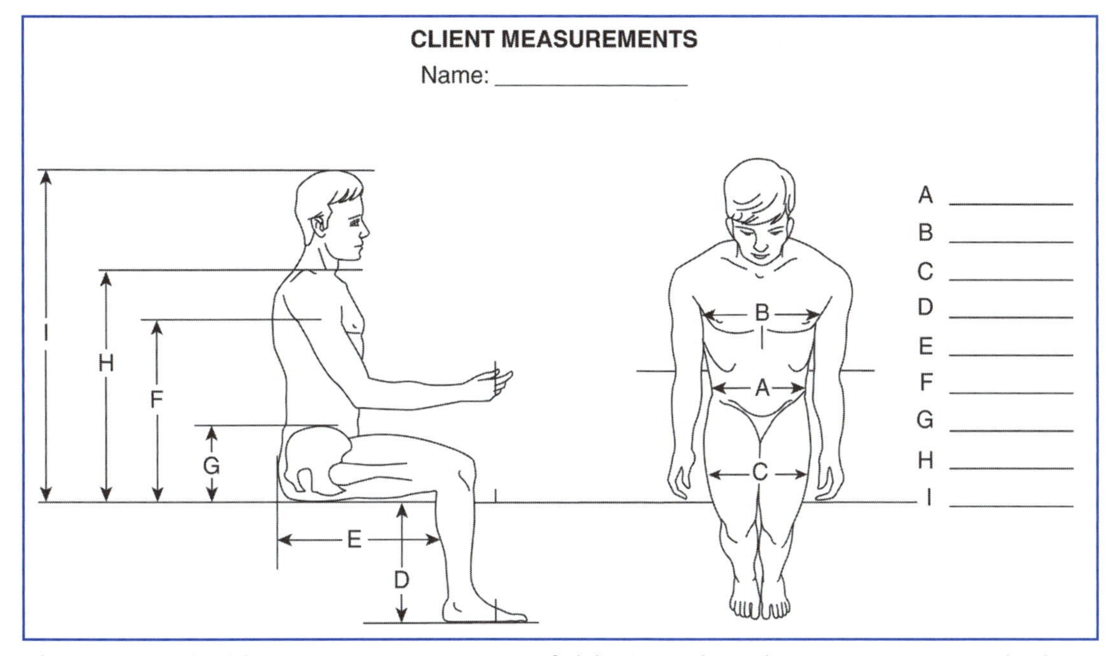


**Figure 26-23.** Wheelchair measurements. Courtesy of Alpha One, Independent Living Program, Portland, ME.

**Figure 26-24.** Measurements for a wheelchair should be made while the client is in the optimal sitting position.

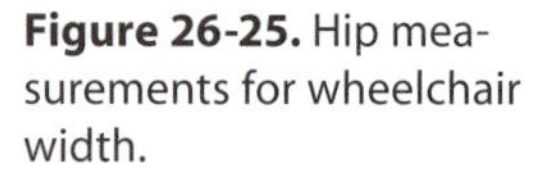

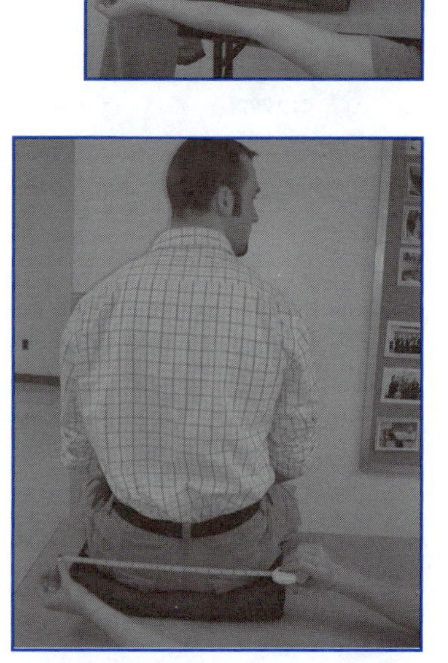

**Figure 26-25.** Hip measurements for wheelchair width.

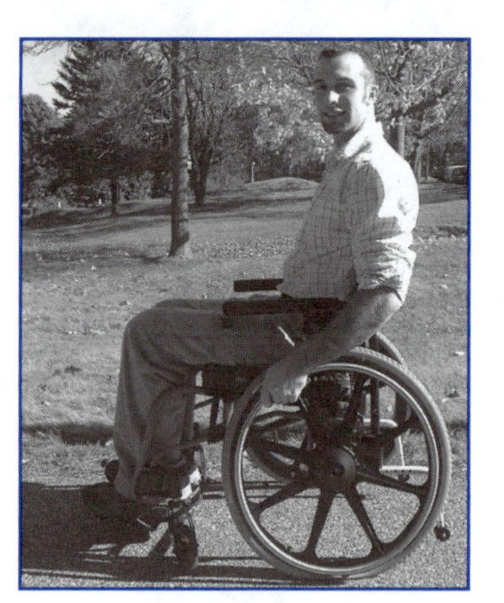

**Figure 26-26.** The proper type and fit of wheelchair is necessary for optimal occupation-based community mobility and participation.

accessibility rights for people with mobility challenges, and this continues to improve (U.S. Department of Justice, n.d.). Both physical and attitudinal accessibility changes in our communities create more opportunities for people with disabilities. Occupational therapy practitioners are at the forefront of these advocacy efforts. Facilitation of clients to return or emerge into the community is an important aspect of a full life and full participation (Baum, 2006). For persons with functional mobility impairment, the first important step is for clients to have insight regarding their own abilities, opportunities, and obstacles. A client who can realistically judge his or her own strength and mobility challenges will have more success in planning for community mobility. For clients with cognitive challenges or lack of insight into their own abilities, the occupational therapy practitioner must help them understand and judge their own needs and abilities. The next step is planning. The occupational therapy practitioner can assist his or her client to plan an outing into the community, such as grocery shopping, visiting a friend, going out to eat, or attending church. Planning includes thinking about transportation, devices, safety and equipment needs, medication management, and many other client-specific factors. Finally, going out into the community in graded steps is achieved. The client should be encouraged to reflect on the experiences and to plan and adjust as he or she progresses in community participation. The occupational therapy practitioner may accompany the client on several community outings in order to foster mobility independence and community participation.

### Transportation

There are many wheelchair-accessible vans, entry systems, and driving controls available to clients with mobility challenges. There is also increasingly more public transportation that provides accessibility to people who use wheelchairs and other mobility devices. Children traveling in school buses should have accessible and safe systems in place for transport. Parents with young children with mobility impairment often transfer their children into a car seat and have portable wheelchairs or push-chairs (strollers) for community mobility. It is important for the occupational therapy practitioner to assist the family to explore their adaptive equipment options as the child grows and needs a more accessible system that allows him or her to stay in the wheelchair.

## Driver Rehabilitation

Driving is an integral part of independent living and essential to a person's success in employment, education, socialization, community participation, and aging in place (American Medical Association [AMA], 2003; Bolding et al., 2006). Occupational therapy practitioners are emerging into the practice of driver rehabilitation for persons with physical disabilities in greater and greater numbers. An entry-level occupational therapy curriculum includes an understanding of driver assessment and vehicle adaptations. Advanced training and certification is available for occupational therapy practitioners to become Driver Rehabilitation Specialists (DRS). A DRS is "one who plans, develops, coordinates, and implements driving services for individuals with disabilities" (AMA, p. 53). Further certification in driving to become a Certified Driver Rehabilitation Specialist (CDRS) is available but not required to practice (AMA). Issues that are red flags for medically impaired driving include the following:

- Acute events: A stroke or brain injury, seizure, surgery, or delirium of any type
- A patient or family member concern
- Medical history that includes chronic conditions, particularly those that affect vision, cardiovascular disease, neurological disease, psychiatric disease, metabolic disease, musculoskeletal disabilities, chronic renal failure, and respiratory disease
- Medical conditions with unpredictable, episodic events
- Medications that can impair performance (AMA, 2003)
- A pattern of motor vehicle accidents

Occupational therapists with specialized training in driving-based occupations will conduct a thorough evaluation that includes vision, perception, mobility, hand and foot function, and cognition. Many independent living centers or rehabilitation centers offer driving assessment and training services. They will assist the client in choosing options such as car or vehicle considerations and the adaptive equipment needed to safely operate a motor vehicle. From there, occupational therapy practitioners will develop a full plan of care to help the client return to driving, begin to drive, or recommend that driving is not a safe option (AMA, 2003; Bolding et al., 2006).

## Issues Related to Driver Rehabilitation

### The Aging Driver

Motor vehicle injuries are the leading cause of injury-related deaths for the 65- to 74-year-old age bracket and the second leading cause (after falls) for the 75- to 84-year-old age bracket (AMA, 2003). Many older drivers begin to change their own habits by limiting driving to familiar places; driving only during the daylight hours; and avoiding busy, congested areas of traffic. Client factors, particularly regarding vision, are important to assess and address as adults age into their elder years. The loss of the ability to drive has been correlated with risk of entering a long-term care facility in the elder population (Freeman, Gange, Munoz, & West, 2006).

### Hand Controls

Clients with paralysis or right-sided impairment may switch to hand controls. These are manufactured and can be used to help a client with paralysis return to the safe occupation of driving. Behind-the-wheel driving instruction is essential for those individuals who are re-establishing their safe driving skills using adaptive devices.

### Driving With Visual Impairment

There are a number of devices now being used to assist the driver who is visually impaired. Most states require a visual acuity of 20/40 to 20/70 or better and visual fields of about 140 degrees, although different states vary in their requirements (AMA, 2003). Bioptic telescopes are legal in many states for people with visual impairment, but the scopes must bring the vision to a level of 20/70 or better (AMA).

### Adapted Vehicles and Lifts

Many companies have a line for adapted vehicles and lifts. These can be very expensive for clients, so it is important to make good decisions for best overall occupational outcomes. There has been an expansion in vehicle adaptations to such a degree that it is imperative occupational therapy practitioners collaborate with durable medical equipment vendors regarding up-to-date equipment options. Behind-the-wheel assessments are vital in order to assess the actual adaptive equipment needs so that money is not needlessly spent. Nationwide, there are alternative financing programs available for low-interest loans so that individuals can borrow the money needed to buy adapted vehicles.

## Summary

Occupational therapy practitioners address occupation-based functional mobility in the contexts in which clients engage in social participation. The occupational therapy practitioner and the physical therapist collaborate in the areas of functional mobility to maximize client potential. Mobility skills progress developmentally from bed and mat mobility to transfers, to community mobility, and finally to driving. Many client factors are involved in occupation-based mobility and should be evaluated and addressed in occupational therapy interventions. Safety is a priority in the mobility-based intervention progression. Intervention planning should include a holistic model and frames of reference. Occupation-based mobility can be addressed within those therapeutic and often interdisciplinary approaches.

ACKNOWLEDGMENTS

The author would like to recognize and thank Kathy Adams, OTR/L for her expertise and content contributions to this chapter. The author is grateful to Sammons, Preston, Rolyan for use of their photographs. Finally, the author thanks Kathy Lemieux, MSOT, OTR/L from Alpha One, the independent living center in Portland, ME, for her input and contributions.

## Evidence-Based Research Chart

| Issue | Description | Evidence |
|---|---|---|
| **Mobility** | | |
| Elders | Elders who fell within 6 months following a hip fracture demonstrate poorer balance, slower gait, and decline in activities of daily living | Restoring elders to full health following a hip fracture is indicated, including addressing mobility and balance deficits (Shumway-Cook, Ciol, Grubon, & Robinson, 2005) |
| Individuals with SCI | Functional mobility found to be one of the top three problems identified by clients with SCI | Client-centered approaches have best results (Donnelly et al., 2004) |
| Seating and mobility for persons with SCI | Model that considers the person, wheelchair, and environments of home, work, and community | Seating and multiple considerations should be used for persons mobilized by a wheelchair (Minkel, 2000) |
| Self-perceived physical independence | Activity limitations correlate with perceptions of independence | Community mobility and coping efficacy improve self-perception of independence (Wang, Badley, & Gignac, 2004) |
| Wheelchair design | Wheelchair performance was tested on a community obstacle course | Differences in wheelchair design affect performance, and wheelchair choice is important to community mobility (Rodgers, Berman, Fails, & Jaser, 2003) |
| Wheelchair users at home | Researchers found that of 525 respondents, 37.9% of wheelchair users fell in the last 12 months. 17.7% suffered a fall-related injury. | Structural modifications and functional mobility-based therapy services for safety are needed (Berg, Hines, & Allen, 2002) |
| Wheelchair and mobility-related assistive services | Users' opinions on mobility devices and satisfaction | Positive effect on activity, transportation, security, and participation in social activities (Wresstle & Samuelsson, 2004) |
| Severely disabled people and powered wheelchairs | Quantitative study on perceived quality of life following use of powered wheelchair | Improvements in mobility and reduction in pain and discomfort were reported (Davies, Souza, & Frank, 2003) |
| Children | Children with cerebral palsy (CP) were compared across environmental settings in their gross motor performance | Results show differences across settings, indicating use of the natural context is important in therapy (Tieman, Palisano, Gracely, & Rosenbaum, 2004) |
| Spirituality and occupation-based mobility | Attendance at church by people with functional disabilities correlated with improved functioning | Church-related community mobility is important (Idler & Kasl, 1997) |
| | Using prayer as a modality for healing is more common among people with mobility limitations | Practitioners should facilitate a client's own spiritual expression and connection to a higher power: "religious pluralism" (Hendershot, 2003) |
| **Driving** | | |
| Nonstandard controls for disabled drivers | Large study of people with acquired disability. 79% had returned to driving. Significantly higher proportion had accidents. | Problems associated with nonfamiliar controls (Prasad, Hunter, & Hanley, 2006) |
| Safety and mobility of people with disabilities in adapted cars | Safety and perceptions of safety, as well as confidence in adapted car were reported | One out of 10 had accidents, a small number attributed to special equipment in the car (Henriksson & Peters, 2004) |
| Effects of fatigue on driving for people with multiple sclerosis (MS) | People with MS report fatigue, leg problems, numbness, and eye problems | MS population reports driving short distances with shorter driving times due to fatigue (Chipchase, Lincoln, & Radford, 2003) |
| Older nondrivers (never drivers and former drivers) | Correlated as an independent risk factor for entering long-term care facilities | Freeman et al., 2006 |
| Driving abilities and skills | Different driving situations require different skills and abilities | Driving is a complex task (Galski, Ehle, & Williams, 1997) |
| People with Parkinson's disease | Effects of cognitive abilities | Cognitive abilities were found NOT to be associated with fitness to drive (Radford, Lincoln, & Lennox, 2004) |

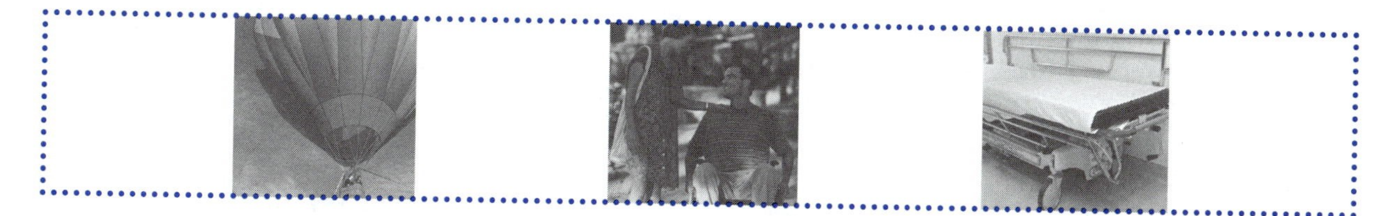

# Student Self-Assessment

1. Body mechanics: The students should put a necklace on with string and a bolt around the string. The necklace should be long enough to hang at the navel of the student. Instruct students to bend and lift items such as books. They should bend with their legs, and the necklace should not go further than 1 or 2 inches forward as they bend. You can also practice keeping the body stable and not allowing any rotation, and pulling versus pushing for bed mobility.
2. Wheelchair experience: Each student should spend one day using a wheelchair. Students should go to class, go out in the community, and perform other typical activities. They will then write a journal entry regarding the challenges and changes they experienced and their psychosocial responses to the wheelchair experience. It is very important for students to take this experience seriously and to not get out of the wheelchair in public, as this could be disrespectful to people who are mobilized by a wheelchair.
3. Bed mobility practice: Students should practice bed mobility for clients with the following diagnoses; hemiplegia, SCI paraplegia, and hip fracture/replacement. They should practice different teaching models in this process.
4. Transfer practice: Students should practice all of the transfer methods reviewed in this chapter. They should progress from bed or mat to wheelchair, from wheelchair to toilet or tub-chair, and finally from wheelchair to car.

# References


Alnaser, M. Z. (2007). Occupational musculoskeletal injuries in the health care environment and its impact on occupational therapy practitioners: A systematic review. *Work, 29*(20), 89-100.

American Medical Association. (2003). *Physicians guide to: Assessing and counseling older drivers*. Chicago, IL: Author.

American Occupational Therapy Association. (2008). Occupational therapy practice framework: Domain and process (2nd ed.). *American Journal of Occupational Therapy, 62*(6), 609-639.

Baum, M. C. (2006). Centennial challenges, millennium opportunities: Presidential address, 2006. *American Journal of Occupational Therapy, 60*, 609-616.

Berg, K., Hines, M., & Allen, S. (2002). Wheelchair users at home: Few home modifications and many injurious falls. *American Journal of Public Health, 92*(1), 48.

Bolding, D., Adler, C., Tipton-Burton, M., & Lillie, S. M. (2006). Mobility. In H. M. Pendleton & W. Schultz-Krohn (Eds.), *Pedretti's occupational therapy practice skills for physical dysfunction* (6th ed., pp. 195-247). St. Louis, MO: Mosby Elsevier.

Brookside Associates Multi-Media Edition. (2007). Nursing Fundamentals I. Retrieved August 6, 2009, from http://www.brooksidepress.org/Products/Nursing_Fundamentals_1/Index.htm

Chipchase, S. Y., Lincoln, N. B., & Radford, K. A. (2003). Measuring fatigue in people with multiple sclerosis. *Disability & Rehabilitation, 25*(14), 778-784.

Creel, T. A., Adler, C., Tipton-Burton, M., & Lillie, S. M. (2001). Mobility. In L. W. Pedretti & M. B. Early (Eds.), *Occupational therapy practice skills for physical dysfunction* (5th ed., pp. 172-178). St. Louis, MO: Mosby.

Davies, A., Souza, L. H., & Frank, A. O. (2003). Changes in the quality of life in severely disabled people following provision of powered indoor/outdoor chairs. *Disability & Rehabilitation, 25*(6), 286.

Donnelly, C., Eng, J. J., Hall, J., Alford, L., Gianchino, R., Norton, K., et al. (2004). Client centered assessment and the identification of meaningful treatment goals for individuals with a spinal cord injury. *Spinal Cord, 42*, 302-307.

Freeman, E. E., Gange, S. J., Munoz, B., & West, S. K. (2006). Driving status and risk of entry into long-term care in older adults. *American Journal of Public Health, 96*(7), 1254-1259.

Galski, T., Ehle, H. T., & Williams, J. B. (1997). Estimates of driving abilities and skills in different conditions. *American Journal of Occupational Therapy, 52*(4), 268-275.

Hendershot, G. E. (2003). Mobility limitations and complementary and alternative medicine: Are people with disabilities more likely to pray? *American Journal of Public Health, 93*(7), 1079-1080.

Henriksson, P., & Peters, B. (2004). Safety and mobility of people with disabilities driving adapted cars. *Scandinavian Journal of Occupational Therapy, 11*, 54-61.

Idler, E. L., & Kasl, S. V. (1997). Religion among disabled and non-disabled persons, II: Attendance at religion services as a predictor of the course of disability. *Journal of Gerontology, 52*(B), S306-S316.

Loukas, K. M. (2008). The evolution of language and perception of disability in occupational therapy. *Education Special Interest Section Newsletter, 18*(2), 1-4.

Matthews, M. M., & Jabri, J. L. (2001). Documentation of occupational therapy services. In L. W. Pedretti & M. B. Early (Eds.), *Occupational therapy practice skills for physical dysfunction* (5th ed., pp. 91-100). St. Louis, MO: Mosby.

Minkel, J. L. (2000). Seating and mobility considerations for people with spinal cord injury. *Physical Therapy, 80*(7), 701-709.

Pierce, S. (2002). Restoring competence in mobility. In C. A. Trombly & M. V. Radomski (Eds.), *Occupational therapy for physical dysfunction* (5th ed., pp. 665-693). Philadelphia, PA: Lippincott Williams & Wilkins.

Prasad, R. S., Hunter, J., & Hanley, J. (2006). Driving experiences of disabled drivers. *Clinical Rehabilitation, 20*(5), 445-450.

Radford, K. A., Lincoln, N. B., & Lennox, G. (2004). The effects of cognitive abilities on driving in people with Parkinson's disease. *Disability & Rehabilitation, 26*(2), 65-70.

Rodgers, H., Berman, S., Fails, D., & Jaser, J. (2003). A comparison of functional mobility in standard versus ultralight wheelchairs as measured by performance on a community obstacle course. *Disability & Rehabilitation, 25*(19), 1083-1088.

Runyan, C. (2006). Neuro-developmental treatment of adult hemiplegia. In H. M. Pendleton & W. Schultz-Krohn (Eds.), *Pedretti's occupational therapy practice skills for physical dysfunction* (6th ed., pp. 769-790). St. Louis, MO: Mosby.

Sammons Preston Rolyan. (2006). *Professional rehab catalog.* Bolingbrook, IL: Patterson Medical Company.

Sammons Preston Rolyan. (2009). Professional online catalog. Retrieved April 20, 2009, from http://www.sammonspreston.com

Shumway-Cook, A., Ciol, M. A., Grubon, W., & Robinson, C. (2005). Incidence of risk factors for falls following hip fracture in community dwelling older adults. *Physical Therapy, 85*, 648-655.

Tieman, B. L., Palisano, R. J., Gracely, E. J., & Rosenbaum, P. L. (2004). Gross motor capability and performance of mobility in children with cerebral palsy: A comparison across home, school and outdoors/community settings. *Physical Therapy, 84*(5), 419-427.

U.S. Department of Justice. (n.d.). Americans with Disabilities Act. Retrieved October 6, 2006, from http://www.ada.gov

Wang, P. P., Badley, E. M., & Gignac, M. (2004). Activity limitation, coping efficacy and self-perceived physical independence in people with disability. *Disability & Rehabilitation, 26*(13), 785-793.

Wheelchair Net. (2006). Wheelchair and seating evaluations. Retrieved October 15, 2006, from http://www.wheelchairnet.org/wcn_ProdServ/Consumers/evaluations.html

Wresstle, E., & Samuelsson, K. (2004). User satisfaction with mobility assistive devices. *Scandinavian Journal of Occupational Therapy, 11*(3), 143-150.

Wilson, P. E., Lange, M. L., & Mandac, B. R. (2006). Seating evaluation and wheelchair prescription. Retrieved August 6, 2009, from http://emedicine.medscape.com/article/318092-overview

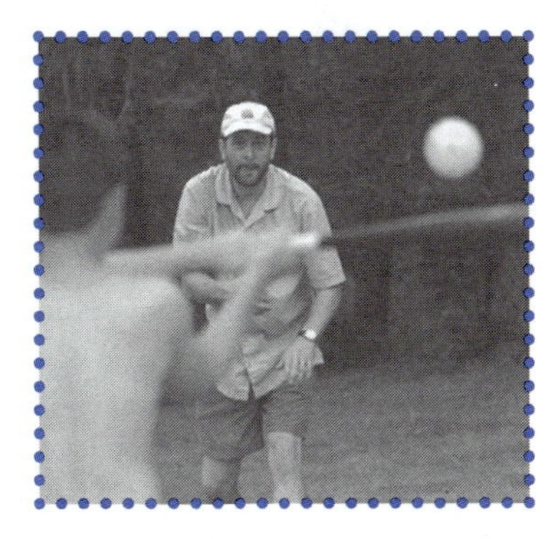

# 27

# PHYSICAL AGENT MODALITIES

*Alfred G. Bracciano, EdD, OTR/L, FAOTA*

## ACOTE Standards Explored in This Chapter

B.5.13-5.14

## Key Terms

| | |
|---|---|
| Deep thermal agents | Physical agent modalities |
| Electrotherapeutic agent | Superficial thermal agent |

## Introduction

The profession of occupational therapy has long debated the role and use of physical agent modalities. There has often been heated dialogue over whether physical agent modalities were "occupational" in nature or were the purvue of other disciplines and had no role in intervention. There have been controversies regarding training, preparation, and competency, with wide variability in academic and clinical preparation and training (Cornish-Painter, Peterson, & Lindstrom-Hazel, 1997; Glauner, Ekes, James, & Holm, 1997). To some extent, the debate continues between academics, theoreticians, and clinicians. The American Occupational Therapy Association (AOTA) clarified and strengthened the definition of physical agent modalities and their role and use as preparatory agents in the AOTA 2008 Position Statement. Partially driven by the need to strengthen regulatory oversight of physical agent modalities, the AOTA revised its position statement to assist regulatory bodies, and clinicians outline and define physical agent modality use. The revised ACOTE standards (B.5.12-5.14, in particular) reinforced the need and responsibility of academic institutions and occupational therapists to provide basic education and theory behind physical agent modality use. This chapter will provide a broad overview of the different categories of physical agent modalities and their clinical use, but it is beyond the scope of this chapter to provide the physiological basis and depth of knowledge necessary to safely integrate physical agents into clinical practice. The reader is encouraged to research other information and data related to physical agents before using them and to review specific regulatory requirements for the state in which he or she will be practicing. The terms *physical agent modality*, *physical agent*, and *physical modality* can be used interchangeably.

Physical agent modalities are one component of the intervention process and should always be used preparatory to engagement in occupational activities and tasks. Physical agent modalities have been defined as those interventions or technologies that produce a change in soft tissue through the use of light, water, temperature, sound, electricity, or mechanical devices. It is important for the occupational therapist to understand the classification system of physical agents and their mechanism of action in order to select the appropriate intervention based on the clinical condition and need of the client. Physical agent modalities are used as part of clinical intervention in order to enhance engagement in occupation and to facilitate healing and performance. Many



K. Sladyk, K. Jacobs, & N. MacRae (Eds.).
*Occupational Therapy Essentials for Clinical Competence* (pp. 295-310).

occupational therapists appear to view the application of physical agents as an external, artificial method, which has a "generalized" reaction that may decrease pain or improve client comfort. There is little recognition by these clinicians that, in fact, by using physical agents, we are able to manipulate the healing tissue at the cellular level or at the level of the "client factor," and with appropriate timing and application, facilitate the healing process and ultimately occupational performance. Physical agents can be powerful adjuncts to intervention and will facilitate outcomes and speed recovery. Physical agents should never be used singularly or in and of themselves. To do so is not considered occupational therapy.

Physical agents are often used in the intervention of musculoskeletal injuries, or by therapists whose primary practice is "hands." This concept is both limiting to the profession and to the client. The fundamental physiological principles related to healing and the influence of physical agents on that process are consistent whether the tissue is located in the hand, shoulder, knee, or back. An appreciation of the impact physical agents can have on the physiological and systemic processes will facilitate clinical reasoning and generalization of the interventions to other conditions and injuries. Occupational therapists bring the unique perspective of occupation and performance to the use and application of these agents as part of the intervention process. There have been dramatic advances in technology, equipment, and research related to physical agents, and to neglect their use as a part of intervention or to overlook their impact to facilitate healing and performance is both limiting to the profession and to the client.

## Regulatory Issues and the Role of the Occupational Therapy Assistant

As physical agent modalities have taken on greater significance as an adjunct to occupational therapy intervention, so too have regulatory restrictions. Many states such as Georgia, Florida, Minnesota, Kentucky, Tennessee, Nebraska, Montana, California, and others have specific requirements and separate licensing regulations that must be met before physical agents can be used by occupational therapists. Most of these states require a specific number of continuing education hours or experience that must be met before physical agents can be used. It is the responsibility of therapists to know what their respective state requires before utilizing physical agents in their clinical practice. Occupational therapy assistants must also meet these regulatory requirements. To date, Nebraska is the only state that restricts occupational therapy assistants to only using superficial thermal agents. In all other states with licensing regulations, occupational therapy assistants can apply physical agents under the direction and supervision of the occupational therapist. Some hospitals or clinical settings may also have restrictions or require additional institutional credentialing before using physical agents. It is the ethical and legal responsibility of the therapist to be aware of all regulatory issues prior to including physical agents as a part of clinical practice.

The AOTA position paper on physical agent modalities (AOTA, 2008) outlines the role responsibilities of the occupational therapist and occupational therapy assistant. The occupational therapist is responsible for determining physical agent modality use for the specific clinical condition being treated. The occupational therapy assistant can administer physical agent modalities as a part of the intervention plan under the direction and supervision of the occupational therapist. It is important to remember that both the occupational therapist and assistant must meet all institutional and state regulatory requirements for supervision, licensure, and competency in order to use physical agents as an adjunct to occupational therapy intervention (AOTA, 2008).

## Physical Agent Modality Classifications

There are four classifications of physical agents commonly used by occupational therapists: superficial thermal agents, deep thermal agents, electrotherapeutic agents, and mechanical devices. The classifications describe the depth of penetration or mechanism of action and provide a convenient method of initial selection of agent for the clinician. Superficial thermal agents are the therapeutic application of any modality that elevates or lowers the temperature of the skin and superficial subcutaneous tissue to a depth of 1 cm. Common superficial thermal agents include hydrotherapy/whirlpool, cryotherapy, hot packs, paraffin, water, and infrared heating. Many of these modalities are historically the most commonly used agents by occupational therapists and are viewed as being relatively "safe" in application and effect. In fact, many of these agents can cause serious burns or injuries, and care should be used with these applications and will be discussed further. Deep thermal agents include therapeutic ultrasound and phonophoresis and are categorized according to their depth of penetration. Deep thermal agents will affect tissue to a depth of approximately 5 cm and may exert both a thermal or mechanical effect. Electrotherapeutic agents are those electrical agents that possess electromagnetic properties and include biofeedback, electrical muscle stimulation (EMS), neuromuscular electrical stimulation (NMES), functional electrical stimulation (FES), transcutaneous electrical nerve stimulation (TENS), electrical stimulation for tissue repair (ESTR), high voltage galvanic stimulation, and iontophoresis. Mechanical devices may include vasopneumatic devices and continuous passive motion (CPM) devices that exert a mechanical force on the underlying tissue (AOTA, 2008).

This chapter will review the mechanism of action and clinical applications of the most commonly used physical agent modalities. The reader is encouraged to continue learning about physical agents through academic preparation, continuing education, reading, and research. Clinicians who will be using physical agents should ensure that they have a thorough grounding in the precautions, indications, and contraindications of the physical agents used. Failure to integrate the theory and application of physical agents as part of the clinical reasoning process will make clinicians mere technicians in using physical agent modalities.

## Biophysiology of Wound Healing—An Occupational Perspective

Occupational therapists have become adept at assessing the client holistically and providing interventions and adaptations to facilitate independence and performance. These interventions and activities are very often "visual" to therapists in that we can actually "see" what we or the client are doing. We can visually "see" how the client is responding in a very concrete, global fashion. In effect, we have immediate feedback on our selection of therapeutic intervention or adaptation in an almost linear fashion. As occupational therapists, we assess and address the performance skills, patterns, context, and demands of the client, which have been impacted by the disease or disorder.

Because of our holistic view of the client's function, we often overlook the ability to influence the unique client factors, body functions, or physiological processes that underlie all performance and function (World Health Organization [WHO], 2001, p. 10). Because of our theoretical and philosophical approach to illness, injury, or disability, we often fail to take into consideration the primary component of performance, that of cellular and physiological function, and how our selection of appropriate physical agents, preparatory to occupation, can facilitate and influence the healing process in the client. We have become adept at providing holistic adaptations to performance deficits but have failed to appreciate the concept that we may actually be able to "heal" and manipulate at a cellular and physiological level those tissues and structures that have been affected. This may be due, in part, to our historical evolution and moving away from the "medical model," which was viewed as limiting and reductionistic to the profession.

This view has become anachronistic with the dramatic advances in technology, neuroscience, and medicine that allow us to appreciate the basic components and details of cellular and physiological functioning and the interrelationship with health and function. To overlook or neglect our ability to influence these physiological processes and healing, which ultimately facilitates occupational performance and independence, is both ethically incongruent and inconsistent with our professional development. Failure to actively embrace and engage these emerging technologies and interventions as a component of the occupational process will lead to the void being filled by other disciplines willing and able to incorporate these techniques into an integrated program of intervention leading to improved performance and outcomes.

Physical agent modalities are those clinical interventions that are used to produce a specific response in soft tissue. These interventions include the use of light, water, temperature, sound, electricity, or mechanical devices to influence the healing process. This chapter will focus on superficial thermal, deep thermal, and electrotherapeutic agents. The AOTA, in their 2008 position statement, identified the specific physical agents that correspond to the categories.

Because of the impact physical agents have at the cellular and physiological level, it is crucial for occupational therapists to have a foundational understanding of the healing process. Any injury to vascularized tissue causes a series of systemic responses that are distinct but overlapping, including inflammation, proliferation, and remodeling. This physiological response occurs in order to rid the area of any micro-organism, foreign material, or dead tissue so that the repair process where new tissue will be formed can occur. Wound healing is an overlapping process of repair that involves a series of events that encompass chemotaxis, cell division, neovascularization, synthesis of new extracellular matrix (ECM) components, and the formation and remodeling of scar tissue (Enoch & Harding, 2003). Wounds or injuries can be caused by disease; by vascular insufficiency due to compromised venous or arterial flow, leading to ischemia or insufficient blood flow; or by trauma such as abrasions, lacerations, avulsions, punctures, burns, or even surgery. These wounds and injuries are often accompanied by pain, limited motion, and decreased motor function. Chronic inflammation, infection, and scarring may also cause complications, preventing a full return to function and performance.

The phases of healing are overlapping and vary in length. A healing wound or injury may demonstrate all three phases at the same time. The three phases of healing include the inflammatory phase, proliferation, and remodeling or maturation (Andreadis, 2006; Bolton & van Rijswijk, 1991). Injury to soft tissues below the skin is dependent upon the nature of the causative factor, the location (either superficial or deep), and the material properties of the tissue. Therapists should understand these phases of healing as the appropriate physical agent will facilitate or modify the response of the tissue, ultimately impacting outcomes. Improper application of physical agents may negatively influence the healing process and lead to further complications and potential tissue damage (Figure 27-1).

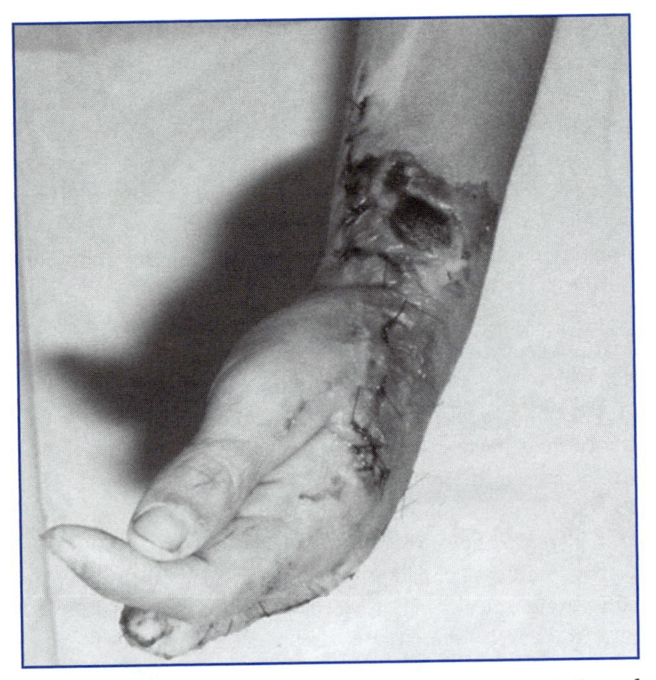

**Figure 27-1.** 11-year-old male—status-post ray amputation of little, ring, and partial middle finger; skin graft in place on dorsal aspect of the hand and wrist; sutures in place. Note the eschar and different phases of healing.

# Wound Healing

## Inflammatory Phase

The inflammatory phase is the initial response of the body to injury. Inflammation is primarily a vascular response to the injury. The initial response to an injury is vasoconstriction, which decreases blood flow to the area, followed by vasodilation and the release of chemicals, nutrients, oxygen, and specialized cells to the site. There are a number of histochemical changes that occur and promote capillary permeability and chemotaxis, which is cell movement along a chemical concentration gradient, positively or negatively. A number of histochemical mediators are released into the tissue at this time, which facilitate formation of the fibrin clot and include histamine, prostaglandins, growth factors, and others that stimulate the inflammatory process and facilitate migration of fibroblasts, macrophages, and other specialized cells that form the "granulation tissue." A combination of blood exudate and serous transudate creates a reddened, hot, swollen, painful environment in the vicinity of the damaged tissue and wound. The inflammatory edema fills all spaces within the wound, surrounding all damaged or repaired structures, thereby binding them together as a one-wound structure. Some swelling in a wound is necessary to trigger the inflammatory process. However, if too little inflammation occurs, the healing response is slow; if too much inflammation occurs, an excessive scar is produced (Hardy, 1989).

## Proliferative Phase

During the proliferative phase of healing, granulation tissue matures to form scar tissue. There are two primary processes that are occurring during this phase: fibroplasia and angiogenesis. Fibroblasts migrate to the area in order to repair the connective tissue of the skin and are mediated by chemicals released from the macrophages. At the same time, new capillary growth in the damaged tissue is growing in an effort to establish blood flow through the region and to remove the metabolic and repair wastes. Fibroblasts lay down collagen fibers that modify and change as the repair matures. Myofibroblasts are responsible for wound contraction and the early strength of the repair by drawing the outer edges of the wound together. Importantly, the collagen fibers are oriented in response to local stress that is applied to them and provide the tensile strength in the appropriate or required direction. This stress can occur internally or externally and is one of the reasons why occupational therapists use dynamic or static splinting as well as physical agent modalities. The intention is to manipulate these healing structures through splinting or physical agents, which can facilitate and enhance the healing process and strength and speed of the repair (Kloth & McCulloch, 1995).

## Remodeling Phase

The remodeling phase of the healing process is sometimes also referred to as epithelialization or the maturation phase. Epithelialization is an important component of the remodeling phase of healing so that the wound has sufficient skin coverage. During this phase, there is continued fibroblastic activity and deposition of the collagen fibers. During this period, there is a balance between the synthesis of the collagen fibers and the subsequent lysis, or breakdown of the collagen. It is during this period the collagen fibers and healing scar and tissue continue to realign themselves and differentiate in function based on the tension and stress applied to the healing area. Remodeling overlaps the proliferative phase of healing and can continue for up to a year or more. The process of scar remodeling is responsible for the final orientation and arrangement of collagen fibers. Remodeling is influenced by both synthesis-lysis balance and fiber orientation. When the balance between synthesis and lysis is out of sync, the probability of keloid or hypertrophic scarring increases and may be problematic (Cuzzell, 2002; Gogia, 1995).

During this period of maturation, the remodeling of the collagen results in the early, randomly deposited scar tissue arranged in both a linear and lateral orientation, approximating the tissues that surround it. During the remodeling phase of healing, the original wound, which resulted in a single scar, now has to differentiate itself to provide a function, such as tendon, muscle, or skin. As occupational therapists, we attempt to modify this process through our interventions, including physical agents and splinting. Induction theory states that the tissue will attempt to mimic the characteristics of the tissue that is surrounding it, while tension theory states that a low load; long duration; stress on the healing tissue through the application of pressure, dynamic splinting, mobilization, soft tissue loading, and unloading; and other techniques account for the differentiation in the healing tissue. It is through the correct and timely selection and application of the physical agent and "stress" to the tissue that is crucial in effecting positive clinical outcomes (Ankrom et al., 2005).

## Superficial Thermal Agents

Superficial thermal agents are those interventions that cause a temperature change in the underlying tissue. Tissue temperature can be modified through the application of heat to increase tissue temperature, or it can be cooled through the application of cold agents. The use of heat or cold to decrease pain and improve function has a long history. It is important to understand the physiological response to these modalities in order to determine how they can be used as part of the intervention process. Heat or cold is transmitted to the underlying tissue through five primary principles:

1. Conduction refers to heat transfer through direct contact with the underlying tissue. The heat loss or gain occurs when there is contact between materials that possess different temperatures. For example, heat will be absorbed by the body when a hot pack is applied, while a cold pack will conduct heat away from the skin. Both methods of heat transfer through the process of conduction.
2. Convection refers to the transfer of heat or cold to the body through the movement of air, matter, liquids, or particles over the extremity or body part. An example of a form of convection is fluidotherapy, where the air temperature can be adjusted and the cellulose particles are circulated by the force of the air around the treated extremity.
3. Radiation occurs when the radiant energy transfers heat through the air from a warm source, such as an infrared lamp, to a cooler source. The infrared lamps that are often seen in restaurants are an example of this. Infrared lamps are rarely used in rehabilitation anymore.
4. Conversion occurs when there is a temperature change resulting from the transformation of energy from one form to another. Clinically, this can be seen when thermal ultrasound is used to heat tissue—the sound energy is transformed to thermal or heat energy as the cells respond to the sound waves by vibrating, changing the sound energy into kinetic energy.
5. Evaporation is the transformation of a liquid into a gaseous state. During this change, there is an exchange of energy with the byproduct of heat being released when the liquid is transformed into a gas. The most common clinical form of evaporation occurs with the use of vapocoolant sprays, which cause a decrease in skin temperature due to the evaporative effects of the spray.

Suzanne was a very active and dynamic 85-year-old female. Her medical history was unremarkable, though she complained of having trouble hearing at times. Suzanne lived independently in a one-floor senior citizens condominium complex, and though she no longer drove, she did use the public transportation extensively to shop, visit her friends for lunch, and attend church services. She was very active in her church and enjoyed socializing with her friends. One wintry day while shoveling snow off the walkway to her door, she slipped and fell. In an attempt to "catch" herself, she put out her arm, extending it fully. When she landed on the ground, she fractured her radius. She was taken to the emergency room where she was placed in a soft splint to accommodate for the swelling and, 2 days later, she underwent closed reduction of the fracture and was placed in a cast. X-rays indicated good apposition (alignment of the two fragments) of the fractured ends. She healed quickly and the cast was removed at 7 weeks.

Following removal of the cast, her skin was flaky, dry, and macerated. Even though her physician reassured her that the break was "solid" and she should move her wrist and use her hand as much as possible, Suzanne was apprehensive and protective of the extremity. She kept the fingers of her hand closed and, when moving, had a tendency to hold her hand at the wrist. She was referred for occupational therapy "evaluation and intervention." On the initial visit, the occupational therapist reviewed the X-rays and report to ensure the fracture was solidly healed and in good alignment and confirmed that there were no biomechanical causes for her hesitancy and protection of the wrist and hand. When asked to move her hand and wrist, Suzanne politely, but firmly, replied she "couldn't" and was "afraid it was going to hurt." Suzanne's hesitancy to use the hand was limiting her ability to take care of her daily routines and self-care activities. She was struggling to dress herself and manipulate fastenings and she was having difficulty cooking and cleaning since she would use the extremity as a "wedge" to hold objects against her body and forearm rather than using her wrist and fingers. Passive range of motion appeared to be within functional limits, but Suzanne would not actively use the hand. The occupational therapist was aware that immobilization of the forearm due to the cast would cause disuse atrophy and generalized weakness in the arm and hand and was anxious to get Suzanne moving to prevent fibrosis or adhesions in her shoulder due to lack of movement caused by the guarded position of the arm and hand. The therapist also realized that the prolonged immobilization may have also contributed to a distorted sensory perception in terms of kinesthesia and proprioception, which could make Suzanne "feel" that her arm and hand were not "moving the same" as before the fall.

It was determined by the occupational therapist to prepare the tissue and area before engaging Suzanne in a variety of activities that would ensure her use of the hand and extremity. Suzanne's skin was dry and flaky, and the skin that was under the cast was "smelly." She was motivated to "clean up [her] arm and get rid of the dead skin." The occupational therapist decided to use a warm, hand whirlpool, with the water at a temperature between 102 and 104 degrees with a gentle agitation. Suzanne was given a washcloth with which to "scrub" the dry skin off and was assisted by the occupational therapist in this task. Suzanne diligently "cleaned" the dead slough off her forearm and allowed the occupational therapist to assist. During this time, Suzanne was extending and flexing her fingers and actively moving her wrist in flexion, extension, as well as supination and pronation of the forearm. After 20 minutes, the therapist removed Suzanne from the water, dried the skin, and applied lotion to the forearm and digits, gently mobilizing and manipulating the wrist and fingers in the process. Suzanne mentioned how the warm water "relaxed" her arm and hand and she was instructed to "soak" her hand in warm water at home, rubbing the extremity with a wash cloth to further clean off the dried skin. Suzanne quickly began to use her healed arm and hand more functionally following a few short interventions incorporating the use of the superficial warmth to the tissues, preparing the tissue in order to engage in a variety of activities and exercises to strengthen her arm and hand and to improve her fine motor control and object manipulation. Because of the superficial heating of the tissue, Suzanne was soon riding public transportation again, visiting her friends for lunch, and engaging in her active pre-injury activities and tasks.

# Heat Agents

There are a variety of therapeutic heat agents that are used by occupational therapists and are categorized according to their depth of penetration. These thermal agents are considered either deep or superficial. Superficial heating agents include hot packs, over-the-counter "thermal wraps," fluidotherapy, paraffin, and warm whirlpool. All of these agents increase the superficial temperatures of the skin and subcutaneous tissues to a depth of approximately 1 to 2 cm. Ultrasound, in its thermal mode, has a depth of penetration to approximately 3 to 5 cm. Short wave diathermy is another physical agent that can increase tissue temperature at deeper levels, but it is rarely used by occupational therapists.

The extent of the temperature change on the underlying tissue is dependent on four primary factors: the temperature difference between the physical agent being applied and the underlying tissue, the duration of the exposure of the tissue to the agent, the intensity of the heat agent, and the volume or area of the tissue being treated. The thermal conductivity of the tissue is also a factor that must be taken into consideration as adipose or fat tissue will act as an insulator to the underlying tissue while blood and muscle due to their blood flow and water content absorb and conduct heat more efficiently.

## Tissue Temperature Effect

The degree of tissue temperature elevation is dependent on the following:

- Volume or area being treated
- The duration of the application
- Temperature variation between the tissue and the physical agent
- Thermal conductivity of the tissue

# Physiological Response to Heat

The primary purpose for applying a thermal agent is to increase the temperature of soft tissue to a specific therapeutic range so a certain physiological response will occur. When the temperature of soft tissue is increased between the ranges of 104°F and 113°F, it can have a positive therapeutic effect on the client. If the soft tissue is heated to a temperature of less than 104°F, then the cell metabolism will not be stimulated adequately enough to elicit a therapeutic response. Conversely, if the same tissue is heated to greater than 113°F, then catabolism and cell death may occur. The physiologic response to heat will vary according to the duration of the application, the volume of tissue being treated, and how long the modality is applied. Heating doses are considered either mild or vigorous with the higher temperatures producing more noticeable redness or hyperemia to the underlying tissue. The application of heat causes a number of physiological responses to occur, including increased blood flow to the area due to vasodilation of the blood vessels and increased rate of cell metabolism, oxygen consumption, capillary permeability, inflammation, and muscle contraction velocity. Conversely, the application of heat will decrease fluid viscosity of the tissue, pain, and muscle spasm (Loten et al., 2006). It is important to take into account not only the factors related earlier but also the age of the client. Older clients may have an impaired ability to dissipate the heat effectively, and care must be taken to prevent burns or systemic overheating (Petrofsky et al., 2006).

## Clinical Application and Goals

The application of heat as an adjunct to intervention has many therapeutic goals. The application of heat to an extremity can aid in pain relief and decrease the muscle spasms that a client may be experiencing. Since blood flow increases as a result of the heat, the outcome will be the removal of the local muscle metabolites and the reduction in sensitivity of the muscle spindles, which tend to stretch and cause pain (Michlovitz, Hun, Erasala, Hengehold, & Weingand, 2004). Heat application can also decrease muscle guarding and muscle spasm, which often lead to the pain-spasm-pain cycle and decrease the client's functional abilities and occupational performance. Heat applications placed on soft tissue can also assist in increasing the tissue extensibility (Nadler et al., 2003).

The superficial heating agents used in most occupational therapy clinics are typically capable of providing moderate and vigorous thermal dosages. A moderate dosage involves elevating the tissue temperature to between 102°F and 106°F and will result in only a slight increase of blood flow. This dosage level is very effective when heat is indicated, but edema may occur. A vigorous dosage results in a marked increase in blood flow. The temperature will increase rapidly, the duration will be relatively long, and the temperature elevation at the site of pathology will be high (between 107°F and 113°F). This dosage level is beneficial for ischemic conditions and for when heat is indicated and edema is not a concern. Heat will also increase the viscosity and elasticity of the soft tissue-muscle tendon and joint capsule when combined with positional or dynamic stretch over a period of time. The average length of time for heat application is between 10 and 20 minutes for the physiological effects to occur in the intervention tissue. The length of time is dependent on the factors identified earlier, the area of tissue being covered, the intensity of the heat, and the duration of application. Though there are different methods with which to apply heat, the biophysiological response will always be the same. In addition, it is important to remember there is a 10-minute window of opportunity following the application of heat within which the load or stretch must be applied, though positional stretch during the heat application can also be utilized and is also effective (Kottke, Pauley, & Ptak, 1966; Laban, 1962).

Indications for using superficial thermal agents include the following:

- Stiff joints
- Subcutaneous adhesions
- Soft tissue contractures
- Chronic arthritis
- Sub-acute and chronic inflammation
- Cumulative trauma
- Wounds
- Neuromas
- Sympathetic nervous system disorders

### Precautions and Contraindications

The choice of heat selection is dependent upon the area of tissue being treated and the goals established for the client. If the area is large and requires the medium to contour to the area (e.g., a shoulder), then a hot pack would be an appropriate selection. Hands and wrists can be easily accommodated in either a fluidotherapy unit or through the application of paraffin. The client's skin should be closely monitored during any heat application as the potential for thermal burns can be high if improperly applied. Heat applications should never be used over open lesions, cuts or lacerations, or sutures of the skin. The area being treated should be inspected prior to the application of the thermal agent and the sensation of the area confirmed. The client's cognitive ability and ability to inform the therapist of any discomfort or pain should also be assessed and reviewed. The skin and treated area should be checked after the first 5 minutes of application if possible to ensure that there are no adverse reactions. Close monitoring of the client is crucial as heat applications are the most common method of burning a client.

Precautions and contraindications for superficial thermal agents include the following:

- Peripheral vascular disease
- Acute inflammation
- Cancer or malignancies
- Acute hemmorhage
- Infection
- Primary repair of tendon or ligaments
- Advanced cardiac disease
- Compromised or limited cognitive status
- External pins/plates/hardware
- Sensory deficits
- Pregnancy

## Cryotherapy

Cryotherapy is the application of a cold agent to selected tissue. The physiological response to cold application is essentially the reverse of heat applications. As with heat application, the physiological response to cold application is dependent on duration of application, area or volume of the tissue being treated, and the rate at which the agent is being applied. With application of cold, the initial response in the underlying tissue is one of vasoconstriction. Superficial cooling agents are recommended for the acute phase of healing and most acute conditions producing a decrease in tissue temperature, resulting in an analgesic effect. Cryotherapy can be used clinically to decrease edema, spasticity, muscle spasm, and pain. As the duration of application is increased, the physiological response is one of decreased nerve conduction velocity, decreased delivery of leukocytes and phagocyte, decreased lymphatic and venous drainage, and decreased muscle excitability and muscle spindle depolarization (Barber, 2000; Gracies, 2001; Sanya & Bello, 1999; Welch et al., 2000). With short duration applications, most clinical applications of cryotherapy will penetrate to a depth of approximately 1 cm, although longer durations may penetrate to a depth of 4 cm (Olson & Stravino, 1972). Commonly used cryoagents include commercially available ice packs, ice ups and ice packs made up of crushed ice, and cryopressure units that are effective following surgery to decrease pain and edema (Singh, Osbahr, Holovacs, Cawley, & Speer, 2001). It is important to recognize that muscle and nerve tissue changes will occur when the temperature of the tissue drops below 80.6°F. Care must be taken when cryo modalities are applied for extended periods of time to prevent frostbite and tissue damage from occurring.

## Precautions and Contraindications

Cryotherapy can be an effective and safe modality when used within the appropriate clinical parameters. However, clients with difficulty with thermoregulation, sensory deficits, or hypersensitivity to cold would be contraindicated or require close monitoring of the application. Cryotherapy is contraindicated in those clients with cryoglobulinemia, Raynaud's disease, or cold urticaria. Systemic responses in clients with cold sensitivity include syncope, increased heart rate, flushing, and a drop in blood pressure. Close monitoring of the client's blood pressure and systemic response should be routinely performed with any thermal application, either heat or cold (Nadler, Prybicien, Malanga, & Sicher, 2003).

Precautions and contraindications include the following:

- Impaired circulation
- Peripheral vascular disease
- Hypersensitivity to cold
- Skin anesthesia
- Open wounds or skin conditions
- Infections

# Deep Thermal Agents: Therapeutic Ultrasound

Ultrasound has been used in medicine for diagnosis, in imaging structures for tissue destruction and surgery, and in rehabilitation for its thermal and nonthermal effects. Therapeutic ultrasound uses acoustic energy, which is above the frequency that we can hear. There are two primary uses for ultrasound in rehabilitation: to heat deeper structures and tissue or to facilitate healing of soft tissues. The historical use of ultrasound was to raise the temperature of deep structures such as tendon, ligament, and joint capsules. Ultrasound parameters can be configured to provide either a "superficial" effect, penetrating to a depth of 1 to 2 cm, or a "deep" effect, penetrating to up to 5 cm.

Ultrasound units consist of an ultrasound generator that uses alternating electrical current and creates an acoustic wave at a specific frequency. The ultrasound unit also consists of a power supply, oscillator circuit, transformer, coaxial cable, and transducer and/or sound head, the part that is actually placed on the client to administer the sound energy. The biophysical principle, which is the basis for ultrasound, is known as the piezoelectric effect. Essentially, when an alternating electrical current is passed through the piezoelectric crystal located in the sound head of the ultrasound transducer, the crystal responds by oscillating, expanding, and contracting. As the crystal expands and contracts in response to the electric current, it "vibrates," creating sound waves that are then transmitted through the use of a coupling agent (electrode gel) to the underlying tissue.

As the crystal expands and contracts in response to the electrical current, it produces sound waves that, when the transducer is placed on a body part, compress the underlying molecules lying in the path of the sound energy. This movement of the molecules in the underlying tissue, essentially oscillating back and forth against each other, is known as longitudinal wave propagation. This sound wave and molecular movement will continue to expand until the energy is absorbed. When the sound wave reaches bone, it will be generated along the periosteum and reflected back up toward the surface, creating a shear wave. The sound wave traveling through the body will become attenuated as the energy is either absorbed or dispersed through reflection or refraction (ter Haar, 1978).

Body tissue is not homogeneous, and each layer of the body will transmit or absorb the ultrasound energy according to its own unique properties. Fluid elements of the body have the lowest impedance, or resistance, to the sound energy and lowest acoustic absorption values. Bone has the highest impedance value and the highest acoustic absorption coefficient. This means bone will stop the flow of the energy and absorb the energy from the ultrasound wave, which will lead to physiologic changes. With higher energy levels produced by the ultrasound machine, there will be a concurrent effect of heating the tissues. As the ultrasound is transmitted to the lower tissues coming in contact with the bone, most of the energy will be reflected back, where it will meet the energy that is being transmitted down into the tissue and can produce a "standing wave" or "hot spot," which can be painful and damage the tissue. To prevent the development of standing waves or hot spots, the sound head should be moved in small circular motions (Dyson, 1987).

To control the amount of energy and biophysiological effect in the tissue, there are a number of factors that are considered and adjusted on the ultrasound equipment, including the frequency, duty cycle, and intensity. The frequency of ultrasound determines the number of complete wave cycles that are generated each second. In the United States, there are two frequencies that can be selected on most ultrasound machines: 1 MHz or 3 MHz. As the number of cycles per second increases, the duration of each cycle and wavelength decreases, which accounts for the difference in the depth of penetration. The frequency of the ultrasound will influence the amount of energy that is absorbed with higher frequencies (3 MHz), which will entail more energy being delivered but more superficial in depth. Intervention using a frequency of 3 MHz leads to a more superficial effect than intervention using a frequency of 1 MHz (Fyfe & Bullock, 1985). Areas of the body such as the dorsal aspect of the hand, lateral and medial epicondyles, fingers, and other superficial structures would be more effectively treated using a frequency of 3 MHz. Deeper soft tissue structures such as the shoulder joint should be treated with a frequency of 1 MHz (Bracciano, 2008).

The biophysical effects of ultrasound are dependent on a number of factors, with the primary one being the intensity of the ultrasound. If the intensity is high enough, it will cause heating of the tissues, while low-intensity and pulsed-mode delivery will result in nonthermal changes due to the "mechanical" effect of the ultrasound energy. Tissues are heated through the transfer of the sound energy into kinetic energy due to the oscillation of the molecules in the tissue responding to the sound waves. To increase the total amount of heat delivered to the targeted tissue, the duration of the ultrasound application and/or the intensity must be increased. Thermal effects of tissue heating will do the following (Enwemeka, 1989; Hong, Liu, & Yu, 1988; Rimington, Draper, Durrant, & Fellingham, 1994):

- Decrease pain perception
- Decrease nerve conduction velocity
- Increase the metabolic rate
- Increase blood flow
- Stimulate the immune system
- Decrease the fluid viscosity in the tissue
- Increase tissue extensibility

Factors influencing the physiological effects of ultrasound include the following:

- Frequency (1 or 3 MHz)
- Duty cycle
- Intensity
- Time

The thermal effects of ultrasound can be decreased through either decreasing the intensity of the ultrasound or by "pulsing" the ultrasound. Pulsing the ultrasound refers to the duty cycle, or that period of time that the sound energy is being delivered to the tissue divided by the pulse period, which is the on time and off time. Most of the ultrasound equipment will have a 50%, 20%, or 10% duty cycle setting. The nonthermal or "mechanical" effects of ultrasound result in second-order physiological effects, which are effective for wound healing. These mechanical effects occur through the process of acoustic streaming and micro-massage at the cell membrane. Benefits have been shown for inflammation, proliferation, and maturation processes with the primary site of ultrasound interaction and activity occurring at the cell membrane. From a clinical standpoint, nonthermal ultrasound (pulsed, low intensity) will facilitate tissue repair (Chan et al., 2006; Ebenbichler & Resch, 1994; Fyfe & Bullock, 1985; Giannini, Giombini, Moneta, Massazza, & Pigozzi, 2004; Turner, Powell, & Ng, 1989). Phonophoresis is the therapeutic application of ultrasound using a topical medication. The intent of phonophoresis is to direct the drug delivery directly to the site where the desired effect is sought. Phonophoresis is noninvasive and essentially painless. There is some discrepancy over whether the mechanism of action is thermal or the mechanical effects of the ultrasound. In addition, there are some inconsistencies regarding the effectiveness of ultrasound due to the wide variability of intervention parameters (Casarotto, Adamowski, Fallopa, & Bacanelli, 2004; Klucinec, 1996; Klucinec, Scheidler, Denegar, Domholdt, & Burgess, 2000; Oziomek, Perrin, Herold, & Denegar, 1991; Reshetov, Tverdokhleb, & Bezmenov, 2000).

## Precautions and Contraindications

Prior to application of ultrasound, it is important that the therapist determine which frequency he or she is using as well as whether the intention of the intervention is to "heat" tissue or to "heal" tissue. Many of the contraindications and precautions of therapeutic ultrasound are with thermal, high-intensity applications. As with any physical agent, care must be used when the client has areas of decreased sensation, mentation, or cognitive abilities. Caution should also be used in clients with pacemakers. Ultrasound is contraindicated in clients with malignant tumors, during pregnancy, over epiphyseal plates of children, with joint cement, and with thrombophlebitis. Ultrasound should never be applied over the eyes, reproductive organs, or central nervous system tissue.

Precautions and contraindications of ultrasound include the following:

- Malignant tumors
- Joint cement
- Pacemakers
- Thrombophlebitis
- Reproductive organs
- Eyes
- Central nervous system tissue
- Pregnancy

# Electrotherapy Principles and Applications

There are a variety of therapeutic applications of electrotherapy available to the occupational therapist. Because of the wide variability in applications and language used in the research and by the manufacturers, there is also a great deal of confusion that exists. The American Physical Therapy Association (APTA) has attempted to standardize the terminology related to electrotherapeutic agents by classifying these agents according to their therapeutic goals. These applications are also the ones most frequently used by occupational therapists in clinical practice and include the following:

- *EMS*: Used for denervated muscles
- *NMES*: Used with innervated muscles
- *FES*: Use of electrical stimulation as an orthotic substitute
- *ESTR*: Electrical stimulation for tissue repair
- *TENS*: Used for decreasing pain

The most commonly used applications by occupational therapists include NMES, FES, TENS, high-voltage galvanic stimulation (HVGS) (used for tissue repair and healing), and iontophoresis (used to administer medications to targeted tissue).

Electricity is a form of energy that exhibits magnetic, chemical, mechanical, and thermal effects. Electrical current involves the flow or movement of ions or electrons from one area to another and from a high concentration to a low concentration. This imbalance in electrons, which causes the flow of electrical current, also seeks the path of least resistance. The human body is electrically conductive and the tissue is either excitable and will respond to the electrical current or is nonexcitable and will only be modified by the electrical fields but will not respond to the electrical current flow. When electricity is applied to excitable tissue, there is physiological and physiochemical changes that occur due in part to the water in the tissues. If the electrical current is of sufficient intensity, duration, and frequency, a muscle contraction will occur. A primary difference between electrically stimulated movement and voluntary contractions is the sequence of movements. In a voluntary contraction, small motor nerves are recruited first, then larger motor nerves, and finally muscles in an asynchronous sequence as gradually greater strength is required. In electrically stimulated movement, however, the reverse occurs with the larger fibers and muscles being recruited first in a synchronous, linear fashion. This accounts for the often "robot-like" movements of electrically stimulated muscles.

## Neuromuscular Electrical Stimulation

The choice of the appropriate electrical device is dependent on the goals set by the occupational therapist during the evaluation and intervention. NMES uses a pulsating alternating current with the primary intention of stimulating intact peripheral motor nerves in order to produce a motor response or muscular contraction. This form of stimulation is most often used to decrease muscle spasms, increase muscle strength, and decrease edema through the pumping action of alternating muscle contractions. NMES is indicated to improve muscle strength without increasing cardiovascular output; it can increase range of motion, decrease or inhibit spasticity, and improve strength and endurance; and it is also used for muscle re-education or facilitation (Baker, Parker, & Sanderson, 1983; Billian & Gorman, 1992; Carmick, 1995, 1997; Chae & Hart, 1998; Scheker & Ozer, 2003). Electrodes are placed on the bulk of the muscle belly over the motor nerve with a second electrode placed distal to the first, usually near the muscle attachment. Correct electrode placement is crucial for effective response and it is recommended to practice electrode placement on yourself or a colleague to ensure appropriate location. The amplitude or strength of the electrical current is increased until the nerve becomes depolarized and the muscle reaches tetany, causing a muscle contraction.

NMES can also be used for orthopedic injuries, particularly those conditions that have been immobilized, causing muscle weakness or hesitancy in moving the affected extremity affecting active range of motion. Combining NMES with occupational activities and movements facilitates outcomes, strengthens the response, and increases strength more than just conventional exercise alone (Hesse, Werner, Bardeleben, & Brandl-Hesse, 2002; Weingarden, Kizony, Nathan, Ohry, & Levy, 1997). NMES has also been used to decrease or modulate spasticity in neurologically impaired or orthopedic clients. Success with neurologically involved clients may vary due to the underlying cause. There are two primary methods for improving range of motion and decreasing spasticity: stimulating the spastic muscle to fatigue or stimulating the antagonist muscle to attempt to strengthen it and overpower the spastic muscle. Combining these NMES techniques with static and dynamic splinting, positional stretch, and other "conventional" methods of intervention may facilitate better outcomes (Daly et al., 1996; Detrembleur, Lejeune, Renders, & Van Den Bergh, 2002; Hesse et al., 2002; Scheker, Chesher, & Ramirez, 1999; Scheker & Ozer, 2003).

FES is a form of NMES, but the application is that the targeted stimulation and application is used as a substitute for an orthotic device or to produce a specific motor movement and activity. FES has been used as a substitute for the conventional "slings" that clients with shoulder subluxation frequently have following a stroke. Other applications of FES may be for reaching activities of the upper extremity or to strengthen or enhance grasp and release activities in order to allow the client to pick up and manipulate objects. There is a great deal of research and interest in the use of NMES with clients who have suffered a cerebral vascular accident (CVA) and in the ability to facilitate return and decrease shoulder subluxation and pain in clients at the early stage of recovery (Aoyagi & Tsubahara, 2004; Chae et al., 2005; Liu, You, & Sun, 2005; Yu, 2004). As the technology and research continues to expand and progress, occupational therapists should stay current with these therapeutic applications in order to facilitate occupational performance in clients with CVA. Electrode placements for shoulder subluxation include over the supraspinatus, upper trapezius, with a second electrode over the posterior deltoid. FES can also be configured to target two or more muscles in order to facilitate active movements such as mass extensor patterns or grasp-and-release activities. A creative approach to the intended movement and activity is required to determine where the appropriate electrode placements should be.

# Electrical Stimulation for Wound Healing

It is beyond the scope of this chapter to outline the various parameters of ESTR. It is recommended that the reader interested in this electrotherapeutic application review other materials and information available. There are some factors salient to many of the clinical conditions discussed earlier. Following an injury or surgery, there is a disruption of the body's normally occurring electrical field with the polarity of the adjacent area changing in polarity. The application of electrical stimulation through the use of direct current and high-voltage pulsed current facilitates the transfer of the energy from the electrical current to the wound due to the change in polarity caused by the injury. The electrical current and stimulation affects not only the circulation but also the histochemical effects and functions as well as orienting the cell structures and facilitating the healing process. ESTR is indicated for pressure ulcers (stages I to IV), diabetic ulcers, venous ulcers, traumatic and surgical wounds, ischemic ulcers, wound flaps, and burn wounds. Precautions and contraindications are essentially the same as those discussed for electrotherapy in general (Baker, Chambers, DeMuth, & Villar, 1997; Bayat et al., 2006; Bogie, Reger, Levine, & Sahgal, 2000; Gardner, Frantz, & Schmidt, 1999; Houghton et al., 2003; Langevin et al., 2006).

# Transcutaneous Electrical Nerve Stimulation

It is important to remember that pain is a complex, multifaceted experience that can have unique social and cultural components. The use of electrical stimulation in the form of TENS can be an effective adjunct to conventional intervention. Pain is modulated by the use of TENS by affecting the perception and sensation of pain rather than correcting any underlying clinical condition. There are two primary theories related to the efficacy of TENS to modulate pain: the gate control theory and the endorphin- or opiate-mediated control theory. The reader is encouraged to explore these theories further to familiarize themselves with the intricacies of each. TENS is most often used in the intervention of musculoskeletal disorders, back pain, arthritis, and inflammatory disorders of soft tissue or for postoperative pain. There are a variety of intervention parameters available and most manufacturers have programmed the TENS units with regimens that are the most effective.

TENS uses pulsed or alternating current and the manufacturers have programmed different combinations of stimulation patterns directly into the equipment. There are four common forms of TENS that are used clinically: subsensory level, sensory level, motor level, noxious level stimulation, or a combination of all four.

1. Subsensory-level stimulation is also known as microcurrent electrical neuromuscular stimulation (MENS), microcurrent electrical stimulation (MES), subliminal stimulation, or low-intensity stimulation (LIS). The characteristic of this form of stimulation is that the intensity of the equipment is so low (less than 1 mamp) that it does not stimulate a muscle contraction and is considered "subthreshold." Much of the research generated by this form of TENS has been in fractures and skin wounds and is based on the movement of the ions in the tissues at such low magnitude that there is no cutaneous sensation (Currier & Mann, 1983; Denegar, 1993).
2. Sensory-level stimulation is also known as conventional or high-rate TENS and is primarily used during the acute phase of injuries. This form of stimulation is based on the gate control mechanism or opiate-mediated pain control and uses amplitudes and durations between 50 to 100 pulses per second (Melzack, 1993). This form of TENS activates the cutaneous tactile sensory fibers and causes cutaneous paresthesia or a tingling sensation. The intensity of this form of stimulation does not elicit a motor response, though the client can "feel" the sensation. This form of TENS has a relatively quick response in decreasing pain, but the long-term effects are not usually longer than 1 hour. Extended periods of pain relief may be due to the stimulation interrupting the pain-spasm-pain cycle.
3. Motor-level stimulation is also known as strong low-rate (SLR) or acupuncture-like TENS and uses a high amplitude and low frequency pulse duration. This form of stimulation is also based on the gate control or opiate-mediated theories of pain control. Motor-level stimulation uses amplitude high enough to produce a motor response in the underlying tissue. As the amplitude is increased, greater numbers of muscle fibers and motor axons are recruited and can reach a titanic contraction. Electrode placement for motor level stimulation is directly over the motor point, which correlates with the location of the client's pain

or on the segmental nerve roots. Motor level stimulation is often used to treat chronic pain or pain that is caused by damage to deeper tissues, muscle spasms, and myofascial pain (Al-Smadi et al., 2003; Bjordal, Johnson, & Ljunggreen, 2003; Breit & Van der Wall, 2004; Chang, Lin, & Hsieh, 2002).

4. Noxious-level stimulation is also known as electro-acupuncture, hyperstimulation, or noxious-level TENS. This form of TENS is of motor-level intensity and uses longer pulse durations and frequencies. As the name suggests, noxious-level stimulation is reached when the stimulation amplitude is increased and perceived by the client to be "painful." This intense stimulation activates the ascending neural mechanisms and is based in part on the endogenous opiate theory. Noxious-level stimulation produces relatively high levels of analgesia. However, the effects are short lived and transitory. Most often, this form of stimulation is used prior to surgical procedures or debridement of tissue (Chandran & Sluka, 2003; Chang et al., 2002; Likar et al., 2001).

Most of the current TENS units have two channels with four electrodes. The initial application of electrodes with clients reporting pain is rather simple—the primary choice is to position the electrodes over or around the painful site. Other sites that may be used include the motor points, which correspond with the area of pain; trigger points; or acupuncture points. All of these locations are considered electrically active and will facilitate the current flow into the selected tissue. Other potential stimulation sites include areas along the peripheral nerves, the tissue overlying the painful areas, specific dermatomes, or over the spinal segmental myotomes, which correspond to the clients' reported pain. Clinically, the therapist needs to determine whether the outcome desired will involve a motor response, sensory analgesia, or a noxious level of stimulation for analgesia. If the client does not report any improvement in the pain level or is unable to tolerate the stimulation, the clinician should change the electrode placement or adjust the stimulation parameters. Intervention is continued if the client is able to tolerate the sensation, reports a decrease in pain, and indicates an improvement in occupational performance or movement (Bracciano, 2008).

## Precautions and Contraindications

As with any physical agent modality, a thorough examination and assessment of the client is necessary to identify the source of the client's pain and symptoms. Reviewing the past medical history and history of the current condition assists in clarifying and identifying contraindications or precautions that might be required. Precautions and contraindications are essentially the same as those for any form of electrical stimulation. Precautions include those clients with known cardiac disease or cardiac arrhythmias. These clients should be monitored for any signs of distress or adverse effects. Care should be used if the TENS is being placed over the lumbar paraspinals or abdominal region during pregnancy, except when used during labor and delivery in uncomplicated pregnancies. If a client has been diagnosed with cancer or malignancies, TENS may be used to assist with pain control. Informed consent of the client and attending physician should be obtained when using electrical stimulation or TENS with both the client with cancer and during pregnancy.

TENS and electrical stimulation are contraindicated in clients with demand-type cardiac pacemakers. Electrical stimulation should never be used over the carotid sinus as stimulation over this region of the neck may cause a hypotensive incident and cardiac irregularities. TENS and stimulation should never be applied over the eye or over areas of decreased or abnormal sensation or used in clients with undiagnosed pain, epilepsy, metastasis, or peripheral vascular disease.

TENS contraindications include the following:

- Peripheral vascular disease
- Infection
- Impaired cognition or mentation
- Demand-type pacemakers
- Over carotid sinus
- Over the eye
- Clients with epilepsy
- Cancer malignancies
- Decreased or absent sensation

## Summary

The rehabilitation field has seen dramatic increases in the technology and advancement of physical agent modalities. These physical agents can be used as part of the therapeutic intervention of a variety of clinical conditions that impact occupational function and independence. Because of the impact and call for evidence-based practice, research related to physical agent modalities continues to grow, with research and intervention parameters more standardized and objective. The occupational therapist who is considering using physical agents as an adjunct to engagement in occupation needs to consider the context and unique client factors relevant to the disease or impairment. Rather than using a "technician-like" approach to physical agents, the skilled clinician needs to determine which client factors and which physiological functions are impacted by the impairment or disorder and how best to facilitate the desired healing response that will ultimately facilitate occupational performance and function. The ability to discern the underlying physiological components and cause of the impairment or condition, and the clinical experience and knowledge to determine how best to impact that component, requires additional training and experiential learning to ensure that we use physical agents in a timely, systematic, and effective fashion. Failure to consider physical agents and their potential for benefiting our clients through improved occupational functioning not only limits our effectiveness as occupational therapists and the profession, but it limits our ability to fully help our clients achieve their highest level of independence.

# Student Self-Assessment

## Therapeutic Application of Cold: Determining Clinical Response

*Objective*: The student will determine the effectiveness of different cold applications in decreasing skin temperature, achieving an analgesic response, and in determining its effect on grip/pinch strength. Students will monitor the form of application, duration, and the client's subjective comments during the application of cold. The student will take a pre- and post-grip and/or pinch test in the same upper extremity to which the cold modality will be applied.

*Equipment*: Select from the various methods of administering cryotherapy, including the following:

- Crushed ice bag
- Ice immersion bucket
- Ice massage cup
- Reusable cold pack
- Stop watch or watch with second/minute hand
- Dynamometer and/or pinch gauge

*Procedure*:

1. Select a method of applying cryotherapy. Identify which upper extremity will be targeted for the application. The modality should be applied to the forearm of the selected upper extremity. Before applying the cold modality, take a baseline grip strength using the dynamometer. Apply the cold modality to the body part for a maximum total of 10 minutes, less if using the ice massage method (approximately 4 minutes).
2. Using the Numerical Rating Scale (NRS) (0 = no pain; 10 = unimaginable pain), have the client "rate" his or her pain level at each temperature measurement (each minute).
3. Note the client's response (verbal and behavioral) as well as the skin appearance during each measurement period.
4. Immediately after discontinuing the application, use the dynamometer/pinch gauge and remeasure grip and/or pinch strength in the upper extremity.
5. Using a different area or body part, apply a different application technique and repeat steps 1 through 4.
6. Following completion of the lab and measurements, note any differences in grip/pinch strength. What did you find? Was one type of application more effective than another? What were the client's subjective comments? Did you notice any patterns?

# Electronic Resources

- AliMed: www.alimed.com
- Amrex Electrotherapy Equipment: www.amrex-zetron.com
- Biodex Medical Systems Inc.: www.biodex.com
- Chattanooga Group: www.chattgroup.com
- Empi: www.empi.com
- Medical Science Products: www.medsciencepro.com
- Mettler Electronics Corp: www.mettlerelectronics.com
- North Coast Medical: www.ncmedical.com
- RehabShopper.com: www.gnrcatalog.com
- Vonco Medical: www.voncomed.com
- Omni Medical Supply: www.omnimedicalsupply.com
- Whitehall Manufacturing: www.whitehallmfg.com

**Evidence-Based Research Chart**

| Intervention | Keywords | Evidence |
|---|---|---|
| Superficial thermal agents—cryotherapy | Cryotherapy/instrumentation, pain, analgesics | Hochberg, 2001 |
| Superficial thermal agents—heat | Pain, pain measurement, heat/therapeutic use, intervention outcome | Michlovitz et al., 2004 |
| Therapeutic ultrasound | Ultrasonic therapy, ultrasonic therapy/methods | Citak-Karakaya, Akbayrak, Demirturk, Ekici, & Bakar, 2006; Lazar et al., 2001; Uhlemann, 1993 |
| Electrotherapy—NMES, TENS | Electric stimulation therapy, hemiplegia/therapy/etiology, TENS | Aoyagi & Tsubahara, 2004; Bjordal et al., 2003; Bogie & Triolo, 2003; Breit & Van der Wall, 2004; Kesar & Binder-Macleod, 2006; Paci, Nannetti, & Rinaldi, 2005; Shields, Dudley-Javoroski, & Cole, 2006; Sullivan & Hedman, 2004; Van Til, Renzenbrink, Groothuis, & Ijzerman, 2006 |

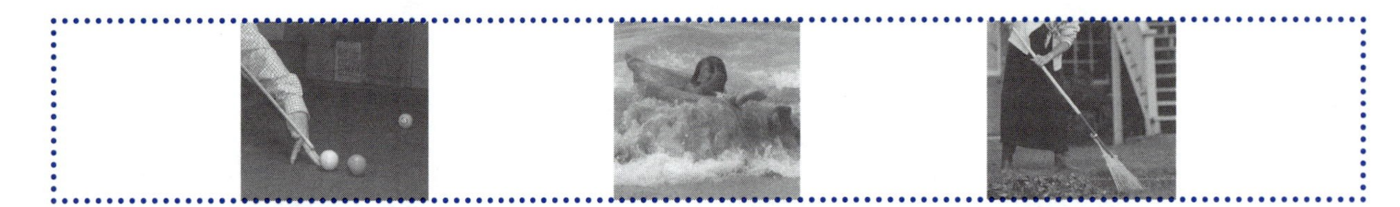

# References


Al-Smadi, J., Warke, K., Wilson, I., Cramp, A. F., Noble, G., Walsh, D. M., et al. (2003). A pilot investigation of the hypoalgesic effects of transcutaneous electrical nerve stimulation upon low back pain in people with multiple sclerosis. *Clinical Rehabilitation, 17,* 742-749.

American Occupational Therapy Association. (2008). Physical agent modalities: A position paper. *American Journal of Occupational Therapy, 62,* 691-693.

Andreadis, S. T. (2006). Experimental models and high-throughput diagnostics for tissue regeneration. *Expert Opinion on Biological Therapy, 6,* 1071-1086.

Ankrom, M. A., Bennett, R. G., Sprigle, S., Langemo, D., Black, J. M., Berlowitz, D. R., et al. (2005). Pressure-related deep tissue injury under intact skin and the current pressure ulcer staging systems. *Advances in Skin & Wound Care, 18,* 35-42.

Aoyagi, Y., & Tsubahara, A. (2004). Therapeutic orthosis and electrical stimulation for upper extremity hemiplegia after stroke: A review of effectiveness based on evidence. *Topics in Stroke Rehabilitation, 11,* 9-15.

Baker, L. L., Chambers, R., DeMuth, S. K., & Villar, F. (1997). Effects of electrical stimulation on wound healing in patients with diabetic ulcers. *Diabetes Care, 20,* 405-412.

Baker, L. L., Parker, K., & Sanderson, D. (1983). Neuromuscular electrical stimulation for the head-injured patient. *Physical Therapy, 63,* 1967-1974.

Barber, F. A. (2000). A comparison of crushed ice and continuous flow cold therapy. *American Journal of Knee Surgery, 13,* 97-101; discussion 102.

Bayat, M., Asgari-Moghadam, Z., Maroufi, M., Rezaie, F. S., Bayat, M., & Rakhshan, M. (2006). Experimental wound healing using microamperage electrical stimulation in rabbits. *Journal of Rehabilitation Research and Development, 43,* 219-226.

Billian, C., & Gorman, P. H. (1992). Upper extremity applications of functional neuromuscular stimulation. *Assistive Technology, 4,* 31-39.

Bjordal, J. M., Johnson, M. I., & Ljunggreen, A. E. (2003). Transcutaneous electrical nerve stimulation (TENS) can reduce postoperative analgesic consumption. A meta-analysis with assessment of optimal treatment parameters for postoperative pain. *European Journal of Pain, 7,* 181-188.

Bogie, K. M., Reger, S. I., Levine, S. P., & Sahgal, V. (2000). Electrical stimulation for pressure sore prevention and wound healing. *Assistive Technology, 12,* 50-66.

Bogie, K. M., & Triolo, R. J. (2003). Effects of regular use of neuromuscular electrical stimulation on tissue health. *Journal of Rehabilitation Research and Development, 40,* 469-475.

Bolton, L., & van Rijswijk, L. (1991). Wound dressings: Meeting clinical and biological needs. *Dermatology Nursing/Dermatology Nurses' Association, 3,* 146-161.

Bracciano, A. G. (2008) *Physical agent modalities: Theory and application for the occupational therapist* (2nd ed.). Thorofare, NJ: SLACK Incorporated.

Breit, R., & Van der Wall, H. (2004). Transcutaneous electrical nerve stimulation for postoperative pain relief after total knee arthroplasty. *Journal of Arthroplasty, 19,* 45-48.

Carmick, J. (1995). Managing equinus in children with cerebral palsy: Electrical stimulation to strengthen the triceps surae muscle. *Developmental Medicine and Child Neurology, 37,* 965-975.

Carmick, J. (1997). Use of neuromuscular electrical stimulation and [corrected] dorsal wrist splint to improve the hand function of a child with spastic hemiparesis. *Physical Therapy, 77,* 661-671.

Casarotto, R. A., Adamowski, J. C., Fallopa, F., & Bacanelli, F. (2004). Coupling agents in therapeutic ultrasound: Acoustic and thermal behavior. *Archives of Physical Medicine and Rehabilitation, 85,* 162-165.

Chae, J., & Hart, R. (1998). Comparison of discomfort associated with surface and percutaneous intramuscular electrical stimulation for persons with chronic hemiplegia. *American Journal of Physical Medicine & Rehabilitation, 77,* 516-522.

Chae, J., Yu, D. T., Walker, M. E., Kirsteins, A., Elovic, E. P., Flanagan, S. R., et al. (2005). Intramuscular electrical stimulation for hemiplegic shoulder pain: A 12-month follow-up of a multiple-center, randomized clinical trial. *American Journal of Physical Medicine & Rehabilitation, 84,* 832-842.

Chan, C. W., Qin, L., Lee, K. M., Zhang, M., Cheng, J. C., & Leung, K. S. (2006). Low intensity pulsed ultrasound accelerated bone remodeling during consolidation stage of distraction osteogenesis. *Journal of Orthopaedic Research, 24,* 263-270.

Chandran, P., & Sluka, K. A. (2003). Development of opioid tolerance with repeated transcutaneous electrical nerve stimulation administration. *Pain, 102,* 195-201.

Chang, Q. Y., Lin, J. G., & Hsieh, C. L. (2002). Effect of electroacupuncture and transcutaneous electrical nerve stimulation at hegu (LI.4) acupuncture point on the cutaneous reflex. *Acupuncture & Electro-Therapeutics Research, 27,* 191-202.

Citak-Karakaya, I., Akbayrak, T., Demirturk, F., Ekici, G., & Bakar, Y. (2006). Short and long-term results of connective tissue manipulation and combined ultrasound therapy in patients with fibromyalgia. *Journal of Manipulative and Physiological Therapeutics, 29,* 524-528.

Cornish-Painter, C., Peterson, C. Q., & Lindstrom-Hazel, D. K. (1997). Skill acquisition and competency testing for physical agent modality use. *American Journal of Occupational Therapy, 51,* 681-685.

Currier, D. P., & Mann, R. (1983). Muscular strength development by electrical stimulation in healthy individuals. *Physical Therapy, 63,* 915-921.

Cuzzell, J. (2002). Wound healing: Translating theory into clinical practice. *Dermatology Nursing, 14,* 257-261.

Daly, J. J., Marsolais, E. B., Mendell, L. M., Rymer, W. Z., Stefanovska, A., Wolpaw, J. R., et al. (1996). Therapeutic neural effects of electrical stimulation. *IEEE Transactions on Rehabilitation Engineering, 4,* 218-230.

Denegar, C. (1993). The effects of low-volt microamperage stimulation on delayed onset muscle soreness. *Journal of Sports Rehabilitation, 1,* 95-102.

Detrembleur, C., Lejeune, T. M., Renders, A., & Van Den Bergh, P. Y. (2002). Botulinum toxin and short-term electrical stimulation in the treatment of equinus in cerebral palsy. *Movement Disorders, 17,* 162-169.

Dyson, M. (1987). Mechanisms involved in therapeutic ultrasound. *Physiotherapy, 73,* 116-120.

Ebenbichler, G., & Resch, K. L. (1994). Critical evaluation of ultrasound therapy. *Wiener Medizinische Wochenschrift (1946), 144,* 51-53.

Enoch, S., & Harding, K. (2003). Wound bed preparation: The science behind the removal of barriers to healing. *Wounds, 15,* 213-229.

Enwemeka, C. S. (1989). The effects of therapeutic ultrasound on tendon healing: A biomechanical study. *American Journal of Physical Medicine & Rehabilitation, 68,* 283-287.

Fyfe, M. C., & Bullock, M. (1985). Therapeutic ultrasound: Some historical background and development in knowledge of its effects on healing. *Australian Journal of Physiotherapy, 31*, 220-224.

Gardner, S. E., Frantz, R. A., & Schmidt, F. L. (1999). Effect of electrical stimulation on chronic wound healing: A meta-analysis. *Wound Repair and Regeneration, 7*, 495-503.

Giannini, S., Giombini, A., Moneta, M. R., Massazza, G., & Pigozzi, F. (2004). Low-intensity pulsed ultrasound in the treatment of traumatic hand fracture in an elite athlete. *American Journal of Physical Medicine & Rehabilitation, 83*, 921-925.

Glauner, J. H., Ekes, A. M., James, A. E., & Holm, M. B. (1997). A pilot study of the theoretical and technical competence and appropriate education for the use of nine physical agent modalities in occupational therapy practice. *American Journal of Occupational Therapy, 51*, 767-774.

Gogia, P. (1995). *Clinical wound management*. Thorofare, NJ: SLACK Incorporated.

Gracies, J. M. (2001). Physical modalities other than stretch in spastic hypertonia. *Physical Medicine and Rehabilitation Clinics of North America, 12*, 769-92, vi.

Hardy, M. A. (1989). The biology of scar formation. *Physical Therapy, 69*, 1014-1032.

Hesse, S., Werner, C., Bardeleben, A., & Brandl-Hesse, B. (2002). Management of upper and lower limb spasticity in neuro-rehabilitation. *Acta Neurochirurgica, 79*(supplement), 117-122.

Hochberg, J. (2001). A randomized prospective study to assess the efficacy of two cold-therapy treatments following carpal tunnel release. *Journal of Hand Therapy, 14*, 208-215.

Hong, C. Z., Liu, H. H., & Yu, J. (1988). Ultrasound thermotherapy effect on the recovery of nerve conduction in experimental compression neuropathy. *Archives of Physical Medicine and Rehabilitation, 69*, 410-414.

Houghton, P. E., Kincaid, C. B., Lovell, M., Campbell, K. E., Keast, D. H., Woodbury, M. G., et al. (2003). Effect of electrical stimulation on chronic leg ulcer size and appearance. *Physical Therapy, 83*, 17-28.

Kesar, T., & Binder-Macleod, S. A. (2006). Effect of frequency and pulse duration on human muscle fatigue during repetititve electrical stimulation. *Experimental Physiology, 91*(6), 967-976.

Kloth, L. C., & McCulloch, J. M. (1995). The inflammatory response to wounding. In J. M. MuCulloch, L. C. Kloth, & J. A. Feedar (Eds.), *Wound healing: Alternatives in management* (2nd ed., p. 3). Philadelphia, PA: F.A. Davis.

Klucinec, B. (1996). The effectiveness of the aquaflex gel pad in the transmission of acoustic energy. *Journal of Athletic Training, 31*, 313-317.

Klucinec, B., Scheidler, M., Denegar, C., Domholdt, E., & Burgess, S. (2000). Transmissivity of coupling agents used to deliver ultrasound through indirect methods. *Journal of Orthopaedic and Sports Physical Therapy, 30*, 263-269.

Kottke, F. J., Pauley, D. L., & Ptak, R. A. (1966). The rationale for prolonged stretching for correction of shortening of connective tissue. *Archives of Physical Medicine and Rehabilitation, 47*, 345-352.

Laban, M. M. (1962). Collagen tissue: Implications of its response to stress in vitro. *Archives of Physical Medicine and Rehabilitation, 43*, 461-466.

Langevin, H. M., Storch, K. N., Cipolla, M. J., White, S. L., Buttolph, T. R., & Taatjes, D. J. (2006). Fibroblast spreading induced by connective tissue stretch involves intracellular redistribution of alpha- and beta-actin. *Histochemistry and Cell Biology, 125*, 487-495.

Lazar, D. A., Curra, F. P., Mohr, B., McNutt, L. D., Kliot, M., & Mourad, P. D. (2001). Acceleration of recovery after injury to the peripheral nervous system using ultrasound and other therapeutic modalities. *Neurosurgery Clinics of North America, 12*, 353-357.

Likar, R., Molnar, M., Pipam, W., Koppert, W., Quantschnigg, B., Disselhoff, B., et al. (2001). Postoperative transcutaneous electrical nerve stimulation (TENS) in shoulder surgery (randomized, double blind, placebo controlled pilot trial). *Schmerz, 15*, 158-163.

Liu, J., You, W. X., & Sun, D. (2005). Effects of functional electric stimulation on shoulder subluxation and upper limb motor function recovery of patients with hemiplegia resulting from stroke. *Di Yi Jun Yi Da Xue Xue Bao, 25*, 1054-1055.

Loten, C., Stokes, B., Worsley, D., Seymour, J. E., Jiang, S., & Isbistergk, G. K. (2006). A randomized controlled trial of hot water (45 degrees C) immersion versus ice packs for pain relief in bluebottle stings. *Medical Journal of Australia, 184*, 329-333.

McPhee, S. D., Bracciano, A. G., Rose, B. W., Brayman, S. J., & Commission on Practice. (2003). Physical agent modalities: A position paper. *American Journal of Occupational Therapy, 57*, 650-651.

Melzack, R. (1993). Pain: Past, present and future. *Canadian Journal of Experimental Psychology, 47*, 615-629.

Michlovitz, S., Hun, L., Erasala, G. N., Hengehold, D. A., & Weingand, K. W. (2004). Continuous low-level heat wrap therapy is effective for treating wrist pain. *Archives of Physical Medicine and Rehabilitation, 85*, 1409-1416.

Nadler, S. F., Prybicien, M., Malanga, G. A., & Sicher, D. (2003). Complications from therapeutic modalities: Results of a national survey of athletic trainers. *Archives of Physical Medicine and Rehabilitation, 84*, 849-853.

Nadler, S. F., Steiner, D. J., Erasala, G. N., Hengehold, D. A., Abeln, S. B., & Weingand, K. W. (2003). Continuous low-level heatwrap therapy for treating acute nonspecific low back pain. *Archives of Physical Medicine and Rehabilitation, 84*, 329-334.

Olson, J. E., & Stravino, V. D. (1972). A review of cryotherapy. *Physical Therapy, 52*, 840-853.

Oziomek, R. S., Perrin, D. H., Herold, D. A., & Denegar, C. R. (1991). Effect of phonophoresis on serum salicylate levels. *Medicine and Science in Sports and Exercise, 23*, 397-401.

Paci, M., Nannetti, L., & Rinaldi, L. A. (2005). Glenohumeral subluxation in hemiplegia: An overview. *Journal of Rehabilitation Research and Development, 42*, 557-568.

Petrofsky, J. S., Lohman III, E., Suh, H. J., Garcia, J., Anders, A., Sutterfield, C., et al. (2006). The effect of aging on conductive heat exchange in the skin at two environmental temperatures. *Medical Science Monitor, 12*, CR400-408.

Reshetov, P. P., Tverdokhleb, I., & Bezmenov, V. A. (2000). The use of hydrocortisone combined with ultrasound with gonarthrosis patients. *Voprosy Kurortologii, Fizioterapii, i Lechebnoi Fizicheskoi Kultury, 4*, 47-48.

Rimington, S. J., Draper, D. O., Durrant, E., & Fellingham, G. (1994). Temperature changes during therapeutic ultrasound in the precooled human gastrocnemius muscle. *Journal of Athletic Training, 29*, 325-327.

Sanya, A. O., & Bello, A. O. (1999). Effects of cold application on isometric strength and endurance of quadriceps femoris muscle. *African Journal of Medicine and Medical Sciences, 28*(3-4), 195-198.

Scheker, L. R., Chesher, S. P., & Ramirez, S. (1999). Neuromuscular electrical stimulation and dynamic bracing as a treatment for upper-extremity spasticity in children with cerebral palsy. *Journal of Hand Surgery (Edinburgh, Lothian), 24*, 226-232.

Scheker, L. R., & Ozer, K. (2003). Electrical stimulation in the management of spastic deformity. *Hand Clinics, 19*(4), 601-606, vi.

Shields, R. K., Dudley-Javoroski, S., & Cole, K. R. (2006). Feedback-controlled stimulation enhances human paralyzed muscle performance. *Journal of Applied Physiology: Respiratory, Environmental and Exercise Physiology, 101*(5), 1312-1319.

Singh, H., Osbahr, D. C., Holovacs, T. F., Cawley, P. W., & Speer, K. P. (2001). The efficacy of continuous cryotherapy on the postoperative shoulder: A prospective, randomized investigation. *Journal of Shoulder and Elbow Surgery, 10*, 522-525.

Sullivan, J. E., & Hedman, L. D. (2004). A home program of sensory and neuromuscular electrical stimulation with upper-limb task practice in a patient 5 years after a stroke. *Physical Therapy, 84*, 1045-1054.

ter Haar, G. (1978). Basic physics of therapeutic ultrasound. *Physiotherapy, 64*, 100-103.

Turner, S. M., Powell, E. S., & Ng, C. S. (1989). The effect of ultrasound on the healing of repaired cockerel tendon: Is collagen cross-linkage a factor? *Journal of Hand Surgery, 14*, 428-433.

Uhlemann, C. (1993). Pain modification in rheumatic diseases using different frequency applications of ultrasound. *Zeitschrift Fur Rheumatologie, 52*, 236-240.

Van Til, J. A., Renzenbrink, G. J., Groothuis, K., & Ijzerman, M. J. (2006). A preliminary economic evaluation of percutaneous neuromuscular electrical stimulation in the treatment of hemiplegic shoulder pain. *Disability and Rehabilitation, 28*, 645-651.

Weingarden, H. P., Kizony, R., Nathan, R., Ohry, A., & Levy, H. (1997). Upper limb functional electrical stimulation for walker ambulation in hemiplegia: A case report. *American Journal of Physical Medicine & Rehabilitation, 76*, 63-67.

Welch, V., Brosseau, L., Shea, B., McGowan, J., Wells, G., & Tugwell, P. (2000). Thermotherapy for treating rheumatoid arthritis. *Cochrane Database of Systematic Reviews, 4*, CD002826.

World Health Organization. (2001). *International classification of functioning, disability, and health (ICF)*. Geneva, Switzerland: Author.

Yu, D. (2004). Shoulder pain in hemiplegia. *Physical Medicine and Rehabilitation Clinics of North America, 15*, vi-vii, 683-697.

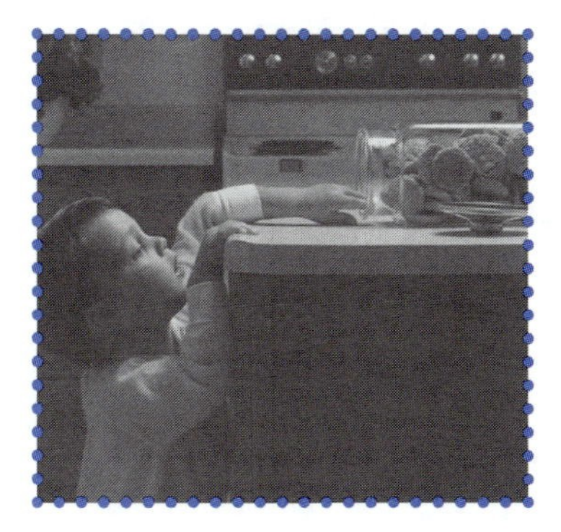

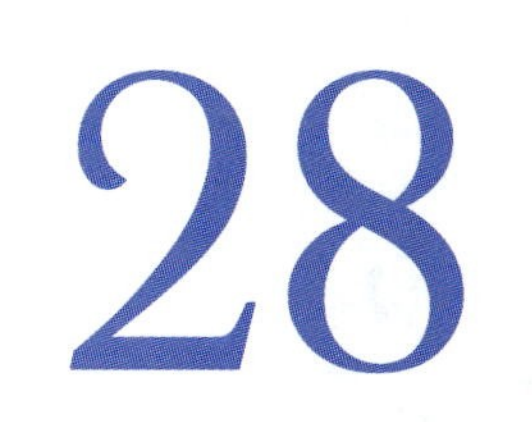

# 28

# FEEDING AND EATING

*Kristin Winston, PhD, OTR/L and Kathryn M. Loukas, MS, OTR/L, FAOTA*

**ACOTE Standard Explored in This Chapter**

B.5.12

**Key Terms**

| | |
|---|---|
| Aspiration | Gastrostomy tube (G-tube) |
| Bolus | Jejunostomy tube |
| Deglutition | Nasogastric tube |
| Dysphagia | NPO (nil per os) |
| Eating | Parenteral tube feedings |
| Enteral tube feedings | Ph probe |
| Feeding | Positioning |
| Gastroesophageal reflux disease (GERD) | Suck, swallow, breathe synchrony |
| Gastroesophageal scintigraphy | Videofluoroscopy |

## Introduction

Feeding and eating are important occupational performance skills across the lifespan that can be interrupted through a number of neurological, developmental, or orthopedic conditions.

Kedesdy and Budd (1998) stated, "No human activity has greater biological and social significance than feeding" (p. 1). The occupations of feeding and eating therefore have great significance in terms of occupational therapy intervention. Across the lifespan, feeding and eating are necessary to support nutritional intake and hydration that in turn support growth and overall health (Baer, 2005). For infants and young children, success in the occupations of eating and feeding satisfy their sense of hunger, provide pleasure related to taste and textures of foods, and create opportunities for parent-child bonding (Kedesdy & Budd). For the parents of young children, success in the occupations of eating and feeding signifies competence in the role of caregiver and in turn facilitates the bonding experience between parent and young child (Kedesdy & Budd). From early childhood through adulthood, the occupations related to eating and feeding continue to fulfill a nutritional need, but these occupations also begin to take on strong social and cultural significance (Baer; Jenks, 2002). Food and eating is frequently a part of celebrations large and small; cultural events; and other social activities at home, at school, in the workplace, as well as within the community (Figure 28-1).



K. Sladyk, K. Jacobs, & N. MacRae (Eds.).
*Occupational Therapy Essentials for Clinical Competence* (pp. 311-322).

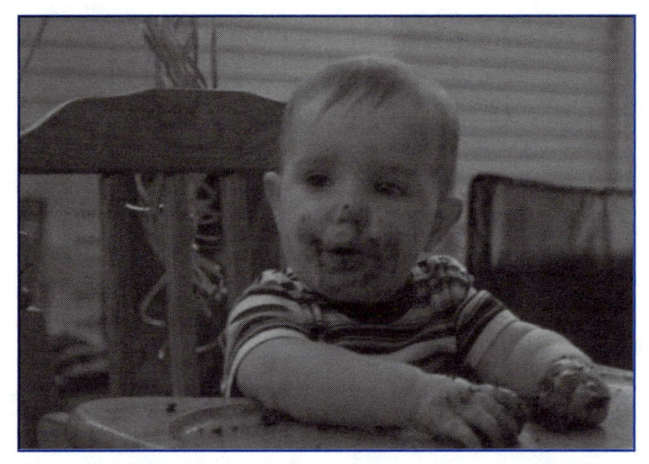

**Figure 28-1.** Enjoying a first birthday cupcake as part of a family celebration.

Secondary to the complex nature of concerns within the occupations of feeding and eating, practice regarding feeding and eating has varying skill levels and varying levels at which therapists are able to intervene (American Occupational Therapy Association [AOTA], 2003, 2007). Intervention is dependent on a thorough assessment and evaluation of factors relating to the person, the environment, and occupation. Occupational therapy practitioners should understand not only the sensory and motor concerns that might be influencing the feeding and eating process but also complex cognitive, perceptual, and psychosocial factors that influence occupational performance in the areas of feeding and eating. The progression from entry-level practitioner to advanced practitioner in this area of practice is unique for each individual therapist and his or her practice setting. Competence in feeding and eating intervention may involve continuing education, on the job training, mentoring, independent study, and practice for the occupational therapy practitioner.

As entry-level practitioners, occupational therapists are educated to address many concerns related to feeding and eating as guided by the theoretical principles that are the foundation for practice. Occupational therapy practitioners provide intervention in this area that relates to occupational performance, performance skills, performance patterns, context, activity demands, and client factors facilitating a holistic approach to intervention (AOTA, 2008). Entry-level practitioners should refer to AOTA's paper entitled *Specialized Knowledge and Skills in Eating and Feeding for Occupational Therapy Practice* (2007) for guidelines related to specific roles for each practitioner.

Occupational therapy practitioners are especially skilled to address the performance of feeding and eating because of the emphasis on occupation, function, motor skills, postural control, sensory processing skills, as well as cognitive and perceptual skills. The occupational therapy practitioner must also understand and apply the importance of trunk and head control, use of the upper extremity and hands, and oral motor functions to the process of feeding and eating.

Occupational therapy practitioners work with individuals who receive their nutritional intake through oral or non-oral means. The following information seeks to clarify issues related to intervention for individuals receiving oral nutrition, non-oral nutrition, or a combination of methods. Non-oral nutrition may be via enteral systems that feed directly into the gastrointestinal tract or via parenteral feeding where nutrition is supplied intravenously.

# Oral Feeding

Oral feeding encompasses the process of gaining nutrition through the intake of fluids and solids by mouth. In the young child, the parent or caregiver facilitates feeding as the young child is dependent in many feeding/eating skills until the motor, sensory, cognitive, and perceptual skills necessary for independence in the area of feeding and eating develop (Case-Smith & Humphry, 2005). Once young children develop the necessary skills, independence in these occupations continues through adulthood, unless illness or disability affects the skills necessary to maintain independence.

Whenever possible, occupational therapy practitioners should work with the client to feed him- or herself to facilitate occupational performance and promote independence. The occupational therapy practitioner should be aware of the possible stigma of being fed for adults, elders, and older children and move toward self-feeding as soon as possible if this is a meaningful goal.

Examples of adaptive equipment that can facilitate self feeding include but are not limited to the following (these items can be found in adaptive equipment catalogues):

- Dycem to stabilize the plate or bowl
- Plate guards to assist getting food onto a utensil
- Weighted, bendable, strapped, or built-up utensils or self-feeding systems such as the Neater Eater (Sammons Preston, Bolingbrook, IL) or Stable Slide (Sammons Preston) self-feeding system.
- Rocker knives can be helpful to cut food when bilateral coordination is compromised
- Universal cuffs can be helpful for those with limited hand control
- A cup with a cut-out (nosey cup) can assist those with difficulty with head control

Independence and occupational performance may also be promoted in feeding and eating for those who are dependent upon a caregiver for nutritional intake. This is accomplished by assisting the individual with difficulty in these areas to become an active participant in the relationship that forms between the individual and the caregiver. Expanding the individual's options for making choices about types of foods/liquids eaten, times of meals, and other contextual or environmental factors related to feeding and eating fosters independence in these occupations.

This, in turn, facilitates independence as individuals are encouraged to make decisions regarding their own lives (Crittenden, 1990).

# Four Phases of Oral Eating

## The Anticipatory/ Oral Preparatory Phase

This phase is described as a process in which the food or drink is brought to the mouth either by the person engaged in eating or by the feeder (AOTA, 2003). This phase includes a combination of motor and sensory skills that include how the food looks and smells as well as the person's ability to reach for the food and bring it to his or her mouth. This phase also includes the sensory processing skills necessary to assist in determining taste, texture, and temperature of foods and the initial motor skills needed to prepare and position the food for swallowing.

Intervention in this phase may be directed at assisting with sensory, motor, cognitive, or perceptual skills that inhibit an individual's occupational performance in the areas of feeding and eating.

Examples of intervention techniques in this phase include the following:

- To address weakness of lips or cheeks, use tapping; vibration; quick stretch, ROM, resistive sucking; and blowing exercises (Jenks, 2002; Jenks & Smith, 2006).
- For the presence of abnormal oral reflexes, train caregivers to avoid stimulation of the reflex through positioning and adaptive techniques, position with stability (Avery-Smith, 2002).
- For postural control to support muscle efficiency, position with stability in the trunk and pelvis (Avery-Smith, 2002; Jenks, 2002).
- For concerns related to oral hypersensitivity, try deep pressure or proprioceptive input in and around the mouth, work with food textures that are comfortable for the individual (some with hypersensitivity prefer smooth textures while others prefer crunchy), develop sensory diet activities that calm and organize the oral area before and during a meal or snack (Logemann, 1998).
- For concerns related to oral hyposensitivity, use warmer/colder and more flavorful food to stimulate sensation, develop sensory diet techniques that are alerting to increase input to the oral area before and during a meal or snack (Arvedson, Brodsky, & Reigstad, 2002; Logemann, 1998).

## The Oral Phase

This phase is described as the phase in which the bolus of food or liquid is propelled by the tongue; masticated by the teeth and gums; and manipulated by the lips, cheeks, and tongue (AOTA, 2003; Jenks, 2002). In this phase, the action is to move the food to the back of the mouth in preparation for initiating the swallow. This phase of the swallow is voluntary and typically takes about 1 second to complete (Jenks).

Intervention in this phase for individuals who are considered safe for oral feeding is typically directed at assisting with sensory and motor skills that inhibit an individual's occupational performance in the areas of feeding and eating.

Examples of intervention techniques in this phase include the following:

- For concerns with slow oral transit time, use cold or sour boluses, infuse sour into food (lemon). The occupational therapy practitioner may try thermal stimulation; cold temperatures may facilitate the initiation of the swallow (Avery-Smith, 2002; Logemann, Kahrilas, Kobara, & Vakil, 1989).
- For concerns related to positioning of the head and neck for a safe swallow, encourage a chin tuck, which moves the base of the tongue back and protects the airway when the larynx is low and swallow is weak (Case-Smith & Humphry, 2005; Ohmae, Logemann, Kaiser, Hanson, & Kahrilas, 1996).
- The occupational therapy practitioner may also try encouraging the individual to use an effortful swallow that helps to elevate the base of the tongue and then encourage the individual to squeeze hard with throat muscles while swallowing (Avery-Smith, 2002; Pouderoux & Kahrilas, 1995).
- Encourage the use of the Mendelsohn Maneuver (following training and supervision in the use of this technique), where the individual pushes the tongue to the roof of the mouth and tries to keep the Adam's apple up while swallowing (Avery-Smith, 2002; Logemann et al., 1989).
- For clients with hemiparesis, suggest using neck rotation to turn the head toward the weaker side, which can help to close the weaker side of the pharynx, utilizing the stronger side (Avery-Smith, 2002; Logemann et al., 1989).

Additional references for assessment and intervention in the oral phase include Arvedson & Brodsky, 2002; Case-Smith & Humphry, 2005; and Wolf & Glass, 1992.

## The Pharyngeal Phase

This phase is described as the phase in which the swallowing response is initiated and breathing is briefly interrupted (Avery-Smith, 2002; Jenks, 2002). Intervention in this phase is typically directed toward working with the individual's team to determine the ability to safely swallow.

This intervention is typically accomplished through facilitated head and neck positioning, including a chin tuck for safe swallowing. Diagnostic testing is frequently recommended to examine the individual's ability to safely swallow a variety of food and liquid consistencies without risk of aspiration (i.e., videofluroscopy). Intervention may involve working with the team to train an individual and his or her caregivers as to what types of foods/liquids are recommended and safe. For example, it may be recommended that the individual have no thin liquids. Strategies would then be discussed to avoid thin liquids, meltables (ice cream, popsicles, or ice), or to thicken liquids to an appropriate consistency as determined by the individual's intervention team (Jenks & Smith, 2006).

Individuals with concerns in this phase frequently are diagnosed with dysphagia. If the client has swallowing problems or an inability to swallow, the occupational therapy practitioner should be aware that continuing education and specialized training is necessary for competent interventions in this area. Specialized medical intervention in addition to individualized precautions are often indicated when a client is experiencing dysphagia. Speech pathologists and occupational therapy practitioners may work collaboratively with the client with dysphagia after diagnostic testing is performed. Additional team members may include the physician, a radiologist, nursing, and nutrition or dietary services (AOTA, 2003, 2007).

## The Esophageal Phase

This phase is described as the phase in which the bolus enters the esophagus and travels through the esophagus and into the stomach (Jenks & Smith, 2006).

Occupational therapy practitioners do not provide direct intervention for concerns identified in this area. However, as a team member working on concerns related to feeding and eating, occupational therapy practitioners need to be aware of concerns that could arise in this phase of eating. Occupational therapy practioners may assist in developing interventions focusing on positioning or other factors to improve safety and comfort. In addition, occupational therapy practitioners may assist in team decisions regarding further diagnostic assessment to determine concerns in this phase of eating (AOTA, 2007).

# Non-Oral Feeding

Non-oral feedings are utilized to support nutritional intake when risk of aspiration is a concern and it does not appear to be safe for the individual to eat by mouth. Non-oral feeding may also be utilized to support nutritional intake when the individual is not able to effectively and efficiently take in enough calories by mouth to support growth and overall health (Morris & Klein, 2000). Feeding tubes or enteral nutrition may be a temporary or a permanent solution to nutritional intake concerns. Occupational therapy practitioners work with individuals and teams to facilitate the transition from non-oral to oral feedings. In addition, occupational therapy practitioners work closely with individuals and their families/caregivers to integrate tube feedings into the habits and routines that exist around mealtimes (Jenks & Smith, 2006; Morris & Klein, 2000).

Non-oral feedings are delivered through various tube placements. A few types as defined in the glossary include nasogastric tubes, gastrostomy tubes, and jejunostomy tubes. A nasogastric tube is inserted through the nasal cavity into the stomach, a gastrostomy tube bypasses the mouth and is inserted surgically directly into the stomach, and a jejunostomy tube is surgically inserted into the jejunum (a branch of the small intestine). For some individuals, non-oral feedings will continue secondary to structural issues or neurological issues that prevent safe oral feedings. For others, the goal is to transition from non-oral feedings to oral feedings. The process of weaning from non-oral to oral feedings is complex. Schauster & Dwyer (1996) suggest that promoting a positive relationship between the individual and caregiver is an important first step in promoting the transition to oral feedings. In addition, the transition is facilitated by intervention aimed at normalizing feeding and eating through safe and structured exploration of oral experiences (Figure 28-2).

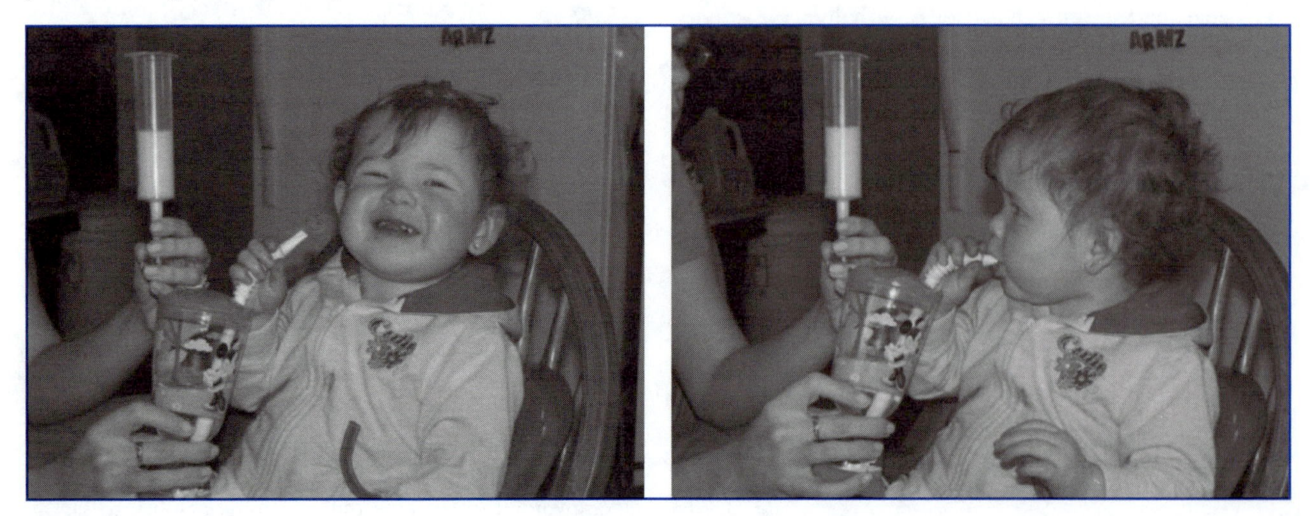

**Figure 28-2.** Providing oral opportunities during non-oral feedings

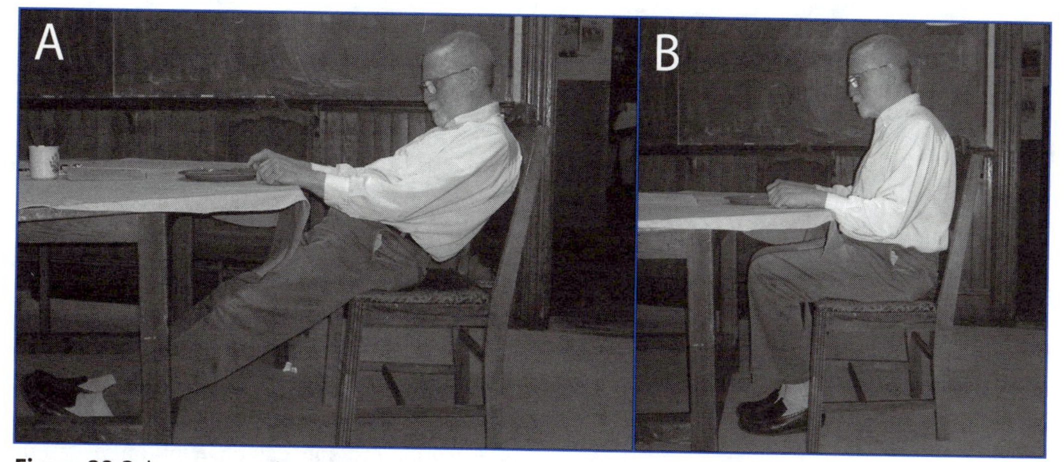


**Figure 28-3.** Improper eating position (A) versus proper eating position (B).

# General Factors to Consider

## Developmental Progression

The infant is born with a small oral cavity. The fatty cheek pads and tongue are in close proximity to each other and nearly fill the oral cavity such that a typically developing infant can easily achieve suction and compress a nipple because of the tight fit when placed in the mouth (Case-Smith & Humphrey, 2005; Morris & Klein, 2000; Wolf & Glass, 1992). The structures of the throat in the infant are also in close proximity to one another. This arrangement of structures allows for the flow of liquid to pass safely from the base of the tongue to the esophagus. Protection of the trachea from liquid occurs as the larynx elevates the epiglottis and falls over the trachea. The structure of the oral cavity allows for a safe swallow when held in a reclined position for early breast and bottlefeeding. Aspiration is unlikely in the first 4 months due to these structural arrangements, allowing the safe feeding of infants in a reclined position (Case-Smith & Humphrey; Morris & Klein). This factor becomes important when working with young children with feeding concerns as structural changes begin to occur between 4 and 6 months and continue through the first year of development (Morris & Klein). This is important in terms of intervention, as therapists need to assist parents in developing options for upright feeding and eating to support safe swallowing without aspiration.

## Positioning

Because the position of the trunk, head, and neck directly affects the ability to swallow safely in children and adults, the first and most important aspect of feeding and eating intervention is assuring that the client is in the proper position for eating (Jenks, 2002). When positioning a client, you should typically begin at the pelvis. "What happens at the lips begins at the hips" (anonymous). The client should be positioned symmetrically from the head through the neck, trunk, and to the hips. A firm surface is best with the knees and ankles at 90 degrees. The pelvis can be in a slight anterior pelvic tilt with the hips at about 100 degrees (Jenks). The trunk should be flexed slightly forward with the back straight. The head should be slightly forward with the chin slightly tucked. Arms can be supported on the table if necessary for support. It should be noted that in some cases, due to structural or neurological impairments, it might be difficult to achieve symmetry. However, this should be the overall goal to encourage safe swallowing, facilitate postural alignment, and prevent structural deformity (Figure 28-3).

## Suck, Swallow, Breathe Synchrony

An infant as well as a client recovering from neurological insult must begin with a suck, swallow, breathe synchrony. The smooth coordination between sucking, swallowing, and breathing is what allows the individual to eat effectively and efficiently (Wolf & Glass, 1992). This is evident as seen with infants suckling from the breast or bottle. It involves a rhythm and is necessary to the development of oral structure for proper eating. It should be noted that clients with breathing difficulties might experience feeding and eating difficulties because of the necessary breathing component in the rhythm of this synchrony of eating.

## Diet Selection

This is an important component of the feeding and eating program. Precautions for clients with suspected swallowing difficulties may include avoiding foods with multiple textures; fibrous or stringy vegetables, meats, or fruits; crumbly or flakey foods; foods that liquefy; and foods with skins or seeds (Jenks, 2002). Diet selection is a team decision that must be determined following comprehensive evaluation of the individual's feeding and eating skills (Jenks, 2002).

## Diet Progression

After making a good diet selection, developmental and rehabilitation approaches suggest the diet should move in the following order (Jenks, 2002):

1. Pureed
2. Mechanical soft
3. Chopped or ground
4. Thick/thin liquids

Ongoing assessment is indicated when considering changing or progressing a client's diet. The decision to move an individual to the next consistency should be a team decision based upon diagnostic assessment and clinical reasoning. The decision to move an individual to the next dietary consistency should be a team decision based upon diagnostic assessment and clinical reasoning. It should be noted that thin liquids are typically the most difficult texture to swallow and the easiest to aspirate. Thin liquids should only be given if you are certain the client has an intact swallow. A safe swallow can be determined through videofluroscopy or a modified barium swallow. Signs and symptoms of possible aspiration include, but are not limited to, the following (Avery-Smith, 2002):

- Prolonged or inefficient cough
- A wet, gurgly quality to the individual's voice before, during, or after eating
- Any color change in the individual during or after eating
- Breathiness or loss of voice when eating

If the occupational therapy practitioner has any concerns regarding the individual's ability to swallow safely, he or she should seek further assessment prior to intervention.

# Additional Issues for Feeding and Eating

## NPO

The Latin term for "nothing by mouth" is a very important and strict precaution. Any occupational therapy practitioner should check a client's chart and adhere to this very important precaution.

## No Thin Liquids

Difficulty with thin liquids is common with people after a neurological insult such as a cerebral vascular accident (CVA) or brain injury. The individual with aspiration precautions should be watched carefully. Liquids can be thickened with applesauce or Thick-It (Precision Foods, Inc., St. Louis, MO) as recommended following medical tests and team discussion. The client should be closely monitored while eating.

## Special Diets

Clients with diabetes, food allergies, or special precautions will be on special diets. The occupational therapy practitioner should be vigilant about knowing precautions and making sure that the client and caregivers fully understand the precautions as well.

## Sensory Impairment

An assessment of the client's sensory processing skills is often an important component of a feeding and eating evaluation. Clients with hyposensitivity or decreased sensation will often be unaware of foods in their cheeks or under their tongue. It is important to work with these clients on sensory re-education to increase awareness when eating and drinking. Clients with hypersensitivity or increased sensitivity are often defensive or hyperaware of temperature, taste, and other sensory properties of foods. A sensory-based intervention program can be helpful to overcome these eating difficulties (Case-Smith & Humphry, 2005).

## General Intervention Techniques

Next is an example of a few general feeding techniques that might be recommended for caregiver carryover of feeding and eating strategies. Caregiver programs are individualized and should be developed based upon the individual's current areas of need.

- Assure proper positioning while feeding and eating by providing the caregiver a picture or diagram
- Provide necessary external supports to help facilitate or maintain proper positioning. This might include pillows, cushions, or other supports as determined by the intervention team
- Follow specifics related to dietary consistency and food choices for each individual's nutrition and safety
- Tactile and sensory input prior to and during feeding to improve sensory awareness in and around the mouth as long as the input is not aversive to the client
- Tuck chin to better align the head and neck for a safe swallow
- Provide tactile cues to encourage use of the correct movement patterns to facilitate eating
- Use adapted equipment as needed to facilitate safety and independence
- Teach to clear throat of food and liquid by coughing

# Professional Reasoning

What are the questions the occupational therapist should ask that begin to guide his or her choice of intervention strategies? The framework (AOTA, 2008) outlines the domain of practice of occupational therapy. "A profession's domain of concern consists of those areas of human experience in which practitioners of the profession offer assistance to others" (Mosey, 1981, p. 51). "The domain of occupational therapy frames the arena in which occupational therapy evaluations and interventions occur" (AOTA, 2008, p. 626).

Professional reasoning and evidence-based practice should guide the occupational therapist in planning and the occupational therapy practitioner in implementing intervention in the area of feeding and eating using the framework (AOTA, 2008). This process is not intended to be prescriptive as each individual occupational therapy practitioner will bring unique areas of strength and areas of concern to be considered. It is also not exhaustive in nature and, as stated above, is intended to provide a guide for assisting occupational therapy practitioners and the individuals with whom they work in planning intervention.

# Occupational Performance

## Performance Skills

What motor skills are influencing the individual's ability to feed him- or herself or participate in the process of being fed?

- Example: There is difficulty with stability and postural control of the trunk, neck, head, and upper or lower extremities while eating.
  - Intervention strategies:
    - Remediation/restoration
    - Therapeutic positioning
    - Neurodevelopmental treatment techniques or other facilitation/inhibition techniques
    - Graded participation in functional activities to increase occupational performance
    - Compensation/adaptation
    - Addition of lateral supports, head/neck supports, or other positioning aides
    - Mobile arm supports
    - Foot supports
- Example: There is decreased strength, coordination, and/or ROM necessary to bring a cup or a spoon to the mouth.
  - Intervention strategies:
    - Remediation/restoration
    - Therapeutic activities to promote active ROM as indicated
    - Therapeutic activities to facilitate muscle strength
    - Neuromuscular facilitation or inhibition techniques to facilitate active use of the upper extremities in feeding and eating
    - Compensation/adaptation
    - Adaptive equipment such as a universal cuff, built-up spoon, or adaptive cup
    - Self-feeding devices
- Example: The individual is demonstrating concerns regarding the ability to swallow safely. This area requires advanced skills and knowledge to intervene. The entry-level practitioner should refer this individual to a more experienced team member or seek consult with a feeding and eating specialist.

What process skills, including level of arousal, attention to task, perceptual awareness, impulse control, and cognitive functioning, are influencing the individual's ability to feed him- or herself or to be fed?

- Example: The individual does not have the necessary energy, endurance, and/or breath support to facilitate occupational performance in the areas of eating and feeding.
  - Intervention strategies:
    - Remediation/Restoration
    - Postural control activities
    - Activities designed to improve breath support
    - Activities designed to build endurance
    - Compensation/Adaptation
    - Positioning
    - Adaptation of the context to facilitate reduced activity, promote relaxation when eating
    - Teach the use of energy conservation techniques and pacing techniques
- Example: The individual lacks the necessary skills to motor plan and sequence the actions needed for occupational performance in the areas of feeding and eating.
  - Intervention strategies:
    - Remediation/restoration
    - Provide consistent instruction during feeding and eating
    - Establish routines for the individual and his or her caregivers around feeding and eating
    - Compensation/adaptation
    - Provide checklists for visual cues
    - Design verbal, written, and/or visual cues to facilitate feeding and eating
- Example: For a client who is dependent on a caregiver for physical assistance or cueing during feeding and eating, there is a concern related to the relationship between the individual and the caregiver that does not support occupational performance.
  - Intervention strategies:
    - Remediation/Restoration
    - Role model the appropriate level of assistance for the caregiver using a coaching model
    - Assist the client to be assertive in the feeding and eating process
    - Compensation/Adaptation
    - Give the caregiver a checklist of appropriate steps

- Put verbal cues on a tape recorder
- Provide adaptive equipment such as a self-feeder to eliminate the need for assistance

Please note that client factors should be individually evaluated and addressed in the occupational therapy process. Many client factors vary and require advanced practice skills for intervention.

## Performance Patterns

As the occupational therapy practitioner, use or develop the individual's habits to assist in facilitating his or her occupational performance in the areas of feeding and eating. Establish or facilitate routines that positively influence occupational performance in the areas of feeding and eating. Establish or facilitate roles to positively impact the individual's occupations related to feeding and eating. Integrate cultural or religious rituals or functions that are important to this individual's occupational performance in the area of feeding and eating into intervention.

## Context

The practitioner should assess the environment for maximal function for each individual client concerning noise and distractions, visual stimuli, room temperature, and olfactory input. Some clients enjoy the company of others, while others prefer to be alone, especially if eating is challenging for them. A typical, natural setting is usually best for clients of all ages.

Context includes the following considerations for intervention:

- *Cultural context*: What are the beliefs, values, or attitudes related to feeding and eating? Examples include consideration of religious holidays and family roles for the occupations of feeding and eating.
- *Physical context*: What are the qualities of the environment or objects within the environment as they relate to feeding and eating? Examples include the use of utensils and the ability to eat in noisy or distracting environments.
- *Social context*: What are the relationships that are important in terms of feeding and eating? Examples include who the individuals are that make up the family table at meals and how relationships change when eating at home versus eating out.
- *Personal context*: Who is the individual receiving intervention for concerns related to feeding and eating? Examples include how intervention differs for a parent versus a child.
- *Spiritual context*: What might inspire or motivate the individual receiving intervention? Examples include the natural environment of the individual and special meals/foods.
- *Temporal context*: What factors related to time might influence performance in the areas of feeding and eating? Examples include considering when the client is used to eating meals—do they prefer a big meal at noon or at 5pm?

## Activity Demands

Consideration of activity demands is an important part of intervention planning for feeding and eating. The occupational therapy practitioner should carefully consider the demands of each activity chosen to ensure that a "just-right challenge" is achieved during the therapeutic process.

## Client Factors

Client factors include body functions and body structures (AOTA, 2008). Body functions include but are not limited to motor, sensory, cognitive, and perceptual functions. Body structures include but are not limited to the structures of the nervous system, structures related to sensory receptors, structures related to movement, and structures related to digestive, cardiovascular, and respiratory systems.

These factors should be considered individually to determine how the factors might affect occupational performance in feeding and eating. Intervention would then be directed at restoration or remediation of areas of concern or at developing compensatory or adaptive strategies to improve performance.

For example, restoration or remediation would be actually improving the ability to bring hand to mouth, whereas compensation would be implementing the use of an assistive device to bring hand to mouth.

## Summary

Feeding and eating are necessary and pleasurable occupations of daily life. Because of the potential risk of aspiration, the occupational therapist should carefully evaluate and plan intervention for each client in relationship to the model of intervention chosen. The occupational therapy practitioner can carry out that plan with interdisciplinary input for effective eating and feeding interventions. Independence or effective interdependence in safe feeding and eating are important components of occupational therapy intervention planning.

## Student Self-Assessment

1. Break up into small groups and discuss how context is important to you, your friends, and your family in terms of eating and feeding. Now consider how you would include contextual factors in your intervention

| Food Type | Motor Patterns Needed (discuss and document motor patterns for the lips, tongue, jaw, cheeks) | Sensory Considerations of Each Food (taste, texture, visual, olfactory, proprioceptive) |
|---|---|---|
| Cracker | | |
| Applesauce | | |
| Milkshake | | |
| Carrot stick | | |
| Rice | | |
| Gummy bear | | |

planning for individuals across the lifespan who are experiencing concerns in the area of eating and feeding. Refer to the framework (AOTA, 2008).

2. Working in pairs or small groups as an experiential learning exercise, complete an activity analysis of the sensory/motor patterns that are necessary for eating different textures. Fill out the chart above with your findings. (This chart can be expanded for classroom purposes.)
3. Using Thick-It, thicken water and juice to each of the following thicknesses: honey, nectar, and pudding. Try the same activity with applesauce or another fruit puree. What are the differences between Thick-It and fruit puree? Are there other foods you might be able to use to thicken thin liquids or purees for a modified diet? Discuss the team members and assessment procedures that will determine what modifications need to be made to an individual's diet.
4. The instructor will need tables and chairs with armrests, applesauce, graham crackers, lollipops, vibration devices, adaptive equipment of all types, spoons, and paper or nosey cups. Students should be instructed to wash their hands and use protective gloves. Hand washing and gloving should be emphasized. Be sure to ask if any students have latex or food allergies. Students will work in pairs, each taking a turn at being a "client" and a "therapist." Students should actually do hands-on positioning, feeding, and facilitation of eating. This can be a fun activity. For each of the two case studies that follow, fill out the table below and actually perform the tasks to help your client eat.
   - Client A: Your client, Bob Brown, is a 65-year-old man who had a CVA about 1 month ago. He is a friendly, kind man who served as a police officer until his recent retirement. Bob has right-sided flaccid hemiparesis with overall low tone and a low level of alertness. He is right dominant, has some language-based expressive aphasia, and enjoys being with his wife but is overwhelmed with too much stimulation. Bob sometimes seems embarrassed when he dribbles food in front of his wife. He has impaired sensation on the right side of his face and is having difficulty with lip closure on the right side of the mouth. He has hypotonia and poor postural control of the trunk. His head control is weak but responds well to facilitation techniques. You are beginning an eating and feeding program and know that there are no swallowing problems. Mr. Brown hopes to return home in 2 weeks.
   - Client B: Susan Smith is a 28-year-old woman who sustained a brain injury 3 months ago. Susan was a blackjack dealer in Las Vegas until her car accident. Susan has overall high muscle tone, has ataxia, and is hyper-alert. She is easily over-stimulated,

| | Client A | Client B |
|---|---|---|
| Environment or context | | |
| Positioning: hips, trunk, head, neck, and jaw | | |
| Adjunctive methods | | |
| Hand-to-mouth technique | | |
| Diet progression/types of food | | |
| Cues or assistance needed | | |
| Adaptive equipment or devices that may be helpful | | |
| Handling ideas | | |
| Observations needed | | |

| Evidence-Based Research Chart | |
|---|---|
| **Topic** | **Evidence** |
| Behavioral approaches to feeding and eating intervention | Babbitt et al., 1994; Linscheid, 2006 |
| Refusal to eat | Bazyk, 2000 |
| General feeding intervention | Bober, Humphry, Carswell, & Core, 2001; Case-Smith & Humphrey, 2005 |
| Management of drooling | Brei, 2003; Domaracki & Sisson, 1990; Iammatteo, Trombly, & Luecke, 1990 |
| Sensory motor concerns related to feeding and eating | Case-Smith, 1989; Palmer & Heyman, 1993 |
| Feeding tube dependency | Schauster & Dwyer, 1996; Tarbell & Allaire, 2002 |

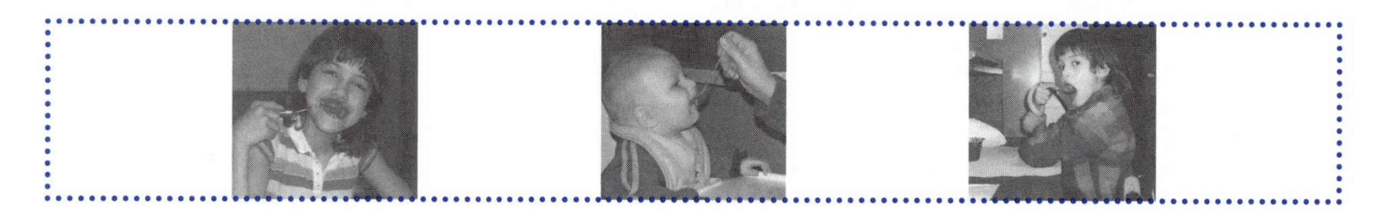

becoming irritated with noise or too many verbal instructions. She has a very short attention span and is impulsive. Susan is able to use her arms, but has difficulty with coordinated hand function. She tends to eat all the time and to stuff her mouth too full, causing her to choke or spit out food. She is restless and moves around as she eats, sometimes even getting up out of the chair. Susan may be discharged to a group home in the near future.

5. Have your students watch a DVD of a videofluoroscopy. These are often available through medical centers with swallowing programs. Watch a typical swallow and have the students discuss what they are seeing in the progression. Watch an atypical swallow and see if the students can see the areas of difficulty. Discuss the case and why swallowing deficits are dangerous and need to have special attention and a team approach. Occupational therapy practitioners should note the signs and symptoms of an abnormal swallow and make appropriate referrals. Occupational therapy practitioners require further education to perform dysphagia intervention.

## References


American Occupational Therapy Association. (2003). Specialized knowledge and skills in eating and feeding for occupational therapy practice. *American Journal of Occupational Therapy, 57*, 670-678.

American Occupational Therapy Association. (2007). Specialized knowledge and skills in eating and feeding for occupational therapy practice. *American Journal of Occupational Therapy, 61*, 686-700.

American Occupational Therapy Association. (2008). Occupational therapy practice framework: Domain and process, second edition. *American Journal of Occupational Therapy, 62*, 625-683.

Arvedson, J. C., & Brodsky, L. (2002). *Pediatric swallowing and feeding assessment and management*. Albany, NY: Singular Publishing Group.

Arvedson, J. C., Brodsky, L., & Reigstad, D. (2002). Clinical feeding and swallowing assessment. In J. C. Arvedson & L. Brodsky (Eds.), *Pediatric swallowing and feeding assessment and management* (2nd ed., pp. 283-340). Albany, NY: Singular Publishing Group.

Avery-Smith, W. (2002). Dysphagia. In C. A. Trombly & M. V. Radomski (Eds.), *Occupational therapy for physical dysfunction* (pp. 1091-1109). Philadelphia, PA: Lippincott Williams & Wilkins.

Baer, C. T. (2005). Addressing feeding with adults with developmental disabilities: A team approach part 1. *Developmental Disabilities Special Interest Section Quarterly, 28*, 1-3.

Babbitt, R. L., Hoch, T. A., Coe, D. A., Cataldo, M. F., Kelly, K. J., Stackhouse, C., et al. (1994). Behavioral assessment and treatment of pediatric feeding disorders. *Developmental and Behavioral Pediatrics, 15*(4), 278-291.

Bazyk, S. (2000). Addressing the complex needs of young children who refuse to eat. *OT Practice, 17*, 10-15.

Bober, S. J., Humphry, R., Carswell, H. W., & Core, A. J. (2001). Toddler's persistence in the emerging occupations of functional play and self-feeding. *American Journal of Occupational Therapy, 55*(4), 369-376.

Brei, T. (2003). Management of drooling. *Seminars in Pediatric Neurology, 10*(4), 265-270.

Case-Smith, J. (1989). Intervention strategies for promoting feeding skills in infants with sensory deficits. *Developmental disabilities: A handbook for occupational therapists*. Philadelphia, PA: Haworth Press.

Case-Smith, J., & Humphry, R. (2005). Feeding intervention. In J. Case-Smith (Ed.), *Occupational therapy for children* (5th ed., pp. 481-520). St. Louis, MO: Elsevier Mosby.

Crittenden, P. M. (1990). Toward a concept of autonomy in adolescents with a disability. *Child Health Care, 19*, 162-168.

Domaracki, L. S., & Sisson, L. A. (1990). Decreasing drooling with oral motor stimulation in children with multiple disabilities. *American Journal of Occupational Therapy, 44*(8), 680-684.

Iammatteo, P. A., Trombly, C., & Luecke, L. (1990). The effect of mouth closure on drooling and speech. *American Journal of Occupational Therapy, 44*(8), 686-691.

Jenks, K. (2002). Dysphagia. In L. W. Pedretti & M. B. Early (Eds.), *Occupational therapy skills for physical dysfunction* (5th ed., pp. 730-766). St. Louis, MO: Mosby.

Jenks, K. N., & Smith, G. (2006). Eating and swallowing. In H. M Pendleton & W. Schultz-Krohn (Eds.), *Pedretti's occupational therapy practice skills for physical dysfunction* (6th ed., pp. 609-645). St. Louis, MO: Mosby.

Kedesdy, J. H., & Budd, K. S. (1998). *Childhood feeding disorders biobehavioral assessment and intervention*. Baltimore, MD: Paul H. Brookes Publishing Co.

Linscheid, T. (2006). Behavioral treatments for pediatric feeding disorders. *Behavior Modification, 30*(1), 6-23.

Logemann, J. A. (1998). *Evaluation and treatment of swallowing disorders*. Austin, TX: Pro-Ed.

Logemann, J. A., Kahrilas, P. J., Kobara, M., & Vakil, N. B. (1989). The benefit of head rotation on pharyngoesophogeal dysphagia. *Archives of Physical Medicine and Rehabilitation, 70*, 767-771.

Morris, S. E., & Klein, M. D. (2000). *Pre-feeding skills: A comprehensive resource for mealtime development* (2nd ed.). Austin, TX: Therapy Skills Builders.

Mosey, A. C. (1981). *Occupational therapy: Configuration of a profession*. New York, NY: Raven.

Ohmae, Y., Logemann, J. A., Kaiser, P., Hanson, D. G., & Kahrilas, P. J. (1996). Effects of two breath-holding maneuvers on oropharyngeal swallow. *Annals of Otology, Rhinology & Laryngology, 105*, 123-131.

Palmer, M. M., & Heyman, M. B. (1993). Assessment and treatment of sensory- versus motor-based feeding problems in very young children. *Infants and Young Children, 6*(2), 67-73.

Pouderoux, P., & Kahrilas, P. J. (1995). Deglutitive tongue force modulation by volition, volume, and viscosity in humans. *Gastroenterology, 108*, 1418-1426.

Schauster, H., & Dwyer, J. (1996). Transition from tube feedings to feedings by mouth in children: Preventing eating dysfunction. *Journal of the American Dietetic Association, 96*, 277-281.

Tarbell, M. C., & Allaire, J. H. (2002). Children with feeding tube dependency: Treating the whole child. *Infants and Young Children, 15*(1), 29-41.

Wolf, L. S., & Glass, R. G. (1992). *Feeding and swallowing disorders in infancy: Assessment and management*. San Antonio, TX: Therapy Skill Builders.

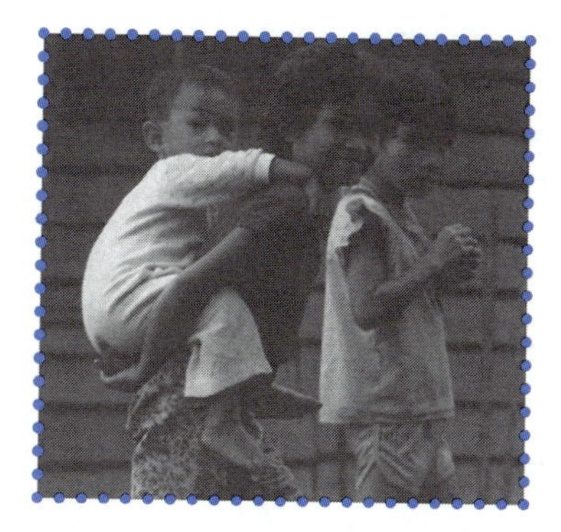

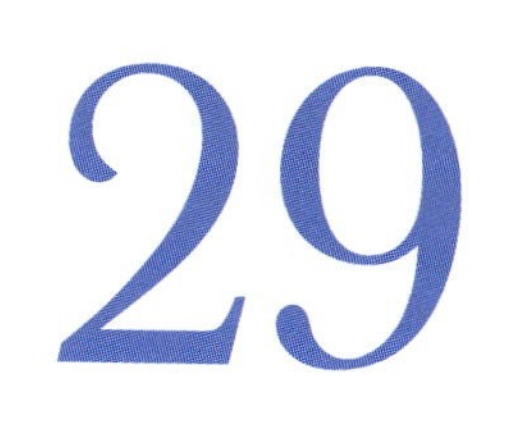

# 29

# USE OF THE NATURAL ENVIRONMENT

*Kathryn M. Loukas, MS, OTR/L, FAOTA*

**ACOTE Standard Explored in This Chapter**

B.5.15

**Key Terms**

| | |
|---|---|
| Context | Natural environments |
| Inclusion | Nonlinear dynamics |
| Interdependence | Real life |
| Least restrictive environment | Simulation |

## Introduction

Occupational therapy has evolved in the use of context in intervention planning. Through the history of occupational therapy, we have moved from the context of institutional settings that began with the moral intervention paradigm (Letts, Rigby & Stewart, 2003), to a focus on occupation (Kielhofner, 1992), to the development of the Person-Environment-Occupation Model of occupation (Law et al., 1996). Early in our history, occupational therapy primarily occurred in the institutional setting. This institutionalization provided a closed system that discouraged individuals from participating in real-life situations in natural settings—it kept our clients and our work invisible to society and it inhibited occupational performance (Reed, 2006; Whalley Hammell, 2003). In her landmark Eleanor Clark Slagle lecture, Grady (1995) encouraged occupational therapy practitioners to reach out and build inclusive communities through accessibility, adaptations, hope, and social supports. Our profession continues to move forward toward this ultimate goal.

Today, engagement in purposeful, real-life occupations has become the goal of occupational therapy intervention in most practice settings. The framework advocates engagement in occupation to support participation in context (American Occupational Therapy Association [AOTA], 2008). Occupational therapy has made a paradigm shift from the medical model to the community model in order to help clients participate in the occupations of "real life" (Scaffa, 2001). Increasing the level of independence is a factor in intervention planning but not always the ultimate goal. Occupational therapy practitioners need to also recognize and embrace the concept of interdependence. A client who wishes to live in his or her own natural environment may need the assistance of family or caregivers, and that is a worthy goal in achieving occupational life satisfaction. A client who is functioning in the natural rhythm of life, even with assistance, may be achieving an individual goal of occupational performance (Hinojosa & Blount, 2000).

Occupational therapy practitioners often use simulation in clinical settings to achieve occupation-based goals. A rehabilitation-based occupational therapist might use the



K. Sladyk, K. Jacobs, & N. MacRae (Eds.).
*Occupational Therapy Essentials for Clinical Competence* (pp. 323-330).

therapy room kitchen to help a client prepare to return home, a therapist in work re-entry therapy might use devices that simulate work tasks such as driving or lifting, and a therapist working in early intervention may simulate a play environment in the occupational therapy room to prepare a child to use a playground in the future. Simulations prepare clients for real life, but use of the actual environment is always best for the final goals and discharge planning (Letts et al., 2003). Natural environments are those where the client would actually engage in the occupation in context. These occupations carry with them important social meaning and occupational roles (Pierce, 2003). Typical natural environments include the following (Hinojosa and Blount, 2000; Perr & Bell, 2000):

- The home
- The outdoor environment
- The workplace
- Daycare settings, head-start programs, developmental preschools for early intervention
- School-based inclusion in the least restrictive environment
- Community resources for play and leisure, recreation, worship, shopping, dining, and social and community events
- Private and public transportation

## Chaos, Complexity, and Nonlinear Dynamics

Chaos theory and the study of nonlinear dynamics is an emerging perspective in the social sciences (Chamberlain & Butz, 1998; Kelso, 1995) and in occupational therapy (Champagne, 2008; Lazzarini, 2004; Royeen, 2003). Dynamic systems theory reflects the importance of the interaction of the complex internal and external systems that make up the whole human being (Case-Smith, 2005; Humphry & Wakeford, 2006; Thelen, 2000). Zoltan (2007) describes the dynamic interactional approach to cognition as "an ongoing production or outcome of the interaction among the individual, the task, and the environment" (p. 16). The environment plays a very significant role in the occupations and occupational development of human beings, leading emerging occupational therapy approaches to emphasize contextualism (Humphry & Wakeford). This contextualism emphasizes the interconnected and inseparable nature of human beings with their environment. According to nonlinear dynamic theory, human beings and behavior are unpredictable, self-organizing systems, each with their own unique initial conditions (Chamberlain & Butz, 1998; Champagne, 2008; Kelso, 1995; Lazzarini, 2004; Royeen, 2003). The person, environment, and occupation are engaged in a transactional relationship, much as the Person-Environment-Occupation Model elucidates (Law, et al., 1996), but in a more interactive, holistic, and unpredictable manner. It is essential that occupational therapy practitioners understand the science of chaotic, complex, nonlinear dynamic systems in natural environments. Through this understanding, practitioners can facilitate meaningful self-organization of clients in the context of their everyday occupations throughout the lifespan (Champagne, 2008; Lazzarini, 2004; Royeen, 2003).

## Occupational Therapy Applications

### Early Intervention

Early intervention programs are designed to enhance the development of children in occupational tasks. The Individuals with Disabilities Education Act (IDEA) mandates that these services occur in "natural environments" and in a family-centered context (AOTA, 2006; Stephens & Tauber, 2005).

Natural environments in early intervention include kangaroo care of the newborn infant resting on the parents' abdomen (Figure 29-1); play environments including play groups, daycare centers, pre-school and developmental groups; cultural and religious activities and contexts; and community settings such as shopping or service appointments. The most natural setting occupational therapy could address for a client in the 0- to 3-year-old age range is the family and home environment. Understanding the initial conditions, context, culture, and occupational patterns of the dynamic family system is important and should influence the occupational therapy intervention plan.

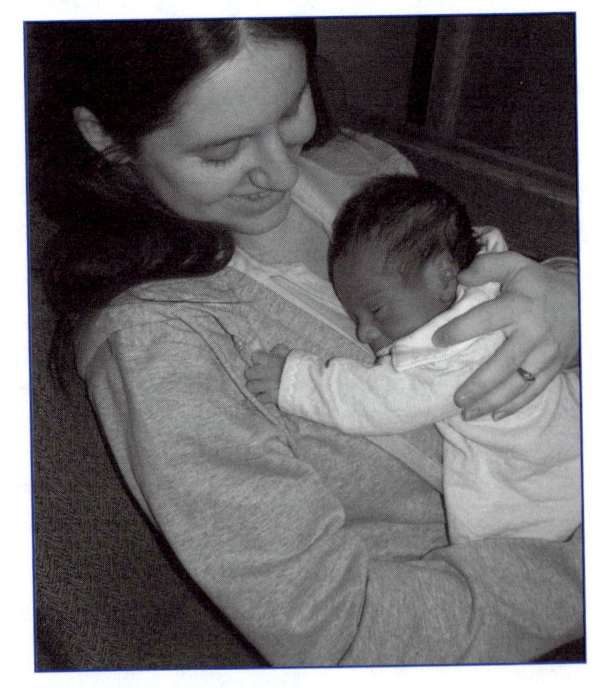

**Figure 29-1.** Kangaroo care.

Lola is the 9-month-old child of Celeste, a 19-year-old single mother living in a small house with her mother. Lola is a child who is developmentally delayed and just beginning to sit up and roll over. Lola also has some difficulty with eating and feeding and does not sleep well. Samantha, the occupational therapist, facilitated Celeste to self-organize a routine for the day, including times for feeding, developmental play, and sleep. As a therapeutic activity, Celeste and Samantha worked together to establish a realistic and meaningful routine and put this schedule on the refrigerator with magnets. Samantha's gentle influence regarding the nature of developmental activities facilitated Celeste to find a playgroup for Lola. The dynamic, social, and interactive nature of the playgroup of children and parents began to transform their isolation and improved community participation for both mother and child. The occupational therapy practitioner helped Celeste embed specially selected, developmental play activities to enhance motor development into Lola's environment. This served to establish an interconnected bond between mother and child. The context of this play included setting up environments that facilitate development in the living room and outdoors. Sensory modulation input was natural and was included to facilitate Lola's nervous system prior to feeding, and to inhibit her system prior to bedtime. As the natural environment of the home became child development-centered, Celeste began to grow in her role as a confident and nurturing mother, while Lola began to thrive.

## School-Based Practice

Current IDEA legislation requires that therapy occur in natural environments and for education to occur in the least restrictive environment (AOTA, 2006; Case-Smith & Rogers, 2005). The school has many natural environments, all of which are dynamic contexts for occupational performance. These include the classroom, the school bus, the playground, the cafeteria, the gym, the art room, the computer room, and the library. Occupational therapy intervention can occur in all of these contexts as direct inclusive therapy or in a consultative approach. The schools have evolved from a model of specialized schools such as the school for the deaf or the cerebral palsy center, to "mainstreaming," which put children under the same roof as their typical peers, and then to seeing children in their typical classroom environment and routine, which is now termed *inclusion*. Inclusion means that all children engage in the same activities in the same environments, although some may need assistance or adaptations in order to participate. Occupational therapy is a profession committed to inclusion in philosophy and practice (Dunn et al., 1995a). In order to be effective in this nonlinear dynamic system, the school-based occupational therapy practitioner must evaluate and effect change in complex and unpredictable ways. This requires facilitating the child, teacher, occupations, and natural environments to support learning and social development in context.

Curtis is a child in the second grade. He is full of life and loves to have fun with other children. He is a child who is living with cerebral palsy that affects his left side with hemiparesis, but cognitively, he is on grade level. Curtis has functional mobility difficulties negotiating the playground, sitting on the backless benches of the cafeteria, and getting on and off the school bus. He also has fine motor difficulties rendering handwriting and art projects frustrating and very difficult. The occupational therapist was committed to including Curtis in all activities and settings of the school, and adopted an adaptation/compensation contextual approach in his Individual Education Plan (IEP) to enable Curtis to participate successfully in all aspects of the school curriculum. John, the occupational therapy assistant, played with Curtis and his peers on the playground, facilitating Curtis to make good choices in equipment selection and offering ideas on how to safely get on and off the swings and slides. A chair was used at the end of the cafeteria table enabling Curtis to have supportive seating but still eat with his peers. Curtis was provided physical assistance on and off the bus for safety reasons. This was facilitated by the occupational therapist in a manner that was meaningful and social to Curtis, his family, and other children involved. Curtis' classrooms were equipped with a computer with a key guard and elbow supports for school-based written work and some art projects. Dynamic occupational therapy intervention occurred in all school contexts and included the interdisciplinary team, teachers, parents, and other children in the second grade curriculum for social participation in natural activities of daily living, play, and work contexts.

## Work-Based Programs

Return to work programs, workplace safety initiatives, ergonomics, sheltered work, employment coaching, and overall rehabilitation can occur in natural environments. The workplace is where many of us spend most of our weekday hours engaging in productive activities (see Chapters 12 and 17). Clients who are interested in employment may find the natural environment of the workplace to be stimulating and motivating. In addition, the occupational therapy practitioner can see how the environment can be adapted, do an actual task analysis of the work to be done, and engage the client in the natural positions and conditions needed for the job. This is an effective way to address work-based goals in occupational therapy. Due to time and distance constraints, many times occupational therapy practitioners cannot bring their clients to the workplace. If this is the case, the best alternative is to simulate the work situation as closely as possible in order to maximize the therapeutic impact of intervention. Occupational therapy practitioners should also consider using a volunteer position as a precursor to the work role. This may serve as a vehicle toward self-actualization and productivity for people with disabling conditions.

Ralph is a 54-year-old plumber who lost his left (nondominant) thumb and index finger at the proximal interphalangeal (PIP) joint in a work-related accident. He is now 2 months post-amputation, participating in outpatient rehabilitation, and has quite a bit of hypersensitivity in the stump areas of his left hand. Ralph is a man who values work at home and the workplace. He is concerned that he will not be able to support his family and is anxious to return to his job. Doris, his occupational therapist, noticed he is not motivated by use of simulations in the outpatient clinic. She tried to set up make-shift plumbing projects, but Ralph insists they are not close to realistic. Doris decides to set up a work-based program on the pipes in Ralph's home. Ralph becomes motivated to use his left hand as a functional assist and the hypersensitivity begins to diminish. As Ralph shows he can still do many plumbing tasks, his wife, Mary, begins to ask about different jobs needed around the house. Ralph complains to her in a good-natured way, but the therapist can see he is pleased to be back in the role of "Mr. Fix-It" in his home. Doris sets up further sessions in the plumbing shop and home environments to facilitate Ralph's return to former performance patterns of work and functional use of the left hand. This dynamic approach to work improves Ralph's relationships, self-image, and mood as his life roles and routines become meaningful again.

## Aging in Place

Elders who wish to age in natural environments, thus "aging in place," may turn to occupational therapy for assistance in that goal (Clark et al., 1997). Occupational therapy can occur in this natural environment while facilitating elders to participate in community programs such as adult day programs, in-home assistance, religious or culturally based activities, and social networks. It is important for elders to stay in their natural environment in order to maintain the habits, routines, and memories associated with their own home and lifestyle. Changing locations can cause an elderly person, particularly those with cognitive impairments, to regress in their overall functioning and quality of life, and may even affect mortality (Edvardsson & Nordvall, 2008). Aging in place allows elders to maintain their habits, familiar surroundings, and social networks for occupational performance. The occupational therapy practitioner adopting an adaptation/compensation contextual approach can assist elders to function in their home through home adaptations, cueing systems, self-organization of the day, and memory enhancement. An emphasis on safety and supported functioning should be established. An occupational therapy practitioner can also train family members or other caretakers on how to best assist elders in their independent or interdependent functioning (Dunn et al., 1995b).

Marjorie is a 68-year-old woman in the mid stages of Alzheimer's disease. Her husband, George (age 70), has been very distraught with his wife's behavior and forgetfulness. George works part time as a sales representative and would like to continue his work. The family sought occupational therapy through a center on aging. Nancy, the occupational therapist at the center, helped the family find resources in the community to assist them. They found an adult daycare center for the days George works and through this became involved with a support group for caretakers of people with Alzheimer's disease. As George learned more about the importance of taking care of himself, his wife, and his home, he began to self-organize. He hired someone to clean the house, as that had really become a burden for him. In addition, they were able to hire an attendant to sleep over to deal with Marjorie's night wandering and allow George to sleep. Nancy helped George and Marjorie maintain previous routines through a picture calendar for Marjorie. This also helped George effectively engage and interact with his wife in meaningful home tasks that used to be delegated only to her such as cooking and gardening. While engaging in these occupational tasks, Nancy is able to role-play ways of dealing with Marjorie when she becomes disoriented, belligerent, or confused. These new interactions facilitate George and their children to deal with Marjorie in social and community settings. Due to this occupational therapy intervention, George and Marjorie are able to participate in their home and community in an interdependent manner further into the future.

## Best Practice and Safety Considerations in Natural Settings

Because natural settings are not as structured or predictable as those performed in a clinic, they can pose more of a safety risk for clients both physically and psychosocially. It is important to consider a number of recommended practices to assure positive outcomes. The following recommendations are adapted from Noonan and McCormick (2006) in their work with young children in natural environments:

- Specialize instructional techniques to the client in the natural environment. This can be accomplished by goals that embed meaningful activities in the client's natural environment, making sure the challenges are not dangerous or too difficult. Task analysis and careful planning is needed for successful therapy in natural environments.
- Assure that interventions are culturally sensitive and relevant. This may require outside investigation and questions to the client and family members.
- Cultivate team and family involvement. Positive outcomes are more likely to occur when supported by the team and the family. Build strong relationships with the therapy team and work collaboratively to support this practice.
- Ecological and contextual assessment. The occupational therapy practitioner should do a thorough ecological assessment for the safety of the client and the therapist. Questions to ask include the following (Noonan and McCormick, 2006, p. 21):
  - What are the intervention goals and objectives?
  - Where should the intervention be provided?
  - How should the intervention be provided?
  - When should the intervention be provided?
  - How can the intervention be evaluated?
- Positive behavioral support—The occupational therapy practitioner should not provide therapy alone in a natural environment when the behavior of the client/family or when safety considerations are questionable. Be sure support is present in any situation that warrants it. Relationship difficulties can also make for difficult or unsafe situations for the client or therapist and should be closely examined prior to the planning of the context of intervention.

Recommendations for establishing an ethical climate for privacy and confidentiality in a community-based practice setting include the following:

- Know and follow the Health Insurance Portability and Accountability Act (HIPAA) and Family Educational Rights and Privacy Act (FERPA) regulations, and encourage others to do the same, including notification of privacy procedures to clients and client families.
- Avoid all "hall talk." Establish confidential places to discuss private client matters, and remember that casual conversations can quickly turn into conversations with confidential information sharing.
- Make sure your clients understand what is private and what is not as research indicates many clients do not understand confidentiality (Sankar, Moran, Merz, & Jones, 2003). For our young clients, involve them in decisions using language they understand.
- Make all efforts to keep private, professional information confidential. Do not carry confidential reports or files casually, and do not leave them in the bathroom or your open car. Transport confidential items only when absolutely necessary. Keep your computer encrypted or password sensitive for all client-related information.
- Respond "naturally" to questions that occur in typical settings but be careful to not violate privacy or confidentiality. Make sure paraprofessionals understand their obligations to privacy and do not give them more information than they need.
- Communicate with your clients and their family about what you need in order to provide best practice as a therapist and what participation in natural environments might entail. Ask about mentioning the disability or educating others, and involve them in decisions and discussion. Help clients and parents understand your need for full disclosure of medical information.
- Implicit consent and reasonable expectations of privacy are part of practice when the client and family are involved in a community-based environment. The family and client need to be informed and "agree" to the setting and approach to intervention through an Individual Education Plan (IEP), Individual Family Service Plan (IFSP), or other legal document (J. Boyden, personal communication, July 10, 2006).
- Establish an ethical climate in the community through modeling, educating, and sponsoring workshops with experts. Consider establishment of an ethics program. Use an ethical decision-making model to assist with difficult decisions (Solum & Schaffer, 2003).

## Summary

Occupational therapy has historically been practiced in a number of contexts including institutions, hospitals, schools, and the client's home. However, emergent best practice indicates that the closer we can get our intervention to the natural environment, the more meaningful and effective the occupational performance of our clients will be. This can be accomplished in many settings by finding the best "real-life" context for the occupation in which our client is engaging or wishes to engage. It is important to make sure the safety of the client and therapist are in place through environmental analysis and/or team collaboration. The chaos, complexity, and nonlinear dynamics of interactive systems are essential to consider when using the natural context in intervention planning. Finally, mandatory privacy and confidentiality issues must be respected in the natural environment. This can be challenging and confusing in the dynamic, unpredictable natural setting but should be highly respected for ethical practice.

## Student Self-Assessment

1. Think about some of your favorite pastimes and write down three of them. Include the activity and the context in which you like to do that activity. Describe how your therapist could best simulate that activity if you ever had occupational therapy. Describe how an occupational therapist could modify or assist you to perform that activity in the context you most enjoy it, if you were experiencing:
   - Hemiparesis of your dominant side
   - Severe visual impairment
   - Social anxiety and panic attacks
   - Cognitive impairments, including impulsivity and short-term memory deficits
2. Name some potential safety risks inherent in the following settings:
   - The kitchen of a client's home
   - Community mobility with an elder who has Parkinson's disease
   - The playground
   - A school field trip to another town
   - The school bus
   - The YMCA pool
   - A summer camp
   - A group home
   - A shelter for battered women

   Now think critically and problem-solve potential precautions to put in place in each of the above settings to assure safety and best practice.
3. Class discussion: Why is privacy and confidentiality more of a concern in natural, "uncontrolled" environments? Please give specific examples.
4. Name three ways that a practitioner can help to achieve an ethical climate of privacy in a natural setting during an activity that promotes real-life social participation.

### Evidence-Based Research Chart

| Program/Context | Intervention | Evidence |
|---|---|---|
| Inclusive preschool | Outdoor play guided by the interdisciplinary Ecology of Human Performance model | Anecdotal and occupational objectives achieved; parent satisfaction (S. Ideishi, R. Ideishi, Gandhi, & Yuen, 2006) |
| Family involvement in intervention with clients who have physical disabilities, developmental disabilities, and mental health | Questionnaire to occupational therapists about family involvement | Family involvement needs to be expanded. Scheduling is the biggest obstacle. More continuing education and articulation of occupational therapy work with families in mental health is needed (Humphrey, Gonzalez, & Taylor, 1993) |
| The effect of context on skill acquisition | Students without disabilities were taught to use chop sticks in and out of context | Natural context elicited improvement of success significantly. Natural context found to facilitate motor learning (Ma, Trombly, & Robinson-Podolski, 1998) |
| Constructing daily routines of mothers with young children with disabilities | Qualitative research in naturalistic environments on daily routines in self-care or skill performance | Development of self-care is shaped by eco-cultural influences and anticipation of future possibilities (Kellegrew, 2000) |
| Family routines and rituals | Family daily routines, interviews of stories, daily routines, and occupation focuses on morning activities | Family routines are important for organization and meaning in self-care of children (Segal, 2004) |
| Occupational therapy role in keeping community-based elders in their homes | Use of assistive devices and focus on safety in functional mobility and overall home-based tasks | Seventeen efficacy studies focusing on decreasing falls and increasing home safety, social participation, and quality of life (Stuetjens et al., 2004). |
| | Group of 361 culturally diverse, independent-living elders participated in occupational therapy groups over a 9-month period. Results were favorable when compared to control group | Preventive occupational therapy benefits independent-living elders across the domains of health, function, and quality of life (Clark et al., 1997). |

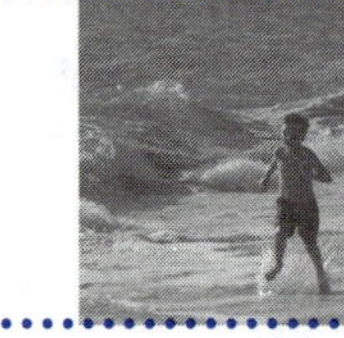
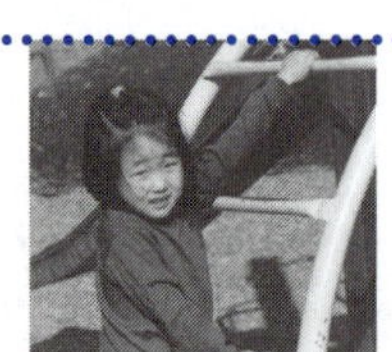
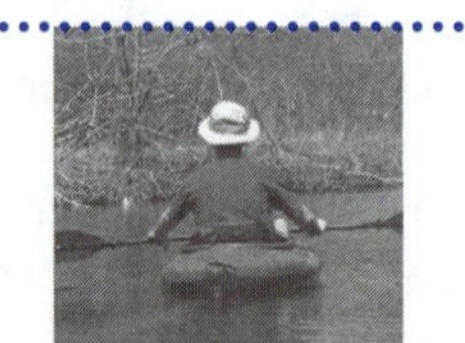

# References


American Occupational Therapy Association. (2006). The new IDEA: Summary of the Individuals with Disabilities Education Improvement Act of 2004 (P.L. 108-446). Retrieved July 5, 2006, from www.aota.org

American Occupational Therapy Association. (2008). Occupational therapy practice framework: Domain and process, second edition. *American Journal of Occupational Therapy, 62*, 625-683.

Case-Smith, J. (2005). Development of childhood occupations. In J. Case-Smith (Ed.), *Occupational therapy for children* (5th ed., pp. 88-116). St. Louis, MO: Elsevier Mosby.

Case-Smith, J., & Rogers, J. (2005). School-based occupational therapy. In J. Case-Smith (Ed.), *Occupational therapy for children* (5th ed., pp. 795-826). St. Louis, MO: Elsevier Mosby.

Chamberlain, L. L., & Butz, M. R. (1998). *Clinical chaos: A therapist's guide to nonlinear dynamics and therapeutic change*. Philadelphia, PA: Brunner/Mazel.

Champagne, T. (2008). *Sensory modulation & environment: Essential elements of occupation* (3rd ed.). Southampton, MA: Champagne Conferences & Consultation.

Clark, F., Azen, S. P., Zemke, R., Jackson, J., Carlson, M., Mandel, D., et al. (1997). Occupational therapy for independent-living older adults. *Journal of the American Medical Association, 278*(16), 1321-1326.

Dunn, W., Foto, M., Hinojosa, J., Boyt-Schell, B., Thomson. L., & Hertfelder, S. (1995a). Independence position paper: The American Occupational Therapy Association broadening the construct of independence. *American Journal of Occupational Therapy, 49*, 1014.

Dunn, W., Foto, M., Hinojosa, J., Boyt-Schell, B., Thomson. L., & Hertfelder, S. (1995b). Occupational therapy: A profession in support of full inclusion. In *Reference manual of the official documents of the American Occupational Therapy Association, Inc.* Bethesda, MD: AOTA Press.

Edvardsson, D., & Nordvall, K. (2008). Lost in the present but confident of the past: Experiences of being in a psycho-geriatric unit as narrated by persons with dementia. *Journal of Clinical Nursing, 17(4)*.

Grady, A. P. (1995). Building inclusive community: A challenge for occupational therapy. *American Journal of Occupational Therapy, 49*, 300-310.

Hinojosa, J., & Blount, M. L. (2000). *The texture of life: Purposeful activities in occupational therapy*. Bethesda, MD: AOTA Press.

Humphrey, R., Gonzalez, S., & Taylor, E. (1993). Family involvement in practice: Issues and attitudes. *American Journal of Occupational Therapy, 47*(7), 587-593.

Humphry, R., & Wakeford, L. (2006). An occupation-centered discussion of development and implications for practice. *American Journal of Occupational Therapy, 60*, 258-267.

Ideishi, S. K., Ideishi, R. I., Gandhi, T., & Yuen, L. (2006). Inclusive preschool outdoor play environments. *School System Special Interest Section Quarterly, 13*(2), 1-4.

Kellegrew, D. H. (2000). Constructing daily routines: A qualitative examination of mothers with young children with disabilities. *American Journal of Occupational Therapy, 54*, 252-259.

Kelso, J. A. S. (1995). *Dynamic patterns: The self-organization of brain and behavior.* Cambridge, MA: The MIT Press.

Kielhofner, G. (1992). *Conceptual foundations of occupational therapy.* Philadelphia, PA: F.A. Davis.

Law, M., Cooper, B., Strong, S., Stewart, P., Rigby, P., & Letts, L. (1996). The person-environment-occupation model: A transactive approach to occupational performance. *Canadian Journal of Occupational Therapy, 63*, 9-23.

Lazzarini, I. (2004). Neuro-occupation: The nonlinear dynamics of intention, meaning and perception. *British Journal of Occupational Therapy, 67*(8), 1-11.

Letts, L., Rigby, P., & Stewart, D. (2003). *Using environments to enable occupational performance*. Thorofare, NJ: SLACK Incorporated.

Ma, H., Trombly, C. A., & Robinson-Podolski, C. (1998). The effect of context on skill acquisition and transfer. *American Journal of Occupational Therapy, 53*, 138-144.

Noonan, M. J., & McCormick, L. (2006). *Young children with disabilities in natural environments*. Baltimore, MD: Brookes Publishing Co.

Perr, A., & Bell, P. F. (2000). Moving from simulation to real life. In J. Hinojosa & M. L. Blount (Eds.), *The texture of life purposeful activities in occupational therapy* (pp. 234-257). Bethesda, MD: AOTA Press.

Pierce, D. (2003). *Occupation by design: Building therapeutic power.* Philadelphia, PA: F.A. Davis.

Reed, K. L. (2006). Occupational therapy values and beliefs, the formative years: 1904-1929. *OT Practice, April 17*, 21-25.

Royeen, C. B. (2003). Chaotic OT: Collective wisdom from a complex profession. *American Journal of Occupational Therapy, 57*(6), 609-624.

Sankar, P., Moran, S., Merz, J. F., & Jones, N. L. (2003). Patient perspectives on medical confidentiality. *Journal of General Internal Medicine, 18*(8), 659-669.

Scaffa, M. (2001). *Occupational therapy in community-based settings.* Philadelphia, PA: F.A. Davis.

Segal, R. (2004). Family routines and rituals: A context for occupational therapy interventions. *American Journal of Occupational Therapy, 58*, 499-508.

Solum, L. L., & Schaffer, M. A. (2003). Ethical problems experienced by school nurses. *Journal of School Nursing, 19*(6), 330-337.

Stephens, L. C., & Tauber, S. K. (2005). Early intervention. In J. Case-Smith (Ed.), *Occupational therapy for children* (5th ed., pp. 771-793). St. Louis, MO: Elsevier Mosby.

Stuetjens, E. M., Dekker, J., Bouter, L. M., Jellena, S., Bakker, E. B., van den Ende, C. H. M. (2004). Occupational therapy for community dwelling elderly people. A systematic review. *Age and Aging, 33*, 453-460.

Thelen, E. (2000). Motor development as foundation and future of developmental psychology. *International Journal of Behavioral Development, 24*(4), 385-397.

Whalley Hammell, K., (2003). Changing Institutional environments to enable occupation among people with severe physical limitations. In L. Letts, P. Rigby, & D. Stewart (Eds.), *Using environments to enable occupational performance* (pp. 35-53). Thorofare, NJ: SLACK Incorporated.

Zoltan, B. (2007). *Vision, perception, and cognition: A manual for the evaluation and treatment of the adult with acquired brain injury* (4th ed.). Thorofare, NJ: SLACK Incorporated.

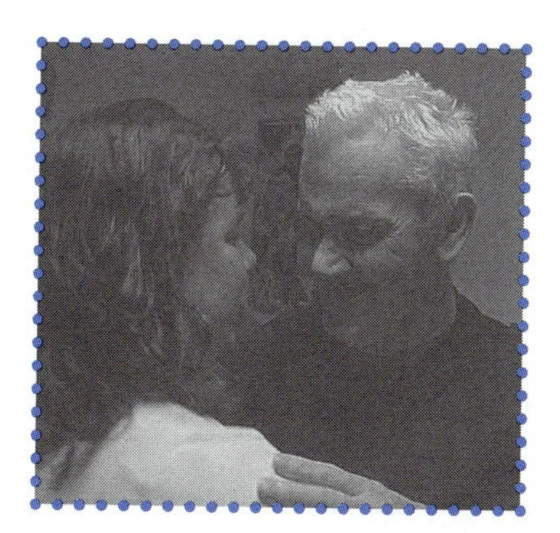

# 30

# EFFECTIVE COMMUNICATION

*Jan Froehlich, MS, OTR/L*

**ACOTE Standard Explored in This Chapter**

B.5.18

**Key Terms**

| | |
|---|---|
| Cultural competence | Nonverbal communication |
| Effective communication | Reflective listening |

## Introduction

Effective communication enables the occupational therapy process, yet communicating well with a wide range of both clients, family, significant others, colleagues, and other health providers and the public can be challenging. Every occupational therapy practitioner, like every human, has undoubtedly experienced many successes and failures in communication. Nonetheless, much can be learned about how to make the communication process increasingly effective. The artful interplay between listening and speaking, coupled with awareness and sensitivity to human diversity, is at the heart of effective communication. For some occupational therapy practitioners, listening comes more easily than speaking. For others, listening is the greater challenge. For still others, the greater challenge is to communicate with confidence and ease when they are with someone from a background that is different from their own.

## The Challenge to Truly Listen

While listening appears to be a simple skill, it has many complexities that are worth exploring. Client-centered therapy requires good listening (Law, Baptiste, & Mills, 1995). Only when the therapist can listen well enough to his or her clients to understand what their real concerns are can client-centered therapy occur. On a basic level, listening involves learning to not interrupt the individual to whom we are listening. In everyday interactions between people, interruptions are frequent (H. Jackins, 1981). This occurs because, as humans, we all want and need to be listened to. Not surprisingly, it is also true that as humans, we all need and want to listen to others. Sometimes, we find ourselves in relationships where there is a natural balance between listening and being listened to. Other times, we find ourselves in relationships where we are the listener or the talker most of the time. Unless these are client/therapist relationships in which we expect to be the primary listener, imbalanced relationships may not be as rewarding as those where there is a natural balance between listening and talking.

Even in relationships where there tends to be a fairly equal balance between listening and talking, if examined closely, we will find there is often frequent interrupting going on in the communication process. Interruptions often take the form of telling one's own story that is similar or giving unsought advice. With this in mind, step number 1 in becoming an effective communicator is first noticing how much we interrupt others as we communicate, and step 2 is to stop doing this. Unfortunately, this may be easier said



K. Sladyk, K. Jacobs, & N. MacRae (Eds.).
*Occupational Therapy Essentials for Clinical Competence* (pp. 331-344).

than done. It may be particularly challenging to do this, unless we know that we too will get a turn to be listened to without interruption. Listening partnerships can assist with this challenge.

# Listening Partnerships

Enhancing all facets of the communication process for occupational therapy practitioners will be addressed in this chapter through listening partnerships. Listening partnerships, which involve taking turns listening and speaking with a peer for a mutually agreed upon amount of time, are borrowed from the theory and practice of co-counseling, also known as re-evaluation counseling (H. Jackins, 1981; Kauffman & New, 2004). The author has used listening partnerships extensively in a communication seminar she has instructed for 18 years (Froehlich & Nesbit, 2004), and occupational therapy students have generally found them to be an invaluable learning tool.

Since it is not possible to become a better communicator without actual practice, the reader will gain the most from this chapter if he or she sets up a listening partnership with a peer or peers who are also reading this text. Pairs are ideal, but small groups can work as well. Meeting with different partners for each meeting over the course of several weeks is recommended for optimal skill development. Then, establishing an agreement to meet with the same person on a regular basis (a regular listening partner) can further enhance the development of effective communication skills. In addition, these partnerships will only go well if the listener keeps time and notifies the speaker when time is up, and if both parties can agree to two kinds of confidentiality:

1. Nothing said in the listening partnership will be shared with anyone outside the listening partnership with the person's name attached.
2. Once a listening partnership is completed, the listener needs permission from the speaker to bring up anything said in the listening partnership.

Focused questions are provided for 16 listening partnerships on the following topics:

1. Not interrupting
2. Nonverbal communication
3. Asking questions and allowing for silences
4. Listening to emotions
5. Self-awareness/life story
6. Restatement, reflection, clarification/more life story
7. Developing cultural competence
8. Gender
9. Sex and sexual orientation
10. Disability
11. Ageism
12. Religious/spiritual beliefs and heritage
13. Ethnicity and culture
14. Socioeconomic class
15. Racism
16. Conflict resolution and assertiveness

Time allotments are recommended for listening partnerships, but the learners may increase or decrease the suggested meeting times as they see appropriate. Discussion/journal questions are also provided so that at the end of each listening partnership, pairs will have an opportunity to reflect both orally and in writing on what they have learned from their exchange and to provide feedback to each other on their communication skills. Although discussions will not be timed exchanges, it will be important to ensure each person is listened to without interruption during discussions. Journaling will offer an opportunity for students to express and clarify their thinking. Murphy (2004) found that focused reflection and articulation actually promotes clinical reasoning. Furthermore, Elbow (2000) documented that journaling can enhance writing skills—another important form of communication for occupational therapists.

## Listening Partnership 1: Not Interrupting (2 Minutes Each Way)

Starting with a 2-minute each way exchange may be enough for an initial listening partnership. Because many of us are not used to being given another person's full attention, it may feel quite awkward to have someone listen to us without interrupting. On the other hand, others of us will feel a great sense of relief to have finally had someone listen to us without interruption. It may also feel very hard to listen without saying anything for 2 "whole" minutes. We may want to say things to reassure the other person, to give him or her advice, or to let him or her know we have been through a similar experience so he or she knows that we are indeed listening. As hard as it may be, it is important to simply listen and say nothing in this first listening partnership and to then discuss how it went afterwards with your partner. It will be important to take turns listening not only during the formal listening partnership but during the discussion as well. Discussions will differ from the partnerships in that no one will be timing the shared exchanges.

### Partnership Topics

1. What were/are communication patterns like in your family?
2. Are you more comfortable listening or speaking?

### Discussion/Journal Questions

1. What was it like to listen for 2 minutes without interrupting?
2. Were you able to be successful at not saying anything?

3. What was it like to be listened to for 2 minutes without interruption?
4. Would you have preferred more or less time?
5. Would you have preferred that your listener say something? If so what?
6. What kind of nonverbal communication did you use that was effective at conveying to your partner that you were listening?

## Listening Partnership 2: Nonverbal Communication (2 to 5 Minutes Each Way)

This leads us to the next important skill necessary for effective communication. In addition to learning to not interrupt, one needs to learn effective nonverbal communication (Purtilo & Haddad, 1996). Tone of voice, posture, body language, touch, eye contact, and facial expressions often speak louder than our words to the person we are assisting. The more we can show we care about the person who is speaking, the more he or she is likely to open up and share what is on his or her mind and heart. Eye contact is a good place to begin. Offering our eye contact to someone who is sharing what is on his or her mind is one important way to let the person know you are there and you are listening. This can be hard for the beginning therapist to do, especially if making eye contact was not done much in one's family of origin or cultural group. As many people speak and share what is on their minds, they themselves do not maintain eye contact, but it is important for them to know that if they do look out, the listener's gaze is available. With practice in listening partnerships, this skill can be obtained very quickly.

Beyond eye contact, the facial expression of an effective listener will show approval, respect, and interest toward the person sharing. A relaxed, confident attitude toward the speaker will enable the person to open up to us. Some of us are not aware of what our facial expressions communicate to others. We may convey an attitude of tension and criticism without being aware of this. Seeking feedback on our facial expressions from those who will give us honest feedback on how we are perceived will assist us in refining our nonverbal communication. Again, listening partnerships are a good way to seek feedback and refine our nonverbal communication skills.

### Partnership Questions

1. What have you noticed about your nonverbal communication?
2. What is it like to make eye contact as a listener or a speaker?
3. What have you noticed about the nonverbal communication of others?
4. Have there been times when you did not feel listened to because of someone's nonverbal behavior?
5. What kinds of nonverbal communication have enabled you to open up to a friend, family member, or professional?

### Discussion/Journal Questions

1. Was this listening partnership any easier than the first one?
2. Were you conscious of your nonverbal behavior as you were the listener?
3. What did your partner do well in terms of nonverbal communication?
4. Were you able to continue practicing not interrupting?

## Listening Partnership 3: Asking Questions and Allowing for Silences (5 Minutes Each Way)

Naturally, beyond learning not to interrupt and learning to provide effective nonverbal communication, the artful communicator learns to ask relevant questions to draw out the talker. A good question to use at the beginning of each listening partnership sessions is, "What is new and good?" Many of us go through much of our lives with our attention on our worries and our frustrations rather than on what is going well in our lives. It is useful to take a few moments to notice what is going well in our lives. There may be times when it is hard to come up with something new and good in our lives, yet the patient listener will give the speaker time to think about something that is new and good. An equally important follow-up question to "What is new and good?" is "What is upsetting or challenging in our lives?"

As we try out these two questions, we may note that the speaker pauses or runs out of things to say. Many beginning listeners have a hard time allowing for silences and feel compelled to say something when a speaker pauses. In fact, when we allow for silences, the person talking often has more to say with no more prompting than simply having a listener at hand who can stay relaxed around silences. After allowing for a few seconds of silence, if the speaker is struggling with what else to say, the simple phrase, "Tell me more" or "What else?" may be all that the speaker needs to hear in order to continue talking about what is on his or her mind.

### Partnership Questions

1. What is new and good in your life?
2. Is there anything else new and good? What is hard or challenging in your life right now? Tell me more.

### Discussion/Journal Questions

1. What went well in this listening partnership?
2. What could have made it even better for both individuals?

## Listening Partnership 4: Listening to Emotions (5 Minutes Each Way)

As listening partners feel increasingly comfortable with each other, more and more emotions may be shared. Emotions are neither good nor bad; they just are. However, it has been found that expression of emotions can decrease stress and tension and foster re-evaluation of one's situation. Crying can release grief and depression; laughter can release fear, tension, and embarrassment; yawning can release physical tension and exhaustion; trembling and shaking can release fear; and raging can release anger and indignation (H. Jackins, 1981). Despite the emotional healing and re-evaluations that can occur with emotional release, other than young children, most humans are somewhat inhibited from emotional expression. Many of us grew up in households where emotions were not welcome or where only certain emotions were allowed. For example, in some families, it was acceptable for women to show grief and sadness and for men to show their anger. Others of us learned to only express our emotions privately, and others grew up in families where they were encouraged to express a whole range of emotion. In order for occupational therapy practitioners to be effective with a wide range of clients, it is important for them to be comfortable listening to a wide range of emotional expression. In addition, they may find it helpful to vent to a good listener so they can think more flexibly about each new situation they are in.

### Partnership Questions

1. What was emotional expression like in your family as you were growing up?
2. Were there any gender differences in the expression of emotion?
3. What do you currently do when you feel upset? Is there anyone you can turn to if you need to cry?
4. What have you noticed when you have had a chance to laugh, cry, shake, or rage? Have you been able to listen to someone when they cried hard?
5. Which emotions are the easiest for you to listen to?

### Discussion/Journal Questions

1. Would you feel comfortable venting painful emotions with your listening partner?
2. What positive feedback and suggestions for improvement can you offer your listening partner at this point?

## Listening Partnership 5: Self-Awareness/Life Story (15+ Minutes Each Way)

Occupational therapy practitioners generally listen to pieces of our client's life story, yet on some occasions, we listen to long narratives about the ups and downs of our client's life (Frank, 1995; Kielhofner, 2002). In order to listen well to life stories, we need to first have opportunities to share and reflect upon our own life story (Davis, 2006). Because our lives are filled with both wonderful experiences and many hardships, it may only feel safe to share certain pieces of our life story with certain people. Each person gets to choose what they feel safe sharing with whom. A good way to begin to share life stories is to reflect on positive memories from childhood first. As increased safety is created within listening partnerships, it will be useful to share some of the things that were hard when we were young. The more relaxed our listening partner is in listening to the hardships we have endured, the more we will be able to share with him or her. Additionally, the more our listening partner can listen to a range of emotional experiences, the more we will feel comfortable sharing the difficulties we have faced.

### Partnership Questions

1. What are some pleasant memories of your childhood?
2. What are some pleasant memories of elementary school?
3. What did you love to play?
4. Who did you like to play with?
5. What was difficult or challenging about your childhood within your family, school, or neighborhood?

### Discussion/Journal Questions

1. What made this partnership go well?
2. What could have made it even better?
3. Could you have talked longer?
4. What was it like to listen for 15 minutes?
5. Were you able to stay in roles as listener and speaker?
6. Were you able to allow for silences?
7. Were there emotions shared? If so, were the listener and speaker comfortable with the emotions shared?

## Listening Partnership 6: Restatement, Reflection, Clarification/More Life Story (15+ Minutes Each Way)

In addition to learning to ask relevant questions, the skilled communicator offers restatement, reflection, and clarification so the listener knows they are being listened to (Davis, 2006). Restatement, or stating back almost exactly what the speaker has said, is used when the listener wants the speaker to know that a very important piece of information they shared has been clearly heard. It is often used as a question so the client can report whether the listener heard exactly what was being communicated. For example, one out of many events a client shared about his or her adolescence may have been, "Things were so bad that I ran away from home." Using restatement, the listener might say, "Things were so bad that you ran away from home." This invites the speaker to confirm the information and to say more. Many of us use restatement without even thinking about it in our everyday conversations. Naturally, restatement can be overused and, if so, it can be annoying to anyone speaking. The beginning listener will want to begin to notice when he or she uses restatement in everyday interactions as well as listening partnerships and evaluate its effectiveness.

A more complex skill is reflective listening. In reflective listening, the listener listens not only to the content being shared but also for the emotions that underlie that content (Davis, 2006). This requires that the listener be very attentive to not only what a person is sharing verbally but also what is being shared nonverbally. Nonverbal communication, including tone of voice, posture, facial expression, and eye contact, gives us great insight into what a person might be feeling. When our speaker pauses, it may be helpful to reflect back to them both the content of what they said and the emotions that we detected. For example, if in sharing her life story, our listening partner looks sad and discloses she felt left out in high school because she did not make the cheerleading squad, you might reflect this back by saying, "It sounds like it was really hard for you when you didn't make the cheerleading squad."

Reflection such as this may invite an outpouring of even more emotion than our partner had previously shared. The beginning listener often refrains from such reflective questions exactly for this reason. They know their speaker will feel more emotion if such a statement is made. Yet, this type of statement conveys a real empathy for what our partner has experienced and may deepen the trust within the listening partnership. Furthermore, as was noted earlier, despite all of the societal taboos on crying, a release of old grief and resentments can clear up our thinking and compel our lives forward in a positive direction (H. Jackins, 1981).

A natural follow-up to the listening skill of reflection is clarification. As we listen closely to our listening partner, we may notice that he or she has shared a great deal of information. Clarification involves summarizing the key issues the individual has expressed and focusing the individual on what is most important or most significant (Davis, 2006). Often, there will be a ring in the voice of the speaker as he or she discusses his or her most significant experiences. The skilled listener listens for this "ring" and refers back to the content that generated the "ring" for clarification and more information.

### Partnership Questions

1. What are some pleasant memories of your adolescence?
2. What was your favorite activity?
3. Talk about your first job.
4. What was difficult or challenging about being an adolescent within your family, school, church, community, or neighborhood?
5. What is/was great/challenging about being a young adult? What is great/challenging about being an adult?

### Discussion/Journal Questions

1. Was it helpful to continue to discuss life stories?
2. Did you use restatement, reflection, or clarification as you listened to your partner?
3. If so, did it work well from your partner's point of view?
4. Are you comfortable receiving both positive and constructive feedback from your partner?

## Listening Partnership 7: Developing Cultural Competence (15+ Minutes Each Way)

As humans, we are much more alike than we are different. Yet the societies that we live in tend to emphasize our differences in the areas of gender, race, class, culture, religion, physical ability/disability, country or origin, languages, body size, sexual orientation, etc. (Rothenberg, 1998). Although some of us may feel proud of our different identities, many of us are mistreated and made to feel badly about our differences through social conditioning and oppression. H. Jackins (1997) defines oppression as "the systematic mistreatment of a group of people by the society and/or by another group of people who serve as agents of the society, with the mistreatment encouraged or enforced by society and its culture" (p. 151). Internalized oppression occurs when groups of oppressed people begin to believe the negative messages, lies, and misinformation the society has placed on them. They invalidate not only themselves, but other members of their group (Kauffman & New, 2004).

As listening partners begin to feel more comfortable with each other, they will find it useful to explore diversity within themselves. In doing so, they can look at both what has been positive about being a member of a particular group and what has been challenging about being a member of a particular group. Ultimately, by engaging in this type of self-examination with a supportive listener, they can heal from any mistreatment they have endured as members of different groups and take fuller pride in all aspects of themselves (Brown & Mazza, 1997). In addition, as Wells and Black (2000) have pointed out, engaging in this type of self-reflection is an important step in becoming a culturally competent therapist. One cannot be responsive and sensitive to diversity in others if one has not first looked at diversity within one's self. Therefore, the next several listening partnerships will give the reader many opportunities to explore diversity within themselves and learn about diversity within their peers. In addition, since knowledge gathering is an essential component of cultural competence, many sources are cited in this chapter for additional information on human diversity.

### Partnership Questions

1. Were you ever in the minority in your neighborhood, school, church, or social situation as you were growing up? If so, what was this like?
2. Were there ever times that you felt mistreated as a member of a particular group? What was this like?
3. Talk about times that you made friends with someone that crossed a line of gender, race, class, culture, sexual orientation, age, physical ability or disability, language, country of origin, etc.

### Discussion/Journal Questions

1. What was it like to dialogue about diversity?
2. How much time did you need for this partnership?

## Listening Partnership 8: Gender (15+ Minutes Each Way)

The beauty of listening partnerships is that both individuals agree to take turns listening to one another. Knowing you will have a turn to be heard enables many a beginner listener to refrain from sharing his or her life story while listening to the life story of another. Yet the question always arises, "Might it not be helpful for me to share my life story with the person I am listening to while I am listening?" The answer is, "Sometimes." Sometimes when we are listening to someone share their life story, it reminds us of similar experiences of our own. We feel eager to let the speaker know that we have been through something similar. On occasion, by sharing a little bit about our experience that is similar to the person speaking, we enable them to keep sharing about their experience. What we need to be mindful of is not turning this into our own listening turn. Again, knowing that we will get our chance when our listening partner has finished telling their story can enable us to wait for our turn.

When men and women begin to dialogue on gender in listening partnerships, they often have quite a bit to say on the subject. It can be challenging in listening partnerships to listen without sharing our own experience. An important question for the listener to always consider is, "Is what I am saying helping my partner to continue to do most of the talking?" Another important fact to keep in mind is that listening does not mean agreement. We can listen to someone for a long time and not agree with what they are saying.

The forces of gender oppression attempt to ascribe rigid roles to both men and women (Froehlich, Hamlin, Loukas, & MacRae, 1992). Both groups are mistreated by gender oppression but in different ways. Some of the key features of women's oppression include the assumption that women are less intelligent or less capable than men, lower pay for equal work (Froehlich, 2005; MacRae, 2005), obsession with appearance, lack of pay or recognition for the significant work of mothering (Crittenden, 2001; Pierce & Frank, 1992; Primeau, 1992), violence and sexual abuse, limited access to positions of influence within businesses and governments, discrediting for being too emotional, and the assumption that mothering and care giving is our ultimate contribution.

The society has only recently begun to recognize that men are also oppressed—not by women but by society as a whole (H. Jackins and others, 1999). Socialization to be violent and competitive begins early in the lives of boys within the family, and it is reinforced in the media. At an early age, boys learn that they may be called upon to kill other men for their country. In preparation for this role, boys are systematically humiliated when they show their grief or tenderness. They are hardened early. Many boys also learn at an early age that it will be their job to dominate and control women. Males are also socialized to believe they can only have closeness with one significant partner and that sex is the ultimate closeness.

Even though individual families work hard to break all of this conditioning for males and females, society continues to oppress us in these ways. As was mentioned previously, one of the worst consequences of oppression is internalized oppression. Once we internalize gender conditioning about ourselves, we oppress ourselves and members of our own group.

Listening partnerships offer an opportunity to free ourselves from internalized oppression, especially when we can first share about our experiences with someone from a similar background (i.e., women with women and men with men). By listening well to each other's experience, we can challenge and dispel the internalization of oppression. After we have shared with someone from a similar background, it is often rich and rewarding to hear the perspective from other groups.

### Partnership Questions

1. What is great about being male/female?
2. What is challenging about being male/female?
3. What do you not like about your own gender?
4. When have you stood up to gender oppression?
5. When have you been an effective ally to the other gender?

### Discussion/Journal Questions

1. What was it like to engage in this listening partnership?
2. Were you able to listen to your partners without interrupting?
3. Did you or your partner find that it was useful to share any of your own story as your partner was speaking?
4. Can you decide to ask these questions of someone of the other gender who is not a listening partner?

## Listening Partnerships 9: Sex and Sexual Orientation (15+ Minutes Each Way)

Regardless of one's sexual orientation, we all grow up with some confusions and embarrassments about sex and sexuality. In attempting to communicate with us about sex when we were young, family members, clergy, and teachers did their best to share helpful information but generally also shared some embarrassment, awkwardness, and perhaps even misinformation. Because sexuality is a part of life that many occupational therapy practitioners address in their interventions with clients, it is important to work toward increasing comfort with the subject so open communication can occur.

In addition, increased comfort with the subject of human sexuality will most likely increase one's comfort in discussing sexual orientation. A number of occupational therapy practitioners have identified that homophobia is a barrier to gay, lesbian, bisexual, and transgendered (GLBT) individuals in receiving optimum occupational therapy services (Jackson, 1995; Kelly, 2000; Kingsley & Molineux, 2000). Because gay oppression continues to threaten the security of people who are GLBT, many choose not to be "out" about their sexual identity in their communities. Therefore, as occupational therapy practitioners, it is important for heterosexuals not to make assumptions about the sexual orientation of people with whom they are interacting.

Listening partnerships between two individuals who are GLBT can provide a safe place for venting about discrimination or hurtful experiences. Internalized oppression, which places divisions between them, can be challenged. It will be useful for heterosexual people to get together with other heterosexual people to talk about all of their experiences with GLBT individuals so they are less awkward in relating to them. As increased safety is gained, it will be richly rewarding for GLBT people to be able to share about their experiences with heterosexuals and for heterosexuals to be strong allies for GLBT individuals in combatting gay oppression.

### Partnership Questions

1. While you were growing up, what attitudes were communicated to you about sex by family, clergy, teachers, and friends?
2. Were you able to talk openly about sex with anyone?
3. Share your experiences with people who are GLBT. If you are gay, lesbian, or bisexual and out, talk about what has been good about your identity and what has been challenging.
4. If you are heterosexual, talk about what has been good about this identify and what has been challenging.

### Discussion/Journal Questions

1. If you have a friend who is gay, lesbian, or bisexual, what would it be like for you to ask him or her what it has been like to his or her identity?
2. What do you and your listening partner appreciate about each other?

## Listening Partnership 10: Disability (15+ Minutes Each Way)

Studies have shown that occupational therapy practitioners tend to have positive attitudes toward people with disabilities, yet there is still room for improvement (Coffey & Velde, 2001; White & Olson, 1998). Occupational therapy practitioners who have had people with disabilities in their lives as friends or family members tend to have the most positive attitudes toward people with disabilities (Benham, 1988). People with positive attitudes toward people with disabilities easily notice the shared humanity between themselves as able-bodied people and their friends with disabilities.

The inclusion movement has created many more opportunities for people with disabilities and able-bodied people to form relationships. People from the United States can be particularly proud of the Americans with Disabilities Act (ADA) of 1990. Enacting a law that ensures people with disabilities receive reasonable accommodations in employment, telecommunications, transportation, and public services has increased the inclusion of people with disabilities in the United States. This field of disabilities studies (Craddock 1996a, 1996b; Kielhofner, 2005) promises to move us all toward an even greater inclusion of people with disabilities in all facets of society.

### Partnership Questions

1. Talk about a disability you currently have or an accident, injury, or disability you have had in the past, describing both positive and challenging aspects to your situation.
2. Share all of your experiences—both positive and challenging—with people with disabilities. What disability would be the most challenging for you to have and why?
3. What client population will be the hardest for you to work with and why?

### Discussion/Journal Questions

1. Have you noticed any students with disabilities on your campus?
2. What would it be like to reach out to this person or people?

## Listening Partnership 11: Ageism (15+ Minutes Each Way)

It is actually great to be any age we are, yet the societies we live in parcel out respect differentially according to age. Young people, teenagers, young adults, and older adults experience less respect than adults in their 30s and 40s. Although adults in their 30s and 40s experience greater respect than people of other ages, they tend to be overburdened with work and family responsibilities. Thus, there are certain hardships associated with being any age.

Examining any mistreatment we have experienced for being a particular age can assist us in being mindful of not perpetuating disrespect toward others because of their age. Since most occupational therapists work with elders, it behooves us to reflect on our experiences with elders so we can build on any positive experiences we had and leave behind any negative experiences.

### Partnership Questions

1. Have you ever been mistreated for being a particular age?
2. What concerns you about growing older?
3. What have been your experiences (positive and negative) with elders?
4. How would you like to be treated as an elder?

### Discussion/Journal Questions

1. Would you like to have a regular listening partner at this point?
2. What have you noticed about yourself as a listener and talker now that you have engaged in many listening partnerships?

## Listening Partnership 12: Religious/Spiritual Beliefs and Heritage (15+ Minutes Each Way)

Religion and spirituality can be a powerful source of hope, inspiration, connection, and meaning in people's lives. Yet at the same time, humanity remains divided around religion. People are oppressed for their particular religious or spiritual beliefs, wars continue to be fought on the basis of these differences, and some religious and spiritual traditions enforce hurtful rigidities upon its participants.

Egan and Swedersky (2003) noted that despite considerable literature describing the potential place of spirituality in occupational therapy practice, many occupational therapists continue to be uncomfortable with the concept of spirituality in practice. In a survey of occupational therapists from Canada and the United States, Farrar (2001) found that the majority of occupational therapy respondents felt that spirituality is appropriate for occupational therapy practice, and one-third felt that religion was appropriate, yet most were unsure how to address either. Those who did address spirituality did so by focusing on self-esteem, locus of control, and hope and purpose in life. Religion was often addressed by addressing functional ability to participate in worship. Many respondents were concerned with how to address spirituality without imposing their own beliefs.

Listening partnerships can help occupational therapy practitioners become more comfortable discussing religion and spirituality. As we become more aware of any strengths and challenges associated with our own religious or spiritual heritage, the more we can listen to others and understand the strengths and challenges of their traditions.

### Partnership Questions

1. Describe your religious/spiritual heritage and current practices.
2. What are the strengths of your religious heritage and what are any challenges or hardships that are part of your religious background?
3. What has it been like to develop relationships from people of other religious/spiritual backgrounds?

### Discussion/Journal Questions

1. What do you want to know about other religions or spiritual practices?

## Listening Partnership #13: Ethnicity and Culture (15+ Minutes Each Way)

We all have a rich cultural heritage that is important to recognize. The United States has historically forced people to give up their cultural/ethnic heritage in favor of assimilating and becoming an "American." People have lost connections with their language and many fine cultural traditions as a result of assimilation. As with religion and spirituality, as we each deepen our awareness and appreciation of our cultural/ethnic heritage, we can appreciate the cultural heritage of others. This will be important in occupational therapy interactions with people from diverse backgrounds (Awaad, 2003; Black, 2002; Chiang & Carlson, 2003; Forwell, Whiteford, & Dyck, 2001; Iwana, 2003; Odawara, 2005; Richardson, 2004; Velde & Wittman, 2001; Wells & Black, 2000; Whiteford & St. Clair, 2002; Wittman & Velde, 2002). For those of us who identify as citizens of the United States, it is also important to fully claim this identity and any nuances related to being from a particular part of the United States.

### Partnership Questions

1. What is your cultural/ethnic background?
2. Why did you or your ancestors come to the United States?
3. What can you take pride in from your cultural heritage?
4. What are some challenges associated with your cultural background?

5. What makes you proud to be an American, and how would you like the United States to be different?

### Discussion/Journal Questions

1. If you have a regular listening partner at this point, how has this changed your listening partnerships?

## Listening Partnership 14: Socioeconomic Class (15+ Minutes Each Way)

Jackins (1990) described how classism has existed as long as humans have functioned in organized societies. The vicious classism that existed under slavery gave way to a slightly less vicious form of classism under feudalism. Despite a few attempts at alternatives, feudalism was eventually replaced by capitalism, or owning class/working class societies worldwide. Under capitalism, a small percentage of the population owns and controls most of the wealth and means of production, while the rest of the population works for a living. In the United States, the wealthiest 1% owns more than the bottom 95% (Galbraith, 2003).

The working class has many subdivisions that include the middle class, blue/pink collar workers (or what has been traditionally thought of as the working class), working poor people, and unemployed people. None of the divisions between classes is clear cut. People can often identify with more than one class background, so individual stories become more meaningful than labels associated with class background.

As Hawes (1996) pointed out, class society permeates everything, and the contradictions of capitalism are manifested in the lives of all individuals. People within the working class are often pitted against one another—the middle class is given a few extra privileges and some status over the working class and poor people in exchange for carrying out oppressive roles. An example is Jewish people, who transcend all classes, yet have historically been used by owning class leaders as scapegoats. They have been made to appear as the controllers of wealth and power by the owning class so that whenever working class people organize and fight their own oppression, they target Jews rather than the real owning class (H. Jackins, 1990). Jewish oppression persists in the forms of stereotyping, denial of anti-Semitism, and continued scapegoating of Jewish people.

Regardless of their class background, most occupational therapists function in the middle class as professionals, but class is very fluid under capitalism. Job cuts, disability, medical issues, divorce, single parenting, etc. can change one's socioeconomic class status virtually overnight. Increased awareness related to class will be beneficial to future occupational therapy practitioners on both a personal and professional level (Baum, McGeary, Pankiewicz, Braford, & Edwards,1996; Bottomley, 2001; Finlayson, Baker, Rodman, & Hertzberg, 2002; Froehlich, 2005; Humphrey, 1995; Neufeld & Lysack, 2004; Padilla, Gupta, & Liotta-Kleinfeld, 2004; Tryssenaar, Jones, & Lee, 1999; Von Zuben, Crist, & Mayberry, 1991). For the occupational therapy practitioner who was raised poor or working class, dialoguing about class can promote pride in one's heritage and assist the transition to the middle class. For the occupational therapy practitioner who was raised middle class, dialoguing about class can increase awareness of the strengths and challenges present in middle class life. Sensitivity and awareness of class can promote open communication between professional occupational therapists and clients of all class backgrounds.

### Partnership Questions

1. Talk about your class background, including the educational level and type of work in which your grandparents and parents engaged.
2. Did your family have enough, more than enough, or less than enough when you were growing up?
3. Did your family's financial resources fluctuate?
4. What are the strengths and challenges associated with your class background?
5. Have you ever encountered anti-Semitism? If so, talk about it. Did you or anyone else stand up against it? What do you remember about learning about the Holocaust?

### Discussion/Journal Questions

1. What was it like to talk about class background?
2. Were there taboos in your family regarding the discussion of money and class?

## Listening Partnership 15: Racism (15+ Minutes Each Way)

There is really only one human race, yet racism would have us believe otherwise. Racism is a vicious form of classism whereby people of color are treated as less than White people. In terms of global economics, people who reside in the southern hemisphere of the world are mostly people of color and tend to be the poorest people in the world (Udayakumar & powell, 2000). The United States, founded on the enslavement of people of African heritage and the genocide of Native American people, continues to struggle with enduring effects of racism and internalized racism.

Many of the effects of racism on people of color, particularly those of African heritage, are obvious in terms of media stereotyping, racial profiling, poverty, violence, lack of access to higher education, poor access to health care, and poor health. Occupational therapy practitioners have begun to acknowledge and dismantle racism within occupational therapy (Black, 2002; Cena, McGruder, & Tomlin, 2002; David, 1995; Evans, 1992; Matlala, 1993; Wells & Black, 2000). The effects of racism on White people are also damaging but in different and less obvious ways. It is damaging for White people to grow up in a society where they are bombarded with negative stereotypes about people of color and told they cannot be close to people of color. No White child was born racist, but when White children first learn about race, they are often confronted with awkwardness and guilt on the part of White adults who are challenged to communicate about race. They grow up to be young adults and adults who also feel bad about racism and awkward about discussing it (T. Jackins and others, 2002). Listening partnerships on racism can foster new awareness about racism, assist in healing from internalized racism, and deepen relationships between White people and people of color.

### Partnership Questions

1. How has racism affected you?
2. What is your earliest memory of noticing someone with a skin color other than yours?
3. Scan all of your memories of Native Americans, Asians, Latinos/Latinas, Arabs, people of African heritage, and people of European heritage.
4. Have you ever witnessed racism or oppression? Did you stand up against it?
5. If so, what was it like to take a stand against racism? If not, what held you back from taking a stand against racism?
6. Can you envision a world without racism?

### Discussion/Journal Questions

1. What conditions enable you to talk freely about racism?
2. What has it been like, overall, to engage in listening partnerships on diversity?

## Listening Partnership 16: Conflict Resolution and Assertiveness (15+ Minutes Each Way)

Conflict is a challenging aspect of human relationships that occurs both between members of a particular group and between people from different groups. Internalized oppression plays a role in conflict as members of oppressed groups mistreat each other (i.e., women versus women or poor people targeting other poor people). Conflict between people in different groups (i.e., men versus women) is also prevalent. Fortunately, increased awareness of the experiences of people from groups other than our own, combined with increased awareness of the mechanism of internalized oppression, can begin to decrease conflict and assist in its resolution (Brown & Mazza, 1997).

Many of us have negative associations with conflict, yet in reality, conflict can be an opportunity for increased communication, brainstorming, problem-solving, and new learning. Negative associations with conflict often stem from our early experiences with conflict in our families and can be re-evaluated in listening partnerships. When we free ourselves from some of the negative emotions associated with early conflict, we can more skillfully handle conflict in the present (Brown & Mazza, 1997).

Each conflict one encounters requires flexible, on-the-spot thinking. Some conflicts are best ignored, some require assistance from a third party, and some require intervention from policy or law enforcement personnel. When appropriate, the skilled communicator knows how to use listening as a conflict resolution skill. As was noted earlier, listening does not mean agreement. Listening means seeking to understand another point of view. If the reader has indeed practiced the listening partnerships in this chapter, he or she may be ready to not only listen to someone he or she is in conflict with, but also to assert that he or she deserves to be listened to as well. It may be necessary to teach the party one is in conflict with to truly listen without interruption.

Finding our voice in situations of conflict can be challenging, particularly for oppressed groups. Davis (2006) underscored the challenges females face in asserting themselves in the presence of males. Venting aggressive feelings we have toward an individual with a supportive listening partnership and noting whether this person reminds us of someone from our past can clear our mind so we can act assertively in the present (Brown & Mazza, 1997)

Davis (2006) described the work of Bower and Bower in identifying a process (DESC) for asserting one's self that involves the following steps:

- Describing the specific behavior that is bothersome
- Expressing how this behavior made you feel
- Specifying the desired changes in behavior
- Sharing the consequences that will occur as a result of the behavioral change

Now that the reader has learned to listen well to others, it might be important to assert that others learn to listen to you. For example, using the DESC formula you might say:

- *Describe*: I have noticed you interrupt me when I am trying to speak.
- *Emotions*: I am bothered when I do not get to complete a thought.
- *Specify*: How about if you listen to me for 5 minutes without saying anything?
- *Consequence*: Then I will listen to you for 5 minutes without interruption and we might get along better.

### Partnership Questions

1. How was conflict handled in your family as you were growing up?
2. Talk about times when you successfully handled conflict. What is challenging for you in situations of conflict? How would you like to handle conflict differently?
3. Are you able to assert yourself, or do you tend to be passive and quiet in situations of conflict?

## Discussion/Journal Questions

1. Can you make a decision to use listening skills as conflict resolution skills?
2. Do you have a goal regarding assertive communication?

# Summary

As Ueland (2006) concluded, "When we are listened to, it creates us, makes us unfold and expand. Ideas actually begin to grow within us and come to life." Eighteen years of experience teaching occupational therapy students to use listening partnerships for the enhancement of their communication skills has enabled me to witness the unfolding and expansion of my students. Students who have had the opportunity to engage in multiple listening partnerships report in journals and papers that not only do they become much better listeners, but they also become more confident as thinkers, speakers, and writers. Although they initially find it difficult to stay in the role as listener or speaker, over time, this becomes natural. Students generally report as the class progresses that they notice how much others do not listen, and many decide to teach friends and family to listen to them.

In addition, listening partnerships focused on diversity have a positive impact on students' awareness and comfort with human diversity within themselves and their peers. Often times, students from oppressed groups find enough caring, trust, and safety in their listening partnerships to vent about their experiences of mistreatment and discrimination. Students from dominant groups such as heterosexual, gentile, White middle class men and women report that they have been deeply enriched by the stories of students of color, students from countries outside of the United States, students with disabilities, students raised poor and working class, and students who are Jewish or Buddhist. Male and female students are riveted by what each other has to say about their experiences. The occupational therapy student who applies weekly time and practice to listening partnerships will make great steps toward becoming an effective, culturally competent communicator—a necessity for forming effective relationships with clients, family, significant others, colleagues, and other health providers and the public.

**Evidence-Based Research Chart**

| Area | Component(s) | Evidence |
|---|---|---|
| Listening skills | Nonverbal and verbal communication | Davis, 2006; Froehlich & Nesbit, 2004; H. Jackins, 1981; Kauffman & New, 2004; Purtilo & Haddad, 1996; Taylor, 2008 |
| Self-awareness/ knowledge of others | Life story/narrative | Davis, 2006; Frank, 1995; Kielhofner, 2002; Taylor, 2008 |
| | Gender | Crittenden, 2001; Froehlich, 2005; Froehlich et al., 1992; H. Jackins and others, 1999; MacRae, 2005; Primeau, 1992; Pierce & Frank, 1992 |
| | Sexual orientation | Jackson, 1995; Kelly, 2000; Kinglsey & Molineaux, 2000 |
| | Disability | Benham, 1988; Coffey & Velde, 2001; Craddock, 1996a, 1996b; Kielhofner, 2005; White & Olson, 1998 |
| | Religion/spirituality | Egan & Swedersky, 2003; Farrar, 2001 |
| | Culture and ethnicity | Awaad, 2003; Chiang & Carlson, 2003; Iwana, 2003; Odawara, 2005; Richardson, 2004; Velde & Wittman, 2001; Wells & Black, 2000; Whiteford & St. Clair, 2002; Wittman & Velde, 2002 |
| | Class | Baum et al., 1996; Bottomley, 2001; Finlayson et al., 2002; Froehich, 2005; Galbraith, 2003; Hawes, 1996; Humphrey, 1995; H. Jackins, 1990; Neufeld & Lysack, 2004; Padilla et al., 2004; Tryssenaar et al., 1999; Von Zuben et al., 1991 |
| | Race | Black, 2002; Cena et al., 2002; David, 1995; Evans, 1992; T. Jackins and others, 2002; Matlala, 1993; Udayakumar & powell, 2000; Wells & Black, 2000 |
| Cultural competence | Awareness/knowledge/skills | Awaad, 2003; Black, 2002; Chiang & Carlson, 2003; Iwana, 2003; Odawara, 2005; Richardson, 2004; Velde & Wittman, 2001; Wells & Black, 2000; Wittman & Velde, 2002; Whiteford & St. Clair, 2002; |
| Writing | Journaling | Elbow, 2000; Murphy, 2004 |

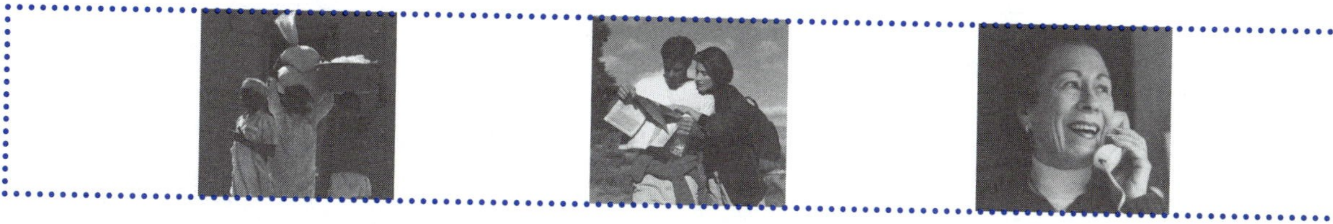

## Student Self-Assessment

1. Reflect on how your communication skills have changed as a result of reading this chapter and engaging in listening partnerships and journaling. Describe any changes you have noticed in your listening skills, with attention to both verbal and nonverbal behavior. Have peers, family, or co-workers given you any feedback on your communications skills? If so, what have they said? Have you noticed any changes in your ability to express your ideas verbally and in writing? If so, describe these changes.
2. What in particular stands out in your mind with regard to journaling and engaging in listening partnerships on diversity? Can you identify some next steps with regard to becoming a culturally competent communicator? If so, what are they?
3. Describe your thoughts regarding the concept of internalized oppression, and reflect upon any of your own struggles with self-invalidation and invalidation of members of your own group.
4. Have you attempted to teach other people to refrain from interrupting you or others as they are speaking? If so, what has this been like?
5. Have you used either listening or the DESC approach to conflict resolution? If so, what were your results? If not, discuss your feelings about potentially using either of these approaches.

## References

Awaad, T. (2003). Culture cultural competency, and occupational therapy: A review of the literature. *British Journal of Occupational Therapy, 66*(8), 356-362.

Baum, C., McGeary, T., Pankiewicz, R., Braford, T., & Edwards, D. (1996). An activity program for cognitively impaired low-income inner city residents. *Topics in Geriatric Rehabilitation, 12*(2), 54-62.

Benham, P. K. (1988). Attitudes of occupational therapy personnel toward persons with disabilities. *American Journal of Occupational Therapy, 42*, 305-311.

Black, R. M. (2002). Occupational therapy's dance with diversity. *American Journal of Occupational Therapy, 56*, 140-148.

Bottomley, J. M. (2001). Health care and homeless older adults. *Topics in Geriatric Rehabilitation, 17*(1), 1-21.

Brown, C. R., & Mazza, G. J. (1997). *Healing into action: A leadership guide for creating diverse communities*. Washington, DC: National Coalition Building Institute (NCBI).

Cena, L., McGruder, J., & Tomlin, G. (2002). Representations of race, ethnicity, and social class in case examples in the *American Journal of Occupational Therapy. American Journal of Occupational Therapy, 56*, 130-139.

Chiang, M., & Carlson, G. (2003). Occupational therapy in multicultural contexts: Issues and strategies. *British Journal of Occupational Therapy, 66*(12), 559-567.

Coffey, D. M., & Velde, B. P. (2001). The experience of being an occupational therapist with a disability: What about being a student? *American Journal of Occupational Therapy, 55*(3), 352-353.

Craddock, J. (1996a). Responses of the occupational therapy profession to the perspective of the disability movement, part 1. *British Journal of Occupational Therapy, 59*(1), 17-24.

Craddock, J. (1996b). Responses of the occupational therapy profession to the perspective of the disability movement, part 2. *British Journal of Occupational Therapy, 59*(2), 73-78.

Crittenden, A. (2001). *The price of motherhood: Why the most important job in the world is still the least valued*. New York, NY: Henry Holt and Company.

David, P. A. (1995). Service provision to black people: A study of occupational therapy staff in physical disability teams within social services. *British Journal of Occupational Therapy, 58*(3), 98-102.

Davis, C. M. (2006). *Patient practitioner interaction: An experiential manual for developing the art of health care*. Thorofare, NJ: SLACK Incorporated.

Egan, M., & Swedersky, J. (2003). Spirituality as experienced by occupational therapists in practice. *American Journal of Occupational Therapy, 57*(5), 525-533.

Elbow, P. (2000). *Everyone can write: Essays toward a hopeful theory of writing and teaching writing*. New York, NY: Oxford Press.

Evans, J. (1992). What occupational therapists can do to eliminate racial barriers to health care access. *American Journal of Occupational Therapy, 46*, 676-766.

Farrar, J. E. (2001). Addressing spirituality and religious life in occupational therapy. *Physical & Occupational Therapy in Geriatrics, 18*(4), 65-85.

Finlayson, M., Baker, M., Rodman, L., & Hertzberg, G. (2002). The process and outcomes of a multimethod needs assessment at a homeless shelter. *American Journal of Occupational Therapy, 56*, 313-321.

Forwell, S., Whiteford, G. & Dyck, I. (2001). Cultural competence in New Zealand and Canada: Occupational therapy students' reflections on class and fieldwork curriculum. *Canadian Journal of Occupational Therapy, 68*(2), 90-103.

Frank, G. (1995). Life histories in occupational therapy clinical practice. *American Journal of Occupational Therapy, 50*, 251-263.

Froehlich, J. (2005). Steps toward dismantling poverty for working poor women. *Work: A Journal of Prevention, Assessment & Rehabilitation, 24*(4), 401-408.

Froehlich, J., Hamlin, R. B., Loukas, K. M., & MacRae, N. (1992). Special issue on feminism as an inclusive perspective. *American Journal of Occupational Therapy, 46*, 967-1044.

Froehlich, J., & Nesbit, S. (2004). The aware communicator: Dialogues on diversity. *Occupational Therapy in Health Care, 18*(1/2), 171-182.

Galbraith, J. K. (2003). Why Bush likes a bad economy. *Progressive, 67*(October), 26-29.

Hawes, D. (1996). Against postmodernism: A Marxist perspective. *British Journal of Occupational Therapy, 59*(3), 131-132.

Humphrey, R. (1995). Families who live in chronic poverty: Meeting the challenge of family-centered services. *American Journal of Occupational Therapy, 49*, 687-693.

Iwana, M. (2003). The issue is: Toward a culturally relevant epistemologies in occupational therapy. *American Journal of Occupational Therapy, 57*, 582-588.

Jackins, H. (1981). *The art of listening*. Seattle, WA: Rational Island Publishers.

Jackins, H. (1990). *Logical thinking about a future society*. Seattle, WA: Rational Island Publishers.

Jackins, H. (1997). *The list*. Seattle, WA: Rational Island Publishers.

Jackins, H., and others. (1999). *The human male: A men's liberation draft policy*. Seattle, WA: Rational Island Publishers.

Jackins, T., and others .(2002). *Working together to end racism: Healing from the damage caused by racism*. Seattle, WA: Rational Island Publishers.

Jackson, J. (1995). Sexual orientation: Its relevance to occupational science and the practice of occupational therapy. *American Journal of Occupational Therapy, 49*, 669-679.

Kauffman, K., & New, C. (2004). *Co-counselling The theory and practice of re-evaluation counseling*. New York, NY: Brunner-Routledge.

Kelly, G. (2000). Rights, ethics and the spirit of occupation. *British Journal of Occupational Therapy, 58*(4), 176.

Kielhofner, G. (2002). *Model of human occupation* (3rd ed.). Philadelphia, PA: Lippincott Williams & Wilkins.

Kielhofner, G. (2005). Special issue: Disability studies. *American Journal of Occupational Therapy, 61*, 481-600.

Kingsley, P., & Molineux, M. (2000). True to our philosophy? Sexual orientation and occupation. *British Journal of Occupational Therapy, 63*(5), 205-210.

Law, M., Baptiste, S., & Mills, J. (1995). Client-centered practice: What does it mean and does it make a difference? *Canadian Journal of Occupational Therapy, 62*, 250-257.

Matlala, M. R. (1993). Race relations at work: A challenge to occupational therapy. *British Journal of Occupational Therapy, 56*(12), 434-436.

MacRae, N. (2005). Women and work: A ten year retrospective. *Work: A Journal of Prevention, Assessment & Rehabilitation, 24*(4), 331-340.

Murphy, J. (2004). Using focused reflection and articulation to promote clinical reasoning: an evidence-based teaching strategy. *Nursing Education Perspectives, 25*(2), 226-231.

Neufeld, S., & Lysack, C. (2004). Allocation of rehabilitation services: Who gets a home evaluation. *OT Practice, 9*(16), Supplement: CE1-CE-8.

Odawara, E. (2005). Cultural competency in occupational therapy: Beyond a cross-cultural view of practice. *American Journal of Occupational Therapy, 59*, 325-334.

Padilla, R., Gupta, J., & Liotta-Kleinfeld, L. (2004). Occupational therapy and social justice: A school-based example. *Occupational Therapy Practice, 9*(16 suppl), CE1-CE8.

Pierce, D., & Frank, G. (1992). A mother's work: Two levels of feminist analysis of family-centered care. *American Journal of Occupational Therapy, 46*, 972-980.

Primeau, L. A. (1992). A woman's place: Unpaid work in the home. *American Journal of Occupational Therapy, 46*, 981-988.

Purtilo, R., & Haddad, A. (1996). *Health professional and patient interaction* (5th ed.). Philadelphia, PA: WB Saunders.

Richardson, P. (2004). How cultural ideas help shape the conceptualization of mental illness. *Mental Health Occupational Therapy, 9*(1), 5-8.

Rothenberg, P. S. (1998). *Race, class and gender in the United States: An integrated study* (4th ed.). New York, NY: St. Martin Press.

Taylor, R. (2008). *The intentional relationship model: Occupational therapy and use of self.* Philadelphia, PA: F.A. Davis Company

Tryssenaar, J., Jones, E. J., & Lee, D. (1999). Occupational performance needs of a shelter population. *Canadian Journal of Occupational Therapy, 66*(4), 188-196.

Udayakumar, S. P., & powell, j. a. (2000). Race, poverty, and globalization. *Poverty & Race*, May/June. Retrieved August 5, 2009, from http://www.prrac.org/full_text.php?text_id=291&item_id=1805&newsletter_id=50&header=Race+%2F+Racism

Ueland, B. (2006). *The art of listening*. Retrieved August 3, 2006, from http://traubman.igc.org/listenof.htm

Velde, B. P., & Wittman, P. P. (2001). Helping occupational therapy students and faculty develop cultural competence. *Occupational Therapy in Health Care, 13*(3/4), 23-32.

Von Zuben, M. V., Crist, P. A., & Mayberry, W. (1991). A pilot study of differences in play behavior between children of low and middle socioeconomic status. *American Journal of Occupational Therapy, 45*, 113-118.

Wells, S. A., & Black, R. M. (2000). *Cultural competency for health professionals*. Bethesda, MD: AOTA Press.

White, M. J., & Olson, R. S. (1998). Attitudes toward people with disabilites: A comparison of rehabilitation nurses, occupational therapists, and physical therapists. *Rehabilitation Nursing, 23*(2), 126-131.

Whiteford, G., & St. Clair, V. W. (2002). Being prepared for diversity in practice: Occupational therapy students' perceptions of valuable intercultural learning experiences. *British Journal of Occupational Therapy, 65*(3), 129-37.

Wittman, P., & Velde, B. P. (2002). Attaining cultural competence, critical thinking and intellectual development: A challenge of occupational therapists. *American Journal of Occupational Therapy, 56*(4), 453-456.

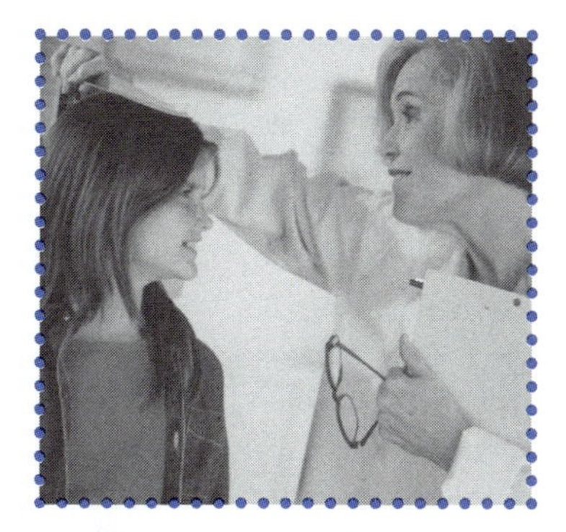

# 31

# Consultation, Referral, Monitoring, and Discharge Planning

*Julie Savoyski, MS, OTR/L*

**ACOTE Standards Explored in This Chapter**

B.5.22-5.25, 5.27

**Key Terms**

| | |
|---|---|
| Consultation | Monitoring |
| Discharge | Referral |

## Introduction

The client has been evaluated and an intervention plan has been established. At this point, it is not just day-to-day intervention that occupies the mind of a competent occupational therapist or occupational therapy assistant. Continual monitoring and reassessment of goals in the intervention plan will ensure the client is working toward the achievement of a desired level of function at discharge. As changes occur in the client's functional status, an alteration of the intervention plan may become necessary. Such a change may require consultation with another professional from within the occupational therapy field or an expert from a different discipline. As intervention nears an end, the role of the occupational therapy practitioner is to coordinate services that relate to the client's occupational performance needs. At times, a referral to community agencies suited to meet the unique needs of the client is necessary. The end of the therapeutic relationship between the client and occupational therapy practitioner occurs at discharge. At this point, the course of intervention is documented in a discharge summary to pass on to other professionals the client may work with in the future.

## Monitoring and Reassessment

Throughout the course of intervention, the client should be consistently monitored and reassessed in order to gauge the effectiveness of intervention. Monitoring is the act of observing a client's response to intervention. These actions will ensure that the client's areas of need are being addressed appropriately. After the initial evaluation has been completed and the intervention plan is in place, progress continues to be documented. This documentation ensures goals and objectives concerning appropriate performance areas, performance components, and performance contexts are in place. Refer to Chapter 32 for more information about progress notes.

Periodic reassessment is also an important part of tracking a client's progress. Reassessment can occur on a formal or informal basis. Under the supervision of an occupational therapist, occupational therapy assistants should participate in the process of reassessment (American Occupational Therapy Association [AOTA], 1994a). As the client transforms throughout the course of intervention, hopefully gaining skills, the occupational therapist makes changes to the intervention plan as necessary. Occupational therapy



K. Sladyk, K. Jacobs, & N. MacRae (Eds.).
*Occupational Therapy Essentials for Clinical Competence* (pp. 345-352).

assistants should be a part of such alterations under the supervision of an occupational therapist (AOTA, 1994a). The supervising occupational therapist maintains the discretion to determine the extent to which the occupational therapy assistant participates in various processes. The occupational therapist's responsibility is to establish that the occupational therapy assistant has the skills and knowledge necessary to complete such tasks (known as determining "service competency"). In some situations, the occupational therapy assistant may have more experience than the occupational therapist and would certainly be incorporated in the process as much as possible. In other situations, the occupational therapy assistant may make suggestions while the occupational therapist does a majority of the task. Each occupational therapist/occupational therapy assistant relationship is different. However, it is important that a sense of mutual respect be maintained at all times (Dillon, 2001).

# The Consultative Process

Although occupational therapy education is broad in scope, occupational therapy practitioners may not have all of the knowledge necessary to address every facet of a client's needs. It is the responsibility of the occupational therapy practitioner to acknowledge this and seek the expertise of other specialists when necessary (Table 31-1) (AOTA, 1994a). This may result in consultation or referral. Consultation is the exchange of ideas with an expert who is called on for professional advice (AOTA, 1994a). There are many niches within the field of occupational therapy in which an individual may specialize (Table 31-2). As a result, there may be times when the occupational therapy practitioner is called on as a consultant for his or her expertise.

The first step in the consultative process is to identify the need for consultation (West, 1973). For example, Tamari is a 12-year-old boy in a residential intervention facility for children with emotional and behavioral disturbances. He works with an occupational therapy assistant who is the activity director and is also exploring self-regulation strategies with Tamari that will prevent him from becoming assaultive when he is upset. The occupational therapy assistant has recognized that Tamari becomes frustrated when he is unable to communicate what he wants and needs to others, which is a result of significant speech impairment. There is no speech therapist at the residential facility.

Table 31-1. Specialists Outside of Occupational Therapy

| Professional | Roles and Responsibilities |
|---|---|
| Speech and language pathologists | Specialize in intervention of physical and/or cognitive disorders resulting in difficulty with verbal communication, speech, and language and feeding/swallowing disorders |
| Physical therapists | Concerned with the assessment and intervention of disabilities through physical means, including strength, endurance, coordination, balance, and mobility |
| Physicians (MD; DO) | Medical doctors or doctors of osteopathy |
| Pediatricians | Physicians who specialize in treating children |
| Neurologists | Physicians who specialize in treating disorders of the nervous system |
| Orthopedists | Physicians who specialize in treating disorders of the musculoskeletal systems |
| Psychiatrist (MD; DO) | A medical specialist whose primary goal is the intervention of mental illness through medication, psychotherapy, and psychosocial interventions |
| Social worker (LCSW; LICSW) | Involved in coordinating clients with agencies that will meet their psychosocial needs, psychotherapy, human services management. Social welfare policy analysis, community organizing, advocacy, teaching, and social science research are also areas of interest in social work |
| Nurses (LPN; RN) | Responsible for the care and safety of well and ill individuals in institutional and community settings |
| Physician assistants (PA); advanced practice registered nurses (APRN) | Medical professionals with advanced training who, under the supervision of an MD or DO, can assess, implement, and coordinate medical intervention |
| Teachers | Responsible for developing and implementing curriculum in a school setting to educate students |
| Therapeutic recreation | Professionals who promote health through engagement in recreational activity |
| Architects | Involved in the planning, designing, and oversight of a building's construction. Familiar with Americans With Disabilities Act (ADA) codes and universal design specifications for private and public structures |
| Administrators | Individuals or groups who assure implementation of policies and procedures in a health care organization |
| Dietician (RD; DTR) | An expert in food and nutrition who promotes good health through proper eating |

**Table 31-2. Specialties Within the Field of Occupational Therapy**

- Administration and management (including private practice subsection)
- Developmental disabilities
- Education (including faculty and fieldwork)
- Gerontology
- Hand therapists (not a special interest section)
- Home and community health (including home modification network)
- Mental health
- Physical disabilities (including hand subsection and driving/driver rehabilitation network)
- School systems
- Sensory integration
- Technology
- Work programs

Based on AOTA special interest sections

Once the client's needs have been identified, the next step is to locate a group, program, organization, or community that can provide the service (West, 1973). In the example of Tamari, the occupational therapy assistant locates a company that provides speech and language pathologists as consultants to residential intervention programs. The consultants should be experts in their field and comfortable with giving advice while having limited exposure to the client or environment (West).

When a suitable organization has been determined, the availability of both parties is then established. A consultation referral should be drawn up, including the services that will be provided by the consultant, as well as when and where the services will be provided. Referral is the practice of directing an initial request for service or changing the degree and direction of service (Agnes, 1999). The consultative referral provides a picture of the necessary case details to be sure the details of the consultative relationship are understood. The expectations of both parties should be clearly outlined to eliminate confusion. At this point, an agreement can been made for the arrangement of services (Jaffe & Epstein, 1992). Tamari's occupational therapy assistant shares his developmental history and the concerns of his grandmother, who is his primary caretaker outside of the program, with the speech and language pathologist assigned to the case. Services are arranged to be delivered on a weekly basis at the facility. Through this early process of information exchange, rapport is established, fostering a sense of trust and respect that can be helpful in the course of the partnership. Consultative relationships can take on a number of different dynamics. A partnership is the preferred and most cooperative type. However, there are times when the interaction may either be consultant lead or consultee lead (Jaffe & Epstein, 1992).

**American Occupational Therapy Association Statement of Occupational Therapy Referral**

The American Occupational Therapy Association, Inc (AOTA) presents this statement to clarify its official position in reference to referral. Referral is the practice of directing initial request for service or changing the degree and direction of service.

AOTA does not maintain that a referral is required for the provision of occupational therapy services. AOTA does maintain that occupational therapy practitioners must be aware of and adhere to the referral requirements of federal, state, and local governmental agencies, third party payers, regulatory and state agencies, and individual facilities.

Registered occupational therapists respond to requests for services whatever their sources. They may accept and enter cases at their own professional discretion and on the basis of their own level of competency.

Certified occupational therapy assistants, under the supervision of and in collaboration with registered occupational therapists and in compliance with AOTA'S Standards of Practice for Occupational Therapy (1994a) and Occupational Therapy Code of Ethics (1994b), acknowledge requests for services, whatever their source. Certified occupational therapy assistants do not accept and enter cases at their own professional discretion without the supervision and collaboration of registered occupational therapists. A certified occupational therapist assistant, in collaboration with a registered occupational therapist, may identify and screen individuals for potential referral. Both certified occupational therapy assistants and registered occupational therapists should educate current and potential referral sources about the process of initiating occupational therapy services.



Once the details of consultation have been identified in the referral, both parties can discuss expectations and a plan can be made for achieving the desired outcomes. Tamari's occupational therapy assistant and speech and language pathologist develop goals to assist him in slowing down his speech so others are able to understand him more easily. Throughout the course of the partnership, reassessment should take place to ensure that progress is being made toward the predetermined intervention goals. Tamari's speech and language pathologist monitors his progress every time they meet and also does formal reassessment on a regular basis.

When goals have been achieved or the client has made as much progress as he or she is able, the case may be closed. In our example, Tamari's discharge from the residential program at the age of 13 is the natural end point for his speech services. The consultative relationship between the occupational therapy assistant and speech and language pathologist does not end there, however, because a few weeks later, a resident is admitted who needs communication services that the occupational therapy assistant is unable to provide.

Throughout the consultative relationship, adequate communication is necessary to be sure that both parties are in agreement about the course of action. Consultation can take place in person or via telephone, e-mail, faxed documentation, and/or meetings. The consultant may be called in regard to a specific case for direct services, as with Tamari's case, but may also provide education to other team members or lend program development ideas (Dudgeon & Greenberg, 1998; Jaffe & Epstein, 1992; West, 1973).

It is helpful to be familiar with resources in the community that may be potential sites for referral or consultation. Maintaining positive relationships with various organizations can be helpful when setting up services for clients (AOTA, 1994a). Examples of such organizations include vocational rehabilitation programs, assisted living communities, psychiatric day programs, medical equipment vendors, and recreational organizations.

At times, the services that may be best for a client are not feasible due to socioeconomic, cultural, or psychosocial barriers. Once such a barrier has been identified, there may be community organizations that provide assistance in that specific area of need. For example, a client being discharged home from a rehabilitation hospital may not have the means to purchase a necessary piece of adaptive equipment. With the work of a diligent occupational therapy practitioner, the equipment could be provided by a community organization that does outreach to low-income individuals in need (AOTA, 1994a).

Consultation is a popular way to provide occupational therapy services, but it is not always easy. At times, there are barriers that can get in the way of services being delivered. This is especially true when working with larger programs, organizations, and communities rather than individuals. Often, the occupational therapy practitioner experiences a lack of power when working with these larger entities. Many people still do not know what occupational therapy is or the role occupational therapy practitioners may have in a specific setting. While this is an excellent opportunity for enlightening the public, it can also stand in the way of efficiency. Poor carry over can also have an impact, as well as issues when recommendations may conflict with the operating policies and procedures of the specific facility. At times, there may be a lack of resources in the program that may make it difficult to fulfill the recommendations made by the occupational therapy practitioner. Lastly, how the facility wants things done may conflict with the advice given by the occupational therapist. Ultimately, it is the program's decision as to whether and how to apply the knowledge they gain from this consultation. This application may not always be exactly how the occupational therapy practitioner envisioned it.

# Discharge

Discharge details are formulated from the time of initial evaluation and throughout intervention in order to set realistic goals and allow adequate time for all necessary services to be arranged (AOTA, 1994a). As with the entire intervention process, the client and his or her family members, caregivers, and significant others should participate in the discussion to determine the most feasible options for discharge.

Considerations should include where the client will go, whether the environment will support the client, environmental changes that may be necessary, what services will be needed, how the services will be paid for, and the establishment of home programs. From this conversation, a clear discharge plan can be determined that will best meet the needs of the client in the next phase of his or her life. For example, the discharge plan for a client in a rehabilitation setting may involve being discharged home in the care of a significant other. A referral for occupational therapy home care service will be sent to the client's insurance company. A planned home visit may reveal that a raised toilet seat will better support the client's ability to be independent. The seat is ordered from a vendor, paid for out of pocket by the client, and will be installed prior to the date of discharge. A home exercise program will be developed and taught to the client and other caregivers. On the day the client leaves the rehab facility, all services will be in place to ensure a smooth transition.

The life roles of the client must also be taken into account during transition planning. The occupational therapy practitioner, the client, and relevant caregivers must examine the client's level of independence and if he or she is capable of community living. It should be determined if the client is capable of self-care. Additionally, the occupational therapy practitioner, in collaboration with the client, must establish that he or she is able to perform the tasks necessary to engage in work, play, and leisure activities (AOTA, 1994a).

As part of the intervention team, the occupational therapy practitioner facilitates the transition process in cooperation with the client. The wishes of his or her family members and loved ones are also considered. At this time, it may be appropriate to refer to the services of other professionals within the field and outside of occupational therapy (see Tables 31-1 and 31-2). Referrals can be arranged to appropriate community agencies for psychosocial, cultural, and socioeconomic barriers and limitations that may need modification (AOTA, 1994a).

There are multiple factors that can determine where a client will go when he or she leaves the care of an occupational therapist or occupational therapy assistant. For example, did the client live alone prior to intervention? Does the client have a person who can serve as a caretaker or were they providing care to another person prior to the event that brought them to this level of care? What is the next functional level? Depending on the setting, there are many paths to choose from when determining the next step for a client. In mental health arenas, clients may move from an inpatient setting to a day program or to their home with wrap-around services. Wrap-around services are supports implemented to allow a client to live at home with as much independence as possible. Wrap-around services may include a phone number to call for peer or professional support. This line may be designated for crisis or non-crisis situations. Other wrap-around services include safe houses, case management, home visits, peer advocacy, and other programs designed to support an individual as needed. Following knee replacement surgery, a client may move from an acute inpatient hospital to a rehabilitation hospital to learn how to perform her occupations safely with a new joint. From the rehabilitation hospital, the client may go on to an assisted living facility, return to her home with regularly scheduled home care occupational therapy services, or return home with a relative.

## Termination of Services and Discharge Summary

A number of events may precipitate the transition process and termination of services. One event is an alteration in the client's abilities, such as achievement of all intervention goals. Also, the client may be discharged from one facility to be admitted to another. For example, a client may be discharged from an acute care setting after a certain time period, only to be admitted to a rehabilitation facility. Lastly, a change in environment may necessitate the transition process. An elementary school student receiving occupational therapy services eventually must move on to middle school. (AOTA, 1994a).

Ideally, discharge occurs when the client has achieved all intervention goals and is no longer in need of occupational therapy services. Sometimes this is not the case when the therapeutic relationship comes to an end. If a client is unable to achieve the goals after a pre-determined period of time, a third party payer may require that the services cease (AOTA, 1994a).

As with all forms of documentation, the structure of a discharge summary may be different depending on the particular setting. However, there are important pieces of information that should be included, as the note is a measure of the therapist's time with the client. Depending on the site, an occupational therapy assistant may be responsible for the entire process or contribute to the process under the supervision of an occupational therapist. In an outpatient or rehabilitative setting, a discharge letter should include the initial presenting problems and referral source. Baseline measurements of function and gains or losses should be noted (AOTA, 1994a). Assessments that were completed and their results should be documented. It is helpful to include the number of intervention sessions and a summary of the course and outcomes of intervention. The model of practice and frame of reference used is helpful information to include. Finally, recommendations should be made regarding areas of concern such as work, driving, level of supervision needed, safety, living placement, further therapy, or other programs that may be appropriate. Recommendations for additional future services such as follow up or re-evaluation should be included in the discharge summary (Figure 31-1) (AOTA, 1994a).

Summary of Intervention

Date:________________

Client name:________________

Reason for admission:________________

Number of sessions:________________

Status at initial evaluation:

Status at discharge:

Assessments:

Intervention Summary (including relevant model of practice and frame of reference):

Plan:

Therapist Signature:________________

**Figure 31-1.** Sample discharge summary.

## Summary

In addition to developing and conducting each occupational therapy session, the occupational therapy practitioner must simultaneously consider numerous other processes. The discharge plan is developed from the very first time the client interacts with the occupational therapy practitioner. Throughout the course of intervention, the occupational therapy practitioner engages in a conversation about discharge options with the client and his or her family members and significant others to determine the best course of action. During intervention sessions, the occupational therapy practitioner engages in monitoring and reassessment to determine that goals in the intervention plan are accurate and achievable. At some point, a consultation or referral may be necessary to meet all of the client's needs. Finally, a discharge summary of the course of intervention highlights the outcome of occupational therapy services.

## Student Self-Assessment

1. Write a consultation referral for Tamari's case.
2. Write a discharge summary about a client you have seen during an observation or fieldwork opportunity. Include all necessary information.
3. Read and summarize two evidence-based articles about occupational therapy and consultation, referral, monitoring, or discharge.

### Evidence-Based Research Chart

| Subjects | Measure/Method | Results |
|---|---|---|
| Clients on an orthopedic ward in one London teaching hospital with fractured femur heads | Interviews, interprofessional audits, and analysis of variance from interdisciplinary integrated care pathways | Integrated care pathways led to improved outcomes for the health care trust with little evidence suggesting that interprofessional relationships and communication were enhanced (Atwal & Caldwell, 2002). |
| 814 pediatric clients received inpatient rehabilitation during 1996 to 1998 | Retrospective cohort design using WeeFIM measures of self-care, mobility, and cognition. Amount of discipline-specific intervention and functional gains were analyzed | Largest gains were made by children with traumatic injuries who were older than age 7. Functional gains were related to the amount of discipline-specific intervention received (Chen, Heinemann, Bode, Granger, & Mallison, 2004). |
| Adult psychiatric clients | Case study of a program that teaches clients stress management and coping skills as inpatients and continues after discharge on an outpatient basis | Courtney & Escobedo, 1990 |
| 20 children aged 3 to 5, diagnosed with developmental delay | Between group design: One group of 10 children received group/consultation intervention from both an occupational therapist and physical therapist, while the other group of 10 children received individual intervention from the occupational therapist and physical therapist. Peabody Developmental Motor Scales, Vineland Adaptive Behavior Scales (Interview Edition), and the Central Institute for Deaf Preschool Performance Scale were used | Both intervention methods proved to be beneficial in this study. Results of the Peabody indicate that group/consultation and individual intervention helped to improve fine motor and gross motor skills in the participants ($p < 0.01$, both groups). The means for both study groups were compared for the Vineland. The results for communication, social skills, and motor skills were all significant with $p < 0.01$. The results for the daily living portion were not significant. The results of the Preschool Performance Scale showed that individual intervention was significant ($p < 0.01$), but the group/consultation intervention was not (Davies & Gavin, 1994). |
| 22 pairs of occupational therapist/occupational therapy assistant teams that work together in PA, OH, and WV | Qualitative study based on interview responses | Three major themes emerged as having an impact on the quality of the occupational therapist/occupational therapy assistant relationship (Dillon, 2001):<br>1. Effective two-way communication<br>2. The need for mutual respect<br>3. The importance of professionalism |
| 20 children aged 3 to 5 with fine motor, gross motor, and/or visual motor delays | Between group design: One group received only consultation from an occupational therapist while the other group received direct-indirect intervention from an occupational therapist. Direct-indirect intervention consisted of direct intervention with consultation when necessary. Goal Attainment Scaling was used to measure the attainment of goals apart from which intervention was being used | This study showed that both consultative intervention and direct-indirect intervention are beneficial. The consultation group met 22 out of 39 goals (56%), while the direct-indirect group met 28 out of 56 goals (50%). When compared with each other, no statistical difference ($p = 0.724$) was shown between the groups (Dreiling & Bundy, 2003). |

## Evidence-Based Research Chart (continued)

| Subjects | Measure/Method | Results |
|---|---|---|
| Seven boys and 3 girls aged 5 to 7 with a primary condition of developmental delay, behavior disorder, or learning disability, and poor sensory processing; four occupational therapists with at least 5 years of school-based experience and 2 years of sensory integration experience; nine classroom teachers in the public school system | Sample of convenience: Teacher/occupational therapist consultation pairs were set up and met once weekly for 60 minutes every week during the school year. During this meeting, one specific performance area was addressed and either a remedial or compensatory strategy was developed by the pair and used by the teacher in the following week. It was then documented if the goal was met. Intervention Documentation Form (IDF) developed with specific guidelines by the first author | Overall success of the consultation was 63%. It was found that 59% of the time, the pairs chose a compensatory strategy, and only 36% of the time, a remedial strategy was chosen (Kemmis & Dunn, 1996). |
| 86 children aged 12 to 70 months with a referral for cerebral palsy, medical conditions, and/or developmental delay.<br>Six physical therapists, five occupational therapists, and three speech and language pathologists comprised of the rehabilitation team | Sample of convenience: The rehabilitation team received initial training in behavioral and monthly consultations from the mental health specialists while providing services to the children and families involved. The families were given questionnaires and assessments to measure levels of stress, perceptions of the child, and the child's adaptive behavior. Bayley Scales of Infant Development, Vineland Adaptive Behavior Scales—Interview Edition/Survey, The Questionnaire on Resources and Stress—Short Form (QRS), and the Child Behavior Checklist (CBCL) for ages 2 to 3 were used at baseline, and at least once again at 6 month or 1 year follow-up, with the exception of the Bayley, which was only used during baseline | This consultation model proved to be effective in some ways. Scores for the Vineland significantly improved ($p < 0.01$) from baseline to 1-year follow-up. No significant change ($p = 0.99$) for CBCL at 1 year. One part of QRS (respondent attitudes) showed significance ($p < 0.05$) at one-year follow-up, while the other two parts (client problems [$p = 0.79$] and family problems [$p = 0.75$]) did not (McDermott et al., 2002). |
| Timeline of legislative mandates for vocational rehabilitation | Discussion of impact on occupational therapy | Presents an example of a successful prevocation program for students with disabilities (Mitchell, Rourk, & Schwarz, 1989). |
| Metanalysis of studies published after 1980, which include a sample of participants with Parkinson's disease who were treated within the scope of occupational therapy with adequate quantitative data to determine effect size with an experimental or quasi-experimental design | Studies were coded by the level of evidence, year of publication, purpose of study, research design type, outcome measures, mean age of subjects, progression of Parkinson's, and the number of participants overall and in intervention and control groups | The outcomes of persons with Parkinson's disease suggest small-to-moderate positive effects of occupational therapy-related interventions (Murphy & Tickle-Degnen, 2001). |

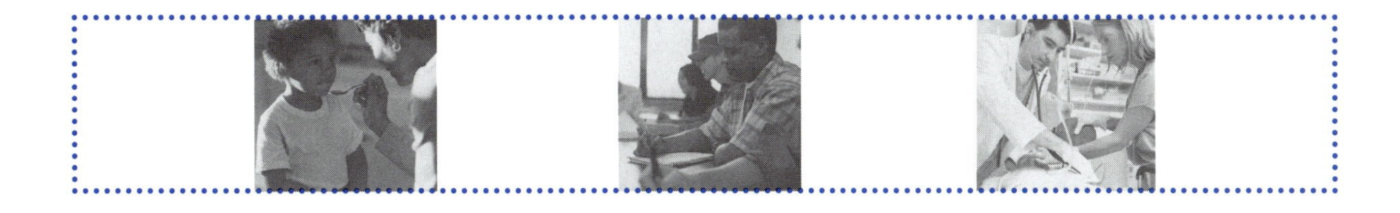

# References


Agnes, M. (Ed.). (1999). *Webster's new world college dictionary* (4th ed.). New York, NY: Macmillan.

American Occupational Therapy Association. (1994a). Standards of practice for occupational therapy. *American Journal of Occupational Therapy, 48*, 1039-1043.

American Occupational Therapy Association (1994b). Occupational Therapy Code of Ethics. *American Journal of Occupational Therapy, 48*, 1037-1038.

American Occupational Therapy Association (1994c). Statement of occupational therapy referral. *American Journal of Occupational Therapy, 48*(11), 1034.

Atwal, A., & Caldwell, K. (2002). Do multidisciplinary integrated care pathways improve interprofessional collaboration? *Scandinavian Journal of Caring Sciences, 16*(4), 360-367.

Chen, C. C., Heinemann, A. W., Bode, R. K., Granger, C. V., & Mallison, T. (2004). Impact of pediatric rehabilitation services on children's functional outcomes. *American Journal of Occupational Therapy, 58*(1), 44-53.

Courtney, C., & Escobedo, B. (1990). A stress management program: Inpatient-to-outpatient continuity. *American Journal of Occupational Therapy, 44*(4), 306-310.

Davies, P., & Gavin., W. (1994). Comparison of individual and group/consultation treatment methods for preschool children with developmental delays. *American Journal of Occupational Therapy, 48*(2), 155-161.

Dillon, T. H. (2001). Practitioner perspectives: Effective intraprofessional relationships in occupational therapy. *Occupational Therapy in Health Care, 14*(3/4), 1-15.

Dreiling, D., & Bundy, A. (2003). A comparison of consultative model and direct-indirect intervention with preschoolers. *American Journal of Occupational Therapy, 57*(5), 566-569.

Dudgeon, B. J., & Greenberg, S. L. (1998). Preparing students for consultation, roles, and systems. *American Journal of Occupational Therapy, 52*(10), 801-809.

Jaffe, E. G., & Epstein, C. F. (Eds.). (1992). *Occupational therapy consultation: Theory, principles and practice*. St. Louis, MO: Mosby.

Kemmis, B., & Dunn, W. (1996). Collaborative consultation: The efficacy of remedial and compensatory interventions in school. *American Journal of Occupational Therapy, 50*(9), 709-717.

McDermott, S., Nagle, R. J., Wright, H., Swann, S. S., Leonhardt, T., & Wuori, D. (2002). Consultation in pediatric rehabilitation for behaviour problems in young children with cerebral palsy and/or developmental delay. *Pediatric Rehabilitation, 5*(2), 99-106.

Mitchell, M., Rourk, J. D., & Schwarz, J. (1989). A team approach to vocational services. *American Journal of Occupational Therapy, 43*(6), 378-383.

Murphy, S., & Tickle-Degnen, L. (2001). The effectiveness of occupational therapy-related treatments for persons with parkinson's disease: A meta-analytic review. *American Journal of Occupational Therapy, 55*(4), 385-392.

West, W. (1973). Principles and process of consultation. In L. Llorens (Ed.), *Consultation in the community: Occupational therapy in child health* (pp. 51-58). Dubuque, IA: Kendall/Hunt Publishing Company.

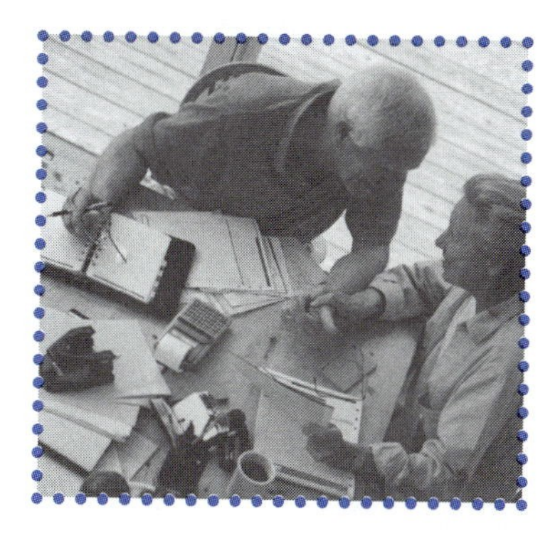

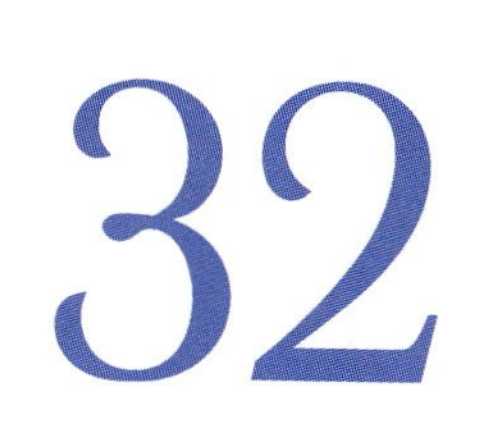

# 32

# Data Collection and Documentation

Nancy MacRae, MS, OTR/L, FAOTA and William R. Croninger, MA, OTR/L

**ACOTE Standards Explored in This Chapter**

B.5.26, 5.28

**Key Terms**

| | |
|---|---|
| DAP format | FIP format |
| Discontinuation note | SOAP note format |

## Introduction

Documentation is an important part of the communication process in occupational therapy and serves a number of goals:

- Documentation provides a record of interventions and a client's reaction to those interventions. Documentation is an important means to verify that an intervention session has occurred. It is also crucial for stating the goals of intervention, listing baseline data, a description of the plan and the implementation, and a detailing of the outcomes. Complete documentation provides a view of intervention and can be used for retrospective research, comparing the course and outcomes of similar cases.
- Documentation promotes communication across the disciplines charged with a client's care. Occupational therapy documentation provides a tool for communicating with other disciplines. It notifies the referring physician about the progress of intervention and other disciplines about what goals are being pursued and what specific techniques and media are being used. Reinforcement of these can occur in other disciplines' sessions as a way to promote the transfer of learning and/or the ability to generalize. Documentation can also specify and/or validate the times a splint or adaptive device needs to be worn and/or used.
- Documentation provides a record of care and is thus a legal document that can and often is used in court. If an intervention session is not documented, it did not occur from the viewpoint of the reimbursor, the administration, and the legal system. Since a client note is part of the client record, it is also a legal document. Should a client be involved in a legal case and need practitioner testimony, documentation is essential for such testimony to be reliable. As the time span between intervention and a legal case may be long, documentation also provides a memory reference to the testifying practitioner.
- Documentation is part of the clinical reasoning process. It can also be fodder for prospective research, providing data for the success or failure of certain intervention approaches. Additionally, it helps the therapist recall what transpired during the last session, can promote reflection on the course of intervention, and can encourage adaptations to sessions. Thus, client notes can be a part of professional growth in improving the clarity of what is written, in assessing the intervention's effectiveness, and in refining clinical reasoning skills.



K. Sladyk, K. Jacobs, & N. MacRae (Eds.).
*Occupational Therapy Essentials for Clinical Competence* (pp. 353-360).

The documentation process is a reflection of the clinical reasoning process. It is represented by a circular diagram (Figure 32-1). During the occupational therapy process, there are various needs for documentation.

An initial note documents the first meeting and interview of a client. The progress note details the continuing and changing status of a client. A discontinuation note summarizes the course of intervention, the model of practice, the frames of reference, strategies and/or activities used, the participation of the client, outcomes realized, and recommendations for the future. The latter kind of documentation becomes particularly important to the next practitioner. A discontinuation note needs to provide a history of intervention with the client, detailing what has occurred and providing recommendations for future intervention to make for a smooth transition for continuing therapy.

Documentation can take a number of other forms depending on the setting, such as an educational, business, or industrial setting and area of practice (e.g., industrial rehabilitation and ergonomics). The Individual Educational Plan (IEP) is found in an educational setting along with a report written to a parent, teacher, special education administrator, principal, superintendent, etc. In the area of industrial rehabilitation and ergonomics, documentation can take other forms, such as a written job site analysis. In a community setting, it will often take the form of a report of findings to include recommendations. In any context, a commonality is that all documentation, when done properly, promotes and justifies the value of occupational therapy.

# The "Language" of Documentation

Formats may vary in different settings and practice areas, but components of good documentation remain the same: it needs to be clear, accurate, relevant, and list exceptions. Additionally, documentation should be succinct, written simply and in an active voice. The writer needs to consider the audience for whom a document is being written. Particularly, when written for nonmedically trained readers, documentation needs to make sense for the designated readers, and it must contain specificity in goals and directions to make it useful. Thus, an official client note in a client chart would likely differ from a progress note sent home to a parent or family member. The content might be similar, but the way it is expressed would differ.

- *Example of note in chart*: Rose was able to endure a 20-minute session in the kitchen. She demonstrated a 15 degree increase in shoulder extension, allowing her to access items in cabinets above eye level. She was able to gather supplies to make a light lunch.
- *Example of note sent to family*: Rose is showing improvement in her ability to independently prepare a light lunch for herself.

Another example would be a home program written for an outpatient client with deficits in fine motor control of the hand. The program could include suggestions for using every day activities (folding clothes, washing and drying dishes) to help improve functional use.

# Process of Documentation

Documentation could be thought of as taking three general forms: initial notes, intervention notes, and discontinuation notes such as discharge, reports, or letters to physicians.

## Basics

Basics need to be included in any client note. Many of them are common sense, but reminders are needed to ensure inclusion. The basics are as follows:

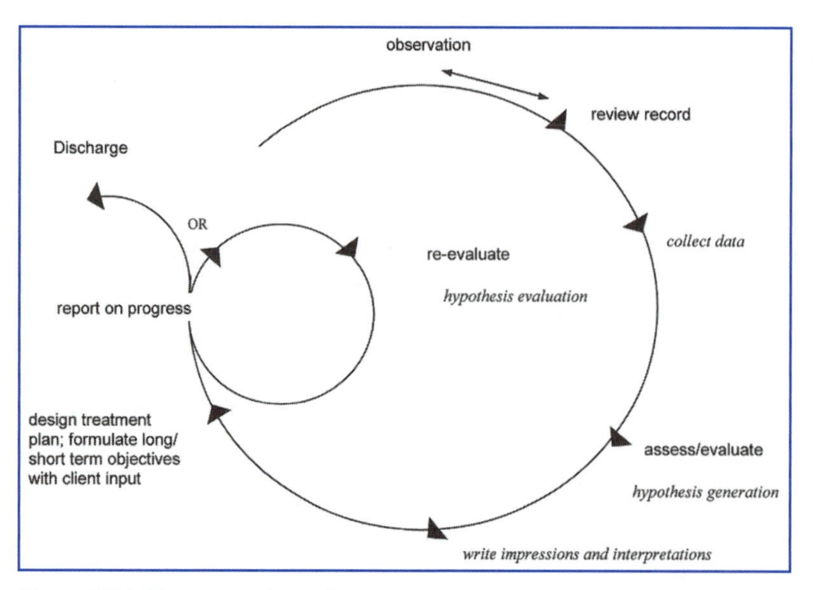


**Figure 32-1.** The occupational therapy process.

- Name of client
- Date of session
- Diagnoses of concern for intervention
- How goals have been addressed, with progress or difficulty noted
- Remember to include any unusual happenings during the session
- Use ink (with appropriate color when designated by site) when writing notes
- Remember to sign name with appropriate initials included
- Most sites do not allow erasures. If you need to correct an error, draw a single line through the mistake and write the correction above, then initial the correction.
- Write note as soon after the session as possible
- Be accurate, clear, and relevant

## Initial Notes

Initial notes are essentially evaluation notes with the specific form varying between entities: general medical, mental health, home health, public education, etc. The initial documentation process can be divided into three stages: actions prior to meeting the client, the client interview, and actions following the interview.

### Actions Prior to Meeting the Client

Data collection begins prior to the client interview. Table 32-1 provides an overview of what and where a therapist working in an acute care physical disabilities setting would look to gather data during an initial assessment. The clinician begins by examining medical records, reports of previous assessments, results of educational testing, and other pertinent documents. At this stage, the clinician needs to form a mental "picture" of the client and an idea of what the clinician is being asked to do.

- Who is the referral agent (a physician, a parent, a classroom teacher, another therapist)?
- What is being asked of the therapist (a splint, a safety evaluation, a fine motor writing evaluation)?
- Using the framework (American Occupational Therapy Association [AOTA], 2008), the clinician gathers data related to the individual's highest level of performance on each of the domains: activities of daily living/instrumental activities of daily living, education/work, play/leisure, and social participation.
    - If a problem exists, the clinician then looks for any information on the client's performance skills or performance patterns.
    - The clinician also looks for information on the client's contexts and any pertinent client factors.

**Table 32-1. Chart Review**

| Criteria | Components |
|---|---|
| Basic information to be retrieved from a chart review | • Date of onset<br>• Admitting diagnosis<br>• Medical history (pertinent medical problems, procedures, pre-existing conditions that may affect evaluation and/or intervention<br>• Current medical intervention (medications, procedures, rehabilitation efforts, and progress)<br>• Current medical status (client getting better/deteriorating, intervention plan, discharge plan, results of recent tests, DNR status, etc.; information can be found in nursing and medical notes)<br>• Personal information (age, marital status, family configuration, residence, work history, financial information)<br>• Medication lists (will any meds affect intervention?) |
| Components pertinent to occupational therapy (where you'll find the information) | • Medical section (physician notes, pertinent past medical history, general information on social situation, response to intervention, course of intervention, referrals to specialists, upcoming surgeries/procedures, precautions, complications during acute phase that might affect recovery such as infection, hydrocephalus, respiratory distress, or seizures)<br>• Nursing section (day-to-day status, response to intervention/disability, often report response to splinting, positioning, ADL, and mobility performances)<br>• Test section (lab reports, X-ray, CT scan, MRI)<br>• Medication lists (sometimes grouped in this section are vital signs, weights, calorie counts)<br>• Professionals section (PT, ST, SW, TR, Neuropsych, VR evaluations, and progress notes); some institutions have continuous problem-oriented records, and these reports are within the body of the medical section |

Reprinted with permission from York, C. D., & MacRae, N. (1993). Class handout. Biddeford, ME: Occupational Therapy Department, University of New England.

- The clinician continues to review documents, looking for information about diagnoses, any precautions, the client's support systems, and the suspected disposition of the client (return to home, discharge to skilled nursing facility, unknown).
- An experienced clinician will also look for information concerning the client's history, interests, experiences, etc. Although not absolutely necessary, sharing this information with the client often helps build rapport and trust during the next stage.

### The Client Interview

Two "interviews" take place during the first meeting. The clinician is interviewing and assessing the client. At the same time, the client is conducting a silent interview, determining whether the clinician is competent, able to be trusted, and whether the client can or even wants to work with the therapist. Not all clients will want to work with you. It may be pain, nausea, fear, or simply a mismatch of personalities. However, in those first few minutes, the weight is on the clinician to demonstrate competency and approachability and develop trust.

Data collection in the client interview begins "at the door," with the therapist noting performance factors such as posture, balance, body symmetry, eye contact, bilateral upper extremity use, and cognition. Following the protocol of the hosting agency, the therapist records the client's responses to questions and assessments related to occupational therapy domains. Of equal importance is the client's perception of strengths, problems, and his or her goals. Prior to leaving the client, the therapist usually discusses findings and any anticipated occupational therapy interventions. In other settings, the therapist may not discuss the findings with the involved individual as the "client" may be a disability insurance company, an organization such as a school system, or another professional.

### Actions Following the Interview

The therapist now has a clear view of the reasons for referral, the desired outcomes, the expected outcomes, as well as client strengths and problem areas. The therapist must now summarize findings, develop a list of strengths and problem areas, and develop appropriate goals and activities, that will help the client achieve those goals and collaboratively determine goals and activities that meet the client's needs.

## Progress Notes

Usually, each intervention session requires a progress note, also called a "contact" note. It is much shorter than the initial note and commonly details only the date, duration, therapeutic activities used, client reactions, and plan of the next intervention.

## Discontinuation Notes

Known also as "discharge notes," this type of note represents a melding of both the initial and progress note. Included is the background information that provides an overview of the reason for referral as well as expected outcomes. Next, a synopsis of problem areas and goals, along with progress, is detailed. The therapist ends by noting any ongoing problems and recommendations for addressing them.

# Documentation Formats

Initial, progress, and discontinuation are types of documentation, but there are other documentation formats. The types of notes occur across all areas of specialization with formats simply providing different methods of organizing data.

## SOAP

A universally accepted format that organizes findings from each of the note types is the SOAP or problem-oriented format (Weed, 1969) for the Problem-Oriented Medical Record system (Borcherding, 2000). The SOAP format has become the preferred format in many facilities (Sames, 2005).

This format is composed of the following four sections, each with specific areas that need to be addressed and included to have a complete document:

- "S" or subjective portion includes the reason for referral and any of the following information given to the practitioner by the client or a designated member of the family.
  - History, including prior level of functioning
  - Lifestyle or home situation
  - Emotions or attitudes
  - Client's goals
  - Client's complaints
  - Client's response to intervention
  - Any other information relevant to case or present condition(s)
- "O" or objective portion includes measurable or observable information.
  - Objective measurements or observations
  - Part of intervention already given to client
  - Relevant client history taken from medical charts (may be setting dependent)
- "A" or assessment portion includes five sections that together provide the reader with the practitioner's clinical reasoning for goals and intervention. These sections are as follows:
  1. *Assets*: The strengths of the client, any areas without normal limits. This is an incredibly important

section as the identification of client strengths facilitates viewing the client as a whole person, not just as one with problems and deficits. Strengths can then be used to assist in intervention.

2. *Problem list*: Listing of areas of deficit for occupational performance with a goal to address prioritized problem areas.
3. *Long-term goals*: Goals that address the functional outcome of the client, worded "in order to..."
4. *Short-term goals*: Behavioral objectives with a listing of specific methods and activities employed.
5. *Summary of intervention*: Impressions with a succinct correlation between all of the parts; the reader should be able to determine quickly what the course of intervention has been and what outcomes have been achieved just by reading the summary.

- "P" or plan for the future; includes a number of items:
  - Frequency and amount of time client needs to be seen by the occupational therapist
  - Location of intervention session
  - Intervention progression
  - Client and family education
  - Equipment needs and equipment ordered/sold to client
  - Plans for future assessment or reassessment
  - Plans for discharge
  - Referral to other services

The original SOAP format includes goals in the "A" section; other authors (Kettenbach, 2004; Sames, 2005) now place goals in the "P" section.

## Description, Assessment, Plan and Findings, Interpretation, Plan

These other forms vary somewhat from the SOAP version, but they all incorporate the skeletal underpinnings of the SOAP version. The DAP notes combine the subjective and objective portions into the "D" portion or the description of the client. The "A" section is the assessment or summary portion, while the "P" part is for the plan. A variation of this type of note is the FIP note, standing for findings (both subjective and objective), interpretation (similar to the summary or assessment), and plan.

## Individualized Educational Plan

The IEP is a standardized format that documents the information determined at an IEP meeting for a specific student. The IEP is a formal process to plan what services and programs are needed for the child to meet educational goals. Guidelines of Individuals with Disabilities Education Act (IDEA) (U.S. Department of Justice, 2005) establish the format. Elements of an IEP are as follows (Case-Smith, Roger, & Johnson, 2004):

- Present levels of educational performance
- Annual goals and short-term objectives (usually 3 months in length)
- Special education and related services
- Explanation of nonparticipation
- Participation in assessments
- Dates, frequency, location, and duration of services
- Transition services—begin at age 14 and annual after that
- Measuring and reporting student progress

Areas of focus in schools include movement-based participation, meal or snack-time, school-based self-care, classroom-based fine motor activities, and vision in the classroom (K. Loukas, personal communication, June 15, 2006). IDEA requires evaluations every 3 years, while IEP goals are set annually, usually meeting four times a year to check on the status of children in reaching outcomes of intervention. An example of an IEP is found in Appendix E.

## Checklists

This format allows for a quick recording of a client's problems and progress using preselected categories. The organization makes it easy for a second therapist to "step in" if the primary therapist is not available. There are, however, disadvantages in that often there is little room to record observations. Some checklists do not allow the therapist to add problems to the prescribed list (Sames, 2005) (Table 32-2).

**Table 32-2. Sample Checklist Format**

| Date/Intervention | 9/1 | 9/2 | 9/3 |
|---|---|---|---|
| Minutes taken to complete dressing (upper and lower body) | 30 | 28 | 27 |
| Verbal cues needed to don shoes | 10 | 9 | 8 |

## Narrative

As implied, this format has data written directly into the client record, as soon after intervention as possible. Narrative notes are commonly free-form as there is no universally accepted structure or model for writing them. Although preferred by many therapists, the result is all too often a wordy and poorly organized note. The lack of organization makes it extremely hard for a therapist unfamiliar with the client to step in and provide therapy. It is time consuming and often inefficient to trace back through prior notes in an effort to learn of the client's problems, progress, and clinician's goals. If the organizational sequence provided by the SOAP note structure is used as a guide, this format can be informative and effective.

## Professional Letters

Letters are also often required in the occupational therapy process. The practitioner may need to write a letter to a physician, documenting the progress of a client or requesting an extension of a prescription for continued therapy. A letter of referral to a professional colleague may be considered good protocol for getting the kind of information requested. Providing the specifics and detailing concerns help the other professional do a better and more thorough job. A letter may be necessary to a reimbursing agency to document the reasons for a piece of adapted equipment. Photographs of a client with that specified piece of adapted equipment can graphically help demonstrate the difference that piece of equipment will make in the client's life (Figure 32-2). Another reason for a professional letter may be to ask for a donation or to thank a donor.

Letters of reference are requested by new professionals and colleagues who are changing practice sites or jobs or applying for licensure. Being able to clearly and accurately reflect on a colleague's job performance provides the prospective hiring agency the information needed to make a good decision. Elements that should be included are the dates you have worked with the colleague and/or student, examples of work with clients and team members, personal characteristics, ethical behavior, potential for growth and strengths, and areas in need of improvement in job performance. A grading of your endorsement or lack of it should end the letter.

## Medical Abbreviations

Knowing how information should be reported in a medical record is as important as knowing what information to include. Historically, health care professionals have used medical abbreviations as a means to shorten the length of time spent in note writing while maintaining thorough

7 August 2006

To: Eleanor Small, D.O.
Hand Surgical Associates
Anywhere, USA

From: Daniel Williams, OTR/L
Regional Hospital
Anywhere, USA

Re: Splint fabrication for Rita Newman

Mrs. Newman was seen in occupational therapy on this date following her recent skiing accident in which she injured the ulnar collateral ligament of her dominant hand. Per your order, a thumb-based, carpo-metacarpal (CMC) immobilization splint was fabricated. The client was provided with written wear and care information.

She was able to perform a simulated housekeeping task with report that the splint fit well and that she experienced a decrease in pain while performing these activities.

I will continue to monitor her comfort and document decrease in pain via telephone for one month. She has been advised to call with any incidence of increased pain or loss in motion. For your review, we have enclosed a picture of the splint that you ordered.

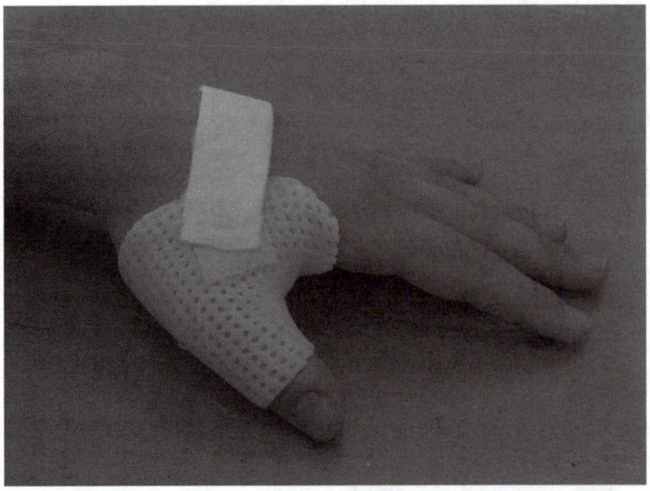

**Figure 32-2.** Sample physician's letter.

patient care records. However, there is no universally accepted set of medical abbreviations, thus abbreviations accepted at one facility may not be accepted by another. More importantly, an abbreviation may not have the same meaning at different facilities. In 2001, the Joint Commission on Accreditation of Healthcare Organizations (JCAHO) issued an alert related to dangerous medical abbreviations. This was followed in 2005 by the creation of a "Do NOT Use" list (JCAHO). The use of medical abbreviations by health care professionals continues to be both common and controversial. It is, therefore, imperative that clinicians use only the abbreviations accepted at their work site.

## Goal Writing

Effective goal writing is a vital part of documentation. It is also one of the more difficult skills for the new clinician to perfect. Occupational therapy values a collaborative relationship between therapist and client. Therefore, the goals should be developed by the client and therapist working together. Goals help prioritize intervention, measure the effectiveness of intervention, and assist with keeping health care costs in line.

Goals are composed of a number of components. An easy way to understand the components is by use of an "A-B-C-D" approach (Kettenbach, 1990).

- A represents who or the audience and is always client oriented.
- B represents the what or the functional behavior; action words need to be used in this portion of the goal.
- C represents the how, with a description of the situation and the circumstances under which the behavior will be accomplished.
- D is represented by some form of measurement, such as percentage, number, or time (i.e., how will the outcome be measured).

An example of each portion of a goal follows:

- Observing hip precautions 100%, the client will don her socks using a sock-aide within two intervention sessions.
- Observing hip precautions 100% <measurement>, the client <who> will don her socks <what> using a sock-aide <how> within two intervention sessions.

Another helpful acronym for effective goal writing is RUMBA, a goal-writing method developed by the AOTA in the 1970s (Sames, 2005):

- *Relevant*: The goal must be relevant to the client.
- *Understandable*: The goal must be easily understood.
- *Measurable*: The goal must be able to be measured—you must be able to know when and how well the goal has been met.
- *Behavioral*: The goal must be observable.
- *Achievable*: The goal must be able to be accomplished by the client.

If these descriptors are used as references by the goal writer, goals have a much better chance of being clear and concise.

## Functional Outcomes

Outcomes identify what the client will be able to do functionally as a result of the intervention. They have resulted from the managed care push in our health care system, with managed care companies scrutinizing costs to make sure they are receiving value for their expenditures. Outcomes also notify the third-party reimbursor of the functional reason behind the goal formation. More importantly, particularly to reflect the framework (AOTA, 2008), a functional outcome should be seen as contributing to an improved occupational performance that promotes social participation by the client. This exemplifies a shift from focusing on improved strength or range of motion, or components, as the goal of intervention to a more top-down, holistic approach that aims for improved occupational performance. An example of a functional outcome is improved upper extremity functioning to assist in the independence in the activity of daily living of dressing.

## Administrative Outcomes

Documentation of clients' functional outcomes can also be used to gather administrative outcome data to support research and quality assurance activities of the department.

## Occupational Therapist/ Occupational Therapy Assistant Differentiation

Occupational therapy assistants collaborate with occupational therapists throughout the occupational therapy process, from screening and evaluation to discontinuation of services. Assistance is always done under the supervision of the occupational therapist. The same is true of documentation. Dependent on site, the occupational therapy assistant may contribute to the documentation note or may write the entire note. If the latter is the case, it is most often a progress note and an occupational therapist's signature is usually required by reimbursors. Since both practitioners contribute to the documentation process, both need to understand what is entailed in the process and how to do it effectively and efficiently.

## Summary

For many practitioners, new and experienced, being able to write well-organized and concise documentation is a major challenge. Well-crafted assessments and notes help the practitioner organize, deliver, assess, and demonstrate occupation-centered interventions. This skill is at the core of clinical reasoning. Effective documentation enhances client care and protects both the practitioner and agency should litigation occur. Finally, effective documentation allows a "trail" of thinking and actions that can be later analyzed to demonstrate the efficacy of the profession by research that supports our evidence-based practices. The rewards, therefore, are worth the effort needed to learn this skill.

## Student Self-Assessment

1. Place the following into its proper location in the SOAP note:
   - Activities to include active assistive range of motion (AAROM) and activities of daily living concentrating on dressing.
   - AROM R UE 0-150 flexion.
   - Using a rolling walker, was close supervision from bed to bathroom and return.
   - Nursing reports patient spent a "restless night."
   - Client seen x 30 minutes in room to concentrate on lower body dressing.
   - Ability to perform dressing independently continues to be decreased secondary to inability to remember sequence.
   - "I hate this."
   - With distant supervision, patient will be able to gather and don all clothing (I) within 20 minutes.
   - Client has been seen in occupational therapy x 20 since admission and has met all goals, no further occupational therapy intervention warranted at this time.
2. Reorganize and reformat the following narrative note, shortening it while being concise and thorough. Use approved abbreviations and medical terminology where appropriate.
   "Mr. Jones is a 35-year-old, married male who was involved in a motor vehicle accident 24 hours ago. He is complaining of quite a bit of pain in both legs. His car was struck in the driver's side. He broke his left leg and has quite a few bruises and abrasions on the right. He broke his left arm. He has some facial cuts and a concussion. I saw him in his room for about 30 minutes to start the evaluation, but he did not know where he was or what day it was. He does remember his name and what happened to him. I think my goals are to make him independent in dressing by discharge. He should also be independent in mobility during activities of daily living using that walker physical therapy provided. He can only put as much pressure on the left leg so as to not break an eggshell at this time. The nurse also said he was in a lot of pain. He rates it as an 8 on a scale of 10. In the memory assessment, he can remember 5 numbers forward and 3 numbers backwards. I think he will eventually be able to go home, but I'm not sure if he will need rehab first."
3. From the scenario above, create two properly formatted goals for Mr. Jones.
4. Write a letter to the attending physician assuming goals have been met and that Mr. Jones is ready for discontinuation from occupational services.

## Electronic Resource

- For further clarification of documentation for occupational therapy: www.aota.org/pubs/otp/1997-2007/columns/capitalbriefing/2004/cb-071204.aspx

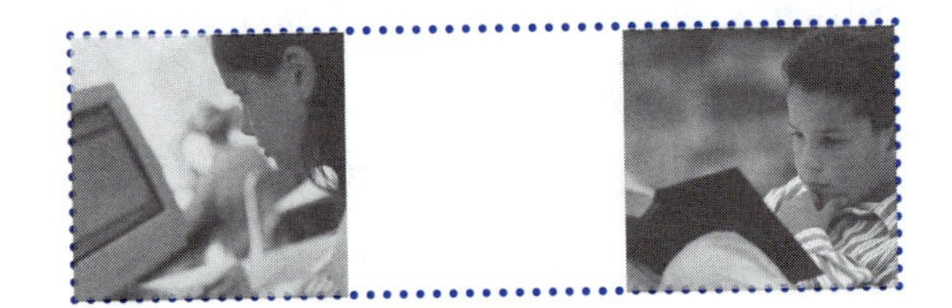

## References


American Occupational Therapy Association. (2008). Occupational therapy practice framework: Domain and process, second edition. *American Journal of Occupational Therapy, 62*, 625-683.

Borcherding, S. (2000). *Documentation manual for writing soap notes in occupational therapy.* Thorofare, NJ: SLACK Incorporated.

Case-Smith, J., Roger, J., & Johnson, J. (2004). School-based occupational therapy. In J. Case-Smith (Ed.), *OT for children* (5th ed., pp. 758-709). St. Louis, MO: Elsevier Mosby.

Joint Commission on Accreditation of Health Care Organizations. (2005). Do not use list. Retrieved July 13, 2006, from http://www.jointcommission.org/PatientSafety/DoNotUseList

Kettenbach, G. (1990). *Writing S.O.A.P. notes.* Philadelphia, PA: F.A.Davis Company.

Kettenbach, G. (2004). *Writing SOAP notes: With patient/client management formats* (3rd ed.). Philadelphia, PA: F.A. Davis.

Sames, K. (2005). *Documenting occupational therapy practice.* Upper Saddle River, NJ: Prentice Hall.

U.S. Department of Justice. (2005). A guide to disability rights laws. Retrieved July 13, 2006, from http://www.usdoj.gov/crt/ada/cguide.pdf

Weed, L. L. (1969). *Medical records, medical education and patient care: The problem-oriented record as a basic tool.* Cleveland, OH: Case Western Reserve University Press.

York, C. D., & MacRae, N. (1993). Class handout. Biddeford, ME: Occupational Therapy Department, University of New England.

# Section VI
## Context of Service Delivery

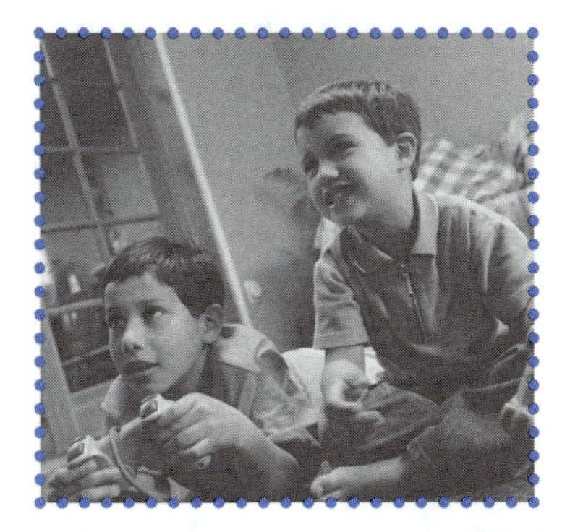

# Changes and Trends in Education Research and Practice

*Jeffrey L. Crabtree, MS, OTD, FAOTA*

**ACOTE Standards Explored in This Chapter**

B.7.1-7.2

**Key Terms**

Client-centered practice
Evidence-based occupational therapy
Moral treatment
Neuroscience-based treatment
Technology

## Introduction

The purpose of this chapter is to discuss some of the significant changes or trends within the profession and the impact of demographic changes and technology.

Many would agree the world, society, the occupational therapy profession—virtually everything—changes. On the other hand, few would agree whether a particular change was good or would agree on the meaning of that change. The concept of a trend is no more objective. Statistically, we know it takes several data points to establish a trend. For example, in the case of consumer spending, when one has data on a dozen holiday seasons of consumer spending, one can estimate a trend. But it is quite another thing to understand why the trend line went in one direction or another, whether the trend will continue, or whether any cause-effect relationship between the trend and forces can be established. The field of occupational therapy is no different. We see changes and we have glimpses of what are likely trends, but it is still quite difficult to understand the forces behind those trends or to predict whether the trends will continue. Consequently, the changes and trends discussed here are a combination of the author's personal biases and literature that supports those biases.

## A Professional Perspective

In this section, select changes and trends occurring in occupational therapy within the United States, within other Western English-speaking countries, and—to a lesser extent—within other countries are reviewed. To do this, the author focused on selected American Occupational Therapy Association (AOTA) documents and English-speaking journals. In most cases, the journals are instruments of national professional associations. Consequently, these journals contain not only scholarly works but also information about the professional association and its members.

It is important to keep in mind that, as the world shrinks because of technology such as the Internet, traditional distinctions between national and international ideas become blurred. So in the strict sense of the word, and from an American perspective, the Canadian, British, and Australian



K. Sladyk, K. Jacobs, & N. MacRae (Eds.).
*Occupational Therapy Essentials for Clinical Competence* (pp. 363-374).

journals of occupational therapy could be considered foreign or international journals, yet a search of English-speaking literature on a particular topic would likely yield pertinent articles in at least one if not all occupational therapy journals from Canada to Australia. These journals publish authors from a variety of countries, and the studies and evolving ideas published in these journals have become an integral part of Americans' notions of occupational therapy.

Two significant examples show the international quality of our current domestic notions about effective occupational therapy. One is the concept of client-centered practice (Canadian Association of Occupational Therapists [CAOT], 1997; Law, Baptiste, & Mills, 1995). In addition to many articles published in the *Canadian Journal of Occupational Therapy* (the developers of this concept are Canadian), client-centered practice has been discussed in the *Indian Journal of Occupational Therapy* (Morgan, Kelkar, & Vyas, 2002), the *British Journal of Occupational Therapy* (Unsworth, 2004), the *Scandinavian Journal of Occupational Therapy* (Hammell, 1995), *Occupational Therapy International* (Rigby, Ryan, From, Walczak, & Jutai, 1996), *Scandinavian Journal of Occupational Therapy* (Mckinnon, 2000), and the *American Journal of Occupational Therapy* (*AJOT*) (Tickle-Degnen, 2002), just to cite one example from each of these journals.

The other example is a measure called the Canadian Occupational Therapy Measure (COPM) (Law et al., 1998). This measure, too, was originated by Canadian occupational therapists, but the measure has been used and statistically verified in a variety of countries, and the results of the research have been published in the *British Journal of Occupational Therapy* (Warren, 2002), the *Scandinavian Journal of Occupational Therapy* (Wressle, Samuelsson, & Henriksson, 1999), *Occupational Therapy International* (Chen, 2002), *Occupational Therapy in Mental Health* (Boyer, Hachey, & Mercier, 2000), the *Australian Occupational Therapy Journal* (Farnworth, 2003), *World Federation of Occupational Therapists Bulletin* (Jansa, Sicherl, Angleitner, & Law, 2004), and *AJOT* (Simmons, Crepeau, & White, 2000) to name a few.

# Change and Trends Within Occupational Therapy in the United States

To put into perspective the changes and trends that have led to what we understand as occupational therapy today, it will be useful to briefly describe the social and medical context of the turn of the 20th century when occupational therapy was a fledgling profession (see Chapter 3). By the late 1800s, the Civil War and reconstruction periods were over. "Moral treatment of the mentally ill" was a specific approach to treating people in the mental hospitals of the day (Bockoven, 1971).

Medicine and health care during the decades before and after 1900 were changing at a fast rate. On July 9, 1893, a black surgeon, Dr. Daniel Hale Williams, performed the world's first open heart surgery (Wikipedia, n.d.); the Curies shared their Nobel prize for physics with Henri Becquerel for their work on radioactivity; vitamins were discovered; Robert Kotch discovered the tubercle bacillus; Wilhelm Konrad Röntgen discovered X-rays (Sutcliffe & Duin, 1992); and only a few "resurrectionists," or grave robbers, were still supplying some medical schools with cadavers. Hospital care changed rapidly during this time. These discoveries, activities, and new approaches to health care only just begin to characterize the changes that took place in medicine and health care around the turn of the 20th century.

The early years of the 20th century were a time when the founders of occupational therapy in the United States, and their supporters, were nurturing the infant profession that essentially came from what has been called the moral treatment era (Bockoven, 1971; Lilleleht, 2002; Luchins, 1992; Peloquin, 1989, 1994; Tuke, 1813). Moral treatment of the mentally ill started in the 19th century at about the same time in England, France, and Italy (Lilleleht). It was then brought to the United States.

Furthermore, Licht (1949) noted that around the turn of the 20th century, occupational therapy was being provided by teachers and crafts persons. The educational programs were composed of a few weeks post-high school training until the early 1920s when the education grew to one year post-high school (West, 1978). In March 1917, a group of supporters met in Clifton Springs, New York to form the National Society for the Promotion of Occupational Therapy (Quiroga, 1995). By 1921, the name was changed to the American Occupational Therapy Association, and the association started publishing the *Archives of Occupational Therapy* in that year. Furthermore, the types of clients seen by occupational therapists was becoming more diversified so that by the early 1900s, practitioners were providing services to those clients with physical problems such as arthritis and tuberculosis as well as those with mental illness (Bing, 1981; Quiroga).

In the fall of 1978, the AOTA's Representative Assembly invited a number of the leaders of the profession to develop a framework that addressed issues affecting the profession (AOTA, 1979a). The presenters' topics included the following:

- A historical perspective of the profession
- A discussion of practice, education, and research issues
- A discussion of the occupational therapy professional identity
- A review of the external influences impacting the profession
- An exploration of traditional and nontraditional practice arenas

All of the critical concerns of that era fit into three areas: education, research, and practice. Some of the presenters were concerned about the quality of professional education and the influence of formal education on practitioners (Gillette, 1979; Johnson, 1979; Wiemer, 1979). Others expressed the need for developing client assessments that were unique to occupational therapy (West, 1979), and for developing research upon which to base our interventions (Yerxa, 1979). It is important to note that education, research, and practice compose dynamic parts of a whole. To be a practitioner, one must be educated in the theories and skills of the profession. Sound theories and skills are founded on evidence from research and on clinical expertise that comes from practice. Therefore, the following sections are arbitrarily divided into education, research, and practice only to be able to highlight some of the changes that have occurred in those areas during the last few decades.

# Education

One of the overarching concerns noted in *Occupational therapy: 2001 AD: Papers presented at the special session of the Representative Assembly, November 1978*, which touched upon research, education, and practice, was concern about our professional status. During the 1970s and 1980s, there were many discussions about what constituted being a profession as opposed to a semiprofession or a technical field (AOTA, 1979a; Fleming, Johnson, Marina, Spergel, & Townsend, 1987). Fidler (1979) identified and compared the various characteristics of these levels of professionalism (technical, semiprofession, and profession), and suggested that for several reasons, occupational therapy was a semiprofession. The reasons included that because of our level of education, we did not have adequately evolved specialized knowledge abstracted and codified into a specific body of theories and principles, and we lacked full control over our practice. Fidler cited our educational training of the time as being "less vigorous or substantive than, for example, the art therapist, the special education teacher, the dance therapist, the nurse, social worker, or therapeutic re-creator (sic)" (p. 35).

The first education for occupational therapists in the second decade of the 20th century was composed of a few weeks post-high school; then it grew to 1 year post-high school by 1923; and then to 34 months with a diploma by 1938 (West, 1979). According to the Council on Medical Education and Hospitals of the American Medical Association, the occupational therapy accrediting body in 1947, there were 18 approved schools that offered either a diploma, certificate, or bachelor's degree in occupational therapy (Council on Medical Education and Hospitals of the American Medical Association, 1947, p. cover 3). In the 1970s, of those graduating from professional programs, 90% received a bachelor's degree, while the others received certificates in occupational therapy (Jantzen, 1979). According to the AOTA (1974), by 1974 there were 51 accredited professional programs in the United States and Puerto Rico. Of those, 10 offered a master's degree to those who had bachelor's degrees in other fields, and 17 programs offered a master's degree for occupational therapists. It is interesting to note that New York University (NYU) was the only school that offered a doctoral degree at that time. Occupational therapists wishing to get a degree beyond the master's level either went to NYU or received degrees in education, psychology, or other areas outside of occupational therapy.

As of June 2008, there were 157 accredited occupational therapy master's level programs in the United States and Puerto Rico, and of these programs, 48 offered postprofessional master's degrees for those already practicing occupational therapy (AOTA, n.d.a). This increase to the master's level of education represents a significant change in occupational therapy education that was mandated by the AOTA (1999) and that required that by 2007, all entry-level occupational therapy professional programs in the United States be at the postbaccalaureate level.

An indication of the continuing national and international trend in acquiring higher degrees, as of June 2008, 25 programs in the United States offered postprofessional doctoral degree programs (AOTA, n. d. a). Canada, Australia, and the United Kingdom initiated master's level entry programs at the University of Western Ontario, Canada and the University of Sydney in 1998 and a program in Scotland in 1999 (Allen, Strong, & Polatajko, 2001).

According to Hilton's (2005) analysis of the current transition to postbaccalaureate entry, there were five documented expectations of that transition (p. 67):

1. Elevate the status of the profession
2. Increase research competency, contributions to professional literature, and accountability to the public
3. Expand to incorporate the growth of knowledge and practice
4. Increase doctorally prepared occupational therapists
5. Increase enrollment of the professional level therapist

It is interesting to note that these expectations, in various forms, are also often put forth as justification for the occupational therapy profession moving to the entry-level doctorate.

As stated earlier, as of June 2008 there were 25 occupational therapy doctoral programs in the United States (AOTA, n.d.a). Some are entry-level clinical doctoral programs and others are postprofessional doctorates. A variety of degrees are offered from the doctor of philosophy (PhD) and doctor of science (ScD) degrees to the doctor of occupational therapy (OTD), a clinical degree. The number of doctoral programs seems to be increasing. This suggests that there will be more changes ahead for occupational therapy education.

Of the occupational therapy doctoral programs, the OTD is most controversial. The results of a recent study of academic occupational therapy programs (Griffiths & Padilla, 2006) suggest that there are several reasons for this controversy. However, there seems to be as many different opinions about the degree as there are people with opinions. The reasons for controversy identified in the study ranged from some respondents thinking there is little support within the profession for the degree, to there being little evidence of the need for the degree in the health care system, to there being too little research, and therefore, an insufficient knowledge-base in the profession to justify the degree.

# Research

The need for research within occupational therapy has existed from the early years of the profession. For example, Licht (1947), when addressing some of the challenges facing occupational therapy in the mid-1940s, said that "little or no statistical data which are suitable for scientific scrutiny and evaluation have been published" (p. 455), and there was only one answer to that challenge—research. The state of research in our profession in the 1970s was characterized by Ethridge and McSweeney's (1970) assessment that "experimental research has thus far been quite rare in occupational therapy literature" (p. 491). Johnson (1979) suggested that the profession relied more on theory based on "a system of beliefs or a philosophy... than upon research that provides confidence in the knowledge we acquire" (p. 60).

To the extent that professional journals reflect the profession's academic structure and professional maturity, Madhill, Brintnell, & Stewin's (1989) review of the number and content of occupational therapy journals may exemplify the growth of research in our profession over the past several decades. Although *AJOT* existed from the beginning of the profession, these researchers found an increase in the number of professional journals internationally as well as in the number of research articles reflecting professional maturity.

The *Occupational Therapy Journal of Research* (*OTJR*) was one of the professional journals initiated in the 1980s. The journal represented one of several initiatives by the American Occupational Therapy Foundation (AOTF) to stimulate research in the United States. In addition to launching the *OTJR*, the AOTF funded an ambitious and enlightening study called the Clinical Reasoning Study (Mattingly & Fleming, 1994). In her editorial in the 10th anniversary issues of *OTJR*, Gillette (1990) reported that the AOTF had been successful in meeting those mandates.

Bonder and Christiansen (2001), at the *OTJR's* 20th anniversary, reported that, based on the number of manuscripts submitted to *OTJR*, "occupational therapy has more active researchers now than ever in its history" (p. 5). While they saw great progress in the profession's research endeavors, they noted that there were at least two goals yet to be reached. First was to create an occupational therapy culture rich in research traditions. The second was to place research emphasis on "activity and participation rather than body structure and function" (p. 10). An important part of the research is its application to practice. By the 21st century, occupational therapy was becoming committed to evidence-based occupational therapy—further proof of the profession's growth and maturity.

# Practice

As suggested earlier, education, research, and practice are all facets of the same concept. Evidence-based occupational therapy is an approach that blends research and practice. Evidence-based occupational therapy evolved from the awareness that best practice requires that practitioners use the best available evidence to support their intervention, and that education, research, and practice compose dynamic parts of a whole. However, occupational therapy practice also has a strong tradition in what has been referred to as the era of humane intervention for the mentally ill and has always rested on a strong humanistic foundation. Entry into the 20th century and the rigors of evidence-based practice in the latter part of the 20th century has brought occupational therapy face-to-face with positivistic science in which measurement and objectivity are valued over intuition and subjectivity.

Johnson (1979) analyzed why education seemed not to bridge the education-practice gap or bring about the changes she felt would help the profession meet its potential. She speculated that "the emotional impact upon young students in the clinical setting is so great that they turn almost immediately to the models of practice they see being demonstrated rather than to the theoretical models they studied but have seldom seen incorporated in practice" (p. 60). This education-practice gap is likely common to other practice professions and not just occupational therapy. Efforts to both maintain high educational standards and to strengthen the relationship between professional education in occupational therapy and practice have traditionally been the role of each national professional association and of transnational organizations such as the World Federation of Occupational Therapists (WFOT), the European Network of Occupational Therapy in Higher Education (ENOTHE), and the Council of Occupational Therapists for the European Countries (COTEC).

"The aim of the Council [COTEC] is to enable National Associations of Occupational Therapists of the European Countries to develop, harmonize, and promote standards of professional practice and education of Occupational Therapists and to advance the science of occupational therapy throughout Europe" (COTEC, n.d.). The ENOTHE aims to unite European occupational therapy educational programs and proposed programs to advance the education and the body of knowledge of occupational therapy and to work with COTEC to promote occupational therapy education in Europe (ENOTHE, n.d.). The mission of the WFOT is to promote occupational therapy as an art and science internationally. The Federation supports the development, use, and practice of occupational therapy worldwide, demonstrating its relevance and contribution to society (WFOT, n.d.).

In the United States, the role of maintaining high educational standards has been taken by the AOTA Accreditation Council for Occupational Therapy Education (ACOTE). The AOTA Commission on Practice has the role of establishing high standards of practice, and over the years, has produced official documents meant to help practitioners maintain best practice. Of these documents, the AOTA *Uniform Terminology for Occupational Therapy* exemplifies the national association's efforts to establish best practice standards. The first edition of the uniform terminology document was published in 1979 (AOTA, 1979b). It was revised two times (AOTA, 1989, 1994). The third edition was modified and the product is called the *Occupational Therapy Practice Framework: Domain and Process* (AOTA, 2008). To assure that these documents would help other health professions understand the scope of occupational therapy, the framework uses the terminology and language of the *International Classification of Functioning, Disability and Health* (ICF) (AOTA, 2008). All of the documents were meant to provide practitioners with a description of the domain of occupational therapy, which "grounds the profession's focus and actions" (p. 609), and to outline the process of evaluation and intervention or interventions.

Over the years, AOTA has developed and published other significant documents affecting practice, including the *Occupational Therapy Code of Ethics* (2005), *Guidelines for Supervision, Roles, and Responsibilities During the Delivery of Occupational Therapy Services* (2004), *Standards for Continuing Competence* (2005), and the *Standards of Practice for Occupational Therapy* (2005) to name a few. The AOTA web site (www.aota.org) has a complete listing of its official documents.

In terms of specific practice approaches, the early 21st century could be called the "dash-based era" of health care. That is, current occupational therapy practice is influenced by the concept of occupation-based therapy, and virtually all health care professions—including occupational therapy—espouse client-centered practice, evidence-based occupational therapy, and neurology-based practice. Furthermore, we treat in hospital-based, school-based, or community-based settings. The following section briefly describes these current approaches to practice.

## Client-Centered Practice

This client-centered practice approach was developed in Canada over the last couple of decades (CAOT, 1997). As Law et al. (1995) stated, this approach "is a philosophy of practice built on concepts that reflect changes in the attitudes and beliefs of clients and occupational therapists" (p. 253). These attitudes and beliefs include the notion that clients need to express their needs and to make choices regarding their occupations, that clients share responsibility for the therapeutic process, that the client-centered approach represents a shift from seeing the person as disabled to seeing the person as enabled, that clients' "roles, interests, environments, and culture are central to the occupational therapy process..." (Law et al., p. 252).

## Occupation-Based Practice

It is important to note that the concept of occupation as a special form of doing has been part of the occupational therapy ethos since the profession's infancy. Just to cite examples from one of the early proponents of occupational therapy, Dr. Adolf Meyer maintained that "occupation is, with good right, called the most essential side of hygienic treatment of most insane patients" (Meyer & Winters, 1951, p. 46). When speaking of his efforts to organize medical work in large state hospitals, Meyer said that "since most mental disorders are, to a large extent, disorders of conduct, a regulated existence with occupation is, on the whole, the...most efficient form of treatment..." (p. 95). Meyer believed that the intervention of people with gastrointestinal disturbances, which he felt also caused mental disorders, should include

> "Occupation treatment [over] mere talking...due to the fact that, after all, we have not yet as excellent control over the things that form the fancy and the thought life of the individual; whereas we look upon performance and activity as the actual functioning and the test of the working of the individual's drives and life" (p. 629).

While the notion of the power of occupation is a part of our early history, it fell into disfavor between World War I to about the 1980s when occupational therapy was dominated by the traditional, reductionistic, medical model, health care system of the day. Mattingly and Fleming (1994), in their study of occupational therapist clinical reasoning, capture the essence of this period of our history when describing what it means to be a "good therapist" in the eyes of non-occupational therapists. They found that occupational therapists needed "to ensure that services were billable, therapists were driven to narrow the scope of treatment goals and activities along more biomedical lines—to treat the physical body" (Mattingly & Fleming, p. 296) without concern for the phenomenological side of their practice. Yet these researchers saw that their subjects seemed naturally drawn to understanding their clients' disabling experience and the broader meanings of disrupted or lost occupations but could not formally incorporate interventions that would help "patients to formulate, either through words or actions, deeper understandings of themselves and their experiences" (p. 296).

A number of current models exist that espouse the notion that occupation should form the basis of occupational therapy intervention, and that, in addressing occupations, therapists address not only functional deficits but broader issues of meaning, purpose, and spirituality—issues that must be addressed if we are going to assist in a client's construction or reconstruction of the self (Baum & Christiansen, 1997; Christiansen, 1999; Crabtree, 2003; B. Howard & J. Howard, 1997; Mattingly & Fleming, 1994). These include the Canadian Occupational Performance Model (CAOT, 1997) and the Occupational Performance Model (Australia) (Chapparo & Ranka, 1997). In addition, the concept of occupational performance forms the core of the framework (AOTA, 2008). Suffice it to say, these models place occupation, or purposive doing, at the center of occupational therapy intervention and assume that humans are occupational beings who express their meaning and purpose through their occupations. These models are discussed in more depth in other chapters.

## Evidence-Based Occupational Therapy

As discussed earlier, evidence-based occupational therapy has received the attention of most health care professionals around the world. This approach started with the advent of evidence-based medicine, which was defined as "the conscientious, explicit, and judicious use of current best evidence in making decisions about the care of individual patients" (Sackett, Rosenberg, Muir Gray, Haynes, & Richardson, 1996, p. 71). As one might imagine, the application of evidence-based medicine across all health care disciplines, many of which have limited research-based knowledge, can be challenging at best and discouraging at worst. Consequently, each profession needs to identify an appropriate match of evidence and clinical reasoning to its practice. The Joint Position Statement on Evidence-Based Occupational Therapy was endorsed by the 2004 AOTA Online Representative Assembly (AOTA, n.d.b) and applies the best concepts from evidence-based medicine to the needs of occupational therapy. Recognition of the need for evidence-based occupational therapy has now reached an international level (Ilott, Taylor, & Bolanos, 2006). Essentially, evidence-based occupational therapy is a collaborative effort between the client and the therapist in which the client (or patient) contributes what is uniquely his or hers to offer, and the therapist contributes his or her expertise (Table 33-1).

## Neuroscience-Based Treatment

The 1990s was designated as the "Decade of the Brain" "to enhance public awareness of the benefits to be derived from brain research" (Library of Congress, n.d.a, n.d.b). During that decade, the Library of Congress and the National Institute of Mental Health of the National Institutes of Health sponsored a number of initiatives to advance the goals set forth by the President. This proclamation stimulated scientific research across the globe (Tandon, 2000).

During and since the Decade of the Brain, in addition to breakthroughs in specific diseases such as stroke, Parkinson's, and Alzheimer's, and in the development of imaging technologies such as the positron emission tomography (PET) scan, magnetic resonance imaging (MRI), and functional magnetic resonance imaging (fMRI), scientists have come to understand the plasticity of the nervous system—an important characteristic of the nervous system for occupational therapists to appreciate, study, and apply to their practice. Simply put, neuronal plasticity conceives the nervous system to be dynamic and capable of cortical reorganization (Curt, Schwab, & Dietz, 2004; Hamzei, Liepert, Dettmers, Weiller, & Rijntjes, 2006; Liepert, 2006; Taub, 2004) and the regenerating nerve tissues. Animal model

**Table 33-1. Contributions of the Client and Therapist in Evidence-Based Occupational Therapy**

| Client's Contributions | Therapist's Contributions |
|---|---|
| Knowledge, beliefs, hopes, etc. necessary for determining meaningful occupational intervention priorities | Knowledge of client's environment and other information relevant to enabling occupational performance |
| Beliefs about what medical, developmental, or social problems prohibit meaningful occupational performance | Using evidence-based occupational therapy principles and professional expertise, assists client to identify and prioritize occupational performance goals |
| Subjective evaluation of present occupational performance | Offers suggestions and encourages client to explore new ways of viewing occupational performance deficits |
| Knowledge and perceptions of personal and environmental resources and limitations | Offers suggestions and encourages client to consider new uses of personal and environmental resources |
| Hopes for outcomes and agreement with possible therapy plans and measures of success | |
| With the therapist, identifies intervention outcomes and commits to the proposed intervention and measures of desired outcomes | |

Adapted from Canadian Association of Occupational Therapists. (1999). Joint position statement on evidence-based occupational therapy. Toronto, ON: CAOT Publications. Retrieved August 14, 2009, from http://www.caot.ca/default.asp?ChangeID=166&pageID=156

researchers, in particular, have discovered a number of examples of plasticity from dendritic arborization (generation of new dendrites) (McAllister, 2000) to axonal regeneration (Curt et al.). Clinical application of these findings holds great promise for occupational therapy. Constraint-induced movement therapy (CIMT) is an example of neuroscience-based therapy. In this approach, the non-affected limb is constrained, and for a period of time, the client must practice using the affected limb to perform various tasks, often to perform activities of daily living (ADL). The frequency and duration of the intervention and the means of constraining the nonaffected limb vary depending on the severity of the disability, the intervention setting (outpatient clinic, home, hospital, etc.) and other factors.

## Emerging Practice Areas

According to the 1973 AOTA member data survey, most occupational therapists (about 55%) practiced in traditional settings such as acute hospitals, rehabilitation hospitals, and school systems (Jantzen, 1979), but there have likely always been occupational therapists who have provided services for which they treat nontraditional clients. For example, in 1973, about 8% of registered occupational therapists worked in community programs such as community mental health centers and day care centers. In this era, a little over 1% of the members stated that they were in private practice. About 30 years later, hospitals and rehabilitation units, skilled nursing and other long-term care facilities, and school systems including early intervention make up over 80% of the settings in which occupational therapists work (AOTA, 2001). Throughout the years, occupational therapists have always worked in what might be called nontraditional or emerging practice areas.

The AOTA has identified a number of emerging practice areas that fit well within the occupational therapy scope of practice in the United States (AOTA, n.d.c). This section identifies only a few of these areas of practice. The reader is encouraged to go to the AOTA members area Web site (www.aota.org) for detailed information about these emerging practice areas. These areas include psychosocial needs of children and youth, health and wellness consultation, assistive device consultation, and many others. With each area, the Web site includes hot links to more detailed information useful to the practitioner. To cite one example, under Driver Rehabilitation, there is a link to the American Medical Association's recommendation that "its members consider occupational therapy for clients whose impaired driving ability poses a threat to public safety" (AOTA, n.d.c).

## Demographics and Technology

The practice of occupational therapy does not exist in a vacuum. Practitioners and what they practice are situated in political, cultural, social, geographical, religious, and many other contexts. Of the many possible contexts to consider, this chapter focuses on demographics and technology. These appear to likely have significant implications for occupational therapists in this century.

### Demographics of the United States

Hiemstra (2003), a futurist, has identified five demographic trends that will have a significant impact on the United States, and by extension, will have important implications for occupational therapists:

1. Americans are getting older.
2. Americans are becoming more ethnically diverse.
3. The Baby Boomers are retiring and generation Y is reaching adulthood.
4. Americans will move back to urban-inner cities.
5. The U.S. population will likely peak in the mid- to late 21st century.

There is no way of knowing today whether these trends will come to pass exactly as predicted, but regardless of the precision of these trends, demographic changes in the United States are likely to have a significant impact on occupational therapy in varying degrees and ways. The aging and increased ethnic diversity of Americans, in particular, will have an impact on occupational therapy in that the increase in the number of older adults will create an increased demand for occupational services, and the increase in the ethnic diversity of our clients will require increased skill on the part of practitioners to be culturally proficient (Royeen & Crabtree, 2006). When you add the increasing numbers of U.S. citizens with disabling conditions to this equation, the demand for occupational therapy services increases even more (U.S. Census Bureau, 2005).

Related to the aging of Americans, "activity limitation" statistics are an indication of the need for occupational therapy. According to the National Center for Health Statistics (NCHS) (2005), activity limitation refers to "limitations in handling personal care needs (activities of daily living), routine needs (instrumental activities of daily living), having a job outside of the home, walking, remembering, and other activities" (p. 50). The NCHS reported that in 2003, over a third of those community-dwelling people 65 years of age and over reported activity limitations. The chronic conditions most common to those 65 years and older are heart or other circulatory conditions and arthritis and other musculoskeletal conditions. The other conditions that caused activity limitations included "senility," diabetes, vision, and hearing disorders. While these data were not related directly to the need for occupational therapy services, it is fair to say that the demand for occupational therapy will increase as more Americans enter these age groups.

As our nation becomes increasingly ethnically diverse, so will our clinics, hospitals, schools, and other occupational therapy service settings. With this diversity comes differences between therapists and clients or clients' basic values, attitudes, and beliefs about what it means to be an individual, the importance (or lack of importance) of independence or the ability to make decisions, and many other aspects of culture. Disagreement concerning such values and beliefs need not confound the occupational therapist's efforts to provide effective services. However, to minimize the chances of such conflicts undermining therapy, occupational therapists need to be culturally proficient, as discussed in Chapter 2.

# Technology

In this section, there is a focus on technology in general, not on the technology that is available for use in therapy. For specific information on assistive technology, please see Chapter 25. In addition, there is a focus on the possible problems related to technology since, as occupational therapists, we are most likely to treat people who are negatively affected by technology rather than those who benefit from technology.

As consumers of technology, we may seldom give a critical thought to the worth of technology, let alone its possible problems. After all, because of technology, we can see and speak in real time to someone on the other side of the globe, we can prepare a tasty meal in only minutes, we can listen to our favorite music, we can communicate with our friends from virtually anywhere and anytime, and our automobiles can tell us where we are and how to get to our destination. Furthermore, if we need a vital organ, because of modern technology, we can receive either a synthetic organ or an organ transplant.

There is no question that technology has made doing some things easier (Smith, 2000), but has it contributed to the good of humanity, and how is a person's occupational performance affected by technology? These are both philosophical and practical questions—the sort of critical questions occupational therapists need to ask themselves if they are to make sound clinical judgments about the effect of technology on their clients and society. To make these clinical judgments, it is important to be able to distinguish between the concepts of positive and negative benefits of technology. A negative benefit is the removal or decrease of something considered bad or negative (Rescher, 1980). For example, using a gas-powered automobile to drive to work might be a negative benefit compared to walking because walking to work takes 2 hours compared to 15 minutes to drive and walking requires much more human energy. Another example of a negative benefit, again saving time and energy, could be using a microwave oven to prepare a frozen meal compared to preparing a meal from scratch and using a conventional stove or oven. In both examples, the negative benefit is found in reducing the amount of time and energy required to perform the activity.

A positive benefit is one that involves an intrinsic good or a positive condition like happiness, joy, pleasure, and the like (Mejias, 2006; Rescher, 1980). No number of negative benefits, on their own, adds up to a positive benefit. In other words, one can have the latest automotive technology that keeps you safe from injuries and technology that cooks a delicious meal and washes, dries, and stacks the dishes without effort, and still be unhappy or still feel unfulfilled. By the same token, people can be very happy and lead a meaningful life and have these magnificent labor and time-saving devices. Peoples' happiness is not directly related to technology. From the occupational therapist's perspective, peoples' happiness is related to being able to perform in ways that meet their goals and help them live productive and satisfying lives.

There are two classes of implications of technology for occupational therapists—one is the obvious, physical, effects of using technology. These include a variety of repetitive stress injuries, many of which are discussed elsewhere in this text book (Amini, 2006). The second is the not-so-obvious implication in which people, as a result of a poor match of technology to the individual's needs, may develop "Internet addiction" (Beard & Wolf, 2001; Hansen, 2002; Michaels, 1988), can have a sense of alienation, of being disenfranchised, or of having no meaningful goals or purpose in life. It is important to note that technology can be very useful and rewarding for some. However, for others, having the latest and best technology may mask their need to be connected to others and to be engaged in meaningful occupations (Bakhtin, Liapunov, & Holquist, 1993; Gergen, 1991; Hall, 1981; Jonas, 1982, 1984; Rivers, 1993, 2005).

When we consider that doing, or occupational performance, is critical to peoples' health and ability to make meaning and quality in their life, occupational therapists need to be able to critically evaluate their client's knowledge and use of technology. As Rogers (1983) stated, "Therapeutic action must be the right action for...[the]... individual. This implies that it must be as congruent as possible with the patient's concept of the 'good life'" (p. 602). For many, the use of technology can make the difference between isolation and participation and between independence and dependence. However, what might be a liberating technology helping one live the good life for one person might be a form of subtle enslavement for another. Take the simple case of a woman who loves to bake desserts from scratch and who has pleased her multigenerational family for years with her cooking skills. After a stroke that leaves her paralyzed on one side, her occupational therapist might be tempted to include preparing frozen desserts as part of the intervention because such an approach would be easy and take less therapy time. The older woman might not criticize the therapist or complain about using microwave technology, but she might be very disheartened to think that she may never return to cooking in the manner to which she is accustomed. In this case, technology has perhaps offered a negative benefit by reducing a burden (clumsy, frustrating, and unsafe cooking techniques) but inadvertently has taken from the woman one of her reasons for living. A more appropriate approach to therapy might be to take the time necessary to help the woman relearn how to bake "the old-fashioned way" using an oven.

# Summary

This chapter discussed some of the significant changes, or trends, within the profession, and situated occupational therapy in the broad context of the 21st century. The author addressed changes in education, research, and practice. While there have been some significant changes in the numbers of occupational therapy practitioners in the United States, the level of education and the amount of research undertaken, the scientific basis of our intervention and intervention, and other factors, many elements of our practice remain essentially the same. At the very least, we continue to provide services to those who have been seriously disabled due to illness, accidents, disease, and other factors. These people, as Jennings suggested, still need "the restoration of wholeness and integrity...and the preservation of a meaningful life..." (1993, p. S25)—the essence of occupational therapy.

There have been significant changes since the 20th century. But again, the people we serve remain essentially the same. They are people who want to be happy, well, and satisfied with their life; to participate in the daily course of social and economical events; and to be able to construct worthy goals and meet those goals. As the occupational therapy profession has grown and matured, it has become more able than ever to meet the needs of those people.

# Student Self-Assessment

1. Search the literature on an occupational therapy assessment or intervention and identify how many professional journals from other countries have published articles on that topic. Were there significant differences in the ways the topic was addressed? If so, how were they different or similar?
2. Compare and contrast two journal articles on a given occupational therapy topic—one from an article published prior to 1950 and one from an article published after 1990.
3. Using Census data, examine the demographics of your state or county. Explain the implications of your findings related to the need for occupational therapy services in your area.
4. Find examples of people's need for assistive technology in your local newspaper. What were the needs, and who provided the services or applied the technology? Did an occupational therapist provide the service? If not, speculate why.
5. Considering the current trends in practice, education, and research, explain how you think the trend will continue in each of those areas and explain why.

# Electronic Resources

- Evidence-based occupational therapy resources, AOTA official documents, and emerging practice areas: www.aota.org
- Information about the American Occupational Therapy Foundation and the Wilma West Library: www.aotf.org
- Client-centered practice resources: www.caot.ca
- Information about international resources and international occupational therapy programs: www.wfot.org.au

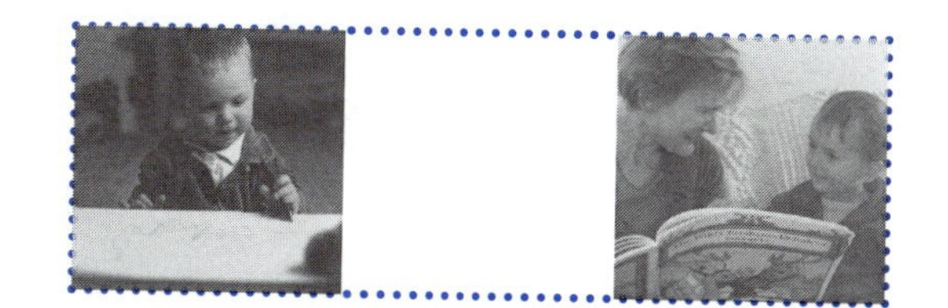

# References


Allen, S., Strong, J., & Polatajko, H. J. (2001). Graduate-entry masters' degrees: Launch pad for occupational therapy in this millennium? *British Journal of Occupational Therapy, 64*(11), 572-576.

American Occupational Therapy Association. (1974). *The 1974-1975 yearbook*. Rockville, MD: Author.

American Occupational Therapy Association. (1979a). Occupational therapy: 2001 AD: Papers presented at the special session of the Representative Assembly, November 1978. Rockville, MD: Author.

American Occupational Therapy Association. (1979b). Uniform terminology for occupational therapy—First edition. *Occupational Therapy News, 35*, 1-8.

American Occupational Therapy Association. (1989). Uniform terminology for occupational therapy—Second edition. *American Journal of Occupational Therapy, 43*, 808-815.

American Occupational Therapy Association. (1994). Uniform terminology for occupational therapy—Third edition. *American Journal of Occupational Therapy, 48*, 1047-1054.

American Occupational Therapy Association. (1999). ACOTE sets timeline for post-baccalaureate degree programs. *OT Week, 13*(33), i & iii.

American Occupational Therapy Association. (2001). *AOTA 2000 Member compensation survey*. Bethesda, MD: Author.

American Occupational Therapy Association. (2008). Occupational therapy practice framework: Domain and process, second edition. *American Journal of Occupational Therapy, 62*, 625-683

American Occupational Therapy Association. (n.d.a). Schools, June 2008. Retrieved June 9, 2008, from http://www.aota.org/Educate/Schools.aspx

American Occupational Therapy Association. (n.d.b). Top 10 emerging practice areas to watch in the new millennium. Retrieved August 2, 2009, from http://www.aota.org/nonmembers/area1/links/link61.asp

Amini, D. (2006). Repetitive stress injuries and the age of communication. *OT Practice, 11*(9), 10-15.

Baum, C., & Christiansen, C. (1997). The occupational therapy context: Philosophy-principles-practice. In C. Christinasen & C. Baum (Eds.), *Occupational therapy: Enabling function and well-being* (pp. 27-45). Thorofare, NJ: Slack Incorporated.

Bakhtin, M. M., Liapunov, V. (Trans. & Ed.), & Holquist, M. (Ed.). (1993). *Toward a philosophy of the act.* Austin, TX: University of Texas Press.

Beard, K. W., & Wolf, E. M. (2001). Modification in the proposed diagnostic criteria for Internet addiction. *Cyberpsychological Behavior, 4*(3), 377-383.

Bing, R. K. (1981). Occupational therapy revisited: A paraphrastic journey. *American Journal of Occupational Therapy, 35*(8), 499-518.

Bockoven, J. S. (1971). Legacy of moral treatment—1800's to 1910. *American Journal of Occupational Therapy, 25*(5), 223-225.

Bonder, B., & Christiansen, C. (2001). Editorial: Coming of age in challenging times. *Occupational Therapy Journal of Research, 21*(1), 3-11.

Boyer, G., Hachey, R., & Mercier, C. (2000). Perceptions of occupational performance and subjective quality of life in persons with severe mental illness. *Occupational Therapy in Mental Health, 15*(2), 1-15.

Canadian Association of Occupational Therapists. (1997). *Enabling occupation: An occupational therapy perspective.* Toronto, Ontario: CAOT Publications.

Canadian Association of Occupational Therapists. (2009). Joint Position Statement on Evidence-based Occupational Therapy. Retrieved August 2, 2009, from http://www.caot.ca/default.asp?ChangeID=166&pageID=156

Chapparo, C., & Ranka, J. (1997). *Occupational performance model* (Australia), Monograph 1. Sydney, Australia: Total Print Control.

Chen, Y-H. (2002). Experiences with the COPM and client-centered practice in adult neurorehabilitation in Taiwan. *Occupational Therapy International, 9*(3), 167-184.

Christiansen, C. H. (1999). Eleanor Clarke Slagle Lectureship—1999; Defining lives: Occupation as identity: An essay on competence, coherence, and the creation of meaning. *American Journal of Occupational Therapy, 53*(6), 547-558.

Council of Occupational Therapists for the European Countries (COTEC). (n.d.). History of COTEC: Introduction. Retrieved July 29, 2006, from http://www.cotec-europe.org

Council on Medical Education and Hospitals of the American Medical Association. (1947). Approved schools for occupational therapy technicians. *Occupational Therapy & Rehabilitation, 26*(3), cover 3.

Crabtree, J. L. (2003). On occupational performance. *Occupational Therapy in Health Care, 17*(2), 1-18.

Curt, A., Schwab, M. E., & Dietz, V. (2004). Providing the clinical basis for new interventional therapies: Refined diagnosis and assessment of recovery after spinal cord injury. *Spinal Cord, 42*, 1-6.

Ethridge, D. A., & McSweeney, M. (1970). Research in occupational therapy part 1. *American Journal of Occupational Therapy, 24*(7), 490-494.

European Network of Occupational Therapy in Higher Education (ENOTHE). (n.d.). Organization: Introduction. Retrieved July 30, 2006, from http://www.enothe.hva.nl

Farnworth, L. (2003). Sylvia Docker Lecture: Time use, tempo and temporality: Occupational therapy's core business or someone else's business? *Australian Occupational Therapy Journal, 50*(3), 116-126.

Fidler, G. (1979). Professional or nonprofessional. In Occupational therapy: 2001 AD: Papers presented at the special session of the Representative Assembly, November 1978 (pp. 31-36). Rockville, MD: AOTA Press.

Fleming, M. H., Johnson, J. A., Marina, M-H., Spergel, E. L., & Townsend, B. (1987). Occupational therapy directions for the future. Report of the Entry-Level Study Committee of the American Occupational Therapy Association. Rockville, MD: AOTA Press.

Gergen, K. J. (1991). *The saturated self: Dilemmas of identity in contemporary life.* New York, NY: Basic Books.

Gillette, N. (1979). Practice, education and research. In Occupational therapy: 2001 AD: Papers presented at the special session of the Representative Assembly, November 1978 (pp. 18-25). Rockville, MD: AOTA Press.

Gillette, N. (1990). Guest editorial: 10th anniversary volume of OTJR: An update of research programs. *Occupational Therapy Journal of Research, 10*(6), 67-73.

Griffiths, Y., & Padilla, R. (2006). National status of the entry-level doctorate in occupational therapy (OTD). *American Journal of Occupational Therapy, 60*(5), 540-550.

Hall, E. T. (1981). *Beyond culture.* New York, NY: Anchor Press.

Hammell, K. W. (1995). Application of learning theory in spinal cord injury rehabilitation: Client-centered occupational therapy. *Scandinavian Journal of Occupational Therapy, 2*(1), 34-39.

Hamzei, F., Liepert, J., Dettmers, C., Weiller, C., & Rijntjes, M. (2006). Two different reorganization patterns after rehabilitative therapy: An exploratory study with fMRI and TMS. *Neuroimage, 31*(2), 710-120.

Hansen, S. (2002). Excessive Internet usage or 'Internet Addiction'? The implications of diagnostic categories for student users. *Journal of Computer Assisted Learning, 18*(2), 235-236.

Hiemstra, G. (2003). Population myths, trends and transportation planning. FuturistNews. Retrieved June 11, 2006, from http://www.futurist.com

Hilton, C. L. (2005). The evolving postbaccalaureate entry: Analysis of occupational therapy entry-level master's degree in the United States. *Occupational Therapy in Health Care, 19*(3), 51-71.

Howard, B. S., & Howard, J. R. (1997). Occupation as spiritual activity. *American Journal of Occupational Therapy, 51*(3), 181-185.

Ilott, I., Taylor, M. C., & Bolanos, C. (2006). Evidence-based occupational therapy: It's time to take a global approach. *British Journal of Occupational Therapy, 69*(1), 38-41.

Jansa, J., Sicherl, Z., Angleitner, K., & Law, M. (2004). The use of Canadian Occupational Performance Measure (COPM) in clients with an acute stroke. *World Federation of Occupational Therapists Bulletin, 50*, 18-23.

Jantzen, A. (1979). The current profile of occupational therapy and the future—professional or vocational? In Occupational therapy: 2001 AD: Papers presented at the special session of the Representative Assembly, November 1978 (pp. 71-75). Rockville, MD: AOTA Press.

Jennings, B. (1993). Healing the self: The moral meaning of relationships in rehabilitation. *American Journal of Physical Medicine and Rehabilitation, 72*, 401-404.

Johnson, J. (1979). Reorganization in relation to the issues. In Occupational therapy: 2001 AD: Papers presented at the special session of the Representative Assembly, November 1978 (pp. 60-68). Rockville, MD: AOTA Press.

Jonas, H. (1982). *The phenomenon of life.* Chicago, IL: University of Chicago Press

Jonas, H. (1984). *The imperative of responsibility.* (H. Jonas & D. Herr, Trans.) Chicago, IL: University of Chicago Press.

Law, M., Baptiste, S., Carswell, A., McColl, M. A., Polatajko, H., & Pollock, N. (1998). *The Canadian occupational performance measure* (3rd ed.). Toronto, Ontario: CAOT Publications.

Law, M., Baptiste, S., & Mills, J. (1995). Client-centered practice: What does it mean and does it make a difference? *Canadian Journal of Occupational Therapy, 62*, 250-257.

Library of Congress. (n.d.a). The decade of the brain 1999-2000. Retrieved August 4, 2006, from http://www.loc.gov/loc/brain

Library of Congress. (n.d.b). Presidential Proclamation 6158. Retrieved August 4, 2006, from http://www.loc.gov/loc/brain/proclaim.html

Licht, S. (1947). Modern trends in occupational therapy. *Occupational Therapy & Rehabilitation, 26*(6), 455-460.

Licht, S. (1949). The changing role of the occupational therapist. *Occupational Therapy & Rehabilitation, 28*(3), 260-264.

Liepert, J. (2006). Motor cortex excitability in stroke before and after constraint-induced movement therapy. *Cognitive and Behavioral Neurology, 19*(1), 41-47.

Lilleleht, E. (2002). Progress and power: Exploring the disciplinary connections between moral treatment and psychiatric rehabilitation. *Philosophy, Psychiatry, & Psychology, 9*(2), 167-182.

Luchins, A. S. (1992). The cult of curability and the doctrine of perfectibility: Social context of the nineteenth century American asylum movement. *History of Psychiatry, 3*, 203-220.

Madhill, H., Brintnell, S., & Stewin, L. (1989). Professional literature: One view of a national perspective. *Australian Occupational Therapy Journal, 36*, 110-119.

Mattingly, C., & Fleming, M. H. (1994). *Clinical reasoning: Forms of inquiry in a therapeutic practice*. Philadelphia, PA: F.A. Davis Company.

McAllister, A. K. (2000). Cellular and molecular mechanisms of dendrite growth. *Cerebral Cortex, 10*(10), 963-973.

Mckinnon, A. L. (2000). Client values and satisfaction with occupational therapy. *Scandinavian Journal of Occupational Therapy, 7*(3), 99-106.

Mejias, U. A. (2006). Technology without ends: A critique of technocracy as a threat to being. Retrieved August 2, 2009, from http://blog.ulisesmejias.com/2006/06/03/technology-without-ends-a-critique-of-technocracy-as-a-threat-to-being

Meyer, A., & Winters, E. E. (Eds.). (1951). *The collected papers of Adolf Meyer* (Vol. 2). Baltimore, MD: Johns Hopkins Press.

Michaels, R. J. (1988). Addiction, compulsion, and the technology of consumption. *Economic Inquiry, 26*(1), 75-88.

Morgan, S. B., Kelkar, R. S., & Vyas, O. A. (2002). Client-centered occupational therapy for acute stroke patients. *Indian Journal of Occupational Therapy, 34*(1), 7-12.

National Center for Health Statistics. (2005). *Health, United States, 2005 with chart book on trends in the health of Americans*. Hyattsville, MD: Author.

Peloquin, S. M. (1989). Moral treatment: Contexts considered. *American Journal of Occupational Therapy, 43*, 537-544.

Peloquin, S. M. (1994). Moral treatment: How a caring practice lost its rationale. *American Journal of Occupational Therapy, 48*, 167-173.

Quiroga, V. A. M. (1995). *Occupational therapy: The first 30 years: 1900 to 1930*. Bethesda, MD: AOTA Press.

Rescher, N. (1980). *Unpopular essays on technological progress*. Pittsburgh, PA: University of Pittsburgh Press.

Rigby, R., Ryan, S., From, W., Walczak, E. & Jutai, J. (1996). A client-centered approach to developing assistive technology with children. *Occupational Therapy International, 3*(1), 67-79.

Rivers, J. R. (1993). *Contra technologiam: The crisis of value in a technological age*. Lanham, MD: University Press of America.

Rivers, J. R. (2005). An introduction to the metaphysics of technology. *Technology in Society, 27*, 551-574.

Rogers, J. C. (1983). Eleanor Clarke Slagle Lectureship—1983; Clinical reasoning: The ethics, science, and art. *American Journal of Occupational Therapy, 37*(9), 601-616.

Royeen, M., & Crabtree, J. L. (2006). *Culture in rehabilitation: From competency to proficiency*. Upper Saddle River, NJ: Prentice Hall.

Sackett, D. L., Rosenberg, W. M. C., Muir Gray, J. A., Haynes, R. B., & Richardson, W. S. (1996). Evidence-based medicine: What it is and what it isn't. *British Medical Journal, 312*, 71-72.

Simmons, D. C., Crepeau, E. B., & White, B. P. (2000). The predictive power of narrative data in occupational therapy evaluation. *American Journal of Occupational Therapy, 54*(5), 471-476.

Smith, R. O. (2000). The role of occupational therapy in a developmental technology model. *American Journal of Occupational Therapy, 54*(3), 339-340.

Sutcliffe, J., & Duin, N. (1992). *A history of medicine*. New York, NY: Barnes & Noble Books.

Tandon, P. N. (2000). The decade of the brain: A brief review. *Neurology India, 48*(3), 199-207.

Taub, E. (2004). Harnessing brain plasticity through behavioral techniques to produce new treatments in neurorehabilitation. *American Psychologist, 59*(8), 692-704.

Tickle-Degnen, L. (2002). Client-centered practice, therapeutic relationships, and the use of research evidence. *American Journal of Occupational Therapy, 56*(4), 470-474.

Tuke, S. (1813). *Description of the retreat, an institution near York, for insane persons*. London, England: Oxford University. [Digitized May 3, 2007].

United States Census Bureau. (2005). Facts for features: 15th anniversary of Americans with Disabilities Act: July 26, 2005. CB05-FF.10-2. Washington, DC: Author.

Unsworth, C. A. (2004). Clinical reasoning: How do pragmatic reasoning, worldview and client-centredness fit? *British Journal of Occupational Therapy, 67*(1), 10-19.

Warren, A. (2002). An evaluation of the Canadian Model of Occupational Performance and the Canadian Occupational Therapy Measure in mental health practice. *British Journal of Occupational Therapy, 65*(11), 515-522.

West, W. (1979). Historical perspectives. In Occupational therapy: 2001 AD: Papers presented at the special session of the Representative Assembly, November 1978 (pp. 9-17). Rockville, MD: AOTA Press.

Wiemer, R. (1979). Traditional and nontraditional practice arenas. In Occupational therapy: 2001 AD: Papers presented at the special session of the Representative Assembly, November 1978 (pp. 42-53). Rockville, MD: AOTA Press.

Wikipedia. (n.d.). Daniel Hale Williams. Retrieved January 9, 2009, from http://en.wikipedia.org/wiki/Daniel_Hale_Williams

World Federation of Occupational Therapists. (n. d.). History. Retrieved July 30, 2006, from http://www.wfot.org.au

Wressle, E., Samuelsson, K., & Henriksson, C. (1999). Responsiveness of the Swedish version of the Canadian Occupational Performance Measure. *Scandinavian Journal of Occupational Therapy, 6*(2), 84-89.

Yerxa, E. (1979). The philosophical base of occupation. In Occupational therapy: 2001 AD: Papers presented at the special session of the Representative Assembly, November 1978 (pp. 26-30). Rockville, MD: AOTA Press.

# Section VII
## Management of Occupational Therapy Services

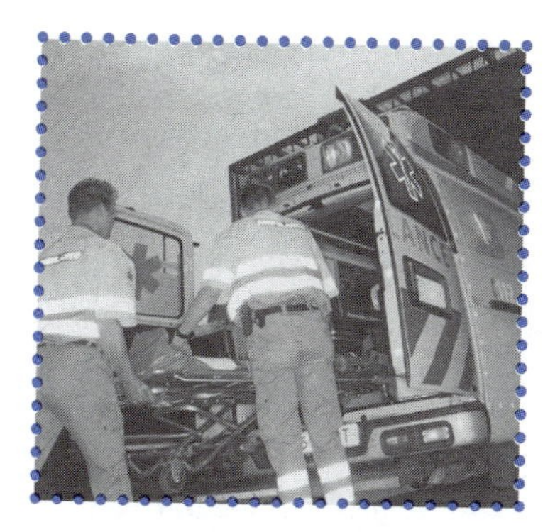

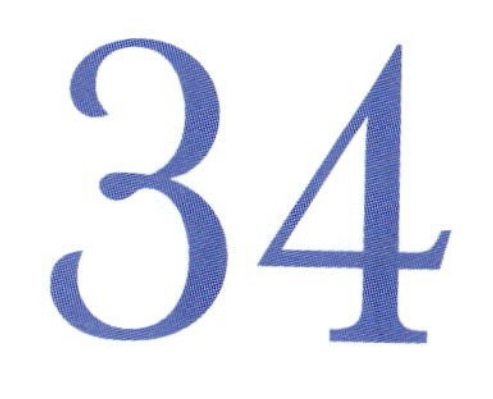

# Laws, Credentials, and Reimbursement

*Dory E. Holmes, MPH, OTR/L and Lisa L. Clark, MS, OTR/L*

**ACOTE Standards Explored in This Chapter**

B.7.3-7.6

**Key Terms**

Case mix groups
Durable medical equipment
Prospective payment system
Resource utilization groups
Utilization review

## Introduction

Twenty-five years ago, it was considered somewhat unethical for an occupational therapist or occupational therapy assistant to ask about a client's reimbursement mechanism. In the last few years, it has become increasingly common to ask and to be aware of how services will be compensated. Indeed, it is almost unethical, now, not to have information about payment. Many hospitals, outpatient settings, and private practices hire people whose sole purpose in the organization is to access reimbursement information. The practitioner is expected to maximize this reimbursement for the client's benefit. This information is now added to the already existent complexities in providing care to consumers in this evidence-based health system. This chapter will introduce the basics of reimbursement systems. It is important to understand that for every rule, there is an exception, and for every payment system, there is a large amount of additional information that cannot be included in an introductory chapter.

For new practitioners, the world of payment can be overwhelming. However, the following is a simple formula to consider:

Reimbursement = Location of Service + Coding + Documentation + Payer

Each section of the formula will be discussed in this chapter.

## Reimbursement

Reimbursement is the fee received for a service rendered. That fee may be paid in several ways: a fee schedule, fee-for-service, discounts, per diem rate, or per episode of care rate. Fees are based on a formula and may be paid in many different ways. These formulas consist of a relative value unit (RVU) and a monetary conversion factor. Components of the RVU are time used by the provider, expenses of running a practice, and professional liability expenses. The conversion factors are determined by geographic cost differences. Set by agreement between the contractor/facility (provider) of service and the payer, the reimbursement payment is typically determined in advance.



K. Sladyk, K. Jacobs, & N. MacRae (Eds.).
*Occupational Therapy Essentials for Clinical Competence* (pp. 377-388).

## Location of Service

It is occupational therapy's good fortune that services are reimbursed today in so many settings. From hospitals, skilled nursing facilities, outpatient settings, home health and community settings, schools, and private practice, the occupational therapist is viewed as a skilled professional health care provider. These various locations have separate and distinct regulatory rules that govern the facilities' operation, billing, and reimbursement practices. The sites of service will be examined in depth in this chapter.

## Coding

Coding is a fundamental to reimbursement (Practice Management Information Corporation [PMIC], 2005). It can involve three parts: the diagnosis code (ICD-9-CM), procedural code (current procedural terminology [CPT]), and procedure code (Healthcare's Common Procedure Coding System [HCPCS]). The primary diagnosis determination is the responsibility of the physician. Occupational therapy practitioners do not typically set the diagnosis code. These diagnosis codes are found in the ICD-9-CM manual (PMIC, 2005). The ICD-9 manual categorizes a client's medical condition by anatomical systems. Coding must match the diagnosis written on the physician's referral/prescription. You or your facility/agency will be ensuring that this is on the bill.

Occupational therapy practitioners should become very familiar with the CPT. CPT codes are the primary set of codes practitioners use and should understand (Centers for Medicare & Medicaid Services [CMS], 2006a). They help allocate charges to the occupational therapy intervention program. The CPT manual provides a uniform language for reliable national communication and makes reporting easier (American Medical Association [AMA], 2005). It facilitates claims processing, guides medical review, and contributes to education and research (Fearon, 2004).

Within the CPT manual is a chapter titled "Physical Medicine and Rehabilitation." The Physical Medicine and Rehabilitation codes describe the majority of interventions provided by occupational therapy personnel. Occupational therapy personnel may also use the HCPCS-II codes. These codes describe supplies, procedures, and services not listed in the CPT manual. An example would be the "L" codes, which are used for orthotics and splinting services billing.

## Documentation

As noted in the chapter on documentation (Chapter 32), written documentation is the true and legal record of the occupational therapy evaluation, plan of care, interventions, and outcomes. It is a tool to support and manage reimbursement. The occupational therapy practitioner's documentation will be examined by auditors or reviewers for the following (Fearon, 2004):

- Medical necessity
- Appropriateness of interventions for the diagnosis
- Appropriate frequency and duration for a client's rehabilitation potential
- Expectation of functional improvement
- The client's response to the service
- The level of staff rendering the service

The documentation, whether narrative or computerized, must support the codes billed to receive the payment expected (AMA, 2006). It must be concise, clear, and should minimize abbreviations. Different plans may have specific documentation criteria such as requiring specific forms or mandating a schedule for progress updates. They may also require pre-approval for the stay and limit the length of stay according to setting. On a rare occasion, a client's insurance plan may not pay for occupational therapy services. Therefore, it is important to ascertain the coverage that is (and is not) provided with each policy. Under most circumstances, it is the provider who is responsible for knowing whether the service is covered. Payers' expectations are that documentation justifies the purpose of occupational therapy and reports the benefits of the intervention specific to the client's goals. Therefore, learning the documentation for each setting is essential.

## Payer

Occupational therapy is a commonly covered benefit. The common payment sources are Medicare, Medicaid, private health insurance, Workers' Compensation, and federally-funded programs such as for veterans, railroad workers, and other federal employees. These payers will reimburse for "skilled" therapy. Skilled means that the intervention requires the unique professional abilities of occupational therapy personnel. Simply stated, only an occupational therapist or occupational therapy assistant under the supervision of an occupational therapist can safely and effectively provide the complexity of service. The occupational therapy practitioner should never assume coverage and should always inquire about a client's benefit.

One example of the importance of understanding reimbursement is Medicare, which is divided into Part A and Part B. Part A covers inpatient hospitals, home health agencies (HHA), and skilled nursing facilities. Part B, a voluntary and supplemental benefit, covers physician services, outpatient services, and durable medical equipment (American Occupational Therapy Association [AOTA], 2005). It is possible that a client could have coverage for occupational therapy in settings covered by Part A but not Part B. Often, individuals make insurance coverage choices and decisions based on the ability to pay without realizing what might be forfeited in the long term.

Another example of the need for the practitioner to be informed about benefits is illustrated in Medicaid programs, which are administered by individual states. Since Medicaid is funded jointly by the state and federal governments, the federal government mandates that states provide a minimum set of specific services. Regrettably, occupational therapy is an "optional" service in these mandates and may not be covered in the state where you work.

A third example of practice limitations is Tricare, the federal insurance program for active military. Occupational therapy is defined in the Tricare Policy Manual (Tricare, 2008). Practitioners must be aware of how services are defined so as to practice and document in a way that follows payer guidelines. Tricare has selected CPT Procedure Codes they approve for reimbursement. Notably, they exclude vocational assessment and training, sensory integration training, and cognitive retraining, despite the fact that these are within occupational therapy's scope of practice.

In an effort to control national health expenditures, the majority of the payers today are managed. Health care expenditures spiraled upward as a result of increasing population, growth in health care personnel, the explosion of medical technology, growth in pharmaceutical advancements, and the growth in financing health care (Bernstein et al., 2003). Therefore, managed care was created to decrease the growing cost of national health care expenditures and to keep the Medicare Trust Fund solvent. Regardless of the payer group, all managed care systems possess some or all of the following characteristics: precertification, preauthorization, concurrent review, utilization review, and predischarge planning. These concepts will be reviewed as we examine the various settings in the continuum of care.

Occupational therapy practitioners should possess a grounded understanding of the basics of reimbursement. They should also understand that it is important to access information directly from the source as much as possible. At times, even employers and billing supervisors cannot follow the intricacies of every system. If a practitioner has a question, she should take time to get to the source and find someone who will explain the issue in understandable language. Though intimidating, asking for information to be clear and understandable is not an unreasonable request. Regardless of payer, the occupational therapy practitioner's focus is upon skilled intervention. The practitioner is ethically bound to provide services that are reasonable and necessary.

Now that some basics of reimbursement concepts have been introduced, this chapter will continue with discussion about payment options typically available in each setting within the continuum of care. Introductory reimbursement information will be highlighted for each practice setting. This will organize the information in a way that mirrors how practitioners must understand it in the context of practice settings.

# Acute Hospital Care

Hospitals are the cornerstone of the American health care system. They differ in size, ownership, mission, financing, and population served. All hospitals are designed to serve communities on a bed-to-population ratio. Some types of hospitals include community hospitals, teaching hospitals, specialty hospitals, public hospitals, and multihospital systems. Hospitals consume 31% of national health care expenditures (Cowan, Catlin, Smith, & Sensenig, 2004). They focus on client care as well as cost-containment, decreasing length of stay, managing utilization of resources, and staff performance. Regardless of type, the mission of any hospital is curing and caring. Hospitals are licensed by the individual states and may voluntarily participate in regulatory accreditations as Joint Commission on Accreditation of Healthcare Organizations (JCAHO) and Commission on Accreditation of Rehabilitation Facilities (CARF). Individual state licensing may require that occupational therapy is provided as a service.

## Medicare

With the increasing number of elderly in all our communities, the predominant payer for hospital care is Medicare. As mentioned previously, inpatient hospital stays are paid by Part A. Medicare is a federally funded program that is available to people 65 and over, individuals with disabilities and their dependents, and those with chronic kidney disease.

Occupational therapy services are "bundled" into an inclusive rate that Medicare pays the hospital. This daily rate is based on the person's diagnosis. Medicare has designed "diagnosis related groups" (DRGs), which take into consideration how much medical care a person usually needs given each particular diagnosis. The payment is to cover the usual and customary hospital stay. If the person needs to stay longer than usual, the hospital may lose money. If the person is able to leave the hospital and return home, or move to another level of care earlier than usual, the hospital may make money on the stay. Occupational therapy is part of what the hospital provides, for which they receive a payment related to the diagnostic group under which the client falls.

## Medicaid

Medicaid is the state and federally funded program for health care. Each state has its own program. There are federal guidelines that mandate a minimum set of services that states must provide with their Medicaid programs (CMS, 2005a). As noted previously, occupational therapy falls under "optional" services, meaning individual states may decide whether their Medicaid programs will cover occupational therapy services. Not all states have opted for occupational therapy coverage. Practitioners must learn about their own states' coverage in order to practice knowledgeably. They can do this via their state occupational therapy membership organizations, or they can get on their states' Web sites and search for occupational therapy- and rehabilitation-covered services.

## Private Health Insurance

Hospitals have contractual agreements with the various private health insurance companies. Contracts typically denote a percent discount on the cost of care, a fee schedule, and/or a predetermined payment amount for an episode of care. Inpatient acute care that is managed may require pre-certification for someone to be admitted from the emergency room to the hospital or to have a surgical procedure performed. While an inpatient, the individual's case is monitored by an external case manager who is reviewing the medical record for daily progress. Utilization review often occurs internally and examines the efficiency of the facility or how services are being utilized. Pre-discharge planning will coordinate the transfer of the client to the next level of care. These subsequent locations usually also have contracts with the payer.

# Inpatient Rehabilitation Facilities

Inpatient rehabilitation facilities (IRFs) are either freestanding hospitals or rehabilitation units in acute care hospitals. Their role is to provide intensive rehabilitation services for an inpatient population. They differ from an acute care hospital because of the focus on function and rehabilitation. Clients who are admitted must be able to tolerate 3 hours of intense therapy per day. Occupational therapy is identified as one of those essential services for a client's recovery.

## Medicare

Just like the acute care hospital, which is paid by Part A, an IRF is reimbursed on a predetermined rate system that classifies client discharges into categories called the case mix groups (CMGs) (CMS, 2006b). These are based on the top most common diagnostic groups admitted to IRFs. The CMG is based upon "rehabilitation impairment categories, functional state (both motor and cognitive), age, and other co-morbidities. The CMG determines the payment the facility receives for an episode of care.

On admission, data are collected on the client using the Minimum Data Set for Post Acute Care (MDS-PAC) client assessment instrument. The assessment instrument emphasizes client care needs. Reimbursing the facility based upon the resources used, the CMG is designed just like the DRG that is used in acute hospital care. The focus is on efficiency and coordinating the care within a timeframe. IRFs also operate under the "75% Rule." This means a certain percentage of the facilities' admissions must require intensive multidisciplinary rehabilitation services. This compliance percentage was designed to ensure that IRFs are distinct from other levels of care (i.e., acute care or skilled care).

## Medicaid

Medicaid is seldom the primary payer on a skilled unit. There are instances where it is used as a secondary payer.

## Private Health Insurance

This payer responds similarly in the IRF setting as it does in the skilled nursing facility (SNF) (see following section).

# Skilled Nursing Facilities

Occupational therapy services are often provided in SNF. The SNFs are typically designed to take clients who are medically stable but require additional ancillary and/or nursing care. They are designed to transition the client to a community setting or to a lower level of care such as a long-term care setting. In the mid- to late 1980s, SNFs were the fastest growing settings for the employment of occupational therapy practitioners (Kane, Chen, Blewett, & Sangl, 1996) (Figure 34-1). In 1985, 55.7% of the nursing homes in the United States offered occupational therapy services, rising to 87.2% in 1995, and then adjusting to 94% in 1999 (Bernstein et al., 2004). This growth was attributed to payment policies reducing acute hospital stays (Torrens, 1993), improvement in technological and pharmaceutical advances, and the passage of the Balanced Budget Act (BBA) of 1997.

## Medicare

Partly as a result of this growth, Medicare (which is the primary payer for rehabilitation in this setting) decided that costs needed to be controlled. The BBA of 1997 was passed and significantly changed how payment was made to these facilities. Medicare enacted a Prospective Payment System (PPS) in 1999 as a result of the BBA. Prior to 1999, sites were reimbursed retrospectively via a formula including how much it cost them to provide rehabilitation services. With the onset of PPS, payments were made based on a daily rate (per diem).

This rate is figured by performing an assessment (minimum data set [MDS]) for the client that helps determine the resources needed to serve him or her. The client is then placed in a resource utilization group (RUG) category based on how much service he or she appears to need (CMS, 2005b). Occupational therapists sometimes assist in the determination of which RUG the client will fall under. The RUG is very important as it determines the per diem payment rate the skilled nursing facility will receive for the client's stay. The RUG is directly related to the total number of minutes of therapy the consumer receives for the week. This is a total of the weekly minutes occupational, physical, and speech therapists have spent with the person. Thus, it behooves the facility from a financial standpoint to offer therapies seven days per week (CMS, 2009a).

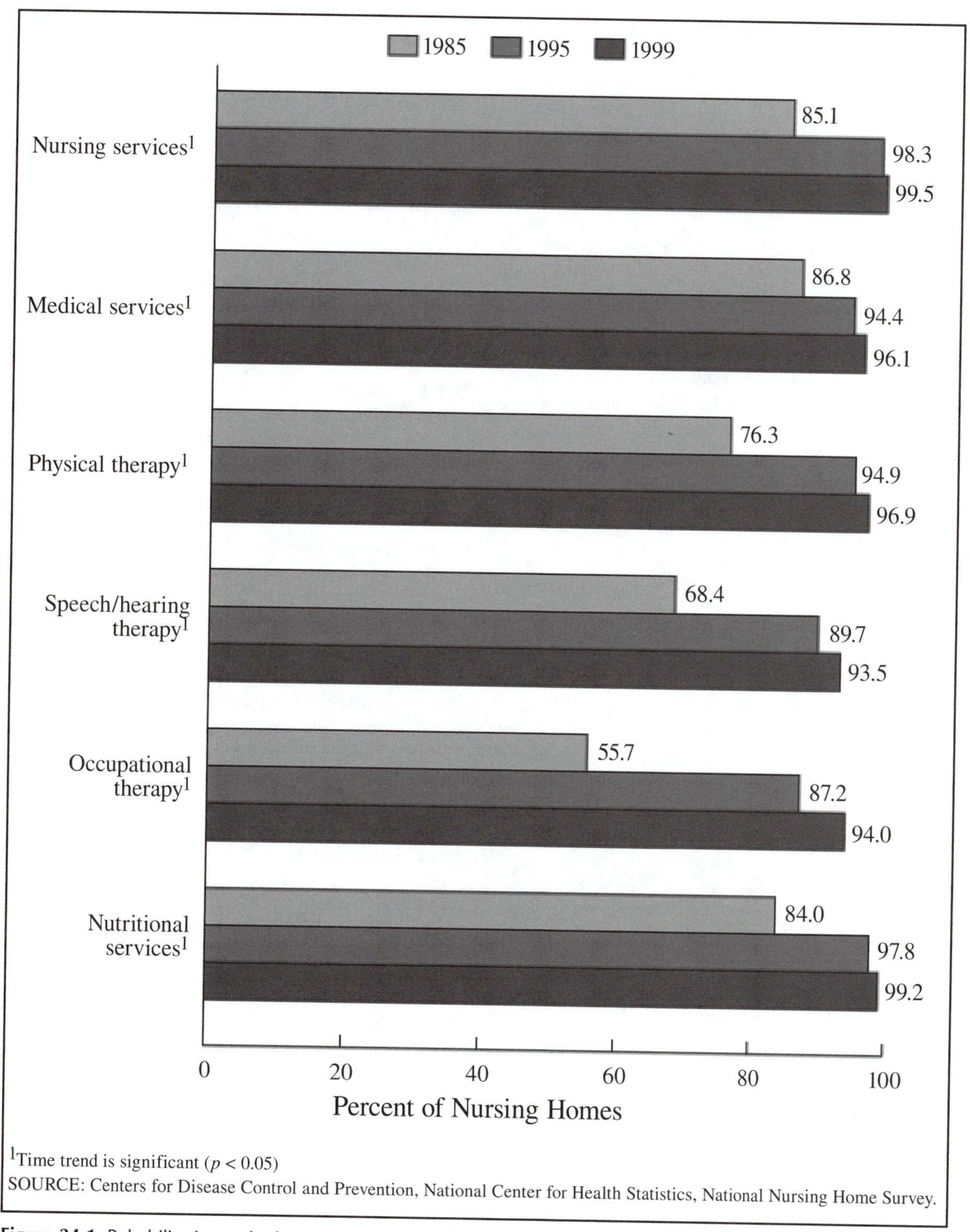


**Figure 34-1.** Rehabilitative and other services offered by nursing homes: United States, 1985, 1995, 1999. Reproduced with permission from the National Center for Health Statistics.

## Medicaid

As with IRFs, Medicaid is seldom the primary payer in this setting. There are instances where it is used as a secondary payer.

## Private Health Insurance

As noted in the acute hospital section, a client may have been transferred to a specific SNF because of contractual agreements. The therapy plan of care will need to be reviewed by a case manager to determine if it is reasonable and necessary. Often, the length of stay is determined by the diagnosis and the limits of the plan. Progress notes will be reviewed concurrently by the external reviewers and internal utilization review team. Occupational therapy practitioners may find durable medical equipment (DME) purchases may only be made through vendors who are approved by the insurance company and who may not be local.

## Comprehensive Outpatient Rehabilitation Facilities

"A CORF is a facility that engages in diagnostic, therapeutic, and restorative services to outpatients for the rehabilitation of the injured and disabled or to clients recovering from illness" (CMS, 2004). It is located in an outpatient setting and the program must be comprehensive, coordinated, and skilled. Minimum services required by regulation are physicians' services, physical therapy, and social or psychological services. Occupational therapy is considered a skilled service, but it is optional. Most comprehensive outpatient rehabilitation facilities (CORFs) employ occupational therapy practitioners.

### Medicare

CORF services are paid under Medicare Part B. Payment is made under the Medicare Physician Fee Schedule (MPFS) for all services except biologicals (i.e., specialized wound dressings) and drugs. It is mandated by Medicare that adequate space and equipment are necessary for any service offered. Generally, all services must be delivered onsite. Exceptions are home evaluations, physical therapy, occupational therapy, and speech-language pathology. Home assessments occur in the client's residence. Coverage is limited to the services of only one professional who is selected by the CORF.

### Medicaid and Private Health Insurance

For information regarding Medicaid and private insurances, refer to the following section. The mechanisms are similar for both settings.

## Outpatient—Hospital-Based

As cost containment and prospective payment have reduced hospital stays, more hospital services are delivered in outpatient settings, often called "ambulatory care." Subsequently, outpatient therapy departments have experienced enormous growth over the past decade. These therapy departments can offer a single service or provide multidisciplinary interventions. For an occupational therapy practitioner, these settings offer opportunities for those who are generalists or specialists.

### Medicare

Outpatient occupational therapy services are reimbursed by Medicare Part B. However, depending on the service site, reimbursement can pay for two distinct sets of services. Occupational therapy personnel can work in either behavioral health partial hospitalization programs (PHPs) or in physical rehabilitation outpatient therapy departments.

Clients eligible for Medicare Part B coverage of PHPs are those who were discharged from an inpatient psychiatric intervention program or those who, in absence of available partial hospitalization, would require inpatient hospitalization. The PHP can also be provided at a community mental health center. The reimbursement system that pays for partial hospitalization is called outpatient prospective payment system (OPPS). OPPS was designed for ambulatory care procedures and pays a per diem rate for the total resources used for a single outpatient visit. Occupational therapy can be one of those resources in a PHP, but it is not mandated. Although prevocational and vocational assessments are within the occupational therapy scope of practice, services primarily related to employment opportunities, work skills, or work settings are not covered.

In hospital-based outpatient therapy departments, occupational therapy is paid for by procedure on the Medicare fee schedule. Medicare will pay 80% of the fee after the client has paid the annual deductible. Medicare administration has developed local coverage determination (LCD) policies to interpret the provisions as they apply to different geographic jurisdictions. The LCD includes consideration for local and regional practice norms. Occupational therapy services are payable under the following conditions (CMS, 2009b):

- Medically necessary
- A plan for furnishing services has been established by a physician/nonphysician practitioner (NPP). A NPP is a physician assistant, clinical nurse specialist, or nurse practitioner. The physician must be a doctor of medicine, osteopathy, podiatric medicine, or optometry. Doctors of dental surgery, dental medicine, or chiropractors cannot refer nor establish a plan of care under Medicare Part B.
- The individual is under the care of a physician
- Care is provided on an outpatient basis

Reimbursement of a therapy claim is provided when an outpatient plan of care for therapy is certified by a physician/NPP every 90 days (CMS, 2008). CMS has printed forms called the 700 and 701 forms for the initial certification and ongoing certification process, respectively. These must be completed by an occupational therapist and not an occupational therapy assistant. The therapist must be able to produce required approved intervention information for the Medicare intermediary upon request.

### Medicaid

Medicaid payments for outpatient occupational therapy services vary by state if the service is a covered service for that state. It is the practitioner's responsibility to acquire information about Medicaid payment in his or her state. If occupational therapy services are reimbursed, it is often at a reduced fee schedule or for a limited number of visits.

### Private Health Insurance

In the outpatient setting, the primary care physician is the gatekeeper to referrals and services. In most situations, the physician must make a request to the insurer for services. Once this is confirmed, the occupational therapy provider will evaluate the client and submit the plan of care to the insurer. The insurer will review for medical necessity and certify a specific number of visits within a timeframe. It is the provider's responsibility to track the number of visits and timeframe. Should the plan of care exceed the limits without prior authorization, the practitioner will not be reimbursed and it may become the client's responsibility to pay. The practitioner may use a variety of methods to track the number of visits or time frames, such as specialized scheduling systems, customized flow sheets for documentation, and appointment logs.

## Outpatient—Private Practice

Clinics or practices owned by private individuals are considered to be private practices. These businesses often specialize in a particular area of rehabilitation, or even one or two particular areas of the occupational therapy scope of practice. Settings can vary widely in the services they offer—from wellness or alternative therapy sites to more traditional orthopedic or ergonomic interventions. Some practitioners act as private practices and contract their services out to schools or nursing homes, for example.

### Medicare

Many guidelines for occupational therapy reimbursement in a private practice clinic are similar to a hospital-owned clinic. One significant difference is that Medicare has passed a cap on rehabilitation services provided in non-hospital outpatient settings. There is a combined cap for physical therapy and speech therapy services, and an equivalent cap for occupational therapy services alone. The CMS Web site is helpful in tracking this (see Electronic Resources). AOTA has also tracked the delays and reinstatement of the outpatient therapy cap on a regular basis.

Practitioners who have private practices with Medicare reimbursement must apply for provider numbers through Medicare. No payment for services will be made without an assigned provider number. Medicare requires proof of a practitioner's credentials before they will issue a provider number.

### Medicaid

Providing occupational therapy services in a private practice and receiving Medicaid payment also requires a provider number be procured from the state. Practitioners will need to ensure that occupational therapy is a reimbursed service in their state and research what services are paid for and at what rate. As a Medicaid provider, therapists should be aware that Medicaid has the right to perform an audit of the practice's financial records at any time.

### Private Health Insurance

Often, these payers will negotiate contracts with outpatient clinics for a predetermined reimbursement amount. This amount can be based on the number of visits, amount paid per visit, or types of intervention that are approved.

## Home Health Care

Home is the setting of choice for recuperation for many individuals, and it has become an integral part in the continuum of comprehensive health care. It integrates health, social, and supportive services that nurture the health and well-being of an individual. The passage of the BBA of 1997 had the opposite effect on HHAs as it did with skilled nursing facilities. During the time when the utilization of SNFs was growing, HHAs experienced a reduction in the length of time clients remained in home health care and the average number of visits.

### Medicare

Eligibility for home care is clearly defined in the Medicare Part A regulations. The client must meet four qualifying criteria. The individual must be the following (CMS, 2005c):

1. Homebound
2. Require intermittent skilled services
3. Have a physician-established plan of care
4. The HHA must be Medicare certified

The definition of homebound is critical. It has five components (CMS, 2005c):

1. A defined place of residence
2. Normal inability to leave home
3. Leaving takes considerable and taxing effort
4. Absences are infrequent and of short duration
5. The client may attend a certified/licensed day care program

Absences from the home should be of short duration and include, for example, attending a religious service; occasional trip to physician or barber; or a unique event such as a family reunion, funeral, or graduation.

Place of residence is defined as a house/apartment, an assisted living facility, group home, or a relative's home. Services cannot take place in a hospital, SNF, or long-term care facility. "Inability to leave home" means that leaving is medically contradicted, and it requires a supportive device or support from another. By definition, taxing effort to leave the home results in shortness of breath, dyspnea on exertion, or weakness.

Homebound status is evaluated on admission and throughout the episode of care. A HHA uses the Outcome and Assessment Information Set (OASIS), which sets the payment rate for each 60 days of service. Rates are based on skilled need. After a period of time, the client may switch from Medicare Part A coverage to his or her Part B benefits. Skilled need must include intermittent skilled nursing, physical therapy, speech pathology, or a continued need for occupational therapy. Only nursing, physical therapy, or speech pathology can initially qualify a client for home care services. Qualifying means that the client must have at least one of these three needs prior to receiving occupational therapy. Once the case is established, occupational therapy can continue as a sole service. The plan of care must be certified by the physician, and the course of care must have a finite and predictable ending period.

### Medicaid

Medicaid is most often a secondary payer for home health services, if accessed at all, and not a primary payer. Some states have created certain provisions for Medicaid reimbursement for certain populations, such as children.

### Private Health Insurance

Each private health insurance policy or managed care policy will allow for different amounts (duration/payment rates) of home health care or may not provide for care in the home setting at all. The occupational therapy practitioner must know what each policy will cover.

## Community Settings

Some community settings offer services that may be paid for on a "fee-for-service" basis. In this instance, the site decides the cost for each service and charges consumers accordingly. In these cases, consumers are funding their own health and wellness care.

School services are often covered by federal Department of Education funds. Legislation over the past 30 years has guaranteed the funding and dramatically changed the provision of services to young children. In 1975, The Education For All Handicapped Children Act (Cengage Learning, n.d.) guaranteed a free and appropriate public education for all handicapped children. Within the law, occupational therapy was defined as a "related" service since it enabled a child to access his or her education. Services needed to be educationally relevant for the school setting. In 1986, the law was amended to include special education and related services to handicapped preschoolers. This amendment focused on family training and education. The significance for our profession was that occupational therapy was clearly identified as a primary early intervention service.

The Individuals with Disabilities Education Act (IDEA) of 1990 was the new name for the 1975 act and was a reauthorization of the earlier commitment to public education for children with disabilities. It defined the minimum amount of services that a state must provide to various student groups (i.e., infants, toddlers, children, and older youth with disabilities). In 1997, IDEA was amended to include rights and protection for children with disabilities. It also stressed learning results for children (U.S. Department of Education, n.d.).

As the price of public education has increased with the expansions and federal education funds have been reduced, some states are also choosing to access Medicaid funds for eligible children in the schools. This can be complex, and practitioners will need to explore the regulations in each state.

## Military Health Services

Our military health system is unique. The system is divided into two groups: active military and retired/disabled. The active military system provides health care wherever enlisted personnel are assigned. This can be anywhere around the world. It has a focus on wellness and is highly organized and integrated. The most unique feature of the military system is the master client record, which travels with the enlistee. The military has developed the most comprehensive medical record in the United States health system. Should a health issue become long-term and the enlistee cannot return to active duty, the individual receives a medical discharge and is referred to the Veterans' Administration (VA). VA hospitals have seen a huge increase in clients as aging veterans have developed medical issues. Originally designed as hospitals, the VAs have experienced growth in their outpatient programs that parallels civilian health care.

Dependents and family members of active military have a separate health system that combines the active military system with the general health care system. Previously known as CHAMPUS, it is today called the U.S. Family Health Care Program. Dependents of military personnel receive routine services at military clinics and are referred to local community providers for specialty services. This system is managed and adheres to the Tricare provision of care.

Occupational therapy is an essential service in both military hospitals and VA hospitals. Therapists and assistants are serving around the globe. Although reimbursement is not the focus, our military health system was the first national movement toward managed care.

## Social Justice Issues and Advocacy

As may have become obvious, there are considerable ways for ethical, moral, and social policy issues to arise in the world of reimbursement. Chapters 2, 40, and 47 provide more information on these topics.

Occupational therapy practitioners are bound by the *Code of Ethics* developed by AOTA and by the code from their places of employment, but how do these play out when there is no funding for someone to receive needed services? Conversely, if organizations consistently provide services for no or minimal payment, how do they stay viable in order to help the most number of people in need of health care? In our culture, we have struggled with the terms we use for people who need health care (patients, clients, consumers, etc.). Kronenberg and Pollard (2006), pointed out that these terms that we strive to use to adequately reflect who our consumers are have a common denominator. They all imply that the person is someone who can pay for our services. How is this consistent with our professional beliefs about social justice and who "deserves" intervention? Occupational therapy practitioners must continue to engage in the struggle of how, where, and why people receive services.

In instances where consumers have no health care coverage, there are some options. Facilities may opt to set up payment plans for clients. In some cases, organizations decide to write off payment for care rendered.

Occupational therapy practitioners should possess strong knowledge about their communities and supports that are available. Help might come from community religious or fraternal organizations who offer financial support to people with significant health care needs. Contacting local agencies such as The United Way can inform the practitioner of myriad community offerings.

Occupational therapy practitioners act as advocates for clients. This includes having awareness of over-arching public health issues and working to be part of the solution. As a member of the larger health care team, it is occupational therapy's responsibility to participate in public health education campaigns to urge consumers to follow recommendations (e.g., weight control, exercise, smoking cessation, backpack safety) and intervention regimens (e.g., medication schedules).

## Meaning for the Practice of Occupational Therapy

In present times, all care is managed in some form. There have been benefits to managed care. The expansion of outpatient and community services has opened up new employment opportunities for practitioners. The cost-saving tenets of managed care have made occupational therapy assistants in greater demand. The early emphasis on quality assurance has fueled the profession's efforts for evidence-based practice and the publication of new professional journals. It has promoted specialty certification and the development of new practice parameters. Cost savings have come from limiting unneeded care and keeping people healthy through prevention.

For every benefit there is a drawback. Care today has benefit limitations, whether in cost, time frame, or choice. These limitations have created role conflicts within some settings. They have affected access and availability. They have also created increased concerns about confidentiality and "indirect" intervention time. In response to these concerns, the Health Insurance Portability and Accountability Act (HIPAA) of 1996 was passed to establish national standards for electronic health care transactions and to assure privacy and security for health data (CMS, 2005d).

From a historical and public health perspective, reimbursement issues have fueled many changes in practice over the years. The push to move care from acute hospital settings to other (less expensive) levels of care has significantly shortened the length of stay (LOS) in acute settings. This shift has also increased the medical acuity of clients moving on to skilled or rehabilitative care, home health care, and even nursing home care. Occupational therapy practitioners have had to learn new skills, reflect on practice, and adapt to new documentation as these changes infiltrated their work places.

Shrinking reimbursement has forced occupational therapy practitioners, and others, to offer 7-days-a-week coverage in settings, while "Monday through Friday" used to be a more typical routine. It has also asked practitioners to ensure that interventions are effective. Evaluation skills are crucial in skillfully setting appropriate interventions that meet clients' needs for service and attend to the parameters of the payment system. Productivity standards have shifted over the years in order to meet the financial needs of provider institutions. This can be stressful in many settings and requires the occupational therapy practitioner to be flexible and creative with scheduling.

Practitioners must understand the big picture of health care reimbursement. It is easy to forget the other part of the reimbursement equation as occupational therapy practitioners work in the "helping" professions. Money for payment has to come from somewhere. Insurance companies, Medicare, or the state Medicaid reimbursement systems are not always adversarial in the sometimes limited services they cover. At times, these organizations are working with limited funds themselves. For example, consider that state Medicaid funds come from people's tax dollars. Someone, somewhere, makes hard decisions about how and where those funds are spent. At times, occupational therapy practitioners need to advocate about insurance coverage. Self-advocacy and consideration for people's best interest from a social justice standpoint is core to the profession's espoused ethics and philosophy. Principle 1 of the Occupational Therapy Code of Ethics requires practitioners show concern for the well-being of the people they serve (see Appendix F).

## Summary

The occupational therapy consumer ultimately pays all health care costs. Over a lifetime, the consumer pays premiums for health care insurance through an employer, payroll taxes under Social Security for Medicare in later years, insurance premiums for private secondary coverage, general out-of-pocket expenses, and state taxes to support the Medicaid system. Consumers of occupational therapy services include clients, insurance companies, vendors, and employers, and they are all demanding quality. It is tantamount that each professional is committed to the standards of practice set by AOTA and is knowledgeable about and using evidence-based interventions.

Occupational therapists derive benefits from engaging with their state and national membership associations (see Chapter 41). These groups advocate for the profession and provide education regarding reimbursement considerations. Encouraging clients to be active participants, valuing lifelong learning in the profession, refining teaching skills, and thoughtfully promoting wellness are key characteristics of practitioners who are able to effectively meet the payment challenges of today's health care continuum. The important issue for the practitioner is to be responsibly informed, provide services thoughtfully and responsibly, and have the confidence to ask questions about reimbursement.

## Student Self-Assessment

1. Explore your own and a family member's insurance policies. Can you understand them? Do they provide for occupational therapy service reimbursement?
2. Review the case in Chapter 25. In pairs, work on coding the diagnostic information in the case using the CPT codes for rehabilitation.
3. Access the AOTA Web site and discuss at least 3 of the questions listed under the Reimbursement section's Frequently Asked Questions. What are the current issues/trends in reimbursement?
4. Break into groups of four or five. Discuss:
    - Why occupational therapy is not a primary or covered service in some insurance plans or settings.
    - What steps can be taken by the profession to remedy this?

## Electronic Resources

- Center for Disease Control, National Center for Health Statistics: www.cdc.gov/nchs
- Center for Medicare and Medicaid Services, Department of Health and Human Services—Valuable resource for manuals, transmittals, and education: www.cms.hhs.gov
- Health Net Federal Services provides provider manuals for military beneficiaries: www.hnfs.net
- Oasis Training provides CMS-sponsored traing for home health care providers and surveyors: www.oasistraining.org
- PT Manager—Resource on management for private practitioners: www.ptmanager.com
- American Occupational Therapy Association: www.aota.org
- National Technical Information Services—Largest resource for government funded scientific, technical, engineering, and business information: www.ntis.gov
- Blue Cross Blue Shield Association—Resources for health plans: www.bluecares.com
- U.S. Department of Veteran Affairs—Resource for helath benfits and services: www.va.gov

**Evidence-Based Research Chart**

| Topics | Evidence |
|---|---|
| History of health care | Torrens, 1993 |
| Health care economics | Harrington & Estes, 2004 |
| Health care utilization | Bernstein et al., 2003 |

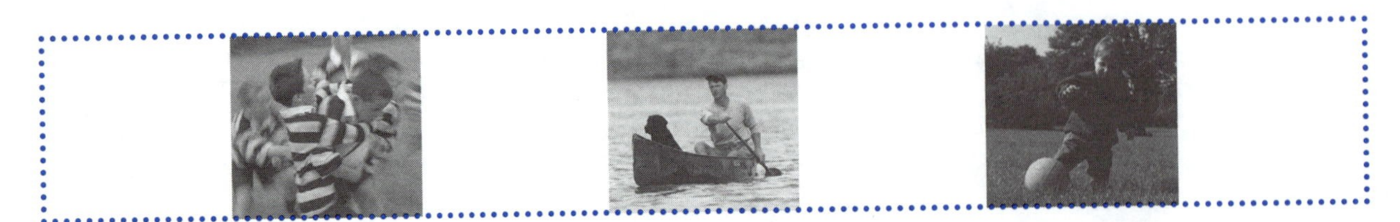

# References

American Medical Association. (2005). *CPT standard edition—2006: Current procedural terminology.* Clifton Park, NY: Thomson Delmar Learning.

American Occupational Therapy Association. (2005). Fact sheet: Medicare basics. Retrieved August 14, 2009, from http://aota.org/Practioners/Reimb/Pay/Medicare/FactSheets/37788.aspx

Bernstein, A. B., Hing, E., Moss, A. J., Allen, K. F., Siller, A. B., & Tiggle, R. B. (2003). *Health care in America: Trends in utilization.* Hyattsville, MD: National Center for Health Statistics. Retrieved August 13, 2009, from http://www.cdc.gov/nchs/data/misc/healthcare.pdf

Cengage Learning. (n.d.). The Education For All Handicapped Children Act (PL 94-142) 1975. Retrieved July 31, 2009, from http://college.cengage.com/education/resources/res_prof/students/spec_ed/legislation/pl_94-142.html

Centers for Medicare and Medicaid Services. (2004). Comprehensive outpatient rehabilitation facility (CORF) coverage, section 20.1: Required services. In *Medicare benefit policy manual.* Retrieved August 13, 2009, from http://www.cms.hhs.gov/manuals/Downloads/bp102c12.pdf

Centers for Medicare and Medicaid Services. (2005a). Medicaid-at-a-glance 2005. Retrieved August 13, 2009, from http://www.cms.hhs.gov/medicaiddatasourcesgeninfo/02_maag2005.asp

Centers for Medicare and Medicaid Services. (2005b). Medicare program; prospective payment system and consolidated billing for skilled nursing facilities for FY 2006. Final rule. *Federal Register, 70*(149), 45025-45127.

Centers for Medicare and Medicaid Services. (2005c). Home health services, section 30.1: Confined to the home. In *Medicare benefit policy manual.* Retrieved August 13, 2009, from http://www.cms.hhs.gov/manuals/Downloads/bp102c07.pdf

Centers for Medicare and Medicaid Services. (2005d). HIPPA Overview. Retrieved August 13, 2009, from http://www.cms.hhs.gov/hipaa-GenInfo

Centers for Medicare and Medicaid Services. (2006a). CMS manual system: Pub 100-04 Medicare claims processing, transmittal 805. Retrieved August 13, 2009, from http://www.cms.hhs.gov/Transmittals/Downloads/R805CP.PDF

Centers for Medicare and Medicaid Services. (2006b). Certification and compliance: Inpatient rehabilitation facilities. Retrieved August 13, 2009, from http://www.cms.hhs.gov/CertificationandComplianc/16_InpatientRehab.asp#TopOfPage

Centers for Medicare and Medicaid Services. (2008). Therapy personnel qualifications and policies effective January 1, 2008. *MLN Matters, MM5921.* Retrieved August 13, 2009, from http://www.cms.hhs.gov/MLNMattersArticles/downloads/MM5921.pdf

Centers for Medicare and Medicaid Services. (2009a). Hospital services covered under part B, section 70.3: Partial hospitalization services. In *Medicare benefit policy manual.* Retrieved August 13, 2009, from http://www.cms.hhs.gov/manuals/downloads/bp102c06.pdf

Centers for Medicare and Medicaid Services. (2009b). Covered medical and other health services, section 220.1: Conditions of coverage and payment for outpatient physical therapy, occupational therapy, or speech-language pathology services. In *Medicare benefit policy manual.* Retrieved August 13, 2009, from http://www.cms.hhs.gov/Manuals/downloads/bp102c15.pdf

Cowan, C., Catlin, A., Smith, C., & Sensenig, A. (2004). National health expenditures, 2002. *Health Care Financing Review, 25*(4), 143-166.

Fearon, H. (2004). Tools for managing reimbursement in the outpatient physical therapy setting. APTA Conference, Maine Chapter, September 24, 2004.

Harrington, C., & Estes, C. L. (2004). *Health policy: Crisis and reform in the U.S. health care delivery system* (4th ed.). Boston, MA: Jones & Bartlett Publishers.

Kane, R. L., Chen, Q., Blewett, L. A., & Sangl, J. (1996). Do rehabilitative nursing homes improve the outcomes of care? *Journal of the American Geriatrics Society, 44*(5), 545-554.

Kronenberg, F., & Pollard, N. (2006). Political dimensions of occupation and the roles of occupational therapy. *American Journal of Occupational Therapy, 60*(6), 617-625.

Practice Management Information Corporation. (2005). ICD-9-CM International Classification of Diseases, clinical modification (9th rev., 6th ed.). Los Angeles, CA: Author.

Tricare. (2008). Chapter 7–Medicine: Section 18.3, occupational therapy. In *Tricare policy manual 6010.57-M, February 2008.* Retrieved August 13, 2009, from http://manuals.tricare.osd.mil

Torrens, P. R. (1993). Historical evolution and overview of health services in the United States. In S. Williams & P. R. Torrens (Eds.), *Introduction to health services* (5th ed., pp. 3-35). Clifton Park, NY: Delmar Cengage Learning.

U.S. Department of Education. (n.d.). Building the legacy: IDEA 2004. Retrieved July 31, 2009, from http://idea.ed.gov

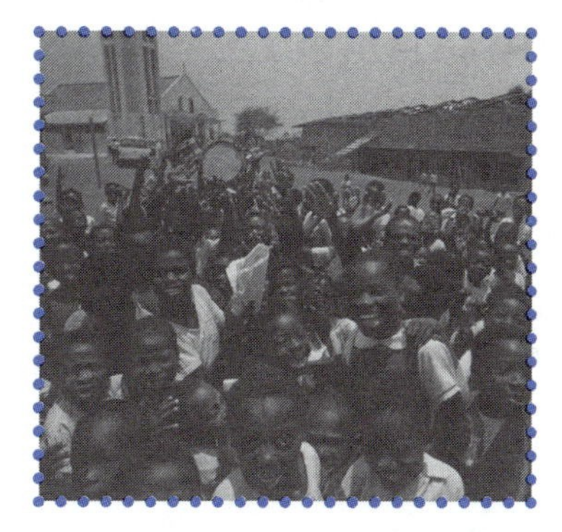

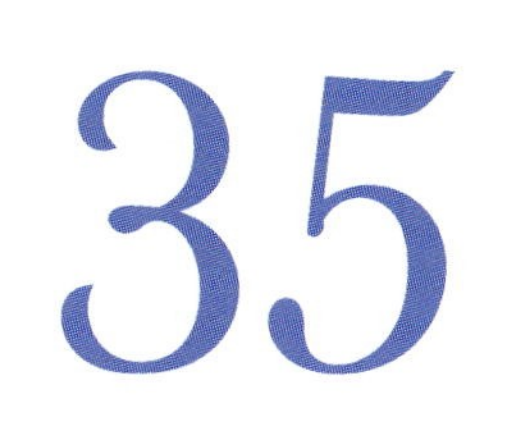

# 35 Systems to Organize and Market Occupational Therapy

*Karen Jacobs, EdD, OTR/L, CPE, FAOTA*

**ACOTE Standard Explored in This Chapter**

B.7.7

**Key Terms**

Advertising
Demographics
Marketing

## Introduction

"We are on the verge of an era when the needs for our services are so great as to push us to the brink of glory, if we can only deliver; or we may stumble, because we shall, I fear, cling tenaciously to what we have done without looking at what we might do if we were to take bold new directions" (Cromwell, 1968). If the concept of marketing had been applied to the profession of occupational therapy 40 years ago, just imagine how much more of a significant role we may have been playing in the health care marketplace today.

The need for occupational therapy practitioners and students to have a good understanding of and apply the concepts of marketing has become more critical today. Marketing can play an important part in the success of the occupational therapy profession. Indeed, it will help us reach the American Occupational Therapy Association's (AOTA) Centennial Vision for the profession: "We envision that occupational therapy is a powerful, widely recognized, science-driven, and evidence-based profession with a globally connected and diverse workforce meeting society's occupational needs" (AOTA, n.d.).

## What Is Marketing?

Marketing has been a misunderstood term, most often used synonymously with public relations, selling, fundraising, or development. However, according to marketer Peter Drucker, "The aim of marketing is to make selling superfluous" (Kotler & Murray, 1975).

Marketing consists of meeting people's needs in the most efficient and, therefore, profitable manner (Cromwell, 1968). Kotler and Clarke (1987) defined marketing in the following manner:

> "Marketing is the analysis, planning, implementation, and control of carefully formulated programs designed to bring about voluntary exchanges of values with target markets for the purpose of achieving organizational objectives. It relies heavily on designing the organization's offering in terms of the target markets' needs and desires, and on using effective pricing, communication, and distribution to inform, motivate, and service the markets."



K. Sladyk, K. Jacobs, & N. MacRae (Eds.).
*Occupational Therapy Essentials for Clinical Competence* (pp. 389-396).

Successful marketing planning begins with an idea that serves as the framework for all marketing efforts. It is an orientation that makes satisfying the customer's needs the integrating organizational principle. While the first impulse of the marketing novice is to design a program, such as a school-based, work-related occupational therapy program, and then look for customers (e.g., adolescents with developmental disabilities), effective marketing dictates that the process be reversed. One first looks at the market and listens carefully to potential customers and then designs the program to match the needs and desires of these potential customers.

## Marketing Planning

The main benefits of marketing planning can be summarized as follows (Branch, 1962):

- Encourages systematic thinking ahead
- Leads to better coordination of organizational efforts
- Leads to the development of performance standards for control
- Causes the individual/organization to sharpen its guiding objectives and policies
- Results in better preparedness for sudden developments

Marketing planning can be viewed as a three-step process. Figure 35-1 delineates this process with planning as the first step. It encompasses identifying attractive markets, developing marketing strategies and programs. Execution is the second step. It includes carrying out the action programs. The third and final step involves marketing control. This final step requires measuring results, analyzing the causes of poor results, and taking corrective action. Adjustments in the plan, its execution, or both would include corrective actions that could be implemented.

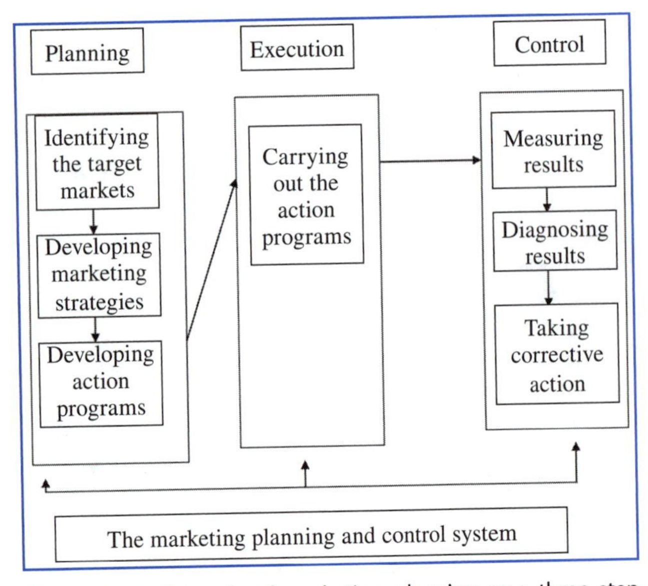


**Figure 35-1.** Example of marketing planning as a three-step process.

# Identifying Attractive Target Markets

Identifying the demands of the market is the first step in marketing. The market is defined as all actual or potential buyers of a product, service, or idea and can be considered in its entirety, such as all referral sources to an early intervention program, or divided into relevant segments according to variables, such as types of professionals (e.g., physicians, special education teachers, or nurses). Identifying attractive target markets includes the analysis of marketing opportunities. This analysis consists of the following:

- A self-audit
- Consumer analysis
- An analysis of other providers of similar services
- An environmental assessment

## Self-Audit

A self-audit assesses the strengths, weaknesses, opportunities, and threats (SWOT analysis) of your department and/or specific program. Factors to be assessed may include the following:

- The reputation of your facility in the community
- The staff and their qualifications, such as certification as a hand therapist, or board-certified professional ergonomist (BCPE)
- Physical size of the program
- Location of the program (e.g., hospital/rehabilitation setting, community based)
- Convenience of your location to mass transit, highways, and parking
- Type and quality of equipment
- Available budget
- Support from administration

This self-audit assists in understanding how well or poorly prepared you are to meet the marketplace demands. Ascertaining what you do well and maintaining that product (service) at an optimal level is part of marketing.

## Consumer Analysis

It is important to assess the potential consumers of your occupational therapy department's services within your catchment area. An analysis of some of the consumers who might use your products may include the following:

- Physicians
- Rehabilitation managers and consultants
- Nurses
- Vocational counselors
- Special education teachers
- Attorneys

- Administrators
- Workers with injuries
- Social workers
- Business and industry
- Third-party payers
- Colleagues, such as physical therapists, athletic trainers

## Analysis of Other Providers of Similar Services

How adequately the needs of the marketplace are being met, what areas are not being served, where duplication and overlap are occurring, and where opportunities for collaboration or joint venture exist can be ascertained through an analysis of other providers of similar services. One simple way to obtain information is to place your name on the mailing list of facilities/companies providing a similar product line. Reading through newsletters and brochures from the competition can be very insightful.

## Environmental Assessment

The changes and trends that may have an impact on occupational therapy services and perhaps the future of the profession compose an environmental assessment. These include the following:

- Demographic variables
- Political and regulatory systems
- Cultural environment
- Economic/financial environment
- Psychographics
- Technological developments

### Demographic Variables

Demographics is the study of human populations according to variables such as age, sex, family size, family life cycle, income, occupation, education, religion, race, and nationality. For example, the increasing number of aging "baby boomers" is a demographic trend that is having an impact on occupational therapy services.

### Political and Regulatory Systems

Both political and regulatory systems may have an impact on occupational therapy services. For example, the Americans with Disabilities Act (ADA) provides opportunities for occupational therapists to be advocates and assist in implementing the ADA, which provides comprehensive civil rights protection from discrimination in employment, transportation, public accommodations, telecommunications, and the activities of state and local government for individuals with disabilities. Specifically, Title 1-Employment provides the occupational therapists with the opportunity to provide assessments and devise reasonable accommodations so that the individual with a disability can perform the essential functions of the job (U.S. Department of Justice, 2007).

### Cultural Environment

Culture is a force that affects individuals within society's behaviors, values, perceptions, and preferences. The United States is becoming a more multicultural society, and it becomes imperative that occupational therapy practitioners and students develop an understanding of and sensitivity to the culture profiles of clients within their catchment area. Having practitioners and students who are bilingual can be most beneficial and may be the variable that assists in making our services even more successful.

### Economic/Financial Environment

An analysis of the economic/financial environment is important because it allows occupational therapy practitioners and students to target occupational therapy services to trends. Important trends include the following:

- Total health care spending represented 16% of the gross domestic product (GDP) in 2005 and is anticipated to increase to 20% by 2015 (Borger et al., 2006; Catlin, Cowan, Hellfer, Washington, & National Health Expenditure Accounts Team, 2006).
- Fourteen percent of children aged 3 to 21 years old are served in federally supported programs under Chapter I and Individuals with Disabilities Education Act (IDEA) (National Center for Education Statistics, n.d.).

### Psychographics

Psychographics is the technique of measuring consumers' social class, lifestyle, and personality characteristics and can provide information on activities, interests, and opinions of these individuals. Understanding the psychographic profile of your clients helps provide information to assist in strategizing products and services to them.

### Technological Developments

The technology arena is greatly advancing and has an almost daily impact on the type of assessment and intervention used by occupational therapy practitioners. Specifically, information technology allows for information to be exchanged in a more efficient manner.

# Selecting Target Markets and Market Segments

Once analysis is completed, there are three steps in target marketing. Market segmentation refers to the act of dividing a market into distinct groups of buyers who might require separate products and marketing mixes. For example, physicians can be segmented into pediatricians or neurologists; health and rehabilitation professionals can be segmented into speech pathologists, physical therapists, and athletic trainers. Market targeting is the act of evaluating and selecting one or more of the markets to enter. An example of this is targeting orthopedic surgeons as the main referral source for a hand therapy program. Product positioning is the act of formulating a competitive position for the product and a detailed marketing mix.

# Developing Marketing Strategies

Developing marketing strategies includes the development of objectives for each identified target market and their implementation. The 4 Ps—product, place, price, and promotion—are the strategies that can be used to influence the demand for a product (Kotler, 1983a; McCarthy, 1999). Here is how each of these "Ps" is used in the marketing mix.

## Product

Simply stated, what we do as occupational therapy practitioners is our product. That is, we help people, organizations, and populations through engagement in occupation.

Ideally, the goal is to offer a product line—a variety of products associated with one another by an overall theme. For example, an occupational therapy department may have an industrial rehabilitation or occupational health program whose product line includes post-offer screening, functional capacity evaluation, and ergonomics consultation. A school-based occupational therapy program may offer product line identifying assessment accommodations for the No Child Left Behind mandate and violence prevention programs.

How a product is packaged may influence its success. It is important to make sure all paperwork (e.g., brochures, business cards, stationary, and reports) have a professional appearance. The ability to access information quickly and be able to present it in a professional manner to the target markets is an asset.

Many new product ideas are generated by understanding our client's needs and wants through direct surveys, projective tests, focus group discussions, and letters and complaints received. It is important to note that for every unhappy customer, you lose 50 others, and that 80% of your business is coming from 20% of your customers (Baum & Luebben, 1986).

## Place

Occupational therapy services can be provided in a variety of places. Some of these include the following:

- Free-standing facilities located in professional buildings, industrial parks, and shopping centers
- Free-standing facilities affiliated with outpatient service departments, rehabilitation centers, or hospitals
- As part of a comprehensive rehabilitation or acute care facility/program/hospital
- At work site programs provided by a company to serve the needs of a specific business or industry
- Schools
- Skilled nursing facilities (SNF)
- Sub-acute/transitional care unit

When analyzing the place aspect of marketing planning, other variables that should be considered are the hours the program is offered for business. For example, is your program open during hours convenient to your markets or your staff?

## Price

The price or fee schedule for occupational therapy services (products) should be based on cost, competitive factors, geographic area, and what the consumer is willing to pay. It is important for the price to be commensurate with perceived value (Miller & Jacobs, 2007).

## Promotion

Promotion is the vehicle of communicating information to your markets about the product's merits, place, and price. Instruments of promotion are advertising, sales promotion, publicity, and personal selling.

### Advertising

Advertising involves the use of a paid message presented in a recognized medium and by an identified sponsor, with the purpose to inform, persuade, and remind. Some advertising vehicles include the following:

- Print ads found in newspapers, journals, and magazines
- Brochures
- Direct mail
- Broadcasts
- Transits
- Billboards
- Quarterly newsletters
- Business cards

### Sales Promotion

Sales promotion is the use of a wide variety of short-term incentives to encourage the purchase of the product. This approach is most effective when used in conjunction with advertising. For example, at an open house for an occupational therapist in a solo ergonomics practice, a successful sales promotion was giving out mouse pads with tips for setting up a computer workstation. Of course, the occupational therapist's contact information was printed on the mouse pad, too.

### Publicity

Publicity is often a relatively underused aspect of promotion in relation to the real contribution it can make (Kotler, 1983b). The most positive aspect of publicity is that it is free. However, one has little control over the placement of it and thus it becomes difficult to focus publicity on specific target markets. An example of publicity might be to contact the local media through a press release about an upcoming event at your facility (e.g., activities to celebrate AOTA's National Backpack Awareness Day). If the media finds the event newsworthy and they are not understaffed, they will often send a reporter to cover the event. Whether the reporter writes a story can be dependent on variables out of your control, such as available time and space in the newspaper, television, or radio. However, a successful strategy in utilizing publicity more effectively has been to develop a rapport with the media personnel. Personally contact your local newspaper, radio, and television stations and introduce yourself. Let them know about occupational therapy and what you do as an occupational therapy practitioner or student and offer to be available to them if they need a resource. Follow up your e-mail/telephone call with your résumé and biosketch for their files (Figure 35-2).

### Personal Selling

Face-to-face communication between you and your audience is the most effective form of promotion, the most expensive, and also the method most used by occupational therapy practitioners (Jacobs, 1987). Word-of-mouth recommendation by staff and consumers of occupational therapy products and services is a powerful sales pitch. Other successful personal selling methods include the following:

- Exhibiting at various conferences
- Developing a free speakers' bureau
- Presenting in-service training to physicians and health and rehabilitation professionals
- Presenting continuing education workshops
- Lecturing
- Attending professional meetings for various organizations
- Holding an open house
- Holding continuing education seminars for referral sources

## Focus Groups

Focus groups have been found to be an effective marketing technique. These techniques can be used with primary referral sources, such as physicians and employers, or with reimbursement agencies or the direct recipient of our services to provide feedback on current programming efforts and recommendations for future program modifications. The use of focus groups allows you to quickly incorporate this feedback into the delivery of your product and services or the product itself. This in turn should generate an increased commitment on the part of the referral sources to the program.

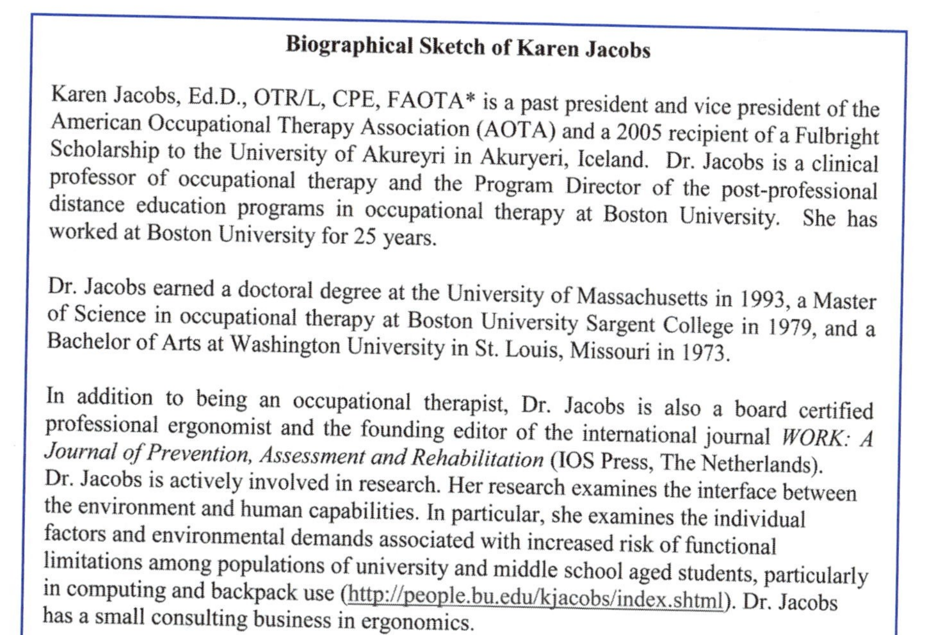

**Biographical Sketch of Karen Jacobs**

Karen Jacobs, Ed.D., OTR/L, CPE, FAOTA* is a past president and vice president of the American Occupational Therapy Association (AOTA) and a 2005 recipient of a Fulbright Scholarship to the University of Akureyri in Akuryeri, Iceland. Dr. Jacobs is a clinical professor of occupational therapy and the Program Director of the post-professional distance education programs in occupational therapy at Boston University. She has worked at Boston University for 25 years.

Dr. Jacobs earned a doctoral degree at the University of Massachusetts in 1993, a Master of Science in occupational therapy at Boston University Sargent College in 1979, and a Bachelor of Arts at Washington University in St. Louis, Missouri in 1973.

In addition to being an occupational therapist, Dr. Jacobs is also a board certified professional ergonomist and the founding editor of the international journal *WORK: A Journal of Prevention, Assessment and Rehabilitation* (IOS Press, The Netherlands). Dr. Jacobs is actively involved in research. Her research examines the interface between the environment and human capabilities. In particular, she examines the individual factors and environmental demands associated with increased risk of functional limitations among populations of university and middle school aged students, particularly in computing and backpack use (http://people.bu.edu/kjacobs/index.shtml). Dr. Jacobs has a small consulting business in ergonomics.

*Ed.D--doctorate in education, OTR/--registered, licensed occupational therapist, CPE-certified professional ergonomist, FAOTA—Fellow of the American Occupational Therapy Association.

**Figure 35-2.** Example of a biosketch.

Focus group interviewing is one of the major marketing research tools for gaining insight into consumer thoughts and feelings (Kotler, 1983a). Focus group interviewing consists of inviting 6 to 10 participants to spend a few hours with a skilled interviewer to discuss any designated subject matter, such as the feasibility of developing a school-based occupational therapy work program. Focus group practitioners are usually paid a small sum for attending the meeting. These are typically held in pleasant surroundings, with refreshments served. The interview begins with broad questions such as, "What do you think about occupational therapy services for elementary school-aged students?" leading to focusing in on more specific questions on the subject matter such as, "What do you think about the feasibility of an occupational therapy ergonomics program addressing the use of information and communication technical being established at Butler Elementary School?" The interviewer encourages free and easy discussion among participants, hoping that the group dynamics will bring out deep feelings and thoughts (Kotler & Clarke, 1984). Although the results cannot generalize the market as a whole due to its small sample size, the information gathered can provide insight into participants' perceptions, attitudes, and satisfaction. Information obtained can help define what issues need to be researched more formally or may provide the foundation for being able to develop a product that will meet the consumer's needs (Kotler & Clarke).

# Execution of the Marketing Plan

Once you have selected your target market, develop a specific marketing mix (product, price, place, and promotion) for your market that stresses the benefits of your product(s). When executing action programs, a timeline should be delineated, such as a 12-month period, to measure whether objectives and goals are being met. The action plan should be dynamic and able to be changed throughout the year as new opportunities and problems arise. Ideally, actions should be assigned to specific individuals who are given exact completion dates. For example, an action that might be assigned to an occupational therapy practitioner can include developing a single paragraph description of the violence prevention programs provided by the occupational therapy department. The practitioner is given a 1-week timeline to complete this action. Once the description is completed, the supervisor has 2 weeks to incorporate this information into a brochure being developed to promote the expanded product line of occupational therapy to potential referral sources. In this case, as in all aspects of promotion, it is important to communicate in a language that is familiar to your market. Avoid professional jargon!

# Marketing Control

Marketing is an area where rapid obsolescence of objectives, policies, strategies, and programs is a constant possibility (Kotler & Clarke, 1984). Marketing control attempts to circumvent this dilemma and assists in maximizing the probability that a product will achieve its short- and long-term objectives. It is important to measure program results, diagnose these results, and take corrective action, if necessary. There are three types of marketing control (Kotler & Clarke):

1. Annual plan control consists of the steps used during the year to monitor and correct deviations from the marketing plan to ensure that annual sales and profit goals are being achieved.
2. Profitability control refers to the efforts used to determine the actual profit or loss of different marketing entities such as the products (services) or market segments.
3. Strategic control is a systematic evaluation of the organization's market performance in relation to the current and forecasted marketing environment.

# Summary

A bright future can be a certainty for occupational therapy practitioners and students who are prepared to accept the reality of today's and tomorrow's health care environment. It will be increasingly competitive with various professions vying for control of limited resources increasingly complex and increasingly controlled by third-party payers and the government.

Occupational therapy practitioners and students' abilities to market their skills and knowledge to those that control the dollars will be an ever-present requirement for success. It will likely make the difference between encroachment by other professions and a resulting second-class specialty, and a proud and effective profession placed squarely in a leadership position within the health care industry (Pickelle & Ramos, 1991). We need to rally to this cheer!

Having access to an expert in marketing to assist in the development of a marketing plan would be the ideal situation, but this is not always the case. On the other hand, the worst possible scenario would be one where even an informal market analysis does not precede product or service development. If this is the case for you, a word of caution: remember that designing a program and then looking for customers typically leads to facing an uphill battle to success. At the very least, before investing a great deal of useless time, effort, and money, attempt to perform a market analysis on your own following the guidelines presented in this chapter and in other available literature.

## Student Self-Assessment

1. Describe, design, and discuss content for a Web page promoting occupational therapy to high school students.
2. Write a biosketch about yourself using Figure 35-2 as an example.
3. Create a brochure about the occupational therapy's contribution to any of the six broad areas of practice: mental health; productive aging; children and youth; health and wellness; work and industry; or rehabilitation, disability, and participation.

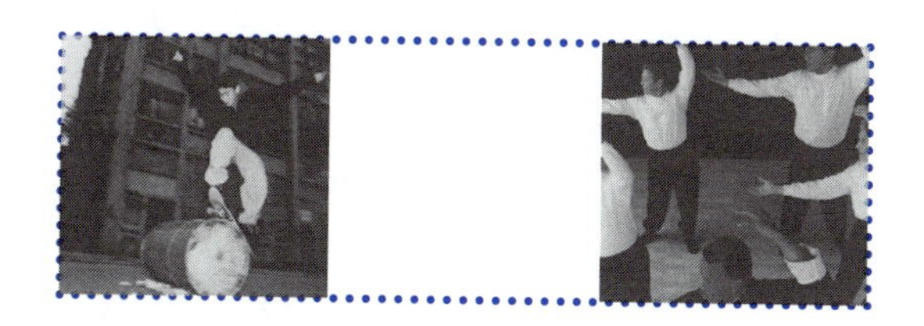

## References


American Occupational Therapy Association. (n.d.). The road to the centennial vision. Retrieved August 6, 2007, from http://www.aota.org/News/Centennial.aspx

Baum, C. M., & Luebben, A. J. (1986). *Prospective payment systems: A handbook for health care clinicians*. Thorofare, NJ: SLACK Incorporated.

Borger, C., Smith, S., Truffer, C., Keehan, S., Sisko, A., Poisal, J., et al. (2006). Health spending projections through 2015: Changes on the horizon. *Health Affairs, 25*(2), w61-w73.

Branch, M. (1962). *The corporate planning process*. New York, NY: American Management Association.

Catlin, A., Cowan, C., Heffler, S., Washington, B., & National Health Expenditure Accounts Team. (2006). National health spending in 2005: The slowdown continues. *Health Affairs, 26*(1), 142-153.

Cromwell, F. (1984). The changing roles of occupational therapists in the 1980s. *Occupational Therapy in Health Care, 1*(1), 8.

Jacobs, K. (1987). Marketing occupational therapy. *American Journal of Occupational Therapy, 41*(5), 315-320.

Kotler, P. (1983a). *Principles of marketing* (2nd ed.). Englewood Cliffs, NJ: Prentice Hall.

Kotler, P. (1983b). *Principles of marketing—Instructor's manual with cases*. Englewood Cliffs, NJ: Prentice Hall.

Kotler, P., & Clarke, R. (1984). *Marketing management* (5th ed.). Englewood Cliffs, NJ: Prentice Hall.

Kotler, P., & Clarke, R. (1987). *Marketing for health care organizations*. Englewood Cliffs, NJ: Prentice Hall.

Kotler, P., & Murray, M. (1975). Third sector management: The role of marketing. *Public Administration Review, 35*(5), 469.

McCarthy, E. J. (1999). *Basic marketing: A managerial approach* (13th ed.). Homewood, IL: Irwin.

Miller, D., & Jacobs, K. (2007). Economics and marketing of ergonomic services. In K. Jacobs (Ed.), *Ergonomics for therapists*. St. Louis, MO: Elsevier.

National Center for Education Statistics. (n.d.). National Center for Education Statistics Web site. Retrieved August 10, 2009, from http://nces.ed.gov

Pickelle, C., & Ramos, T. (1991). Publishers' message. *Rehab Management, 9*.

United States Department of Justice. (2007). U.S. Department of Justice Web site. Retrieved August 10, 2009, from http://www.usdoj.gov

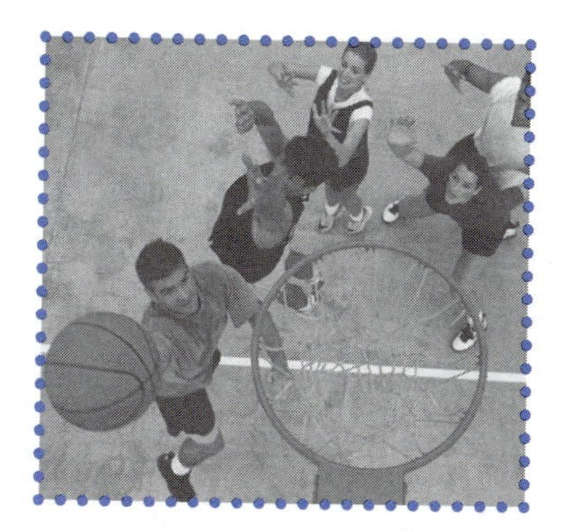

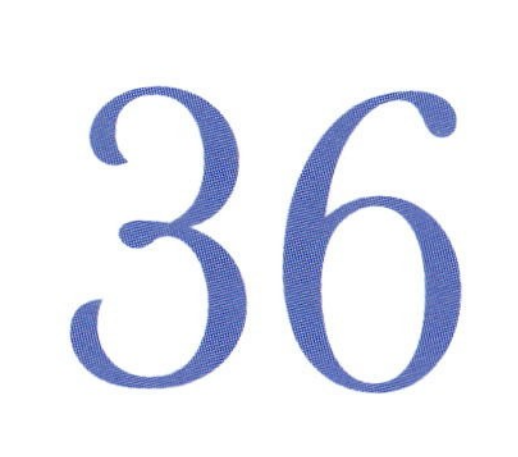

# Quality Improvement

Jennifer Kaldenberg, MSA, OTR/L, SCLV, CLVT;
Nancy MacRae, MS, OTR/L, FAOTA; and Karen Jacobs, EdD, OTR/L, CPE, FAOTA

**ACOTE Standard Explored in This Chapter**

B.7.8

**Key Terms**

Benchmark
Quality assessment
Quality improvement

## Introduction

"Quality starts with the person, not with the product/service, not with the work process that creates it" (Albrecht, 1993, p. 54). Quality is an extremely complex construct and can be defined in many ways. It is dependent on the context in which it is used and measured. It has a value component, which is typically the relationship between cost and quality. Health care players (clients, providers, and payers) define quality differently, usually from their unique perspectives. Some of the possible defining concepts of quality include safety, timeliness, courtesy, availability, technical support, accessibility, reliability, economic impact, accuracy, waste, durability, flexibility, and follow-up. Service is also a likely consideration, with the following five dimensions often cited as important (Parasuraman, Berry, & Zeithaml, 1991):

1. Reliability of service
2. Tangible product or service
3. Responsiveness of service to client/customer
4. Assurance of quality to consumer
5. Empathy exercised toward consumer

Quality improvement is a management philosophy and method for structuring problem solving. Its goal is to meet/exceed customer/client requirements for quality services through a process of improvement. The process is a continuous, nonlinear process. The data gathered are used to make decisions, just as it is with evidence-based practice. A frequently used model, developed by Donabedian (1980), lists three portions of a quality improvement program:

1. *Structure*: The resources available within the specific environment are used to do this
2. *Process*: The actual delivery of services
3. *Outcomes*: The final result of the program

All aspects of the model are complementary. Additionally, quality for practitioners can be understood from a micro as well as a macro view. The micro view deals with clinical aspects of care and the technical quality with which they are delivered. Geographic differences may impact this view. Interpersonal aspects of care have significance for clients—the provider's interest in and concern for the client makes an indelible impression. Quality-of-life definitions usually involve the client's sense of overall well-being and ability to participate in those activities/occupations found meaningful.



K. Sladyk, K. Jacobs, & N. MacRae (Eds.).
*Occupational Therapy Essentials for Clinical Competence* (pp. 397-406).

The macro view of quality includes a broader view of the system-wide efficiencies and outcomes, such as cost, access, and population health status (Shi & Singh, 2008, pp. 515-517). National initiatives as well as state and community actions are required to address these concerns.

For a quality improvement process to be successful, a number of components need to be in place. They are as follows:

- Administrative support of this philosophy
- Training of all staff on the concepts, strategies, tools, and techniques of quality improvement
- Adoption of the norm of customer preferences being the primary determinant of quality (Table 36-1)
- Support for a team approach that encourages all to work together to improve quality; motivation must be apparent for this approach to process analysis and change and be effective

Successful quality improvement efforts work because consumers discern a greater value from the service/product than from that of the competition and a number of the following components. Five "C" components of valid customer requirements are as follows (Braveman, 2006):

1. Product is current
2. Outcome is calculable
3. Plan can be completed
4. Plan is consumer based
5. Plan is consistent with organizational goals

Quality improvement plans are often associated with less waste and improved services, resulting in lower costs and leading to a higher profit margin, asset utilization, and competitive position. All of this improves the "bottom line," satisfying shareholders and key supporters as well as consumers.

## Stages and Principles

The outcome assessment process is a critical part of evaluating and improving quality. The process consists of the following:

- Identifying goals for organization, program, client, or self
- Developing a plan to achieve goals
- Implementing the plan
- Measuring and reporting outcomes

Another way to understand this process is to explain the one Deming (2000) has created. It is a quality chain reaction consisting of a four part cycle:

1. *Plan*: Determine what will be measured
2. *Do*: Collect data on chosen indicators
3. *Check*: Analyze data and identify areas for improvement
4. *Act*: Implement improvements, first in pilot program; provide rewards and recognition for the team

Deming insisted these domains were integrated and needed to be used together. Additionally, users of this system needed to have an appreciation for a systems approach, the likelihood of variation of performance, the theory of the scientific method of knowledge generation, and an understanding of both intrinsic and extrinsic factors affecting motivation and participation in change within an organization (Braveman, 2006).

In addition to following Deming's organized cycle, the rationale for such a plan needs to address queries as the following:

- Who are the stakeholders?
- How do you improve responsiveness of the program?
- How do you insure high quality standard?

## Application to Clinical Settings

In an environment of constant change, cost containment, mergers, and managed health care, professionals must strive to provide quality care. Examining efficiency, effectiveness, and adherence to standards of quality management (QM) in health care is a systematic process for evaluating health care services (Joint Commission on Accreditation

Table 36-1. Client-Driven Actions

| Becoming a Client-Driven Entity Means Moving | |
|---|---|
| **From** | **To** |
| Motivation through fear and loyalty | Motivation through shared vision |
| An attitude of "It's their problem" | Ownership of every problem that affects the client |
| "That's the way we've always done it" | Continued improvement |
| Making decisions based on assumptions | Making decisions based on client data |
| Everything begins and ends with management | Everything begins and ends with the client |
| Organizational foxholes | Cross-functional cooperation |
| Being good at crisis management and recovery | Doing it right the first time |

Adapted from Whiteley, R. C. (1993). *The customer-driven company: Moving from talk to action.* New York, NY: Basic Books.

of Healthcare Organizations [JCAHO], 1996). Efficiency refers to services that are both cost effective and timely in their delivery. Clinical services must be effective in achieving set objectives or outcomes for care.

Quality improvement or management programs are designed to measure and assess performance to ensure adherence to pre-established standards. These standards are established by state, federal, and accreditory organizations such as the JCAHO and Commission on Accreditation of Rehabilitation Facilities (CARF). Hospitals and other health care facilities refer to this process in many terms: *continuous quality improvement, total QM, quality assurance*, and *performance improvement*. The processes of quality assurance, quality improvement/assessment, and performance are all methods of assessment. Motivations (external versus internal), focus (problem based versus quality processes), delegation (departmentally versus interdepartmentally), and outcomes (hiding problems versus improvement) may vary (Jacobs & Logigian, 1994).

Table 36-2 provides the differences among quality assurance, similar to quality improvement but a step beyond quality assessment; quality assessment, a measure of quality against standards; and performance improvement, a combination of both.

There are many methods for evaluating quality such as:

- Clinical audits refer to a group of peers working collectively to review case records for adherence to established standards pre-established by the peer group.
- Peer review is a type of record review based on criteria established by the individual department, for what is determined to be quality care (JCAHO, 1996; Rakich, Logest, & Darr, 1992). Maslin (1991, p. 177) stated: "Common to both peer review and clinical audit procedures is the term process criteria, referring to the activities or procedures undertaken as part of good patient care."
- Accreditation is sought by many hospitals and health care organizations as proof of providing services that meet established minimum standards for Medicare reimbursement (Jacobs & Logigian, 1994; JCAHO, 1997). When performance fails to meet these standards, the organization must assess the performance and attempt to improve the areas of deficit. Changes can occur organizationally, departmentally, or individually. When discussing QM, we must not only look to the organization, but to each individual occupational therapy practitioner, whether a registered occupational therapist or a certified occupational therapy assistant, providing the services.

## Data Collection Methods

Data collection methods include qualitative or quantitative methodology or the combination of both, as well as the use of benchmarks. Benchmarks are the quantifiable measures of the outcomes of a process used as comparisons to current performances or targets for an improved outcome (Braveman, 2006). Many methods can be used to collect data. They include observation, interviews, surveys/questionnaires, and focus groups.

Data analysis drives change. It closes the loop of quality improvement. A determination about whether the data support the focus on the goals of an organization or whether it supports its view of success must be determined with an adjustment plan conceived based on the data. Data can also be utilized to indicate the effectiveness of a practitioner's performance.

The ultimate goal of QM programs is to have a continuous focus on quality to become the way of doing business. Success occurs when there is a constant focus on clients and their satisfaction, a constant readiness for change and process improvement, the daily use of quality improvement tools, an abiding belief that use of data to make decisions

**Table 36-2. Differences Among Quality Assurance, Quality Assessment, and Performance Improvement**

| Quality Assurance | Quality Assessment | Performance Improvement |
|---|---|---|
| Externally driven | Internally motivated | Internally and externally motivated |
| Self-oriented | Customer driven | Customer/data driven |
| Vertical | Horizontal | Organization wide |
| Delegated to a few | Embraced by all | Embraced by all |
| Focused on people | Focused on processes | Focused on processes, systems, and functions |
| Hiding problems | Seeking problems | Seeking opportunities for improvement; utilizes benchmarking or comparative data |
| Seeks endpoints | Has no endpoints | Has no endpoints |

Adapted from Rakich, J. S., Logest, B. B., & Darr, K. (1992). *Managing health services organizations* (3rd ed.). Baltimore, MD: Health Professions Press.

is the right way to proceed, and a commitment to balance these tasks with those of the needs of people as standard operating procedures (Braveman, 2006).

# Exemplary Quality Improvement Accrediting Agencies

In this chapter, we will discuss JCAHO's quality improvement 10-step program. This is used as an exemplar due to its popular use by many health care agencies. This is the process with which most occupational therapy practitioners will come in contact. CARF is another accrediting agency with which practitioners may be familiar, but its processes will not be discussed in this chapter.

# JCAHO

JCAHO is a private organization developed to survey hospitals, mental health care, home care, ambulatory care, and long-term care facilities. These facilities are evaluated based on standards established by committees composed of peer experts within the Joint Commission. JCAHO (1997, p. 5) stated that its mission is "to improve the quality of care provided to the public through the provision of health care accreditation and related services that support performance improvement in health care organizations."

Most health care organizations in the United States seek accreditation from JCAHO in order to prove that they meet the minimum standards necessary for Medicare reimbursement eligibility. Since the 1990s, JCAHO has placed greater emphasis on the evaluation of quality health care and has established a process for monitoring and evaluating quality standards, which has been shown to be helpful in developing or improving QM programs (JCAHO, 1997).

## JCAHO's 10-Step Process

The 10-step process established by JCAHO provides the necessary steps for monitoring and evaluating quality standards. This is a comprehensive process designed to assess and improve the quality of client care, staff performance, and interactions. The process may be completed departmentally or interdepartmentally, as increased emphasis has been placed on a collaborative or interdepartmental process. If we look at health care delivery in rehabilitation, it is not an individual effort but a team working together to maximize the client's outcomes. If services are performed as a team, evaluation should also be collaborative. JCAHO stated that "through collaboration, it aligns the vision of the organization with the work and goals of the individuals responsible for the organizations success" (1996, p. 19).

1. The first step is to "assign responsibility" for monitoring and evaluating the specific activities. Responsibility for the overall quality improvement process generally falls under the director of occupational therapy services. However, it is important that the individuals responsible for the direct care also assist in the process.
   Because certified occupational therapy assistants are highly involved with client care, they are in a prime position to collect data for QM purposes. The certified occupational therapy assistant's level of involvement will depend on years of experience, knowledge in a particular area of practice and setting, and service competency. Not only does the occupational therapy practitioner working directly with the client have a greater understanding of the aspects of care, but he or she can also integrate the findings of the quality improvement process into future interventions (Griffin, 1993).
2. The second step is to "delineate the scope of care," including the primary functions of the department, such as hours of operation, types of services provided, types of clients treated, and who is providing the care (Hinojosa et al., 1998).
   For example, the inpatient occupational therapy department for the rehabilitation unit provides care Monday through Sunday from 7:30 a.m. to 5:00 p.m. for all clients admitted to the rehabilitation unit. This is a 26-bed unit, and clients are seen in the occupational therapy clinic for a wide variety of diagnoses, all having rehabilitative needs. The staff is composed of three occupational therapists, two certified occupational therapy assistants, and an occupational therapy aide.
3. The third step is to "identify the important aspects of care," which includes the key functions, interventions, and processes that may be categorized as high risk, high volume, or problem prone (Jacobs & Logigian, 1994). These important aspects of care are the ones most appropriately evaluated by QM activities.
   a. High-risk activities include the various aspects of care that place clients at risk for serious consequences if care is not received (e.g., bed and wheelchair positioning and upper and lower extremity splinting and orthotics) due to clients being at risk for contractures, edema, or skin breakdown.
   b. High-volume activities are those services that occur frequently within the department, such as client education, client assessment, and home safety education.
   c. Problem-prone care might include those aspects of care that are found to lack compliance with standards (e.g., timeliness and completeness of client documentation or infection control).
4. In step 4, "indicators are identified" for the important aspects of care to be monitored by the occupational therapy department. Indicators established should identify the desired activity and outcomes of care. Refer to Table 36-3 for an example.

| Table 36-3. Indicators and Thresholds | | | |
|---|---|---|---|
| **Indicator** | **Threshold** | **Data Collection Method** | **Possible Causes for Thresholds Not Being Met** |
| Falls prevention education was completed and thoroughly documented as evidence by: | 95% | • Quarterly chart review of 30 records by the occupational therapist<br>• Reports to occupational therapist director and QM committee | • Short length of stay<br>• Illness<br>• Family<br>• Client refusal |
| Clients received: | 95% | • Falls assessment | |
| Documentation: | 95% | • Documentation of education and client/family understanding | |
| Treatment: | 98% | • Testing/procedures 3 hours of therapy daily to include occupational therapy and physical therapy and at times, Speech-Language Pathology (SLP) as documented in client's chart | |

5. In step 5, "thresholds are established for evaluation." In determining how each indicator will be measured, establish the benchmark or target for expected performance of the function, process, or service provided by the department. For the indicator of falls prevention, a threshold of 95% was established. This means that of all the cases reviewed, a minimum of 95% of all clients received falls prevention education and that education was completed and thoroughly documented.
6. The next step is then to "monitor the important aspects of care by collecting and organizing the data for each indicator" (Rakich et al., 1992, p. 459). As seen in the example in Table 36-3, data collection can be completed through chart review, client and physician surveys, attendance records, etc. In order to appropriately collect and organize the data, the department or organization must first determine what standards or criteria to utilize to determine adherence to the indicator.
7. Once data is organized, indicators are evaluated.
   a. When thresholds are met, the department or organization may look for other areas for improvement or evaluation.
   b. If thresholds are not met, further evaluation is completed to determine possible causes. Possible causes can be developed into further indicators.
8. Once the data are collected, organized, and analyzed, the next step is to "take action," determining what actions need to take place in order to improve care. In the example of falls prevention education, if thresholds are not met, the department supervisors may decide to hold education sessions for all staff, outlining the importance of education and proper documentation.
9. After implementation or action, the department must assess the effectiveness of the action. This will determine if improvement may be maintained over time. This would be assessed by continued evaluation of the indicator in the following quarter.
10. The final step is "communicating the results of the findings." The information gathered will be shared with the occupational therapy department and QM committee. The QM committee is usually composed of administrators, QM personnel, and department coordinators. The director of occupational therapy services generally presents the results to the QM committee in writing and at quarterly meetings. The QM committee may make further recommendations for remediation.
    Departmental communication is essential in fostering team development and motivating staff members to maximize efficiency and effectiveness of intervention. Occupational therapy practitioners who are involved in the QM process will have increased understanding of the indicators and their potential effects on the client, the department, and the organization.

Table 36-4 provides an outline of a similar process for monitoring and evaluating assessment and improvement programs.

With a strong QM program, departments and organizations will show improved efficiency with decreased cost and waste and improved productivity and effectiveness, with positive outcomes and client satisfaction. Quality care should always be thought of as an ongoing process for the organization as a whole and for each individual working within the organization.

## Impact on the Profession

Quality improvement processes are important to the profession of occupational therapy. The principles mirror those of evidence-based practice and support a strengthening and growth of our profession and its foundation of occupation. Our profession maintains a unique definition of quality outcomes: occupational therapy outcomes need to

| Table 36-4. The Monitoring and Evaluation Process for Assessment and Improvement | |
|---|---|
| Assign responsibility | The organization leaders oversee the design and foster and approach to continuously improve quality including the use of intradepartmental and extradepartmental activities |
| Delineate the scope | The organization, as a whole or as a department, delineates its scope of care and service |
| Identify importance | The organization, as a whole or as a department, identifies high-priority key functions, processes, activities, etc. to be monitored |
| Identify indicators | Teams of experts, inter- or intradepartmental, identify indicators for the important aspects of care and service. Indicators pertaining to structures of care are no longer emphasized |
| Establish evaluation | Teams of experts establish the level, pattern, or trend triggers in data for each indicator that will trigger intensive evaluation. Statistical methods are emphasized, as is the fact that thresholds are not the only way evaluation is triggered |
| Collect and organize | The data collection methodology often includes a data means by which feedback from sources other than ongoing monitoring is used to indicate areas for evaluation and improvement |
| Initiate evaluation | When thresholds are reached and when other feedback (e.g., client reports) identifies other opportunities for improvement, leaders set priorities for evaluation and establish teams, which evaluate the client care or service function in question |
| Take action | Greater emphasis is placed on focusing actions on processes, especially the hands off between departments and services |
| Assess effectiveness | A greater emphasis is placed on assuring that improvement is sustained over time |
| Communicate results | Findings of those performing monitoring and evaluation of the findings are forwarded to the leaders and affected individuals and groups |
| Other feedback | Receive surveys, comments, suggestions, and complaints |

be based on engagement in occupation (O'Sullivan, 2004). Measures can include the following (Case-Smith, 2005, pp. 8-9):

- Occupational performance
- Client satisfaction
- Role competence
- Adaptation
- Health and wellness
- Prevention
- Quality of life

Clinical assessment tools need to be critically analyzed with a determination made as to what they assess, how they will be used, and what their limitations are. Tools also need to be reliable, valid, and sensitive. Some examples of currently used tools are as follows:

- *FIM*: Functional Independence Measure; a national tool used in rehabilitation settings
- *MDIS*: Minimum Data Information Set; used to determine level of intervention needed in nursing homes
- *OASIS*: Outcomes Assessment Information Set; home health standardized assessment
- *SF-36*: National quality of life assessment
- *COPM*: Canadian Occupational Performance Measure; can be used with multiple populations

# Outcome Measures

Quality outcome measures also need to be applied at the individual practitioner level to assure quality care for the clients and the continuing competence of practitioners. Looking at quality care, the occupational therapy practitioner must look at the overall outcomes of client intervention and their individual professional competence as an occupational therapy practitioner. Hinojosa et al. (1998) defined continuing competence as "a dynamic multidimensional process in which the professional develops and maintains the knowledge, performance skills, interpersonal abilities, critical reasoning skills, and ethical reasoning skills necessary to continue in his or her evolving roles throughout a professional career" (p. 4). This process requires the occupational therapy practitioner to understand that this is a continuous process of improvement (Griffin, 1993).

The AOTA, the national organization for occupational therapy practitioners, is committed to assisting its members in keeping abreast of advancements in the profession and establishing standards that define quality services. The AOTA has established a council to address the issue of continued competence in occupational therapy, standards of which were adopted by the AOTA Representative Assembly in 1999. With financial and time constraints commonly experienced by many occupational therapy practitioners, the AOTA has developed continuing education (CE) articles, self-paced clinical courses, workshops on disk, and online courses to assist its members in meeting

CE requirements and obtaining CE units (CEUs) to the resources to keep current in a growing profession.

Occupational therapy practitioners must maintain and demonstrate the appropriate knowledge and skill level for client intervention in varied roles. Many state licensure boards require documentation of CE (refer to your state licensure laws) in order to maintain current licensure. These CE credits should be related to the occupational therapy practitioner's individual roles within the organization.

As of 2002, the National Board for Certification in Occupational Therapy (NBCOT) requires practitioners to accrue 36 hours of professional development units (PDUs) over a 3-year period in order to maintain certification and to use the credentials of certified occupational therapy assistant or registered occupational therapy. The requirement is intended to complement state licensure terms. Of the 36 units, 50% (18 PDUs) must be directly related to the delivery of occupational therapy services (NBCOT, 2003).

CEUs are converted to PDUs based on a formula established by NBCOT. In addition, NBCOT offers a listing of a wide variety of professional activities that may be applied to PDUs (NBCOT, 2003). Practitioners must keep records, usually in the form of a portfolio, of their professional development activities. At re-certification time, NBCOT will randomly audit re-certification applicants for the required PDUs (NBCOT, 2003).

## Skills Needed by Practitioners

Occupational therapy practitioners must be able to demonstrate appropriate communication, interpersonal abilities, and problem solving in order to maintain professional relations with clients, family members, peers, and other health care professionals. Being able to adapt in order to meet the needs of the client, family, or health care professional will foster greater understanding and may improve overall intervention outcomes. Lastly, occupational therapy practitioners must always adhere to the *Code of Ethics* established by the AOTA. This code guides our practice and allows occupational therapy practitioners to make appropriate decisions and actions. Each occupational therapy practitioner is responsible for his or her own ethical practice.

Given the demand for accountability within the health care field, the rapid changes within the profession of occupational therapy and areas of technology, it becomes essential for occupational therapy practitioners to continuously update individual skills and knowledge level (Griffin, 1993; Punwar, 1998). As a new graduate or an advanced practitioner, it is important to have a professional development plan in order to compete in an ever-changing health care environment. The professional development plan enables the occupational therapy practitioner to assess his or her own strengths and weaknesses, develop goals and objectives to improve skills or knowledge, and identify possible resources to meet the goals (Griffin).

Skills that you will apply include the following:

- Effective communication is necessary in organizing, implementing, and reporting QM activities. Practitioners need to share information with colleagues who are also involved in the study, with the head of the QM study team, and possibly with facility administration.
- The tasks of management are frequently a part of a QM study. Therefore, knowledge of their procedures and purpose will be of benefit to the practitioner who participates in QM activities.
- Leadership can be displayed in a number of ways. Occupational therapy practitioners may lead the entire study or a portion of it. Certified occupational therapy assistants are encouraged to assume a leadership role by noting areas in practice that could benefit from quality monitoring.

QM activities are frequently a requirement of accrediting bodies and state regulatory boards. Assessing and improving the quality of care to the clients we serve is an ethical responsibility as is continually improving and upgrading our own skills. Results of QM activities provide a sound basis for change, improvement, and growth. Practitioners' participation in QM activities will hopefully make the resultant changes easier to implement.

## Summary

Keys to success in a quality improvement endeavor are to consider it as a continuous circular process, not a one-time deal nor solely as a cost-cutting maneuver. Such a process requires a culture change and a full buy-in from all concerned. Devising the end results (outcomes) can lead to increased satisfaction for the stakeholders and makes the task even more worthwhile.

QM is an ongoing, circular process that includes administration, professionals, and consumers. The process is completed to ensure the highest quality care possible. To sustain quality, administration and professionals must communicate and actively participate in the QM process. The 10-step process provided by JCAHO demonstrates how the development of a comprehensive QM program can be used to monitor and evaluate quality standards. Assessment of quality does not stop at the clinic or organization; occupational therapy practitioners must strive to provide quality and ethical services and take the responsibility for their professional development.

Remembering that "the moment of truth is an episode in which the customer (client) comes into contact with the organization and gets an impression of its service" (Albrecht, 1993, p. 116) underscores the critical importance of the occupational therapy profession investing in continually improving the quality of their services.

## Student Self-Assessment

1. Identify the 10-step process for monitoring and evaluating quality standards.
2. Further discuss possible solutions to remedy the intervention minutes problem within the department.

The occupational therapy department in a 16-bed inpatient rehabilitation unit has developed a quality management program to review the following:

- Splinting schedules and adherence to the schedules by the staff
- Falls prevention education and carry-over of the information for the clients
- Intervention minutes

The department, including the occupational therapy director, registered occupational therapists, and certified occupational therapist assistants, collected data and completed a chart review. Splinting schedules were to be placed in the chart and documented in the nursing daily sheets for adherence to the schedule. Falls prevention education was to be documented in the occupational therapy daily notes, including client understanding and carry-over. Intervention documentation was to be documented in the daily notes and billing records for a minimum of 45 minutes twice a day (BID). Goals were established as follows:

- Splinting schedules and adherence to the schedule were documented 95% of the time.
- Falls prevention education was completed and thoroughly documented with client understanding 95% of the time.
- Clients received occupational therapy intervention in 45-minute sessions BID 95% of the time; if therapy was missed, thorough documentation was included for missed session 100% of the time.

Thresholds for splinting and falls prevention were met at 95%, while thresholds for intervention minutes were not met and achieved 85% compliance. The occupational therapy department held a meeting to discuss the results. The occupational therapy department has two full-time registered occupational therapists, two full-time occupational therapy assistants, and an occupational therapy aide. Department hours are from 8 a.m. to 5 p.m. Monday through Saturday, and Sunday from 8 a.m. to noon.

### Evidence-Based Research Chart

| Topic | Evidence |
|---|---|
| Health care economics | Rosenthal, Fernandopulle, Song, & Landon, 2004 |
| Health care performance | Jencks, Huff, & Cuerdon, 2003 |
| Evidence-based quality improvement | Lindenauer et al., 2007 |
| Effectiveness of quality improvement strategies and programs | Grimshaw et al., 2003; Mittman, 2004; Shojania & Grimshaw, 2005 |

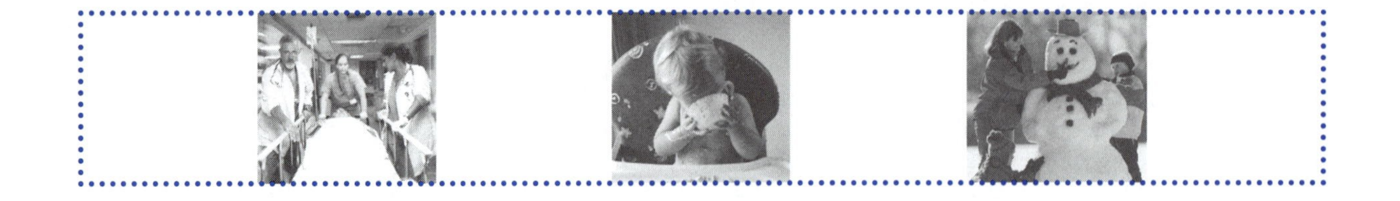

# References

Albrecht, K. (1993). *The only thing that matters: Bringing the power of the customer into the center of your business* (p. 54). New York, NY: Harper Paperbacks.

Braveman, B. (2006). *Leading & managing occupational therapy services: An evidence-based approach*. Philadelphia, PA: F.A. Davis.

Case-Smith, J. (2005). Using client outcome data to guide your professional development. *OT Practice, 10*(4), 8-9.

Deming, D. E. (2000). *Out of crisis*. Cambridge, MA: The MIT Press.

Donabedian, A. (1980). *Explorations in quality assessment and monitoring: The definition of quality and approaches to its assessment* (Vol. 1.). Ann Arbor, MI: Health Administration Press.

Griffin, R. W. (1993). *Management* (4th ed.). Boston, MA: Houghton Mifflin.

Grimshaw, J., McAuley, L. M., Bero, L. A., Grilli, R., Oxman, A. D., Ramsay, C., et al. (2003). Systematic reviews of the effectiveness of quality improvement strategies and programmes. *Quality and Safety in Health Care, 12*, 298-303.

Hinojosa, J., Bowen, R., Epstein, C., Scwope, C., Davis Rourk, J., Berg Rice, V., et al. (1998). *Continuing competency task force report to the executive board*. Bethesda, MD: AOTA Press.

Jacobs, J. S., & Logigian, M. K. (Eds.). (1994). *Functions of a manager in occupational therapy* (Rev. ed.). Thorofare, NJ: SLACK Incorporated.

Joint Commission on the Accreditation of Healthcare Organizations. (1996). *Using performance improvement tools in home care and hospice organizations*. Oakbrook Terrace, IL: Author.

Joint Commission on the Accreditation of Healthcare Organizations. (1997). *Performance improvement in home care and hospice*. Oakbrook Terrance, IL: Author.

Jencks, S., Huff, T., & Cuerdon, T. (2003). Change in the quality of care delivered to Medicare beneficiaries, 1998-1999 to 2000-2001. *Journal of the American Medical Association, 289*, 305-312.

Lindenauer, P., Remus, D., Roman, S., Rothberg, M., Benjamin, E., Ma, A., et al. (2007). Public reporting and pay for performance in hospital quality improvement. *New England Journal of Medicine, 356*(5), 486-496.

Maslin, Z. B. (1991). *Management in occupational therapy*. San Diego, CA: Singular Publishing Group.

Mittman, B. (2004). Creating the evidence base for quality improvement collaboratives. *Annual of Internal Medicine, 140*(11), 897-901.

National Board for Certification in Occupational Therapy. (2003). Certification renewal handbook. Retrieved August 9, 2009, from http://www.nbcot.org/webarticles/anmviewer.asp?a=66&z=13

O'Sullivan, G. (2004). Leisure activity programming: Promoting life satisfaction and quality of life for residents in long-term care. *New Zealand Journal of Occupational Therapy, 51*(2), 33-38.

Parasuraman, A., Berry, L. L., & Zeithaml, V. A. (1991). Understanding customer expectations of service. *Sloan Management Review, 32*(3), 39-48.

Punwar, A. J. (1998). *Occupational therapy: Principles & practice*. Baltimore, MD: Williams & Wilkins.

Rakich, J. S., Logest, B. B., & Darr, K. (1992). *Managing health services organizations* (3rd ed.). Baltimore, MD: Health Professions Press.

Rosenthal, M., Fernandopulle, R., Song, H., & Landon, B. (2004). Paying for quality: Providers' incentives for quality improvement. *Health Affairs, 23*(2), 127-141.

Shi, L., & Singh, D. (2008). *Delivering health care in America: A systems approach*. Boston, MA: Jones & Bartlett Publishers.

Shojania, K., & Grimshaw, J. (2005). Evidence-based quality improvement: The state of the science. *Health Affairs, 24*(1), 138-150.

Whiteley, R. C. (1993). *The customer-driven company: Moving from talk to action*. New York, NY: Basic Books.

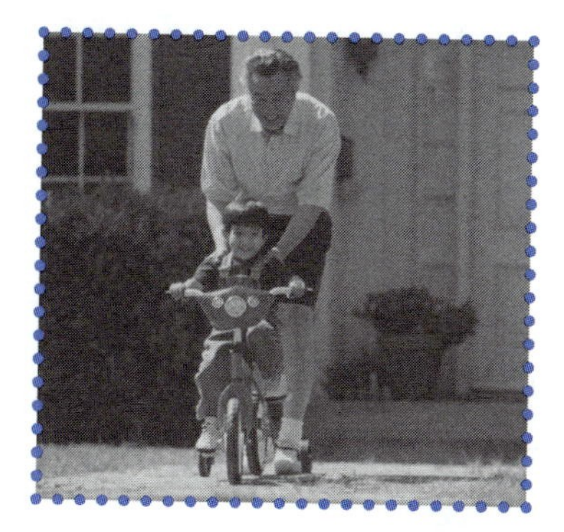

# Supervision and Fieldwork

*Amy Jo Lamb, OTD, OTR*

**ACOTE Standards Explored in This Chapter**

B.7.9-7.10

**Key Terms**

| | |
|---|---|
| Clinical education | Occupational therapy practitioners |
| Clinical instructor | Site |
| Level I fieldwork | Supervisee |
| Level II fieldwork | Supervision |

## Introduction

The advancement of the occupational therapy profession is multifaceted. At the heart of this advancement is the clinical education of the future generation of occupational therapy students as well as the effective, competency-based, legal, and ethical supervision of occupational therapy and non-occupational therapy personnel.

This chapter will begin by providing an overview of strategies for effective, competency-based, legal, and ethical supervision of occupational therapy and non-occupational therapy personnel. It will discuss clinical education in occupational therapy and the criteria for becoming a fieldwork educator.

## General Supervision Issues

Supervision is a continuing and dynamic process that encourages professional development in both the supervisee and supervisor. Supervision is considered a professional responsibility and, therefore, an important aspect of good clinical practice. Both the occupational therapy assistant and occupational therapist should seek supervision according to the *Code of Ethics* and good clinical judgment. (Sladyk, 2005).

### Functions of a Supervisor

The functions of a supervisor are in three areas: educational, administrative, and supportive.

### Supervision Levels

The American Occupational Therapy Association (AOTA) defines four levels of supervision (AOTA, 2005):

1. *Close*: Daily, direct contact at the work site
2. *Routine*: Direct contact at least two times per week at the work site with phone or written contact in addition
3. *General*: Direct monthly contact with phone or written contact as needed
4. *Minimal*: Provided only on an as-needed basis.



K. Sladyk, K. Jacobs, & N. MacRae (Eds.).
*Occupational Therapy Essentials for Clinical Competence* (pp. 407-412).

## Supervision of the Occupational Therapy Assistant

Supervision of the occupational therapy assistant by an occupational therapist is a requirement both professionally and likely legally. A new graduate occupational therapy assistant is required to have direct supervision by an occupational therapist or intermediate/advanced occupational therapy assistant under the direction of an occupational therapist. Intermediate or advanced occupational therapy assistants may have routine or general supervision as their competency level develops.

## Supervision of the Occupational Therapist

Although no supervision is required, supervision by an occupational therapist with advanced skills is recommended and will enhance clinical practice.

## Performance Evaluations

Almost all facilities require a minimum yearly written review of work productivity. Often, the supervisor completes a form and schedules a meeting with the supervisee to review his or her work. Feedback on this form should not come as a surprise to the supervisee as a good supervisor has talked about the issues well before a formal written evaluation is completed. Feedback should be specific, balanced, and focused on behaviors. The supervisee should develop professional goals for the next review period that fit the program's mission statement. Together, the supervisor and supervisee should develop a plan to meet (Sladyk, 2005).

# Overview of Supervision

The supervision of occupational therapy students is a process by which both the clinical instructor and the student are learning from the other. Students are able to help their clinical instructor and others stay up to date on current intervention techniques, professional advancements, and evidence supporting practice. Clinical instructors allow students the opportunity to learn via application. It is this immersion into practice under the tutelage of an experienced clinical instructor that students develop the clinical practices they will take with them on their professional journey.

There are multiple models of fieldwork supervision. Some sites employ a 1:1 model where the student is with the same clinical instructor for the duration of the experience. This clinical instructor gradually turns his or her caseload over to the student. However, in most cases, the clinical instructor is directly with the student throughout the affiliation. Other sites employ a multisupervisory model in which a student has two supervisors who share the student, and each gives part of their caseload to the student as time progresses. In this model, as the student increases in his or her comfort and competencies, he or she may have more autonomy and spend time with patients without a supervisor in the room. Neither method is better than another, although some students may find they are a better match for one model over another. Thus, this is good information to have when matching a student to a site.

A key factor in supervision is found in understanding the generational differences currently found in the clinic and in our upcoming generation of occupational therapists and occupational therapy assistants.

When examining generations, we look at the commonalities among individuals from hugely different backgrounds within a defined period of time (Raines, 2003). How does this information play a role in occupational therapy education? Consider who we are often pairing together as a clinical instructor and a student. Clinical instructors must have a minimum of 1 year of practice experience to supervise a Level II student. Many, however, average between 5 and 20 years of practice. What has changed in occupational therapy in the last 20 years? Perhaps the better question is, what has not changed in the last 20 years? Areas of practice have shifted, educational programs have evolved, and the current generation of student is different than the student of 20 years ago. For this discussion, we will focus on three generations, all of which are key players within occupational therapy clinical education: the baby boomers, generation X, and millennial generation. Table 37-1 explores these generations further.

**Table 37-1. Traits Across the Generations**

| Generation (Born between) | Outlook | Work Ethic | View of Authority | Leadership Through | Perspective |
|---|---|---|---|---|---|
| Baby Boomers (1940 to 1960) | Optimistic | Driven | Love/hate | Consensus | Team |
| Generation X (1960 to 1980) | Skeptical | Balanced | Unimpressed | Competence | Self |
| Millennial (1980 to 2000) | Hopeful | Ambitious | Relaxed, polite | Achievers | Civic |

Adapted from Raines, C. (2003). *Connecting generations.* Melo Park, CA: Crisp Publications

Generational differences cannot go ignored as we examine the supervisor/supervisee relationship. Let us examine the supervisor/supervisee concept further and then look at case studies that include the generational mixes found in today's clinics and educational programs.

## Supervisor

Being a clinical instructor for a student is a process that is sure to spark development and growth in both the supervisor and the supervisee. The first step in examining one's fit for taking this step is often found in self-assessment. There are several tools for such self-assessment that can be found in the resources at the end of this chapter.

Communication is another key factory in the supervisory process. It is often the supervisor who takes the lead in initiating this process with the student. This is best done by scheduling time to sit together and discuss how each of you communicates. For example, if the supervisor is very direct in his or her communication, a student who is more timid may read that as a lack of openness and may refrain from engaging in dialogue or asking questions out of fear. Opening the lines for communication allows for each party to share how they communicate up front before any issues emerge and grow. These open lines also provide a good avenue to offer feedback. Frequent feedback is essential to student learning. How does your student prefer feedback? Perhaps he or she prefers it immediately or perhaps all lumped together at the end of the day in a summary session. Does he or she prefer the nuts and bolts of what he or she needs to work on, or does he or she prefer the positive to cushion his or her areas of development? This information can all be discovered via open communication lines.

## Supervisee

Putting your best foot forward first is a great way to build a strong relationship with your clinical instructor. Prior to the experience, examine what it is you need and expect from the affiliation. Share this information with your clinical instructor to help define what you are hoping to gain from the experience in conjunction with the site's expectations for you on your path to developing entry-level competency. This is often best done during the orientation on your first day. You can request to have some time to sit and talk with your clinical instructor on the first day in advance when you are calling to get details regarding the logistics of the experience.

Know what to expect. Review the materials the site has for this student program, including weekly objectives and expectations. If you have questions, ask—do not assume. Utilize these documents for your own reflection as to your progress and what areas you feel you need more exposure to in an effort to be more comfortable.

Positive attitudes are fundamental to success. When students approach an experience with a positive attitude, are open to feedback, and participate in the supervisory relationship with open communication, good things happen. Supervision is fundamental to your skill development and learning and being open to the process is the first step toward success.

## Strategies

Utilize the Fieldwork Experience Assessment Tool. This document has a section for both the clinical instructor and the student to complete. Completing the respective session prior to the start of the clinical experience and establishing a time to discuss the similarities and differences will set a strong foundation on which this newfound relationship can build. Clinical sites can request students to complete their section prior to arrival so that the clinical instructor can incorporate this dialogue as part of the orientation process.

Create multifaceted mechanisms for delivering feedback. Feedback is essential to learning and development. However, each of us processes information differently. Provide avenues to reach the student in multiple ways. Written feedback can be provided in weekly progress forms and given to the students. Feedback in writing allows the student to reflect back on your comments. Verbal feedback can be provided in conjunction with the weekly written forms and reviewed with the student in a weekly meeting. Verbal feedback can also occur immediately after intervention sessions by asking students to reflect on what happened, what went well, and what they would have done differently. This sparks their development of clinical reasoning and opens the door for you to offer feedback after they have shared their reflections with you. Finally, demonstrations can serve as feedback as well. If a student is struggling with sliding board transfers, demonstrating it and having them practice on you is a good avenue for learning.

Establish opportunities for students to learn from one another. If your facility frequently has multiple students at a time, engage them together and allow them to learn from one another. This can be done by weekly meetings with a lead therapist in the department or more informally by having students work together on projects for the site.

Maria is an occupational therapist with 10 years of experience and has just begun supervising Erin in a level II experience in a fast-paced pediatric private practice.

Maria enjoys balance to her life. She uses her time at work very efficiently so she can have time to enjoy her family when she leaves. Maria is straightforward in communication and prefers to have others say what they are thinking up front and to have data to support their thoughts. Maria's biggest pet peeve is people who have not done their homework for a meeting or project, meaning time is wasted. Maria delegates projects and expects best effort at all times.

Erin is on her second level II fieldwork and wants to have her experience tailored to her personal goals. She has a high level of confidence and self-assurance, but, at times, others misinterpret that as attitude. Erin has grown up in an era of technology and is turned off by the bland patient education information available at the facility. Erin likes others to recognize and show respect for her achievements. She does not like to make decisions on the spot and prefers discussions to explore concepts before making decisions. Erin prefers people to tell her what their expectations are of her performance so she can meet the standard set.

This is a fairly typical example of what the clinical instructor and student relationship may look like. The differences in generations could result in challenges or perhaps opportunities depending upon how the individuals involved approach this new collaboration.

With an understanding of generational differences, there are several ways the clinical instructor and student can foster a good learning experience. Maria can schedule regular meetings between herself and Erin to ensure there is time for the exploration of concepts that Erin craves to learn. Erin can be cognizant of Maria's nonverbal cues and refrain from asking questions while she is on her way into a meeting or intervention session, but write down the questions to ask at their scheduled meeting or when Maria looks more open to dialogue. Maria could ask Erin to do a site enhancement project to update the patient education handouts using her technological skills. Erin can look at assignments and projects and perform to the best of her ability at all times rather than ask for an assignment guideline, or ask Maria to look at the project at midterm for feedback. These suggestions may help to blend the generational lines that may otherwise create interpersonal challenges between the student and clinical instructor and ultimately overshadow the learning experience.

# Clinical Education in Occupational Therapy

Clinical education is a true opportunity for current practitioners to participate in the educational process of students as well as to learn about developing areas that academic institutions are integral in establishing. Such experiences may include clinical opportunities students have in conjunction with didactic courses, Level I fieldwork, Level II fieldwork, and any other experiential components embedded within a curriculum. Throughout clinical education experiences, there are multiple parties who have active roles in a successful experience.

## University's Role

Each university has an Academic Fieldwork Coordinator. This person is integral to an optimal learning experience just as the clinical instructor and student are. This individual can serve all parties in different ways. The Academic Fieldwork Coordinator provides education to sites regarding the curriculum to assist each facility in understanding what knowledge students come with. They can assist both clinical instructors and students in communication and strategies for success. In essence, this person is a resource and a coach at any given time.

## Clinical Instructor's Role

Many clinical instructors enjoy having students and learning from them while assisting the students in developing their practice skills. Clinical instructors would most likely benefit from doing a self-analysis of their supervisory skills to allow for reflection on how they can create an optimal learning environment for students. Education of students in the clinic, so they are able to demonstrate competence in practice, indicates that learning in the workplace needs to be intentional (Hook & Lawson-Porter, 2003). Self-analysis of supervisory skills is the first step in taking an intentional step to the educational process. The American Occupational Therapy Association (AOTA) Self-Assessment Tool for Fieldwork Educator Competency is a valuable resource examining professional competence, education, supervision, evaluation, and administration, offering strategies to continue development in each area (AOTA, 2002a).

## Student Role

Students should recognize that fieldwork is not something that happens to them. It is a part of their clinical education in which they can take an active role in structuring to create the learning experience they desire. Positive professional behaviors in the academic setting seem to be related to fieldwork success (Scheerer, 2003). Professional behaviors include a variety of factors, one of which is communication skills. Communication is essential to the fieldwork experience. Students communicate with other health care team members, peers, supervisors, clients, family members, non-health care personnel, and reimbursement agencies.

# Fieldwork

"Fieldwork education is a crucial part of professional preparation" (AOTA, 2006, p. 11). Such integration into the clinic serves as one method for learning the skills of practice while learning how to navigate the greater health care system with which we are surrounded.

### Level I

"The goal of Level I fieldwork is to introduce students to the fieldwork experience, to apply knowledge to practice, and to develop understanding of the needs of clients" (AOTA, 2006, p. 12). These experiences are valuable exploratory opportunities for students to examine a variety of areas of practice, including emerging areas of practice to better understand the role of occupational therapy in the respective setting.

### Level II

"Level II fieldwork's primary goal is to develop competent, entry-level, generalist occupational therapists" (AOTA, 2006, p. 12). The Level II experience allows students to develop their skills in preparation for practice after graduation. These experiences often have a fundamental role in how a student plans his or her career path.

### Other Clinical Affiliations

Other clinical affiliations or experiences are found within several of the entry-level doctoral programs offered across the country. These experiences vary by name and title and may be referred to as Level II fieldwork, residencies, or professional rotations, to name a few. The common thread these affiliations share is the effort to develop competency with an advanced skill set.

## Competency-Based Fieldwork

Competency refers to the skill set required for entry-level practice as either an occupational therapy assistant or an occupational therapist. There are several tools that can be utilized to document the progression of competencies related to occupational therapy practice.

*The Competency-Based Fieldwork Evaluation for Occupational Therapists* measures seven core competencies for practice and is relatively easy to use (Bossers, Miller, Polatajko, & Hartley, 2001). A unique feature to this document is the inclusion of a learning contract associated with each section to be utilized if needed to develop structure for the student to achieve competency.

The Fieldwork Performance Evaluation is another valuable tool to measure competencies and can be done at intervals throughout the experience to offer concrete information to the student. The Fieldwork Performance Evaluation for the Occupational Therapy Student (AOTA, 2002b) and the Fieldwork Performance Evaluation for the Occupational Therapy Assistant Student (AOTA, 2002a) are commonly used by universities to gather information about students' competency development as they progress. These tools are most frequently used at midterm and finals. There are additional ways in which this tool can be utilized to assist in fieldwork education. One method is to examine monthly progress to offer students with frequent written feedback on the expectations of their devilment. This may be especially beneficial for a student who needs consistent, concrete feedback in writing to be able to develop their skills. Another method is to have students complete the form separately from the clinical instructor and then compare them during a meeting. This allows the student an opportunity for self-reflection, it allows the clinical instructor to gauge where the student views his or her performance compared to where the clinical instructor rated the student's performance, and it allows the academic fieldwork coordinator to have concrete information to build from should problems arise.

## Ethical Dilemmas in Fieldwork

It is inevitable that students and clinicians will encounter ethical challenges. When ethical issues emerge during these experiences, each person is watching for the other to see how they will handle it.

There are models of decision making related to ethics that can be of use in demonstrating the process of handling ethical dilemmas. Gervais (2005) identified six steps to assist in this process. These steps include gathering background knowledge of the situation; examining the case based on its facts and context; completing a self-assessment, including the personal capacity for your decision, weighing options for what is most right, acting on the option you feel is ethically correct, and evaluating via reflection to examine what you learned in your review and handling of this situation; and what you would do the same or what you would do differently should the situation arise again.

Modeling ethical reasoning to students is essential to their learning and often plays a key role in how they will approach ethical situations that arise in their practice. There are several ways that this modeling can occur. If an ethical issue should arise with a patient on the student or clinical instructor caseload, you can engage them with you as you navigate your decision making. Clinical instructors can provide students with written examples or case studies of ethical issues as an assignment for the student to document how he or she would handle the issue.

Offering students the opportunity to practice looking at ethical situations in clinical practice under the guidance of a clinical instructor allows real world opportunities for learning.

## Summary

Fieldwork education allows students the opportunity to learn and establish the necessary competencies to fully engage in practice. This valuable piece of education is vital to the growth and development of occupational therapy practice. The opportunities that lie within fieldwork education and supervision far outweigh any challenges that may be present.

## Student Self-Assessment

1. Explore what you would like to accomplish in your upcoming fieldwork experiences.
2. In pairs, practice verbalizing what you would like to learn from your fieldwork experience in preparation for talking with your on-site clinical instructor.
3. Identify in writing what your learning style is, how you prefer feedback, and what your communication style is.

## Electronic Resources

- Fieldwork survival guide: www.aota.org/Students/Current/Fieldwork/Tools/38207.aspx
- Center for Teaching Excellence: http://cte.umdnj.edu/clinical_education/index.cfm
- AOTA fieldwork education resources: www.aota.org/Educate/EdRes/Fieldwork/Supervisor.aspx
- Kennedy Institute: http://bioethics.georgetown.edu
- Self assessment tool: www.aota.org/Educate/EdRes/Fieldwork/Supervisor/Forms/38251.aspx
- Fieldwork Evaluation Assessment Tool: www.aota.org/Educate/EdRes/Fieldwork/StuSuprvsn/38220.aspx

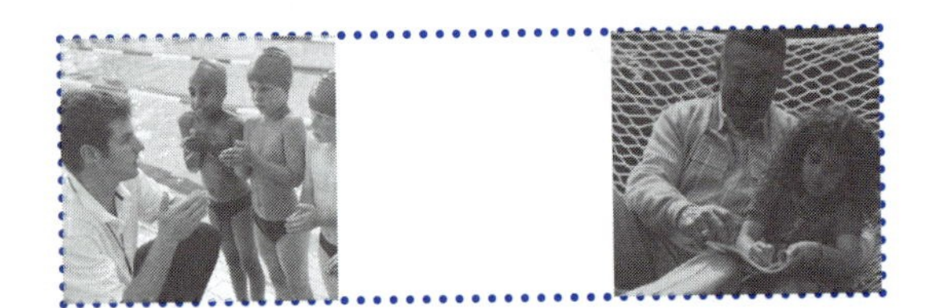

## References

American Occupational Therapy Association. (2002a). Fieldwork Evaluation Assessment Tool. Retrieved September 1, 2006, from http://www.aota.org/Educate/EdRes/Fieldwork/StuSuprvsn/38220.aspx

American Occupational Therapy Association. (2002b). Accreditation Council for Occupational Therapy Education Standards and Interpretative Guidelines. Retrieved October 10, 2006, from http://www.aota.org/Educate/Accredit/StandardsReview/guide/42369.aspx

American Occupational Therapy Association. (2005). Standards of practice. Retrieved October 10, 2006, from http://www.aota.org/Practitioners/Resources/OTAs/ScopeandStandards/36194.aspx

American Occupational Therapy Association. (2006). Accreditation Standards for the Master's Degree Level Educational Program for the Occupational Therapist. Adopted July 2006, Effective January 1, 2008. Retrieved on October 10, 2006, from http://www.aota.org/Educate/Accredit/StandardsReview.aspx

Bossers, A., Miller, L. T., Polatajko, H. J., & Hartley, M. (2001). *Competency-based fieldwork evaluation for occupational therapists CBFE-OT.* Albany, NY: Delmar.

Gervais, K. G. (2005). A model for ethical decision making to inform the ethics education of future health care professionals. In R. B. Purtilo, G. M. Jensen, & C. B. Royeen (Eds.), *Educating for moral action: A sourcebook in health and rehabilitation ethics.* Philadelphia, PA: F.A. Davis.

Hook, A., & Lawson-Porter, A. (2003). The development and evaluation of a fieldwork educator's training program for allied health professionals. *Medical Teacher, 25*(5), 527-536.

Raines, C. (2003). *Connecting generations: The sourcebook for a new workplace.* Menlo Park, CA: Crisp Publications.

Scheerer, C. (2003). Perceptions of effective professional behavior feedback: Occupational therapy student voices. *American Journal of Occupational Therapy, 57*(2), 205-213.

Sladyk, K. (Ed.). (2005). *OT study cards in a box.* Thorofare, NJ: SLACK Incorporated.

## Suggested Reading

Costa, D. (Ed.). (2004). *The essential guide to occupational therapy fieldwork education: Resources for today's educators and practitioners.* Bethesda, MD: AOTA Press.

Sladyk, K. (Ed.). (2002). *The successful occupational therapy fieldwork student.* Thorofare, NJ: SLACK Incorporated.

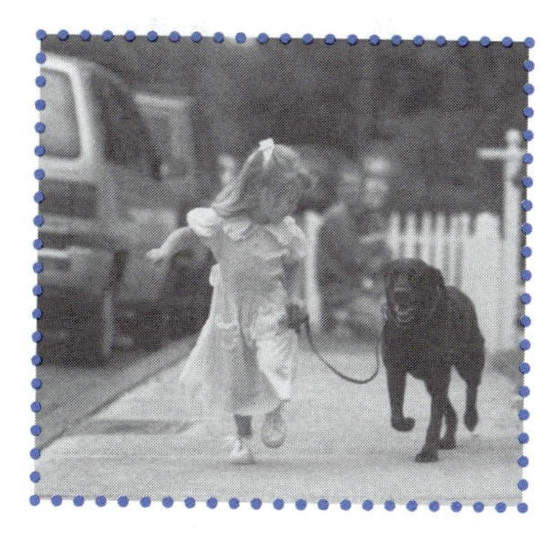

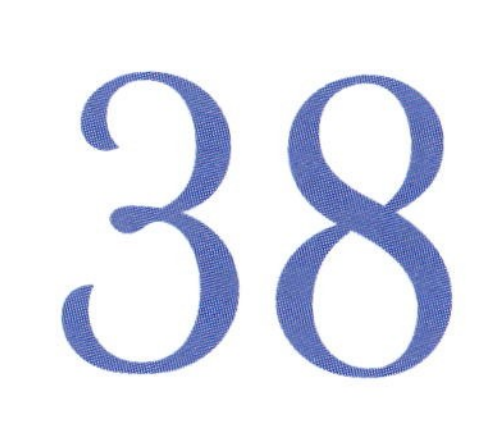

# 38

# LEADERSHIP

Lisa L. Clark, MS, OTR/L and James Marc-Aurele, MBA, OTR/L

**ACOTE Standards Explored in This Chapter**

B.6.4, 7.2, 7.6, 9.1-9.2, 9.7-9.8

**Key Terms**

Context
Leadership
Manager

## Introduction

*The growth and development of people is the highest calling of leadership.*
—Harvey S. Firestone

When we first think of leadership, what comes to mind? Do we think about world leaders, whose position of power influences national and international public policies? Do we think about impassioned advocates who bring about sweeping social change against the odds of convention and misplaced conviction? Often, particular people come to mind: Golda Meir, Ghandi, Martin Luther King, Jr., Winston Churchill, etc. They embody what we think of as leaders—people who create a vision, move others to believe in it, and aspire to achieve it.

At first thought, leadership is a descriptor of the actions of those who have achieved exceptional status and influence as a result of accomplishments credited to their efforts. While this is often the case, leadership in its truest sense is far more common. Opportunities for leadership present themselves every day. As occupational therapy practitioners, we are in a position to be leaders in our profession, our communities, and in our day-to-day interactions with others.

This chapter will explore the importance of leadership in the profession. We will discuss different types of leadership as a necessary background to thinking about effective leadership. Personal, social, and cultural contexts are important influences in leadership abilities and styles. Being a leader can be an occupation. The framework will be utilized to examine the contexts that define leadership (American Occupational Therapy Association [AOTA], 2008). Although leadership occurs in political, community, and global settings, it is also very present in occupational therapy practitioners' daily work. This chapter will illustrate several forms of leadership and make it clear that leadership opportunities, and even obligations, exist for all occupational therapy practitioners in all settings. Finally, the chapter will close with an emphasis on how leadership in occupational therapy can play an important role in promoting social justice and social change.

## Leadership as Occupation

*Leadership and learning are indispensable to each other.*
—John F. Kennedy



K. Sladyk, K. Jacobs, & N. MacRae (Eds.).
*Occupational Therapy Essentials for Clinical Competence* (pp. 413-420).

The framework (AOTA, 2008) informs internal and external audiences of the unique scope of service of occupational therapy, and replaces the *Uniform Terminology III* document. The framework uses the following definition of occupation: "Activities...of everyday life, named, organized, and given value and meaning by the individuals and a culture. Occupation is everything people do to occupy themselves, including looking after themselves...enjoying life...and contributing to the social and economic fabric of their communities..." (Law, Polatajko, Baptiste, & Townsend, 2002). The occupation of leadership can be described using the framework as a background.

Acting as an effective leader involves performance skills, motor and process abilities, as well as communication/interaction skills. Leadership influences and is influenced by individual roles, habits, and routines. There are particular activity demands involved in leadership, and these demands differ in each situation. Context significantly influences leadership. The framework names several types of context: cultural, social, physical, temporal, virtual, and personal. Below is a brief exploration of each context and its relation to leadership.

1. *Cultural context*: The culture in which leadership takes place is important. This context includes beliefs, customs, standards of behavior, and laws that are all part of an accepted culture, of which an individual is a member (AOTA, 2008). These are generally factors that are external to the person. However, much of a cultural context can be internalized by the person as well. Laws that govern employee/employer relations can be part of a leader's cultural context. The internal culture of an organization will also influence how leadership is performed.
2. *Social context*: Social context includes expectations of other people who are important to the individual, as well as accepted norms of larger social groups (AOTA, 2008). Leaders may have particular ways of dressing or using specific words or language as part of their social context. The social context can significantly influence leading.
3. *Physical context*: Physical context is the "environment" factor typically thought of when discussing context. It includes nonhuman aspects of the environment such as tools, plants, furniture, objects, animals, and natural terrain (AOTA, 2008). The physical context of where an individual engages in leading can greatly influence performance of leadership abilities. A concrete example of this is Martin Luther King, Jr.'s opportunity to use a microphone when leading/speaking to large groups. In this example, his physical context greatly enhanced his ability to lead effectively.
4. *Temporal context*: This "time" context refers to the influence time can have on the performance of occupations (AOTA, 2008). A leader who holds meetings at the end of a long workday may find his or her effectiveness limited by the temporal context. Some leaders may feel influenced in their work by the time of year.
5. *Virtual context*: This term refers to communication that occurs without physical contact and takes place over the airways or with a computer (AOTA, 2008). The virtual context has greatly influenced how and when communication takes place, as well as how effective it is. Leadership involves a great deal of communication (Hamm, 2006). Leaders must pay attention to the influence of the virtual context on the effectiveness of their leading.
6. *Personal context*: According to the framework, personal context is made up of personal factors about the individual—age, gender, and other demographic information such as educational status and socioeconomic status. One example of this is studies where gender is examined as an influence on leadership styles (George & Jones, 2002).

The framework also describes a specific factor about the person that is important in the consideration of leadership, and that is spirituality. Spirituality takes into account what motivates or is inspirational to an individual. All leaders, in large or small ways, must be in touch with what is meaningful to them (Sadler-Smith & Shefy, 2004). Kouzes and Posner (2002) discussed exemplary leadership as having five important components. One of these is "Encouraging the Heart." They maintained that leaders need to "hear the heart and see the soul" (Kouzes & Posner, p. 329). Spirituality is an important factor to consider in terms of how each person participates in leadership behaviors.

Leadership as an occupation can be analyzed using the framework (AOTA, 2008), the latest written work describing what occupational therapy practitioners do and how and where they do it. It informs us about what motor, process, and communication abilities are helpful in leading, and it promotes discussion on the importance of contexts as they influence occupations.

# Theories of Leadership

In developing leadership abilities, it is useful to understand how leadership theories and models have evolved over time. In some ways, the movement of leadership models to ones of more participatory, or shared, philosophies more closely mirrors the way occupational therapy practitioners have been working to interact with people for the last century.

## Trait Theories

There are many definitions and interpretations of leadership. In the past 75 years, countless theories have been espoused in an attempt to identify and explain the characteristics of leaders and effective leadership. DeYoung

(2005) described how Lewin proposed that most leaders engaged in three leadership styles based on personality traits. These included authoritarian, democratic, and *laissez-faire*. Additional studies (George & Jones, 2002) focused on specific traits or characteristics displayed by leaders. Researchers identified several traits thought to have the strongest correlation with effective leadership. These included intelligence, task-relevant knowledge, energy, tolerance for stress, integrity, emotional maturity, and self-confidence. These traits were thought to be relatively fixed and not amenable to change. This view implies a predetermined ability to lead based on the possession of certain traits.

### Behavioral Theories

DeYoung (2005) identified the specific behaviors engaged in by leaders to promote organizational effectiveness, as he refered to the Ohio State research, which has been cited by many authors in leadership. According to these studies, leadership behavior can be classified as either consideration behaviors or as initiating structure behaviors. Consideration behavior is defined as behavior indicating a leader trusts, respects, and values good relationships with his or her followers. Initiating structure behaviors are defined as actions a leader performs to make sure the work gets done. It is important to recognize that these leadership behaviors are not mutually exclusive. Leaders can and do engage in both initiating structure and consideration behaviors. The behavioral models provide insight into leader characteristics but do not address how and why leadership happens (George & Jones, 2002).

## Leadership and Context

One of the early theorists credited with considering the context of leadership was Frederick Fiedler (1978). He attempted to explore the interrelationship between leader characteristics and the specific situation in which leadership takes place. The framework would refer to this as the influence of context. Fiedler defined the situation as having three specific dimensions: leader-follower relations, task structure, and the position power of the leader. In Fiedler's view, these three relationships, identified as contingency dimensions, significantly impacted leadership effectiveness (Fiedler, 1967). These characteristics were thought of as existing on a continuum from low to high. Together, the characteristics would determine "situational favorableness" for a particular leadership style (George & Jones, 2002). According to Fiedler, leaders engaged in two specific styles of leadership: relationship oriented and task oriented (DeYoung, 2005). Relationship-oriented leaders placed primary value on establishing positive working relationships with those they were leading. Leaders who were task-oriented primarily emphasized task completion. Fiedler suggested that leaders are most effective in situations that most closely match their leadership styles. It is significant that he viewed leadership styles to be relatively fixed, such that leaders could not easily move from one style to the other. Thus, in his view, leadership style was a first-order variable with the situation (or context) as a determinant as to how effective a leadership style would be.

Fiedler's work began to look at situational factors and gave rise to the Situational Leadership Model. Developed by Hersey and Blanchard, the Situational Leadership Model examined the relationship among three dimensions: task behavior, relationship behavior, and the maturity of the individuals being led. The task behavior refers to the degree of structure and clarity that the leader provides (clearly defined work roles and responsibilities). The relationship dimension refers to the emotional and psychological relationship between the leader and the individual being led (Hersey & Blanchard, 1982). According to Hersey and Blanchard, these first two dimensions are greatly influenced by the maturity level of the individual being led. The maturity level is characterized by three specific criteria: level of motivation, willingness to assume responsibility, and the individual's experience and education level. Based on these criteria, the leader modifies his or her leadership approach. For example, when working with an entry-level occupational therapy practitioner, a leader will likely provide more structure for a given task to promote success, whereas a practitioner with considerable experience in the same situation may require less direction from the leader. Likewise, the leader must consider the level of motivation of the individual in altering his or her leadership behavior.

## Leadership and Intuition

More recently, the role of intuition has gained increased attention. Some leadership abilities can be innate (Sadler-Smith & Shefy, 2004). Intuition is formed by individual feelings based on experience. Once regarded as anything but useful, intuition is being recognized as a component to leadership. The role of intuition is supported by some researchers who postulate "much if not most of cognition occurs automatically outside of consciousness" (Sadler-Smith & Shefy, p. 78). Some studies indicate that senior leaders lead more intuitively than middle managers, highlighting the impact of experience in developing intuition.

## Participatory Leadership

As the evolution of leadership continued over the decades, participatory leadership models gained increasing acceptance (McLagen & Nell, 1995). Given the multitude of societal and cultural change factors in organizations, participatory leadership models have become more popular. "With these changes, coaching and commitment cultures have replaced the command, control, and compartmentalization orientations of the past" (Kets de Vries, 2005,

p. 62). Participatory leadership embraces change and readily involves others (Kouzes & Posner, 2007). Leadership in day-to-day work can move from person to person depending upon the tasks involved and competencies needed. The leader facilitates and guides transitions (Ackerman & MacKenzie, 2006; McLagen & Nell). Participatory leaders readily defer to others' expertise. The parallels with occupational therapy client-centered practice are easily discerned. Engaging in participatory leadership is a powerful way to help people grow their strengths and enable future leaders. In participatory leadership, the focus is on collaboration, commitment, and context. Participatory leadership incorporates much of the multi-faceted tenets of previous leadership theories. Pearce (2004) advocates that the more complex a task is, the more there is a need for shared/participatory leadership. This model is less a body of new work than a coming together of earlier approaches, melding traits, behaviors, and contextual factors.

In this brief review of leadership theories, it is noted that early theories focused on individual traits and characteristics. This was followed by a study of specific behaviors, and more recent work has focused on the context of leadership. Although this review is limited, the theories here were chosen to provide a degree of insight into the components of leadership to help us begin to understand the what, why, and how of leadership. The effectiveness of leadership is a complex and ongoing field of study. The most effective leaders are able to utilize knowledge, experience, and consideration of personal and contextual factors when determining a style of interaction. The issue is not to excel at one particular type of leadership but to determine which approach is best given each particular scenario and context (Pearce, 2004; Shortell & Kaluzney, 2000).

## Case Example

Ann is the manager of occupational therapy at a community medical center. Ann has 18 years of experience as an occupational therapist. Her specialty area of practice has been working with people with repetitive strain injuries. Ann possesses a very strong work ethic and believes that others should embrace this as well. She is responsible for overseeing the delivery of occupational therapy services in three different settings at two different locations. Her job responsibilities include scheduling and supply inventories. She initially found both tasks overwhelming without administrative support. She is now thankful that she enrolled in a continuing education course to learn to use software that helps to manage work schedules and inventories.

The level of experience of the staff Ann supervises is mixed. Brad is a new graduate occupational therapist. He is a father to two toddlers. He struggles occasionally to juggle his important roles of father, husband, and professional. Jennie has 25 years of experience as an occupational therapy assistant in rehabilitation with people experiencing neurological deficits. She has a strong belief in self-advocacy and at times finds herself working in opposition to established systems. Juliette is an occupational therapist with 8 years of general experience with people who have physical disabilities. She is Franco-American and works long hours to complete her work to her own high standards.

The organizational culture of the medical center is one of careful consideration of problems. The leadership values employee contributions for many, but not all, tasks. Some issues are clearly handled in a directive style. Many middle managers are allowed to lead in the manner they see fit.

## Problem #1

In order to comply with new insurance regulations, a directive has come down from senior management that billing documentation from each department must be on the same form. Ann's preferred leadership style is one of participatory leadership. However, this is an example of an issue that requires a directive leadership approach.

- *Virtual context*: Virtual communication may negatively influence Ann's ability to lead around this issue. Ann may find sending out a blanket e-mail about this relatively large change in documentation does not engender effective communication with staff.
- *Temporal context*: This change needs to be implemented immediately. This temporal context constrains Ann's effectiveness as a leader in making this change.
- *Cultural context*: The organization understands the value of communicating directives when needed. They believe that the leader (Ann) can give these directives in whatever style she prefers.
- *Personal context*: Ann's years of experience may help her leadership with staff when delivering the billing form information.
- *Social context*: Ann's family values include a strong work ethic, and she realizes that some things just need to happen to keep organizations working effectively. Ann's staff members' contexts become part of her social context at work and do influence her leading abilities around this problem. She will have to consider Brad's time constraints and Jennie's penchant for questioning the system.
- *Physical context*: The fact that the staff Ann leads are in different physical locations influences her effectiveness in leading them to work with this new form.

Ann's sense of spirituality and her understanding of this in her own life can influence how she performs her leadership role. Her fundamental orientation to life is one of a belief in calm centeredness. This part of her person positively influences her leading, especially in potentially stressful times.

## Problem #2

The occupational therapy staff wishes to infuse the framework into their daily documentation. The first step will be to revamp the initial assessment form for the outpatient department. Ann's preferred participatory leadership style can be put into play more in this scenario.

- *Virtual context*: The use of e-mail can enhance Ann's leadership here, as suggestions and drafts of assessment forms may be easily shared among occupational therapy staff in different physical locations.
- *Temporal context*: This context will not significantly influence Ann's leading, as there are no time constraints to the project.
- *Cultural context*: The organization values employee input for some projects. This context will help Ann lead her team to a successful conclusion in changing their assessment.
- *Personal context*: No change from the previous problem.
- *Social context*: Again the staffs' contexts become part of Ann's social context at work. She will need to be cognizant of Brad's work schedule. Jennie will probably be helpful because her input is included in this project. Ann's appreciation of a strong work ethic leads her to value employees in all categories and will assist her in positive leading with the occupational therapy assistant and the occupational therapists alike. This will enhance her leadership and thus the outcome of the project. Ann values Juliette's attention to detail and this will also help the project.
- *Physical context*: Ann chooses a conference meeting that contains plush chairs, good lighting, and plenty of work space room for their first brainstorming meeting. Healthy snacks are provided. Ann knows that the physical context can greatly influence success in occupational performance.

## Conclusion

The contexts of the leading, which are part of each problem, are important, despite the fact that Ann must use different leadership styles in each scenario. Her effectiveness as a leader is greatly enhanced when she carefully considers the influences of the different contexts. Her abilities as a reflective leader help her consider the influence that context can have on her leading. She also recognizes when she needs to utilize different management strategies. By engaging her staff in a participatory fashion in the second scenario, Ann is able to capitalize on the strengths and experiences of the staff. Their participation, along with her leadership skills, combines to create an ultimately successful project.

# Management Versus Leadership

*Management is efficiency in climbing the ladder of success; leadership determines whether the ladder is leaning against the right wall.*
—Stephen R. Covey

Leadership and management are often thought of as synonymous terms, implying that leaders manage, and managers lead. While this may be the case in some instances, it is arguably more complex than this. Effective leaders readily embrace change—they facilitate and guide transitions. Leaders involve others and are aware of their own limitations. Leaders are able to create a shared vision among people.

Managers are often described in terms of the tasks to which they ably attend. They are responsible for resource allocation (staffing and budgets), generating reports, and managing programs (Borkowski, 2005; Grady, 2003).

Let us go back to our case study. Ann was in a position of leadership. In the first scenario, it could be said that she was managing. The new billing form information came in the form of a directive, which needed to be communicated. In the second scenario, she was able to lead more effectively. She valued input, understood and had thought about her own limitations, and inspired a shared vision with her coworkers around their project.

It is important to note that management and leadership are not mutually exclusive entities, nor is the comparison meant to diminish the functions of a manager. Management functions provide necessary parameters for operations to take place. Leaders may or may not be responsible for managerial components within their situations of leadership.

# Leadership from Occupational Therapy Practitioners

Leadership should be, and is, undertaken by occupational therapists and occupational therapy assistants, as well as students. Some leadership skills can be similar to skills that practitioners use in their daily practice (McCormack, 2003; Strzelecki, 2007). Practitioners recognize that leadership skills and abilities can be present in everyone. Many state occupational therapy member associations, such as Maine and New York, are free to elect occupational therapists and occupational therapy assistants as President or other executive board positions. The New York State Occupational Therapy Association elected an occupational therapy assistant for a second term as President, starting in

June 2005 (AOTA, 2005a). There are many other examples of occupational therapists and occupational therapy assistants providing exemplary leadership within and outside of the profession.

## Occupational Therapy Code of Ethics

Another key document for the profession that can shed light on leadership is the *Occupational Therapy Code of Ethics*. The Code is covered in greater detail in Chapter 40 but will be briefly mentioned in this chapter.

The Occupational Therapy Code of Ethics (AOTA, 2005b) is a list of seven important principles that define how occupational therapy practitioners should conduct themselves in practice of the profession. Many of the principles seem to strictly apply to working with clients at first glance. However, the preamble to the document asks that we understand that "this commitment extends beyond service recipients to include professional colleagues, students, educators, businesses and the community" (AOTA, 2005b, p. 639). The creators also stated that "occupational therapy personnel have an ethical responsibility first and foremost to recipients of service as well as to society" (AOTA, p. 639). It is clear that occupational therapy practitioners are asked to be responsive to individuals, communities, and beyond. Leadership can be an effective occupation to help accomplish this. Occupational therapy practitioners can practice leadership in far-reaching, even political, ways and can thoughtfully recognize that every therapeutic interaction with another can be an act of leadership. Our professional Code of Ethics calls us to "virtuous practice of artistry and science…and to noble acts of courage" (AOTA, p. 639).

Leadership is not merely an opportunity but an obligation. By carefully increasing awareness and intentional concern for context, all practitioners can engage in leadership. Opportunities for leadership may present themselves in formal ways such as holding a position as manager or supervisor, but there are other equally important opportunities for leadership (Strzelecki, 2007). Using the information presented about the framework and how leadership can be analyzed as an occupation and having a better understanding of leadership models can engender a discussion about the influence of context on each individual's leadership abilities. Occupational therapy practitioners and students can think about their leadership abilities and desires by reflecting on their process and communication skills, in addition to pondering their own individual contextual influences.

Personal context, such as age and education level, can affect how someone leads. Some of these individual factors are also influenced by the social context (society) and the cultural context (see Chapter 2). How do we tend to respond to a leader who has recently graduated from college? Or a leader who is in his or her 80s? Do we have societal or cultural expectations of how old or young a person must be to lead effectively? If so, does it behoove us to reconsider these perceived limitations? According to the framework, laws and societal changes are all part of the cultural context. Reflective leaders will need to consider how laws and changes occurring in the larger community (e.g., changes in reimbursement) are affecting their leadership. How do these influences change what leaders must do and how they do it?

On a smaller scale, individual leaders should also examine the influence of expectations and norms of their closer circles. These would include beliefs, behavioral standards, or norms, and can have an enormous effect on how people communicate and process information. Is the leader's family supportive of achievement? Do friends encourage or disparage moral standards? People who lead effectively reflect on what strategic tasks and occupations have been successful in the past. Also, has the use of virtual communication methods been a hindrance or a help in leading others? Leadership may also be influenced by the spiritual context, and this is an important area to ponder. The final context considered here in personal reflection of leaders is the physical. The physical environment (furniture, plants, objects, etc.) can stifle or encourage leading and the activities that accompany it. Each person should determine the importance of each of these contexts in his or her leadership practices.

The ways in which the framework breaks out different contextual influences can be a start in helping individuals assess their leadership abilities and experiences. Most occupational therapy practitioners will find that, upon reflection, many of the tasks they already complete can be seen in a leadership frame. Leadership theories and models can be infused into this complex weave of leading as an occupation. This weaving is a mechanism for individuals to reflect on how, where, and when leadership interfaces with their own lives. Occupational therapy practitioners understand people as occupational beings (Jarman, 2004). We can contemplate ourselves as occupational beings and become aware of how leading is an occupation that is important to the profession. Leadership in occupational therapy is an adventure in which all can participate in some way.

Spreier, Fontaine, and Malloy (2006) recognized that teams working together are more effective than individuals moving toward a goal on their own. This is part of participatory leadership. Every time an occupational therapy practitioner works with someone, he or she is leading in a participatory sense. Once we embrace this realization, it is a small step to move to leading in a community or global context. Occupational therapy practitioners are especially well positioned to create and influence systems of care and wellness (social and cultural contexts) because of our client-centered beliefs and the leadership abilities that we exemplify every day.

## Leadership as an Ingredient of Social Change and Justice

Clearly, occupational therapy practitioners are uniquely situated to practice effective leadership. This can create social change. We can lead in our daily interactions with others as well as in the larger community. The framework clarifies how context and abilities are important in influencing occupations. Our Code of Ethics demands that we consider individuals and communities in our professional activities. Discovery about leadership philosophies and models informs our learning and reflection on different beliefs and styles.

Kronenberg and Pollard (2006) reminded us that, globally, the largest number of occupational therapy practitioners reside and work in the United States. This national group "significantly influences thinking, practice, education, and research of OT practitioners all over the world" (Kronenberg & Pollard, p.1). Perhaps in the United States, we are especially obligated to think outside of the box. We must critically assess our core professional values and how well they do or do not fit with our social and cultural contexts. Kronenberg and Pollard asserted that our profession's work is "always under construction" and "essentially never finished" (p. 1). He went on to suggest that with our expertise in occupations, perhaps we need to "problematize situations in which 'occupations' contribute to the construction of communities and societies that are exclusive" (Kronenberg & Pollard, p. 2).

Townsend and others discussed the term *occupational justice* as a way to think about social justice issues through the lens of occupation (Townsend & Whiteford, 2005; Townsend & Wilcock, 2004). If we understand that occupations are key in the health and wellness of human beings, then it is a short journey to realizing that occupations and people's opportunities to participate in them are very much part of social justice considerations (Sinclair, 2006). Conversely, there are occupational justice issues in communities where some occupations may be forced on people. In the wake of Hurricane Katrina in the southern United States in 2005, many people who experienced the force of the storm probably found themselves participating in the occupations of acquiring food and shelter in a very different manner than before the storm. News stories chronicled the socioeconomic issues about which strata of the population was more likely to be caught in the storm, versus the socioeconomic status of the people who moved to safer ground.

Kronenberg and Pollard (2006) asked us to consider how continued study in occupational therapy and occupational science can inform "societies' responses to these complex and global realities" (p. 2). Consideration of occupational justice is a leadership issue in the occupational therapy profession.

## Summary

*Never doubt that a small group of thoughtful,*
*concerned citizens can change the world.*
*Indeed, it is the only thing that ever has.*
—Margaret Mead

This chapter has explored leadership by discussing different leadership theories and analyzing the occupation of leading using the framework. The framework emphasis was on the role of context and the importance of reflection in developing leadership abilities. Participatory leadership offers particular benefits to occupational therapy practitioners in many situations. Ultimately, leaders should possess abilities in various types of leadership and employ them based on situation and context. Finally, issues of occupational justice are crucial ones to address in occupational therapy leadership. Leadership occurs every day in the profession. Once we recognize and name these happenings, we are in a position to respond to our obligation to lead in community and global arenas.

## Student Self-Assessment

1. Construct a personal leadership plan that addresses a particular task (simple or complex), the type of leadership you plan to employ in completing the task, and the strengths and weaknesses of the chosen style.
2. In groups of four to eight, choose a leadership scenario from a national or global incident that is in the news. Discuss the social justice implications of people's leadership and participation in the incident. What leadership styles/skills were used? Were they effective? Why or why not? What other leadership abilities could have been used that might have been more effective?
3. Consider one leadership experience you have witnessed or of which you have been a part. Discuss and analyze the different contexts, according to the framework, and how each of them influenced the leadership scenario.

| Evidence-Based Research Chart | |
|---|---|
| **Topic** | **Evidence** |
| Leadership theories/models | Borkowski, 2005; George & Jones, 2002; Hamm, 2006 |
| Leadership contexts, as occupational therapy practitioners think of them | AOTA, 2008 |
| Reflective leadership | Kets DeVries, 2005; Kouzes & Posner, 2002; Sadler-Smith & Shefy, 2004 |
| Social justice implications in leadership | Kronenberg, Algado, & Pollard, 2005; Townsend & Wilcock, 2004 |

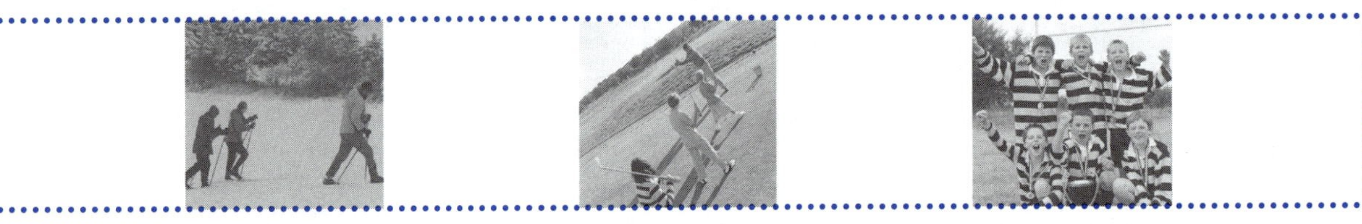

# References


Ackerman, R., & MacKenzie, S. (2006). Uncovering teacher leadership. *Educational Leadership, 63*, 66-70.

American Occupational Therapy Association. (2005a). OTA exchange. *OT Practice, 10*(4), 23.

American Occupational Therapy Association. (2005b). Occupational Therapy Code of Ethics. *American Journal of Occupational Therapy, 59*, 639-642.

American Occupational Therapy Association. (2008). Occupational therapy practice framework: Domain and process, second edition. *American Journal of Occupational Therapy, 62*, 625-683.

Borkowski, N. (2005). *Organizational behavior in health care*. Sudbury, MA: Jones & Bartlett Publishers.

DeYoung, R. (2005). Behavioral theories of leadership. In N. Borkowski (Ed.), *Organizational behavior in health care* (pp. 173-185). Boston, MA: Jones and Bartlett.

Fiedler, F. E. (1967). *A theory of leadership effectiveness*. New York, NY: McGraw-Hill.

Fiedler, F. E. (1978). The contingency model and the dynamics of the leadership process. In L. Berkowitz (Ed.), *Advances in experimental psychology*. New York, NY: Academic Press.

George, J., & Jones, G. (2002). *Organizational behavior* (3rd ed.). Upper Saddle River, NJ: Prentice Hall.

Grady, A. (2003). From management to leadership. In G.H. McCormack, E. Jaffe, & M. Goodman-Levy (Eds.), *The occupational therapy manager* (4th ed., pp. 331-347). Bethesda, MD: AOTA Press.

Hamm, J. (2006).The five messages leaders must manage. *Harvard Business Review, 84*, 114-123.

Hersey, P., & Blanchard, K. (1982). *Management of organizational behavior: Utilizing human resources*. Upper Saddle River, NJ: Prentice Hall.

Jarman, J. (2004) What is occupation?: Interdisciplinary perspectives on defining and classifying human activity. In C. Christiansen & E. Townsend (Eds.), *Introduction to occupation: The art and science of living* (pp. 47-61). Upper Saddle River, NJ: Prentice Hall.

Kets de Vries, M. F. R. (2005). Leadership group coaching in action: The zen of creating high performance teams. *Academy of Management Executive, 19*, 61-76.

Kouzes, J., & Posner, B. (2002). *The leadership challenge* (3rd ed.). San Francisco, CA: Jossey-Bass.

Kouzes, J., & Posner, B. (2007). *The leadership challenge* (4th ed.). San Francisco, CA: John Wiley & Sons.

Kronenberg, F., & Pollard, N. (2006). Political dimensions of occupation and the roles of occupational therapy. *American Journal of Occupational Therapy, 60*(6), 617-625..

Kronenberg, F., Algado, S. S., & Pollard, N. (Eds.). (2005). *Occupational therapy without borders: Learning from the spirit of survivors*. Philadelphia, PA: Elsevier.

Law, M., Polatajko, H., Baptiste, S., & Townsend, E. (2002). In American Occupational Therapy Association. *Occupational therapy practice framework: Domain and process*. Bethesda, MD: AOTA Press.

McCormack, G. (2003). Historical and current perspectives of management. In G. H. McCormack, E. Jaffe, & M. Goodman-Levy (Eds.), *The occupational therapy manager* (4th ed., pp. 331-347). Bethesda, MD: AOTA Press.

McLagan, P., & Nell, C. (1995). *The age of participation—New governance for the workplace and the world*. San Francisco, CA: Barrett-Koehler.

Pearce, C. (2004). The future of leadership: Combining vertical and shared leadership to transform knowledge work. *Academy of Management Executive, 18*, 47-57.

Sadler-Smith, E., & Shefy, E. (2004). The intuitive executive: Understanding and applying "gut feel" in decision making. *Academy of Management Executive, 18*(4), 76-91.

Shortell, S., & Kaluzney, A. (2000). *Health care management: Organizational design and behavior*. Florence, KY: Delmar Cengage Learning.

Sinclair, K. (2006) Occupational therapy worldwide: WFOT. *Australian Occupational Therapy Journal, 53*, 49-150.

Spreier, S., Fontaine, M., & Malloy, R. (2006.) Leadership run amok: The destructive power of overachievers. *Harvard Business Review, 84*, 72-82.

Strzelecki, M. (2007). Leaders of the pack. *OT Practice, 12*(7), 16-19.

Townsend, E., & Whiteford, G. (2005) A participatory occupational justice framework. In F. Kronenberg, S. Algado, & N. Pollard (Eds.), *Occupational therapy without borders: Learning from the spirit of survivors* (pp. 110-125). London, England: Elsevier.

Townsend, E., & Wilcock, A. (2004). Occupational justice. In C. Christiansen & E. Townsend (Eds.), *Introduction to occupation: The art and science of living* (pp. 243-273). Upper Saddle River, NJ: Prentice Hall.

# Section VIII
## Research

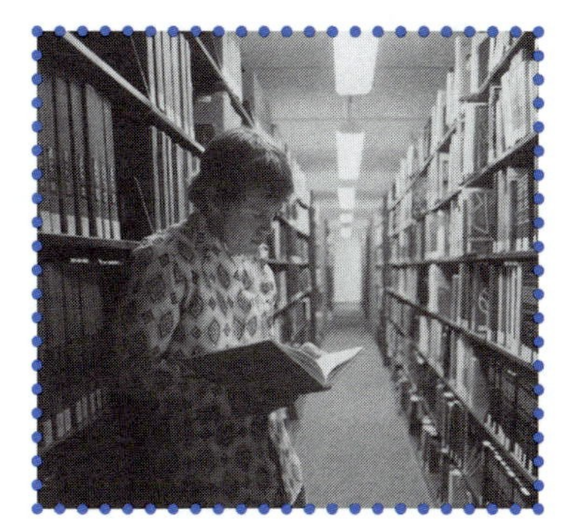

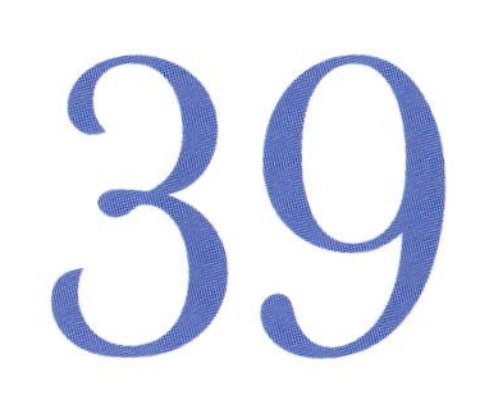

# 39 The Beginning Researcher

*Karen Sladyk, PhD, OTR/L, FAOTA*

**ACOTE Standards Explored in This Chapter**

B.8.1-8.9

**Key Terms**

| | |
|---|---|
| Effect size | Quantitative research |
| Probability | Reliability |
| Qualitative research | Validity |

## Importance of Research in Occupational Therapy

Sometimes new graduates are in such a hurry to start practicing occupational therapy that they focus only on client intervention. The standards for accreditation of both occupational therapy and occupational therapy assistant programs require colleges to teach beginning research skills, but students may not be interested. For an occupational therapy program, these skills include an appreciation for research, the components of research including statistics, the interpretation of studies related to occupational therapy, and the application of evidence to occupational therapy. Occupational therapy assistant programs are required to address the importance of research, the skills to use professional literature, and the role of the occupational therapy assistant in research, evaluation, and documentation. Despite the lack of specific research exam questions on the National Board for Certification in Occupational Therapy (NBCOT) exam, students will be more competent in practice skills with an understanding of research and will therefore be best practitioners.

New graduates may be overwhelmed with the research being published in the *American Journal of Occupational Therapy* (*AJOT*) or other research journals. It is easy to be afraid of too much information. Despite the fact that occupational therapy has several research publications and the American Occupational Therapy Foundation (AOTF) supports research, as a profession, we pale compared to our peers. Unfortunately, we are often ignored as a profession because of our lack of research, and other disciplines can use this to broaden their interests and encroach upon our domains of practice. Therefore, it is important for all occupational therapy assistants and occupational therapists to participate in research to further the profession of occupational therapy. Failure to do so could result in occupational therapy being left behind as a profession. The American Occupational Therapy Association (AOTA) (2006) feels so strongly about this issue that the Centennial Vision calls practitioners to action in growing our future. The Centennial Vision is the roadmap for the association's preparation for the profession's 100th birthday in 2017. Our leaders envision occupational therapy as a "powerful, widely recognized, science-driven, and evidence-based profession." Research is the key to this growth.



K. Sladyk, K. Jacobs, & N. MacRae (Eds.).
*Occupational Therapy Essentials for Clinical Competence* (pp. 423-432).

### Research Opportunities

Many practitioners feel they do not have the time in the clinic to conduct research, but the time can take as little as 5 minutes per day (Gillette, 1997). In a clinical setting, research design can evaluate if occupational therapy is effective by studying clients before and after occupational therapy intervention. The data used can be part of the documentation system, requiring no additional work until the data are collected at the end. Important data can be summarized and presented at a conference or in a publication. Practitioners can work in a group or share the responsibilities within an academic setting. Quality assurance plans, program evaluations, outcome reports, utilization data, and the current documentation system can all provide opportunities for research in occupational therapy. An appropriate beginning is writing a research protocol.

### Research Protocol

The protocol is written before the study begins and is designed to provide a road map for the soundness of the research. This protocol or proposal includes the following:

- Identification of the problem
- Review of literature of what other authors have found concerning this problem
- Identification of the sample to be studied
- Description of the method of selection
- Identification of the hypothesis to be tested with the dependent and independent variable
- Description of the procedure for intervention

### Research Results

The final presentation of the study can take several forms. If it is part of college work, your school will have specific criteria to follow. If your intention is publication, each journal has author's guides to shape your paper. In general, the results can be presented as the following:

- Introduction
- Problem statement
- Purpose and significance
- Literature review
- Research design and methods
- Results and interpretation
- References

## Role of the Occupational Therapy Assistant in Research

The occupational therapy assistant can actively participate in the design and data collection of a research protocol. Occupational therapy assistants with interests beyond their current skill should be supported to develop further skills under the direction of an occupational therapist or other research professional. Support might include assistance with understanding the meaning of statistical information in journal articles, understanding research vocabulary, or calculating effect size data from information included in older journal articles.

### Suggested Research Activities for an Occupational Therapy Assistant

- Evaluation of current admission and discharge scores on selected activities of daily living (ADL) evaluations
- Client satisfaction of intervention practices
- Evidence-based practice article review and summary
- Changes in health status pre- and post-occupational therapy intervention
- Use of occupational therapy modalities in changes in health status in clients
- Specific technique or adaptive equipment evaluation
- Chart reviews of critical incidences
- Issues related to the department's quality assurance goals

Supervision meetings between the occupational therapy assistant and occupational therapist can provide the opportunity to address research issues. Documenting this process in supervision notes helps meet accreditation and continuing education requirements. As research can be intimidating to those without formal training, supportive supervision techniques can help the occupational therapy assistant feel like part of the research team.

## Reading a Research Article

Research articles in peer-reviewed journals are considered one of the most reliable evidence available to a profession. A peer-reviewed process has readers reviewing the article for strengths without knowing the identity of the author. This blind review process of selection for publication helps assure only the best quality articles are published. Articles published on the Internet should be viewed with caution, as much of the posting on the Internet has not been professionally reviewed by respected peers. To assure the research is viable, the author will include complete details of the statistical analysis of the data. It is often the statistics that scare the reader and make the reader question their understanding. Some basic understanding of statistics makes reading the article more meaningful.

### Interpretation and Application of Research

Reading a research article is a challenge to a novice and may require the use of a research textbook to understand each quantitative detail. Of first importance is the significance of the results (Kranzler, 2007). Almost all studies report the significance, usually .05 or lower, when the results are significant. This means if the study were repeated 100 times, it would report different results less than 5 times.

The second important factor is the effect size. Effect size is fairly new in research and tells the magnitude of the results. Large effect sizes are best because the study not only found something significant, but it was a large result. An analogy: A researcher doing a study is like a fisherman going fishing. The significance score, the $p = .05$, tells you that if you cast your fishing pole 100 times, you likely will have a fish 95 times and a tire only 5 times. The effect size will tell you how big the fish is on the end of the line (a guppy or a whale).

Also important is information about the reliability and validity of the research or the tools/assessments used to measure the change reported in the research. Reliability looks at the accuracy and stability of the test. This score should be high. Validity asks about the ability to generalize the information to another population. This can be a challenge when the sample was small or very specific to a diagnosis.

Novice research readers may find that reading an article in a study group or journal club is helpful as others can help figure out difficult language. For further help in the study's interpretation and application, write the author of the study for additional information. The study's primary author's contact information is usually included on the paper.

# Types of Research

Depending on the focus of the textbook, you will find different disciplines categorize research in different ways. Below are different comparisons of types of research (Kielhofner, 2006; Leary, 2001; Royeen, 1997).

## Quantitative Versus Qualitative

Quantitative research involves numbers as the data source while qualitative involves words as the data source. Quantitative is more valued by evidence-based practice researchers, while qualitative research is valued by others for describing the richness of an experience. Quantitative research uses statistics to analyze and then interpret data. Qualitative data analyzes words for themes and patterns. Both data can use computer software for analysis of data.

## Basic Versus Applied

Basic research develops evidence to accumulate knowledge, but it often does not seek to answer a specific clinical question. Applied research has meaning that can be applied to functional use in real-world situations. Often, applied research develops from basic research as basic research provides foundational relationships.

# Categories of Research

Often, research types are described by the purpose of the research. The following are research types often seen in occupational therapy:

- *Correlational*: The focus of correlational research is to examine relationships between two factors such as ADL functioning and self-esteem. The research question is often posed as, "Is there a relationship between X and Y?" Although correlations show the strength of relationship such as smoking and lung cancer, readers should always assume that causation cannot be determined by a strong correlation. In the first example of ADL and self-esteem, one could argue that poor self-esteem causes poor ADL, and one could also argue that poor ADL cause poor self-esteem.
- *Descriptive*: The purpose of descriptive research is just that—to describe a situation. This may include quantitative measures such as mean, mode, median, range, or standard deviation (Table 39-1) but does not include statistical analysis. Descriptive research is very common but lacks the rigor of experimental or quasi-experimental research and is considered less valuable to the evidence-based practice researcher.
- *Evaluative*: Evaluative research evaluates the effectiveness of a program, service, intervention, or method. Typically, using both quantitative and qualitative methods, evaluative research seeks data to either develop new programs or summarize the effectiveness of current programs. Often, quality assurance or continuous quality improvement programs are evaluative in nature.
- *Experimental*: Using controlled, randomized research methods, experimental research is the closest to pure research available to occupational therapy. Highly valued by evidence-based practitioners, this research seeks to control error variance to maximize the findings of the research results. Internal and external validity are important in experimental research because controlling for problems increases the power of the results. Controlled groups of intervention and non-intervention, randomly assigned, increase the power of the findings.
- *Historical*: We can often learn from the study of our history. Historical research seeks to study past experiences to impact current behaviors. By studying trends and effects, researchers can predict present practices. The major challenge in historical research is the availability of reliable data, considered the "sample" in this type of research. The best sources of data are primary sources such as first-hand reports (e.g., diaries) over secondary sources (e.g., stories passed on from generation to generation).

| Table 39-1. Commonly Used Terms in Research | | |
|---|---|---|
| ABA design | Face validity | Pearson correlation coefficient |
| Abstract | Frequency | Pilot test |
| Analysis of variance (ANOVA) | Independent T-test | Post hoc tests |
| Annotated bibliography | Independent variable | Pretest sensitization |
| Cluster sampling | Internal validity | Psychometrics |
| Concurrent validity | Mean | Range |
| Confounding variable | Measures of central tendency | Sample |
| Construct validity | Measures of variability | Sampling error |
| Content analysis | Median | Standard deviation |
| Control group | Meta-analysis | Statistical significance |
| Convenient sample | Mode | T-test |
| Correlational coefficient | Multiple regression analysis | Test-retest reliability |
| Data | Naturalistic observation | Type I error |
| Dependent variable | Outlier | Type II error |
| Error variance | *p* value | Variability |
| External validity | Paired T-test | Variance |
| F-test | | |

*For definitions, please see the Glossary

- *Methodological*: The purpose of methodological research is to investigate the reliability and validity of materials developed in occupational therapy. Similar to evaluative research, methodological research can be used to investigate the strength of adaptive equipment, assessments, and intervention modalities. This research is common as a new occupational therapy assessment is developed and marketed. A significant contributor to occupational therapy research, methodological research is also valued by evidence-based practice researchers.
- *Naturalistic*: Sometimes called ethnographic research, naturalistic research seeks to study human behavior in its natural environment without the controls of an experimental design. The strength of naturalistic research lies in the fact that the environment is not manipulated. However, this research gives up control over confounding variables.
- *Quasi-experimental*: Quasi means "near." Quasi-experimental tries to use the pure design of experimental by controlling as many factors or variables as possible, but also to have the experiment be as "real world" as possible. By attempting to strike a balance between control and real life, the research acknowledges that some variables may interfere with the strength of the results. True randomization is often not done in this type of research since it may be unethical. For example, testing safety belts with real people assigned to a control group would put their lives at risk.
- *Single-subject research design (SSRD)*: Different from a case study done in hindsight and lacking rigor, a SSRD is a planned experimental designed with a sample of one. This type of research is very effective in studying rare conditions or when done as a cluster of samples. Baseline measurements are followed by intervention and another measurement. This process can continue over time with several measurements. In single-subject research, the research participants act as their own control.

# Language of Research

Often, the vocabulary of research and statistics is the most intimidating aspect of understanding research. Remember that all disciplines have their own language. For example, when you first started your occupational therapy studies, *ADL*, *range of motion* (ROM), and *MMT* did not make sense, but with time, the use of such language becomes comfortable. The same is true of research vocabulary. Once you use it, the language becomes natural. Table 39-1 includes some common terms seen in research articles. The definitions are intended to help develop an understanding of the concept, not to fully explain the term (Sladyk, 2003).

# American Psychological Association Format Summary

As a general rule, many professional occupational therapy papers or proposals follow "APA format." The American Psychological Association (APA) has developed a detailed format on writing papers. You can purchase the Publication Manual of the American Psychological Association (APA, 2009) at your local bookstore.

This summary includes the basics of APA format for occupational therapy. If the journal or conference committee requires full APA format, use the 350 plus-page APA publication manual for specifics. This summary will focus on the citations in the text and the reference page.

## In Text Citations

There are 3 ways to cite a reference in the body of the text. All 3 include the author's last name (surname) and the year of publication. First names are rarely included to remain gender free.

**Examples**

Christiansen (2007) discussed the role of occupational performance related to dysfunction.

In 2007, Christiansen discussed the role of occupational performance related to dysfunction.

The role of occupational performance was related to dysfunction (Christiansen, 2007).

If the information you are referencing is written by 2 authors, you must include both surnames. Notice how the word "and" or "&" is used.

**Examples**

Struther and Schell (1991) addressed the effect of public policy on performance.

In 1991, Struther and Schell discussed the effect of public policy on performance.

Public policy has had an effect on performance (Struther & Schell, 1991).

If the information you are referencing is written by 3, 4, or 5 authors, you must include all of the names the first time you cite them. After the first citation, use only the surname of the first author followed by "et al.". Notice that et al. has a period after al. In addition, pay attention to how commas are used. In APA format, a comma is always before the word "and" in text with 3 or more words, but not with 2.

**Examples**

Allen, Earhart, and Blue (2000) used a cognitive approach to psychosocial illness. Allen et al. believed this approach was helpful to understanding mental illness and functioning.

In 2000, Allen, Earhart, and Blue used a cognitive approach to psychosocial illness. Allen et al. believed this approach was helpful to understanding mental illness and functioning.

A cognitive approach to psychosocial illness was used (Allen, Earhart, & Blue, 2000). Allen et al. believed this approach was helpful to understanding mental illness and functioning.

Other unique citations in the text of the paper include:

- Group as the author: (American Occupational Therapy Association, 2006).
- Unknown author: (Anonymous, 2005).
- Same last name: (P. Smith & R. Smith, 2007).

## Reference Page Citations

The reference page has some rules. Center the word "reference" on top of the page, then use the following typing format:

- Do not indent the first line. Indent the second line and all other lines
- Type the author's surname followed by a comma. Example: Smith,
- Type first initial, period, space, then second initial, period, space. Example: Smith, H. J.
- Use an "&" to separate 2 or more names. Example: Smith, H. J., & Melling, B. S.
- Use a comma to separate several names. Example: Law, M., Baum, C. M., & Baptiste, S.
- Type the year in parenthesis followed by a period. Example: (2007).
- Type the title in lower case followed by a period. Example: Reliability of the BaFPE.
- If the title is a book, italicize. Example: *Elder care.*
- If the title is a journal article, do not underline. Example: Reliability of the BaFPE.
- If the title is a journal, type italicized journal name followed by a comma, the volume number, and a period. Example: *American Journal of Occupational Therapy, 49.*
- Only books and journal names are italic.
- If the title is a book, follow the title with the city of publication, comma, the state, colon, publisher, and period. Example: Thorofare, NJ: SLACK Incorporated.
- Use only official two-letter post office-approved state abbreviations. Both letters are capitalized and there are no spaces or periods in them, unlike first name initials, which have spaces.
- Finish the citation with page numbers if appropriate, followed by a period. Example: 763.

**Example**

Law, M., Baum, C. M., & Baptiste, S. (2005). *Occupation-based practice: Fostering performance and participation.* Thorofare, NJ: SLACK Incorporated.

- Alphabetize the names, letter by letter.

**Examples**

American Occupational Therapy Association. (2002). *Occupational therapy practice framework*. Bethesda, MD: Author.

Burke, J. P., & DePoy, E. (1991). An emerging view of mastery, excellence, and leadership in occupational therapy practice. *American Journal of Occupational Therapy, 45*, 1027-1032.

Christiansen, C., & Baum, C. (Eds.). (2003). *Occupational therapy: Enabling function and well being*. Thorofare, NJ: SLACK Incorporated.

- If several works are by the same person, arrange oldest first.

**Examples**

Fleming, M. (1989). The therapist with the three-track mind. In American Occupational Therapy Association. *AOTA Practice Symposium*. Bethesda, MD: Author.

Fleming, M. (1991). Clinical reasoning in medicine compared with clinical reasoning in occupational therapy. *American Journal of Occupational Therapy, 45*, 988-996.

- Use lowercase letters to separate same author, same year works.

**Examples**

Fleming, M. (1991a). Clinical reasoning in medicine compared with clinical reasoning in occupational therapy. *American Journal of Occupational Therapy, 45*, 988-996.

Fleming, M. (1991b). The therapist with the three-track mind. *American Journal of Occupational Therapy, 45*, 1007-1014.

- Put one-author works before multiple authors.

**Examples**

Crepeau, E. B. (1991). Achieving intersubjective understanding: Examples from an occupational therapy session. *American Journal of Occupational Therapy, 45*, 1016-1025.

Crepeau, E. B., & Leguard, T. (1991). *Self paced instruction for clinical education and supervision*. Bethesda, MD: AOTA Press.

There are a few other helpful tips for writing an occupational therapy paper using APA format. Generally, headings for each section are in uppercase letters centered across the line. In most cases, do not use abbreviations. Write out the whole word. Try to remain gender bias-free in your writing by using only the author's last name. When citing an Internet site, use the complete Web address.

Important information: Just because a student has cited a source does not mean it cannot be plagiarized. Copying text word for word with a cite but without quotes is not acceptable.

Information adapted from Sladyk, K. (1997). *OT student primer: A guide to college success*. Thorofare, NJ: SLACK Incorporated.

# Evidence-Based Practice

An evidence-based practice is when a practitioner reviews research on a specific topic, synthesizes the research meaning, and applies the research meaning to a specific individual or group (Law, 2002). Evidence-based practice has faced challenges in being integrated into current occupational therapy practice because occupational therapy practitioners tend to be more hands-on in their intervention approach selections (Holm, 2000, 2001). Evidenced-based practice can be supportive of the profession's basic foundations by reinforcing the value of meaningful occupation.

Changes in health care at both the governmental and insurance provider levels have demanded that all health care providers provide care in the most effective and efficient manner. This does not necessarily mean cookie-cutter approaches, but it does mean the practitioner provides services based on the evidence available in the literature.

To evaluate the literature, the reader must be able to know what is good research and what is less valued. The experts in evidence-based practice have put several systems of ranking the value of evidence. A current project at the AOTA (Lieberman, Arbesman, & Scheer, 2006) uses four levels to rank the literature that focuses on quantitative research using random controlled trials as the highest level (level 1). SSRD over time is the lowest ranked level and is assigned level 4. Case studies, narrative, and qualitative research are not ranked. The AOTA system is typical and valued in the scientific community. Other systems are similar but may contain an additional level that provides greater diversity in the types of research accepted as evidence. However, the focus in evidence-based practice is always on solid research designs that control for a maximum amount of variance. The focus on quantitative research and the lack of acceptance of qualitative research is typical in evidence-based practice, although debated by some. Qualitative research may not have statistical analysis, but it often contains rich details not available in quantitative data and is gaining more acceptance in the profession.

A practitioner reviewing the evidence needs skills in searching for, evaluating, applying, and communicating the evidence to the individual. Tips for the management of these stages follow.

## Searching for the Evidence

Choose one library with electronic searching resources to begin searching.

Form a relationship with the library staff and explain your long-term plans.

Use a standard outline for reviewing all articles such as the following:

Citation:

Level of research:

( ) Meta analysis or complete review of several well-designed studies

( ) Well-designed randomized controlled trial

( ) Well-designed non randomized trial

( ) Nonexperimental studies, descriptive evidence

( ) Other: Opinions of individual experts or panels, qualitative reports

Purpose of the study or the research question(s):

Sample characteristics:

Interventions:

Independent variable(s) (what is being manipulated):

Dependent variable(s) (what is being measured):

Results and significance:

## Evaluating the Research

Review research vocabulary, techniques, and textbooks for novice researchers.

## Apply the Research to Individuals

Evaluate similarities and differences between and among the research participants with your current clients.

Evaluate similarities and differences between the intervention methods and the needs of your current clients.

## Communicate the Research With Your Clients

Use good communication skills. Communicate effectively in volume and pace for the client. Begin the communication at the consumer's current level of understanding. Empower the client to be the leader of his or her intervention by helping to analyze the research meaning from his perspective.

## Case Study on Evidence-Based Practice

Using the case "Maddy" in Chapter 40, the occupational therapists asks the evidence-based practice question, "What does the literature say is helpful for reassuring a frightened client about her future when she is in inpatient intervention and not in her familiar home? In addition, what is the best assessment for discharge discussion making?"

As the occupational therapist is a member of AOTA, she has access to the evidence-based practice (EBP) resources of the Association and begins there. After signing in online, the occupational therapist begins in the practice section of the Web site. She begins first with the reviews on how to do an EBP review as a refresher, and then looks at the Critically Appraised Topics (CAT). She is excited to find information she needs in this area as well as suggestions for further research.

The occupational therapist then signs onto the hospital library online and does an initial search on ERIC and CINEAL. The initial hits of over 10,000 overwhelm her. The occupational therapist then sees the importance of making a specific clinical question and narrows her search to "memory strategies for confused client" and "independent living discharge assessment." These searches result in specific recommendations of a memory book and the Kohlman Evaluation of Living Skills (KELS). The occupational therapist, knowing the client's reading level and eye sight challenges, adapts the memory book to a large, high contrast poster that hangs in the client's room. For the KELS, the occupational therapist uses the client's home as the site of the assessment, and the client scores high enough that the occupational therapist is confident she can live independently without assistance. This makes Maddy happy.

## Recommended Beginning Readings in Evidence-Based Practice

Holms, M. B. (2000). Our mandate for the new millennium: Evidence-based practice, 2000 Eleanor Clarke Slagle lecture. *American Journal of Occupational Therapy, 54*, 574-585.

Holm, M. B. (2001). Our mandate for the new millennium: Evidence-based practice (AOTA Continuing education article). *OT Practice, July*, CE1-CE13.

Law, M. (2002). *Evidence-based rehabilitation: A guide to practice.* Thorofare, NJ: SLACK Incorporated.

## Living the Life of a Researcher

Making research an integrated aspect of your professional life is not difficult. If you are committed to your profession and your professionalism, then you are automatically committed to being a research consumer and practitioner. Consider the following suggestions:

- Use research in your practice. Make a commitment to be an evidence-based practitioner.
- Develop a research portfolio/file on topics of interest. Copy and file articles of interest in folders. Maintain an annotated bibliography on the outside of the

folder or attached to the article. After graduation, arrange notes and handouts by topics. Avoid storing articles in notebooks as they are space limited. A filing cabinet or plastic filing container has flexible space to allow your collection to grow.

- Join or form a journal club. Each member of the club agrees to read an article and summarize the topic for the club members. Schedule regular meetings. The added benefit of networking will strengthen your practice.
- Participate in peer review at your facility or volunteer to do peer review at another agency. Welcome peer review of your own work instead of being guarded. In addition, journals are often looking for expert peer reviewers. National and state associations are looking for peer reviewers for conference papers.
- Refresh your research skills from time to time by reviewing school notes or textbooks. Attend local conferences on research skills or ask your local occupational therapy programs to offer a research conference for beginners. Take another research class.
- Write for publication. Begin with simple tasks such as letters to the editor, commentaries about an issue of concern, or a program description for the state occupational therapy newsletter. Consider doing basic comparisons of pre- and post-admission data from your facility. This outcome research can be accepted in many different journals.
- Conduct a SSRD study. Partner with other therapists who treat the same disability and each do SSRD on one client. Write the results as a group.
- Be on the lookout for unusual groups of participants or data. For example, hobby or social groups you participate in, such as church or clubs, may provide convenient samples and unusual events such as town celebrations or weather events that may provide interesting data.
- Develop an assessment or piece of equipment for clinical use. Evaluate the effectiveness using a rigorous approach.
- Investigate concurrent validity of two assessments or adapt an existing instrument to a different population. Evaluate the effectiveness.
- Replicate a study in your clinical setting or with different populations.
- Team with faculty from a local research university to participate in a funded grant research project.
- When ready, write a grant to apply for funding yourself from a local/regional agency or foundation.

Living the life of a researcher is not an all-or-nothing choice. Practitioners involved in research, as well as service provision, will find their practice enriched with research projects. Informed practice is the ultimate practice for the therapist and the client.

# Grant Writing

A review of current occupational therapy textbooks found very little reference to grant writing in any index. Grant writing is not a difficult task but, like research, it often scares students and practitioners. The key to successful grant writing is planning and a mixture of management and research skills (Kielhofner, 2006).

One of the most serious problems faced by occupational therapists in grant writing is "jumping" into the activity planning section before laying the grant foundation. The second most common problem is not following the rules of the grant program. Almost every grant-funding agency will have some type of training available. If these are conference style, go to the meetings as much as possible as the meetings are strong networking opportunities.

Planning process for grant writing includes the following:

- *Foundation*: Begin with your program's underlying purpose, mission, philosophy, and goals as the foundation of the grant.
- *Objectives*: Ask yourself several questions. What are the measurable goals of the program? How can the grant support your objectives? At the end of the grant, what evidence will you be able to provide the funders to show that your program worked?
- *Needs assessment to justify program*: Too many times grants are developed without an evaluation of the needs of the program. What good is a grant without a solid need for the program? Use multiple sources for the needs assessment, including key informants, research, and surveys.
- *Program development*: The fourth step can be the most fun. Too often people who write grants start here and ignore the first three steps. What will make your program different and more effective?
- *Policies and procedures*: Help to control the effects of the grant like internal validity helps control error variance in research.
- *Operational goals and evaluation system*: Now that you have the grant money, how do you know it works?

## Tips for Grant Writing

- Start small—several student grants are out there for research.
- Try often because most grant writers submit many grants before they are successfully funded.
- Team up with a researcher who has been funded.
- Put unfunded attempts on your résumé until you get a funded grant, then drop the inclusion of unfunded grants.

Many student service organizations offer grants for small projects. For example, Rotary Club often funds local projects. Check these when you are doing your graduate work. Use their procedures when writing your grant. If a specific format is not provided, a modified version of your research paper can be a guide for your grant application.

- *Introduction*: Very short and to the point
- *Problem statement*: Why this is a problem and how funding will help
- *Shorten literature review*: What has been done already (aim for no more than two pages)
- *Program goal and plan of action*
- *Program evaluation*: The three program parts are like the method and result sections

See Appendix G for a sample of a grant proposal.

## Summary

Research skills are essential to good practice and professional development. Research and grant writing skills enhance the quality of client care and provide a solid foundation to our profession. Mastery of research language and reading evidence will lead to an effective practice, better client intervention, and a fulfilling lifetime career in occupational therapy.

## Student Self-Assessment

1. Make flash cards of research vocabulary for studying.
2. Proofread peer articles for APA errors; cite and quote as needed.
3. Volunteer 1 hour per week in your academic support department to assist other students writing research papers.
4. Scan the library shelves for journals unrelated to occupational therapy to see what topics the journal covers that might be converted to an occupational therapy topic. For example, an art journal may address the art of a specific culture. How does this art provide meaning and occupation to its people?

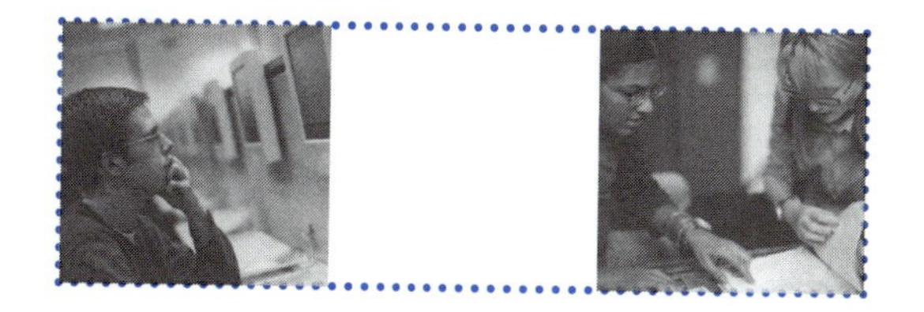

## References

American Occupational Therapy Association. (2006). *AOTA's Centennial Vision*. Bethesda, MD: Author.

American Psychological Association. (2009). *Publication manual of the American Psychological Association* (6th ed.). Washington, DC: Author.

Gillette, N. (1997). *Academic faculty supporting problem-based learning*. American Ocupational Therapy Foundation Conference in Newark, NJ.

Holms, M. B. (2000). Our mandate for the new millennium: Evidence-based practice, 2000 Eleanor Clarke Slagle lecture. *American Journal of Occupational Therapy, 54*, 574-585.

Holms, M. B. (2001). Our mandate for the new millennium: Evidence-based practice (AOTA Continuing education article). *OT Practice, July*, CE1-CE13.

Kielhofner, G. (2006). *Research in occupational therapy*. Philadelphia, PA: F.A. Davis.

Kranzler, J. H. (2007). *Statistics for the terrified*. Upper Saddle River, NJ: Prentice Hall.

Law, M. (2002). *Evidence-based rehabilitation: A guide to practice*. Thorofare, NJ: SLACK Incorporated.

Leary, M. R. (2001). *Introduction to behavioral research methods*. Boston, MA: Allyn and Bacon.

Lieberman, D., Arbesman, M., & Scheer, J. (2006). *Utilizing AOTA's evidence-based practice products and resources*. Presentation at AOTA Annual Conference, Charlotte, NC. April 26, 2006.

Royeen, C. B. (1997). *A research primer in occupational and physical therapy*. Bethesda, MD: AOTA Press.

Sladyk, K. (1997). *OT student primer: A guide to college success*. Thorofare, NJ: SLACK Incorporated.

Sladyk, K. (2003). *OT study cards in a box*. Thorofare, NJ: SLACK Incorporated.

# Section IX
## Professional Ethics, Values, and Responsibilities

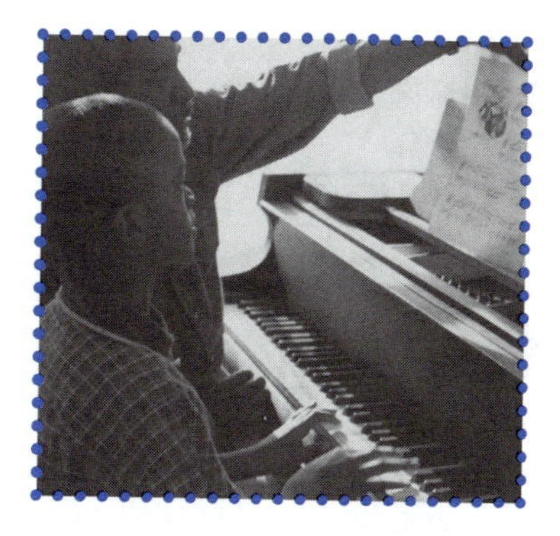

# 40

# Ethics and Its Application

*Gail M. Bloom, OTD, MA, OTR/L*

**ACOTE Standards Explored in This Chapter**

B.7.3-7.4, 9.1, 9.5, 9.10-9.11

**Key Terms**

Ethics
Judgment
Morality
Values

## Introduction

Occupational therapy and the study of ethics share common ground because both are concerned with meaningful choices for the individual. The practice of occupational therapy is established upon an emphasis on autonomy and occupation that is meaningful to the individual. Occupational therapy has a long tradition of caring about morality-based social values. Occupational therapy professional values are linked to the promotion of maximum independence by adapting the environment and/or enhancing functional ability fundamental to promoting quality of life. Central to the practice of occupational therapy is a commitment to quality-of-life issues.

The ethical decision-making process and the clinical problem-solving approach of occupational therapy both rely on a process for function-based analysis. The process involves the identification of the principles specific to the particular case situation, contemplation, negotiation, and reaching a resolution. Ethical decision making is, of necessity, woven among the threads of clinical decision making.

Ethical decision making is about the process. Ethical action is the product of ethical decision making. Ethical decision making is a mandatory component of clinical problem solving. Critical thinking requires carefully weighing alternatives. Deliberate analysis is a part of problem solving. The conceptual understanding of ethics is critical to decoding the complexity of specific situations. The occupational therapist practitioner should take all case-specific factors into consideration prior to making a reasoned decision. An understanding of ethics can assist in sorting out complicated health and social issues. Ethical reasoning is a part of clinical decision making. Daily clinical issues provide opportunity for the direct application of ethics in everyday practice.

The same ingredients can be useful for ethical problem solving in clinical, corporate, and academic settings. Perhaps the secret recipe is seeking a balance of theoretical knowledge, science-based evidence, and practical application—well seasoned with humanistic empathy and caring.

"All I really need to know about how to live and what to do and how to be I learned in kindergarten," wrote Robert Fulghum, with his rules for everyday living (1988).

"Share everything.
Play fair.
Don't hit people.
Put things back where you found them.
Clean up your own mess.
Don't take things that aren't yours.
Say you're sorry when you hurt somebody.



K. Sladyk, K. Jacobs, & N. MacRae (Eds.).
*Occupational Therapy Essentials for Clinical Competence* (pp. 435-450).

Wash your hands before you eat.

Flush.

Warm cookies and cold milk are good for you.

Live a balanced life—learn some and think some and draw and paint and sing and dance and play and work every day some.

Take a nap every afternoon.

When you go out into the world, watch out for traffic, hold hands, and stick together.

Be aware of wonder. Remember the little seed in the Styrofoam cup: The roots go down and the plant goes up and nobody really knows how or why, but we are all like that.

Goldfish and hamsters and white mice and even the little seed in the Styrofoam cup—they all die. So do we.

Remember the Dick-and-Jane books and the first word you learned—the biggest word of all—LOOK.

Everything you need to know is in there somewhere: the Golden Rule, love, basic sanitation, ecology, politics, equality, and sane living" (From *All I Really Need to Know I Learned in Kindergarten* by Robert L. Fulghum, copyright © 1986, 1988 by Robert L. Fulghum. Used by permission of Villard Books, a division of Random House, Inc.).

It is tempting to stop there. Everything the occupational therapy practitioner needs to know about ethics is in Fulghum's Credo.

Altruism is another way to express the importance of sharing; and "holding hands and sticking together" reflects an obligation to community. Equality and justice are based on fairness. Act with goodwill, show compassion, and treat others with integrity and respect, or in other words, beneficence. Do not cause harm and do not hurt anyone. Know the rules and follow them. In the rapidly changing health care environment, the occupational therapy practitioner is confronted with complex ethical issues. As a professional, the occupational therapy practitioner must take responsibility for understanding applicable policies, federal and state laws, and association principles. The occupational therapy practitioner must maintain high standards of professional competence mandating an understanding of ethics.

In the interest of adding comprehensive knowledge, we will continue with a fuller exploration of ethics. The moral aspects of practice require professionalism. Professional competencies include knowing how to obtain informed consent, knowing what to do if a client refuses intervention, and knowing how to communicate confidential material. An understanding of ethics will help the occupational therapy practitioner know how to cope with quality-of-life issues and quality of care problems. Development of skills will assist the occupational therapy practitioner make ethical decisions for moral behavior.

We will begin by establishing a foundation of understanding through an examination of some basic ethical concepts. We will look at the structure of societal groups and organizations as the structural hallmarks or characteristic building blocks toward the implementation of ethical principles. We will show how everyday practice provides opportunity for the direct application of ethics.

## A Foundation of Understanding

The practical application of knowledge is as fundamental to the study of ethics as it is to the practice of occupational therapy. A study of ethics examines how an individual thinks and behaves toward others. Philosophers place an emphasis on concepts like fairness, equality, goodness, justice, consequence, and obligation. These traditional moral concepts provide a foundation to create a practical, function-based approach to ethics.

The honorable occupational therapy practitioner must have self-awareness. There is an obligation to examine one's own personal values and belief system with recognition and insight of oneself as a moral agent. Concepts of right and wrong can be gathered from a variety of sources. Morality is the accepted standard of right or wrong that directs the conduct of a person or a group. Morality is learned early. The social environment is filled with influences, including family, schools, religion, and the media. Adherence to ethical principles will influence choices. For example, a choice to participate in an activity could be influenced by ethical rules learned in school or, conversely, avoidance of a particular activity might be influenced by moral rules learned as a child in the home. Essentially, ethics are a set of value-based principles to assist the individual in making moral decisions.

A basic rule of conduct is known as an ethical principle. A principle that sets a standard of quality or a worthwhile ideal is a value. Most people consider certain values such as caring, honesty, and respect to be morally worthy. Tradition and custom have assigned worth to certain actions. There is an obligation to consider the consequences of one's actions. The moral individual must focus on the questioning that results in decision making. The moral occupational therapy practitioner must focus on the case-specific human factors to employ a process of clinical reasoning resulting in ethical decision making. A decision is a thoughtful judgment resulting in the production of action. Judgment is the act of deciding after considering alternatives. The organization of ethical principles into an orderly system of beliefs can assist the individual in determining rightness, morality, and praiseworthy behavior from wrongness, immorality, and blameworthy behavior. Ethics is the study of right and wrong conduct as determined by means of a reasonable thought process.

## Theories of Fundamental Characteristics

There are some philosophical schools of thought that accept belief systems based on basic rules. This type of deontological theory of reasoning relies on an acceptance of universal laws or accepted truths. The fundamental principles of morality are examined for guidance to determine the best plan of action. An action is judged either "good" or "bad" because of the intrinsic nature of the action to be good or bad. There is an objective understanding of what is accepted as good or bad. There is an obligation for action or inaction simply because some deeds are praiseworthy or blameworthy. Action is either right or wrong. One is obligated to a course of action that promotes goodness. There is an explicit call to duty.

Awareness of moral standards is necessary in order to choose in accordance with inherent moral guides. The correct course of action can be determined by applying the appropriate obligatory rule to the situation.

Rules based on universal imperatives include "natural order" and the Golden Rule. Goodness or worth does not change with the circumstances of a specific situation. For example, consider the concept of "fairness." In order to be "fair," all decisions must be based on the acceptance of a rule to treat all persons in an equitable, impartial way independent of any particular circumstances those persons might be facing. A standard of "justice" will not tolerate unfair discrimination because ethical action requires a duty to be fair and equitable, or it is "unjust" by definition. Therefore, fairness does not change with the circumstances of a specific situation.

## Theories of Comparative Characteristics

There are many philosophical schools of thought without an acceptance of a belief system based on fundamental universal rules and they oppose a reliance on objective principles. These moral systems demand a comparative evaluation of the particular unique circumstances of a specific situation for guidance. These thinkers ask if any rule can be valid for every possible application. Black or white thinking is avoided with an exploration of all the gradations of gray.

Theories of teleological ethics apply a methodical process of reasoning to assess the subjective nature of goodness and badness. Focus is placed on defining what is meant by "good" and determining which action will result in the most good. Additionally, "bad" is defined and thought is given to determining which action will result in the most harm. There is a duty to weigh the benefits and costs of any potential action. It is assumed that some options will be more beneficial than others, while other actions are more likely to produce more harm. An action is worthwhile if the resulting consequences are valued with more good consequences than bad consequences.

A justification for action or inaction is derived from a review of options. Predictions are made to determine relative benefits (or utility). Ethical dilemma occurs with the acknowledgment that undesirable choices may lead to less-than-ideal alternatives. There is awareness of a need to choose between the lesser of unappealing options.

Moral worth is determined by the social consequences of an action in a community. This approach to ethics requires careful weighing of all of the social benefits and costs of an action and choosing whichever action maximizes good relative to harm.

Utilitarian reasoning is one type of teleological approach. Actions have multiple consequences and consequences are compared. Utilitarian thinking compares benefits and costs with an emphasis on utility, something that provides a useful purpose. Decision making using utilitarian reasoning will opt for the choice that promotes the greatest good for the greatest number of people.

Examination of the consequences of an action to determine if its outcome is primarily good or bad is one method to decide on a course of action. The goals (or ends) are evaluated. Quite literally, "the ends justify the means" is founded in this line of reasoning.

Another type of ethical reasoning examines the process rather than the final goal. In this almost mathematical approach, either a quantitative or a qualitative value is assigned to situational variables. Resolution of an ethical dilemma is based on the assumption that moral value can be determined during the decision-making process with the creation of a list, the counting of the pros and cons, or the categorization of the arguments for and against an action. Analysis following a separation of the whole into its elemental parts can reveal the goodness and badness of each component variable.

An occupational therapy intervention decision can be viewed as an ethical decision when one thinks about factors such as the allocation of scarce resources. Time is often a scarce resource in a clinic. Consider the ethical dilemma presented if an occupational therapy practitioner devotes time to fabricate a splint for one client, and then without sufficient time in the workday several other clients will not be seen that day. Let us solve the problem using a quantitative analysis. The action (splinting) is assessed to have two good components (pro) and five bad components (con) in our example dilemma. The larger amount of situational variables on the con side of the equation necessitates a suggested ethical resolution to avoid the action in consideration. The quantitative process for decision making can be illustrated with a simple chart (Table 40-1).

Our dilemma can be resolved with a different type of method. Rather than a quantitative analysis, we will see that switching to a qualitative analysis might obtain a very different result. A quality rating is used to indicate relative benefit. The comparative numerical weight indicates whether an action should be pursued. Our situational variables are assessed on a 10-point maximum quality rating scale for each factor. The qualitative numerical equation with a total of 19 favorable (pro) points compared to a total of 13 against (con) points indicates more benefit if the action (splinting) is pursued. The larger value assigned to the situational variables on the pro side of the equation obligates us to pursue the action in consideration. Again, the qualitative process for decision making can be illustrated with a simple chart (Table 40-2).

**Table 40-1. Quantitative Process for Ethical Decision Making**

| Action | Pro | Con |
|---|---|---|
| Splint | • Avoid contractures<br>• Maintain skin integrity | • Amount of fabrication time<br>• Several clients will not get therapy<br>• Cost of material<br>• On/off assistance needed<br>• Cleaning assistance needed |

**Table 40-2. Qualitative Process for Ethical Decision Making**

| Action | Pro | Quality Value | Con | Quality Value |
|---|---|---|---|---|
| Splint | • Avoid contractures<br>• Maintain skin integrity | 10<br>9 | • Amount of fabrication time<br>• Several clients will not get therapy<br>• Cost of material<br>• On/off assistance needed<br>• Cleaning assistance needed | 4<br>5<br>2<br>1<br>1 |
| Total value | | 19 | | 13 |

## Theories of Relative Standards

Another philosophical school of thought asks if any rule can be valid for all people all the time. Ethical relativism is formed around the assumption that rules to guide behavior should change relative to time and place. Principles are expected to change over the course of time. Morality does not remain static but changes according to the accepted standards of a specific society at a specific point in time. Actions regarded as praiseworthy or blameworthy may be different within various cultures, religions, and other segments of society. Some cultures accept certain practices as acceptable, while other cultures condemn the same type of action. Morality does not come with a set of absolute rules everyone follows automatically. Values can differ because judgments of praiseworthy and blameworthy actions are a function of the social order.

The circumstances of history have instances of certain actions socially acceptable in their time but judged immoral from our perspective looking back in time. This type of reasoning can lead to incendiary debates such as, "Was child labor a rational socioeconomic product of its time?" Historical perspective can stimulate dialogue on the appropriateness of the massive legislative and institutional changes leading to the deinstitutionalization and community integration efforts of persons with mental illness during the 1970s and 1980s. Well-intentioned people can disagree as to what is right or wrong. For example, there are societal and cultural differences when judging the moral acceptability of euthanasia, abortion, or numerous other topics of controversy. There is no easy determination of good behaviors.

One view toward ethical decision making advocates a neutral position or having no judgment about anything. Ironically, this requires a judgmental decision. Saying "I don't want to judge" is a judgment. A course of action or inaction will result even without an acknowledgment of moral beliefs. Ethics obligates one to judge.

## Making a Distinction Between Ethical and Legal

It is important to note that legal and ethical considerations are not necessarily the same. There are historical examples of legislation with unintended ramifications resulting in major unexpected ethical problems. There are examples of legal action that does not seem ethical. Choices can be legally acceptable but not ethically appropriate. Widespread commercial advertising promoting cheaply made toys to children is legal but not necessarily ethical in motivation. Conversely, illegal activity can be morally defensible. The story of Robin Hood robbing the rich to give to the poor is a classic example of an illegal action that can be defended as ethically acceptable. Of course, there are instances when illegal and unethical are the same. Unequal pay based on gender discrimination is both against the law and unethical.

Federal, state, and municipal governments have the power to pass legislation and implement regulations. The forces of government have jurisdiction within their own borders. Each monitors for compliance and develops methods of enforcement. Consequences for noncompliance include a wide variety of sanctions, penalties for infractions handed down in the form of fines, or prison time. Compliance based merely on rule recognition rather than an internalized system of values has a focus on the threat of detection and punishment. Drivers who do not obey posted speed limits on interstate highways but slow down in the presence of a marked police vehicle demonstrate this observable truth.

A number of laws differ from state to state. State licensure laws for guiding the practice of occupational therapy practitioners are somewhat different from state to state. Some state laws are intended to protect the rights of persons in need of special protection such as minors (age of maturity will vary) and other categories of persons deemed most at risk.

Both medical law and medical ethics (bioethics) are in dynamic change. New legislation and the latest court decisions create a need for up-to-date interpretation of law. Federal and state judicial systems consider and then rule on court cases creating revised interpretation of Constitutional rights or other laws. On occasion, the rights of the individual will conflict with the rights of society. For example, courts have decided that society has an obligation to protect life, and courts have ordered life-saving medical intervention for young persons with parents who refuse intervention. Legal concerns and ethical issues often overlap in the delivery of health care. Courts analyze specific questions and make an official ruling based on the particular situation presented in the case. Precedent is set with interpretation of influential cases and subsequent generalization to similar situations. Past dilemmas offer guidance for handling current dilemmas.

## The Structural Hallmarks: Groups, Organizations, and Resource Distribution

Medical ethics can be a hodgepodge of incompatible values. Medical ethical dilemmas reflect the moral conflicts in society. Proponents and opponents can logically and passionately argue contradictory viewpoints on life and death issues.

Social policy often cannot keep pace with scientific discoveries and demographic change. Funding initiatives fluctuate depending on external macro-environmental conditions and shifting environmental priorities. For example, innovations in biotechnology (i.e., new medications, experimental testing), civil emergencies due to the threat of terrorism or epidemic (i.e., tuberculosis, polio, influenza, measles), and weather-related disasters (i.e., hurricanes, floods) have had an impact on the amount of dollars available for public health programs as well as the types of health services funded. The overburdened health care system struggles with limited resources and rising expenses. In many places, "business as usual" means doing more with less. The perception of danger or crisis could legitimize organizational behavior the larger society would judge as unethical. Price controls have resulted in some agencies padding allowable expenses by ordering authorized but unnecessary procedures after changes to third-party reimbursement guidelines. An organization's values may be compromised or abandoned when threatening external forces influence decisions to conduct business outside of the accepted values and standards of society. There is a temptation to increase profits while decreasing quality of service. Some facilities unable to recruit skilled professionals have been known to hire untrained workers to fill the gaps for skilled therapeutic services due to staffing shortages. Advances in medical technology influence change in medical ethics. Technology now lets us do the unimaginable. In the old days, when your heart or breathing stopped, you were dead. Technological advances have led to new possibilities. Clients, family members, and health care professionals have to sort through complex issues as they make important bioethical decisions for themselves, for loved ones, or for recipients of services.

Ultimately, decisions are always made. At least in part, medical decisions are based on somebody's value judgment. The values that guide behavior in society at large are the basic standards used to make decisions in medical ethics. Generally accepted social principles form the philosophical foundation for medical ethics. If fairness is an esteemed value in society as a whole, then fairness will also be an important factor for the resolution of medical ethical dilemmas. If compassion is an important social value, then empathy and caring will guide medical ethical decision making. A process of moral decline can be halted. Praiseworthy efforts can create solutions. "Superior quality" is a value judgment with an expectation for excellence.

Public policy establishes social infrastructure. Essential commodities such as housing, food, water, and education are considered basic rights in modern society. The quality and methods of distribution of fundamental commodities vary widely. It should be noted that health care access and service allotment are not always defined as a basic right. At this time in history, society does not grant equal access to health care services or equality to service delivery. For example, certain parts of the population have limited access to health care due to financial limitations or geographic location.

The moral agents expected to provide the structure for health care benefits and services are governments, business, and philanthropic organizations. Value-based concepts such as dignity and respect can provide a health care facility with a foundation for service delivery. Organizations in the business of health care service delivery are expected to provide quality services in an equitable way. As a society, we expect a health care business to conduct operations in a manner that creates some good, has social responsibility, and does not harm the greater community.

How do decisions about health care cost, program access, and service quality get made and who should make them? Who is covered? What is covered? Who pays for it? How much is paid? An ethical society must strive to create a fair system because of a social obligation to maximize justice and equitable consequences. There must be an attempt to form a balance of more good over less harm. Equitable distribution refers to the moral concept of justice; benefits should be distributed in fair proportions. How is "fair" determined? Course of action is planned after weighing the competing interests in terms of the benefits and costs to all stakeholders including the client, facility, insurers, advocacy groups, lawyers, legislators, and society as a whole. Access to health care is determined by public policy. Some provisions have been made for some segments of the population. As an example, changes in Medicare can modify service access as well as amend programmatic costs. Medicare reimburses costs of approved services for eligible enrollees; however, not all services are covered as Medicare reimbursable expenses, and Medicare eligibility guidelines must be met for program participation.

Ethical issues focus on questions of entitlement (who can get service), access (which types of services are covered), and allotment (how many visits). Like other economic-based commodities, our present society has decided that health care is not a right or entitlement—some would say that health care is rationed. Many wonder if health care can be rationed effectively or efficiently. Whether health care is rationed fairly is a question dependent on ethical judgment. Universal health care coverage has been the source of fierce political debates.

One approach for allocation of health care resources through rationing is managed care. The system of managed care was intended to structure cost-effective practices, an attempt to encourage efficiency by increasing productivity while simultaneously limiting costs. Almost all health care insurers have limits placed on types and amounts of health care services. Managed care program enrollees have limits placed on types and amounts of health care services with restricted access for services provided outside of the managed care network. A criticism of managed care is that it limits choice. For example, a client might be required to assume out-of-pocket, private payment costs for choosing occupational therapy services if occupational therapy is not provided at the in-network facility.

The passage of time has brought changes and will continue to bring changes to the provision of health care in America. Incremental changes will provide models of health care reform providing lessons for what to do and what not to do. Successes will be replicated and deficiencies will be improved. As Americans searched for a fair and affordable system of health care delivery, some states crafted creative solutions toward providing increased health care services. Oregon is an example of taking a step toward health care reform by developing an innovative managed care structure designed to provide greater health care prevention and service access. Oregon was confronted with problems shared by all states throughout the United States with large numbers of the population either uninsured or underinsured and Medicaid budgets expanding (Medicaid is an entitlement program regulated by the federal and state governments to provide health care for persons with low income). The Oregon Health Plan established a prioritized list of health services providing payment for a coordinated health network inclusive of "Healthy Living" prevention services, primary care, acute care, mental health programs, addiction treatment, long-term care, and assistance with prescription drug coverage. When creating the Oregon Health Plan, a diverse coalition of citizens agreed upon principles worth noting in terms of entitlement, access, and allotment (Oregon Department of Human Services, 2006) (Table 40-3).

# Direct Application in Everyday Practice

## Codes and Standards for Occupational Therapy

From corporations to street gangs, an adoption of group values is an expected obligation of group membership. All groups of all types assume members' acceptance of group values. Group membership implies compliance with

**Table 40-3. Oregon Health Plan Principles**

The Oregon Health Plan model was created with an emphasis on collaboration and negotiation among a variety of health care stakeholders. The Oregon Health Plan is based on a set of ethical principles:

- All citizens should have universal access to a basic level of care
- Society is responsible for financing care for poor people
- There must be a process to define a "basic" level of care
- The process must be based on criteria that are publicly debated, reflect a consensus of social values, and consider the good of society as a whole
- The health care delivery system must encourage use of services and procedures which are effective and appropriate, and discourage over-treatment
- Health care is one important factor affecting health; funding for health care must be balanced with other programs which also affect health
- Funding must be explicit and economically sustainable
- There must be clear accountability for allocating resources and for the human consequences of funding decisions

Reproduced from Oregon Department of Human Services. (2006). The prioritized list—an overview. Retrieved September 5, 2009, from http://www.oregon.gov/DHS/healthplan/priorlist/main.shtml

fundamental principles of the group. A sense of belonging to a group will foster adoption of group norms as personal values.

Either an implicit agreement or an explicit contract is established between an organization and its members. Guidelines govern individual action with corresponding penalties levied against any individual who violates a norm. Behavioral norms are established through either formal or informal systems. The degree of formal structure does not determine the amount of internalization of values or the extent of compliance to rules. Custom and tradition are relatively informal methods of sharing group values, and yet they have compelling authoritative commands for observance of principles. Regulations and laws are examples of formal methods of sharing group values with strong incentives for compliance.

Private entities such as professional associations or corporations create standards of conduct. We can assume that just like individuals, organizations will rely on more than one type of value-based principle. It is not unusual for an organizational policy to go beyond the minimum requirements set by legal standards. Customs, principles, and regulations blend to define ethical behavior unique to an organization. Attitudes and traditions are a part of organizational culture.

Cooperative creation of an ethical work environment sets the tone for an organization. Constructing an ethical climate is most effective when the people who implement the policies and procedures participate in their formation because a realistic, yet rigorous, set of ethical standards is more likely to be adhered to if there is a "buy-in" from those who must live under its authority. A proactive management can support ethical behavior by adopting a policy to lead by example. If management clearly supports ethical behavior, employees will be more likely to view an unethical practice as unacceptable. Employees can reasonably expect a safe workplace environment, fair work conditions, and an equitable salary with benefits. There is an advanced expectation of job satisfaction. It is incumbent upon employees to utilize skills and perform a fair amount of work in return.

A code of ethics creates recognition of the behaviors deemed good or bad within a group context. A code of ethics is a collection of value-based rules forming an impartial guide for making moral decisions by an identified group. Typically, secondary documents are created to assist in interpretation and implementation of the code of ethics. Generally, safeguards are built into the system to encourage compliance and provide mechanisms for sanctions to deal with ethical misconduct in violation of principles specified in the code of ethics. A code of ethics is an explicit statement of values and principles. It provides an organization's membership guidance on how to avoid penalties. Any formal statement can serve as a code of ethics if it provides an organization's membership with an outline of what is right and valued, defines underlying beliefs, and highlights important values. In many cases, a code of ethics is integrated into the organization's mission statement.

Both the National Board for Certification in Occupational Therapy (NBCOT) and the American Occupational Therapy Association (AOTA) have responsibility for protection of the public interest. In service of that mission, they both specify criteria for the practice of occupational therapy and define the responsibilities of occupational therapy professionals (Figure 40-1).

NBCOT standards emphasize the necessity for avoidance of any behavior or action that "reasonably could be expected to result in harm to recipients of occupational therapy services" (NBCOT, 2009). Consumers of occupational therapy services are protected from unqualified practitioners and "those practitioners whose behavior falls short of these standards" (NBCOT, 2008). Violations can result in certification ineligibility for a specified time or specified actions such as monitoring or supervision. The NBCOT has the authority to impose sanctions up to indefinite revocation of certification.

The AOTA has developed and adopted a series of documents to provide guidance for the occupational therapy practitioner. These documents of the AOTA represent an attempt to design a comprehensive ethics plan for the profession and a guide for practitioners. A set of principles is given in the Occupational Therapy Code of Ethics (Reitz et al., 2005). Guidelines to the Occupational Therapy Code of Ethics (Reitz et al., 2006) presents an outline that correlates professional behaviors with principles from the code. Standards of Practice for Occupational Therapy (AOTA, 1998) provides practice guidelines for the delivery of occupational therapy services. It defines minimum practice standards, giving the occupational therapy practitioner guidance for application of values and principles. Enforcement Procedures for the Occupational Therapy Code of Ethics (AOTA, 2005) establishes a complaint process and sanctions as well as outlining the AOTA ability to penalize AOTA members who violate the ethics standards. Appropriate authorities inclusive of licensing and regulatory bodies, employers, and certification boards are recognized as properly having jurisdiction over occupational therapy practitioners.

Core Values and Attitudes of Occupational Therapy Practice (Kanny & Hansen, 1993) is a document occupational therapy practitioners can use as a guide to ethical decision making in support of the Occupational Therapy Code of Ethics (Reitz et al., 2005). A combination of deontological beliefs and teleological application principles are offered as a method to sort through conflicting priorities. Seven ethical values and morality-based attitudes form the core foundation for the practice of occupational therapy (Kanny & Hansen) (Table 40-4).

The Occupational Therapy Code of Ethics was created by the AOTA for occupational therapy professionals. It is meant to assist in ethical decision making when moral conflict exists. The Occupational Therapy Code of Ethics implies recognition that members of the profession will be called upon to make decisions regarding ethical issues

## NBCOT® Candidate/Certificant Code of Conduct

**Preamble**

The National Board for Certification in Occupational Therapy, Inc. ("NBCOT," formerly known as "AOTCB") is a professional organization that supports and promotes occupational therapy practitioner certification. This Candidate/Certificant Code of Conduct enables NBCOT to define and clarify the professional responsibilities for present and future NBCOT certificants, i.e., OCCUPATIONAL THERAPIST REGISTERED OTR® (OTR) henceforth OTR, and CERTIFIED OCCUPATIONAL THERAPY ASSISTANT COTA® (COTA) henceforth COTA.

It is vital that NBCOT certificants conduct their work in an appropriate and professional manner to earn and maintain the confidence and respect of recipients of occupational therapy, colleagues, employers, students, and the public.

As certified professionals in the field of occupational therapy, NBCOT certificants will at all times act with integrity and adhere to high standards for personal and professional conduct, accept responsibility for their actions, both personally and professionally, continually seek to enhance their professional capabilities, practice with fairness and honesty, abide by all federal, state, and local laws and regulations, and encourage others to act in a professional manner consistent with the certification standards and responsibilities set forth below.

Where the term "certificant" is used, the term "applicant or candidate" is included in its scope.

**Principle 1**

Certificants shall provide accurate and truthful representations to NBCOT concerning all information related to aspects of the Certification Program, including, but not limited to, the submission of information:

- ✓ On the examination and certification renewal applications, and renewal audit form
- ✓ Requested by NBCOT for a disciplinary action situation
- ✓ Requested by NBCOT concerning allegations related to:
  - » test security violations and/or disclosure of confidential examination material content to unauthorized parties;
  - » misrepresentations by a certificant regarding his/her credential(s) and/or education;
  - » the unauthorized use of NBCOT's intellectual property, certification marks, and other copyrighted materials.

**Principle 2**

Certificants who are the subject of a complaint shall cooperate with NBCOT concerning investigations of violations of the *Candidate/Certificant Code of Conduct*, including the collection of relevant information.

**Principle 3**

Certificants shall be accurate, truthful, and complete in any and all communications relating to their education, professional work, research, and contributions to the field of occupational therapy.

**Principle 4**

Certificants shall comply with laws, regulations, and statutes governing the practice of occupational therapy.

**Principle 5**

Certificants shall not have been convicted of a crime, the circumstances of which substantially relate to the practice of occupational therapy or indicate an inability to engage in the practice of occupational therapy safely, and/or competently.

**Principle 6**

Certificants shall not engage in behavior or conduct, unlawful or otherwise, that cause(s) them to be, or reasonably perceived to be, a threat or potential threat to the health, well-being, or safety of recipients or potential recipients of occupational therapy services, students or colleagues.

**Principle 7**

Certificants shall not engage in the practice of occupational therapy while one's ability to practice is impaired due to chemical (i.e., legal and/or illegal) drug or alcohol abuse.

Approved June 2002
Revised February 2003
Revised June 2006
Revised October 2008



**Figure 40-1.** NBCOT Candidate/Certificant Code of Conduct (revised 2008). Reproduced with permission from NBCOT. For Procedures for the Enforcement of the NBCOT Candidate/Certificant Code of Conduct, see Appendix H.

**Table 40-4. The Core Foundation for the Practice of Occupational Therapy**

| |
|---|
| **Altruism** is concerned with creating benefit for others. |
| **Equality** is the basis for impartial fairness. |
| **Freedom** is reflected in self-determination and the right to choose. |
| **Justice** is being objective and evenhanded while conforming to righteous obligations. |
| **Dignity** places emphasis on the unique characteristics of each person as valuable and worthy of respect. |
| **Truth** is a requirement for honesty and a seeking of realistic appraisals. |
| **Prudence** asks for the practitioner "to temper extremes, make judgments, and respond on the basis of intelligent reflection and rational thought." |

Adapted from Kanny, E., & Hansen, R. A. (1993). Core values and attitudes of occupational therapy practice. *American Journal of Occupational Therapy, 47,* 1085-1086.

that are situation-specific. The existence of the Code of Ethics reflects the profession's longstanding commitment to a set of values. Occupational therapy practitioners have a duty to know the collection of principles that form the Occupational Therapy Code of Ethics.

Principle 1 is based on the concept of beneficence—maximize possible benefits. It calls for compassionate goodwill. Occupational therapy practitioners are expected to provide services in a fair way without discrimination. This includes a call to justice for fair distribution of services. There is an expectation to become advocates for individual well-being and community safety.

Principle 2 is based on the concept of nonmaleficence—minimize or avoid causing harm. Occupational therapy practitioners are called upon to refrain from poor judgment or limited objectivity.

Principle 3 is based on double obligations. The first is autonomy—free will decision making. Autonomy or self-determination demands respect for individuality. There is an obligation to collaborate and to follow the standards of informed consent. The second is confidentiality—protecting private information.

Principle 4 requires occupational therapy practitioners to be aware of professional standards and maintain proficiency, a duty to assume responsibility for continued competency.

Principle 5 mandates compliance with laws, institutional rules, and association policies through procedural justice and adherence to the Code of Ethics.

Principle 6 places an obligation for being truthful—veracity. Accurate and honest disclosure of information is a requirement. There is a responsibility to maintain the public's trust in occupational therapy.

Principle 7 identifies a need for fidelity, professional interactions to be handled with integrity and fairness. There is an obligation to protect the rights of others.

# Confidentiality

Occupational therapy practitioners have a duty to protect the privacy of recipients of services. This requires the establishment of a trusting relationship and guarding information shared in confidence. Discussions must be protected, taking care that conversations will not be overheard. Records are not to be disclosed except under conditions of authorized access in compliance with regulations. Computer security measures must be observed.

# Informed Consent

Informed consent is a process that acknowledges the service recipient's right to be directly involved in health care decisions. Although facility procedures may focus on signing an informed consent form, the key to true informed consent is the process of educating with appropriate, relevant, and truthful information so a reasonable person can make a decision regarding the risk (harm) and options for success (benefits). The informed consent process protects against unwanted intervention and makes active participation a requirement.

The concept of informed consent is based on the principle of autonomy. Respect for the individual is fundamental to the concepts of self-determination and autonomy. Principle 3 of the Occupational Therapy Code of Ethics states that occupational therapy personnel must "collaborate" with recipients of services "in setting goals and priorities throughout the intervention process, including full disclosure of the nature, risk, and potential outcomes of any interventions" (Reitz et al., 2005). The occupational therapy practitioner must include the recipient of services as a full participant in the decision-making process. There is an obligation upon the occupational therapy practitioner to insure understanding before initiating any intervention.

Closely linked to beneficence, the process of informed consent relies on the recognition of self-determination in health care decision making. A minimum of three components is widely recognized as necessary for informed consent: sufficient knowledge for decision making (disclosure), sufficient capability to understand information (competency), and freedom to choose (voluntary).

A dynamic plan for communication should be standard procedure in order to dutifully fulfill the obligations of obtaining informed consent. Information must be shared in a manner that will facilitate communication. Efforts need to be made to reduce anxiety to allow in a complete manner the asking and answering of questions for maximum comprehension. The feelings, hopes, and fears of the individual must be considered within an environment that fosters open communication. Although the practitioner has an obligation to clearly describe the preferred clinical alternative, the practitioner should avoid prejudicing the selection process or creating coercive influence. Many times, the authoritarian image of the caregiving professional can cause a sense of intimidation.

Technical jargon needs to be avoided. At a minimum, terminology must be clearly defined. Whenever possible, layman's terms should be used. Lack of comprehension may be due to language barriers, literacy level, cognitive deficits, or situation-specific anxiety. Health care literacy is generally thought to be at low levels, even among educated, industrialized populations. The demanding medical environment may cause a barrier to understanding due to stress. The health care provider and client may not speak the same language, creating linguistic challenges to obtaining informed consent. Terminology to describe pathology is lacking by Western standards in many cultures (Crigger, Holcomb, & Weiss, 2001). Translators have been known to bias because of dialect or cross-cultural miscommunication (Barnes, Davis, Moran, Portillo, & Koenig, 1998; Crigger et al.). There can be culture-based differences in interpretation of maintaining hope and denial, repression, avoidance, or confrontation (Barnes et al.; Kagawa-Singer, 1993). The presence of unfamiliar translators taking part in personal, emotion-laden conversations can cause additional barriers to communication (Barnes et al.).

The paternalistic sentiment of the health care professional's "knowing what is best" for the client is no longer in vogue. The client has a right to either accept or refuse the recommended intervention. A choice for refusal of intervention should be honored but does not necessarily mean the end of discussions. An exploration of the reason for refusal and consideration of alternatives is not only acceptable, but it is required of an occupational therapy practitioner as a client advocate.

Enough information must be given to allow the making of a choice. The process of obtaining informed consent need not consist of an exhaustive list of every possible risk no matter how slight the probability. The purpose of the recommended intervention must be presented. Available intervention alternatives must be offered. The probability of benefits and risks must be explained for all available options. The occupational therapy practitioner must try to understand the situation from the perspective of the recipient of services.

The ability to give informed consent involves determination of competency by legal or common law standards. Capacity for reason and deliberation is required to understand the alternatives and appreciate the risks or benefits. It is useful to look at "decisional capacity" instead of reliance on legal standards of "competence," which can remove the decision-making responsibility from the recipient of services because of an impaired ability to communicate, degenerating or wavering mental status, or because the person is a minor below the age of consent. Decisional capacity is based on the determination that the individual is capable of making a decision at a given time.

How are decisions made if the person does not have decisional capacity? The question that should be asked in this type of case is, "What would the person do if able to decide independently?" Decisions must be made in the context of knowledge of the individual's past values and preferences in order to make consistent life choices. Conversations with family, friends, and staff at residential centers can lead to insights. If the recipient of services is unable to make a clinical care decision, and if the preferred option remains unknown, then informed consent will need to be obtained from an appropriately designated person. Some states recognize a health care proxy, a family member, or friend designated by the individual to make medical intervention decisions. The designated individual's authority for making decisions is directly derived from the client's free choice because the health care proxy must be identified when the client is considered competent.

When the client's wishes or attitudes are not known because the situation circumstances were never discussed or are not known to the surrogate decision makers, then decisions can be made according to "best interests" decision making. In some cases, the courts will assign a legal guardian to weigh all of the facts and determine what is in the client's "best interest." "Substituted judgment" is a form of decision making that asks, "If the client could tell us, what would the client's choice be in this situation?" The best intervention option is determined by asking, "What would a person do in this specific situation?" It is putting yourself in the client's shoes and contemplating, "What if." Once again, the details of the specific situation must be considered in decision making. The situation-specific details necessitate the weighing of risks and benefits resulting in examination of quality-of-life issues. Decisions should not be based on stereotypical social bias based on age or presence of disability.

Widening global interests have raised interesting questions in regard to informed consent. How informed is "informed?" How can coercion best be avoided when economic and educational power is uneven? The standards, codes, and guidelines common throughout the industrialized world are thought to be representative of moral fundamentalist principles (Crigger et al., 2001). Moral fundamentalism accepts informed consent principles as universal and applicable throughout the world in all clinical and research situations; therefore, the protocol for obtaining informed consent should not be modified. Moral multiculturalism is in contrast to moral fundamentalism. A multicultural ethic does not seek absolutes but accepts a more situational approach that varies among communities. Different cultures have adopted binding principles comparative to place and time; therefore, voluntary informed consent should be modified to meet the needs of the individuals.

Some cultures believe the rights of the bigger community or family override the rights of the individual. In a family, the cultural expectation may motivate a husband to routinely make decisions on behalf of his wife (Crigger et al., 2001). Decisions by a leader are expected as the norm. Often, the client will assume a passive role in decision making by allowing the "expert" health care practitioner to take control (Barnes et al., 1998). The doctor or clinician can take the form of an unintentional source of power and authority figure. Some cultures avoid an overt discussion of dying or life-threatening illness. This cultural norm would lead to medical decision making by a trusted family member rather than directly by the client. "Partial disclosure" or "ambiguity" is widely practiced as a way to share information in an indirect manner (Candib, 2002). Only recently, medical culture in Western traditions adopted the view that disclosure of life-threatening diagnosis was a beneficent act. In 1961, the majority of U.S. doctors did not disclose the diagnosis of cancer directly to clients; however, by the mid to late 1970s, most doctors disclosed as a routine practice (Candib; Gold, 2004).

It is important to avoid stereotypes and generalizations based on ethnicity. Each person and each family will have a unique experience based on family roles, education, immigration, assimilation, and personal patterns (Candib, 2002; Gold, 2004; Ho, 2006). Emphasis should be placed on expressed client values and expectations (Leino-Kilpi et al., 2003). A rational and respectfully humanitarian position accommodates both fundamentalism and multiculturalism by meeting "traditional fundamental standards of ethics while respecting cultural and societal norms" (Crigger et al., 2001, p. 465). Adherence to client autonomy respects the rights of the individual, even if the individual chooses to abdicate decision-making control to another person. Family involvement in decision making can represent an interdependent approach to obtaining informed consent. Allowing professional judgment to form intervention decisions is another valid expression of individual decision making for informed consent. If the client expresses a clear preference for another (or others) to contribute to the decision-making process, then the wish to involve others should be accepted as being as valid as an individualistic decision-making process (Barnes et al., 1998; Ho). Clinical ethics committees have been established in a number of health care facilities. A study showed that facility employees are most likely to look to clinical ethics committees for legalistic guidance on informed consent and recordkeeping (Kerridge, Pearson, & Rolfe, 1998). Authoritarian forcing of individual decision making is another form of paternalism (Candib; Ho). An active listening approach can allow the clinician or researcher to hear the preferences of the participant while avoiding a compromise to the values of the clinician or, more importantly, the client. Autonomy can be preserved with an appreciation of individual needs. A commitment for respect and honesty can be maintained.

Criticism of the informed consent form has become widespread. Much like other medical documents, the informed consent form is viewed as too technical, too complicated, and too lengthy for the typical reader. Studies show that the document is often skimmed or not read in detail (Huntington & Robinson, 2007; Varnhagen et al., 2005). It is hypothesized that in addition to low readability, informed consent documents are not read because of a perception of low risk (Huntington & Robinson; Varnhagen et al.) because the institution or clinician is trusted. True informed consent is not obtained even with a signature on a document when the document is not fully read and understood. Health messages developed according to universal accessibility standards clarify unfamiliar medical terminology and make complex concepts more comprehensible. Improved readability can be created with simpler text, decreased jargon and technological language, choice of font, and format clarity. Creating an informed consent document that meets universal accessibility standards for improving literacy can honor legal requirements and address ethical concerns for process.

Informed consent guidelines can be developed with a focus on research as well as on clinical practice. Although there are aspects of clinical informed consent similar to research informed consent, there are differences and implications to consider. The dual roles of researcher and clinician can cause confusion, conflict of interest, and potential for coercion (Crigger et al., 2001). Universities are required by federal law to develop and implement procedures for research. Informed consent goes beyond the requirements of obtaining a signature on a permission form. Commonly accepted practice understands informed consent to be a process throughout the research participant's experience.

# Quality of Life

Changes in health might cause a reprioritizing of values and standards. Diagnosis of disease, the intervention process, and the side effects of the intervention can disrupt adaptation and occupational balance while challenging coping strategies. When independence is limited or task accomplishment becomes compromised, then occupational roles may be altered. The presence of disability may imply the presence of limitations in functional independence and might decrease opportunities for life satisfaction. Quality of life may be diminished. Alternatively, coping strategies may enhance perceptions of control over situations. A sense of mastery can enhance positive adjustment and improve quality of life.

Good quality of life is determined by the personal values of the individual. Quality of life is a nonspecific criterion that has different meaning for each individual. Quality of life is more than an ability to perform self-care activities. Quality-of-life measurement needs to go beyond fragmentation of component parts. Relative independence in functional activities of daily living is not an adequate measure of quality-of-life factors. An understanding of meaningful engagement in occupation can help assess quality of life beyond generalizations based on cultural or gender implications or the presence of disability.

# Decisions

An awareness of ethics should be integrated into everyday practice. Everyday clinical practice is based on ethical judgment. Always contemplate the relevant ethical implications. Application of ethical knowledge and moral reasoning strategies enhance proficiency of the occupational therapy practitioner when coping with real world concerns. Faced with increasing demands and decreasing resources, the occupational therapy practitioner must cope with issues of quality, quantity, access, and allocation.

Quality care is the primary goal for occupational therapy practitioners and other care providers. Quality care can be defined as the best possible intervention resulting in the best outcome for the individual recipient of care. Who defines "quality?" The recipient of care, the provider of care, and the party who pays for the care determine quality. Ethical concerns occur because health care providers have dual goals that could conflict: to provide quality services and to generate high profits. Serious ethical dilemmas arise when the role of clinical advocate is compromised in conflict against the role of income generator. Pressures for cost containment can influence service delivery to move beyond clinical decision making to a decision based on financial or allocation factors. Dilemmas are created when practitioners feel that clinical excellence or social responsibility is in opposition to economic reality.

Understanding the social environment can clarify expectations for the individual recipient of care as part of the whole community. Community is a source of support representing fundamental access to basic resources. Conversely, community can be a source of barriers limiting access to essential material goods. The setting suggests a context surrounding the individual that can have an influence on choice. Social standards create customs, beliefs, attitudes, expected behaviors, and normative social routines.

Like all medical and human services professionals, occupational therapy practitioners will be faced with ethical dilemmas. In some cases, the occupational therapy practitioner may feel excluded from the decision-making process. Occupational therapy practitioners must assume an active role in the decision-making process. Introduce the pertinent ethical questions and initiate conversations about the relevant moral principles. Liability and fear of malpractice litigation can slow the decision-making process. Decision making in the clinical setting can "get stuck" while everyone with a stake in the process waits for someone else to decide on a direction.

The role of medical ethics is to assist in solving complex problems in health care situations where there is no clear identification of right or wrong, or there is a need to identify the best alternative out of choices. Conflicting and competing agendas, priorities, choices, values, and opinions of stakeholders may make medical ethics seem complicated. Rarely are there clearly defined problems with definitive solutions. An ethical dilemma is a situation where an argument can be made for opposing decisions or conflicting choices. Sometimes there is more than one "right" solution to a problem. There are situations when there is no clear indication of the "right or wrong" accepted course of action. Rules might be vague or not well established. Sometimes partial good can be found in incompatible trade-offs. At times, dubious pathways lead to "good" end results. Other times, none of the available alternatives appear to be acceptable options resulting in a good ending.

Which principle should prevail when deciding on an action? Perhaps the highest standard for medical ethical decision making is a reliance on the principle of beneficence. The virtuous occupational therapy practitioner will strive to maximize possible benefits in a fair way. Is there a fair and just way to sort through conflicting principles to decide on a course of action or inaction? The moral occupational therapy practitioner will identify and analyze ethical problems. An appropriate response to ethical problems is an exploration of choices. No two cases are ever identical—"one size fits all" solutions do not exist. Emphasis cannot be placed on learning the "right" concept or replicating the "correct" action because there may be more than one "right" solution. Responsible decision making depends on thoughtful consideration of competing rights, obligations, values, and interests. Judgments necessitate a clarification of values and ethical principles. How should an occupational therapy practitioner determine the best option when challenged with an ethical dilemma? A process for ethical decision making is derived from clinical practice. A time-honored method to report on clinical progress—the SOAP note—can be borrowed and adapted for resolving ethical dilemmas (Table 40-5).

**Table 40-5. Steps for Writing an Ethical Decision-Making SOAP**

1. Create an initial problem list.
2. **Subjective**: Identify the subjective case-specific issues.
3. **Objective**: Gather objective case-relevant data.
4. **Assess**: Assess the situation.
5. **Plan**: Articulate a plan of action.
6. Implement the plan.
7. Re-evaluate and modify action steps as needed.

- *Step 1*: Create an initial problem list. Define the central problem or most significant problems. What is the conflict? List all stakeholders who are involved.
- *Step 2*: Identify the ethical issues or problems raised by the case-specific situation. It is critical to understand the clinical and social facts of the particular

situation. Are the thoughts and wishes of the participants clear? Recognize the presence of feelings (i.e., acceptance, fear, worry, anger, ambivalence, or other emotions). Clarify your own opinion and biases.

- *Step 3*: Gather objective case-relevant data. Search the literature to identify similar situations. Be aware of clinical standards. Determine the consensus of experts on prior cases. Examine the interpretation of law through court decisions. Find relevant departmental or organizational procedures. List professional association guidelines. Know your code of ethics principles. Identify the core ethical principles.
- *Step 4*: Assess the situation. Contemplate the relevant ethical principles. Articulate the alternative solutions. Think through the issues with systematic analysis. Postulate all of the consequences of each choice. Weigh the competing interests, needs, risks, and benefits of all involved participants. Determine if the options are reasonable. Apply the larger principles to the specific people of the particular situation.
- *Step 5*: Articulate a plan of action for a practical and realistic solution. Formulate an overall plan.
- *Step 6*: Implement the plan.
- *Step 7*: Evaluate the need to modify the plan based on the process and the results.

# Student Self-Assessment

1. Personal Reflection: Where did you get your sense of morality? Write a four- or five- page biographical narrative describing your values and principles linking the evolution of your standards to your personal history of past experiences or events.
2. Personal Credo: Write your own code of ethics. Create a moral credo defining your personal system of philosophical beliefs.
3. Professional Credo: Adapt your personal code of ethics to craft a professional doctrine suitable for clinical use.
4. Small group exercise: Working in teams, think of a situation that raises an ethical dilemma. Do not try to resolve the moral conflict.
    - *Exercise #1*: Brainstorm as many ideas as possible and generate alternative solutions.
    - *Exercise #2*: List the relevant ethical principles and values.
    - *Exercise #3*: Present a role-play and demonstrate the attitudes, opinions, and feelings of the participants.
5. Document review
    - *Exercise #1*: Visit a local health care facility or human services agency. Obtain a copy of a document that includes ethical concepts. Identify the main ethical principles or standards in the document.
    - *Exercise #2*: Search the websites of a local hospital and a major teaching hospital of your choice. Look for a mission statement, code of ethics, or Patient Bill of Rights for both facilities. Compare the documents. Do they refer to the same values? Find and describe two ethics-based components that are the same and two components that are different.

# Ethics Case Study Projects

Answer the following Ethics Case Study Questions for each case:

1. List the most significant ethical considerations. Explain your answer.
2. Which principles in the Occupational Therapy Code of Ethics apply to the case? Explain your answer.
3. Write an ethical decision-making SOAP.
4. Discuss the implications of allocation and distribution of resources.

**Case Study #1—Larry**

Leaving the cafeteria after a late afternoon snack, you are rushing toward the elevator to get to a Utilization Review Meeting when Larry, a nurse, taps your shoulder and with a big, friendly grin says, "I'm so glad that I ran into you. Let's ride back up to the unit together because I want your opinion about Mr. Stone's getting discharged next week." As the doors close on the crowded elevator, Larry looks at you and continues speaking, "So, I want to know if Mr. Stone can dress independently yet?"

**Case Study #2—Edie**

You work in the outpatient unit of a busy rehabilitation hospital. Dropped off in the parking lot by her mom, Edie always arrives promptly for her occupational therapy visits. She is being seen for intervention of a fracture to her left elbow following a slip on the stairs at her piano teacher's home. Her intervention time seems to be shorter than the hour duration because throughout the sessions, she chats about the numerous activities and events typical to an active 16-year-old high school student. Shortly before the end of today's session, Edie confides that she has been using illegal drugs she buys from another student.

## Case Study #3—Maddy

You are a member of a geriatric medical behavioral assessment team in a large suburban hospital. One of your clients is an 80-year-old female recuperating from a fall. The cause of her fall remains unknown. Medical testing is ongoing; all results are inconclusive. She has multiple chronic conditions, including diabetes and arthritis. She is legally blind. Significant hearing loss in both ears is somewhat compensated for with bilateral hearing aids. Never married, Maddy lives alone in the house that had been the family home for three generations. She had dedicated her adult life to caring for her disabled mother who gradually became progressively more frail and incontinent in her last years until she passed away about 10 years ago. Family members (a brother and niece who, coincidentally, is a nurse on another unit) share responsibility of occasional visits, grocery shopping, and helping with mail for bill payments. Her health insurance will not cover long-term home care services. Her small pension combined with her Social Security check make her slightly over-income for subsidized programs. Both relatives describe Maddy as strong, independent, and self-reliant, and proud of it. The brother would like to see Maddy return to independent living in her own home as soon as possible. The niece has asked the assessment team to help decide for long-term planning.

During her stay, Maddy presents as frightened, depressed, and anxious. She has ripped out her IVs repeatedly. She thwarts attempts made by staff to keep her seated in a chair and refuses to stay in her hospital bed. The staff is concerned for her ongoing safety because she has proven to be "a fall risk." Everyone who enters her room is asked the same question, "When can I go home?"

Some of the assessment team are worried about returning Maddy to her own home. They would like her to have more supervision and suggest transfer to a long-term care facility. An assisted living facility, nursing home, or custodial care residence are possibilities being considered. As one staff member said, "Sure she wants to go home but this would be for her own good; she will learn to like it."

The multidisciplinary team looks to you, the occupational therapist, to determine the level of independent functioning with ADL and to assess safety in the home. Will this client be safe at home? Should this client be transferred to a long-term care residential setting for the management of nutritional and health needs? The discharge meeting starts.

## Case Study #4—Sunny Meadows

### Case Study #4A- The College Roommate

Your college roommate's family owns several skilled nursing facilities (SNF) in a metropolitan center. After graduation, your friend's father asks you to work in the main facility where the corporate office is housed.

After a few months of work at Sunny Meadows, it becomes obvious that the amount of actual resident visits to therapy does not match what is documented in the medical record. You are aware that health care insurers generally require termination of services if measurable progress halts. You have been instructed by the program director to provide intervention but document in the medical record slow progress so the residents appear to need more intervention than is actually required.

You have not seen your old roommate since graduation. You are meeting for a casual lunch on the following Sunday.

### Case Study #4B – Michael and Maria

Michael, a 45-year-old resident who experienced a traumatic brain injury, is no longer making measurable therapeutic gains. Michael's wife, Maria, is a frequent visitor at Sunny Meadows and often accompanies her husband to the occupational therapy clinic. Maria is very worried, "I don't want Michael to go downhill and lose his ability to do things. You know he is trying very hard! Can't you help maintain what he can do now? Can you help prevent losing function? Can't you provide services as long as he needs your help? You know he has goals. Is not hope important, even without measurable progress?"

## Case Study #5—Fred

Fred is a 92-year-old man on your caseload. You are providing occupational therapy intervention after a hip fracture secondary to metastatic lung cancer. He has learned that his condition is considered terminal. He is obviously depressed. He has no family. He has outlived his wife of 61 years. A drunk driver in a motor vehicle accident killed his only daughter on Christmas Eve 7 years ago. His best and only friend no longer recognizes him due to Alzheimer's disease. He tells you that he doesn't want occupational therapy, or more surgery, radiation therapy, or chemotherapy: "I just want to be left alone."

### Case Study #6—Juan

Juan is well liked for his quick sense of humor and compassionate demeanor. His obvious empathy for younger kids is frequently shown by his friendly attitude on the school playground. He is an artistically talented 16 year old with strong academic skills who attends the regional non-graded magnet school. Juan lives in a residential group setting because of a shortage of appropriate foster care homes. Often not available for meetings, his mom is known to have addictions with numerous hospital admissions for attempts at recovery. She changes addresses frequently. A social worker from the Department of Social Services (DSS) has custodial control over his care. A volunteer Educational Surrogate Parent (ESP) supervises his educational plans and is authorized to sign all educational documents. A child under the age of 18 will be assigned an ESP if eligible for an Individualized Education Program (IEP) and under DSS custody. An IEP is required under the Individuals with Disabilities Education Act (IDEA) to develop an educational plan to meet the needs of a child with disabilities for appropriate accommodation as needed for classroom and testing situations.

Juan first came to the attention of the DSS when his teacher noticed cigarette burn marks along the insides of his arms. When questioned, he revealed he sometimes thought about suicide. His short attention span and periodic fits of rage were too much for his teacher in the traditional classroom environment. Recently, the outpatient mental health unit intervention team completed retesting and tentatively made the diagnosis of bipolar disorder. Intervention suggestions include medication, individual counseling, and stress management techniques. The suggested intervention plan is to be implemented by staff at the residential facility and the regional magnet school.

After 2 months of intervention, Juan is saying he wants to quit school and he is refusing to take medication. He complains that medication side effects always make him feel tired and thirsty. He says the worst part is no longer feeling "the flow of creativity, his artistic energy is gone." There is a conflict between the course of action the professionals feel is prudent and what Juan wants to do. The residential staff are concerned because Juan is beginning to become "a loner," isolating himself in his bedroom. His specialist teachers in the magnet school agree Juan is more difficult to engage and he seems distracted.

You work for the occupational therapy team of the school department in a large urban community. An invitation to Juan's IEP meeting scheduled for a week from yesterday arrived in today's mail. Shortly before his transfer to the magnet school, the homeroom teacher requested an "occupational therapy consult for handwriting improvement." Initial contact with Juan was made in his old classroom. Sitting in a corner chair slouched into his oversized black hooded sweatshirt, he avoided eye contact. His only comments were, "My handwriting is just fine like it is. I don't want your help."

Knowing occupational therapy can provide a range of interventions that could improve functional abilities in the school environment, you know you have a lot to offer kids like Juan. You look at your desk calendar to discover you already agreed to participate in another IEP meeting scheduled at the same time for a student who attends a different school within your district caseload. Sighing, you decide to write a memo to be read into the official meeting minutes outlining your thoughts and recommendations.

## Electronic Resources

- The American Occupational Therapy Association: www.aota.org
- National Board for Certification in Occupational Therapy: www.nbcot.org
- National Institutes of Health—Bioethics Resources on the Web. This website contains a broad collage of annotated Web links with resources available to those with an interest in bioethics, including education, research involving human participants and animals, medical and health care ethics, and the implications of applied genetics and biotechnology: http://bioethics.od.nih.gov
- The President's Council on Bioethics: http://bioethics.gov
- Office for Protection From Research Risks, Tips On Informed Consent: www.hhs.gov/ohrp/humansubjects/guidance/ictips.htm
- United States Department of Health & Human Services; Includes links for information on policies and regulations as well as specific population resources: www.hhs.gov

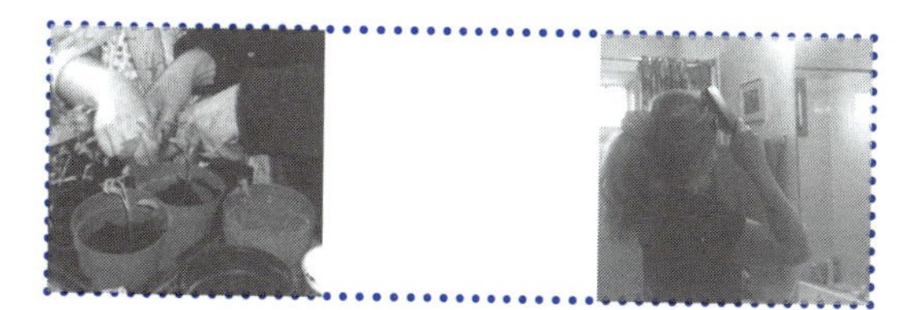

# References


American Occupational Therapy Association. (1998). Standards of practice for occupational therapy. *American Journal of Occupational Therapy, 52*, 866-869.

American Occupational Therapy Association. (2005). Enforcement procedures for the Occupational Therapy Code of Ethics. *American Journal of Occupational Therapy, 59*(6), 643-652.

Barnes, D. M., Davis, A. J., Moran, T., Portillo, C. J., & Koenig, B. A. (1998). Informed consent in a multicultural cancer patient population: Implications for nursing practice. *Nursing Ethics, 5*(5), 412-423.

Candib, L. M. (2002). Truth telling and advance planning at the end of life: Problems with autonomy in a multicultural world. *Families, Systems & Health, 20*(3), 213-228.

Crigger, N. J., Holcomb, L., & Weiss, J. (2001). Fundamentalism, multiculturalism and problems of conducting research with populations in developing nations. *Nursing Ethics, 8*(5), 459-468.

Fulghum, R. (1988). *All I really need to know I learned in kindergarten: Uncommon thoughts on common things* (pp. 6-7). New York, NY: Villard Books.

Gold, M. (2004). Is honesty always the best policy? Ethical aspects of truth telling. *Internal Medicine Journal, 34*, 578-580.

Ho, A. (2006). Family and informed consent in multicultural setting. *American Journal of Bioethics, 6*(1), 26-28.

Huntington, I., & Robinson, W. (2007). The many ways of saying yes and no: Reflections on the research coordinator's role in recruiting research participants and obtaining informed consent. *IRB: Ethics & Human Research, 29*(3), 6-10.

Kagawa-Singer, M. (1993). Redefining health: Living with cancer. *Social Science and Medicine, 37*(3), 295-304.

Kanny, E., & Hansen, R. A. (1993). Core values and attitudes of occupational therapy practice. *American Journal of Occupational Therapy, 47*, 1085-1086.

Kerridge, I. H., Pearson, S., & Rolfe, I. E. (1998). Determining the function of a clinical ethics committee: Making ethics work. *Journal of Quality in Clinical Practice, 18*, 117-124.

Leino-Kilpi, H., Valimaki, M., Dassen, T., Gasull, M., Lemonidou, C., Scott, P. A., et al. (2003). Perceptions of autonomy, privacy, and informed consent in the care of elderly people in five European countries: Comparison and implications for the future. *Nursing Ethics, 10*(1), 58-66.

National Board for Certification in Occupational Therapy. (2008) Procedures for the enforcement of the NBCOT Candidate/Certificant Code of Conduct. Retrieved September 16, 2009, from http://www.nbcot.org/WebArticles/articlefiles/121-enforcement_procedures.pdf

National Board for Certification in Occupational Therapy. (2009). NBCOT Candidate/Certificant Code of Conduct. Retrieved September 16, 2009, from http://www.nbcot.org/WebArticles/articlefiles/64-CodeOfConduct_2007.pdf

Oregon Department of Human Services. (2006). The Prioritized List—An overview. Retrieved September 1, 2009, from http://www.oregon.gov/DHS/healthplan/priorlist/main.shtml

Reitz, S. M., Arnold, M., Franck, L. G., Austin, D. J., Hill, D., McQuade, L. J., et al. (2005). Occupational therapy code of ethics. *American Journal of Occupational Therapy, 59*(6), 639-642.

Reitz, S. M., Austin, D. J., Brandt, L. C., DeBrakeller, B., Franck, L. G., Homenko, D. F., et al. (2006). Guidelines to the Occupational Therapy Code of Ethics. *American Journal of Occupational Therapy, 60*(6), 652-658.

Varnhagen, C. K., Gushta, M., Daniels, J., Peters, T. C., Parmar, N., Law, D., et al. (2005). How informed is online informed consent? *Ethics & Behavior, 15*(1), 37-48.

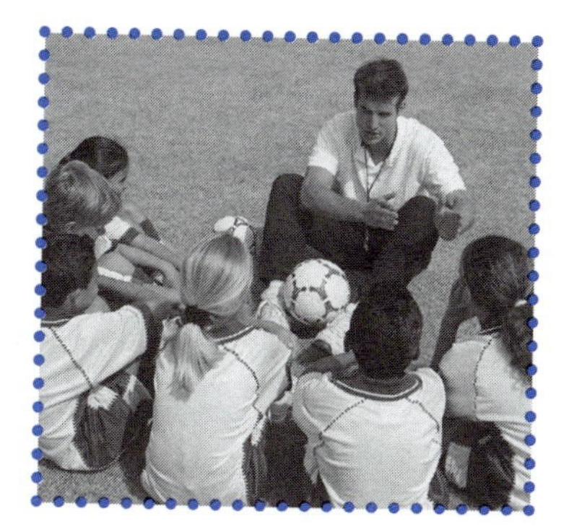

# 41

# International, National, State, Local, and Related Occupational Therapy Associations

*Diane Sauter-Davis, MA ,OTR/L*

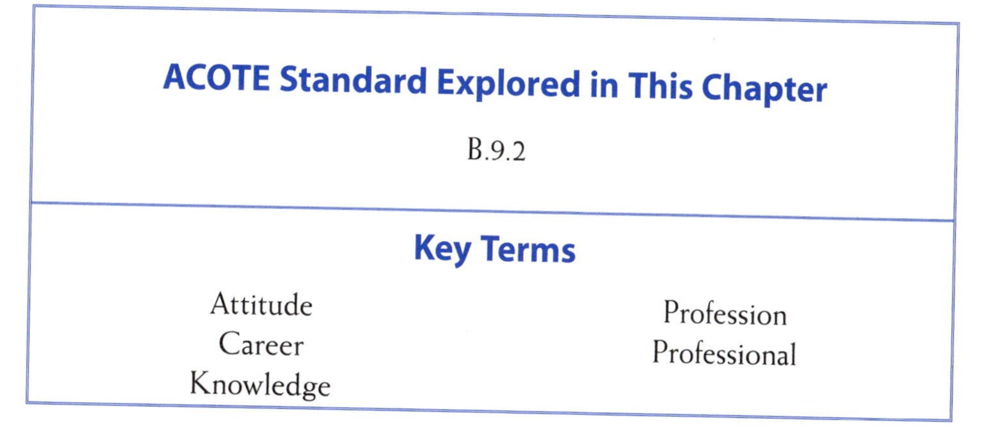

**ACOTE Standard Explored in This Chapter**

B.9.2

**Key Terms**

Attitude
Career
Knowledge
Profession
Professional

## Introduction

*Have you ever really considered what it means to be "a professional?" How is a profession different from a career?*

A career is a line of business or a way of making a living. A career may or may not be a profession. Many people choose careers but not all people choose professions.

The word *profession* is defined as "an occupation requiring extensive education or specialized training" (Encarta, 2006). This stems from the verb *to profess*—to declare public acknowledgement of something. "To profess" has been historically associated with religion and/or adherence to religious beliefs.

A professional is one who is engaged in a profession. Professionals engage in particular ways known and sanctioned by their profession. In occupational therapy, we agree to specific ethics, language, and methods of engagement. Following these principles and employing professional behaviors is called *professionalization.*

If we look at these definitions, we begin to understand that being a professional is more than simply having knowledge and skill. A profession includes shared perspectives in knowledge, attitudes, and behaviors. Professionals demonstrate these shared beliefs and standards.

What is the value of professional knowledge, attitudes, and behaviors relative to being a professional?

Knowledge is what you know, attitude is your mind set or your outlook, and behavior is what you do or your actions. In order to be a "professional," these three things must be aligned. One of these without the other limits an otherwise skillful practitioner.

*How does this connect with the topic of professional associations? Why is participation in professional associations important?*



K. Sladyk, K. Jacobs, & N. MacRae (Eds.).
*Occupational Therapy Essentials for Clinical Competence* (pp. 451-464).

The following words are synonyms for association—*organization, union, alliance, connection,* and *link* (Encarta, 2006). The commonality of these terms leads us to believe that an association is a supportive network for a group of people with a similar declaration. Therefore, the knowledge, attitudes, and behaviors of professional members are shaped, in part, by the professional associations in which they participate. Belonging to an organization that believes in you and understands your mission is vital to your growth as a professional. Professional associations are groups that support, develop, and sustain your growth as a professional. They provide opportunities for networking, contributing, and promoting occupational therapy.

*How are professions shaped?*

Professions are dynamic, interactive entities. They are open systems, much like humans are open systems. Associations affect and are affected by internal and external factors. The internal factors include member issues—member needs, member wants, member attitudes, and member behaviors, to name a few. External factors may include public policy, funding, public perceptions, and environmental demands.

The more diversity within associations increases the opportunities to change and grow. These growth opportunities shape both the internal and external factors. Simply stated, if you want to affect the direction of your profession, an association is a place to begin!

# Occupational Therapy Resources

In this chapter, you will become familiar with associations specific to occupational therapy, some general information about governing bodies and groups within the American Occupational Therapy Association (AOTA), and organizations related to occupational therapy that provide networking functions. You will also learn the process of how a professional begins to participate in their profession. The following is a list of resources that will be discussed.

- Accreditation Council for Occupational Therapy Education (ACOTE)
- AOTA
- The Fund to Promote Awareness of Occupational Therapy
- Affiliated State Association Presidents (ASAP)
- State Occupational Therapy Associations—all 50 states, Washington DC, and Puerto Rico have local associations
- American Occupational Therapy Political Action Committee (AOTAPAC)
- American Occupational Therapy Foundation (AOTF)
- World Federation of Occupational Therapists (WFOT)
- The Canadian Association of Occupational Therapists (CAOT)
- Australian Association of Occupational Therapists (OT AUSTRALIA)
- Council for Occupational Therapists for the European Countries (COTEC)
- National Board for Certification in Occupational Therapy (NBCOT)
- Rehabilitation Engineering and Assistive Technology Society of North America (RESNA)
- American Society of Hand Therapists (ASHT)
- Human Factors and Ergonomics Society (HFES)

# Accreditation Council for Occupational Therapy Education

## Vision Statement

"ACOTE is committed to the establishment, promotion, and evaluation of standards of excellence in occupational therapy education. To this end, ACOTE will lead in the development of effective collaborative partnerships with the communities of interest, both internal and external to the profession of occupational therapy, which are affected by its activities" (AOTA, 2008).

## Mission Statement

"The mission of ACOTE is to foster the development and accreditation of quality occupational therapy education programs. By establishing rigorous standards for occupational therapy education, ACOTE supports the preparation of competent occupational therapy practitioners" (AOTA, 2008).

ACOTE 2006 Standards for an Accredited Master's Level Educational Program for the Occupational Therapist determines that emerging occupational therapy practitioners must understand the value of professional associations. The standard addressed in this chapter is as follows:

- Standard B.9.2: "Discuss and justify how the role of a professional is enhanced by knowledge of and involvement in international, national, state, and local occupational therapy associations and related professional associations" (AOTA, 2008).

To completely appreciate the importance of these standards within the educational context, occupational therapy students must have a basic understanding of each organization and its relationship(s) to occupational therapy.

# American Occupational Therapy Association

## History of the American Occupational Therapy Association

AOTA is the nationally recognized professional association of more than 38,000 occupational therapists, occupational therapy assistants, and students of occupational therapy (AOTA, 2008).

The history of AOTA begins with the National Society for the Promotion of Occupational Therapy founded in 1917 and incorporated under the laws of the District of Columbia. The founders included a passionate group of advocates for occupation: William Rush Dunton, a psychiatrist who coined the term *occupation therapy* and served as the first president of the National Society for the Promotion of Occupational Therapy; Susan Tracy, an "occupational" nurse; George Barton, an architect by profession who contracted tuberculosis as an adult and became a firm believer in the value of occupation and occupational therapy; and Eleanor Clarke Slagle, an educator, social worker, and superintendent of occupational therapy at the Hull House (Padilla, 2005).

The Essentials were the skills deemed necessary for all occupational therapists in 1935. The term *essentials* was used by ACOTE through 1991 to recognize the criteria and guidelines established for all occupational therapy education (occupational therapist and occupational therapy assistant). ACOTE currently uses the term *standards* to connote the educational requirements for all entry-level occupational therapy practitioners.

"At that time, the mission of the Association, as set forth in its Constitution, "shall be to study and advance curative occupations for invalids and convalescents; to gather news of progress in occupational therapy and to use such knowledge to the common good; to encourage original research, to promote cooperation among occupational therapy societies, and with other agencies of rehabilitation."

About 3 years after its incorporation, the Association was urged by several leading physicians and authorities on hospital administration to establish a national register or directory of occupational therapists "for the protection of hospitals and institutions from unqualified persons posing as occupational therapists."

After careful consideration and on the advice of other national organizations in the field of medicine, the Association decided that the first step toward the establishment of a national register or directory was the establishment of minimum standards of training for occupational therapists.

In 1921, the name of the Association was changed to the American Occupational Therapy Association (AOTA). In 1923, accreditation of educational programs became a stated function of the AOTA, and basic educational standards were developed.

AOTA approached the Council on Medical Education of the American Medical Association (AMA) in 1933 to request cooperation in the development and improvement of educational programs for occupational therapists.

The Essentials of an Acceptable School of Occupational Therapy were adopted by the AMA House of Delegates in 1935. This action represented the first cooperative accreditation activity by the AMA. In 1958, AOTA assumed responsibility for approval of educational programs for the occupational therapy assistant. The standards on which accreditation was based were modeled after the Essentials established for baccalaureate programs.

In 1964, the AOTA/AMA collaborative relationship in accreditation was officially recognized by the National Commission on Accrediting (NCA). The NCA was a private agency serving as a coordinating agency for accrediting activities in higher education. Although it had no legal authority, it had great influence on educational accreditation through the listing of accrediting agencies it recommended to its members. The NCA continued its activities in a merger with the Federation of Regional Accrediting Commissions of Higher Education since January 1975. The new organization was the Council on Postsecondary Accreditation (COPA).

In 1990, AOTA petitioned the Committee on Allied Health Education and Accreditation (CAHEA) to include the accreditation of the occupational therapy assistant programs in the CAHEA system. Following approval of the change by the AMA Council on Medical Education, CAHEA petitioned both COPA and the U.S. Department of Education (USDE) for recognition as the accrediting body for occupational therapy assistant education.

In 1991, occupational therapy assistant programs with approval status from the AOTA Accreditation Committee became accredited by CAHEA/AMA in collaboration with the AOTA Accreditation Committee.

On January 1, 1994, the AOTA Accreditation Committee changed its name to the AOTA Accreditation Council for Occupational Therapy Education (ACOTE) and became operational as an accrediting agency independent of CAHEA/AMA.

During 1994, the ACOTE became listed by the USDE as a nationally recognized accrediting agency for professional programs in the field of occupational therapy. The ACOTE was also granted initial recognition by the Commission on Recognition of Postsecondary Accreditation (CORPA). CORPA was the nongovernmental recognition agency for accrediting bodies that was formed when the Council on Postsecondary Accreditation (COPA) dissolved in 1994.

On March 1, 1994, 197 previously accredited/approved and developing occupational therapy and occupational therapy assistant educational programs were transferred into the ACOTE accreditation system.

In a ballot election concluded October 31, 1994, the AOTA membership approved the proposed AOTA Bylaws Amendment that reflected the creation of AOTA's new accrediting body and establishment of the ACOTE as a standing committee of the AOTA Executive Board.

The Council on Higher Education Accreditation (CHEA) is presently the nongovernmental agency for accrediting bodies that replaced the Commission on Recognition of Postsecondary Accreditation (CORPA). In February, 1997, CHEA voted to accept CORPA's recognition status of ACOTE.

Reproduced with permission from American Occupational Therapy Association. (2009a). History of AOTA accreditation. Retrieved September 11, 2009, from www.aota.org/Educate/accredit/overview/38124.aspx

## American Occupational Therapy Association Mission Statement

The American Occupational Therapy Association advances the quality, availability, use, and support of occupational therapy through standard-setting, advocacy, education, and research on behalf of its members and the public" (AOTA, 2006).

## American Occupational Therapy Association Centennial Vision

AOTA advances occupational therapy as the pre-eminent profession in promoting the health, productivity, and quality of life of individuals and society through the therapeutic application of occupation (Padilla, 2005).

With extensive input from the membership over a 2-year period, the Centennial Vision statement adopted by the AOTA Board of Directors in January 2006 was approved by the Representative Assembly (RA) in April 2006.

"We envision that occupational therapy is a powerful, widely recognized, science-driven, and evidence-based profession with a globally connected and diverse workforce meeting society's occupational needs" (AOTA, 2006).

This statement allows us to celebrate our past and to determine our future. In 2017, both AOTA and the profession will turn 100. How will you celebrate 100 years of occupational therapy? Where will occupational therapy be in the 21st century? What will you do to promote the occupational therapy profession of the future?

The mission and the centennial vision both help occupational therapy practitioners to understand the direction of their profession.

We can begin to see what the future holds for occupational therapy. What opportunities and threats face occupational therapy in the years ahead? What strengths do we have to position our profession for the future? What weaknesses must we acknowledge to grow, change, and respond effectively?

Figure 41-1 depicts the strategic efforts of AOTA from 2006-2009. Strategic plans are guiding statements set by organizations to assist them in achieving effective outcomes. This strategic plan describes the priorities that AOTA plans to use to assure that occupational therapy is well positioned for the future.

## American Occupational Therapy Association Governance Structure

AOTA is a nonprofit association that uses a system of paid and volunteer positions to systematically complete the work that needs to be done. AOTA utilizes a governance structure that employs an executive director. This individual is a paid employee with experience running nonprofits and may or may not be an occupational therapy practitioner. An organizational chart helps to define the reporting mechanisms within an organization. The primary governance bodies of AOTA are outlined in Figure 41-2.

### Governance Bodies

AOTA's governance system consists of various and interdependent bodies. It is governed by a structure that includes an executive director. The director is a paid employee who is responsible for the oversight of the total organization.

Members of AOTA vote for all other board of directors officers, including the president, secretary, treasurer, and those who are association directors who serve on the board. The above-listed positions are volunteer positions. Other volunteer positions available in the governance structure include the following:

- *ASAP*: A body of the board of directors comprised of occupational therapy presidents from all 50 states and Puerto Rico
- *ACOTE*: Establishes standards for occupational therapy education and is an associated body of the executive board. ACOTE is recognized by the U.S. Department of Education and the Council for Higher Education Accreditation (CHEA) as the only accrediting body for occupational therapy and occupational therapy assistant educational programs. ACOTE membership includes the following:

## AOTA STRATEGIC GOALS & OBJECTIVES 2006–2009

**1) Building the profession's capacity to fulfill its potential and mission**

a) Prepare occupational therapists and occupational therapy assistants for the 21st century
b) Ensure a diverse workforce for multiple roles
c) Increase the profession's research capacity and productivity
d) Strengthen our capacity to influence and lead
e) Enhance collaboration with international partners and state affiliates

**2) Demonstrating and articulating our value to individuals, organizations and communities**

a) Increase public understanding of the profession and its value in meeting diverse health and participation needs
b) Support traditional occupational therapy roles and foster the development of emerging practice areas to help meet society's health, wellness and quality of life needs
c) Engage proactively with key external organizations and decision makers to assert occupational therapy leadership in essential areas of societal need

**3) Linking education, research and practice**

a) Promote stronger linkages and collaboration among the occupational therapy research, education and practice communities
b) Facilitate dissemination of occupational therapy knowledge to foster innovation in research, education and practice
c) Promote the dissemination and application of evidence-based knowledge

**4) Creating an inclusive community of members**

a) Work to meet the needs of members across the diverse professional roles in practice, education and research and increase member satisfaction
b) Expand outreach to occupational therapists, occupational therapy assistants, and students to grow membership
c) Foster opportunities for active member participation, recognition and leadership, and promote and develop volunteer leadership excellence

**5) Securing the financial resources to invest in the profession's ability to respond to societal needs**

a) Actively monitor internal and environmental trends affecting operations
b) Monitor current and prospective members' needs and expectations
c) Exercise transparency and accountability in management practices
d) Work to expand and diversify revenue streams

Approved by the AOTA Board of Directors 10-06-06

**Figure 41-1.** AOTA Strategic Goals and Objectives 2006-2009. Reprinted with permission from AOTA Press.

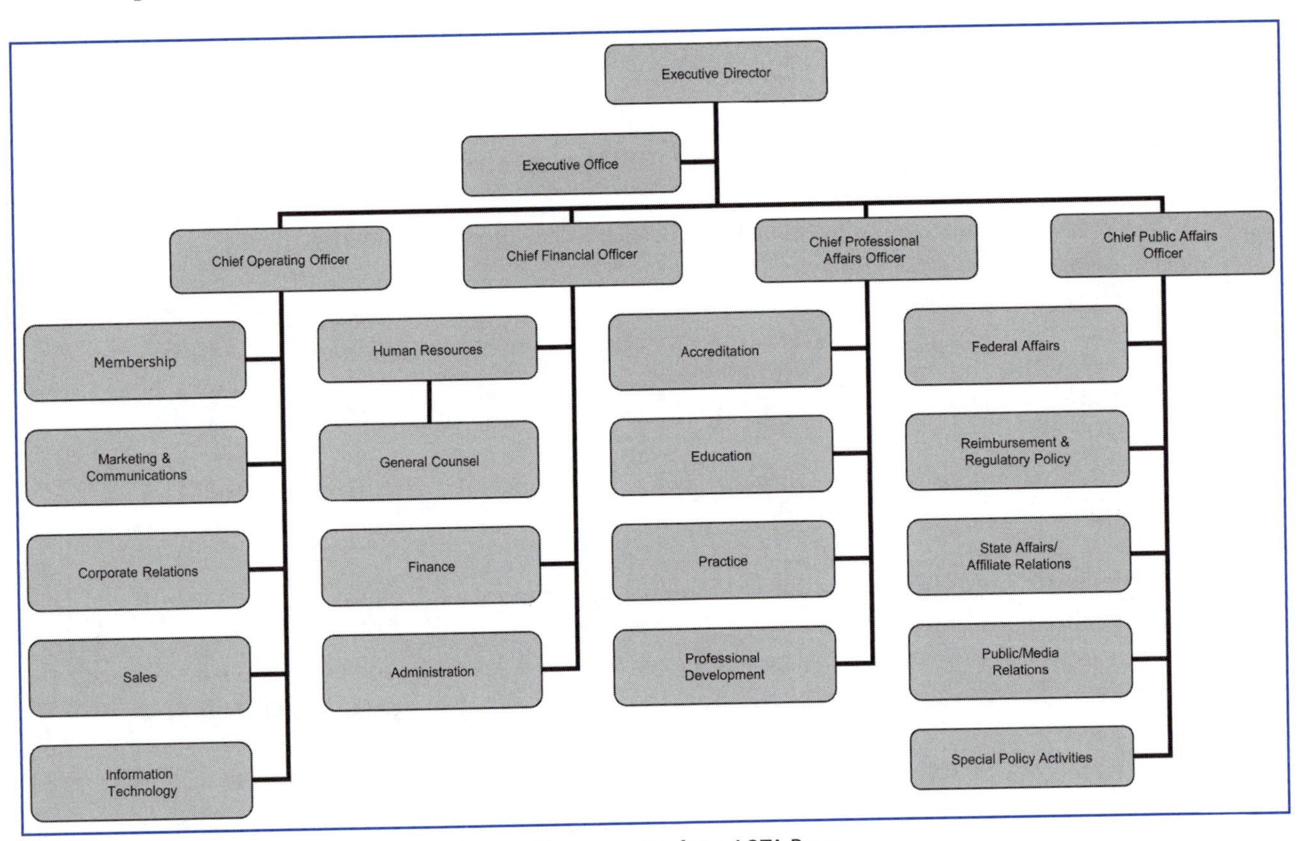


**Figure 41-2.** AOTA organizational chart. Reprinted with permission from AOTA Press.

  - Chairperson
  - Vice-chairperson
  - Council members representing professional and technical programs, public members, and an ex-officio AOTA accreditation staff liaison

  All decisions regarding accreditation of occupational therapy and occupational therapy assistant educational programs are made by ACOTE.
- *The Roster of Accreditation Evaluators (RAE)*: A separate group of occupational therapists and occupational therapy assistants, representing many areas of special expertise, that serve the vital function of assisting ACOTE in the evaluation of occupational therapy and occupational therapy assistant educational programs. To qualify as an accreditor (RAE member), the applicant must:
  - Be either an occupational therapist or occupational therapy assistant
  - Be a member in good standing with AOTA
  - Have at least 5 years experience as an occupational therapy practitioner, including 3 years in education or fieldwork, occupational therapy administration, or another area of expertise

  One cannot hold concurrent positions on any AOTA policy or decision-making body to include RA (Representative or Alternate), Board of Directors, Commission on Standards and Ethics, or Commission on Education. In addition, RAE members may not hold a position in a credentialing capacity (e.g., NBCOT Executive Board member or Certification Examination Item Writer). This position is a 3-year commitment (AOTA, n.d.).
- *RA*: The policymaking body of AOTA. These representatives are elected from each state and Puerto Rico. Chairs of committees and commissions and a public member also serve on the RA.
- *Special Interest Sections Council (SISC)*: Body of the RA organized to meet specific practice-related needs. AOTA's Special Interest Sections (SIS) connect you to vast numbers of colleagues in your field and areas of interest. The special value of SIS participation comes from the depth and breadth of knowledge, experience, and perspective that you gain from your colleagues and from the opportunities you can find to help shape your profession and take an important place within your professional community. The following are the current SIS available to members:
  - Administration and Management (including Private Practice Subsection)
  - Developmental Disabilities Education (including Faculty and Fieldwork Subsections)
  - Gerontology Home and Community Health (including Home Modification Network)
  - Mental Health

- Physical Disabilities (including Hand Subsection and Driving/Driver Rehabilitation Network)
- School Systems
- Sensory Integration Technology Work Programs

- *Commission on Education (COE)*: A group within the RA that focuses on issues of education. They make recommendations about policy needs related to education to be discussed in the RA. They are chosen in a variety of ways depending on position. The chairperson and chairperson elect are elected by AOTA membership. The following members are appointed members of COE:
  - Academic fieldwork coordinator
  - Clinical fieldwork educator
  - Educator who is an occupational therapy assistant
  - Professional level academic educator
  - Technical level academic educator
  - Postprofessional academic educator

  Associated members representing other bodies include:
  - Assembly of Student Delegates (ASD) liaison
  - Education Special Interest Section (EDSIS) liaison
  - Program directors education councils
  - Professional program directors and occupational therapy assistant program directors
- *Commission on Practice (COP)*: Serves in the RA to promote quality practice. They set practice standards for occupational therapy service delivery for occupational therapists and occupational therapy assistants.

## How Can You Get Involved?

How can you become a part of AOTA? What voice will you have in the future of your profession?

You can become a member at any time. The fees are adjusted according to member categories and qualifications. Your membership cycle is unique to you. AOTA will invoice you the same time each year. As a member, you receive the *American Journal of Occupational Therapy* (*AJOT*), *OT Practice*, and access to all SIS networks and subscriptions, as well as member-only Web site information. You can choose one printed *SIS Quarterly*. Students have two choices—Student Plus and Standard Student membership. As a Student Plus member, you receive full member benefits plus the Student Plus fieldwork list serve.

You can be an active member of AOTA through the committee, surveys, or state leadership. It takes a diverse volunteer network to create a successful member association. You may have the skills needed to help your organization.

## American Occupational Therapy Association Annual Conference and Exposition

AOTA holds its national conference and exposition each spring. The conference changes geographically each year to support all members' access. There are workshops, symposiums, and luncheons with experts. The exhibition hall is filled with an array of tools and resources for practitioners. There are opportunities to meet occupational therapy practitioners from around the nation and the world. Conference is a great opportunity to learn, network, and explore. You can find out more about occupational therapy, how to get involved, and about AOTA's conference on AOTA's Web site at www.aota.org.

## Why Get Involved in Any Professional Organization?

There are as many reasons to get involved in professional organizations as there are professions. The following are some of the reasons you will find to get involved:

- To direct health policy for occupational therapy
- To gain political power as a professional unit
- To stay informed and up to date
- To deliver best occupational therapy practice
- To secure occupational therapy as a profession for the future
- To contribute to your profession
- To advocate for your profession
- To share your skills with occupational therapy practitioners and non-occupational therapy practitioners alike

See the sidebar on the next page for personal testimonies about the value of being involved in a professional organization.

## The Fund to Promote Awareness of Occupational Therapy

AOTA created The Fund to Promote Awareness of Occupational Therapy as part of a long-term strategy to raise awareness of occupational therapy. The Fund is a 501(c)(3) organization offering a tax-advantaged venue for donations and other support.

The Fund is committed to ongoing resource development to support targeted education, research, and professional development opportunities that will increase the public's understanding and utilization of occupational therapy services.

## The Value of Belonging to Associations—Personal Testimonies

### *Over a 45-Year Career*

My experience of over 45 years in occupational therapy practice began with studying at the Philadelphia School of Occupational Therapy, newly affiliated with the University of Pennsylvania. Two remarkable professors, Helen Willard and Clare Spackman, introduced me to the profession and the responsibilities of local, state, national, and international involvement. This is what I did, beginning with their firm philosophical base of what occupational therapy was and could provide to society.

My high school and undergraduate liberal arts education led me to interest in health, social issues, psychology, and cultural differences. In my clinical practice following post graduate education and credentialing, I had the opportunity to meet many occupational therapists from other countries working in the United States. Association with them at State Association meetings informed me of programs in their countries and differences in practice perspectives and techniques. All of my classmates joined the AOTA and learned more about different practices on the east and west coasts as well as internationally. I also learned from my participation on the Council on Practice and the International Committee.

Following my independent extended travel in Europe, I received a fellowship to work in France, assisted by the AOTA and the World Rehabilitation Fund. This experience continued my association with AOTA, the French Occupational Therapy Association, and the World Federation of Occupational Therapists (WFOT). On return to the US, I was able to continue all organization and association levels, which led to representing the Maine Occupational Therapy Association at the AOTA Representative Assembly, 2nd Alternate and 1st Alternate of the AOTA to the WFOT, to Chair the WFOT International Committee and to serve eventually as 1st Vice President of the WFOT.

My attention to the colleagues I met at all of these levels enabled me to have the opportunity to teach at two universities, to write for a major textbook, and to give presentations in this country and abroad. A further extension of these levels of occupational therapy experience was my representation of the WFOT to the Pan American Region of the World Health Organization.

My work interactively in this and other countries and my clinical practice has been enhanced by the initial strength of the philosophical base of occupational therapy in school. Working up the levels of organizations was a continual challenge and enlightenment of the possibilities of occupational therapy services to the variety of people and problems we have the privilege to meet. My life has been enriched by my involvement and practice of occupational therapy. I could not have made a better choice.

*E. Anne Spencer, BA, OTR/L, MA, FAOTA*

### *Over a 30-Year Career*

I entered the profession of Occupational Therapy in 1975 in a rural part of central Maine as a solo practitioner. Shortly after starting my job, I knew intuitively that I needed to connect with the occupational therapists practicing in the area.

But, how to find them? Around this time, the Maine Occupational Therapy Association (MeOTA) was forming and that became the avenue for me to find others who had a similar need to connect. Those first Maine state meetings drew fewer than 30 therapists, but we were a hearty bunch—those relationships grew strong and steadfast over many years. We took on many key roles in developing our state association—we served as state officers, created our bylaws, grew our membership, collected dues, started a newsletter, sponsored continuing education opportunities, represented Maine to the AOTA, and worked with AOTA to develop our Maine Occupational Therapy Licensure. Seems like we did it all!

My first "official" duty in our State Association was to represent Maine to the AOTA Representative Assembly. This experience really clarified the very critical connection between the "grass roots" state practitioners with the national organization. From this position, I shifted my State commitment and served a number of years as the MeOTA Legislative Committee Chair. At other points, I served as the Continuing Education Chair and finally as the State Association President.

I believe that networking over the years with my occupational therapy colleagues and having professional relationships based on mutual support and respect has formed the cornerstone of my ongoing competence as an occupational therapy practitioner. Now, 34 years later, I attend and participate at the State Association Annual Conferences and serve Maine consumers on the State Occupational Therapy Licensure Board.

*Kathy Adams, OTR/L, ATP*

***Over a 12-Year Career***

I became an occupational therapy assistant in 1995. I traveled for some time and then resettled in Maine. I became involved with the Kennebec Valley Community College Advisory Board and then MeOTA. My involvement in MeOTA as a member, an executive board member, and as conference chair has allowed me to share with the Maine health care community the power and success of occupational therapy. It has also provided me with foundational education and information to approach occupational therapy interventions with a stronger emphasis on occupation. In September 2006, I was accepted to the roster of ACOTE evaluators. I am excited at the prospects of this challenge. As a clinician, I now bring more ideas, more research, and more experience to each client I provide occupational therapy to.

*Melissa Tilton, COTA/L*

***Over a 10-Year Career***

I am a member of RESNA. When I entered the field of occupational therapy, I was quite intrigued about the prospect of choosing a special interest for my practice. I was very fortunate to become involved with the Technical Exploration Center, an assistive technology lending library in Maine. My exposure to assistive technology gave me the bug for pursuing a more in-depth knowledge of this field. My colleagues encouraged me to look into the certification program that RESNA offers. RESNA raises the bar in standards of practice for assistive technology (AT) practitioners. I am grateful and honored to be a part of the organization. Being involved in this association has certainly taught me the value of organized professional support. The opportunities that have been presented appear limitless as I continue to become more involved in the field of AT.

*Colleen Adams, COTA/L, ATP*

***Over a 5-Year Career***

I graduated from Kennebec Valley Community College in 2004 and was anxious to learn more about how my profession supported its practitioners and communities. Consequently, I became a member of MeOTA as a student, and I continued to be part of my state association after graduation. Being a member of MeOTA gave me the chance to expand my networking and learning opportunities by attending and participating in MeOTA conferences, which led to very positive experiences. I enjoyed the process of meeting other practitioners and learning new skills at these conferences; so much so that in 2006, when an opportunity to become the OTA Representative on MeOTA's executive board came up, I jumped at the chance.

The opportunity of serving my profession through my state occupational therapy association has been incredibly rewarding both professionally and personally. Today, I continue to promote my profession and support occupational therapy assistants as their OTA Representative by identifying their needs and concerns, providing learning and networking opportunities, mentoring, and legislative involvement. Much of this is accomplished through MeOTA's OTA Forum—a group of OT practitioners who gather to learn, share concerns, network, and share their own talents and knowledge with members in monthly meetings. Personally, I have acquired new friends, developed leadership skills, and have found personal satisfaction and meaning by being part of a professional association.

*Rebecca Cirillo, COTA/L*

Their mission statement reads:

> "The fund is committed to ongoing resource development to support targeted education, research, and professional development opportunities that will increase the public's understanding of occupational therapy. The Fund exists to achieve greater understanding, availability, and use of occupational therapy and to promote the profession's contributions to health, wellness, participation, productivity, and quality of life in society" (Fund to Promote Awareness of Occupational Therapy, n.d.).

The Fund's vision statement is: "The Fund to Promote Awareness of Occupational Therapy facilitates society's understanding of and demand for occupational therapy and the profession's capacity to bring its virtues to more people in existing and future practice and policy environments" (Fund to Promote Awareness of Occupational Therapy, n.d.).

Working collaboratively with AOTA is ASAP. States are represented by their state association presidents at ASAP meetings held each year.

# Affiliated State Association Presidents

## History

ASAP is a standing committee in the AOTA Bylaws. It is a body of the AOTA Board of Directors. ASAP began in 2001 with the Standing Committee called Chapter State Association Presidents (CSAP). CSAP and AOTA entered into an affiliation agreement. An affiliate is a professional organization of occupational therapists, occupational therapy assistants, and students that has been recognized by the national association. Affiliates represent members located within an individual state, commonwealth, the District of Columbia, or Puerto Rico (AOTA, 2009b). The name of the standing committee was changed to ASAP to reflect the affiliate status. A state becomes an affiliate of the AOTA through the process described in the *Affiliation Principles for AOTA and State Associations*. Continued recognition is dependent on compliance with the *Affiliation Principles* and termination can occur for the reasons and through the process described in the *Affiliation Principles* (AOTA, 2009b).

### Purpose

The purpose of the affiliation is to foster communication and collaboration between AOTA and state associations (AOTA, 2009b).

### Mission

The mission of ASAP is to be the voice and resource that supports the practice of occupational therapy at the state level by (AOTA, n.d.):

- Representing state affiliate members to AOTA
- Communicating and networking with state affiliates as well as AOTA
- Training and mentoring state affiliate leadership
- Advising AOTA Board of Directors and RA

## State Associations

### Mission

The missions of all state occupational therapy associations are different, but all associations are designed to support members. The action statement of many state associations, similar to AOTA's mission, is to promote, foster, support, and advance occupational therapy within that particular state. State associations do not credential, license, certify, or enforce polices. The following is an example of a state mission:

"The Maine Occupational Therapy Association [MeOTA] is committed to promoting the profession of Occupational Therapy and supporting all Occupational Therapy practitioners in the State of Maine" (MeOTA, 2006).

### Organizational Structure

Organizational structures of many state associations are similar to the organizational structure of AOTA. Some states hire Executive Directors or managers to fulfill leadership duties, but many rely on volunteer leadership elected by membership.

### How Can You Get Involved in Your State Association?

Each state association is different, but all state associations have opportunities for involvement. State associations for occupational therapy provide a professional network for members. They serve the interests of members, represent the profession to the public, and promote access to occupational therapy.

State associations are volunteer organizations run by members, for members. Each membership year is unique to each state. It is important to find out the membership cycle for your state's association.

You can seek out information about how to contact your state association president or RA delegate on the AOTA Web site.

You can also ask any occupational therapy program within your state how you can access your state's association Web site. There are many opportunities at the state level. Most positions within state associations are volunteer positions and all welcome participation from members. If you desire, you can belong to several state associations concurrently.

## American Occupational Therapy Political Action Committee

### What Is a PAC?

A political action committee (PAC) is the legally sanctioned vehicle through which organizations, such as AOTA, can engage in otherwise prohibited political action and work to influence the outcome of Federal elections. The concept of PACs is described more thoroughly in Chapter 47, so we will include a brief description of AOTPAC.

"AOTA hires its own lobbyist to represent occupational therapy issues on Capitol Hill. These people are knowledgeable about the legislative process and OT" (Stephens, 2006).

AOTPAC is a voluntary, nonprofit, unincorporated committee of members of AOTA. AOTPAC was authorized by the RA in 1976 and has been operational since the Spring of 1978. The purpose of AOTPAC is to further the legislative aims of AOTA by influencing or attempting to influence the selection, nomination, election, or appointment of any individual to any Federal public office, and of any occupational therapist, registered, certified occupational therapy assistant, or occupational therapy student member of AOTA seeking election to public office at any level. The committee is not affiliated with any political party (AOTA, 2007a).

## American Occupational Therapy Foundation

The American Occupational Therapy Foundation (AOTF) is a charitable, nonprofit organization created in 1965 to advance the science of occupational therapy and increase public understanding of its value. AOTF gratefully acknowledges the support provided by AOTA in helping the profession build its capacity to engage in research that guides practice.

AOTA and AOTF have jointly funded occupational therapy research and secure competitive grant funding for research endeavors. AOTF offers over 70 scholarships each year through memorial endowments and partnerships with state associations. AOTF publishes *OTJR: Occupation, Participation and Health Journal* and maintains the content and maintenance of OT SEARCH through the Wilma L. West Library, which resides in the Foundation (AOTF, n.d.).

The profession of occupational therapy has networks of member organizations nationally and internationally designed to support and enhance the practice and profession of occupational therapy. These associations are vital to the future of occupational therapy. You can become a part of this integrated community at any time and participate at your comfort level. In turn, these associations will support you in your professional growth.

# International Occupational Therapy Organizations

## World Federation of Occupational Therapists

WFOT is the official international organization for the promotion of occupational therapy. It maintains the ethics of the profession and advances the practice and standards of occupational therapy internationally. It also promotes internationally recognized standards for the education of occupational therapists.

WFOT supports and promotes occupational therapy around the world. Currently, there are 57 member countries, including the United States, one of the founding countries (AOTA, 2007b).

### How Can You Get Involved?

You can contribute to the global development and growth of the profession by joining as an individual member of WFOT through your AOTA membership.

You will receive the WFOT professional journal (*The Bulletin*) twice a year and have an opportunity to engage in international projects. You can join WFOT by paying additional dues that are required with your AOTA membership. You can access the WFOT Web site at www.wfot.org.

## The Canadian Association of Occupational Therapists

CAOT provides services, products, events, and networking opportunities to help occupational therapists achieve excellence in their professional practice. In addition, CAOT provides national leadership to actively develop and promote the client-centered profession of occupational therapy in Canada and internationally.

The mission of CAOT is to advance excellence in occupational therapy. Their vision is that all people in Canada will value and have access to occupational therapy, and their values include integrity, accountability, respect, and equity (CAOT, n.d.). You can access CAOT at www.caot.ca.

## The Australian Association

The vision of OT AUSTRALIA is to be the voice of the occupational therapy profession in Australia. The mission is to promote and represent the profession of occupational therapy as a key element of the allied health sector of Australia. The values include the following (OT AUSTRALIA, n.d.):

- Members and staff as their most important assets
- Occupational therapy has a valuable contribution to make to the health and well-being of all Australians
- Success is dependent upon respect and trust within a strong and unified leadership team involving national council in collaboration with member associations
- The Association is socially responsive and responsible and takes a proactive stance on social issues such as human rights and environment and climate change
- The Association will strive to respond to the needs of consumers and to social changes and developments across the community
- The Association has a role in contributing to the development of occupational therapy internationally

For more information about OT AUSTRALIA go to www.ausot.com.au.

## European Associations

COTEC is made up of delegates from European national associations of occupational therapists and aims to develop, harmonize, and improve standards of professional practice and education, as well as to advance the theory of occupational therapy throughout Europe.

COTEC was initially established as a representative Committee of Occupational Therapists for the European Communities. It was founded in 1986 to coordinate the views of the national associations of occupational therapists of the then-Member States of the European Communities. In May 2001, the Committee passed a motion to change the name to Council for Occupational Therapists for the European Countries in view of the inclusion of countries that are not members of the European Union, but being part of Europe share the same aims.

The current membership of COTEC consists of over 20 national associations of occupational therapists. The national associations of a number of other European countries have observer status. All of these associations send delegates to the council meetings.

The Council meets in plenary session twice a year to plan and coordinate the ongoing work. These meetings are held in different European countries and are arranged by each host association (COTEC, 2006). You can access COTEC at www.cotec-europe.org.

# Resource Organizations

## National Board for Certification of Occupational Therapy

NBCOT is not an association, but it is an important resource for all occupational therapy practitioners. NBCOT is a not-for-profit credentialing agency that provides certification for the occupational therapy profession. NBCOT serves the public interest by developing, administering, and continually reviewing a certification process that reflects current standards of competent practice in occupational therapy. NBCOT works with state regulatory authorities, providing information on credentials, disciplinary actions, and regulatory and certification renewal issues.

NBCOT administers, develops, and continually reviews the certification process that reflects the current ACOTE standards.

The mission of NBCOT is to serve the public interest through the certification of occupational therapy practitioners (NBCOT, 2003).

The vision of NBCOT is to be internationally recognized, by all relevant stakeholders, as the premier organization for certifying occupational therapy practitioners and for promoting quality in the provision of occupational therapy services to consumers through the initial and ongoing certification of occupational therapy practitioners (NBCOT, 2003).

The following list includes some, but not all, of other organizations/associations that might have occupational therapy practitioners as members. There are many associated organizations that support specific areas of interest and expertise.

## Rehabilitation Engineering and Assistive Technology Society of North America

RESNA is an example of an association that supports the needs of people with disabilities. Occupational therapy practitioners with an interest in assistive technology might join RESNA for education and support. RESNA is an interdisciplinary association of people with a common interest in technology and disability. The purpose is to improve the potential of people with disabilities to achieve their goals through the use of technology. They serve that purpose by promoting research, development, education, advocacy, and provision of technology, while at the same time, supporting the individuals engaged in these activities (RESNA, 2009).

## American Society of Hand Therapists

ASHT "advances the science of hand treatment through communication, education, advocacy, research and clinical standards" (ASHT, n.d.). Hand therapists are occupational or physical therapists who "through advanced study and experience specialize in treating individuals with conditions affecting the hands and upper extremities. A hand specialist may also have advanced certification as a Certified Hand Therapist (CHT)" (ASHT, n.d.).

## Human Factors and Ergonomics Society

HEFS's mission is to promote the discovery and exchange of knowledge concerning the characteristics of human beings that are applicable to the design of systems and devices of all kinds. HFES considers how people function effectively in their activities and it advocates the systematic use of this knowledge to achieve compatibility in the design of interactive systems of people, machines, and environments to ensure their effectiveness, safety, and ease of performance (HFES, n.d.).

# Summary

Becoming a professional does not just happen when you receive your occupational therapy credential. Becoming a professional occurs over time. Professional knowledge, attitudes, and behaviors of skillful practitioners shape the profession and are shaped, in part, by the professional associations in which they participate. Belonging to organizations that share your understanding of occupation, your philosophy of self-determination, and your beliefs of health and wellness is vital to your growth as a professional. Your professional associations are member focused, created to support you in your professional quest.

# Student Self-Assessment

Reflection is a continuous process that creates connections and increases engagement. Reflection helps to create the context of experience.

Taking the steps to get involved in your profession occurs best with reflection and commitment. Reflective thinking is part of reflective action. It is the bridge between ideas and fact. It helps to integrate your knowledge, attitudes, and behaviors. Together, these are the characteristics of a reflective professional.

1. Your Readiness Self-Assessment: The chart on the next page is based on reflective thinking. It is the first part of getting involved. It can help you to determine what your role can be in the occupational therapy profession and which level of belonging you may be ready for.

   The following list will help you to determine how to get involved. This is your general action plan. Steps to become involved include the following:

   - Decide to get involved.
   - Determine how much time you can devote to any organization. Will you be a member, active member, leader, etc?

## Readiness Self Assessment

| | Knowledge min/mod/max | Attitude yes/no | Behavior yes/no |
|---|---|---|---|
| 1. Are you excited about occupational therapy? | | | |
| 2. Are you interested in networking? | | | |
| 3. Are you looking for continuing education opportunities? | | | |
| 4. Do you have the need for continuing education? | | | |
| 5. Are you interested in professional development? | | | |
| 6. Do you like to keep abreast of new information in the field? | | | |
| 7. Are you looking to connect with other occupational therapy practitioners who have similar ideas about occupational therapy | | | |
| 8. Do you want to find out more about particular practice issues? | | | |
| 9. Are you interested in developing leadership skills? | | | |
| 10. Do you like small, grassroots organizations? | | | |
| 11. Are you comfortable promoting occupational therapy? | | | |
| 12. Would you like to have a mentor? | | | |
| 13. Would you like to be a mentor? | | | |
| 14. Do you know the difference between licensure, NBCOT and AOTA, and a state association? | | | |
| 15. Do you understand how to pursue AOTA(Plus), NBCOT credentials, and licensure (CEU's)? | | | |
| 16. Are you interested in how public policy affects you as an occupational therapy practitioner? | | | |
| 17. Are you able to budget the needed funds? a.) Can you afford up to $100/year for membership? b.) Can you afford more than $100/year for membership? | | | |
| 18. Do you have multiple competing financial interests? | | | |
| 19. Are you interested in state, national, international issues (in this order)? | | | |
| 20. Are you interested in national, state, international issues (in this order)? | | | |
| 21. Are you interested in international issues and issues focusing on related occupational therapy issues? | | | |
| 22. Are you planning to search for an occupational therapy job? | | | |
| 23. Do you think membership makes a difference to your future employers? | | | |
| 24. Do you think being involved makes a difference? | | | |

**Yes to all**: You are ready to engage in any and all association membership activities.
**No to all**: You may not be ready to engage in your profession as a member. Review your decision to become a professional. Developing your Personal Involvement Plan may help you to determine a direction.
**Yes to 1-9; 11; 14; 17b; 18; 20-24**: You are ready for AOTA or State membership.
**Yes to 1-13; 14; 17a; 19; 21-24**: You may be better off starting at the state level. Build your connections and your financial resources.

## Personal Involvement Plan

| Areas of Interest | Areas to Explore/ Develop | Your Professional Goals | Method/Activity/ Resources to Achieve Goal | Target Date | Date Completed | Outcome |
|---|---|---|---|---|---|---|
| | | | | | | |
| | | | | | | |

Adapted from 2006 ACOTE Standards (Form F)

   - Determine the cost/benefit of belonging. How will you finance your decision? What will you gain from your membership?
   - Contact organization by Web site, mail, email, or phone. Contact an occupational therapy friend, peer, and/or colleague and ask about the benefits of belonging.
   - Fill out an application and pay your membership fee. Note your date of membership cycle on your calendar.
   - Complete your Personal Involvement Plan. Set goals to explore your new role as a member and your new professional organization.
   - Participate as you feel comfortable. Take advantage of the member opportunities. Join committees, contribute your expertise, and mentor a new peer.
   - Provide feedback when asked.
   - Be solution oriented, not problem focused.
   - Enjoy being part of something bigger than yourself.
2. Design your own Personal Involvement Plan. Use the grid on page 463 to help you to determine a path to professional membership.
3. Discuss your readiness assessment with a peer. Develop a dialogue about your plan and your future success as an occupational therapy professional.
4. A. Discuss and justify how the role of a professional is enhanced by knowledge of and involvement in international, national, state, and local occupational therapy associations and related professional associations.

   B. Now explain and give examples of how the role of a professional is enhanced by knowledge of and involvement in international, national, state, and local occupational therapy associations and related professional associations.

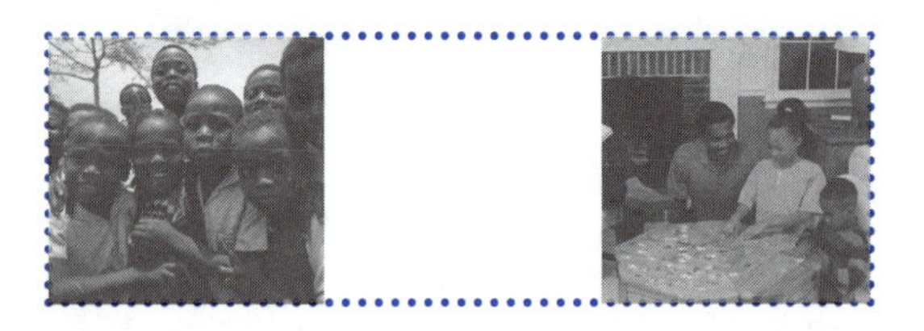

# References

American Occupational Therapy Association. (2004). AOTPAC fact sheet. Retrieved July 22, 2009, from http://www.aota.org/Practitioners/Advocacy/AOTPAC/About/36338.aspx

American Occupational Therapy Association. (2006). About AOTA. Retrieved July 22, 2009, from http://www.aota.org/About.aspx

American Occupational Therapy Association. (2007a). American Occupational Therapy Political Action Committee. Retrieved September 10, 2009, from http://www.aota.org/about/alliances/38593.aspx

American Occupational Therapy Association. (2007b). Frequently asked questions about WFOT. Retrieved September 10, 2009, from http://www.aota.org/Practitioners/Resources/Intl/WFOT/40549.aspx

American Occupational Therapy Association. (2008). ACOTE guidelines and policy statements. Retrieved September 10, 2009, from http://www.aota.org/educate/accredit/policies/policies/38144.aspx

American Occupational Therapy Association. (2009a). History of AOTA accreditation. Retrieved September 11, 2009, from www.aota.org/Educate/accredit/overview/38124.aspx

American Occupational Therapy Association. (2009b). Articles of incorporation: The official bylaws of the American Occupational Therapy Association, Inc. Retrieved July 22, 2009, from http://www.aota.org/About/Core/Bylaws.aspx

American Occupational Therapy Association. (n.d.). Affiliated State Association Presidents (ASAP) and ASAP Steering Committee. Retrieved September 10, 2009, from http://www.aota.org/governance/leadership.aspx

American Occupational Therapy Foundation. (n.d.). About AOTF. Retrieved September 10, 2009, from http://www.aotf.org/aboutaotf.aspx

American Society of Hand Therapists. (n.d.). Consumer education. Retrieved September 8, 2009, from http://www.asht.org/education/consumer.cfm

Braveman, B. (2006). *Leading and managing occupational therapy services*. Philadelphia, PA: F.A. Davis.

Canadian Association of Occupational Therapists. (n.d.). About CAOT. Retrieved September 8, 2009, from http://www.caot.ca/default.asp?pageid=2

MSN Encarta. (2009). "Profession." Retrieved September 15, 2009, from http://encarta.msn.com/dictionary_1861736704/profession.html

Fund to Promote Awareness of Occupational Therapy. (n.d.). About the Fund to Promote Awareness of Occupational Therapy. Retrieved September 12, 2009, from www.promoteot.org/AF_AboutTheFund.html

Hubbard, S. (2005). Professional organizations: Who should join? *American Journal of Occupational Therapy, 59*(1), 113-116.

Human Factors and Ergonomics Society. (n.d.). About HFES. Retrieved September 12, 2009, from http://www.hfes.org/web/AboutHFES/about.html

Maine Occupational Therapy Association. (2006). MeOTA Member handbook. Cumberland, ME: Author.

National Board for Certification in Occupational Therapy, Inc. (2003). About us. Retrieved September 12, 2009, from http://www.nbcot.org/webarticles/anmviewer.asp?a=45&z=12

OT Australia. (n.d.). Vision and purpose. Retrieved September 8, 2009, from http://www.ausot.com.au/inner.asp?relid=5&pageid=35#our20%values

Padilla, R. (2005). *A professional legacy* (2nd ed.). Bethesda, MD: AOTA Press.

Rehabilitation Engineering and Assistive Technology Society of North America. (2009). RESNA. Retrieved September 12, 2009, from www.resna.org

Solomon, A., & Jacobs, K. (2003). *Management skills for the occupational therapy assistant*. Thorofare, NJ: SLACK Incorporated.

Stephens, L. (2006). What would the world be without political action? *OT Practice, 11*(10), 6. Retrieved September 10, 2009, from http://www.aota.org/pubs/otp/1997-2007/columns/capitalbriefing/2006/cb-061206.aspx

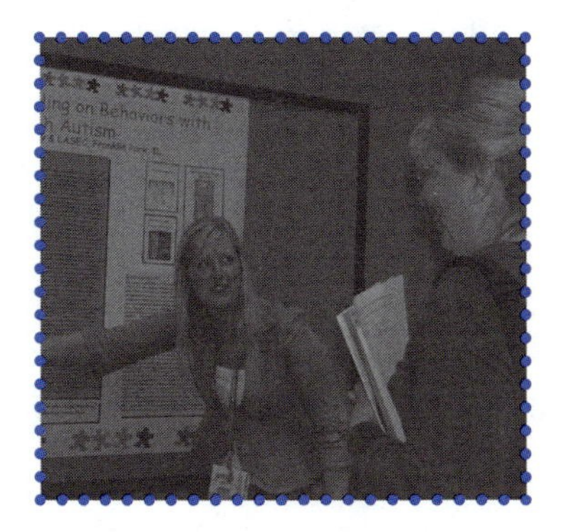

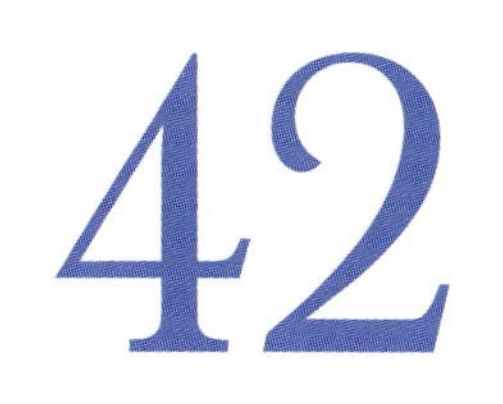

# Promoting Occupational Therapy to Others and the Public

*Jan Rowe, Dr. OT*

**ACOTE Standard Explored in This Chapter**

B.9.3

**Key Terms**

Advertisement
Persuade
Promotion

## Introduction

In this chapter, we will discuss the importance of promoting our profession to survive the changes in health care and to be recognized in community participation. As students and occupational therapy practitioners, we need to be comfortable with our roles within the profession. In our profession, we also need to be able to define occupational therapy, regardless of our niche. Occupational therapy is "fine motor skills," "activities of daily living," "handwriting," and "community transportation," but it is so much more! Occupation is core to our profession. Not using the word *occupation* in our definition of the profession is a big mistake. The framework defines occupation as "goal-directed pursuits that typically extend over time have meaning to the performance, and involve multiple tasks" (American Occupational Therapy Association [AOTA], 2008, p. 672). Students and practitioners alike have the power to educate the public about occupational therapy. Students learn to define occupational therapy for class assignments, during student occupational therapy association activities, in their fieldwork participation, and through state and national events.

Practitioners have daily opportunities to define and promote occupation to clients, stakeholders, organizations, and community members. Just how do we define occupation? Many think of occupational therapy very narrowly. Jamnadas, Burns, and Paul (2001) reported that students from physician assistants and nursing professions had perceived knowledge about occupational therapy, but their awareness of the scope of the profession was very narrow. In fact, most of their knowledge regarded activities of daily living (ADL). These results imply that more information about our profession is needed with other professional programs as well as the general public. Additionally, in 1999, Barnhart interviewed different clinicians as part of her attempt to provide strategies for promotion of the profession. She found that therapists felt the general public had a lack of awareness about occupational therapy, but certainly the specifics of what we do as occupational therapists is unknown to most (Barnhart, p. 26).

This chapter will explore promotion of our profession through the art of persuasion, advertisement, and assessing the profession's image. Two case studies will be used to explore how occupational therapy practitioners and



K. Sladyk, K. Jacobs, & N. MacRae (Eds.).
*Occupational Therapy Essentials for Clinical Competence* (pp. 465-468).

students can promote the profession within society, in the business world, and to communities to answer the age-old question, "What is occupational therapy?"

Finally, this chapter will include a review of the literature to provide the reader with information on what has been done to promote our profession both within and external to our field. We will look at literature from occupational therapy as well as other health professions such as nursing and physical therapy. While some literature does exist on promotion of the profession, the majority of what was found was anecdotal or "tips for promotion." Image is also important to the survival of a profession. As occupational therapy practitioners, we have all had the question, "What is occupational therapy?" posed to us. Promotion of a person, product, or service relies on an image. What is our occupational therapy image? If a consistent, representative, and catchy image is lacking, consumers, colleagues, and communities will have difficulty remembering who we are and will therefore have difficulty establishing loyalty to our profession (Scarborough & Zimmerer, 2003).

# Promotion

In order to effectively promote something, you need to have knowledge or awareness of the item or service, understand what it can do for you, and then believe in it (Barnhart, 1999). Promotion involves savvy persuasion of individuals or groups. Promotion also involves a level of advertisement. Persuasion and advertisement are done in many ways, depending on the personality and skills of the promoter (Scarborough & Zimmerer, 2003).

All occupational therapy practitioners know the value of "selling their goods." Our caseloads, number of community contracts, student recruitments for educational programs, and even number of clients in private practices depend on our skills of "selling." Personal, one-to-one selling does have a significant impact (Jacobs, 1998).

Consider the skills of school children selling candy in their neighborhood to promote and fundraise for a school band. Not all will be promotion savvy, but they believe in the band, and their belief is what drives them. As they make sale after sale, they learn that if you make others believe in your product, they will support it.

# Persuasion

Acts of persuasion are as variable as the persuader. From the skills of a 6 year old to the skills of an educated, experienced occupational therapy practitioner, persuasion is powerful if effectively employed. Persuasion involves promotion and can include "publicity, personal selling, and advertising" (Scarborough & Zimmerer, 2003, p. 317). Timing is also included in the art of persuasion. As an effective persuader, you have to know when to pitch the idea, when to push or sell hard, and then when to quit. Leave the other party with just enough information (and contact numbers) and the feeling that this has all been under his or her control. Of course, there is also the strategy of the school child: "Believe it and they will buy." Do not stop talking until they buy the candy, agree to see an occupational therapy practitioner, or choose your educational program over others!

Is one-to-one selling of ideas, images, or services effective? Are we able to persuade our clients, customers, or communities that they need occupational therapy services? Consider the "partnership" that takes place during client-centered practice. In this relationship, there is mutual respect for both parties and an agreement to work together to achieve agreed-upon goals. In this partnership, there is "buy-in" by the client and therapist in order to meet established goals. This is an example of one-to-one selling (Law & Mills, 1998). We also sell one to one when we provide our clients with the evidence that supports our practice. In this one-to-one selling, the client may have an empowered and positive experience with occupational therapy and become a loyal fan. In our education of communities and organizations, occupational therapy is further promoted. Group selling is possibly more powerful and effective than one-to-one selling. Overall, it seems that persuasion is not enough. Advertising our services has become more popular over the past several years. This has been achieved in the national awareness campaign with advertisements about occupational therapy appearing in *People Weekly, Family Circle, Better Homes and Gardens*, and *USA Today* (Jacobs, 1998, p. 620).

# Advertisement

Advertising can have a significant impact for an individual, company, or profession. Advertisements have an agreed upon message by a paid sponsor (Jacobs, 1998; Scarborough & Zimmerer, 2003). Advertisement includes "calling public attention to something, especially by emphasizing desirable qualities so as to arouse a desire to buy or patronize" (Merriam-Webster, 2006).

You may be aware of the national advertisement campaign launched by AOTA in 1997. In the first phase of the campaign, paid messages appeared in a variety of well-known and common household magazines targeted to women between the ages of 35 and 55. In preparation for the sponsored ads, the marketing agency conducted interviews with occupational therapy practitioners to find out the answer to what their practice involved. The outcome was the byline "skills for the job of living" (Jacobs, 1998; Whiting, 1999). This was in effect a redirection of the question, "What is occupation?" The slogan "Occupational therapy: Skills for the job of living" has provided us mileage as a profession, but do more people actually understand the term *occupation*?

The answer is a resounding yes. According to Whiting (1999), there was a 44% increase in requests for information about occupational therapy from 1998 to 1999. In addition, "more than 16 million people, most of them members of our target audience, saw the ads" (p. 5).

In the second phase of the ad campaign, the target audience included managed care organizations, long-term care facilities, and consumers (again, women between the ages of 35 and 55). The results again were very positive. The advertisements "reached over 2.6 million key decision makers in managed care and long-term care" (Whiting, 1999, p. 12). Hundreds of our practice guidelines were requested by people seeing the advertisements, and almost 1.5 million people saw the internet ads. The advertising agency working for AOTA remarked that "this campaign has been a huge success!" (Whiting, p. 12).

In 2008, AOTA launched a new promotional campaign, which replaced the previous tag line with "Living Life to Its Fullest."

Four years ago, the Nursing Association partnered with Johnson & Johnson (New Brunswick, NJ)—a well-known, family-oriented company. Partnering with a "household name" such as Johnson & Johnson has been a "win-win" situation for both parties. The nursing profession has had significant promotion as a result of the Johnson & Johnson advertisement campaign. Nursing has seen an increase in applicants to the professional educational programs, over 8 million dollars has been raised for nursing scholarships, and the first-ever "men in nursing scholarship" has been developed. Finally, there has been increased visibility for the profession overall (Johnson & Johnson, 2006). AOTA's partnership with L.L. Bean (Freeport, ME) to promote National School Backpack Awareness is one such example of partnership in occupational therapy.

The American Physical Therapy Association (APTA) has a national advertisement campaign as well. They are hoping to recruit physical therapist practitioners to promote their own practice or their company with "expertly crafted TV and radio commercials and corresponding print ad tailor-made for the Baby Boomers and Beyond audience whose lives are hindered by chronic aches and pains" (APTA, n.d.). Physical therapists can obtain copies of these commercials from the APTA with all components of the ad campaign, which can be personalized with therapists' contact information.

# Our Image

When you think of our profession, what image comes to mind? It is one thing to define our profession in words; it is another to define our profession in images. Maybe the AOTA's logo is our profession's image. Or is our image based on the stories we read and pictures we see during AOTA's occupational therapy month each year? Perhaps our image is the annual backpack awareness campaign—Luminie, the lightening bug!

Many occupational therapy practitioners and students often have difficulty stating succinctly what we do in occupational therapy. We must explain to our clients and community what we do, the evidence behind why we do it, and the level of education needed to enter the profession.

In the nursing discipline, Lusk (2000) found that nurses from the 1930s to 1950s were seen by the public as subordinate to physicians and hospital administrators. Overall, the nurses of the 1940s were seen as performing more complex activities when compared to the nurses of the 1930s and 1950s. The important message in this article is that nurses of that era were not seen as professional. In the profession of occupational therapy, we want the public to view us as professionals. Image, pride for the profession, and insuring that people know what occupational therapy is are key.

The old adage "a picture is worth a thousand words" might be useful here. In an *OT Practice* issue, the Oklahoma State Association President, Suzanne Bowman, shows off her "OT Cruiser" (Collins, 2002, p. 11). Promoting occupational therapy visually is powerful. Not only does this type of promotion get people talking, but it also can and will convey pride in our profession. Wearing occupational therapy shirts and using pens, note pads, and drink holders with the occupational therapy logo are powerful ways to convey an image of the pride for our profession. Providing clients, consumers, students, and community stakeholders with visual images and "freebies" is a step in the right direction. To equate the profession with an image is memorable and can lead to building a loyal fan base.

# General Promotion

When promoting anything or anyone, the same three principles apply: publicity, personal selling, and advertising (Scarborough & Zimmerer, 2003). We are all capable of doing any or all of these three things. Consider writing an article for *OT Practice* or a letter to the editor for your local newspaper. Sponsor an in-service or seminar for a local agency to promote occupational therapy or go to your child's school and talk to his or her classmates about occupational therapy. Speaking and "selling" to individuals is another approach.

Personal selling for occupational therapy enlists the client-centered approach, but in general, personal selling is that one-to-one relationship between salesperson and consumer or customer. Developing the relationship is often what gives one company the "edge" over another. Having good interpersonal skills is a must when engaging in personal selling. Let the other person talk while you listen, be enthusiastic, pay attention to all details, and measure your success by the client's satisfaction. These are good strategies for effective practitioners as well, but in the end, we might have to resort to advertising our wares.

Advertising can encompass various media types, including magazines, newspapers, direct mail, radio, television, and now the World Wide Web. We have previously discussed occupational therapy's past approach to advertising. These attempts will need to continue in assorted ways to

| Evidence-Based Research Chart | | |
|---|---|---|
| **Promotion Program** | **Activities** | **Evidence** |
| Recruitment strategy; prospective occupational therapy students | Careers pack | Craik & Ross, 2003 |
| National perspective about occupational therapy | Publication/presentation | Dickinson, 2003; Jacobs, 1998 |
| Promotional ideas | "Mediaspeak;" National Awareness Campaign; OT Cruiser; Mass media to promote nursing | Collins, 2002; Walls, 1999; Whitehead, 2000; Whiting, 1999 |
| Awareness/knowledge of occupational therapy; nursing | Marketing; survey | Barnhart, 1999; Jamnadas et al., 2001; Lusk, 2000 |

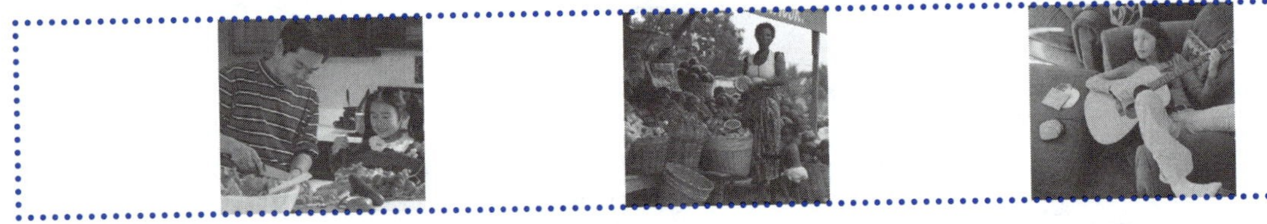

ensure we reach our target populations. The target populations will change over time depending on the message we are sending and, therefore, our media type will have to vary in order to reach our intended audience. Identify your audience and select the most appropriate media to reach them, then go for it!

## Summary

This chapter, along with Chapter 35, provides an overview of promotional strategies that will assist in the marketing of occupational therapy to a broad and complex global community.

## Student Self-Assessment

1. In 15 seconds or less, describe or define occupational therapy. How did you do? Did you get the words *occupation, daily living skills, health promotion,* and *activities of daily living* in there? If you were going to do this activity again, what would you change about your definition?
2. Occupational therapy is a diverse and wide-reaching profession. We often define the profession based on what our role is within the discipline. In order to promote the field of occupational therapy, you need to give your listener a full range of what the profession is and what it can do for them. As another assignment, jot down the first 10 things that come to mind when you think about what an occupational therapist can do for a client, student, resident, community, or organization. What commonalities did you find in your lists? How often do you think about occupational therapy serving communities?

## References


American Occupational Therapy Association. (2008). Occupational therapy practice framework: Domain and process, second edition. *American Journal of Occupational Therapy, 62*, 625-683.

American Physical Therapy Association. (n.d.). Tools & resources. Retrieved July 29, 2009, from http://www.apta.org/AM/Template.cfm?Section=Tools_and_Resources1&Template=/TaggedPage/TaggedPageDisplay.cfm&TPLID=322&ContentID=40239

Barnhart, P. D. (1999). Secrets of success: OTs share their strategies. *OT Practice, 4*(3), 26-30.

Collins, L. (2002). Easy ways to promote occupational therapy. *OT Practice, 8*, 11-14.

Craik, C., & Ross, F. (2003). Promotion of occupational therapy as career: A survey of occupational therapy managers. *British Journal of Occupational Therapy, 66*(2), 78-81.

Dickinson, R. (2003). Occupational therapy: A hidden treasure. *Canadian Journal of Occupational Therapy, 70*(3), 133-135.

Jacobs, K. (1998). Innovation to action: Marketing occupational therapy. *OT Practice, 52*(8), 618-620.

Jamnadas, B., Burns, J., & Paul, S. (2001). Understanding occupational therapy: Nursing and physician assistant students' knowledge about occupational therapy. *Occupational Therapy in Health Care, 14*(1), 13-27.

Johnson & Johnson. (2006). The campaign for nursing's future: A progress report. Retrieved July 29, 2009, from http://www.discovernursing.com/progressreport.pdf

Law, M., & Mills, J. (1998). Client-centered occupational therapy. In M. Law (Ed.), *Client-centered occupational therapy*. Thorofare, NJ: SLACK Incorporated.

Lusk, B. (2000). Pretty and powerless: Nurses in advertisements, 1930-1950. *Research in Nursing and Health, 23*(3), 229-236.

Merriam-Webster. (2006). On-line dictionary, 10th ed. Retrieved June 16, 2006, from http://www.merriam-webster.com

Scarborough, N. M., & Zimmerer, T. W. (2003). *Effective small business management: An entrepreneurial approach* (7th ed.). Upper Saddle River, NJ: Prentice Hall.

Walls, B. S. (1999). Sound bite: OT practitioners learn "mediaspeak." *OT Practice, 4*(7), 7, 20.

Whitehead, D. (2000). Using mass media within health-promoting practice: A nursing perspective. *Journal of Advanced Nursing, 32*(4), 807-816.

Whiting, F. (1999). PromOTing OT: Year two of the national awareness campaign. *OT Practice, 4*(6), 5, 12.

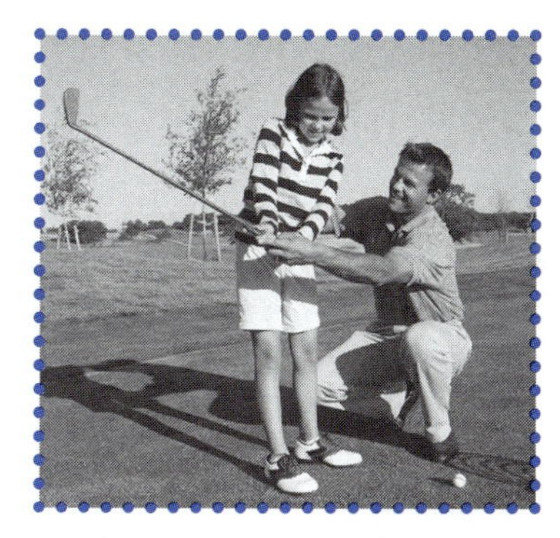

# 43

# Professional Development

*Karen Sladyk, PhD, OTR/L, FAOTA*

**ACOTE Standard Explored in This Chapter**

B.9.4

**Key Terms**

Professional development | Professional portfolio

## Introduction

Celebrations are required when you finish your degree, but those who think that education is finally done are denying themselves and their clients. Learning is lifelong. Those who participate in learning throughout their careers report greater satisfaction and wellness in their personal life (Solovic, 2008).

Graduates report that they feel like both an expert and a total novice at the same time. Occupational therapy education has provided new graduates with the skills to be a competent entry-level practitioner (Accreditation Council for Occupational Therapy Education, 2006), yet competency is a dynamic concept, requiring the updating of an ongoing set of skills (American Occupational Therapy Association [AOTA], 1995). Thus, professional development needs to be a lifelong dynamic goal for all occupational therapy practitioners to assist them in growing professionally.

## American Occupational Therapy Association Membership

Less than half of all occupational therapy practitioners are members of AOTA, yet the answer to almost every professional question you have is likely housed in AOTA. When graduates are asked why they are not members, "money" and "forgetting" are the most common answers. Like all membership organizations, AOTA supports its members. It makes sense that valuable resources are not going to be used answering nonmember questions, so if your peers are not members, they should not be angry when they do not get assistance when they call AOTA for help with a problem. Can you walk into a social club and expect to be served lunch at members' prices? AOTA is a nonprofit organization developed by its members to serve its members. AOTA has a wealth of knowledge and is eager to share with members, so if you forgot to renew your membership, call them and join. If money is your justification, membership is less than 75 cents per day (you cannot even get a cup of coffee for that), and AOTA has a Medicare voice on Capital Hill everyday. With your membership fees, you also get professionals who advocate for occupational therapy to the public; professionals who fight cuts to reimbursements; professionals who work with states to keep occupational therapy practice from being invaded by other disciplines; a full occupational therapy library; a sleek Web site; a place to post your resume; a huge national occupational therapy conference; and access to numerous discounts on insurance, credit cards, or travel costs. An occupational therapist making $45 per hour is really making 75 cents per minute. AOTA membership is equal to



K. Sladyk, K. Jacobs, & N. MacRae (Eds.).
*Occupational Therapy Essentials for Clinical Competence* (pp. 469-474).

1 minute of work per day. If an occupational therapy practitioner tried to just be an advocate, it would take more than one minute a day. It makes financial and time-management sense to pay AOTA 1 minute of your pay per day.

AOTA has a wealth of formal and informal professional development opportunities such as the *American Journal of Occupational Therapy* (*AJOT*), the trade magazine *OT Practice*, numerous self-study programs, a national conference, special traveling regional conferences, the Wilma West Library, a foundation that supports research, a book and publication department, a Web site with up-to-the-minute information, fax-on-demand services, and live people who answer your calls when you need information. Many of these professional development opportunities award certificates for state licensure or workplace requirements. AOTA (1995) has developed a self-appraisal booklet that can guide you in assessing your current skills and developing a professional development plan. In addition, AOTA is working with the national certification organization (www.nbcot.org) to collaborate on future professional development requirements for the profession.

Besides joining AOTA, consider joining your state occupational therapy association. This is a wonderful place to network and develop leadership skills through volunteering. AOTA can provide you with the state association membership contact person, or you can check around at your school—applications are likely posted on a bulletin board.

## Long- and Short-Term Professional Goals

Well, you finally can answer, "What do you want to be when you grow up?" Now the question is, "What occupations are in your life, and what occupations are future goals?" Consider timeline goal writing. What are your personal and professional goals for 1 year, 5 years, 10 years, lifetime? There is no reason to separate personal and professional goals. As we know from the study of occupation (AOTA, 2008), no one role stands alone. A new graduate may have a short-term goal to find a generalist entry-level position in occupational therapy, but may also have plans to marry and start a family.

Career goals change over a lifetime because when you grow, your career goals grow too (Ellis, 2000). Skills developed in an occupational therapy career are helpful in other careers. Many occupational therapy practitioners have opened their own businesses, including play equipment, career coaching, craft supplies, and even a quilt shop.

By reviewing your long- and short-term goals, you can begin to plan your professional development. A specific professional development plan will be the ladder to accomplishing your goals. Finding the right combination of educational opportunities becomes the foundation to your professional development. Keep records of your journey in planning and implementing your professional development in a professional portfolio (see Chapter 44).

## Formal Versus Informal Education

More education? Think about what it is like when you go away on vacation. You eat all of your favorite foods and do all kinds of fun stuff. Oddly, by the end of your vacation, you are looking forward to getting home. Once you are home, you wonder what it would be like to go back on vacation. While you are in school, the thought of more school does not sound appealing, but you may feel differently later.

Formal education is typically a college degree or a formal organizational certificate, while informal education, often called continuing education, includes a variety of learning from having a mentor to attending a local conference. There are many experts in education who will argue that one type of education is better than another type. You will likely get advice on this topic even if you do not seek the advice. The ultimate opinion, of course, is yours. Educating yourself using either informal or formal education will help keep you current in your field. Many options are available to you.

## Formal Professional Development Opportunities

Formal education is less varied than informal education but generally more highly regarded by society as a valued educational experience. Typically, this includes college degrees and specialty certifications from recognized organizations. Although higher in costs and time commitments, formal education is easier to document because of the resulting degree or credential.

Traditional formal education means returning to college or university to seek a higher degree than the one you currently possess. The benefits of another degree might include self-esteem, promotion, pay raise, and mastery of a subject. Some workplaces offer promotion or pay raises with another degree, while others do not. Many workplaces even encourage college study by offering special discounts, time off, or tuition reimbursement programs. If you think you are likely to return to college after you start working, be sure to check into tuition assistance programs with the personnel department when you interview.

In addition, online formal degree programs have shown enormous growth in the last few years. As with anything online, the potential student needs to fully investigate the program. Does the school have accreditation? Is the school nonprofit or for profit? Are the faculty employed by the institution or are they contract teachers? How does the community view the degree? Degrees that are "accelerated" mean different things in different institutions. You need to know what you are buying online.

Returning to college means evaluating your professional development goals and deciding if you want to further your studies in occupational therapy or in a supporting area. In addition, you may be able to move to a new city or may be limited to what is drivable to your current job. You will need to consider your budget and the tuition reimbursement rules of work, if the school is willing to take part-time students, and how the schedule meets your needs.

Almost every school has at least an abbreviated catalog on their Web site, so the traditional way of calling schools and requesting a catalog is now old-fashion. Web sites typically have virtual campus tours and student testimonials that can provide you with information about the college. However, remember that a Web site is really only an advertisement. Screen possible schools by talking with people in your community. Once you view the catalogs, look for programs of interest. Consider the tuition costs and what you can afford.

## Doctoral Degrees

The idea of a doctoral degree may not be appealing at this time. However, many practitioners have thought about this degree for both professional development or career advancement. Doctoral-level work is most certainly a challenge at which many occupational therapists have succeeded. If you hold as your goal a faculty appointment or advance practice in a leading institution, doctoral-level education is highly desirable.

Just like the degrees mentioned previously, doctorates can be in occupational therapy or a related area (Sladyk, 1997). Several universities offer doctoral education in occupational therapy, and some contain online classes that limit required time on campus. For those interested in other related areas, it is possible to combine your love of occupational therapy with a new study area. For example, most doctoral programs will allow you to transfer up to two classes. Most will allow independent studies. So, if you are an occupational therapist studying adult learning, you may be able to transfer a class in clinical reasoning and a class on fieldwork into your program. An independent study can compare and contrast clinical reasoning with theories on critical thinking in adulthood. Lastly, you can use occupational therapy as a component of your dissertation. Check with the doctoral program you are interested in for their rules and regulations.

If you think a doctorate is in your future, consider looking at combination programs that give you a master's degree on your way to your doctorate (Peters, 1997). Also, carefully weigh out the benefits of a PhD, ScD, EdD or clinical doctorate (OTD). Each has its own benefits. Although all require great disciplined study, the PhD has a long history of being well-established and is often privately acknowledged as the preferred degree. In some universities, the PhD is the only acceptable degree for tenure. Lastly, understand the program requirements before you start. Is there a required full-time residency? Are part-time classes available? How is the research component of the degree managed? The more you know before you start, the easier it will be to finish.

## Specialty Certifications

Many professional organizations, including AOTA, offer specialty certificates. Some organizations provide intensive education followed by testing to gain certification such as NDT (neurodevelopment treatment) or SI (sensory integration) training. Other organizations provide strict qualification requirements followed by testing to gain credentials such as "Board certified in..." Each organization can provide you with the requirements of the certification. AOTA has two different programs available for documenting excellence in a specialty or area of practice. Members can access this information online. Having the requirements in mind well before you qualify can help you design your professional development plan to prepare you for future certifications.

## Informal Professional Development Opportunities

If returning for formal education does not fit your style, informal professional development opportunities might better meet your current needs. Continuing education has seen an explosion of ideas in occupational therapy recently. Pick up any occupational therapy trade magazine and you will find pages of educational opportunities. Not only are conferences listed, but AOTA offers members self-study programs, online computer education, and a national occupational therapy conference that attracts over 5,000 people at one time. Many occupational therapy practitioners favor traditional conferences for continuing education, but informal learning can take many forms.

Opportunities for professional development in informal educational experiences include the following:

- *AJOT*, SIS newsletters, *OT Practice* magazine
- AOTA annual conference
- Asking an expert at work to mentor you
- New books recently published
- Online computer conference and online practice support
- Participating in peer review
- Participating in research projects
- Self-study programs
- State occupational therapy association conferences and SIS groups
- Supervising level I or II students
- Trade magazines in occupational therapy
- Volunteering to present a topic
- Work performance review
- Workplace in-services or journal clubs
- Workshops or seminars
- Writing for publication

An important aspect of any educational experience is not just participating, but the resulting knowledge being used effectively in your practice (Hinojosa et al., 2000). Documenting knowledge gained from informal education is more difficult than formal education but equally important. Each conference or program should have established outcome objectives before you sign up. Consider demonstrating your continuing competence through attendance certificates, examinations, work performance reviews, peer reviews, summative paper or presentation, or a professional portfolio.

Many occupational therapy schools offer free or inexpensive conferences related to educational issues such as fieldwork. These conferences allow attendees to enjoy the latest information about education at a greatly reduced price. In addition, occupational therapists can share experiences and educational models that are effective in the clinic. Sometimes, occupational therapy schools offer certificates of advanced training. When you take a cluster of master-level classes, you earn the certificate. Those interested in continuing on to an advanced degree can count the certificate classes toward a master's degree.

Online classes or self-study programs allow practitioners to study a topic at their own pace without leaving their home or workplace. These self-contained conferences award certificates of completion, and some can be accepted for master's degree credits. With these types of continuing education opportunities, rural occupational therapy assistants and occupational therapists can participate without leaving home. Self-study programs can be done in a small group, allowing for questions and feedback, as well as networking. Other online services are available from AOTA, including resources for help on special problems.

Many individual and specialty groups also offer conferences. You will find these listed in the occupational therapy trade magazines. Fees for these conferences vary greatly, and the topics are usually specific with some advanced skills required. The best way to stay up to date on these specialty topics is to scan the conference listings regularly.

Often, continuing education opportunities are mailed directly to your home. *AJOT* provides you with monthly, up-to-date research in occupational therapy. Readers are sometimes intimidated by the level of writing, but the editor and reviewers work hard to make the articles clear. The more you read the journal, the more you will understand. One way to better understand journal articles is to first read about evidence-based practice concepts. Check your college textbooks for an introduction to evidence-based practice. Understanding these foundational skills will make reading the articles helpful.

*AJOT* makes an excellent continuing education opportunity because it is delivered to you, is self-paced, and is available at no additional cost with your membership. *OT Practice* provides a more informal continuing education opportunity by focusing on current practice in a practical format. Like *AJOT*, it comes right to your home and is included with your AOTA membership. Often, *OT Practice* has self-study units included in the magazine. Read the self-study article, take a short multiple-choice test, pay a small fee, and get continuing education credit.

## Self-Appraisal and Action Plan

The endless professional development opportunities available for occupational therapy practitioners make it necessary to develop a personalized action plan to specifically address your professional development needs. Linking your professional goals, your continuing education, and your self-assessment of your new skills is part of the action plan. Once you have your professional development action plan clear, how will you document your skills so you can show potential future employers? Consider developing a portfolio to document your goal, plans, participation, and self-appraisal. This portfolio can be used to store evidence needed for licensure renewals. AOTA can provide assistance in professional portfolio development.

## Summary

It is your professional responsibility to stay current in the practice of occupational therapy because it is important to your consumers of occupational therapy. Furthering your education can take two different roads. First, formal education such as returning to a college or university for another degree can develop or refine skills. Second, less formal continuing education allows learners to be specific in their learning needs. Educational experts disagree as to which type is best. Learners must evaluate their own needs and then establish a professional development action plan specific to their needs. This action plan includes documentation of professional skills developed.

## Student Self-Assessment

1. Draw a time line on rolled paper from graduation day to retirement day. Mark projected milestones in your personal and professional life.
2. Investigate the costs and time commitments of several conferences. Average out the per-hour costs to the participants.
3. Make a list of benefits from AOTA and divide out the current student fees and professional fees per day. List items you can buy for the same per-day fee.

# References


Accreditation Council for Occupational Therapy Education. (2006). *Standards for an accredited educational program for the occupational therapist*. Bethesda, MD: AOTA Press.

American Occupational Therapy Association. (1995). *Developing, maintaining, and updating competency in occupational therapy: A guide to self-appraisal*. Bethesda, MD: Author.

American Occupational Therapy Association. (2008). Occupational therapy practice framework: Domain and process, second edition. *American Journal of Occupational Therapy, 62*, 625-683.

Ellis, D. (2000). *Becoming a master student*. Boston, MA: Houghton Mifflin Company.

Hinojosa, J., Bowen, R., Case-Smith, J., Epstein, C., Moyers, P., & Schwope, C. (2000). Self-initiated continuing competence. *OT Practice*, December, CE1-CE8.

Peters, R. L. (1997). *Getting what you came for: The smart student's guide to earning a masters or a PhD*. New York, NY: The Noonday Press.

Sladyk, K. (1997). Graduate school and continuing education. In K. Sladyk (Ed.), *OT student primer: A guide to college success* (pp. 323-329). Thorofare, NJ: SLACK Incorporated.

Solovic, S. W. (2008). *The girl's guide to building a million-dollar business*. New York, NY: AMACOM American Management Association.

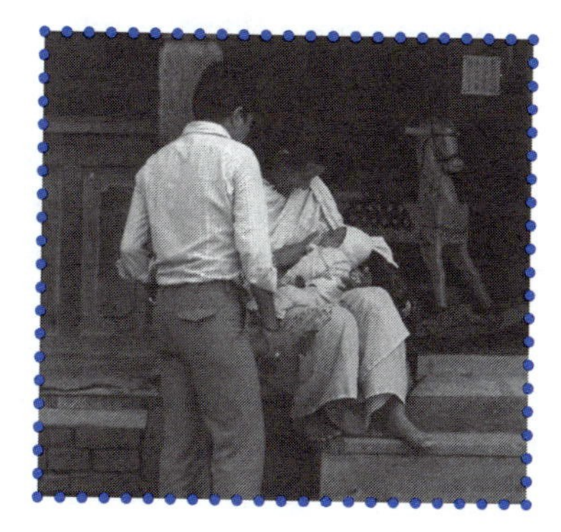

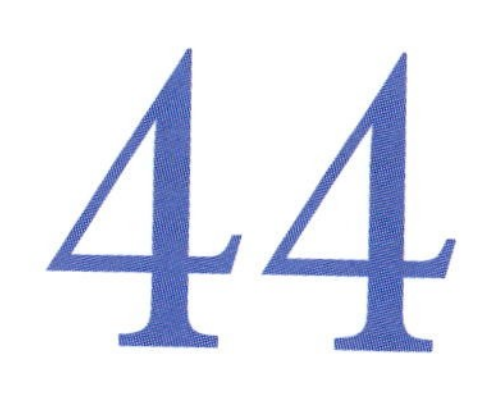

# Competence and Professional Development

*Penelope A. Moyers, EdD, BCMH, OTR/L, FAOTA*

**ACOTE Standard Explored in This Chapter**

B.9.6

**Key Terms**

| | |
|---|---|
| Competencies | Professional development |
| Continuing competence | Professional portfolio |
| Continuing competency | Self-assessment |

## Introduction

"In today's complex world, we must educate not merely for competence, but for capability (the ability to adapt to change, generate new knowledge, and continuously improve performance)" (Fraser & Greenhalgh, 2001).

The stakes for being competent as occupational therapists and occupational therapy assistants continue to rise with the advent of evidence-based practice (Moyers & Hinojosa, 2003). We still need to focus on preventing harm by ensuring that our clients are not seriously injured during implementation of services due to practitioner neglect or malpractice or due to poor risk management. However, harm now has a broader meaning. In addition, harm results when our clients receive ineffective intervention or intervention not as effective as an alternative method in improving occupational performance and participation in daily life. Harm also results from occupational therapy population- or organization-based services that are poorly designed, implemented, and evaluated. The harm that occurs relates to the cost-benefit of services in terms of the expenditures made for poor outcomes. Additionally, the client, organization, or population may have to assume other costs associated with intervention continuing over a longer duration than expected, with the additional burden for care giving resulting from reduced performance in activities of daily living, with the loss of the worker role to support daily living, and with the possible reduction in the economic viability of the community if a large population or organization is negatively affected by ineffective programming. Policy for reimbursement of medically based services is beginning to incorporate the concept of paying for performance or the outcome achieved after intervention (Sautter et al., 2007).

Because of the increasing pressure for accountability related to health care and social service outcomes, employers, third-party payers, community agencies, business, and industry all expect practitioners to remain competent and knowledgeable of the new developments in the field of occupational therapy and in related contextual areas involving local, state, national, and global communities. No longer is it acceptable to believe that an occupational therapist or



K. Sladyk, K. Jacobs, & N. MacRae (Eds.).
*Occupational Therapy Essentials for Clinical Competence* (pp. 475-484).

occupational therapy assistant enters practice thoroughly trained, possessing all of the knowledge needed throughout one's career. The career path taken should be punctuated with learning and knowledge management strategies to enhance professional development and continuing competence and competency.

In this chapter, the framework (American Occupational Therapy Association [AOTA], 2008) will be used to understand the occupation of education, particularly as learning is important for continuing competence and competency and professional development. These terms then are differentiated to highlight the three distinct purposes of the different types of learning. A model proposes how change occurs and describes how assessment links practice performance, career growth, and learning. Based upon any gap between actual and desired practice performance or gap between desired career development and actual career trajectory, a learning plan is developed that includes feasible strategies thought best to narrow these gaps and most likely to produce a measurable change in client daily life participation outcomes and in achievement of the practitioner's career goals. The roles of administrators, organizations, professional organizations, universities, continuing education providers, credentialing bodies, and government in fostering this model are described.

## Education as an Occupation

"Lifelong learning means that education converges with (and is influenced by) work, family, and personal development" (Fraser & Greenhalgh, 2001).

Education in the framework addresses the "activities needed for learning and participating in the environment" (AOTA, 2008, p. 638). One can be a student beyond the formal education years when exploring learning needs and interests and participating in "classes, programs, and activities that provide instruction/training in identified areas of interest" (AOTA, p. 638). This chapter is concerned with the education related to the occupation of work after one has completed entry-level formal education as an occupational therapist or occupational therapy assistant. This lifelong education throughout one's career requires the practitioner to not only possess the necessary underlying motor and praxis, sensory-perceptual, emotional regulation, cognitive, and communication and social performance skills, but also the ability to adapt new knowledge and skills to one's professional roles in order to be a successful learner.

Learning as a part of the educational process is influenced by social, cultural, physical, virtual, temporal, and personal contexts. For instance, the social expectations of the public and the profession are for the practitioner to be competent and up to date in the skills associated with providing a high-quality service. The organization in which one works may have a culture in which learning is left up to the individual practitioner rather than one that values learning as an aspect of organizational performance. The physical environment could be designed where learning is either facilitated or inhibited, depending upon the learning preferences of the learner. Often, virtual synchronous or asynchronous environments, whether in the form of list serves, online courses, blogs, conference calls, and Web sites, are where learning occurs in order to accommodate geographical distance and a variety of schedule differences among learners. Thus, virtual contexts allow learners to individually address the temporal contextual needs of their daily life and biorhythms so that learning can occur at the most opportune time. The personal contextual factors of age, educational level, and socioeconomic status can influence learning in terms of the design of the education (e.g., education with expectations for large amounts of memorization may be difficult for older learners; or learners with young children may have less time to engage in educational offerings occurring over a long duration or requiring travel and overnight stays away from the family) and costs associated with the educational offering (e.g., participating in some offerings may be cost prohibitive for practitioners with little employer support, lower salaries, and family financial pressures).

## Competence, Competency, and Professional Development

The word *continuing* is typically combined with both competence and competency to denote a lifelong learning process. Often, the terms *competence* and *competency* are used interchangeably when, in fact, there is an important difference between these two concepts. Competence "refers to an individual's capacity to perform" professional responsibilities, whereas competency "focuses on an individual's actual performance in a particular situation" (McConnell, 2001, p. 14). Professional development is a process where one plans and achieves excellence, establishes expertise, seeks a change in responsibilities, or assumes more complex professional roles (Moyers & Hinojosa, 2003). Continuing competence and competency are requirements for one's current professional responsibilities in a given role in contrast to professional development, which involves what one aspires to achieve regardless of one's present position or role. Professional development may not focus on what one needs to learn in order to perform better but rather may address what one is interested in learning in order to advance one's career.

Continuing competence is designed to build capacity to perform one's responsibilities in the future for a given role. Occupational therapy practice and health care in general advances rapidly, so a practitioner who does not engage in continuing competence activities will become markedly out-of-date in a short amount of time. For example, if a new documentation system is going to be implemented, training would need to occur to properly prepare for the change. Because neither the systems in which we work nor the external environment will ever be constant (Fraser & Greenhalgh, 2001), educating for capacity is becoming more important.

Continuing competency in contrast ensures that the practitioner performs according to standard given that a distinctive set of variables dynamically interact, resulting in each client situation being unique. It is well known that practitioner performance is highly context dependent, with a practitioner possibly having better outcomes in one situation compared to another similar situation (Handfield-Jones et al., 2002). With continuing competency, there is also an assumption that all practitioner skills and abilities fade with lack of practice, feedback, or administrative/system support.

Another factor important in understanding both continuing competence and competency is that there is not a linear relationship between learning and improved practice performance. Instead, there may be periods of time when there is either no improvement or even a slight decrease in performance. These periods of little change then may be followed by sudden jumps in practice performance (Handfield-Jones et al., 2002). Because most practice is based on cognitively complex tasks, learning typically requires cognitive reorganization that may involve abandonment of previously held ideas and principles. Therefore, the impact of learning on practice appears to occur in sudden leaps rather than through continuous and gradual change. Consequently, while practice performance improves in some areas, it may simultaneously deteriorate in others.

# Self-Assessment Model

The learning of currently practicing occupational therapists and occupational therapy assistants is very different from what occurred when students were in the professional program. The focus at that time was upon learning generalist practice and a core set of competencies, allowing few opportunities to learn any particular interest area in depth. Level II fieldwork and the first 1 or 2 years on the job have typically been the time for specialized learning and, more recently, the entry-level doctorate could allow time for delving into these interest areas. The first several years in a position where intensive job training occurs, however, is now complicated not only by the need to focus learning efforts to enhance performance but by the requirement to simultaneously keep up with advances in these specialty areas. As a result, practitioners are expected to engage in and employers must facilitate a systematic approach to learning that considers learning styles, client populations, career stage, and influence of previous learning, while at the same time understanding the barriers and supports for application of new learning within practice. Learning plans maximize the practitioner's educational efforts to enhance therapy outcomes and to advance one's career (Wilkinson, et al., 2002). Thus, learning is a process to be managed, one necessitating a dynamic approach to target the learning needs that arise from daily practice and from one's goals for career development.

In order to link practice performance with learning, the occupational therapist and occupational therapy assistant have to engage in a self-assessment process (Figure 44-1). "Self-assessment provides the means by which therapists and assistants develop goals and plans for professional growth, reassess current goals, assess performance, analyze demands and resources of the work environment, and interpret information about the consumers' outcomes" (Moyers & Hinojosa, 2003, p. 484). Self-assessment for the development of a learning plan should primarily be formative (i.e., assessments conducted to determine what needs to be learned and how best to learn), as summative assessments (i.e., assessments conducted to determine what has been learned) are mainly used for employee evaluation, certification programs, or licensure. Self-assessment answers the question, "What can I do to improve competence and competency in my job or role?" Self-assessment can also answer what one needs to do to advance one's career (Smith & Tillema, 2001). Self-assessment not only locates discrepancies in current practice compared to some ideal, but it also validates what is going well. In terms of professional development, self-assessment ascertains strengths and how to further develop those strengths in preparation for career advancement.

# Job Responsibilities and Client Outcomes

Self-assessment begins with an analysis of one's job responsibilities and roles, typically answering the following questions:

- What are my main responsibilities and roles?
- Within those roles, what are my most significant job tasks?
- What kinds of expertise are required to produce successful outcomes?
- What are the criteria for successful performance?

Then, the self-assessment incorporates information from one's own work performance, and would include answering such questions as the following:

- How do outcomes data inform my learning needs?
- Is improvement in my performance indicated?
- Are there systems problems I can help modify?
- What can I do to improve efficiency and effectiveness of occupational therapy services?

Self-assessment for professional development is slightly different and includes such questions as the following:

- What are my goals for my career?
- What roles will I need to develop?
- What kinds of tasks might be included in these roles?

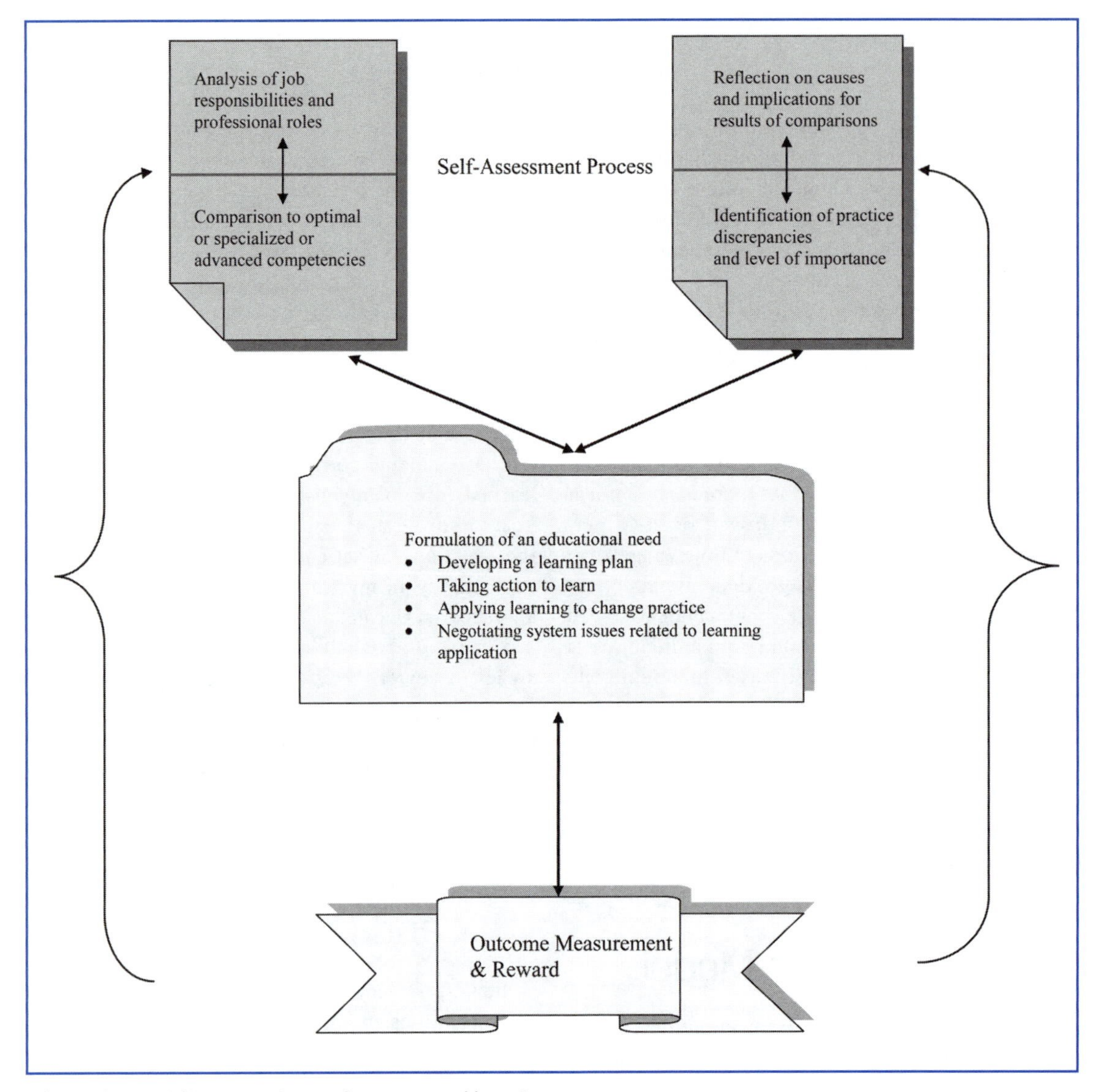


**Figure 44-1.** Linking practice performance and learning.

- What skills and types of reasoning are involved in these tasks?
- What is my current skill level and reasoning ability in comparison to what might be required for these new tasks?
- What are the criteria for successful performance?

Generally, the practitioner learns to compare his or her current practice performance with some ideal or desired result. To be helpful, self-assessment for the practitioner requires the gathering of valid and reliable information about one's appropriateness and adequacy in working with clients in terms of helping them achieve occupational performance and participation goals. Self-assessments may include knowledge tests, skills checkouts, performance observations, case studies, self-reflection, peer ratings, records audits, outcomes data, or consumer feedback (Ward, Gruppen, & Regehr, 2002). Self-assessment for professional development typically requires feedback from a mentor or from someone who is in a similar role in comparison to the one in which one hopes to assume.

The question is, how does one determine what is the desirable practice or desired professional skill development? This requires research into the existence of practice guidelines or standards, protocols, professional benchmarks, expert recommendations, efficacy and effectiveness studies, and meta-analyses or systematic evidence reviews, as well as expectations of employers, clients, third-party payers, and the public.

## Competencies

Competencies are another type of standard guiding self-assessment. Competencies are explicit statements that define specific areas of expertise or competency (Decker, 1999), of which there are four types, including those that are (Decker & Strader, 1997):

1. Generic across all jobs in an organization
2. Related to management, supervision, or leadership roles
3. Threshold or minimum requirements of a job
4. Specific to a job

A sample statement to illustrate how competencies are written is "ability to select the most appropriate assessment instrument given the client's age, health and disability status, values, goals, and preferences for specific occupational performance outcomes." This is a threshold statement that could be written to be more specific to a specialized area of occupational therapy practice by referring to an age range or other demographics, diagnoses, type of occupational performance, or method of intervention.

## Discrepancies

Practice discrepancies uncovered through self-assessment do not always necessitate a change in practice, but careful analysis is needed to determine whether modification is needed. The practitioner reflects upon why the difference exists as perhaps there is system, population, or other key circumstances that explain why one's results are dissimilar to the benchmarks. The size of the gap between what exists and what should occur in practice or in professional development contributes to motivation for change in that a small discrepancy may be overlooked as unimportant and a large discrepancy may appear impossible to resolve (Handfield-Jones et al., 2002). Ultimately, an educational need is identified that prompts development and implementation of a learning plan. The desired change has to be divisible into small, manageable learning steps.

Learning then has to be applied to practice to bring about a change with thought given to how to measure the impact of the learning application upon client satisfaction and outcomes. Application to practice requires removal of system barriers and creation of system supports in which administration plays a key role. For instance, if the occupational therapist has learned how to administer a reliable and valid occupational performance assessment tool that has evidence in its effectiveness in developing occupation-based intervention, but there are no funds available to purchase the instrument, space to administer the evaluation, or time allowed to complete the evaluation, nor an intervention philosophy that supports occupation-based practice, then the practitioner will be unable to apply this new learning. Similarly, learning will be difficult to apply to professional development if the new opportunities or roles are not available in one's employment or within one's professional roles.

## Motivation for Learning

Motivation for learning is complicated and is dependent upon one's understanding of the ethical nature inherent in the learning process. The competence of the occupational therapist and the occupational therapy assistant provides the moral justification for implementing occupational therapy processes and services (Moyers, 2005). Principle 4 of the AOTA *Code of Ethics* (AOTA, 2000) indicates the practitioner's responsibility for maintaining high standards of competence. In many states, mandatory continuing education is an aspect of licensure renewal. Similarly, the National Board for Certification in Occupational Therapy (NBCOT) has requirements for achievement of Professional Development Units (PDUs) in the renewal process for the practitioner to use the initials OTR or COTA, whichever is appropriate. The Joint Commission on the Accreditation of Healthcare Organizations (JCAHO), which accredits hospitals and other health care organizations, has standards that require all employees to update and demonstrate competence to carry out the job tasks assigned.

Motivation to engage in self-assessment and ongoing learning activities, in addition to external requirements of employers and credentialing and accrediting bodies, has an intrinsic component partially related to the virtues of being a "good" occupational therapist or occupational therapy assistant. The practitioner must display the integrity to self-assess as honestly as possible as a part of one's altruistic responsibility for providing optimal client services (Moyers, 2005). Prudence as a virtue facilitates the disciplined pursuit of competence in which there is a sincere effort to learn what will most likely contribute to excellent client outcomes and high levels of service satisfaction (Moyers). The practitioner must also have certain underlying abilities to support learning, such as the "requisite intellectual skill and cognitive complexity to understand and synthesize" information, the emotional ability to take risks in applying learning, and the relational abilities to inform clients and work within the system to implement learning application (Moyers, p. 28). Obviously, learning application that leads to successful practice change in enhancing service outcomes has the potential for creating an iterative self-assessment process as the result of motivation derived from the quality improvement process itself.

## Development and Implementation of the Learning Plan

Given the complexity of the roles occupational therapists and occupational therapy assistants assume, the questions guiding the development and implementation of the learning plan, whether for continuing competency and competence or professional development, are shown in Table 44-1.

The job competencies thought most likely to lead to high-quality client outcomes are addressed in the learning plan. These selected competencies are analyzed through the

| Table 44-1. Learning Questions and Learning Purposes | | | |
|---|---|---|---|
| **Questions** | **Continuing Competence** | **Continuing Competency** | **Professional Development** |
| Trigger for learning | Does trend information or forecasts indicate that a change in my typical practice will be required in the future for my current role? | Is there a gap between my practice outcomes and what is standard or what is ideal? | In order to assume another position, to be promoted, or to undertake professional leadership, what do I need to learn given my current skills and abilities? |
| Timing | When should learning occur given the likelihood that the prediction about future practice is feasible in my practice context? | When should learning occur given the importance of the standard to outcomes and to safety? | When should learning occur given my career goals and opportunities? |
| Content | What specific content for learning that might be applied in my practice context is suggested by the trend data or forecasts? | What specific evidence-based learning content would most likely improve safety or outcomes in my practice? | What specific learning content would best prepare me for my future roles? |
| Learning methods and strategies | How should the learning be organized and delivered given the application feasibility issues? | How should the learning be organized and delivered to ensure application to practice according to standard insuring improvements in outcomes or safety? | How should the learning be organized and delivered to assist me in developing potentially applicable skills and abilities needed for assumption of other roles and responsibilities? |
| Location of learning | How important is learning in the context of my practice given that feasibility of application may or may not yet be determined? | How can I implement learning in the context of my practice so that I am able to apply the new learning to practice more effectively and efficiently? | How can I locate opportunities to apply learning so that skills and abilities will not erode before I reach my career goals? |
| Educational providers and role of employer | Who is producing the most up-to-date information on this trend, and is conducting the latest research applicable to my practice? | How can I work with my employer to create learning opportunities within the context of my practice? | Is my employer supportive of my career goals and should I consider locating a mentor outside of work to help me get started? |
| Application | What aspect of the learning could be applied to practice in the near future? Do I need more education and training before application? | What aspect of the learning must be applied to practice in order to better meet standards for safety and for outcomes? | What aspect of the learning could be implemented if I take advantage of upcoming career opportunities? |
| Context, environment, or system | What aspects of the practice context support or inhibit the feasibility of learning application in the near future? | What barriers in the practice context require removal and what supports should be put in place in order to assist me in meeting standards and achieving outcomes? | What barriers and supports in my professional context exist that would impact application of learning if I seek specific career opportunities? |
| Modifying context | What are the best strategies to enhance feasibility of learning being applied to practice in the near future? | What strategies would be effective in modifying the practice context to support immediate application of learning so that standards are met and outcomes are improved? | What do I need to do to make sure I can take advantage of opportunities to apply new skills and abilities in order to meet my career goals? |
| Evaluation of the impact of learning | How will I know if my learning has made a difference in practice given questions of feasibility of application? Should I target evaluation primarily to change in knowledge? | How and when should the impact of learning on client outcomes be measured, or how will I know my learning has been effective in meeting standards? | What formative and summative skill and ability evaluations should I implement to give me feedback about my progress toward my career goals? |

help of the *Standards for Continuing Competence* (AOTA, 2005), which includes how critical and ethical reasoning, interpersonal and performance skills, and knowledge contribute to successful enactment of each competency. For instance, refer to the sample competency described earlier—select the best assessment given the client's age, health and disability status, and goals for occupational performance. This competency requires knowledge of assessments available to measure the specific occupational performance. Critical reasoning involves the ability to select, according to best evidence, the assessment most likely to accurately and reliably assess the occupational performance of interest given the client's characteristics, values, and needs. The performance skill underlying this competency is the ability to administer the assessment according to standardization. Collaboratively selecting the assessment and explaining the evaluation process to promote client decision making is the requisite interpersonal ability. Weighing pragmatic issues of the evaluation process against client needs includes an ethical reasoning ability.

Also, in order to develop an effective learning plan, one needs to be aware of the best methods for learning performance and interpersonal skills, gaining knowledge, and developing critical and ethical reasoning. For instance, reading may be appropriate for gaining knowledge but does not compare to role playing and simulation strategies that may be more effective in enhancing interpersonal abilities. Learning plans typically include learning goals, target dates for completion of the learning activities, learning activities, resources needed to implement the plan, how one plans to apply the learning to practice, and how one will determine the effectiveness of learning. Learning goals are derived from the learning needs identified in the self-assessment, relate to the job competencies and the *Standards for Continuing Competence* (AOTA, 2005), and lead to learning applied to practice.

In general, learning for competent performance against standards, for developing capacity, and for professional development must address the intricacy of today's practice environment regardless of one's roles within that environment. Because occupational therapists and occupational therapy assistants assume roles where problem solving occurs in complex environments, the cognitive processes are similar to creative thinking (Fraser & Greenhalgh, 2001). Therefore, learning approaches should be designed to facilitate the creative thinking involved in the ability to "appraise the situation as a whole, prioritize issues, and then integrate and make sense of many different sources of data to arrive at a solution" (Fraser & Greenhalgh, p. 801). These creative learning approaches are nonlinear in nature or are designed to help learners capture a situation in its "holistic complexity" (Fraser & Greenhalgh, p. 801). Nonlinear learning methods typically involve storytelling, case histories, reflection, and problem-based learning strategies. There is an emphasis upon self-directed learning where the learner is supported in developing his or her own learning goals, receiving feedback, reflecting, and consolidating one's ideas. These self-directed learning goals avoid rigid and prescriptive content; the subject matter may vary depending on the needs of the learner. There also should be efforts to capture the benefits of informal and unplanned learning. Some examples of these learning methods include the following (Fraser & Greenhalgh, p. 802):

- Experiential learning (i.e., job shadowing or apprenticeships)
- Networking opportunities
- Reflection exercises
- List serves for professional interest groups
- "Teachback" opportunities where newly skilled practitioners teach others their shared understanding
- Feedback on the application of the learning

# Portfolios

Portfolios archive the self-assessment process described in the model, including the reflection on the self-assessment to determine learning needs related to job-related competencies or to professional development aspirations (Tillema, 2001). The learning plan devised to address the learning needs is also housed in the portfolio, along with evidence of engagement in the various learning activities, such as specialty certifications or professional recognition and documentation of continuing education, coursework, publications, or presentations. Each learning activity is carefully appraised to ensure the activity contributes to achievement of the learning competencies. The self-appraisal process answers the question, "What evidence would best indicate my potential for possessing the competencies needed for practice?"

The most complete portfolios are reflective in nature as there is an examination of why one chose a particular learning activity and how participation in that activity affected one's practice relative to the specific competency. Reflection connects learning application to practice with client outcomes. For instance, if the competency is about administering specialized assessments, then why was writing a case study chosen, how did constructing the case study contribute to knowing how and when to administer particular assessments, and how did the client evaluation experience change as the result of applying the learning to practice? Portfolios used to document one's continuing competence or competency or professional development processes are thus quite different in complexity and should not be considered the same as a scrapbook of personal and professional achievements, an archive of all one has ever done in one's life or career, or a collection of random continuing education certificates and program handouts. Portfolios can demonstrate the potential for continuing competence and competency, especially if requiring evidence of the following (Miller, 1990):

- Knowing
- Knowing how (knows the procedures or steps)
- Showing how (can do the procedures or steps)
- Actual doing (actually does the procedures in practice)

Even though portfolios have usefulness in determining potential for continuing competence and competency, safeguards to ensure the quality of the portfolio must be in place because the self-assessment (determining the learning need) and self-appraisal (selecting the best evidence of achieving the competency) skills of a health care professional may be limited under certain conditions. Health care professionals benefit from training in these self-evaluation processes, require experience over time, and need feedback from others who view their performance in order to become more skilled in self-assessment and in self-appraisal (Kruger & Dunning, 1999). Feedback is needed because high achievers tend to underestimate their abilities, and low achievers tend to overestimate their abilities. However, persons who are incompetent may not only reach erroneous conclusions about their level of ability (overestimate), but they may also lack the meta-cognitive ability to realize their incompetence. Inherent within self-assessment and self-appraisal is the ability to accurately reflect on one's own practice to determine where further learning would be beneficial.

# Roles of Stakeholders

A variety of stakeholders are interested in continuing competence and competency and professional development. The stakeholders in the professional community include occupational therapists and occupational therapy assistants, AOTA, state occupational therapy associations, state licensing boards, and NBCOT. Stakeholders in the community at large include clients; the public, state, and federal governments; third-party payers; accrediting bodies; other professional organizations; employers; and educators. Some of these stakeholders, such as occupational therapists and occupational therapy assistants, are interested in continuing competence and competency as equally as they are concerned with professional development. Others are primarily interested in continuing competence and competency, with a secondary focus on professional development. Because of their missions to protect the public, state licensing boards and voluntary credentialing programs like NBCOT have a primary focus on continuing competence and competency. Professional development is encouraged as it intersects with ensuring that the public receives services from competent occupational therapists and occupational therapy assistants.

Providers of continuing education, such as state and national organizations and universities, need to help learners understand the competencies to be addressed in the offering, as well as incorporate learning activities more likely to lead to gains in knowledge, skills, or reasoning abilities. The providers should also help the learner devise a transfer of training plan, or how the practitioner hopes to apply the learning to practice. Suggestions on how to measure the impact of the learning application should be made as well. The learning program should also incorporate time for periodic reflection about what one is learning and how that learning might improve practice.

Employers have a large role in the learning of their employees in terms of facilitating the self-assessment process, the use of portfolios, and the self-appraisal of learning activities. Careful consideration of the resources needed for learning should occur and should be reflected in the budgeting process in terms of ensuring that the employee has time for learning and the money needed to implement the learning plan. Employers are also in the best position to remove barriers to and to create supportive environments for the application of learning. This typically involves changes in the system so new approaches and interventions can be tried and measured. Employers can also help employees obtain and interpret client outcomes data both in terms of identifying learning needs and in terms of assessing the success of learning application. Reward and incentive systems are also an important way employers can facilitate the continuing competence and competency and professional development of their staff. Finally, employers are crucial in determining the competency of their employees as they can use observational methods to compare actual performance to standards.

# Summary

Portfolios are an important aspect of continuing competence and competency and professional development. Portfolios document the self-assessment process where it becomes clear the learning need has arisen following a systematic investigative process. The learning need then leads to careful selection of learning activities thought more likely to produce an improvement in one or more competencies necessary for excellent practice. Achieving these competencies through a focus on obtaining knowledge, skills, and reasoning abilities should result in a significant impact on client outcomes. Portfolios designed in this manner are a powerful tool in facilitating formative assessment and effective learning. However, the challenge is ensuring that sufficient rigor is maintained throughout the portfolio self-assessment and self-appraisal processes. Portfolios are more importantly a way for ensuring all occupational therapists and occupational therapy assistants undertake an active role in identifying and meeting their own learning needs as an aspect of continuous quality improvement within health care and social systems. Widespread rigorous use of portfolios stands to greatly impact the profession in its ability to provide society with quality occupational therapy services.

| Evidence-Based Research Chart | |
|---|---|
| **Topic** | **Evidence** |
| Self-assessment | Hicks & Hennessy, 2000; Kruger & Dunning, 1999; Meretoja & Leino-Kilpi, 2003; Rethans et al., 2002; Wilkinson et al., 2002 |
| Portfolios | Keim, Johnson, & Gates, 2001; Smith & Tillema, 2001; Tillema, 2001; Wilkinson et al., 2002 |
| Learning methods | Gustafsson & Fagerberg, 2004; Happell & Martin, 2004; Hicks & Hennessy, 2000; Khomeiran, Yekta, Kiger, & Ahmadi, 2006; Landers, McWhorter, Krum, & Glovinsky, 2005; McQueen, Miller, Nivison, & Husband, 2006; Nylenna & Aasland, 2000; O'Brien et al., 1997; Welch & Dawson, 2006 |
| System barrier and facilitators | Parks, Hyde, Deeks, & Milne, 2001; Rappolt, Pearce, McEwen, & Polatajko, 2005; Sparrow, Ashford, & Heel, 2005 |

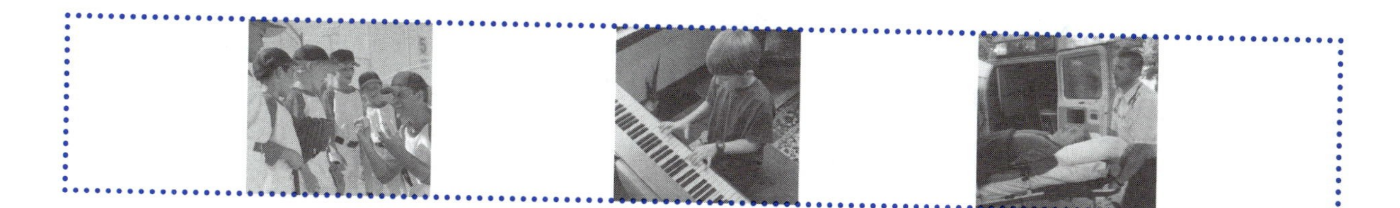

## Student Self-Assessment

1. Spend time reflecting about your career goals 5 years after you graduate. Identify generally what you would need to learn to achieve this career goal, the resources you would need, and how you would obtain these resources.
2. Suggest some ways you could incorporate nonlinear learning and self-directed learning to augment what you are learning in a particular class.
3. Reflect on an unplanned learning event in which you experienced a change in your ability to analyze a client situation. Share this reflection in small groups.
4. If you worked with a practitioner who stated she never had time to read anything about occupational therapy, explain how this would be an ethical dilemma and how you would address this situation as her colleague.

## References


American Occupational Therapy Association. (2000). *Code of ethics.* Bethesda, MD: Author.

American Occupational Therapy Association. (2005). Standards: Standards for continuing competence, AOTA standards for continuing competence. *American Journal of Occupational Therapy, 59*, 661-662.

American Occupational Therapy Association. (2008). Occupational therapy practice framework: Domain and process, second edition. *American Journal of Occupational Therapy, 62*, 625-683.

Decker, P. J. (1999). The hidden competencies of health care: Why self-esteem, accountability, and professionalism may affect hospital customer satisfaction scores. *Hospital Topics, 77*(1), 14.

Decker, P. J., & Strader, M. K. (1997). Beyond JCAHO: Using competency models to improve health care organizations, Part 1. *Hospital Topics, 75*(1), 23.

Fraser, S. W., & Greenhalgh, T. (2001). Complexity science. Coping with complexity: Education for capability. *British Medical Journal, 323*(6), 799-803.

Gustafsson, C., & Fagerberg, I. (2004). Reflection, the way to professional development? *Journal of Clinical Nursing, 13*, 271-280.

Handfield-Jones, R. S., Mann, K. V., Challis, M. E., Hobma, S. O., Klass, D. F., McManus, I. C., et al. (2002). Linking assessment to learning: A new route to quality assurance in medical practice. *Medical Education, 36*, 949-958.

Happell, B., & Martin, T. (2004). Exploring the impact of the implementation of a nursing clinical development unit program: What outcomes are evident? *International Journal of Mental Health Nursing, 13*, 177-184.

Hicks, C., & Hennessy, D. (2000). An alternative technique for evaluating the effectiveness of continuing professional development courses for health care professionals: A pilot study with practice nurses. *Journal of Nursing Management, 9*, 39-49.

Keim, K. S., Johnson, C. A., & Gates, G. E. (2001). Learning needs and continuing professional education activities of professional development portfolio participants. *Journal of the American Dietetic Association, 101*, 692-713.

Khomeiran, R. T., Yekta, Z. P., Kiger, A. M., & Ahmadi, F. (2006). Professional competence: Factors described by nurses as influencing their development. *International Nursing Review, 53*, 66-72.

Kruger, J., & Dunning, D. (1999). Unskilled and unaware of it: How difficulties in recognizing one's own incompetence lead to inflated self-assessments. *Journal of Personality and Social Psychology, 77*(6), 1121-1134.

Landers, M. R., McWhorter, J. W., Krum, L. L., & Glovinsky, D. (2005). Mandatory continuing education is physical therapy: Survey of physical therapists in states with and states without a mandate. *Physical Therapy, 85*, 861-871.

McConnell, E. A. (2001). Competence vs. competency. *Nursing Management, 32*(5), 14.

McQueen, J., Miller, C., Nivison, C., & Husband, V. (2006). An investigation into the use of a journal club or evidence-based practice. *International Journal of Therapy & Rehabilitation, 13*, 311-317.

Meretoja, R., & Leino-Kilpi, H. (2003). Comparison of competence assessments made by nurse managers and practicing nurses. *Journal of Nursing Management, 11*, 404-409.

Miller, G. E. (1990). The assessment of clinical skills/competence/performance. *Academic Medicine, 65*(Suppl), S63-S67.

Moyers, P. A. (2005). The ethics of competence. In R. B. Purtilo, G. M. Jensen, & C. B. Royeen (Eds.), *Educating for moral action: A sourcebook in health and rehabilitation ethics* (pp. 21-30). Philadelphia, PA: F.A. Davis.

Moyers, P. A., & Hinojosa, J. (2003). Continuing competency. In G. McCormack, E. Jaffe, & M. Goodman-Lavey (Eds.), *The occupational therapy manager* (4th ed., pp. 489). Bethesda, MD: AOTA Press.

Nylenna, M., & Aasland, O. G. (2000). Primary care physicians and their information-seeking behaviour. *Scandinavian Journal of Primary Health Care, 18*, 9-13.

O'Brien, M. A., Oxman, A. D., Davis, D. A., Haynes, R. B., Freemantle, N., & Harvey, E. L. (1997). Educational outreach visits: Effects on professional practice and health care outcomes. *Cochrane Database of Systematic Reviews*, Issue 4. Art. No.: CD000409.

Parks, J., Hyde, C., Deeks, J., & Milne, R. (2001). Teaching critical appraisal skills in health care settings. *Cochrane Database of Systematic Reviews*, Issue 3. Art. No.: CD001270.

Rappolt, S., Pearce, K., McEwen, S., & Polatajko, H. J. (2005). Exploring organizational characteristics associated with practice changes following a mentored online educational module. *Journal of Continuing Education in the Health Professions, 25*, 116-124.

Rethans, J. J., Norcini, J. J., Barón-Maldonado, M., Blackmore, D., Jolly, B. C., LaDuca, T., et al. (2002). The relationship between competence and performance: Implications for assessing practice performance. *Medical Education, 36*, 901-909.

Sautter, K. M., Bokhour, B. C., White, B., Young, G. J., Burgess, J. F., Berlowitz, D., et al. (2007). The early experience of a hospital-based pay-for performance program. *Journal of Healthcare Management, 52*(2), 95-107.

Sparrow, J., Ashford, R., & Heel, D. (2005). A methodology to identify workplace features that can facilitate or impede reflective practice: A National Health Service UK study. *Reflective Practice, 6*, 189-197.

Smith, K., & Tillema, H. H. (2001). Long-term influences of portfolios on professional development. *Scandinavian Journal of Educational Research, 45*(2), 183-203.

Tillema, H. H. (2001). Portfolios as developmental assessment tools. *International Journal of Training and Development, 5*(2), 1360-1376.

Ward, M., Gruppen, L., & Regehr, G. (2002). Measuring self-assessment: Current state of the art. *Advances in Health Sciences Education: Theory and Practice, 7*, 63-80.

Welch, A., & Dawson, P. (2006). Closing the gap: Collaborative learning as a strategy to embed evidence within occupational therapy practice. *Journal of Evaluation in Clinical Practice, 12*, 227-238.

Wilkinson, T. J., Challis, M., Hobma, S. O., Newble, D. I., Parboosingh, J. T., Sibbald, R. G., et al. (2002). The use of portfolios for assessment of the competence and performance of doctors in practice. *Medical Education, 36*, 918-924.

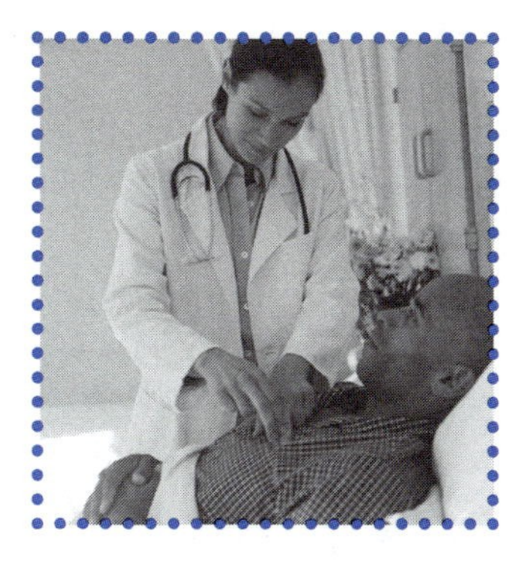

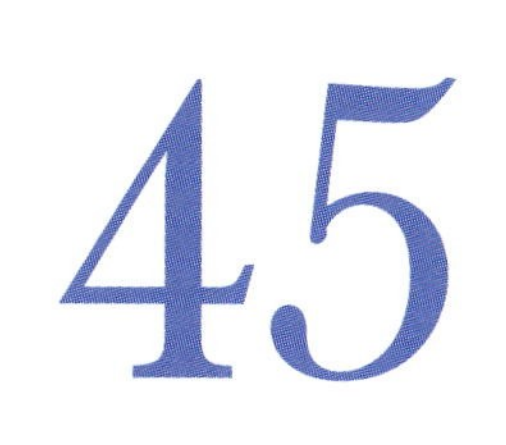

# 45

# Roles of Occupational Therapists

*Thomas F. Fisher, PhD, OTR, CCM, FAOTA*

**ACOTE Standards Explored in This Chapter**

B.9.7-9.9

**Key Terms**

| | |
|---|---|
| Contractor | Fieldwork Educator |
| Educator | Practitioner |
| Entrepreneur | Researcher |

## Introduction

Christiansen and Baum (1997) defined roles as "a set of behaviors that have some socially agreed upon function and for which there is an accepted code of norms" (p. 603). Through the years, occupational therapists' roles have expanded. Some occupational therapists are administrators of hospitals, deans of universities, and case managers (Fisher, 1996). Regardless of which point in the profession's history, the primary focus of the occupational therapist has remained consistent (i.e., identifying strengths and barriers for individuals and/or groups as they function in their daily life roles). An occupational therapist assesses an individual's performance within a given role and designs intervention plans that address the skills needed for those specific roles. Through these interventions, an individual acquires or redevelops the skills necessary for role performance. The skills translate into habits of behavior. Within each role, individuals develop a repertoire of skills and habits necessary for successful occupational performance. An individual performs many different roles during his or her lifetime.

During a professional career, an occupational therapist may assume several roles. Each role is unique and has specific performance expectations. Understanding and appreciating these roles and performance expectations is fundamental to being an occupational therapist in the 21st century. As a profession, we believe that roles not only shape what we do and how we look at the world, but they also allow us to know who we are.

Because of the many roles that shape our lives, we believe that roles provide us with an awareness of social identity and related obligations, as well as a framework for appreciating relevant situations and constructing appropriate behaviors. Roles support us in identifying our unique value and contribution to society (Kramer, Hinojosa, & Royeen, 2003). As occupational therapists, we also address roles with the clients we serve. It is an essential part of the occupational therapy process.

In 1976, Black encouraged occupational therapists to view consumers of occupational therapy as "occupants of roles" (p. 226). She believed occupational therapists have a responsibility to evaluate and provide interventions for clients to help them assume the roles they need to perform. She felt this kept therapists true to the legacy of the profession.

The notion of persons having a variety of roles during their life is true for occupational therapists as well. During



K. Sladyk, K. Jacobs, & N. MacRae (Eds.).
*Occupational Therapy Essentials for Clinical Competence* (pp. 485-496).

a career as an occupational therapist, one has the opportunity to assume several roles such as practitioner, educator, researcher, and entrepreneur.

Shannon (1985) addressed the broadening roles of occupational therapists in the continuity of care in a special edition of *Occupational Therapy in Health Care*. He expanded on an earlier discussion about occupational therapy beyond hospital-based occupational therapy practice. He reminded therapists to understand the political, economic, and cultural environment in which they practice, regardless of their role. He suggested they appreciate their holistic perspective and broad knowledge base, and he emphasized the unique opportunities that community practice brings.

Oakley, Kielhofner, Barris, and Reichler (1986) felt so strongly about this notion of roles, they developed a validated instrument—The Role Checklist. This instrument was developed out of a need for a reliable and valid assessment focusing on the several types of roles in which people engage. The Role Checklist provides the occupational therapist with data about individuals' perception of themselves and their participation in roles throughout their life and the degree to which each role is valued. This instrument is used by occupational therapists in a variety of settings, primarily with adults. It addresses the following four dimensions of roles (Oakley et al., p. 159):

1. *Perceived incumbency*: "An individual's belief that he or she occupies a role"
2. *Occupational role career*: "Progression of roles throughout one's life"
3. *Role balance*: "The ability to maintain sufficient important life roles without conflict or overload of role demand"
4. *Role value*: "Degree of that an individual attaches to a particular role"

Henry and Coster (1997) investigated competency beliefs and occupational role behaviors among adolescents. They used the Model of Human Occupation as their theoretical underpinning and concluded that a person's occupational role behavior, be it adaptive or maladaptive, is dependent on the adolescent's academic ability, social competence, and physical competence. They concluded by showing some implications for occupational therapy with adolescents with mental health disorders.

Kao and Kellegrew (2000) discussed a similar notion of self-concept and academic achievement with adolescents and their role development. They found young people who have successful experiences in their role as student have a better self-concept and outlook on life.

In addition, an occupational therapist has the potential and opportunity to supervise and collaborate with occupational therapy assistants, thus expanding into the role of supervisor. This chapter's focus identifies specific roles, then addresses the role of supervisor and collaborator with occupational therapy assistants. At the end of this chapter, responsibilities of the occupational therapist when service provision is on a contractual basis in the current systems will be addressed.

## Roles

Each occupational therapist's employment setting, method of service delivery, competence, and professional development plan are interdependent and completely individualized. Frequently, an occupational therapist's position with an employer may include more than one role. For example, as an occupational therapy educator, the individual may also function as a researcher and consultant. Another example would be an occupational therapist on an inpatient rehabilitation unit who could be functioning as a supervisor to the other occupational therapists and occupational therapy assistants or as the team coordinator for the unit (i.e., stroke, spinal cord, brain injury, etc.) in addition to providing direct occupational therapy services. Furthermore, this individual could also be fulfilling the role of fieldwork educator.

In each role, the occupational therapist has performance areas as well as essential and marginal job functions. The essential functions are the major purposes of a position, while marginal functions are necessary to support the essential or major functions. The performance areas specify common activities and expectations associated with the role. As a competent contemporary occupational therapist, it is imperative that the individual performance of roles is within the ethical code and standards of the profession (American Occupational Therapy Association [AOTA], 2004a).

Regardless of the employment arrangement (therapist employed by the organization, independent contractor to the organization, consultant to the organization), the professional responsibility of the occupational therapist to perform the role and provide services in an ethical and professional manner cannot be overemphasized.

Because of the profession's belief about roles and the variety of roles occupational therapists assume during a career, the professional organization has addressed this officially. The AOTA has official documents that support occupational therapists in understanding and appreciating the various roles, and they describe the supervision of occupational therapists and occupational therapy assistants. The roles that will be examined include practitioner, field work educator, educator, researcher, and entrepreneur.

## Practitioner

In the United States, "occupational therapy practitioner" refers to both occupational therapists and occupational therapy assistants. For the purpose of this chapter, the discussion will be limited to the occupational therapist, given the text is addressing the educational standards for the entry-level occupational therapist. Typically, occupational therapists progress along a continuum when in clinical practice. They move from entry level to intermediate, and then into advanced level based on experience, education, and practice skills. The essential function of the practitioner is to provide occupational therapy services, which includes assessments, interventions, program planning and implementation, discharge planning, and transition planning (AOTA, 2004a). Services may be provided in direct, indirect, and/or consultative approaches. Within the role of practitioner, the occupational therapist may serve an administrative role or a client educator role in addition to providing direct services.

In some settings, occupational therapy practitioners (therapists and assistants) provide services in groups. In fact, in mental health settings, acute rehabilitation settings, and many community settings (adult day programs, outpatient facilities, developmental disabilities centers, etc.), this is how occupational therapy services are delivered (Scaffa, 2001). Occasionally, the practitioner may also function in the role of supervisor and/or fieldwork educator.

## Fieldwork Educator

With the additional role of fieldwork educator comes additional responsibilities for the therapist. The fieldwork educator needs to not only understand, value, and evaluate the provision of skilled services, but must also understand the components of graduate professional education. This individual assists the student integration of classroom knowledge and application to practice. Performing both roles uses a variety of skills and requires additional knowledge. It is important to note that in occupational therapy, an occupational therapist is not permitted to supervise a Level II fieldwork student until he or she has practiced full-time for 1 year (Accreditation Council for Occupational Therapy Education [ACOTE], 1999). However, he or she can begin taking Level I students soon after graduation. In addition to these two roles, the occupational therapist might also provide an educational offering in the community to families of persons with disabilities, support groups, other health professionals, etc. This assists in explaining the continuum of providing occupational therapy education services to individuals and groups. All of these functions and roles establish the contemporary role of practitioner in occupational therapy. Due to the shortage of educators, universities are presented situations where fieldwork educators just meet the minimum standards to take students. Serving in these additional capacities is making the role of practitioner for occupational therapists increasingly challenging. Many organizations have productivity standards (e.g., long-term care facilities, home health) for their therapists. They must be able to charge for a minimum 6 or 7 hours of service a day. To have that level of client contact is challenging in today's fast-paced health care, social, and educational systems for most therapists. Those therapists who accept an additional role as fieldwork educator demonstrate a true commitment to the future of the profession. This underscores the professionalism of these practitioners. Advocating for administrative support for this additional role may reduce the stress for these involved practitioners.

## Educator

At some point in one's career as an occupational therapist, an individual might consider a role as a faculty member in an academic setting. This is differentiated from being a fieldwork educator as they are frequently considered adjunct faculty by some universities. The profession, through the policymaking body of the organization (Representative Assembly), established a set of standards that articulate the competencies for individuals assuming the role as a faculty member in a professional entry-level occupational therapist academic setting (AOTA, 2004b) or a technical-level occupational therapy assistant faculty member in an academic setting (AOTA, 2004b). Additionally, there are role documents for the program directors and academic fieldwork coordinators as well. These official documents articulate those competencies long suggested by scholars in the field of occupational therapy (Clark, 1987; Fidler, 1981; Jantzen,1974; Mosey, 1998). They too believed that occupational therapists practicing in professional education have critical demands placed on them, and their performance influences practice, education, and research.

In fact, Bondoc (2005) suggested that professional accountability begins in the formative and formal educational years of the occupational therapist, thus making it critical that, as a profession, we recognize that graduate professional education needs to have those individuals who understand evidence-based education and practice. He articulated how education is a connection that binds the profession, and evidence-based education enhances that link. Because of this, it is no surprise there was and still is a belief that therapists functioning in the role of occupational therapy educator should be held to certain standards. These standards are important to recognize and understand. Therefore, they are explicit and are discussed in this chapter. The development of these standards and subsequent approval was not controversial. It was an expectation from the field. In the future, it would be useful to have similar competencies identified for other roles occupational therapists assume (i.e., consultant, researcher, etc.).

There are similar competencies for the role of the academic fieldwork coordinator. Like the faculty competencies, these competencies describe the values, knowledge, skills, and responsibilities needed for this role of academic fieldwork coordinator. The competencies for the faculty members and academic fieldwork coordinator in a professional-level occupational therapy program assist universities and colleges in determining and evaluating those routine functions of a faculty member in a professional entry-level program, when hiring and retaining competent faculty.

Competencies based on AOTA's Standards for Continuing Competence (AOTA, 2004b) describe those skills, responsibilities, obligations, and expertise/content knowledge in an area of occupational therapy service that the educator should possess. The standards are clear. The competencies to meet those standards are general statements that need not always be applied to each situation. Competencies may need to be modified. AOTA encourages universities to consider these guidelines when instructing future occupational therapists. The standards are knowledge, critical and ethical reasoning, interpersonal skills, and performance skills. See Table 45-1 for the standards.

In terms of the standard for knowledge and serving in the academic role, this standard goes on to declare that a faculty member must do the following:

- "Demonstrate the knowledge of how to facilitate student development toward leadership roles
- Develop a plan to continue competency in the breadth and depth of knowledge in the profession to incorporate student learning
- Facilitate effective learning processes that can be used to enhance the learning opportunities for students
- Develop a plan to continue proficiency in teaching through investigation, formal education, continuing education and self-investigation" (AOTA, 2004b, p. 649)

The standard of critical reasoning declares the faculty member must:

- "Facilitate professional development in teaching through continuing education, research, or self-investigation
- Demonstrate the ability to effectively judge new materials, literature, and educational materials that enhance the lifelong learning of future occupational therapy practitioners
- Demonstrate the ability to critically integrate practice, theory, literature, and research for evidence-based practice
- Demonstrate the ability to critically evaluate curriculum and participate in curriculum development" (AOTA, 2004b, p. 649)

The ethical reasoning standard includes acting as a "role model of an occupational therapy advocate and change agent with professional and ethical behavior" (AOTA, 2004b, p. 650).

Interpersonal skills require that the faculty member in an academic setting must: do the following

- "Project a positive image of the program both internally (within the college or university) and externally (within the community)
- Demonstrate a competent and positive attitude that will result in the mentoring of students in the beginning skills of scholarship, research, and/or service
- Effectively mentor and advise students and student groups
- Create a positive presence of occupational therapy in the university/college and community through service, scholarship, and/or educational experiences
- Effectively mentor other faculty members in their development of teaching, scholarship/research, and/or service

**Table 45-1. Standards for Continuing Competence**

| Standard | Description | Example |
|---|---|---|
| Knowledge | "Occupational therapy practitioners shall demonstrate understanding and comprehension of the information required for the multiple roles they assume" (AOTA, 2004b, p. 649). | Regardless of setting, occupational therapists address the roles the client assumes during his or her everyday life. |
| Critical reasoning | "Occupational therapy practitioners shall employ reasoning processes to make sound judgments and decisions within the context of their roles" (p. 649). | When presented with a client who is critically ill and has had multiple roles, the occupational therapist establishes a rapport with the client, and the client's support system determines an appropriate and safe intervention plan. |
| Ethical reasoning | "Occupational therapy practitioners shall identify, analyze, and clarify ethical issues of dilemmas in order to make responsible decisions within the context of their roles" (p. 650). | Billing for services in a manner directed by the employer instead of that decision made by the occupational therapist. |
| Interpersonal skills | "Occupational therapy practitioners shall develop and maintain their professional relationships with others within the context of their roles" (p. 649). | During team meetings (regardless of settings), the occupational therapist presents client-centered, occupation-based, theory-driven, and evidence-based assessments and interventions. |
| Performance skills | "Occupational therapy practitioners shall demonstrate the expertise, attitudes, proficiencies, and ability to competently fulfill their roles" (p. 649). | During one's career, a professional development plan is established and revisited routinely. |

- Demonstrate positive interactions with diverse faculty, students, and others" (AOTA, 2004b, p. 649).

Finally, the standard for performance skills states that the faculty member must do the following:

- "Demonstrate the expertise to contribute to the growing body of knowledge in occupational therapy
- Demonstrate the ability to contribute to the profession, academic community, and/or society through service
- Demonstrate the ability to competently prepare ethical and competent practitioners for both traditional and emerging practice settings" (AOTA, 2004b, p. 649)

Similarly, the academic fieldwork coordinator has specific competencies articulated in the document *Role Competencies for an Academic Fieldwork Coordinator* (AOTA, 2004c).

The competencies identified for each standard for the academic fieldwork coordinator, which could be modified or may not apply to all situations, are different than those for the faculty. The standards are the same. This was intentional by the Commission on Education of the AOTA. The roles and thus the responsibilities and competencies are different. In 2003, the Representative Assembly of the AOTA approved this document. Within the knowledge standard, competencies recognized for the occupational therapist in the role of academic fieldwork coordinator that must be met are as follows:

- "Demonstrate the expertise to be able to facilitate the development of future leaders in occupational therapy through student development in supervised quality fieldwork settings
- Develop a plan to continue competency in the breadth and depth of knowledge in the profession to incorporate into student learning
- Develop a plan to promote effective learning processes for students in the program and associated fieldwork education sites
- Demonstrate competence to develop and maintain accurate and current knowledge of reimbursement issues, federal regulations concerning student services, legal issues concerning fieldwork experiences, and pertinent federal/state regulations such as the Americans With Disabilities Act (ADA)
- Demonstrate the competence to develop and maintain accurate and current knowledge in contractual agreements between colleges/universities and fieldwork sites
- Demonstrate the competence to develop and maintain proficiency in fieldwork coordination skills through investigation, formal education, continuing education, or self study" (AOTA, 2004c, p. 653)

Critical reasoning has the following competencies:

- "Facilitate professional development in teaching/fieldwork coordination through continuing education, research, or self-investigation
- Demonstrate the ability to effectively judge new materials, literature, and educational materials relating to fieldwork that enhances the lifelong learning for future occupational therapists
- Demonstrate the ability to critically integrate practice, theory, literature, and educational materials relating to fieldwork education sites
- Demonstrate the ability to critically evaluate the curriculum, particularly in terms of fieldwork education, for participation in curriculum development
- Demonstrate the ability to evaluate the interpersonal dynamics between occupational therapy practitioners and students to resolve issues and determine action plans" (AOTA, 2004c, p. 653)

Ethical reasoning expects conformance to the following competencies:

- "Act as a role model as an occupational therapy advocate and change agent with professional and ethical behavior
- Clarify and analyze fieldwork issues within an ethical framework for positive resolution
- Identify and represent the educational and fieldwork settings accurately to ensure that legal contracts are appropriately documented" (AOTA, 2004c, p. 654)

As with the faculty standards and competencies, there are performance skills and interpersonal skills standards. The performance skills competencies are as follows:

- "Demonstrate the ability to plan fieldwork experiences that will prepare ethical and competent practitioners for both traditional and emerging practice settings
- Demonstrate the expertise to develop fieldwork course objectives, course materials, and educational experiences that promote optimal learning for students
- Demonstrate the expertise to evaluate students' learning outcomes for fieldwork to meet the objectives of the program and the organization
- Demonstrate the ability to develop and implement a plan that effectively evaluates fieldwork educators and fieldwork sites to meet the objectives of the program and the organization
- Demonstrate the expertise to prepare, develop, and/or coordinate the legal contracts and associated issues for fieldwork establishment and maintenance
- Demonstrate the ability to design and implement a logical and justified system of fieldwork assignment for students and fieldwork educators

- Demonstrate the ability to plan and implement a plan that develops and maintains accurate documentation of student performance, collaboration with fieldwork settings and supervisors, and/or other documentation required for fieldwork experiences" (AOTA, 2004c, p. 654)

Finally, the standard related to interpersonal skills requests the academic fieldwork coordinator must meet these competencies:

- "Projects a positive image of the program both internally (within the college or university) and externally (within the community)
- Demonstrates a competent and positive attitude that will result in the development and mentoring of fieldwork educators
- Effectively mentors and advises students in relation to fieldwork education issues
- Effectively mediates interpersonal issues between students and fieldwork educators
- Demonstrates positive interactions with diverse faculty, fieldwork educators, and practitioners
- Demonstrates positive interactions with appropriate administrators and attorneys to facilitate contract negotiations" (AOTA, 2004c, p. 653)

These role competency documents are the most defined competencies for any role an occupational therapist may assume. The AOTA does have a commission established for developing and maintaining specialty certification and board certification in specific areas of practice. However, those certifications are emerging through the work of the Commission for Continuing Competency. Those programs are discussed elsewhere in this book.

For the AOTA to have engaged in this level of discussion, adoption by the Representative Assembly is evidence supporting the notion that occupational therapists wanting a professional career as a faculty member in an academic setting need to be committed to demonstrating these competencies. The profession has articulated its beliefs about professional occupational therapy education and the competencies occupational therapists in the role of faculty or academic fieldwork educator should demonstrate. Some individuals in the academic setting may make a career in the role of researcher. This role is one all entry-level occupational therapists should understand and value.

## Researcher

Another role occupational therapists perform is that of researcher. Kielhofner (2006) suggested that occupational therapists who become researchers do this because they "find the process of discovery exhilarating and because they see how it enhances occupational therapy practice" (p. xiii). This specific role had less emphasis in earlier educational standards but then became recognized and required in the 1998 ACOTE Standards (ACOTE, 1999). The educational standards affirm this need for research as the profession moves forward with post-baccalaureate entry education (master's or doctorate). The role of researcher has gained focus because of research standards for entry level, the expectation for evidence-based practice, and the advancement of the profession. This particular role should continue to attract individuals with the formal preparation, interest, and commitment to inquiry.

Like other health professionals, occupational therapy acknowledged the need for research and scholarly activity and acquired an appreciation and understanding of the importance of research as entry-level therapists came into the profession. These standards obligate academic programs to recruit and retain faculty with these knowledge and skills who can teach this content and role model the behavior of researcher. As the profession's number of faculty with doctorates increases, the number of faculty assuming the role of researcher should also increase. According to Kielhofner (2006), the intent of the academic standard for entry-level occupational therapists was focused on "designing and implementing an entry-level research study" (p. 20). However, because of these standards, academic programs are expected to provide students with the skills to build evidence for interventions used in occupational therapy as well as to promote further education for those who may be interested in a career as a researcher. The major functions for this role of researcher at entry level are to collect, read, interpret, and apply scholarly information as it relates to occupational therapy. In addition to these functions, entry-level research skills include assuming responsibility for ethical concerns related to research and complying with the various institutional research boards and committees (AOTA, 1994).

As an individual progresses through the research continuum, it is feasible for a therapist to acquire a research degree and assume the role exclusively as a researcher, scholar, or scientist. As a scholar, one possesses advanced knowledge and engages in the conceptualization of a research project, develops the proposal independently, and refines the study as needed. Research scholars in occupational therapy advance the profession of occupational therapy through their discovery, knowledge, and evidence. The Academy of Research, through the American Occupational Therapy Foundation (AOTF), recognizes and inducts individuals who have made substantial contributions to occupational therapy through research and science.

## Entrepreneur

A final role an entry-level occupational theapist should be familiar with is that of entrepreneur. Early in the profession, the role of entrepreneur was not advocated nor addressed in the academic standards for entry-level occupational therapists. Although recognized, it was not a role explicitly identified until the 1998 ACOTE Standards

(ACOTE, 1999). Entrepreneurs are either partially or fully self-employed individuals. They include those in private practice, independent contractors, and consultants. Because of the broad scope of services these individuals may be providing, the structure of their organization may be sole proprietorship, partnership, corporation, group practice, or joint venture (AOTA, 2000). Independent contractors, consultants, and private practice owners are held to the same standard for demonstrating competencies as employees of an organization. This arrangement for demonstrating competence becomes a responsibility for both the contract employee and the employer contracting for the services. Regardless of what the employer or potential employer tells the occupational therapist, it is that individual's responsibility to perform in an ethical and professional manner. This professional responsibility will be discussed in more detail later in this chapter.

In the role of entrepreneur, key performance areas for the entry-level occupational therapist as identified by AOTA (2000) may include the following:

- "Delivering quality occupational therapy services within the scope of endeavor
- Establishing a business organization appropriate to nature and scope of activities
- Negotiating contractual relationships that take into account the setting, services, and reimbursement
- Developing and implementing a business plan designed to ensure viability
- Using financial and legal consultation, establishing and collecting fees for service
- Complying with reimbursement requirements, managing business support services
- Developing and implementing marketing strategies, as appropriate" (p. 319) to mention a few

When discussing common types of businesses as an entrepreneur, typically, five are identified. We will now discuss some of the advantages and disadvantages of each:

1. Sole proprietorship
    - *Advantages*: Easiest and least expensive to organize; can be established, bought, sold, or terminated quickly; size and structure can change and others (family) can be involved according to the proprietor's wishes
    - *Disadvantages*: Both personal and business assets are at risk, mixing personal and business finances can make it more difficult to measure success, and conflicts or disagreements within the family can stagnate the business and delay needed decision making
2. Partnership
    - *Advantages*: Relatively easy to establish, partners may combine resources, greater capacity for obtaining credit by partners as opposed to trying to do it solo
    - *Disadvantages*: Personal assets of all partners are put at risk, business is disrupted upon the death or withdrawal of either partner
3. Limited liability corporation (LLC)
    - *Advantages*: Owners are provided a flexible form of business organization that provides liability protection comparable to the protection provided by incorporation; can be established at a moderate cost in a short time; all members, one or more members, or a nonmember individual may manage an LLC
    - *Disadvantages*: Corporations are monitored by federal, state, and local agencies and so may require more paperwork to comply with regulations and incorporation may have higher taxes
4. S Corporation
    - *Advantages*: Liability of stockholders is limited to their investment in the corporation, personal assets are protected, additional funds can be raised through the sale of stock
    - *Disadvantages*: Personal guarantees from officers/stockholders may be required, conflict can arise if a group of stockholders decide to join together to make change if the corporation has limited credit
5. C Corporation
    - *Advantages*: Fractional ownership interests are easily accommodated in the initial offering of stock; purchase, sale, and gifting of stock make it possible for changes in ownership without disrupting the business and requires separation of finances and records to reduce inequity
    - *Disadvantages*: Conflict with a group of stockholders could stagnate decision making, paid benefits to stockholders may become costly and effect the business and personal guarantees from corporate officers may be required.

Braveman (2005) describes each type in more detail in *Leading and Managing Occupational Therapy Services*, which is supported by current evidence, operational definitions, advantages, and disadvantages for types of businesses. To assume the role of an entrepreneur, one needs to understand the various common types of businesses.

## Sole Proprietorship

Sole proprietorships "merge together the business and its affairs and the owner's personal affairs and, therefore, from the standpoint of nearly all legal rights and responsibilities, the business and the owner are considered to be one and the same" (Braveman, 2005, p. 65). Advantages identified include their ease and expense in forming; quickly established, bought, sold, and terminated; not required to have public notification to start, terminate, or be modified beyond routine permits and licenses; the size and structure can change and others (family, etc.) can be involved according to the proprietor's wishes; and complex business planning or organizational arrangements (bylaws, organizational charter, etc.) are not required (Braveman).

Disadvantages are that personal and business assets are at risk unless they are protected in a trust or some other protective mechanism, combining business and personal finances make it difficult to measure the financial outcomes of the business, and the business ends with the death of the proprietor. A new business would need to be formed if others wish to continue the business. "In family sole proprietorships, each generation must purchase or inherit the business assets, paying any applicable" (Braveman, 2005, p. 65). Finally, because of limited resources, available credit and financial capacities may be hindered for the individual at various times (Braveman).

## Partnership

A partnership "is an association of two or more persons formed to carry on a business for profit" (Braveman, 2005, p. 66). Some of the advantages to this arrangement are that they are relatively easy to establish and partners may combine resources and benefit from the combination of their skills and interests. Because of the combining of resources, a larger credit availability may be possible than would have been on an individual's own. Finally, recordkeeping and income tax filing is only slightly more involved than for individuals (Braveman). Some of the disadvantages of partnerships are that personal assets of all partners are put at risk and business is disrupted when a death or resignation from one of the partners occurs. Depending on the number of partners, when one partner would like to see one thing happen but the other partners do not, the majority decides. Laws related to inheritance and planning for succession are disadvantages. At times, they are difficult to end without financial loss or interpersonal conflict with the partners. In fact, they can lose profitability if disagreements among partners delay business decision making (Braveman).

## Limited Liability Corporation

An LCC "is a form of business that, unlike a sole proprietorship, is separate and distinct from the personal and business affairs of its owners" (Braveman, 2005, p. 66). The advantages of being an LCC are that the owners are protected similar to those in corporation in terms of liability protection and the start-up cost is moderate and done in a short period of time. This type of business can be managed by a variety of individuals, which makes it attractive. And, individuals who are the members of the LCC express the interests of the company through the articles of the organization (Braveman). Like the others, there are disadvantages. To start an LCC, there needs to be a public notification as well as legal assistance. This makes it not as attractive as sole proprietorship or partnership. LCCs are regulated by federal, state, and local agencies and so may require more paperwork. Lastly, LCCs could result in higher overall taxes (Braveman, 2005).

## S Corporations

An S Corporation is "a corporation that is taxed under Subchapter S of the Internal Revenue Code and receives Internal Revenue Service (IRS) approval of its requests for Subchapter S status. Corporation finances and records are established and maintained separate and distinct from the finances and records of its stockholders" (Braveman, 2005, p. 67). Advantages of an S Corporation are that liability of the stockholders is limited to investments; these corporations can raise additional funds through the sale of stock; they can operate even when a death of a stockholder occurs; decision making within the organization is based on the percentage of ownership by the multiple owners; and they allow for communication between stockholders, owners, legal counsel, and other groups and change of ownership through sale or gift without disrupting the business (Braveman).

An S Corporation's disadvantages are that personal guarantees from the officers or stockholders may be required if the corporation has limited credit, a group of stockholders could limit decision making, and minority stockholders may be limited in recovering limited investment in the corporation if it were to have problems. In fact, ownership of stock may be miscommunicated for those not active or knowledgeable when the gift or sale to others occurs. Finally, the corporate shield of limited liability may be lost if procedures and processes are not followed, therefore having the shareholders personally liable in some instances (Braveman, 2005).

## C Corporation

A C Corporation is "a corporation that is taxed under Subsection C of the Internal Revenue Code and receives IRS approval of its request for Subchapter C status. The C corporation is separate and distinct from the owners of the corporation (stockholders)" (p. 67). There are several advantages to this type of business., such as there is a perpetual life of the corporation; ownership interest are accommodated from the onset of stock; purchasing, selling, and gifting can happen at any time without influencing the business; personal life of stockholders is simplified; and annual meetings of the stockholders facilitate communication (Braveman, 2005). Some disadvantages include paying more income tax on the net income before distribution of dividends to stockholders, which results in double taxation of corporate income distributed to stockholders, and a small group of stockholders could stagnate decision making (Braveman, 2005).

# Collaboration With Occupational Therapy Assistants

In the 1950s, because of the demand for occupational therapy services and the time required to prepare professional occupational therapists, the profession created occupational therapy assistants in the United States (Crampton, 1958). Early on, the occupational therapy assistant education was designed for those individuals who were high school graduates or equivalent and employed as an occupational therapy aide. Many of the earlier occupational therapy assistant graduates were prepared to work in mental health occupational therapy. The training went from strictly technical to additional didactic instruction. Supervised clinical work (as it was called in earlier times) was mandatory. Throughout the history of occupational therapy assistant education, occupational therapists have been careful to include the assistant in the discussion but recognize the professional occupational therapist had the formal educational preparation to understand the essence of occupation and its influence on humans (Hirama, 1986). Because of the appreciation of what the occupational therapy assistant brings to practice, the profession has routinely included participation from assistants in discussions of mission, education, practice, and leadership.

Occupational therapy assistants have more inclusion in the profession than other assistants have in their professions (i.e., medicine, physical therapy, nursing). For example, physical therapy assistants who are members of their professional organization are only allowed affiliate membership and have voice about policy through a separate body (APTA, 2007). That separate body has two people in the House of Delegates representing the issues of the assistants. Occupational therapy assistants in the AOTA can run for any office of the professional organization, with the exception of the Chairperson of the Commission on Education. That individual must be an occupational therapist with a doctorate. This is the criteria established by the Nominating Committee of the AOTA and approved by the Representative Assembly. In the *Guidelines for Supervision, Roles, and Responsibilities During the Delivery of Occupational Therapy Services* (AOTA, 2004a) it states, "the occupational therapy assistant delivers occupational therapy services under the supervision of and in partnership with the occupational therapist" (p. 663).

Collaborating with occupational therapy assistants has been and will continue to be a cost-effective method for delivering occupational therapy services. New models of service have emerged over the last decade. Use of occupational therapy assistants by occupational therapists has changed over time. However, regardless of the service model, AOTA purports collaboration between occupational therapists and occupational therapy assistants as fundamental and necessary.

In fact, ACOTE Standard B.9.8 explicitly requires professional entry-level academic programs for the occupational therapist to show evidence of how they are preparing students to collaborate with occupational therapy assistants (ACOTE, 1999, 2006; AOTA, 2000). Throughout the decades, occupational therapists and occupational therapy assistants providing services together has been important to the profession and society (Hirama, 1986). Understanding and valuing this relationship is necessary for every occupational therapist and occupational therapy assistant. Because of this relationship, the need for the occupational therapist to possess supervision skills cannot be overemphasized. As discussed earlier, understanding the importance of the supervisory role and performing those functions competently allow for the successful delivery of occupational therapy services. Being capable of meeting this is an expectation and standard for accrediting an educational program (ACOTE, 1999). To accomplish this important expectation, it becomes necessary for professional entry-level programs to provide examples of the collaborative relationships during the didactic portion of the academic preparation, have occupational therapy assistants on the faculty or as guest lecturers, and facilitate the exposure of student occupational therapists to occupational therapy assistants while doing both Level I and II fieldwork. Over the last decade, many more occupational therapy practitioners are contracting with organizations such as school systems to provide occupational therapy services.

## Contractual Occupational Therapy Services

Understanding the responsibilities of a professional when providing occupational therapy services on a contract basis is paramount in the current environment. Green (2004) reported the vacancy rate for occupational therapists in the past decade is more than 11%. As a result, organizations are willing to contract for services instead of hiring in-house staff. Because of the current environment (more demand than supply), some occupational therapists are transitioning from an employee of the organization to an independent contractor. When making this transition, there are several issues the professional needs to understand. First, and most importantly, the independent contractor needs to adhere to the profession's *Code of Ethics* and *Standards of Practice*. Demonstrating a commitment to providing and continually improving occupational therapy services is a must. In this role as contractor, one needs to understand that not only does contracting allow autonomy, but it also requires the individual to be self-directed and goal-oriented. Promoting the provision of the best possible quality of interventions for clients served is a primary goal of all occupational therapists; doing it also avoids litigation.

In addition, lifelong learning, providing evidence-based interventions, and keeping current with the literature and technology are values that contemporary occupational therapists have.

As previously stated in this chapter, occupational therapists who are independent contractors or in some other way engage in a contractual arrangement to provide occupational therapy services are held to the same standards as permanent employees of an organization. This is such a fundamental practice parameter that the Joint Commission on Accreditation for Healthcare Organizations (JCAHO) requires employers to manage contract services and its employees just as they manage their direct employees (JCAHO, 2004). It is a shared responsibility between the occupational therapist and the agency with whom he or she contracts. Establishing competency-based plans for all therapists, including contract therapists, helps identify the training that is needed and what should be assessed on a routine basis. For example, as an independent contractor to a free-standing rehabilitation hospital providing supplemental occupational therapy services, the contractor should be assessed on knowledge and skill related to the Functional Independence Measure, dysphagia, orthotic design and fabrication, and documentation. Because these are skills and knowledge that full-time in-house staff need, so too should contract employees.

A complete familiarity with and commitment to upholding the profession's *Code of Ethics* and *Standards of Practice* cannot be overemphasized. Obeying the Code and *Standards of Practice* is an expectation. Ignorance is no excuse. Therefore, the contractual professional needs to engage in self-monitoring, perhaps to a greater extent than those employed by an organization. There is some thought that those independently contracting are having less scrutiny than those employed as employees. This is not the case. The Code and Standards are discussed elsewhere in this textbook.

# Summary

Understanding the importance of roles occupational therapists assume is as important as valuing them from a client perspective. In this chapter, the varying roles of practitioner, researcher, educator, and entrepreneur were discussed. In addition, the importance of the collaborative relationship with occupational therapy assistants as well as appreciating the responsibilities associated with providing services on a contractual basis were presented. This chapter provided only an overview of issues related to one's role as an occupational therapist. It is the responsibility of the professional occupational therapist to further explore and investigate his or her role(s) as he or she moves through his or her career trajectory.

# Student Self-Assessment

1. Identify some of the professional roles you can assume as a new graduate occupational therapist. Next, identify the roles you can assume after you have been in practice for two years, five years, and ten years. Discuss why the roles may change over time.
2. There are several roles you will assume as a professional occupational therapist. Identify and discuss the skills and knowledge needed for each role. Finally, develop a professional plan for yourself, identifying the roles you will assume and how you will prepare for each role.
3. Continuing your competency as an occupational therapist is a given. Discuss how you plan to continue your competency as an occupational therapist when you enter the field.

# Electronic Resources

- American Occupational Therapy Association: www.aota.org
- Accreditation Council for Occupational Therapy Education: www. acoteonline.org
- Commission on Continuing Competence and Professional Development: prodev@aota.org
- National Board for Certification in Occupational Therapy: www.nbcot.org

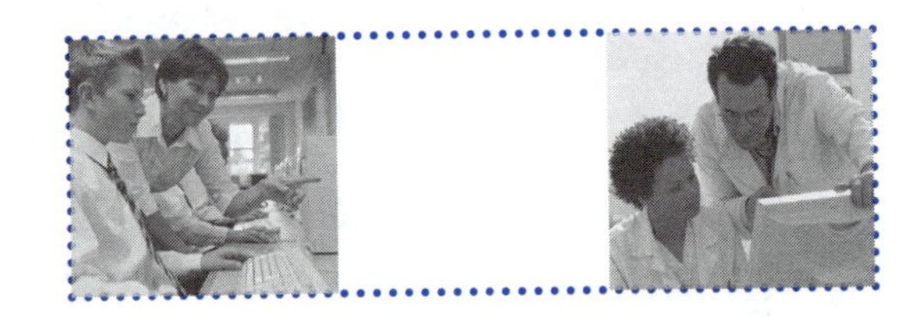

# References


Accreditation Council for Occupational Therapy Education. (1999). Standards for an accredited educational program for the occupational therapist. *American Journal of Occupational Therapy, 53*, 575-581.

Accreditation Council for Occupational Therapy Education. (2006). *The reference manual of the official documents of the AOTA* (11th ed.). Bethesda, MD: AOTA Press.

American Occupational Therapy Association. (1994). Roles papers. *American Journal of Occupational Therapy, 48*, 844-851.

American Occupational Therapy Association. (2000). Occupational therapy roles and career exploration and development : A companion guide to the Occupational Therapy Role Documents. In *The reference manual of the official documents of the American Occupational Therapy Association* (8th ed.). Bethesda, MD: Author.

American Occupational Therapy Association. (2004a). Guidelines for supervision, roles, and responsibilities during the delivery of occupational therapy services. *American Journal of Occupational Therapy, 58*(6), 663-667.

American Occupational Therapy Association. (2004b). Role competencies for a professional-level occupational therapist faculty member in an academic setting. *American Journal of Occupational Therapy, 58*(6), 649-650.

American Occupational Therapy Association. (2004c). Role competencies for an academic fieldwork coordinator. *American Journal of Occupational Therapy, 58*(6), 653-654.

American Physical Therapy Association. (2007). American Physical Therapy Association Web site. Retrieved July 18, 2007, from http://www.apta.org

Black, M. M. (1976). The occupational career. *American Journal of Occupational Therapy, 30*(4), 225-228.

Bondoc, S. (2005). Occupational therapy and evidence-based education. *Education Special Interest Section Quarterly, 15*(4), 1-4.

Braveman, B. (2005). *Leading and managing occupational therapy services: An evidence-based approach*. Philadelphia, PA: F.A. Davis.

Christiansen, C., & Baum, M. C. (1997). Glossary. In C. Christiansen & C. Baum (Eds.), *Occupational therapy: Enabling function and well-being* (2nd ed., pp. 591-606). Thorofare, NJ: SLACK Incorporated.

Clark, B. (1987). *The academic life: Small worlds, different worlds*. Princeton, NJ: The Carnegie Foundation for the Advancement of Teaching.

Crampton, M. W. (1958). The recognition of occupational therapy assistants. *American Journal of Occupational Therapy, 12*, 269-275.

Fidler, G. S. (1981). From crafts to competence. *American Journal of Occupational Therapy, 35*, 567-573.

Fisher, T. F. (1996). Roles and functions of a case manager. *American Journal of Occupational Therapy, 50*, 452-454.

Green, N. (2004). Demand and recruitment. *OT Practice, 9*(5), 48.

Henry, A. D., & Coster, W. J. (1997). Competency beliefs and occupational role behavior among adolescents: Explication of the personal causation construct. *American Journal of Occupational Therapy, 51*(4), 267-76.

Hirama, H. (1986). The COTA: A chronological review. In S. Ryan (Ed.), *The certified occupational therapist: Roles and responsibilities*. Thorofare, NJ: SLACK Incorporated.

Jantzen, A. C. (1974). Academic occupational therapy: A career specialty, 1973 Eleanor Clarke Slagle lecture. *American Journal of Occupational Therapy Association, 28*, 73-81.

Joint Commission on Accreditation of Healthcare Organizations. (2004). Human resource standards applicability to contracted and volunteer personnel. Retrieved October 26, 2009, from http://www.jointcommission.org/AccreditationPrograms/HomeCare/Standards/09_FAQs/HR/Human_Resource_Standards.htm

Kao, C. C., & Kellegrew, D. H. (2000). Self concept, achievement and occupation in gifted Taiwanese adolescents. *Occupational Therapy International, 7*(2), 121-133.

Kielhofner, G. (2006). *Research in occupational therapy: Methods of inquiry for enhancing practice*. Philadelphia, PA: F.A. Davis.

Kramer, P., Hinojosa, J., & Royeen, C. B. (2003). *Perspectives in human occupation: Participation in life*. Philadelphia, PA: Lippincott Williams & Wilkins.

McCormick, G., Jaffe, E., & Goodman-Lavey, M. (Eds.). (2003). *The occupational therapy manager* (4th ed.). Bethesda, MD: AOTA Press.

Mosey, A. C. (1998). The competent scholar. *American Journal of Occupational Therapy, 52*, 760-764.

Oakley, F., Kielhofner, G., Barris, R., & Reichler, R. (1986). The role checklist: Development and empirical assessment of reliability. *Occupational Therapy Journal of Research, 6*(3), 157-170.

Scaffa, M. (2001). *Occupational therapy in community-based practice settings*. Philadelphia, PA: F.A. Davis.

Shannon, P. D. (1985). From another perspective: An overview of the issue. *Occupational Therapy in Health Care, 2*(1), 3-11.

# Suggested Reading

Accreditation Council for Occupational Therapy Education. (2007). Standards and interpretive guidelines. Retrieved July 29, 2009, from http://www.aota.org/Educate/Accredit/StandardsReview/guide/42369.aspx

American Occupational Therapy Association. (2008). Occupational therapy practice framework: Domain and process, second edition. *American Journal of Occupational Therapy, 62*, 625-683.

Bruce, M. A. G., & Borg, B. (2002). *Psychosocial frames of reference: Core for occupation-based practice* (3rd ed.). Thorofare, NJ: SLACK Incorporated.

Coster, W. (1998). Occupation-centered assessment of children. *American Journal of Occupational Therapy, 52*(5), 337-344.

Wilcock, A. A. (2003). Population interventions focused on health for all. In E. B. Crepeau, E. S. Cohn, & B. A. Boyt Schell (Eds.), *Willard and Spackman's occupational therapy* (10th ed.). Haggerstown, MD: Lippincott, Williams and Wilkins.

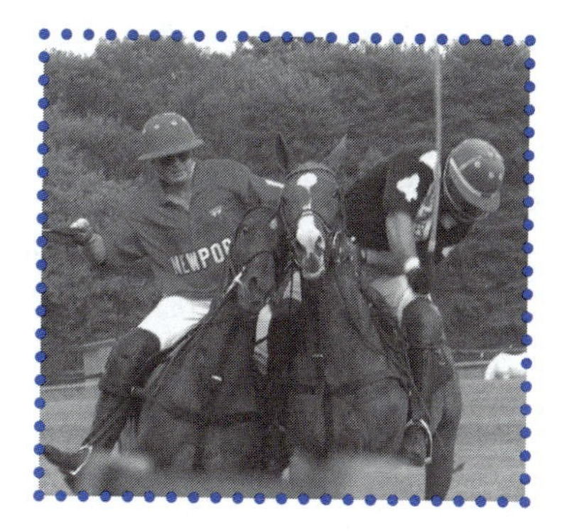

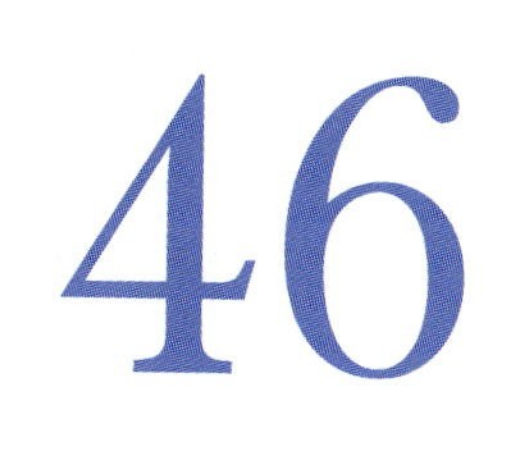

# Conflict Resolution

Jim Murray, SPHR

**ACOTE Standards Explored in This Chapter**

B.9.10-9.11

**Key Terms**

Collaboration
Compromise
Conflict resolution

## Introduction

Is conflict a negative or a positive? Unfortunately, many professionals focus on the negative aspects of conflict as opposed to the positive outcomes of structured resolutions. Conflict is a natural component of the typical workday. How practitioners, whether a recent graduate or a seasoned professional, resolve conflict in the workplace will, along with their clinical skills and aptitude, build their professional reputation and demonstrate how well they will associate with their co-workers, how flexible they will be in their work environment, and how they will address ethical issues that arise during the course of their employment. An occupational therapy practitioner's understanding of how to resolve both interpersonal and organizational ethical conflicts is a skill that will benefit him or her and serve as a building block to future professional success. As the occupational therapy practitioner approaches conflict, an awareness of the positive results will outweigh any perceived negativity.

The negative aspect of conflict, and often the most glaring, is the inevitable confrontation. Confrontation, regardless of how minor, can make any professional uncomfortable and will often cause one to question his or her perspective: "Is it really worth the confrontation? Maybe it will go away? Is it really a big deal?" Feelings of indecision and uncertainty are created by the potential confrontation. These questions and emotions can carry enough weight to dissuade one from resolving the conflict. Occupational therapy practitioners should not allow the negatives to outweigh the positives, but they should instead work toward resolving the situation.

Successful conflict resolution will have an immediate positive impact on the work environment as well as a lasting effect on the occupational therapy practitioner. When a conflict is resolved properly, the occupational therapy practitioner will gain professional respect, will adhere to high ethical standards, and will develop professional competencies, allowing for future growth and maturity. The learned skill of conflict resolution will benefit the occupational therapy practitioner during the immediate issue but will be transferable to future conflicts in the workplace.

This chapter will focus on the following areas:

- What are *conflict* and *conflict resolution*?
- What are the different approaches to resolving conflict?
- What is proactive versus reactive conflict?
- What resources can assist with conflict resolution?



K. Sladyk, K. Jacobs, & N. MacRae (Eds.).
*Occupational Therapy Essentials for Clinical Competence* (pp. 497-506).

## Conflict and Conflict Resolution

According to the Merriam-Webster Online Dictionary, conflict can be defined as a "...struggle resulting from incompatible or opposing needs, drives, wishes, or internal or external demands" (2009). Clinicians will work closely with doctors, nurses, and other practitioners, as well as with patients and families. They may also come into contact with vendors and suppliers of medical goods. Regardless of with whom occupational therapy practitioners associate, different people possess disparate levels of education, perspectives, life views, and opinions. Professionals at different points in their careers also have different priorities and objectives at work. Because of these differences, a certain level of disagreement, or conflict, is inevitable. Practitioners "must work with a staff that may hold a variety of perspectives and values. Inevitably, perspectives clash. And without intervention strategies, these subtle irritations can quickly progress into friction and conflict" (Petrazzi, 2005, p. 38). An occupational therapy practitioner must be aware of the differences that naturally exist in the workplace and that these disparities often result in conflict. Conflict tends to fall into two categories: interpersonal and ethical.

Interpersonal conflicts involve the occupational therapy practitioner and another individual or group. The conflict can be with an occupational therapy practitioner's manager, co-worker, client, or vendor. Due to the large number of people with whom the occupational therapy practitioner comes into contact, the possibility for conflict is great. Different people and different perspectives can be varied. "In healthcare, there are wide gaps in employees' levels of education. Those with more education may be condescending to the less educated workers" (Tyler, 2002, p. 85). Those with more professional experience may not respect a new practitioner's opinion on a diagnosis. An occupational therapy practitioner must be aware of these different perspectives and their impact on the workplace. Often, interpersonal conflicts can be difficult because practitioners can decide how to approach the issue and formulate a plan to resolve the conflict, but they cannot control the other person's perspective or approach. Different approaches to interpersonal conflicts will be discussed later in this chapter.

For ethical conflicts, occupational therapy practitioners may not be in control of the overall situation, but they can control their reactions to the ethical question. For example, if the occupational therapy practitioner is instructed by her manager to incorrectly bill to a health insurance provider, the practitioner cannot control the request, but she can make the decision to react in an ethical manner or to follow the questionable directions from the manager. An occupational therapy practitioner may also be tempted to discharge a difficult patient prior to the completion of his intervention. There are numerous daily decisions an occupational therapy practitioner must make that have ethical components. Different approaches to ethical conflicts will also be reviewed later in this chapter as well as in the chapter on ethics (see Chapter 40).

Overall, "conflict" can arrive in the workplace in many forms. Conflict can be an immediately recognizable event, or it can be a slow-building process that, unless it is addressed at an early stage, will eventually bubble up and overflow. Conflict can be caused by different perspectives, stress in the workplace, or by the desire of the individual to convince others that his or her point of view is correct. Stress in the workplace will affect patience and shorten tempers. Conflict is often construed as a negative event. However, conflict often yields positive and constructive results.

## What Now?

Conflicts do not go away. Whether the conflict exists with a co-worker, professor, or manager, the occupational therapy practitioner needs to resolve each conflict in a professional and ethical manner. As students start their studies and careers in occupational therapy, the approach to conflict resolution is very similar to other professions: understanding conflict, recognizing the conflict, and then formulating an approach. Occupational therapy practitioners must also realize that the resolution of each conflict will have an impact on their co-workers, their professional reputation, and potentially on their employer.

Recognizing a conflict is both an intellectual evaluation as well as a visceral feeling. A conflict could be as overt as a verbal or physical altercation or the purposeful mistreatment of a client. Or, the conflict can be as subtle as a stare or an uncomfortable silence between co-workers, or a dilemma some would view as unethical while others would not. The occupational therapy practitioner's employer may require the practitioner bill a certain number of units per employer expectations. An occupational therapy practitioner may be pressured to bill for individual sessions when it was a group session. An occupational therapy practitioner may be working with individuals who are incompetent or unethical. How does an occupational therapy practitioner decide when to get involved? When is it the occupational therapy practitioner's place to confront the conflict? Or, is the resolution really the manager's problem and not the occupational therapy practitioner's?

However extreme or mild, any situation that is ethically questionable or that causes negativity and tension in the workplace can be defined as conflict and needs to be dealt with as soon as possible. Conflicts do not go away, nor do they resolve themselves. Failure to address a conflict at its early stages typically has negative results. An ignored conflict will often build and develop into a larger and more complex issue. The complexity and seriousness of the issue then will require greater conflict resolution skills for the occupational therapy practitioner. Conflict resolution is often easier during the beginning stages before it is allowed to grow into a more serious issue.

This proactive approach is easier said than done. If occupational therapy practitioners cannot recognize conflict, then how can they resolve the issue? They may feel they are being paranoid or possibly they are being too sensitive. Regardless, a good rule of thumb in recognizing the potential for conflict is that if the perspective of the other is in opposition to or in disagreement from the occupational therapy practitioner's professional and/or personal views, then a conflict most likely exists. If what is being done or said is contrary to his or her training, opinion, or knowledge, then a conflict may occur when practitioners offer their contrary perspective. If a situation does not appear logical or the situation does not "feel" right, these cues will often indicate a conflict exists with the occupational therapy practitioner's perspectives and views. The situation should be addressed as soon as possible, although addressing the situation does not mean practitioners need to win others to their viewpoint. Rather, it means there is something that needs to be addressed that is contrary to the occupational therapy practitioner's perspectives. How the occupational therapy practitioner approaches the conflict will be crucial to resolving it and ensuring it does not worsen.

# Different Approaches to Conflict

"The term 'conflict resolution' commonly refers to the process by which people from opposing positions on issues arrive at mutually acceptable solutions through collaborative problem solving" (Tyler, 2002). There are multiple reactions to conflict, both positive and negative. Most can be useful, while no specific approach is the answer for all occasions. The tactics to conflict resolution depend on the specific situation. Each situation may call for different tactics, but the basic strategy should stay the same. The primary goal for the occupational therapy practitioner is to be heard, understood, and considered. For ethical conflicts, occupational therapy practitioners need to understand the American Occupational Therapy Association's (AOTA) *Code of Ethics* and its principles, and how flexible, if at all, they will be with them.

For both interpersonal and organizational ethical conflicts, the different approaches to conflict vary. This chapter will address several responses that are not productive, and several approaches that will resolve the conflict as well as better prepare the occupational therapy practitioner for future success.

## What Not to Do

### Argument

The argumentative approach is not one of reconciliation or dialogue, but an approach geared to "win" the contrary opinion to the occupational therapy practitioner's side. This strategy builds on the premise that the occupational therapy practitioner has the correct view, regardless of the other's perspective. Argumentative practitioners are not interested in debating the issue or giving merit to the other perspective, but rather the exchange is a monologue focused on the occupational therapy practitioner's solution being the only resolution. This strategy does not resolve conflict but often escalates it. The unwillingness to listen to the other side of an argument can lead to raised voices and heightened sensitivities. If the contrary perspective is not argumentative and can be bullied, the occupational therapy practitioner may "win" the argument and thus resolve that conflict. However, in the workplace, this solution inevitably leads to larger and potentially more explosive issues down the road. If occupational therapy practitioners are viewed as confrontational and unwilling to listen to other's views, they will be viewed negatively in the workplace. Listed below are specific positives and negatives of this approach.

- Positives
  - Can "win" a conflict without giving up any of the occupational therapy practitioner's perspective. Potentially get 100% of what he or she wants.
  - This aggressive approach can get the issues to the forefront.
- Negatives
  - Can alienate other co-workers.
  - Viewed as a "bully" and not a team player.
  - Not conducive to an environment that encourages openness and dialogue.
  - Co-workers are not going to look to compromise or collaborate with the occupational therapy practitioner because they know the practitioner's typical approach is argumentative.

When the positives and negatives are weighed, the argumentative approach is not a consistently productive solution for resolving conflict.

### Avoidance

The avoidance approach is a common tactic utilized by many professionals. It is often the "easy way out" and allows the occupational therapy practitioner, at least for a time, to avoid the conflict. As mentioned earlier, most professionals do not like conflict, which makes the avoidance approach very popular. Practitioners "may be concerned about hurting a co-worker's feelings, creating animosity, or damaging relationships" (Mollica, 2005, p. 114). However, an occupational therapy practitioner should not avoid the conflict, hoping it will disappear. Even if the issue goes away, avoidance is only a temporary solution. Eventually, due to workplace stress or other factors, the same issue will inevitably reappear. Conflicts and ignored issues tend not to solve themselves but rather build and worsen over time. If the conflict is an interpersonal issue, the only way to resolve the conflict through avoidance is if either the practitioner or the other person leaves the company. With this "solution," one may have avoided the current situation, but the occupational therapy practitioner has failed to develop the necessary skills to effectively deal with the next interpersonal conflict that will inevitably arise. Ethical conflict, unlike interpersonal conflicts, cannot simply leave the employer. Ethical conflicts can be indicative of the corporate culture and value system. If the practitioner decides to do nothing, this decision still impacts the events. By avoiding the conflict, the occupational therapy practitioner is making an ethical decision to do nothing. "An unresolved conflict or interpersonal disagreement festers just under the surface on your work environment. It bubbles to the surface whenever enabled, and always at the worst possible moment" (Heathfield, n.d.). Using the avoidance approach means the occupational therapy practitioner is not learning resolution skills. This skill gap will have negative effects on the long-term professional career of the occupational therapy practitioner. Issues are inevitable, and therefore practitioners will eventually have to confront a conflict. They may be questioned by their manager or directly confronted by a co-worker. If a minor issue is evident, occupational therapy practitioners need to address it while the issue is still easily resolved. Ignoring it will be the seed of larger issues. Listed below are the positives and the negatives of this approach.

- Positives
  - Do not have to confront the issue.
  - Potential for the issue to simply go away.
- Negatives
  - Issues do not resolve themselves. Avoided issues typically grow into bigger issues where more advanced conflict management skills are required. Does not get the issue into the open.
  - Co-workers and management may view the occupational therapy practitioner as someone without convictions and values.
  - The occupational therapy practitioner is not viewed as a problem solver.

The avoidance approach is at best a temporary solution for conflict resolution. Avoiding the problem does not solve it, nor does it prepare the occupational therapy practitioner professionally for future conflicts.

## Productive Solutions

### Compromise

Compromising occurs when both parties are unwilling to concede their issue in full. This unwillingness points to a compromise as potentially the only solution. A compromise occurs when both parties work together, but eventually each side concedes a portion of their viewpoint in order to arrive at an agreement and to resolve the conflict. Both parties realize that "winning" the argument or conflict is not the primary goal, but rather being able to work together as a team and arriving at the best possible solution is the desired end result. Conceding part of their issue is the difficult part of the discussions. If both parties are passionate about an issue, then an initial agreement to engage in a dialogue is necessary. The dialogue between the two parties has to be productive and structured. Each side has to acknowledge the validity of the opponent's argument, communicate the most important parts of their arguments, and then acknowledge that the other person, like the occupational therapy practitioner, is compromising their position. Listed below are the positives and the negatives of this approach.

- Positives
  - Builds consensus and teamwork.
  - Promotes dialogue and an understanding of the other perspective.
  - Co-workers will see the practitioner as a listener who is open to others.
  - No one "wins," but no one "loses."
- Negatives
  - If the conflict is ethical in nature, often a compromise solution does not exist.
  - If one person is truly right, then he or she is giving up a portion of the best solution.
  - Difficult to agree on what each side of the conflict should give up to arrive at a compromise.
  - Conceding a component of one's perspective may lead to regret or animosity.

### Collaboration

The first three approaches toward conflict resolution are not the optimal responses. Each scenario contains negative points that could outweigh the positive gains. The collaborative approach occurs when both parties have their perspectives but they put them aside to do what is best for the situation and the organization, not what is best for them. Both parties enter into a partnership mutually beneficial for themselves, as well as the company. Collaboration is a true dialogue where discussion of the best resolution is the focus, not convincing each other that one's solution is the best. The issue is not argued or avoided, and positions are not compromised. For occupational therapy practitioners, communication with collaboration in mind has the goal of learning through dialogue as opposed to convincing the person with the contrary view that his or her opinion is wrong. Listed below are the positives and the negatives of this approach.

- Positives
  - The organization benefits as opposed to the individual.
  - True dialogue and teamwork exist; culture of openness and collaboration is supported.
  - No one has to lose any part of his or her perspective because the views are open to the best possible resolution.

- Co-workers view the practitioner as an active listener who is open to contrary views.
- Negatives
  - None

The best overall strategy is that of collaboration. When both ends of the conflict are open to collaborating, then this is the best option. The focus is no longer on "winning" the conflict but doing what is best for the organization.

How do practitioners convince the alternate view that collaboration is the best approach? Practitioners may approach the conflict with open mindedness and unselfish motives, but the other's approach may be argumentative. Occupational therapy practitioners must strive to guarantee that the contrary method is consistent with their collaborative approach. Gaining this consistency is very difficult. The best method is for occupational therapy practitioners to demonstrate the situation through conversation—a question-and-answer approach. The more occupational therapy practitioners demonstrate a respect for the contrary opinions through active listening and questioning, the more open the other will be to their viewpoints.

# Proactive Versus Reactive Conflict

Within interpersonal and ethical conflicts, there are two basic approaches to resolving the conflict: proactive and reactive. Proactive conflict typically occurs when an occupational therapy practitioner successfully recognizes an issue and has decided to address it before it escalates. Or, based on previous communications, the occupational therapy practitioner understands the expectations from management. The positives of a proactive approach are being able to think about and then plan for the resolution. If occupational therapy practitioners are having an ongoing issue with a client, they can plan their approach, language, and position prior to speaking with the client. However, practitioners need to be careful they do not overanalyze the situation. Having too much time to think about the conflict can also be a negative. Occupational therapy practitioners can "psych themselves out" and actually cause and create a more stressful situation. The opportunity to plan the conflict resolution should and will outweigh any buildup of stress. By formulating a flexible resolution, occupational therapy practitioners can ensure that their words are measured, their approach is confident, and their attitude is positive.

Clear and concise communication skills support proactive problem solving and conflict resolution. Communication is an essential ingredient as the occupational therapy practitioner attempts to resolve a conflict. "Because communication skills are essential in conflict resolution, taking it upon 'themselves' to improve these skills should rank high on 'the practitioner's list of things to do upon entering into today's workplace'" (Kemp-Longmore, 2000, p. 131). Communication in the workplace is buttressed by setting clear expectations. If practitioners understand their role and are allowed to communicate their expectations in return then a starting point to help resolve conflicts will be established based on these expectations. When practitioners start a new position in a company, they should be provided with guidelines on the company's culture, rules of conduct, and best practices. However, practitioners also need to meet with their manager to ensure they understand the company's expectations and have an opportunity to communicate their expectations in turn. If both parties have a mutual understanding of expectations at the start of the employment relationship, then any future conflicts will be easier to address.

Conflict resolution is rendered nearly impossible if proper communication does not exist between occupational therapy practitioners and their co-workers, manager, and company. Though much responsibility rests with the more experienced manager to ensure that communication occurs, an occupational therapy practitioner is a professional who should also be working to develop communication and expectations. If occupational therapy practitioners do not understand their manager's or the company's expectations in ethical and clinical matters, they must take it upon themselves to seek the answers. A passive or reactive approach is not the best option. "I did not know" is not a good excuse for a lack of communication.

The reactive situation to conflict typically occurs when the practitioner is approached by another individual or witnesses a questionably ethical event. Unplanned conflicts provoke a reactive response from the occupational therapy practitioner. It can be a confrontation from a co-worker, a hostile patient, or a simple disagreement with a co-worker on a course of intervention. The area of unplanned conflict is what most individuals classically define as conflict. The "flight" versus "fight" natural response occurs, and occupational therapy practitioners have to react. Do they strike out or step back? If practitioners are aware of and comfortable with the different responses to conflict, a reaction to the unplanned conflict can occur more easily. With more experience in conflict resolution, utilization of the different approaches to conflict resolution will broaden.

## What to Do

Planning for the conflict can be difficult. Occupational therapy practitioners have to recognize conflict, construct an approach, review previous communications, and then determine if and how to act. Practitioners must also learn to develop conflict resolution skills and not abdicate to another party for resolution. For managers, solving their "employee's problems for them hurts their performance by reducing collaboration and making them dependent" (Mollica, 2005, p. 111). To avoid this dependency, practitioners need to review the above sections for guidance in recognizing the conflict and formulating an approach for resolution. A viable strategy for planning the conflict resolution exercise involves the following:

- The practitioner needs to determine the desired outcome from the conflict
    - o What is the end goal?
    - o What does the practitioner wish to achieve with the conflict resolution?
- Once the end goal is identified, the practitioner needs to create a tactical plan with steps designed to achieve the goal. Tactics include the following:
    - o Affirm the relationship. Rather than starting the conversation highlighting the differences, practitioners can act positively. It can be "as simple as saying, 'Greg, our working relationship is important and I'm seeing a problem that could interfere with our rapport...'" (Grensing-Pophal, 2004).
    - o Be prepared to ask questions to learn about the other's perspective; gather facts about the situation. When a practitioner looks at another perspective, he or she has the "tendency to respond to conflict by trying to put one's self in the other person's position and trying to understand their point of view" (Delahoussaye, 2002, p. 20).
    - o Listen to the answers for the questions asked; engage in active listening. Body language will tell the listener as much as the spoken word. Practitioners should be aware of how body language impacts what is being said. If body language is meek or unsure, the attempt at conflict resolution will appear the same.
    - o The practitioner needs to clarify and explain his or her own views. Practitioners need to be convincing about their own views and prepared to act on them accordingly.

The result of the interchange of questions coupled with active listening should result in a resolution to the conflict. Remember, "...the conflict can be simple or complex. It can take no more than a single meeting of the minds, while other conflicts may take an ongoing process and, in some cases, the use of outside mediators" (Kemp-Longmore, 2000, p. 131). For many conflicts, change will not be immediate. The collaborative approach is an ongoing process.

## Example of an Interpersonal Conflict

Practitioner relationships with managers can be both positive and negative. A positive relationship has the manager acting as a mentor and a helping guide. A negative relationship may exist because the day-to-day supervision of new graduates can be trying for managers pressed by multiple priorities. A manager who yells and does not provide clear directions can set up a potential interpersonal conflict. Using the guidance above, the steps would be as follows:

- *Determine the desired outcome*: Achieving better communication with the manager and ensuring the manager understands that yelling at the therapist is not respectful or productive.
- The tactics the practitioner needs to take to reach the desired outcome include:
    - o *Gather facts*: Practitioners need to be aware of company policies regarding dispute resolution and conflict. They can then ask the manager the following questions:
        - ▪ What is your communication style?
        - ▪ What do you feel are the best methods to communicate priorities?
        - ▪ What are your priorities for the day and how does the practitioner supervision fit into your busy schedule?

      These questions will provide the practitioner with a general idea of how the manager perceives his or her communication style as well as a better idea of the work responsibilities of the manager. If practitioners have a better understanding of the manager's role, they can better communicate knowing what causes the pressure and stress in the manager's workday. If the manager is unavailable for an informal meeting, the practitioner needs to schedule a formal meeting with the manager. The conversation should be in private.
    - o *Active listening*: Asking questions and actively listening to the responses also tells the manager the practitioner is interested in his or her day, priorities, and how the occupational therapy practitioners fit into his or her schedule.
    - o *Provide own expectations and perspective*: By asking questions and listening to the manager, the practitioner has opened the door for communication with the manager. He or she is now better able to share his or her perspective on communication and what works or does not work for him or her. By being open to the manager's views, the manager in turn should be more open to the practitioner's perspectives.
    - o In most cases, a conversation using the steps above will resolve the conflict. In those cases where the conflict continues, the practitioner is encouraged to involve a third party, such as a representative from Human Resources (HR), to act as a mediator. The mediator will most likely follow the steps above to ensure a productive dialogue takes place and that expectations are clear moving forward.

## Example of an Ethical Conflict

Typically, billing is done using a code for every 15 minutes, with each 15-minute segment making up one unit. The practitioner is asked by management to bill 3 units for each patient. The practitioner spends 30 minutes, or 2 units, treating a patient. Should the practitioner bill for 2 units covering 30 minutes, or the required 3 units? Using the guidance above, the steps would be as follows:

- *Determine the desired outcome*: Practitioners must be ethical in their billing practices while adhering to the rules of their clinic. The practitioner should only bill for the actual time spent with the patient.
- Gather facts:
  - Review the company's policy, if one exists, on billing practices.
  - Understand the AOTA *Code of Ethics* and its principles.
  - Determine if management understands the time it takes to treat the patient.
    - Assess the impact on you and your work by properly billing.
    - Assess the impact on you and your work by improperly billing.
- Once the practitioner evaluates the manager's perspective, as well as the corporation's policy, a decision can be made on the ethical steps to take. If the decision is contrary to what the company and the manager desire, the occupational therapy practitioner still has to behave ethically according to the standards established by the profession.

Whether the conflict is interpersonal or ethical in nature, "employees who can resolve most of their own conflicts in the workplace are most likely productive and efficient and can be a tremendous asset to a company's bottom line" (Mollica, 2005, p. 112). It is important for clinicians to understand the processes involved in resolving conflicts. The greater this understanding, the more professional success the practitioners will achieve.

## Resources to Assist the Practitioner in Resolving Conflicts

Practitioners need to be able to judge the level of conflict and determine if they are able to resolve the situation on their own. If a conflict arises that occupational therapy practitioners are not able to resolve, or if they desire another opinion on their course of action, then there are several resources to turn to for assistance.

- *Management*: If a practitioner has a conflict with a co-worker or a patient, the manager is often the best resource. The initial step should be to ask for advice instead of letting the manager solve the problem for him or her. If the manager resolves the issues, the occupational therapy practitioner will not learn the skills and tools to solve future issues. Practitioners need to get initial guidance but then implement the course of action themselves. If they are unable to resolve the conflict, or the situation makes them extremely uncomfortable or requires a supervisor's intervention, then the manager can serve as a mediator to the conflict.
- *HR*: Conflicts, such as sexual harassment and more serious issues, should be brought to the immediate attention of HR. Practitioners can always talk to their manager, but if the problem is the manager, then confiding in HR is the best approach. When occupational therapy practitioners join an organization, they need to ensure that during the new hire process or during the first week of their employment, they understand what the processes are in dealing with conflict. Typically, a company's employee handbook will outline the proper steps to take if an issue should arise. If the occupational therapy practitioner works for a small facility that does not have HR, the occupational therapy practitioners should discuss these processes with the manager or with their co-workers prior to issues arising.
- *Professional network*: One of the most important and often ignored professional tools is the development of a professional network. A professional network may consist of current and former co-workers, management, and educators. A network will assist in many ways with professional resources, advice, and career counseling. As occupational therapy practitioners start a career, they should take the time and make the effort to build a professional network. The network will be able to assist them in a variety of ways and offer them clinical, professional, and ethical advice. In dealing with ethical or interpersonal conflicts, speaking with others can be invaluable. For professionals new to the workforce, having a network of peers with which to confer about similar experiences and issues is a valuable tool.

## Summary

*Conflict* is a word that makes most professionals uncomfortable and wary. It is acceptable for practitioners to be wary of conflict. However, it is not acceptable for practitioners to avoid or to ignore conflicts. The inability to deal with conflicts will have a negative impact on practitioners' effective job performance. The preceding chapter defined "conflict," provided guidelines on recognizing conflict in the workplace, and outlined four different approaches to resolving conflict. These tools, along with the examples of interpersonal and ethical conflicts, should better prepare a new professional to handle the conflicts that exist in every work environment. Resolving conflict in the workplace is an essential skill that all professionals must possess. The ability to resolve conflict successfully will separate them from their peers as they grow in their profession.

## Student Self-Assessment

Using the different approaches to conflict resolution outlined previously, evaluate the following learning activities and apply the different possible approaches. What approaches are most effective in the following scenarios?

## Activity #1

The practitioner, Stephannie, is a recent graduate working in a small outpatient rehabilitation clinic owned by two doctors. She works with one other senior practitioner who supervises her, three other practitioners whom are her peers, several administrative staff, and the two doctors. After several months on the job, she is dealing with the following issues:

- Her supervisor's expectations are not clear. Stephannie is unsure if she is doing a good job.
- One of the administrative staff gives her the "cold shoulder" whenever they are in a room together.
- She has a good relationship with one doctor, but the other doctor recently questioned her judgment in front of her peers.
- One of her peers has started using Stephannie's work area to eat her lunch.

### Productive Resolutions

- Stephannie should foster dialogue with her supervisor. Since she is unsure how her job performance is thus far, she should directly ask her supervisor while also requesting specific examples of how she is, or is not, performing. If her supervisor is not providing the feedback, Stephannie needs to seek out the information.
- Stephannie could use avoidance or take the argumentative approach, but those options would not resolve the conflict. If Stephannie desires a productive relationship with the administrative staff, avoiding the situation will not help her understand the staff's motivation. Being argumentative would most likely increase the "cold shoulder" approach from the staff because Stephannie does not understand the issues. The best approach is to collaborate with the staff member to gain understanding of the issues. This could involve a self-assessment by Stephannie to see if she is doing anything to provoke the "cold shoulder" as well as confronting the staff member with non-accusatory questions to determine a resolution to the issues.
- Questioning a superior's behavior is always difficult. This scenario may require the involvement of her supervisor as well as HR. If Stephannie avoids the situation, then the doctor may continue to act inappropriately in front of her peers. If she is argumentative, she could be viewed as "unprofessional" or a "boat rocker." In this scenario, the practitioner should seek support and help from her supervisor and HR to assist her in formulating the most productive solution.
- If Stephannie does not want to share her private work station, then the compromise approach is not the best avenue. The best approach is for Stephannie to engage in a dialogue with her peer and communicate specifically what she desires. This communication should not be argumentative.

## Activity #2

The practitioner, James, is a new graduate working in a large inpatient hospital. He works with a very large team of occupational therapy practitioners from diverse backgrounds and with different levels of experience. After several months on the job, he is dealing with the following:

- James never sees his supervisor. He relies on his peers for guidance and direction. He is unsure if he should be talking with his supervisor because of the hectic environment.
- Most decisions amongst the occupational therapy practitioners are done in groups by voting, with majority vote winning. James does not feel he has a chance to offer his opinions and views.
- Several of the clients treat James like a kid. They seek answers from the more experienced practitioners even though James is qualified to assist.
- The schedule that James now works is changing. James is not sure if the new shift will work with his personal priorities.

### Productive Resolutions

- James should make every effort to find his supervisor and try and create a dialogue with her. James needs to know if he should be relying on his peers for guidance or if his supervisor will be there to coach and train him. If it is the former, the sooner that James understands the supervisory relationship, the more productive he will be. If it is the latter, then James and his supervisor have to do a better job at communicating. Scheduling a weekly meeting or bi-weekly lunch could be a start in developing the communication channels.
- The best solution is not to confront the group's decision-making process as a new practitioner in the hospital but to become familiar with the process. Once familiar with the process, James will be better suited to know when to inject his opinions and views. With a voting scenario, James should have the opportunity to voice his perspective while also questioning and challenging his peers in a collaborative manner on their opinions. If, over time, the decision-making process is still not to James's liking, he should discuss the situation with his supervisor as opposed to bringing his issue to the entire group.

| Evidence-Based Research Chart | |
|---|---|
| **Topic** | **Evidence** |
| Conflict can be positive and should not be avoided | Bannan, 2004; Kemp-Longmore, 2002; Tyler, 2002 |
| Conflict can be the result of different perspectives | Delahoussaye, 2002; Petrazzi, 2005; Tyler, 2002; |
| There are many different approaches to conflict, with collaboration being the most productive | Kemp-Longmore, 2002; Mollica, 2005; Tompkins & Rogers, 2004 |
| Communication is essential to have successful conflict resolution | Bannan, 2004; Gresing-Pophal, 2004; Kemp-Longmore, 2002; Mollica, 2005 |

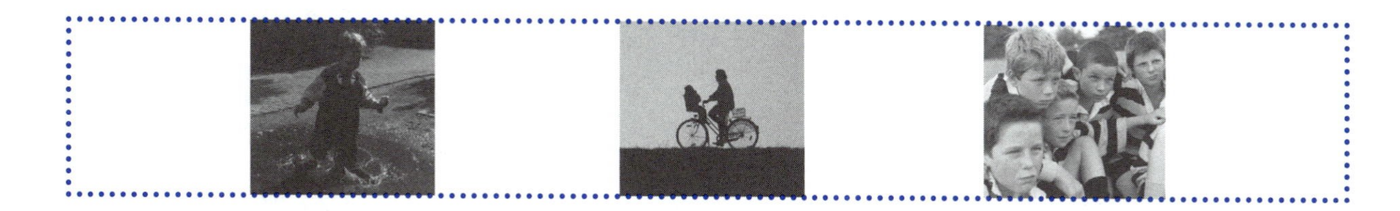

- It may take James some time to gain the respect and confidence from clients. The best solution is not to confront the clients and demand they seek guidance from only him. Rather, James should converse with his peers and ask them to redirect the client's questions to him. This approach, assuming James is helpful, will develop client trust in James's abilities and eventually migrate their concerns from his peers to him.
- If James was hired with his current schedule in mind but that schedule is now changing, he has to decide what route to take. If he is flexible and is able to adjust his schedule, then there is no issue. If he is inflexible because of other commitments outside of work (continuing education, family, etc.), then he has to decide on his next steps. He can consult with his supervisor and see if there is another shift available or he can opt to leave the position. This last scenario is more of a personal decision as opposed to a standard resolution.

## References


Bannan, K. J. (2004). Left unsaid: How ignoring internal conflict can kill your small business. Retrieved August 1, 2006, from http://www.mybusinessmag.com/fullstory.php3?sid=976

Delahoussaye, M. (2002). Don't get mad, get promoted (conflict resolution). *Training, 39*, 20-21.

Gresing-Pophal, L. (2004). Society for Human Resources Management, Resolving client disputes: Deal with it. Retrieved June 11, 2006, from http://www.shrm.org/consultants/library_published/nonIC/CMS_010133.asp

Heathfield, S. M. (n.d.) Workplace conflict resolution: People management tips. Managing your human resources. Retrieved June 11, 2006, from http://humanresources.about.com/od/managementtips/a/conflict_solue.htm

Kemp-Longmore, C. (2002). Conflict resolution in the workplace. *The Black Collegian, 30*(i2), 131.

Merriam-Webster Online Dictionary. (2009). Conflict. Retrieved September 28, 2009, from http://www.merriam-webster.com/dictionary/conflict

Mollica, K. (2005). Stay above the fray: Protect your time—and your sanity—by coaching employees to deal with interpersonal conflicts on their own. *HR Magazine, 50*(4), 111-115.

Petrazzi, A. A. (2005). Sign of the times: Eliminate generational conflict by understanding different perspectives. *Advance Magazine, 21*, 38.

Tompkins, T. C., & Rogers, K. S. (2004). Using conflict to your advantage: Butting heads is not always bad. Retrieved August 1, 2006, from http://gbr.pepperdine.edu/041/learningteams.html

Tyler, K. (2002). Extending the olive branch. Conflict resolution training helps employees and managers defuse skirmishes. *HR Magazine, 47*(11), 85-88.

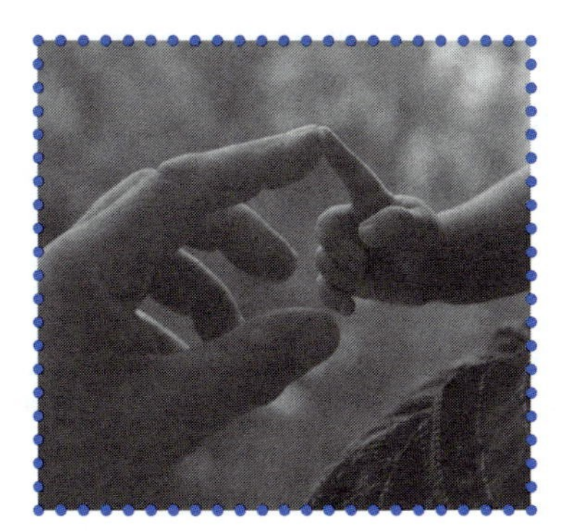

# 47

# Advocacy

*Elisa Marks, MS, OTR/L, CEAS, CHT*

## ACOTE Standards Explored in This Chapter

B.9.12-9.13

## Key Terms

Legislative process
Lobbyist
Moratorium
TriAlliance of Health and Rehabilitation Professions

## Introduction

Advocacy is defined by the American Heritage Dictionary as "the act of pleading or arguing in favor of something, such as a cause, idea, or policy; active support" (2000). Occupational therapy professionals have a responsibility to advocate on behalf of their chosen profession. In this chapter, the role of occupational therapy practitioner and student as advocate will be explored with specific examples of activities the therapy advocate can pursue.

Politics and advocacy play a crucial role in the ability to practice as an occupational therapist and occupational therapy assistant. Legislation that is passed on Capitol Hill defines the way occupational therapy practitioners are reimbursed and the scope of their practice. Federal legislation affects occupational therapy practitioners in all areas of practice, including but not limited to school-based practitioners, skilled nursing facility practitioners, and mental health practitioners. To affect change on the local, state, and Federal level, it is imperative that new graduates integrate grassroots advocacy into their professional goals and development.

Advocacy is important for the viability of occupational therapy. Without advocacy, the profession of occupational therapy would be much more limited in scope of practice as well as in reimbursement. For example, occupational therapy practitioners might not be able to practice in low-vision rehabilitation, splinting and prosthetics, community-based programs, and schools. When therapists take the time—and it does not take much time—to make their voices heard, positive changes happen. There are many ways to be a grassroots advocate both as an individual and as a group of colleagues. Techniques and activities will be explored later in this chapter.

## Occupational Therapy Advocacy

Several examples illustrate both the need for occupational therapy practitioners and occupational therapy students to be advocates and the positive influence advocacy can have on the legislative process. The following section shows how occupational therapy practitioners mobilized and supported the American Occupational Therapy Association (AOTA). In the first part, occupational therapy advocacy directly affected legislative change. In the second part, the need for continued advocacy is illustrated.



K. Sladyk, K. Jacobs, & N. MacRae (Eds.).
*Occupational Therapy Essentials for Clinical Competence* (pp. 507-516).

## Balanced Budget Amendment of 1997

During the Federal budget negotiations of 1997, Congress looked very closely at mechanisms that would save money within the Medicare system. Since it is anticipated that Medicare will not be able to pay all of its obligations by 2018 (Sahadi, 2006), legislators looked for services within Medicare that were costing more than was deemed appropriate. Excessive amounts of therapy were being billed by some providers of occupational, physical, and speech therapies. The rehabilitation therapies became the target of intense scrutiny and the focus of money-saving action. In response to the perceived abuses within the system, Congress looked at ways to limit the amount of services that therapists provided.

Ultimately, Congress passed legislation that allowed $1500 per year of occupational therapy and $1500 per year of physical therapy and speech therapy combined for outpatient therapies received under Medicare Part B. This legislation became known as the "$1500 Therapy Caps" in the rehabilitation community. This was the only "dollar amount" cap for professional services in all of Medicare (AOTA, n.d.a). An exception that was noted in the original version of the legislation was for clients receiving therapy at a hospital-based outpatient rehabilitation department. These programs were exempt from the cap as "fall back" for clients who exceeded the cap at other facilities but had a continued need for rehabilitation. The legislation was notable for what it did not discuss.

The legislation made no exceptions for Medicare recipients who had more than one injury or illness per calendar year. Therefore, if Mrs. Smith had a stroke in January and used $1300 of her therapy benefit and then broke a hip in September of that same year, she would only be allowed another $200 of occupational therapy. Two hundred dollars will not cover an evaluation in many facilities.

The legislation did not address the needs of rural Medicare subscribers who did not have access to a hospital with an outpatient rehabilitation department. These Medicare members would not have a "fall back" mechanism despite distance or limited transportation options.

The legislation also did not address the needs of clients with multiple diagnoses. Clients with complicated medical histories that may include diabetes, dementia, multiple sclerosis, etc. typically used more therapy visits and their recovery was slower. There were no exceptions for progressive illnesses or clients who were medically unstable.

The following scenario will demonstrate how advocacy made a positive difference. When the therapy caps were implemented, many facilities reduced their therapy staffs because reimbursement for therapy services was severely restricted. Practitioners and their professional associations mobilized, and Congress revisited the issue. Over the years, there were short windows when the caps were in place, but thanks to the successful advocacy efforts, multiple moratoriums were placed on the caps. During these times, Congress put a hold on implementation of the caps in order to explore more equitable and meaningful restraints on the system. Unfortunately, in 2006, therapists were again met with an expiring moratorium and a greater likelihood that Centers for Medicare and Medicaid Services (CMS) would find a manageable way to implement the $1500 cap (currently $1740 in inflation-adjusted dollars).

In 2006, Congress and CMS developed an intricate system to implement the caps. Lobbyists from the physical therapy, occupational therapy, and speech therapy professional associations worked together through the TriAlliance of Health and Rehabilitation Professions with legislators to create exceptions to the cap (American Physical Therapy Association [APTA], 2000). These exceptions would help to ensure that the clients with more complicated needs would have access to the services that were medically necessary. A lengthy list of exceptions were written, including clients suffering multiple incidents in one calendar year, clients dealing with a defined list of complex diagnoses, clients needing both physical and speech therapy, and clients having a combination of diagnoses. The provider was charged with requesting the exception in order to continue intervention.

This framework ensured that clients were receiving more of the care that they needed, but these exceptions had their flaws as well. A major flaw included that they were only regulated for 2006.

## Home Health Qualifying Service

As of 2006, in order for a client to receive occupational therapy home health services, he or she must first be assessed by a nurse, speech therapist, or physical therapist. Despite the fact that a client may have been discharged from the hospital the day before with a recommendation for home health occupational therapy only, he or she cannot be seen solely by occupational therapy in the home. Only physical therapy, speech therapy, and nursing are "qualifying services" to identify needed home health care. Overutilization of services occurs when multiple providers must assess a client in order for only one service to be involved. Occupational therapy practitioners continue the hard work of lobbying legislators to include occupational therapy as a home health qualifying service.

## Who Is an Advocate?

Many therapists would say that they do not need to be involved with politics, they are only concerned about their clients' day-to-day health and rehabilitation needs. This belief is mistaken. All therapists and occupational therapy students must be advocates. The involvement in advocacy may vary from practitioner to practitioner, but it is a professional responsibility to be politically aware. One may even involve clients in advocating for occupational therapy.

## Occupational Therapy Practitioner and Student as Advocate

There are many ways to be a grassroots advocate for your profession without studying the minutae of policy. An occupational therapy practitioner advocates for the profession every time he or she explains what the profession of occupational therapy represents. An occupational therapy practitioner is an advocate every time she or he has a client who states that occupational therapy made a difference in his or her lives. These steps toward broader awareness of the profession and its goals lay the groundwork for meaningful advocacy activities.

There are many small projects that a therapist can participate in that have an effect on the legislative process. First, therapists must be aware of who their elected officials are. This information is readily available in the phone book, on the Internet (access www.us.gov and click on "Voting and Elections"), and at the local library. When an issue arises that warrants advocacy, the practitioner and student must know who his or her audience is for sharing information. Sharing examples of client success stories with a legislator can highlight the impact of occupational therapy services. This may illustrate to a legislator the benefit a piece of occupational therapy-related legislation will bring to the legislator's district. Both letter writing and phone calls to a legislator's office can influence the way a legislator considers voting on a piece of legislation. Additional examples of therapist advocacy will follow later in the chapter.

## Lobbyist as Advocate

Professional organizations, such as AOTA, employ lobbyists to help with legislative influence. Lobbyists are professionals who provide legislators and their assistants or legislative aides (LA) with detailed information on focused issues. For example, a legislator may not be an expert on how occupational therapy practitioners can help drivers with disabilities. A lobbyist from AOTA would provide both anecdotal and statistical information about the role of occupational therapy in driver rehabilitation. This may include information such as the dollar savings on caregivers when clients return to independent driving or on the reduced accident and injury rate after clients have completed a driver rehabilitation program. The professional lobbyist provides the solid data that argues for or against legislation that will help the profession obtain client access, reimbursement, and competitiveness.

## Client as Advocate

When a practitioner teaches clients about occupational therapy, it creates stories of the profession that can be shared. Clients who are inspired by their occupational therapy practitioner will share their success story with other members of their community. This creates more people who are aware of the need for occupational therapy in the continuum of care.

Client DM suffered a severe hand injury when she slipped in the laundry room. As she fell, her arm crashed through the glass window on her front-loading clothes dryer. She had significant nerve, tendon, and vessel injury to her dominant hand. As a working mother of two teenagers, she was devastated by her injury but highly motivated to participate in occupational therapy to return to her previous occupational roles. Being out of work had a significant financial impact as her children's private school tuition was significantly discounted due to the many hours she put in as food service manager at the school. DM worked closely with her occupational therapist to first learn adaptive techniques for the protection and healing of her dominant hand. When she was able to progress to functional activities, her occupational therapist identified a variety of graded functional activities that DM could participate in to help her hand heal and get stronger. DM was excited to begin her housework again and drive her kids to school. Her appreciation for occupational therapy was evident in how much she raved about the special care she received from her therapist. DM lived next door to her Representative to the United States Congress. She frequently spoke of her therapists and the impact good access to occupational therapy made in her recovery while sharing coffee in his kitchen. Prior to her injury, her Representative had been unfamiliar with the field of occupational therapy and now was educated by a good friend and client advocate of occupational therapy.

# Types of Advocacy

## Direct Advocacy

Occupational therapy practitioners and students can reach out directly to legislators and members of their staff to share concerns about pending legislation. Additionally, they can build relationships with a legislator's office and become a resource for the staff when issues regarding rehabilitation arise. Examples of direct advocacy include the following:

- *Letter writing*: Personal letters that tell the stories of clients benefiting from occupational therapy. Includes your request for their vote on a particular piece of legislation (Figure 47-1).
- *Phone calls*: Calls to legislators or their LA on health care. Discuss the legislation you are calling about and how you would like the legislator to vote. Include personal client stories.
- *Meeting the legislator in person*: Attend a town hall meeting, invite the legislator to visit your work facility, or visit his or her office in the statehouse or on Capitol Hill (Figure 47-2).

BU College of Health & Rehabilitation Sciences: Sargent College

February 10, 2009

State Representative Marilyn Giuliano
House Republican Office
L.O.B. Room 4200
Hartford, CT 06106

Dear Representative Giuliano:

As an occupational therapy student and constituent of Old Saybrook I am writing this letter in support of bill S.B. 144 Health insurance for parents of children receiving services from the Department of Developmental Services. As an occupational therapy student, I am aware that research has indicated that parents of children and adults who consume services from the Department of Developmental Services have demanding lives and often endure physical and mental distress.

By providing these families with adequate healthcare you would be allowing them to focus on providing the best care possible to their children, and alleviating their personal concerns about becoming sick or being unable to care for their children. By keeping these parents healthy it prevents their children from being placed into residential facilities at the cost of the state. As occupational therapist we are interested in providing the best care possible in the most natural environment, as we know this provides the best quality of life for both the child and the caregiver. These children are mostly likely to have their needs met and to reach their fullest potential in a home with the people they know best to support them.

The parents of these children if unable to stay home would be forced to put their children into residential placements. This can cause undue stress for both the parent and the child. As someone who has worked in residential facilities, I know they are both stressful and emotionally traumatic to the children placed in them. Not only is this an unnecessary stress that could be avoided, but also residential facilities are very costly. It would be more cost effective to keep these children at home and provide insurance for their parents, who could best meet their needs.

For many parents it is not only their primary role to be a parent, but actually it is a defining part of their life. To take this privilege away from them could be devastating, resulting in them requiring more care, and again at the cost of the state due to their lack of insurance. As stated previously parents of children receiving services from the Department of Developmental Services already work hard to take care of their children as well as advocate for getting their needs met. Passing this bill would make it easy for them to take care of themselves and provide the essential care their children require.

Please support bill S.B. 144 Health Insurance coverage for parents of children receiving services from the Department of Developmental Services. Thank you for your consideration and kind attention to this issue.

Sincerely,

Stacey Fulkerson
Boston University Occupational Therapy Student

**Figure 47-1.** Sample letter to legislator.

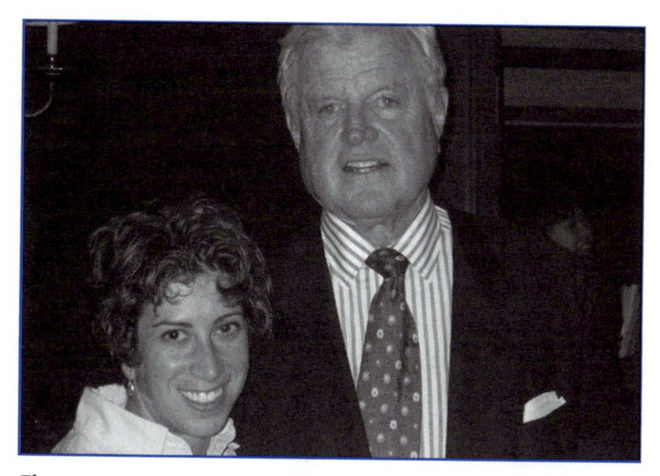

**Figure 47-2.** Author meeting with Senator Edward Kennedy (D-MA).

When speaking with a legislator, the practitioner or student must make certain to state where he or she lives. This allows the elected official to see that the therapist/student is a voter in his or her district. Additionally, the practitioner or students should always refer to him- or herself as an "occupational therapy practitioner" or "occupational therapy student" since the elected official may not be aware what "OT" abbreviates. It is especially important for the practitioner to remember that he or she is the expert. The elected official and his or her staff are NOT occupational therapy practitioners. They do not have the knowledge and depth of understanding regarding occupational therapy theory and the benefits of occupational therapy that a student or practitioner has. Although some may get nervous or anxious about answering questions regarding occupational therapy, the practitioner will be the expert. It is also acceptable to let the staff member know that you do not have the information he or she is asking for and you will get back to him or her. AOTA's public affairs staff can be a resource for getting answers that are beyond the scope of a clinical practitioner.

## Indirect Advocacy

In addition to reaching out to legislators, occupational therapy practitioners and students can practice advocacy through other avenues. Belonging to professional associations is a way for large groups of professionals to make their voice heard in a uniform, forceful manner. Professional associations such as AOTA and state associations rely on member involvement to promote the profession. Additionally, belonging to an affiliated advocacy group that benefits from occupational therapy helps to promote the profession. An occupational therapy practitioner working in an outpatient neurological rehabilitation clinic may find involvement in the Stroke Association to be both professionally beneficial and personally fulfilling. As members of such affiliated groups benefit from occupational therapy, their support of key legislation is helpful.

In 2002, AOTA held its first National Backpack Awareness Campaign (AOTA, n.d.b). The association invited occupational therapy students and practitioners to participate in educating the public about the hazards that can arise from overloaded backpacks children carry to school. According to AOTA, over 7,000 emergency room visits a year are attributed to improper backpack usage. The initiative's success can be measured by the fact that in 2005, over 300,000 students attended various backpack weigh-in events held on a single day by occupational therapy practitioners throughout the country. Media have attended these events and promoted the role of the occupational therapy practitioners in assuring safe backpack use. This indirect advocacy educated the public on the role of occupational therapy.

# Role of a Political Action Committee

Having relationships with politicians and policymakers is crucial if a professional organization hopes to influence the political process. Building this relationship often takes years, and the players frequently change with the election cycle. Elections play a critical role in forming the political playing field. It is during these periods leading up to Election Day that a political action committee (PAC) plays its most important role.

According to the Center for Responsive Politics and Federal Election Commission reports, the most expensive Congressional race in 2004 cost over $36 million. The cost of running television ads, calling voters, creating mailers, traveling to meet voters, and delivering people to the polls on Election Day is beyond the reach of most candidates' personal checkbooks. Therefore, politicians must reach out to interested parties and raise contributions to support their re-election campaign. PACs are a way for groups of individuals of common interest to come together, raise money, and give candidates significant monetary support. The monetary ability to support a wider array of candidates will also impact the ability to build relationships with a wide variety of politicians. AOTA created a PAC known as the American Occupational Therapy Political Action Committee (AOTPAC). This PAC was created in 1976 in order to support candidate/elected officials who are supportive of occupational therapy. AOTPAC is chaired by a volunteer committee of AOTA members who assist in fundraising and vote on distribution of funds to those candidates that may be supportive of the occupational therapy profession.

PACs choose to support candidates based on multiple factors. Frequently, the candidate's experience with promoting the group's issue is instrumental in receiving a donation from the affiliated PAC. Therefore, if a candidate is running for election and is intimately familiar with the issue (e.g., occupational therapy), it is likely that candidate will help support legislative efforts as needed. Additionally, if a politician who sits on a key committee is up for re-election and this candidate has a history of votes in favor of occupational therapy, AOTPAC may choose to support this candidate's re-election. PACs are a way for groups of individuals of common interest to come together, raise money, and give candidates significant monetary support.

# Summary

Advocacy is a professional responsibility throughout an occupational therapy practitioner's career. Occupational therapy practitioners and students have a variety of opportunities to participate in grassroots advocacy, including calling/emailing members of Congress, attending town hall meetings, inviting candidates to their facility, and developing relationships with affiliated advocacy groups. Additionally, PACs (such as AOTPAC) use member donations to provide direct financial support to occupational therapy-friendly candidates who are running for office or re-election. Staying abreast of current legislative issues and speaking proudly of the role occupational therapy practitioners play in rehabilitation is the foundation of being an effective grassroots advocate.

# Student Self-Assessment

1. Identify two relevant health care issues that could affect occupational therapy practice. Utilizing daily newspapers from the current month, identify three to five articles that deal directly with health care policy. Analyze these issues and determine the effects on occupational therapy practice. Submit one or two articles with a brief explanation why the issues will have no impact on occupational therapy services. Select two additional articles and identify the potential impact these policy issues may have on the delivery of occupational therapy services. Consider all aspects of the issue, including access to care, reimbursement, delivery of services, and scope of practice.
2. Plan a legislative action day.

- Step 1: Begin by holding a planning meeting and determine the reach of your group's efforts. Identify the piece of legislation you will use to focus your advocacy efforts. Determine the amount of time and space you will have available for your efforts.
- Step 2: Educate your peers on the main tenets of legislation and its effect on the practice of occupational therapy.
- Step 3: Plan activities for legislative action day. Include at least two of the following activities to maximize the reach of your lobbying:
  - Organize a letter writing team. Provide sample letters for group members to use as a guide. Personalized letters with stories of client success have the most impact. For example, tell the story of a client who was able to return home instead of remain in a skilled nursing facility. Tell the story of a client who no longer needed a caregiver after the intervention of an occupational therapy practitioner.
  - Sample letter (with intro to encourage colleagues to write letters also):

Please call or write your legislator and ask them to support SB 1402. The Business and Professions Committee will hear this bill on April 22, 2002. The physical therapy community is putting up strong opposition—we must let the legislators know that we very much want this bill to move forward. This bill amends our current licensure law to address the following issues:

- Broadens the hand therapy definition to match the HTCC (Hand Therapy Certification Commission) definition, which is more inclusive.
- Allows the Board of Occupational Therapy to develop regulations regarding advanced practice in hand therapy, modalities, and dysphagia.
- Allows entry-level occupational therapists to perform feeding evaluation and intervention, and differentiates this from swallowing.

Two legislators on this committee represent members in the Western Chapter. Members in State Senate District 26 should write to Senator Murray. Members in State Senate District 22 should write to Senator Polanco. A sample letter follows—please be brief and original.

Dear Senator:
I am writing to you as a constituent and occupational therapist. I urge you to strongly support SB 1402 when it comes before the Business and Professions Committee on April 22, 2002. This bill is very important to myself and my colleagues. It strengthens the licensure law that was passed last year. My patients will benefit from having their occupational therapist governed by a clearer, stronger, and more definitive practice act. I have invested many hours in my professional education, clinical skills, and patient care. I assure you that SB 1402 will help my profession grow in a careful and safe manner. Thank you for your time and consideration.
Sincerely,
Ms. Occupational Therapy Practitioner

- Organize a phone-calling team. Call the office of your elected official and explain that you would like him or her to support the piece of legislation. Identify yourself as a constituent and share your personal stories of occupational therapy.
- Invite a legislator to visit your school/program and see firsthand the success of occupational therapy. Let the local media know that you will have a legislator or candidate visiting. When the media covers the event, exposure of occupational therapy increases and the candidate/legislator receives press for his or her campaign.
- Develop an ongoing plan to build your advocacy skills.
- Develop a plan to build a relationship with a staffer in your legislator's office.
- Visit Capitol Hill or your Statehouse. Call the lawmaker's office and request an appointment in advance. You may meet with a staff member, which can be a very effective visit. The LA is the person the lawmaker turns to for the detailed research on an issue. If possible, arrange several visits for different constituencies in your group. Provide feedback to your professional organization at the end of the day.
- Organize a fundraising event for a candidate for elected office. Ideas range from bake sales to cocktail parties. Invite the candidate to attend if possible.
- If you do meet with an elected official, always write a personal thank you and reiterate what support you need. Example:

Dear Ms. Nelson,
Thank you so much for taking the time to meet with me and my fellow occupational therapists on June 5, 2003. We very much appreciate your support on repealing the Medicare cap. Since it seems that the current Medicare legislation on the House floor will contain a provision for a moratorium, please vote for this! Many California consumers will be harmed if the $1590 cap takes effect on July 1 as scheduled. Again, it was a pleasure to meet with you. Please feel free to call me if you need any further input on issues related to rehabilitation. I have enclosed a photo of myself and Congressman Waxman that I took that day. Please pass this along to Rep. Waxman. Thanks again.
Sincerely,
Ms. Occupational Therapy Practitioner

## Electronic Resources

- AOTA: www.aota.org
- Centers for Medicare & Medicaid Services (CMS): www.cms.hhs.gov
- Federal Election Commission: www.fec.gov

**Evidence-Based Research Chart**

| Topic | Evidence |
|---|---|
| Examples of advocacy | AOTA, n.d.a, n.d.c; CMS, 2006; Sahadi, 2006 |
| Role of PAC | Federal Election Commission Reports, 2004 |

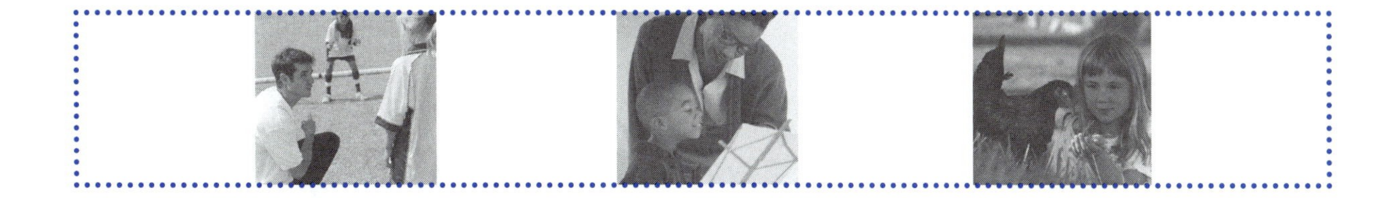

## References

American Occupational Therapy Association. (n.d.a). The Medicare Part B outpatient therapy caps. Retrieved September 1, 2009, from http://www.aota.org/Students/Advocate/AdvocacyFact/40490.aspx

American Occupational Therapy Association. (n.d.b). National school backpack awareness day. Retrieved July 28, 2006, from http://www.promoteot.org/AI_BackpackAwareness.html

American Occupational Therapy Association. (n.d.c). Federal legislative issues update—June 2006. Retrieved June 14, 2006, from http://www.aota.org/Practitioners/Advocacy/Federal/Newsletter/2006/40482.aspx

American Physical Therapy Association. (2000). TriAlliance to Explore Medicare Alternative Payment Methods. Retrieved July 19, 2006, from http://www.apta.org/AM/Template.cfm?Section=Home&TEMPLATE=/CM/ContentDisplay.cfm&CONTENTID=30620

Center for Medicare and Medicaid Studies. (2006). MLN Matters, #MM4364. Retrieved June 14, 2006, from http://www.cms.hhs.gov/MLNMattersArticles/downloads/MM4364.pdf

Centers for Medicare and Medicaid Studies. (2006). Medcare Benefit Policy Manual, Chapter 15. Retrieved June 14, 2006, from http://www.cms.hhs.gov/Manuals/downloads/bp102c15.pdf

Editors of the American Heritage Dictionaries. (2000). *American heritage dictionary of the English language* (4th ed). Boston, MA: Houghton Mifflin.

Sahadi, J. (2006). Social Security, Medicare to run out sooner. Retrieved June 14, 2006, from http://money.cnn.com/2006/05/01/retirement/SStrustees_2006report/index.htm

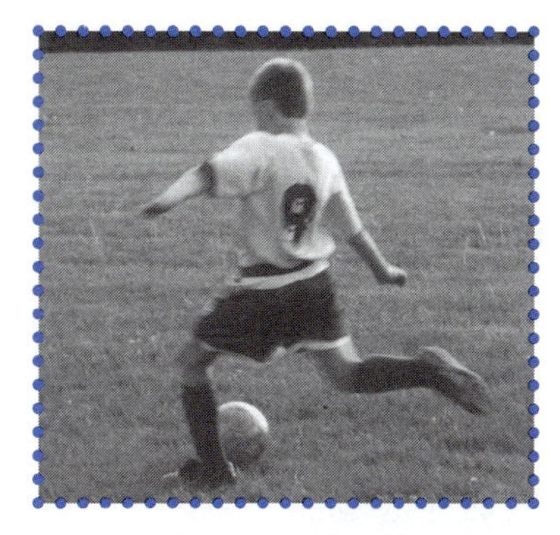

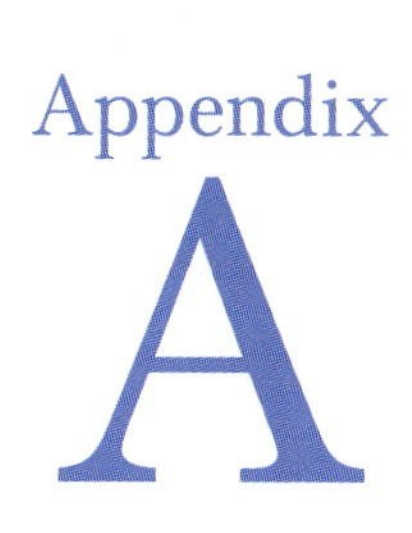

Appendix A

# 2006 ACOTE Accreditation Standards for a Master's-Degree-Level Educational Program for the Occupational Therapist

*Reproduced with permission from the American Occupational Therapy Association.*

ACOTE ACCREDITATION COUNCIL FOR OCCUPATIONAL THERAPY EDUCATION (ACOTE®) of THE AMERICAN OCCUPATIONAL THERAPY ASSOCIATION, INC.

# ACCREDITATION STANDARDS FOR A MASTER'S-DEGREE-LEVEL EDUCATIONAL PROGRAM FOR THE OCCUPATIONAL THERAPIST

Adopted August 2006, Effective January 1, 2008

**The Accreditation Council for Occupational Therapy Education (ACOTE) of the American Occupational Therapy Association (AOTA) accredits educational programs for the occupational therapist. The Standards comply with the United States Department of Education (USDE) criteria for recognition of accrediting agencies.**

*These Standards are the requirements used in accrediting educational programs that prepare individuals to enter the occupational therapy profession. The extent to which a program complies with these Standards determines its accreditation status.*

## PREAMBLE

The rapidly changing and dynamic nature of contemporary health and human services delivery systems requires the occupational therapist to possess basic skills as a direct care provider, consultant, educator, manager, researcher, and advocate for the profession and the consumer.

A graduate from an ACOTE-accredited master's-degree-level occupational therapy program must

- Have acquired, as a foundation for professional study, a breadth and depth of knowledge in the liberal arts and sciences and an understanding of issues related to diversity.
- Be educated as a generalist with a broad exposure to the delivery models and systems used in settings where occupational therapy is currently practiced and where it is emerging as a service.
- Have achieved entry-level competence through a combination of academic and fieldwork education.
- Be prepared to articulate and apply occupational therapy theory and evidence-based evaluations and interventions to achieve expected outcomes as related to occupation.
- Be prepared to be a lifelong learner and keep current with evidence-based professional practice.
- Uphold the ethical standards, values, and attitudes of the occupational therapy profession.
- Understand the distinct roles and responsibilities of the occupational therapist and occupational therapy assistant in the supervisory process.
- Be prepared to advocate as a professional for the occupational therapy services offered and for the recipients of those services.
- Be prepared to be an effective consumer of the latest research and knowledge bases that support practice and contribute to the growth and dissemination of research and knowledge.

| NUMBER | OT MASTER'S-DEGREE-LEVEL STANDARD |
|---|---|
| **SECTION A: GENERAL REQUIREMENTS FOR ACCREDITATION** | |
| **A.1.0. SPONSORSHIP AND ACCREDITATION** | |
| A.1.1. | The sponsoring institution(s) and affiliates, if any, must be accredited by recognized national, regional, or state agencies with accrediting authority. For programs in countries other than the United States, ACOTE will determine an alternative and equivalent external review process. |
| A.1.2. | Sponsoring institutions must be authorized under applicable law or other acceptable authority to provide a program of post-secondary education and have appropriate degree-granting authority. |
| A.1.3. | Accredited occupational therapy educational programs may be established only in senior colleges, universities, or medical schools. |
| A.1.4. | The sponsoring institution must assume primary responsibility for appointment of faculty, admission of students, and curriculum planning. This would include course content, satisfactory completion of the educational program, and granting of the degree. The sponsoring institution must also be responsible for the coordination of classroom teaching and supervised fieldwork practice and for providing assurance that the practice activities assigned to students in a fieldwork setting are appropriate to the program. |

| NUMBER | OT MASTER'S-DEGREE-LEVEL STANDARD |
|---|---|
| A.1.5. | The sponsoring institution or program must<br>• Inform ACOTE of the transfer of program sponsorship or change of the institution's name within 30 days of the transfer or change.<br>• Inform ACOTE within 30 days of the date of notification of any adverse accreditation action taken to change the sponsoring institution's accreditation status to probation or withdrawal of accreditation.<br>• Submit a Letter of Intent to add or change a program degree level at least 1 year prior to the planned admission of students into that level.<br>• Inform ACOTE within 30 days of the resignation of the program director or appointment of a new or interim program director.<br>• Pay accreditation fees within 90 days of the invoice date.<br>• Submit a Report of Self-Study and other required reports (e.g., Biennial Report, Plan of Correction, Progress Report) within the period of time designated by ACOTE. All reports must be complete and contain all requested information.<br>• Agree to a site visit date before the end of the period for which accreditation was previously awarded.<br>• Demonstrate honesty and integrity in all interactions with ACOTE. |
| **A.2.0.** | **ACADEMIC RESOURCES** |
| A.2.1. | The program must have a director who is assigned to the occupational therapy educational program on a full-time basis. The director may be assigned other institutional duties that do not interfere with the management and administration of the program. The institution must ensure that the needs of the program are being met. |
| A.2.2. | The program director must be an initially certified occupational therapist who is licensed or credentialed according to regulations in the state or jurisdiction in which the program is located. The director must hold academic qualifications comparable to the majority of other program directors within the institutional unit (e.g., division, college, school) to which the program is assigned. By July 1, 2012, the program director must hold a doctoral degree. |
| A.2.3. | The program director must have a minimum of 6 years of experience in the field of occupational therapy, including practice as an occupational therapist, administrative or supervisory experience, and at least 2 years of experience in a full-time academic appointment with teaching responsibilities. |
| A.2.4. | The program director must be responsible for the management and administration of the program, including planning, evaluation, budgeting, selection of faculty and staff, maintenance of accreditation, and commitment to strategies for professional development. |
| A.2.5. | The program director and faculty must possess the academic and experiential qualifications and backgrounds (identified in documented descriptions of roles and responsibilities) that are necessary to meet program objectives and the mission of the institution. |
| A.2.6. | The program must document policies and procedures to ensure that the program director and faculty are aware of and abide by the current code of ethics of the profession of occupational therapy. |
| A.2.7. | The program must identify an individual as academic fieldwork coordinator who is specifically responsible for the program's compliance with the fieldwork requirements of Standards Section B.10.0. This individual must be a licensed or credentialed occupational therapist. Academic fieldwork coordinators who hold a faculty position must meet the requirements of Standard A.2.9. |
| A.2.8. | The faculty must include currently licensed or credentialed occupational therapists. |
| A.2.9. | All full-time faculty must hold a minimum of a master's degree. By July 1, 2012, the majority of full-time faculty who are occupational therapists must hold a doctoral degree. |
| A.2.10. | The faculty must have documented expertise in their area(s) of teaching responsibility and knowledge of the content delivery method (e.g., distance learning). |
| A.2.11. | The occupational therapy faculty at each accredited location where the program is offered must be sufficient in number and must possess the expertise necessary to ensure appropriate curriculum design, content delivery, and program evaluation. |
| A.2.12. | Faculty responsibilities must be consistent with and supportive of the mission of the institution. |
| A.2.13. | The faculty–student ratio must permit the achievement of the purpose and stated objectives for laboratory and lecture courses, be compatible with accepted practices of the institution for similar programs, and ensure student and consumer safety. |

| NUMBER | OT MASTER'S-DEGREE-LEVEL STANDARD |
|---|---|
| A.2.14. | Clerical and support staff must be provided to the program, consistent with institutional practice, to meet programmatic and administrative requirements, including support for any portion of the program offered by distance education. |
| A.2.15. | The program must be allocated a budget of regular institutional funds, not including grants, gifts, and other restricted sources, sufficient to implement and maintain the objectives of the program and to fulfill the program's obligation to matriculated and entering students. |
| A.2.16. | Classrooms and laboratories must be provided that are consistent with the program's educational objectives, teaching methods, number of students, and safety and health standards of the institution, and must allow for efficient operation of the program. If any portion of the program is offered by distance education, technology and resources must be adequate to support a distance-learning environment. |
| A.2.17. | Laboratory space provided by the institution must be assigned to the occupational therapy program on a priority basis. If laboratory space is provided by another institution or agency, there must be a written and signed agreement to ensure assignment of space for program use. |
| A.2.18. | Adequate space must be provided to store and secure equipment and supplies. |
| A.2.19. | The program director and faculty must have office space consistent with institutional practice. |
| A.2.20. | Adequate space must be provided for the private advising of students. |
| A.2.21. | Appropriate and sufficient equipment and supplies must be provided by the institution for student use and for the didactic and supervised fieldwork components of the curriculum. |
| A.2.22. | Students must be given access to and have the opportunity to use the evaluative and treatment methodologies that reflect both current practice and practice in the geographic area served by the program. |
| A.2.23. | Students must have ready access to a supply of current and relevant books, journals, periodicals, computers, software, and other reference materials needed to meet the requirements of the curriculum. This may include, but is not limited to, libraries, online services, interlibrary loan, and resource centers. |
| A.2.24. | Instructional aids and technology must be available in sufficient quantity and quality to be consistent with the program objectives and teaching methods. |
| **A.3.0. STUDENTS** | |
| A.3.1. | Admission of students to the occupational therapy program must be made in accordance with the practices of the institution. There must be stated admission criteria that are clearly defined and published and reflective of the demands of the program. |
| A.3.2. | Policies pertaining to standards for admission, advanced placement, transfer of credit, credit for experiential learning (if applicable), and prerequisite educational or work experience requirements must be readily accessible to prospective students and the public. |
| A.3.3. | Programs must document implementation of a mechanism to ensure that students receiving credit for previous courses and/or work experience have met the content requirements of the appropriate master's Standards. |
| A.3.4. | Criteria for successful completion of each segment of the educational program and for graduation must be given in advance to each student. |
| A.3.5. | Evaluation content and methods must be consistent with the curriculum design, objectives, and competencies of the didactic and fieldwork components of the program. |
| A.3.6. | Evaluation must be conducted on a regular basis to provide students and program officials with timely indications of the students' progress and academic standing. |
| A.3.7. | Students must be informed of and have access to the student support services that are provided to other students in the institution. |
| A.3.8. | Advising related to professional coursework and fieldwork education must be the responsibility of the occupational therapy faculty. |
| **A.4.0. OPERATIONAL POLICIES** | |
| A.4.1. | All program publications and advertising—including, but not limited to, academic calendars, announcements, catalogs, handbooks, and Web sites—must accurately reflect the program offered. |

| NUMBER | OT MASTER'S-DEGREE-LEVEL STANDARD |
|---|---|
| A.4.2. | Accurate and current information regarding student outcomes must be readily available to the public in at least one publication or Web page. The following data must be reported as an aggregate for the three most recent calendar years and specify the<br>• 3-year time period being reported,<br>• total number of program graduates during that period,<br>• total number of first-time test takers of the national certification examination during that period,<br>• total number of first-time test takers who passed the exam during that period, and<br>• percentage of the total number of first-time test takers who passed the exam during that period. |
| A.4.3. | The program's accreditation status and the name, address, and telephone number of ACOTE must be published in all of the following used by the institution: catalog, Web site, and program-related brochures or flyers available to prospective students. |
| A.4.4. | Faculty recruitment and employment practices, as well as student recruitment and admission procedures, must be nondiscriminatory. |
| A.4.5. | Graduation requirements, tuition, and fees must be accurately stated, published, and made known to all applicants. When published fees are subject to change, a statement to that effect must be included. |
| A.4.6. | The program or sponsoring institution must have a defined and published policy and procedure for processing student and faculty grievances. |
| A.4.7. | Policies and procedures for handling complaints against the program must be published and made known. The program must maintain a record of student complaints that includes the nature and disposition of each complaint. |
| A.4.8. | Policies and processes for student withdrawal and for refunds of tuition and fees must be published and made known to all applicants. |
| A.4.9. | Policies and procedures for student probation, suspension, and dismissal must be published and made known. |
| A.4.10. | Policies and procedures must be published and made known for human-subject research protocol. |
| A.4.11. | Written policies and procedures must be made available to students regarding appropriate use of equipment and supplies and for all educational activities that have implications for the health and safety of clients, students, and faculty (including infection control and evacuation procedures). |
| A.4.12. | A program admitting students on the basis of ability to benefit (defined by the U.S. Department of Education as admitting students who do not have either a high school diploma or its equivalent) must publicize its objectives, assessment measures, and means of evaluating the student's ability to benefit. |
| A.4.13. | Documentation of all progression, retention, graduation, certification, and credentialing requirements must be published and made known to applicants. This must include a statement about the potential impact of a felony conviction on a graduate's eligibility for certification and credentialing. |
| A.4.14. | The program must have a documented and published policy to ensure students complete all graduation and fieldwork requirements in a timely manner. This must include a statement that all Level II fieldwork be completed within a time frame established by the program. |
| A.4.15. | Records regarding student admission, enrollment, and achievement must be maintained and kept in a secure setting. Grades and credits for courses must be recorded on students' transcripts and permanently maintained by the sponsoring institution. |
| **A.5.0.** | **STRATEGIC PLAN AND PROGRAM ASSESSMENT** |
| A.5.1. | The program must document a current strategic plan that articulates the program's future vision and guides the program development (e.g., faculty recruitment and professional growth, changes in the curriculum design, priorities in academic resources, procurement of fieldwork sites). A program strategic plan must include, but need not be limited to<br>• Evidence that the plan is based on program evaluation and an analysis of external and internal environments.<br>• Long-term goals that address the vision and mission of both the institution and program, as well as specific needs of the program.<br>• Specific measurable action steps with expected timelines by which the program will reach its long-term goals.<br>• Persons(s) responsible for action steps.<br>• Evidence of periodic updating of action steps and long-term goals as they are met or as circumstances change. |

| NUMBER | OT MASTER'S-DEGREE-LEVEL STANDARD |
|---|---|
| A.5.2. | The program director and each faculty member who teaches two or more courses must have a current written professional growth and development plan. Each plan must contain the signature of the faculty member and supervisor. At a minimum the plan must include, but need not be limited to<br>• Goals to enhance the faculty member's ability to fulfill designated responsibilities (e.g., goals related to currency in areas of teaching responsibility, teaching effectiveness, research, scholarly activity).<br>• Specific measurable action steps with expected timelines by which the faculty member will achieve the goals.<br>• Evidence of annual updates of action steps and goals as they are met or as circumstances change.<br>• Identification of the ways in which the faculty member's professional development plan will contribute to attaining the program's strategic goals. |
| A.5.3. | Programs must routinely secure and document sufficient qualitative and quantitative information to allow for meaningful analysis about the extent to which the program is meeting its stated goals and objectives. This must include, but need not be limited to<br>• Faculty effectiveness in their assigned teaching responsibilities.<br>• Students' progression through the program.<br>• Fieldwork performance evaluation.<br>• Student evaluation of fieldwork experience.<br>• Student satisfaction with the program.<br>• Graduates' performance on the NBCOT certification exam.<br>• Graduates' job placement and performance based on employer satisfaction. |
| A.5.4. | The average total pass rate of OT master's program graduates taking the national certification exam for the first time over the three most recent calendar years must be 70% or higher. |
| A.5.5. | Programs must routinely and systematically analyze data to determine the extent to which the program is meeting its stated goals and objectives. An annual report summarizing analysis of data and planned action responses must be maintained. |
| A.5.6. | The results of ongoing evaluation must be appropriately reflected in the program's strategic plan, curriculum, and other dimensions of the program. |
| **A.6.0. CURRICULUM FRAMEWORK**<br>**The curriculum framework is a description of the program that includes the program's mission, philosophy, and curriculum design.** | |
| A.6.1. | The curriculum must include preparation for practice as a generalist with a broad exposure to current practice settings (e.g., school, hospital, community, long-term care) and emerging practice areas (as defined by the program). The curriculum must prepare students to work with a variety of populations including, but not limited to, children, adolescents, adults, and elderly persons in areas of physical and mental health. |
| A.6.2. | The program must document a system and rationale for ensuring that the length of study of the program is appropriate to the expected learning and competence of the graduate. |
| A.6.3. | The statement of philosophy of the occupational therapy program must reflect the current published philosophy of the profession and must include a statement of the program's fundamental beliefs about human beings and how they learn. |
| A.6.4. | The statement of the mission of the occupational therapy program must be consistent with and supportive of the mission of the sponsoring institution. |
| A.6.5. | The curriculum design must reflect the mission and philosophy of both the occupational therapy program and the institution and must provide the basis for program planning, implementation, and evaluation. The design must identify educational goals and describe the selection of the content, scope, and sequencing of coursework. |
| A.6.6. | The program must have clearly documented assessment measures by which students are regularly evaluated on their acquisition of knowledge, skills, attitudes, and competencies required for graduation. |
| A.6.7. | The program must have written syllabi for each course that include course objectives and learning activities that, in total, reflect all course content required by the Standards. Instructional methods (e.g., presentations, demonstrations, discussion) and materials used to accomplish course objectives must be documented. Programs must also demonstrate the consistency between course syllabi and the curriculum design. |

| NUMBER | OT MASTER'S-DEGREE-LEVEL STANDARD |
|---|---|
| **SECTION B: SPECIFIC REQUIREMENTS FOR ACCREDITATION**<br>**The specific requirements for accreditation contain the content that a program must include. The content requirements are written as expected student outcomes. Faculty are responsible for developing learning activities and evaluation methods to document that students meet these outcomes.** | |
| **B.1.0. FOUNDATIONAL CONTENT REQUIREMENTS**<br>**Program content must be based on a broad foundation in the liberal arts and sciences. A strong foundation in the biological, physical, social, and behavioral sciences supports an understanding of occupation across the life span. Coursework in these areas may be prerequisite to or concurrent with professional education and must facilitate development of the performance criteria listed below. The student will be able to** | |
| B.1.1. | Demonstrate oral and written communication skills. |
| B.1.2. | Employ logical thinking, critical analysis, problem solving, and creativity. |
| B.1.3. | Demonstrate competence in basic computer use, including the ability to use databases and search engines to access information, word processing for writing, and presentation software (e.g., PowerPoint). |
| B.1.4. | Demonstrate knowledge and understanding of the structure and function of the human body to include the biological and physical sciences. Course content must include, but is not limited to, biology, anatomy, physiology, neuroscience, and kinesiology or biomechanics. |
| B.1.5. | Demonstrate knowledge and understanding of human development throughout the life span (infants, children, adolescents, adults, and elderly persons). Course content must include, but is not limited to, developmental psychology. |
| B.1.6. | Demonstrate knowledge and understanding of the concepts of human behavior to include the behavioral and social sciences. Course content must include, but is not limited to, introductory psychology, abnormal psychology, and introductory sociology or introductory anthropology. |
| B.1.7. | Demonstrate knowledge and appreciation of the role of sociocultural, socioeconomic, and diversity factors and lifestyle choices in contemporary society. Course content must include, but is not limited to, introductory psychology, abnormal psychology, and introductory sociology or introductory anthropology. |
| B.1.8. | Articulate the influence of social conditions and the ethical context in which humans choose and engage in occupations. |
| B.1.9. | Demonstrate knowledge of global social issues and prevailing health and welfare needs. |
| B.1.10. | Demonstrate the ability to use statistics to interpret tests and measurements. |
| **B.2.0. BASIC TENETS OF OCCUPATIONAL THERAPY**<br>**Coursework must facilitate development of the performance criteria listed below. The student will be able to** | |
| B.2.1. | Articulate an understanding of the importance of the history and philosophical base of the profession of occupational therapy. |
| B.2.2. | Explain the meaning and dynamics of occupation and activity, including the interaction of areas of occupation, performance skills, performance patterns, activity demands, context(s), and client factors. |
| B.2.3. | Articulate to consumers, potential employers, colleagues, third-party payers, regulatory boards, policymakers, other audiences, and the general public both the unique nature of occupation as viewed by the profession of occupational therapy and the value of occupation to support participation in context(s) for the client. |
| B.2.4. | Articulate the importance of balancing areas of occupation with the achievement of health and wellness. |
| B.2.5. | Explain the role of occupation in the promotion of health and the prevention of disease and disability for the individual, family, and society. |
| B.2.6. | Analyze the effects of physical and mental health, heritable diseases and predisposing genetic conditions, disability, disease processes, and traumatic injury to the individual within the cultural context of family and society on occupational performance. |
| B.2.7. | Exhibit the ability to analyze tasks relative to areas of occupation, performance skills, performance patterns, activity demands, context(s), and client factors to formulate an intervention plan. |
| B.2.8. | Use sound judgment in regard to safety of self and others, and adhere to safety regulations throughout the occupational therapy process. |

| NUMBER | OT MASTER'S-DEGREE-LEVEL STANDARD |
|---|---|
| B.2.9. | Express support for the quality of life, well-being, and occupation of the individual, group, or population to promote physical and mental health and prevention of injury and disease considering the context (e.g., cultural, physical, social, personal, spiritual, temporal, virtual). |
| B.2.10. | Use clinical reasoning to explain the rationale for and use of compensatory strategies when desired life tasks cannot be performed. |
| B.2.11. | Analyze, synthesize, and apply models of occupational performance and theories of occupation. |
| **B.3.0. OCCUPATIONAL THERAPY THEORETICAL PERSPECTIVES**<br>**The program must facilitate the development of the performance criteria listed below. The student will be able to** | |
| B.3.1. | Describe theories that underlie the practice of occupational therapy. |
| B.3.2. | Compare and contrast models of practice and frames of reference that are used in occupational therapy. |
| B.3.3. | Discuss how theories, models of practice, and frames of reference are used in occupational therapy evaluation and intervention. |
| B.3.4. | Analyze and discuss how history, theory, and the sociopolitical climate influence practice. |
| B.3.5. | Apply theoretical constructs to evaluation and intervention with various types of clients and practice contexts to analyze and effect meaningful occupation. |
| B.3.6. | Discuss the process of theory development and its importance to occupational therapy. |
| **B.4.0. SCREENING, EVALUATION, AND REFERRAL**<br>**The process of screening, evaluation, and referral as related to occupational performance and participation must be culturally relevant and based on theoretical perspectives, models of practice, frames of reference, and available evidence. The program must facilitate development of the performance criteria listed below. The student will be able to** | |
| B.4.1. | Use standardized and nonstandardized screening and assessment tools to determine the need for occupational therapy intervention. These include, but are not limited to, specified screening tools; assessments; skilled observations; checklists; histories; consultations with other professionals; and interviews with the client, family, and significant others. |
| B.4.2. | Select appropriate assessment tools based on client needs, contextual factors, and psychometric properties of tests. These must be relevant to a variety of populations across the life span, culturally relevant, based on available evidence, and incorporate use of occupation in the assessment process. |
| B.4.3. | Use appropriate procedures and protocols (including standardized formats) when administering assessments. |
| B.4.4. | Evaluate client(s)' occupational performance in activities of daily living (ADL), instrumental activities of daily living (IADL), education, work, play, leisure, and social participation. Evaluation of occupational performance using standardized and nonstandardized assessment tools includes<br>• The occupational profile, including participation in activities that are meaningful and necessary for the client to carry out roles in home, work, and community environments.<br>• Client factors, including body functions (e.g., neuromuscular, sensory, visual, perceptual, cognitive, mental) and body structures (e.g., cardiovascular, digestive, integumentary systems).<br>• Performance patterns (e.g., habits, routines, roles) and behavior patterns.<br>• Cultural, physical, social, personal, spiritual, temporal, and virtual contexts and activity demands that affect performance.<br>• Performance skills, including motor (e.g., posture, mobility, coordination, strength, energy), process (e.g., energy, knowledge, temporal organization, organizing space and objects, adaptation), and communication and interaction skills (e.g., physicality, information exchange, relations). |
| B.4.5. | Compare and contrast the role of the occupational therapist and occupational therapy assistant in the screening and evaluation process along with the importance of and rationale for supervision and collaborative work between the occupational therapist and occupational therapy assistant in that process. |
| B.4.6. | Interpret criterion-referenced and norm-referenced standardized test scores based on an understanding of sampling, normative data, standard and criterion scores, reliability, and validity. |
| B.4.7. | Consider factors that might bias assessment results, such as culture, disability status, and situational variables related to the individual and context. |
| B.4.8. | Interpret the evaluation data in relation to accepted terminology of the profession and relevant theoretical frameworks. |

| NUMBER | OT MASTER'S-DEGREE-LEVEL STANDARD |
|---|---|
| B.4.9. | Evaluate appropriateness and discuss mechanisms for referring clients for additional evaluation to specialists who are internal and external to the profession. |
| B.4.10. | Document occupational therapy services to ensure accountability of service provision and to meet standards for reimbursement of services, adhering to applicable facility, local, state, federal, and reimbursement agencies. Documentation must effectively communicate the need and rationale for occupational therapy services. |
| **B.5.0. INTERVENTION PLAN: FORMULATION AND IMPLEMENTATION** **The process of formulation and implementation of the therapeutic intervention plan to facilitate occupational performance and participation must be culturally relevant; reflective of current occupational therapy practice; based on available evidence; and based on theoretical perspectives, models of practice, and frames of reference. The program must facilitate development of the performance criteria listed below. The student will be able to** | |
| B.5.1. | Use evaluation findings based on appropriate theoretical approaches, models of practice, and frames of reference to develop occupation-based intervention plans and strategies (including goals and methods to achieve them) based on the stated needs of the client as well as data gathered during the evaluation process in collaboration with the client and others. Intervention plans and strategies must be culturally relevant, reflective of current occupational therapy practice, and based on available evidence. Interventions address the following components:<br>• The occupational profile, including participation in activities that are meaningful and necessary for the client to carry out roles in home, work, and community environments.<br>• Client factors, including body functions (e.g., neuromuscular, sensory, visual, perceptual, cognitive, mental) and body structures (e.g., cardiovascular, digestive, integumentary systems).<br>• Performance patterns (e.g., habits, routines, roles) and behavior patterns.<br>• Cultural, physical, social, personal, spiritual, temporal, and virtual contexts and activity demands that affect performance.<br>• Performance skills, including motor (e.g., posture, mobility, coordination, strength, energy), process (e.g., energy, knowledge, temporal organization, organizing space and objects, adaptation), and communication and interaction skills (e.g., physicality, information exchange, relations). |
| B.5.2. | Select and provide direct occupational therapy interventions and procedures to enhance safety, wellness, and performance in activities of daily living (ADL), instrumental activities of daily living (IADL), education, work, play, leisure, and social participation. |
| B.5.3. | Provide therapeutic use of occupation and activities (e.g., occupation-based activity, practice skills, preparatory methods). |
| B.5.4. | Provide training in self-care, self-management, home management, and community and work integration. |
| B.5.5. | Provide development, remediation, and compensation for physical, cognitive, perceptual, sensory (e.g., vision, tactile, auditory, gustatory, olfactory, pain, temperature, pressure, vestibular, proprioception), neuromuscular, and behavioral skills. |
| B.5.6. | Provide therapeutic use of self, including one's personality, insights, perceptions, and judgments as part of the therapeutic process in both individual and group interaction. |
| B.5.7. | Describe the role of the occupational therapist in care coordination, case management, and transition services in traditional and emerging practice environments. |
| B.5.8. | Modify environments (e.g., home, work, school, community) and adapt processes, including the application of ergonomic principles. |
| B.5.9. | Articulate principles of and be able to design, fabricate, apply, fit, and train in assistive technologies and devices (e.g., electronic aids to daily living, seating systems) used to enhance occupational performance. |
| B.5.10. | Provide design, fabrication, application, fitting, and training in orthotic devices used to enhance occupational performance and training in the use of prosthetic devices, based on scientific principles of kinesiology, biomechanics, and physics. |
| B.5.11. | Provide recommendations and training in techniques to enhance mobility, including physical transfers, wheelchair management, and community mobility, and address issues related to driver rehabilitation. |
| B.5.12. | Provide management of feeding and eating to enable performance (including the process of bringing food or fluids from the plate or cup to the mouth, the ability to keep and manipulate food or fluid in the mouth, and the initiation of swallowing) and train others in precautions and techniques while considering client and contextual factors. |

| NUMBER | OT MASTER'S-DEGREE-LEVEL STANDARD |
|---|---|
| B.5.13. | Explain the use of superficial thermal and mechanical modalities as a preparatory measure to improve occupational performance, including foundational knowledge, underlying principles, indications, contraindications, and precautions. Demonstrate safe and effective application of superficial thermal and mechanical modalities. |
| B.5.14. | Explain the use of deep thermal and electrotherapeutic modalities as a preparatory measure to improve occupational performance, including indications, contraindications, and precautions. |
| B.5.15. | Develop and promote the use of appropriate home and community programming to support performance in the client's natural environment and participation in all contexts relevant to the client. |
| B.5.16. | Demonstrate the ability to educate the client, caregiver, family, and significant others to facilitate skills in areas of occupation as well as prevention, health maintenance, and safety. |
| B.5.17. | Apply the principles of the teaching–learning process using educational methods to design educational experiences to address the needs of the client, family, significant others, colleagues, other health providers, and the public. |
| B.5.18. | Effectively interact through written, oral, and nonverbal communication with the client, family, significant others, colleagues, other health providers, and the public in a professionally acceptable manner. |
| B.5.19. | Grade and adapt the environment, tools, materials, occupations, and interventions to reflect the changing needs of the client and the sociocultural context. |
| B.5.20. | Select and teach compensatory strategies, such as use of technology, adaptations to the environment, and involvement of humans and nonhumans in the completion of tasks. |
| B.5.21. | Identify and demonstrate techniques in skills of supervision and collaboration with occupational therapy assistants on therapeutic interventions. |
| B.5.22. | Understand when and how to use the consultative process with groups, programs, organizations, or communities. |
| B.5.23. | Refer to specialists (both internal and external to the profession) for consultation and intervention. |
| B.5.24. | Monitor and reassess, in collaboration with the client, caregiver, family, and significant others, the effect of occupational therapy intervention and the need for continued or modified intervention. |
| B.5.25. | Plan for discharge, in collaboration with the client, by reviewing the needs of the client, caregiver, family, and significant others; resources; and discharge environment. This includes, but is not limited to, identification of client's current status within the continuum of care and the identification of community, human, and fiscal resources; recommendations for environmental adaptations; and home programming to facilitate the client's progression along the continuum toward outcome goals. |
| B.5.26. | Organize, collect, and analyze data in a systematic manner for evaluation of practice outcomes. Report evaluation results and modify practice as needed to improve outcomes. |
| B.5.27. | Terminate occupational therapy services when stated outcomes have been achieved or it has been determined that they cannot be achieved. This includes developing a summary of occupational therapy outcomes, appropriate recommendations and referrals, and discussion with the client and with appropriate others of post-discharge needs. |
| B.5.28. | Document occupational therapy services to ensure accountability of service provision and to meet standards for reimbursement of services. Documentation must effectively communicate the need and rationale for occupational therapy services and must be appropriate to the context in which the service is delivered. |
| **B.6.0. CONTEXT OF SERVICE DELIVERY** **Context of service delivery includes the knowledge and understanding of the various contexts in which occupational therapy services are provided. The program must facilitate development of the performance criteria listed below. The student will be able to** | |
| B.6.1. | Differentiate among the contexts of health care, education, community, and social systems as they relate to the practice of occupational therapy. |
| B.6.2. | Discuss the current policy issues and the social, economic, political, geographic, and demographic factors that influence the various contexts for practice of occupational therapy. |
| B.6.3. | Describe the current social, economic, political, geographic, and demographic factors to promote policy development and the provision of occupational therapy services. |
| B.6.4. | Articulate the role and responsibility of the practitioner to address changes in service delivery policies to effect changes in the system, and to identify opportunities in emerging practice areas. |

| NUMBER | OT MASTER'S-DEGREE-LEVEL STANDARD |
|---|---|
| B.6.5. | Articulate the trends in models of service delivery and their potential effect on the practice of occupational therapy, including, but not limited to, medical, educational, community, and social models. |
| B.6.6. | Use national and international resources in making assessment or intervention choices, and appreciate the influence of international occupational therapy contributions to education, research, and practice. |
| **B.7.0. MANAGEMENT OF OCCUPATIONAL THERAPY SERVICES** **Management of occupational therapy services includes the application of principles of management and systems in the provision of occupational therapy services to individuals and organizations. The program must facilitate development of the performance criteria listed below. The student will be able to** | |
| B.7.1. | Explain how the various practice settings (e.g., medical institutions, community practice, school systems) affect the delivery of occupational therapy services. |
| B.7.2. | Describe and discuss the impact of contextual factors on the management and delivery of occupational therapy services. |
| B.7.3. | Describe the systems and structures that create federal and state legislation and regulation and their implications and effects on practice. |
| B.7.4. | Demonstrate knowledge of applicable national requirements for credentialing and requirements for licensure, certification, or registration under state laws. |
| B.7.5. | Demonstrate knowledge of various reimbursement systems (e.g., federal, state, third-party, private-payer), appeals mechanisms, and documentation requirements that affect the practice of occupational therapy. |
| B.7.6. | Describe the mechanisms, systems, and techniques needed to properly maintain, organize, and prioritize workloads and intervention settings including inventories. |
| B.7.7. | Demonstrate the ability to plan, develop, organize, and market the delivery of services to include the determination of programmatic needs, service delivery options, and formulation and management of staffing for effective service provision. |
| B.7.8. | Demonstrate the ability to design ongoing processes for quality improvement (e.g., outcome studies analysis) and develop program changes as needed to ensure quality of services and to direct administrative changes. |
| B.7.9. | Develop strategies for effective, competency-based legal and ethical supervision of occupational therapy and non–occupational therapy personnel. |
| B.7.10. | Describe the ongoing professional responsibility for providing fieldwork education and the criteria for becoming a fieldwork educator. |
| **B.8.0. RESEARCH** **Application of research includes the ability to read and understand current research that affects practice and the provision of occupational therapy services. The program must facilitate development of the performance criteria listed below. The student will be able to** | |
| B.8.1. | Articulate the importance of research, scholarly activities, and the continued development of a body of knowledge relevant to the profession of occupational therapy. |
| B.8.2. | Effectively locate, understand, and evaluate information, including the quality of research evidence. |
| B.8.3. | Use research literature to make evidence-based decisions. |
| B.8.4. | Understand and use basic descriptive, correlational, and inferential quantitative statistics and code, analyze, and synthesize qualitative data. |
| B.8.5. | Understand and critique the validity of research studies, including designs (both quantitative and qualitative) and methodologies. |
| B.8.6. | Demonstrate the skills necessary to design a research proposal that includes the research question, relevant literature, sample, design, measurement, and data analysis. |
| B.8.7. | Implement one or more aspects of research methodology. These may be simulated or actual and may include, but are not limited to, designing research instruments, collecting data, and analyzing or synthesizing data. These research activities may be completed individually, with a group, or with a faculty member. |
| B.8.8. | Demonstrate basic skills necessary to write a research report in a format for presentation or publication. |

| NUMBER | OT MASTER'S-DEGREE-LEVEL STANDARD |
|---|---|
| B.8.9. | Demonstrate an understanding of the process of locating and securing grants and how grants can serve as a fiscal resource for research and practice. |
| **B.9.0. PROFESSIONAL ETHICS, VALUES, AND RESPONSIBILITIES** **Professional ethics, values, and responsibilities include an understanding and appreciation of ethics and values of the profession of occupational therapy. The program must facilitate development of the performance criteria listed below. The student will be able to** | |
| B.9.1. | Demonstrate a knowledge and understanding of the American Occupational Therapy Association (AOTA) *Occupational Therapy Code of Ethics*, *Core Values and Attitudes of Occupational Therapy Practice*, and AOTA *Standards of Practice* and use them as a guide for ethical decision making in professional interactions, client interventions, and employment settings. |
| B.9.2. | Discuss and justify how the role of a professional is enhanced by knowledge of and involvement in international, national, state, and local occupational therapy associations and related professional associations. |
| B.9.3. | Promote occupational therapy by educating other professionals, service providers, consumers, third-party payers, regulatory bodies, and the public. |
| B.9.4. | Discuss strategies for ongoing professional development to ensure that practice is consistent with current and accepted standards. |
| B.9.5. | Discuss professional responsibilities related to liability issues under current models of service provision. |
| B.9.6. | Discuss and evaluate personal and professional abilities and competencies as they relate to job responsibilities. |
| B.9.7. | Discuss and justify the varied roles of the occupational therapist as a practitioner, educator, researcher, consultant, and entrepreneur. |
| B.9.8. | Explain and justify the importance of supervisory roles, responsibilities, and collaborative professional relationships between the occupational therapist and the occupational therapy assistant. |
| B.9.9. | Describe and discuss professional responsibilities and issues when providing service on a contractual basis. |
| B.9.10. | Explain strategies for analyzing issues and making decisions to resolve personal and organizational ethical conflicts. |
| B.9.11. | Explain the variety of informal and formal ethical dispute–resolution systems that have jurisdiction over occupational therapy practice. |
| B.9.12. | Describe and discuss strategies to assist the consumer in gaining access to occupational therapy services. |
| B.9.13. | Demonstrate professional advocacy by participating in organizations or agencies promoting the profession (e.g., American Occupational Therapy Association, state occupational therapy associations, advocacy organizations). |
| **B.10.0. FIELDWORK EDUCATION** **Fieldwork education is a crucial part of professional preparation and is best integrated as a component of the curriculum design. Fieldwork experiences should be implemented and evaluated for their effectiveness by the educational institution. The experience should provide the student with the opportunity to carry out professional responsibilities under supervision and for professional role modeling. The academic fieldwork coordinator is responsible for the program's compliance with fieldwork education requirements. The academic fieldwork coordinator will** | |
| B.10.1. | Document the criteria and process for selecting fieldwork sites. Ensure that the fieldwork program reflects the sequence, depth, focus, and scope of content in the curriculum design. |
| B.10.2. | Ensure that the academic fieldwork coordinator and faculty collaborate to design fieldwork experiences that strengthen the ties between didactic and fieldwork education. |
| B.10.3. | Provide fieldwork education in settings that are equipped to meet the curriculum goals, provide educational experiences applicable to the academic program, and have fieldwork educators who are able to effectively meet the learning needs of the students. |
| B.10.4. | Ensure that the academic fieldwork coordinator is responsible for advocating the development of links between the fieldwork and didactic aspects of the curriculum, for communicating about the curriculum to fieldwork educators, and for maintaining contracts and site data related to fieldwork placements. |
| B.10.5. | Demonstrate that academic and fieldwork educators collaborate in establishing fieldwork objectives, identifying site requirements, and communicating with the student and fieldwork educator about progress and performance during fieldwork. |

| NUMBER | OT MASTER'S-DEGREE-LEVEL STANDARD |
|---|---|
| B.10.6. | Document a policy and procedure for complying with fieldwork site health requirements and maintaining student health records in a secure setting. |
| B.10.7. | Ensure that the ratio of fieldwork educators to student(s) enables proper supervision and the ability to provide frequent assessment of student progress in achieving stated fieldwork objectives. |
| B.10.8. | Ensure that fieldwork agreements are sufficient in scope and number to allow completion of graduation requirements in a timely manner in accordance with the policy adopted by the program. |
| B.10.9. | For programs in which the academic and fieldwork components of the curriculum are provided by two or more institutions, responsibilities of each sponsoring institution and fieldwork site must be clearly documented in a memorandum of understanding. For active Level I and Level II fieldwork sites, programs must have current fieldwork agreements or memoranda of understanding that are signed by both parties. (Electronic contracts and signatures are acceptable.) |
| B.10.10. | Documentation must be provided that each memorandum of understanding between institutions and active fieldwork sites is reviewed at least every 5 years by both parties. Programs must provide documentation that both parties have reviewed the contract. |
| **The goal of Level I fieldwork is to introduce students to the fieldwork experience, to apply knowledge to practice, and to develop understanding of the needs of clients. The program will** | |
| B.10.11. | Ensure that Level I fieldwork is integral to the program's curriculum design and include experiences designed to enrich didactic coursework through directed observation and participation in selected aspects of the occupational therapy process. |
| B.10.12. | Ensure that qualified personnel supervise Level I fieldwork. Examples may include, but are not limited to, currently licensed or credentialed occupational therapists and occupational therapy assistants, psychologists, physician assistants, teachers, social workers, nurses, and physical therapists. |
| B.10.13. | Document all Level I fieldwork experiences that are provided to students, including mechanisms for formal evaluation of student performance. Ensure that Level I fieldwork is not substituted for any part of Level II fieldwork. |
| **The goal of Level II fieldwork is to develop competent, entry-level, generalist occupational therapists. Level II fieldwork must be integral to the program's curriculum design and must include an in-depth experience in delivering occupational therapy services to clients, focusing on the application of purposeful and meaningful occupation and research, administration, and management of occupational therapy services. It is recommended that the student be exposed to a variety of clients across the life span and to a variety of settings. The program will** | |
| B.10.14. | Ensure that the fieldwork experience is designed to promote clinical reasoning and reflective practice, to transmit the values and beliefs that enable ethical practice, and to develop professionalism and competence in career responsibilities. |
| B.10.15. | Provide Level II fieldwork in traditional and/or emerging settings, consistent with the curriculum design. In all settings, psychosocial factors influencing engagement in occupation must be understood and integrated for the development of client-centered, meaningful, occupation-based outcomes. The student can complete Level II fieldwork in a minimum of one setting if it is reflective of more than one practice area, or in a maximum of four different settings. |
| B.10.16. | Require a minimum of 24 weeks' full-time Level II fieldwork. This may be completed on a part-time basis as defined by the fieldwork placement in accordance with the fieldwork placement's usual and customary personnel policies as long as it is at least 50% of a full-time equivalent at that site. |
| B.10.17. | Ensure that the student is supervised by a currently licensed or credentialed occupational therapist who has a minimum of 1 year of practice experience subsequent to initial certification, and is adequately prepared to serve as a fieldwork educator. The supervising therapist may be engaged by the fieldwork site or by the educational program. |
| B.10.18. | Document a mechanism for evaluating the effectiveness of supervision (e.g., student evaluation of fieldwork) and for providing resources for enhancing supervision (e.g., materials on supervisory skills, continuing education opportunities, articles on theory and practice). |
| B.10.19. | Ensure that supervision provides protection of consumers and opportunities for appropriate role modeling of occupational therapy practice. Initially, supervision should be direct and then decrease to less direct supervision as is appropriate for the setting, the severity of the client's condition, and the ability of the student. |

| NUMBER | OT MASTER'S-DEGREE-LEVEL STANDARD |
|---|---|
| B.10.20. | Ensure that supervision provided in a setting where no occupational therapy services exist includes a documented plan for provision of occupational therapy services and supervision by a currently licensed or credentialed occupational therapist with at least 3 years of professional experience. Supervision must include a minimum of 8 hours per week. Supervision must be initially direct and then may be decreased to less direct supervision as is appropriate for the setting, the client's needs, and the ability of the student. An occupational therapy supervisor must be available, via a variety of contact measures, to the student during all working hours. An on-site supervisor designee of another profession must be assigned while the occupational therapy supervisor is off site. |
| B.10.21. | Document mechanisms for requiring formal evaluation of student performance on Level II fieldwork (e.g., the American Occupational Therapy Association *Fieldwork Performance Evaluation for the Occupational Therapy Student* or equivalent). |
| B.10.22. | Ensure that students attending Level II fieldwork outside the United States are supervised by an occupational therapist who graduated from a program approved by the World Federation of Occupational Therapists and has 1 year of experience in practice. Such fieldwork must not exceed 12 weeks. |

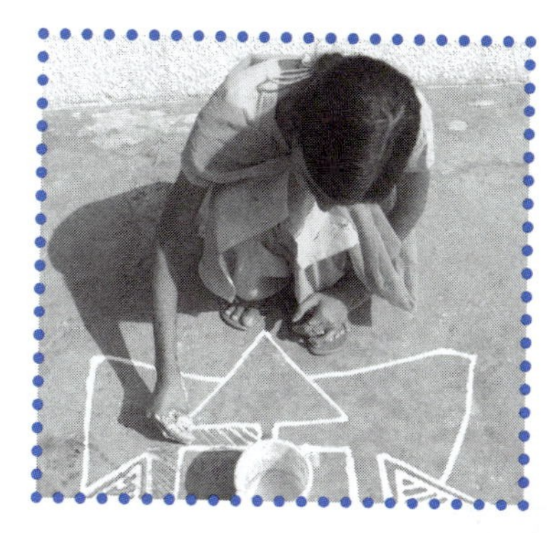

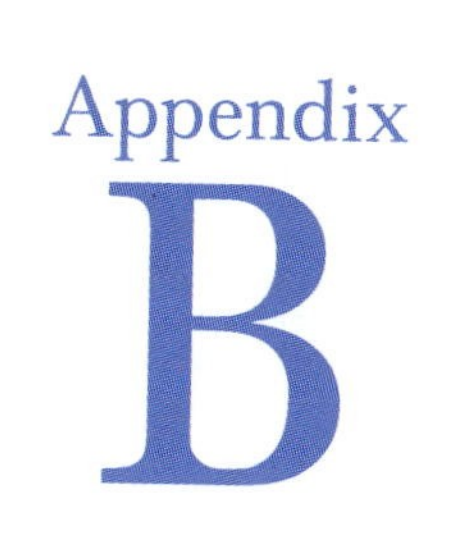

Appendix B

# Assessment Tool Grid

# Assessment Tool Grid

Amy Peluso Burns

Printed with permission from the author.

| Name of Assessment tool, Author, and Publication date | Standardized | Validity/ Reliability | Setting Used | Areas Assessed | Age Group |
|---|---|---|---|---|---|
| **Foundations for Functional Activity** | | | | | |
| **Balance/Posture/Mobility** | | | | | |
| **Berg Scale** *Measures 14 balance items. Includes sitting and standing unsupported, sit-to-stand, transfers, picking up objects from floor, and turning.* | No | Valid and Reliable | Home or clinic setting | Transfers, sitting, standing, balance | Adult/elderly |
| **Functional Reach Test** *Simple way to measure standing balance. Measures the difference between arm's length and maximal forward reach.* | Yes | Valid and Reliable | Wall and tape measure needed | Reaching and balance | Adult/elderly |
| **Modified Gait Abnormality Rating Scale (GARS)** *Seven item assessment of gait, stepping and arm movements, staggering foot contact, hip ROM, shoulder extension, etc.* | No | | Room to walk | Hip ROM, foot contact, staggering, arm/leg symmetry, guarding | Adult/elderly |
| **Timed Get Up and Go (TGUG)** *Measures the overall time to complete a series of functionally important tasks. Helps to identify clients with balance deficits.* | No | Valid and Reliable | Room to walk 10 feet; chair | Balance, posture, mobility | Adult/elderly |
| **Tinetti** *Measures a client's gait and balance.* | No | Inter-rater reliability | Room to walk 10 feet; chair | Balance and gait | Adult/elderly |
| **Cognition** | | | | | |
| **Autobiographical Memory Interview (AMI)** *Interview recalling events from the clients' past including school, wedding, children, etc.* | Yes | Valid and Reliable | Quiet environment with minimal distractions | Memory, retrograde amnesia | Adult/elderly |
| **Bay Area Functional Performance Evaluation (BaFPE)** *Assesses how a client might function in task-oriented settings and settings with social interaction. Uses sea shells, design blocks, and associated items.* | Yes | Valid and Reliable | Seated at table | Memory, organization, attention span | Adult/elderly |
| **Behavioral Inattention Test** *Assesses unilateral visual neglect. Includes card sorting, article reading, figure/shape copying, etc.* | Yes | Valid and Reliable | Quiet environment with minimal distractions | Unilateral visual neglect, picture recalling, line crossing, article reading, phone dialing | Adult/elderly |

| | | | | | |
|---|---|---|---|---|---|
| **Brown ADD Scale**<br>*Assesses executive function impairments associated with ADD/ADHD and related problems.* | Yes | Valid and Reliable | Quiet environment with minimal distractions | Attention, listening skills | Age 3 to adult |
| **Cognitive Assessment of Minnesota (CAM)**<br>*Assesses the cognitive abilities of adults with neurological impairments.* | Yes | Valid and Reliable | Quiet room | Attention, memory, visual neglect | Ages 18 to 70 |
| **Contextual Memory Test**<br>*Assesses awareness of memory capacity, strategy use, and recall in adults with memory dysfunction.* | Yes | Valid and Reliable | Quiet room with minimal distraction | Memory, awareness of memory capacity, recall of line drawings | Adult/elderly |
| **Glasgow Coma Scale**<br>*Measures response of eyes, verbal response, and motor response in numerical levels.* | No | Reliable | In hospital | Alertness, awareness, verbal response, motor response | All ages |
| **King-Devick Test of Oculomotor Speed and Accuracy (K-D)**<br>*Assesses residual oculomotor functions in a clinical setting, and its components can also be used for vision therapy training purposes as well.* | Yes | Valid and Reliable | Quiet environment with minimal distractions | eye tracking skills, general motor skills | Ages 6 to 14 |
| **Leiter International Performance Scale - Revised (Leiter-R)**<br>*A non-verbal test to assess cognitive functions in children and adolescents.* | Yes | Valid and Reliable | Individual setting, comfortable for the client | Intellectual ability, memory, attention | Ages 2 to 20 years, 11 months |
| **Lowenstein Occupational Therapy Cognitive Assessment (LOTCA) (also LOTCA-Geriatric)**<br>*Assesses clients with neurological deficits and mental health issues. Tests orientation, visual/spatial perception, praxis, visuomotor. Includes cards, blocks, pegboard.* | Yes | Valid and Reliable | Quiet environment with minimal distractions | Orientation, perception, praxis, visuomotor, organization, thinking operations | Adult/elderly |
| **Luria-Nebraska Neuropsychological Battery**<br>*Reading numbers, writing words, differentiate hard/soft touch, sounds. Provides a pattern analysis of strengths and weakness across areas of brain function.* | Yes | Valid and Reliable | Quiet environment with minimal distractions | Numbers, reading, writing, touching | All ages |
| **Mini-Mental Status Evaluation (MMSE)**<br>*Used to assess cognitive function.* | Yes | Valid and Reliable | Seated at table | Brain injury, writing, reading, drawing | Ages 18+ |

| | | | | | |
|---|---|---|---|---|---|
| **Ranchos Los Amigos** (Developed at the Rancho Los Amigos Hospital in California by the Head Injury Treatment Team) *Medical scale, assesses the level of recovery of a client with a brain injury and those recovering from a coma.* | No | Reliable | In hospital | Alertness, awareness | All ages |
| **Rivermead Behavioral Memory Test (RBMT-II)** *Assessment of gross memory impairments encountered by clients in their everyday lives. Identifies everyday memory problems and monitors change over time.* | Yes | Valid and Reliable | Quiet environment with minimal distractions | Memory: immediate and recall | Ages 16+ |
| **Severe Impairment Battery** *Evaluates cognitive abilities at the lower end of the range (severely impaired dementia client). Allows for non-verbal and partially correct responses.* | Yes | Valid and Reliable | Quiet environment with minimal distractions | Memory, completing simple actions | Adult/elderly |
| **Test of Everyday Attention** *Measures selective attention, sustained attention, and attentional switching. Includes map search, telephone search, elevator counting, etc.* | Yes | Valid and Reliable | Quiet room; table and chairs | Everyday materials (map searching, phone skills, etc.) | Ages 18 to 80 |
| **Dexterity** | | | | | |
| **Jebsen-Taylor Hand Function Test** *Assesses a broad range of hand functions used in daily activities. A seven-part test that uses common items such as paper clips, cans, pencils, etc.* | Yes | Reliable | Seated, requires adequate lighting | Writing, page turning, lifting small/large objects, simulated feeding | Ages 20 to 94 |
| **Manipulative Aptitude Test** *Measures hand/arm/finger dexterity and speed through sorting and assembling.* | Yes | Valid and Reliable | Seated at a table or desk | Dexterity, manipulative aptitude, dominant hand | Ages 13+ |
| **Minnesota Rate of Manipulation** *Assesses unilateral and bilateral manual dexterity along with eye-hand coordination. Provides information on standing tolerance, sustained neck flexion, weight bearing, and repetitive reach.* | Yes | Valid and Reliable | Table and chair | Manual dexterity, turning, displacing | Ages 13+ |
| **Nine Hole Peg** *Client places nine dowels in nine holes while being timed.* | Yes | Valid and Reliable | Table and chair | Finger dexterity | Ages 20+ |
| **O'Connor Finger Dexterity Test** *Requires hand placement of 3 pins per hole.* | Yes | | Table and chair | Predictor of rapid manipulation | Ages 13+ |

| | | | | | |
|---|---|---|---|---|---|
| **O'Connor Tweezer Dexterity Test**<br>*Measures the speed with which a client can puck up pins with a tweezer, one at a time, and place the pin into a small hole.* | Yes | | Table and chair | Finger dexterity, fine motor coordination, speed, eye-hand coordination | Ages 13+ |
| **Pennsylvania Bi-manual Worksample**<br>*Assesses finger dexterity of both hands, as well as gross movements of both arms.* | Yes | Reliable | Table and chair | Finger dexterity of both hands, gross movements of both arms, eye-hand coordination | Ages 16+ |
| **Purdue Pegboard**<br>*Assesses gross movement of hands/fingers/arms, as well as fingertip dexterity.* | Yes | Valid and Reliable | Table and chair | Gross movement of hands, fingers, and arms; fingertip dexterity | Ages 5+ |
| **Range of Motion**<br>*Measurement of the achievable distance between the flexed position and the extended position of a particular joint or muscle group.* | Yes | Valid, not 100% reliable | Comfortable for client, chair/mat | Biomechanical | All ages |
| **Rosenbusch Test of Finger Dexterity**<br>*Measures the speed of inter-digital manipulation of each hand separately.* | Yes | Valid and Reliable | Table and chair | Manipulation of all parts of the hand | All ages |
| **Strength Testing**<br>*The strength of each muscle group is measured on a scale of 0/5 to 5/5.* | Yes | Valid, not 100% reliable | Comfortable for client, chair/mat | Biomechanical | All ages |
| **Motor/cognition/coping/self-help (Pediatric)** | | | | | |
| **Battelle Developmental Inventory, Second Edition, (BDI-2)**<br>*Developmental assessment for early childhood. Screening, diagnosis, and evaluation of early development.* | Yes | Valid and Reliable | Familiar to child; little to no auditory and visual distractions | Personal-social, motor, adaptive, communication, cognitive (all with sub-domains too) | Birth to age 8 |
| **Bayley Scales of Infant Development (BIDS)**<br>*Measures the mental and motor development and tests the behavior of infants.* | Yes | Valid and Reliable | Quiet environment with minimal distractions | Performance in occupation, performance skills, context, activity demands | Ages 1 to 42 months |
| **Behavioral-Characteristics Progression (BCP)** *Curriculum-based assessment and planning tool for use by special education professionals serving children and adults who are functioning between the developmental ages of 1 to 14 years.* | No | Valid and Reliable | Comfortable for child | Self-help, fine motor, gross motor, academic, etc. | Ages 1 to 14 |
| **Bruininks-Oseretsky of Motor Proficiency**<br>*Comprehensive index of motor proficiency as well as separate measures of both gross and fine motor skills.* | Yes | Valid and Reliable | Gym | Motor | Ages 4.5 to 14.5 |

| | | | | | |
|---|---|---|---|---|---|
| **The Carolina Curriculum for Infants and Toddlers with Special Needs, Second Edition (CCITSN)** *Designed for children who have mild to severe special needs and who function in the birth to 24-month developmental range.* | Yes | Valid and Reliable | Comfortable for child | Cognition, communication, social adaptation, fine motor, gross motor | Birth to age 2 |
| **The Carolina Curriculum for Preschoolers with Special Needs (CCPSN)** *Designed for children who have mild to severe special needs and who function in the 2- to 5-year developmental range.* | Yes | Valid and Reliable | Comfortable for child | Cognition, communication, social adaptation, fine motor, gross motor | Ages 2 to 5 |
| **Coping-Inventory** *Assesses the behavior patterns and skills used by children and adults to meet personal needs and adapt to the demands of their environment.* | No | Self-rated and observation | Variety of environments | Two forms of coping behavior, self and environment | Ages 3+ |
| **First Step (FirstSTEp)** *Screening test for evaluating pre-schooler.* | Yes | Valid and Reliable | Public schools, public health situations, pediatrician's office | IDEA domains: cognition, communication, and motor | Ages 2 years, 9 months to 6 years, 2 months |
| **Early Coping Inventory** *Assesses the coping-related behavior of children.* | No | Observation form | Comfortable for child | Sensorimotor, reactive behavior, self-initiated behavior | Ages 4 to 36 months |
| **Hawaii Early Learning Profile (HELP)** *Test is helpful to see development of child throughout periods of time.* | Criterion referenced | Valid and Reliable | Comfortable for child | Cognition, language, gross motor, fine motor, social-emotional, self-help, regulatory, sensory organization | Birth to age 3 and preschool |
| **Infant-Toddler and Family Instrument (ITFI) and Manual** *Helps to evaluate the strengths and vulnerabilities of children and their families.* | | Valid and Reliable | Family environment, comfortable | Gross and fine motor, social and emotional, language, coping and self-help | Ages 6 months to 3 years |
| **Kent Inventory of Developmental Skills (KIDS)** *Provides a clear picture of a child's development status and relative strengths and needs.* | Yes | Valid and Reliable | Familiar to child; home | Cognitive, motor, communication, self-help, social | Birth to 15 months, or up to age 6 when severe developmental disabilities are present |
| **Mullen Scales of Early Learning** *Provides a complete picture of cognitive and motor ability.* | Yes | Valid and Reliable | Clinic and school setting | Visual, linguistic, motor, distinguish between receptive and expressive processing | Birth to 68 months |

| | | | | | |
|---|---|---|---|---|---|
| **Peabody Developmental Motor Scales, Second Edition, (PDMS-2)**<br>*Measures both gross and fine motor skills.* | Yes | Valid and Reliable | Quiet environment with minimal distractions | Motor (gross and fine) | Birth to age 7 |
| **Pediatric Evaluation of Disability Inventory (PEDI)**<br>*Assesses key functional capabilities and performance.* | Yes | Valid and Reliable | Natural environment for child | Self-care, mobility, social function | Ages 6 months to 7 years |
| **PEERAMID-2**<br>*Assesses a child's performance in five different areas of development.* | Yes | n/a | Quiet, comfortable | Fine motor/ graphomotor function, language function, gross motor function, memory function, and visual processing | School Grades 4 to 10 |
| **Pediatric Examination of Educational Readiness (PEER)**<br>*Assesses the preschooler's performance in six areas.* | Yes | n/a | Quiet, child comfortable, no parents | Orientation, gross motor, visual-fine motor, sequential, linguistic, and preacademic learning | Ages 4 to 6 |
| **Pediatric Extended Exam at Three (PEET)**<br>*Assesses a child's performance in five basic areas of development.* | Yes | n/a | Quiet, comfortable, low visual stim, supportive | Gross motor, language, visual-fine motor, memory, and intersensory integration | Age 3 |
| **Pediatric Early Elementary Exam (PEEX-2)**<br>*Assesses a child's performance in five different areas of development.* | Yes | n/a | quiet, comfortable, sit to left or right of child at table | Fine motor/ graphomotor function, language function, gross motor function, memory function, and visual processing function | Ages 6 to 9 |
| **Posture and Fine Motor Assessments (PFMAI)**<br>*Designed to identify motor delays in infants and to monitor progress in the first year of life.* | Yes | Valid and Reliable | Familiar, child only in diaper | Motor | Ages 2 to 12 months |
| **Quick Neurological Screening Test - II, Revised Edition**<br>*Designed for use in screening for early identification of disabilities* | Norms suggest cutoff scores | Some Validity and Reliability | Table and chairs, room to walk | Hand skill, discrimination, eye tracking, sound patterns, movements | Ages 5+ |
| **Temperament and Atypical Behavior Scale (TABS)**<br>*Early Childhood Indicators of Developmental Dysfunction* | Norm referenced | Valid and Reliable | Parent may be able to complete independently, or with help from professional | Sensory regulation, attachment behaviors | Ages 11 to 71 months |
| **Test of Gross Motor Development (TGMD-2)**<br>*Measures gross motor abilities that develop in early life* | Yes | Valid and Reliable | School (Open and large area) | Gross motor | Ages 3 to 10 |

| | | | | | |
|---|---|---|---|---|---|
| **Toddler Infant Motor Eval (TIME)**<br>*Evaluates children who have atypical motor development.* | Yes | Valid and Reliable | Quiet environment with minimal distractions | Motor | Birth to 42 months |
| **Play** | | | | | |
| **Adolescent Role Assessment (ARA)**<br>*Gathers information on the adolescent's occupational role involvement over time and across domains.* | No | Scores lack internal consistency | Comfortable for client | Social integration, school, roles, play, family | Ages 13 to 20 |
| **Adolesant Leisure Interest Profile**<br>*Asks adolescent to report his or her interest and/or participation in a variety of age-appropriate leisure activities.* | No | Self-report, Valid and Reliable | Comfortable for child | Sports, outdoor, summer, winter, indoor, creative | Ages 12 to 21 |
| **Infant Preschool Play Assessment Scale (I-PAS)**<br>*Systematically observes children at play and in other routines or natural environments.* | Criterion referenced | Valid and Reliable | Comfortable for child | Social, sensorimotor, memory, gross motor, communication, motivation, problem solving | Birth to 5 years |
| **Kid Play Profile**<br>*Asks child to report his or her interest and/or participation in a variety of age-appropriate leisure activities.* | No | Self-report, Valid and Reliable | Comfortable for child | Sports, outdoor, summer, winter, indoor, creative | Ages 6 to 9 |
| **Knox Preschool Play Scale (KPPS)**<br>*Preschoolers can be observed during free play, and a play age can be computed.* | Yes | Valid and Reliable | Comfortable for child, classroom setting | Space management, material management, imitation, participation | Preschoolers |
| **Preteen Play Profile**<br>*Asks preteen to report his or her interest and/or participation in a variety of age-appropriate leisure activities.* | No | Self-report, Valid and Reliable | Comfortable for child | Sports, outdoor, summer, winter, indoor, creative | Ages 9 to 12 |
| **Takata Play History (TPH)**<br>*Probes past and actual play history that relate to sensory integration function.* | No | Valid and Reliable | Comfortable for child | Sensorimotor, symbolic, dramatic, games, recreational | All children |
| **Test of Playfulness (ToP)**<br>*The information gathered provides a clue on inner drive and response to just right challenges, socialization, and play.* | No | Valid and Reliable | Indoors and outdoors | Intrinsic motivation, internal control, freedom to suspend reality | Ages 18 months+ |
| **Transdiciplinary Play-Based Assessment**<br>*Allows children to initiate and engage in play activities that are natural and enjoyable.* | Norm referenced | Valid and Reliable | Environment comfortable to child | Cognitive, social-emotional, communication, language, and sensorimotor | Infancy to age 6 |
| **Sensation/Edema** | | | | | |
| **Tactile Activity Kit**<br>*Versatile tool for sensory integration therapy.* | No | Not Valid, Not Reliable | Table-top | Tactile stimulation, discrimination, and desensitization | All ages |

| | | | | | |
|---|---|---|---|---|---|
| **Volumeter** *Fill container with water, measure the displaced water of both hands.* | No | | Countertop or table; need access to water faucet | Edema, swelling of UE | All ages |
| **Sensory** | | | | | |
| **DeGangi-Berk Test of Sensory Integration (TSI)** *Measures overall sensory integration, as well as postural control, bilateral motor integration, and reflex integration.* | Yes | Valid and Reliable | Environment comfortable for child | Vestibular function; postural control, bilateral motor integration, reflex integration | Ages 3 to 5 |
| **Sensory Integration and Praxis Tests (SIPT)** *Measures sensory processing deficits related to learning and behavior problems.* | Yes | Valid and Reliable | Environment comfortable for child | Visual, tactile, kinesthetic perception, motor performance | Ages 4 to 8 |
| **Sensory Processing Measure** *Provides a complete picture of children's sensory processing difficulties at school and at home.* | Yes | Valid and Reliable | Home Form by caregiver in the home; School Forms by staff in multiple school environments | Sensory processing, praxis, social participation | Ages 5 to 12 |
| **Sensory Profile** *Measures children's responses to sensory events in everyday life.* | Yes | Valid and Reliable | Environment comfortable for child | Modulation of sensory input across sensory systems, behavioral/emotional responses associated with sensory processing | Ages 3 to 10 |
| **Sensory Profile: Infant/Toddler** *Examines patterns in children who are at risk or have specific disabilities.* | Yes | Valid and Reliable | Environment comfortable for child | Modulation of sensory input across sensory systems, behavioral/emotional responses associated with sensory processing | Birth to 36 months |
| **Sensory Profile: Adolescent/Adult** *Identifies sensory processing patterns and effects on functional performance.* | Based on normative information | Valid and Reliable | Environment comfortable for child | Modulation of sensory input across sensory systems, behavioral/emotional responses associated with sensory processing | Ages 11+ |
| **Sensory Profile School Companion** *Assesses children's sensory processing information related to school performance.* | Yes | Valid and Reliable | Environment comfortable for child | Classroom behavior and performance | Ages 3 to 11 |

| | | | | | |
|---|---|---|---|---|---|
| **Test of Sensory Function in Infants (TSFI)**<br>*Objective assessment to determine whether, and to what extent, an infant has sensory processing deficits.* | Yes | Valid and Reliable | Individually administered, simple interaction with the infant, infant can be seated on parent's lap | Deep pressure, visual tactile integration, adaptive motor function, ocular motor control, reactivity to vestibular stimulation | Ages 4 to 18 months |
| **Vision/Visual Perceptual** | | | | | |
| **Benton Visual Form Discrimination**<br>*Assesses the ability to discriminate between complex visual configurations. Book of line drawings.* | No | Valid | Quiet environment with minimal distractions | Neglect, neuropsycho-logical | Adult/elderly |
| **Developmental Test of Visual-Motor Integration (VMI)**<br>*Visuomotor skills are tested as the student copies a series of shapes in a test booklet.* | Yes | Valid and Reliable | Seated at desk/table, lighting, free of distraction | Visual perceptual | Ages 3+ |
| **Developmental Test of Visual Perception (DTVP-2)**<br>*Measures visual perception and motor integration skills.* | Yes | Valid and Reliable | Seated at desk/table, lighting, free of distraction | Pure visual perception (no motor response) and visual-motor integration | Ages 4 to 10 |
| **Hooper Visual Organization Test (VOT)**<br>*Ability to visually integrate information into whole perceptions through the use of line drawings arranged in puzzles.* | Yes | Valid and Reliable | Quiet environment with minimal distractions | Organization of visual stimuli | Ages 13+ |
| **McDowell Visual Screening Kit**<br>*Allows vision testing of very young or severely disabled children.* | Screening | Valid and Reliable | Comfortable for child | Distance visual acuity, near point acuity, ocular alignment, color perception, ocular function | Ages 2.5 to 5.5 |
| **Motor-Free Visual Perception Test (MVPT-3)**<br>*Assesses overall visual perceptual ability.* | Yes | Valid and Reliable | Seated at table Adequate light and free from distraction | Visual perceptual | Ages 4+ |
| **STROOP Color and Word Test**<br>*Reading aloud colored words. The words themselves are names of colors, but the actual color is different than the name.* | Yes | Valid and Reliable | Quiet environment with minimal distractions | Brain function and planning | Ages 15+ |
| **Test of Visual Motor Skills**<br>*Assesses a child's ability to transcribe geometric forms.* | Yes | Valid and Reliable | Seated at desk/table, individually or in groups | Eye-hand coordination skills | Ages 3 to 14 |
| **Test of Visual Motor Skills (UPPER)**<br>*Measures visual motor functioning using 16 geometric figures.* | Yes | Valid and Reliable | Seated at table Adequate light and free from distraction | Visual motor | Ages 12 to 40 |

| | | | | | |
|---|---|---|---|---|---|
| **Test of Visual-Perceptual Skills (non-motor) (TVPS-R)**<br>*Measures seven areas of visual-perception skills.* | Yes | Valid and Reliable | Seated at desk/table, lighting, free of distraction | Visual discrimination/memory, visual spatial relationships, visual form-constancy, visual sequential memory, visual figure ground, visual closure | Ages 4 to 13 |
| **Warren's Brain Injury Visual Assessment Battery for Adults (biVABA)**<br>*Assessment of visual processing ability after a brain injury.* | Yes | Valid and Reliable | Comfortable for client | Visual perceptual processing, oculomotor function, how function is affected | Post CVA or head/brain injury |

| **ADLs and IADL** | | | | | |
|---|---|---|---|---|---|
| **Name of Assessment tool, Author, and Publication date** | **Standardized** | **Validity/ Reliability** | **Setting Used** | **Areas Assessed** | **Age** |
| **Allen Cognitive Level Test (ACL)**<br>*Leather lacing test.* | Yes | Valid and Reliable | Environment with minimal distractions and good lighting | Problem solving, sequencing | Adults/elderly |
| **Arnadottir Occupational Therapy Neurobehavioral Evaluation (A-one)**<br>*Determines the impact of neurobehavioral impairments on activities of daily living and mobility tasks using a five-point scale.* | Yes | Valid and Reliable | Clinic or home setting | ADLs, severity of neurobehavioral impairment, occupational performance | Adults/elderly |
| **Assessment of Motor and Process Skills (AMPS)**<br>*Observational assessment, measures the quality of a person's ADLs. Rates the effort, efficiency, safety, and independence of ADL motor/process skills. *Training required.* | Yes | Valid and Reliable | Various conditions | IADLs, motor skills and processing skills | Adults/elderly |
| **Assessment of Occupational Functioning (AOF)**<br>*Assesses the functional capacity of residents in long-term treatment settings who have physical and/or psychiatric problems.* | Yes | Valid and Reliable | Comfortable for the client | IADLs, MOHO, volition, habituation, performance | Ages 13+ |
| **Barthel Index**<br>*Assesses self-care functions in older adults.* | No | Predictive validity | Individual or group evaluation | Self-care | Adults/elderly |
| **Canadian Occupational Performance Measure (COPM)**<br>*Individualized outcome measure designed to detect changes in self-perception of occupational performance over time.* | Yes, but not norm referenced | Valid and Reliable | Comfortable for client | Occupational performances and perception | All ages |
| **Comprehensive Occupational Therapy Evaluation (COTE)**<br>*Developed in an acute psychiatric setting. Identifies 25 OT-related behaviors within three categories (general behavior, interpersonal behavior, and task behavior).* | Yes | Valid and Reliable | Quiet environment with minimal distractions | Behavior | All ages |
| **Direct Assessment of Functional Abilities (DAFA)**<br>*Direct measurement of the instrumental activities of daily living. Used to determine functional deficits in clients with mild cognitive impairment.* | Yes | Valid and Reliable | Clinic setting, cafeteria, gift shop, and exam room | IADLs | Adults/elderly |

| | | | | | |
|---|---|---|---|---|---|
| **Functional Independent Measure (FIM)**<br>*Scale (range from 1 to 7) that measures a client's ability to function with independence. Collected upon admission to rehabilitation unit, upon discharge, and after discharge.* | Yes | Valid and Reliable | Clinic or home setting | ADLs, self-care, communication, cognitive function | Adults/elderly |
| **Independent Living Scales (ILS)**<br>*Offers assessment, daily living skills, self-advocacy training, and support with issues that challenge the independence of a client.* | Yes | Valid and Reliable | Table and chairs; can be bedside | IADL, memory, orientation, money management, health, safety, etc. | Ages 65+ |
| **Index of Activities of Daily Living (ADL)**<br>*Assesses functional status as a measurement of the client's ability to perform activities of daily living independently. *No longer in print, may still be seen in some clinics.* | Yes | Valid and Reliable | Inpatient observations | ADL, biological and psychological function | Ages 65+ |
| **Kitchen Task Assessment (KTA)**<br>*Measures organization, planning, and judgment skills through common kitchen tasks.* | Yes | Valid and Reliable | Kitchen/ cooking environment | IADL, initiation, organization, sequencing, judgment, safety | Adults/elderly |
| **Klein-Bell Activities of Daily Living Scale**<br>*Assesses age-related changes in activities of daily living ability. *No longer in print, may still be seen in some clinics.* | Yes | Valid and Reliable | General rehabilitation setting | ADLs | Adults/elderly |
| **Kohlman Evaluation of Living Skills (KELS)**<br>*Ability to function in 17 basic living skills. Assesses skills in five areas: self-care, safety and health, money management, transportation/ telephone, and work/leisure.* | Yes | Valid and Reliable | Table and chairs | Self-care, safety and health, money management, transportation, telephone, work, leisure | Adults/elderly |
| **Level of Rehabilitation Scale (LORS-II)**<br>*Evaluates the success of inpatient rehabilitation programs.* | Yes | Valid and Reliable | Hospital rehabilitation units | ADLs | Adults/elderly |
| **Milwaukee Evaluation of Daily Living Skills (MEDLS)**<br>*Information from clients and families; establishes baseline behaviors necessary to develop treatment plans and guide intervention in regard to daily living skills.* | No | Valid and Reliable | Home environment | ADLs, including communication, personal care, clothing care, etc. | Adult/elderly |

| **Occupational Circumstances Assessment and Interview Rating Scale (OCAIRS)** *A 40-minute interview that analyzes the extent and nature of a client's occupational adaptation and participation.* | No | Valid and Reliable | Comfortable for the client | MOHO, volitional, habituation, performance | Ages 13+ |
|---|---|---|---|---|---|
| **Occupational Performance History Interview (OPHI-II)** *Interview that gathers the appreciation of a client's life history, the direction in which they want to take their life, as well as the impact of a disability on their life.* | Yes | Valid and Reliable | Comfortable for client | Occupational roles, daily routine, critical life events | Adolescents and adults |
| **Pre-Feeding Skills Checklist** *Manual for feeding assessment and intervention.* | No | Valid and Reliable | Quiet environment with minimal distractions | Feeding positions, types, quantity, sucking, movements | Ages 1 to 24 months |
| **Performance Assessment of Self-care Skills (PASS)** *Performance-based observation tool covering functional mobility, personal care, and IADLs. Measures short term functional change in elderly after hospitalization. *Requires 2-day training workshop.* | Criterion referenced | Valid and Reliable | Clinic and home version | IADLs | Adult/elderly |
| **Role-Checklist** *Assesses the values that clients place on their occupational roles.* | Yes | Valid and Reliable | Comfortable for client | MOHO, habituation sub-system | Ages 13+ |
| **Routine Task Inventory (RTI-II)** *Measures the level of performance in activities of daily living through observation and questioning.* | No | Valid and Reliable | Clinic or home setting | ADLs, effect of cognitive impairment on task performance | Adult/elderly |
| **Occupational Self Assessment** *This is a self-assessment of perceptions of strengths and weaknesses relative to occupational functioning.* | Yes | Valid and Reliable | Comfortable for the client | MOHO, volitional, habituation, performance | Ages 16+ |
| **Environmental Evaluations** | | | | | |
| **Enabler** *Norm-based environment assessment, developed to assess the accessibility of housing and its close surroundings.* | Yes | Valid and Reliable | Home environment and close surroundings | IADLs, neurological, musculoskeletal, psychological, movement, cognition, physical | All ages |
| **Home Observation for Measurement of the Environment** *Measures the quality and quantity of stimulation and support available to a child in the home environment.* | Yes | Valid and Reliable | Home environment | Interaction, environment | Ages 3 to 15 |

## Education

| Name of Assessment tool, Author, and Publication date | Standardized | Validity/ Reliability | Setting Used | Areas Assessed | Age |
|---|---|---|---|---|---|
| **Occupational Therapy Psychosocial Assessment of Learning (OT PAL)** *Designed to examine the environmental factors to determine the best "fit" between a child and his or her environment.* | No | Content validity | Classroom | Volition, habituation, and environmental fit within the classroom setting | Ages 6 to 12 |
| **School Function Assessment** *Measures school-related functional skills.* | Yes | Valid and Reliable | School setting | Participation, task supports, activity performance, adaptations | School grades 1 to 6 |
| **Handwriting** | | | | | |
| **Denver Handwriting Analysis (DHA)** | No | Valid and Reliable | Classroom | Fine motor, visual motor, auditory | School grades 3 to 8 |
| **Erhardt Developmental Prehension Assessment (EDPA)** *Designed for charting the prehensile development of a child.* | Yes | Valid and Reliable | Quiet environment with minimal distractions | Positional-reflexive, cognitively directed, pre-writing skills | Birth to 15 months |
| **Evaluation Tool of Children's Handwriting (ETCH)** *Evaluates six different areas of children's handwriting.* | Yes | Valid and Reliable | Quiet environment with minimal distractions | Alphabet production, numerical writing, near/far point copying, dictation, sentence composition | School grades 1 to 6 |
| **Minnesota Handwriting Assessment** *Used to analyze handwriting skills.* | Yes | Valid and Reliable | Quiet environment with minimal distractions | Legibility, form, alignment, size, spacing | 1st and 2nd grade |
| **Observation of Handwriting Skills** *Looks at the functional handwriting performance of the student in the classroom. Helps to identify areas that could impact handwriting or academic performance.* | No | Valid and Reliable | Quiet environment with minimal distractions | Gross and fine motor, visual motor, visual memory | Kindergarten and 1st grade-age |

## Work and Retirement

| Name of Assessment tool, Author, and Publication date | Standardized | Validity/ Reliability | Setting Used | Areas Assessed | Age |
|---|---|---|---|---|---|
| **Worker Environment Impact Scale (WEIS)** *Assesses environmental characteristics that facilitate successful employment experiences. Goal is to maximize the "fit" of the worker and his or her skill to the job environment.* | No | Fair Validity and Reliability | Comfortable for the client | Space-related issues, fit of environment | Ages 16+ |
| **Worker Role Interview (WRI)** *Identifies psychosocial and environmental factors that influence a client's ability to return to work.* | Yes | Valid and Reliable | Work, comfortable for client | Physical evaluation, essential job functions, psychosocial capacity to return to work | Ages 16+ |

| Leisure (many ADL/IADL evaluations include leisure) | | | | | |
|---|---|---|---|---|---|
| **Name of Assessment tool, Author, and Publication date** | **Standardized** | **Validity/ Reliability** | **Setting Used** | **Areas Assessed** | **Age** |
| **Adolescent Leisure Interest Profile** *Asks adolescent to report his or her interest and/or participation in a variety of age-appropriate leisure activities.* | No | Self-report, Valid and Reliable | Comfortable for the client | Sports, outdoor, summer, winter, indoor, creative | Ages 12 to 21 |
| **Adolescent Role Assessment (ARA)** *Gathers information on the adolescent's occupational role involvement over time and across domains.* | No | Scores lack internal consistency | Comfortable for the client | Social integration, school, roles, play, family | Ages 13 to 20 |

| Social Participation | | | | | |
|---|---|---|---|---|---|
| **Name of Assessment tool, Author, and Publication date** | **Standardized** | **Validity/ Reliability** | **Setting Used** | **Areas Assessed** | **Age** |
| **Coping Inventory** *Profiles coping styles, as well as behaviors, that facilitate or interfere with adaptive coping. Self-administered and profiled.* | No | Self-report and observation | Comfortable for the client | Sensorimotor, reactive behavior, self-initiated behavior, adaptive coping | Ages 15+ |
| **Life Satisfaction Index** *Looking at five factors that make up total life satisfaction (pleasure, meaningfulness, feeling of success, self-image, happiness).* | Yes | Valid and Reliable | Comfortable for the client | Activity, developmental theory, internal satisfaction | Ages 50 to 90 |
| **Occupational Questionnaire (OQ)** *Self-report assessment. Client documents the main activity in which he or she engages for each half-hour throughout the morning/day/evening and identifies each activity as work, ADL, recreation, or rest. Explores the meaning of leisure from the client's perspective.* | Yes | Valid and Reliable | Clinic or home setting | IADLs, volition, activity pattern, life satisfaction, interests, values, personal causation | Ages 13+ |
| **Social Profile** *Assessment of activity participation, social interaction, and membership roles in a group.* | No | Valid and Reliable; Ongoing research | Activity focused | Individualized to client choices | Adolescents and adults |
| **Volitional Questionnaire** *Observational assessment, gathers information on a client's volition.* | Yes | Valid | Observations are context specific: leisure, work, ADL environments | MOHO, volition subsystem, work, leisure, intrinsic motivation, values, interests | Ages 16+ |

| Wellness | | | | | |
|---|---|---|---|---|---|
| **Name of Assessment tool, Author, and Publication date** | **Standardized** | **Validity/ Reliability** | **Setting Used** | **Areas Assessed** | **Age** |
| **Engagement in Meaningful Activities Survey (EMAS)** *Clients read statements about activities, put an 'X' in the box that best describes them (never to always).* | Yes, for research purposes only | Valid and Reliable | Comfortable for the client | Activities | Adult/elderly |
| **Measure of Sub-Acute Rehabilitation Potential** *Uses a five-point rating scale to assess health status, history, hope, help, health efforts.* | No | | 90-day type clinical setting | Health status, history, hope, help, health efforts | Adult/elderly |
| **Stress Management Questionnaire (SMQ)** *Identification of symptoms linked to stress and coping strategies that aid in the reduction of stress.* | Yes | Valid and Reliable | Comfortable for the client | Coping, stressors, behavioral theory | Adult/elderly |

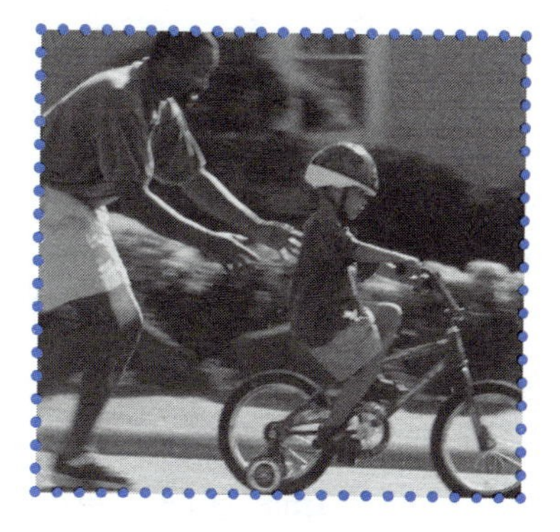

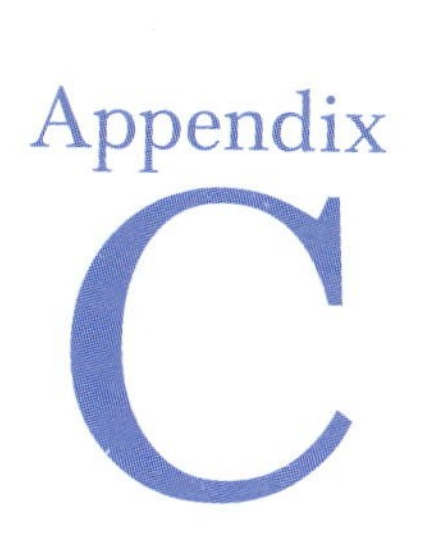

# Appendix C

# ASSESSMENTS IN PLAY AND LEISURE

# Play Assessments

| Child-Initiated Pretend Play Assessment (ChIPPA) | |
|---|---|
| **Ages** | Children 3 to 7 years of age |
| **Purpose** | Measures the quality of spontaneous pretend play (Bundy, 2005) |
| **Format/ Procedure** | Observation of play in two 15-minute sessions. Assesses three items—elaborate play actions, substitutions, and imitated actions. Involves imaginative play with typical toys and symbolic, unstructured play. Author recommends that the administrator should be professionally trained to work with children (Bundy, 2005) |
| **Psychometric Properties** | Scoring manual is unpublished. Internal consistency = not reported. Interrater reliability (involves use of videotapes): elaborate play actions 0.96 or 0.98; substitutions 1.00 or 0.97; imitated actions 0.98 to 1.00; Test-retest reliability: elaborate play actions $r = 0.73$ to $r = 0.85$; substitutions $r = 0.56$ to $r = 0.57$. Distribution of the remaining items was not normal. Content validity has been established via expert review, and play items were tested for developmental sensitivity and gender neutrality; Construct validity = not reported (Bundy, 2005). Interrater reliability also established at kappa 0.7 (Swindells & Stagnitti, 2006) |

| Children's Playfulness Scale | |
|---|---|
| **Ages** | Preschool- and toddler-aged children |
| **Purpose** | Measures the predisposition to be playful |
| **Format/ Procedure** | Twenty-three item instrument categorized into five areas of playfulness: physical spontaneity, social spontaneity, cognitive spontaneity, manifest joy, and sense of humor. Rater scored based on observations |
| **Psychometric Properties** | Interrater reliability ranged from 0.92 to 0.97; Test-retest reliability ranged from 0.84 to 0.88 at 1 month, 0.88 to 0.92 at 3 months, and 0.89 to 0.95 between the two intervals. Internal consistency for the scales ranged from 0.80 to 0.89 and 0.88 overall. Content validity based on playfulness research; Construct validity reported (Asher, 1996) |

| (Revised) Knox Preschool Play Scale (PPS-R) | |
|---|---|
| **Ages** | Children 0 to 6 years of age |
| **Purpose** | Provides child's capacity for play and some information regarding play interests. Has been used for both diagnostic purposes and as an outcome measure for intervention (Bundy, 2005) |
| **Format/ Procedure** | Observation of play inside and outside in familiar settings and with familiar toys and peers. Four dimensions of play are observed: space management, material management, imitation, and participation. Administered in two 30-minute observations (Bundy, 2005; Sturgess, 1997) |
| **Psychometric Properties** | Not standardized as administration occurs in familiar environments. Internal consistency-not reported; Interrater reliability-coefficients ranged from $r = 0.88$ to $r = 0.996$; $p = 0.0001$; Test-retest reliability-coefficients range from $r = 0.91$ to $r = 0.965$; $p = 0.0001$; Content validity has been established via an extensive review of the literature; Construct validity-not reported (Bundy, 2005; Rodger & Ziviani, 1999; Stagnitti, 2004) |

| Penn Interactive Peer Play Scale (PIPPS) | |
|---|---|
| **Ages** | Preschool and kindergarten age in disadvantaged urban areas |
| **Purpose** | Developed to assess peer play interactions in disadvantaged urban children at risk for experiencing disconnection between school and home life (Fantuzzo & Hampton, 2000) |
| **Format/ Procedure** | Parallel versions of parent and teacher rating scales, with preschool and kindergarten versions. The parent versions assess play in the home and neighborhood, and the teacher version examines play in structured and unstructured school activities. Each version is comprised of 32 items indicating the frequency the behavior is observed during free play within the preceding 2 months in three constructs: play interaction, play disruption, and play disconnection (Fantuzzo & Hampton) |
| **Psychometric Properties** | Each construct demonstrated a Cronbach alpha reliability of 0.90, 0.91, and 0.87. Inter-rater reliability of each construct was 0.84, 0.81, and 0.74. Content validity based on theoretical research. Congruence among test items was established (Fantuzzo & Hampton) |

| Play History | |
|---|---|
| **Ages** | 0 to 16 years |
| **Purpose** | Caregiver perspective of children's play; a tool for intervention planning |
| **Format/ Procedure** | Semi-structured interview administered to parents and/or caregivers; Gather information on past play experiences and actual play; Records play in five epochs—sensorimotor, symbolic, and simple constructive; dramatic; complex constructive; pre-game; and recreational. Each section is divided into four elements: materials, actions, people, and setting (Bundy, 2005; Sturgess, 1997; Taylor, Menarchek-Fetkovich, & Day, 2000) |
| **Psychometric Properties** | Test-retest reliability coefficient was 0.77 with section coefficients ranging from 0.41 to 0.78; Inter-rater reliability using videotaped interviews was 0.91 with section coefficients ranging from 0.58-0.85. Reliability was higher for typically developing children than children with disabilities (Behnke & Menarchek-Fetkovich, 1984); content validity based on theoretical research (Bundy; Taylor et al.) |

| Play in Early Childhood Education System (PIECES) | |
|---|---|
| **Ages** | Early Childhood |
| **Purpose** | To develop a standardized procedure for assessment and coding of play in preschoolers |
| **Format/ Procedure** | Still being developed |
| **Psychometric Properties** | Relatively new assessment that is still being developed and standardized. Research is limited. However, initial studies indicate reliability of the assessment. Content validity is reported by the authors secondary to development based on empirical research (Kelly-Vance & Ryalls, 2005) |

| Symbolic Play Test (SPT) | |
|---|---|
| **Ages** | Ages 1 to 3 |
| **Purpose** | Developed to assess functional play skills typically demonstrated in children between 12 and 36 months (Power & Radcliffe, 2000) |
| **Format/ Procedure** | Children are observed in several modes of play, including tactile exploration, self-orientation, and doll orientation. Four sets of toys are presented in a specific manner. Administration takes approximately 15 to 20 minutes, and raw scores are obtained and converted to a developmental age (Power & Radcliffe). Assesses symbolic play to determine whether language development relates to difficulties with symbolism or concept formation (Sturgess, 1997) |
| **Psychometric Properties** | Split-half reliability coefficients were corrected by the Spearman-Brown formula and ranged from 0.52 to 0.92. Reliability coefficients at the 15- and 18-month age levels were low (0.57 and 0.52, respectively), borderline at the 12-, 21-, and 36-month levels (0.74-0.79), and acceptable at the 24- and 30-month levels (greater than 0.90). Test-retest reliability was 0.72 at 3 months. Floor and ceiling effects affect validity. Normative data was obtained on 137 children, with much of the testing occurring on the same children. This included seven age ranges with small sample sizes within each range (Power & Radcliffe) |

| Test of Playfulness (ToP) | |
|---|---|
| **Ages** | 3 months to 15 years |
| **Purpose** | Captures the four playfulness components: intrinsic motivation, internal control, freedom from some constraints of reality, and framing (Bundy, 2005) |
| **Format/ Procedure** | 29 observational items; each item is scored 0 to 3 reflecting extent, intensity, or skill. Administered during 15 to 20 minutes of free play in a familiar environment. Author urges administration in more than one environment (Bundy); The Test of Playfulness continues to be developed and researched (Stagnitti, 2004) |
| **Psychometric Properties** | Internal consistency—Cronbach's alpha was near 1.00; Interrater reliability—Rasch model goodness of fit; Test-retest reliability is being established and is not yet published; Content validity has been established via an extensive review of the literature; Construct validity—28/29 items demonstrate acceptable goodness of fit statistics using Rasch analysis (Bundy) |

The Test of Playfulness (ToP) is not commercially available, but may be obtained by contacting the author, Anita Bundy, ScD, OTR, School of Occupation and Leisure Sciences, University of Sydney, PO Box 170, Lidcombe NSW, Australia, a.bundy@fhs.usyd.edu.au (Bundy, 2005).

| Transdisciplinary Play-Based Assessment (TPBA) 2nd Edition | |
|---|---|
| **Ages** | Children 0 to 6 years of age |
| **Purpose** | Captures the four playfulness components: intrinsic motivation, internal control, freedom from some constraints of reality, and framing (Bundy, 2005; Linder, 2000) |
| **Format/ Procedure** | 29 observational items; each item is scored 0 to 3 reflecting extent, intensity, or skill. Administered during 15 to 20 minutes of free play in a familiar environment. Author urges administration in more than one environment (Bundy; Linder) |
| **Psychometric Properties** | Internal consistency—Cronbach's alpha was near 1.00; Interrater reliability—Rasch model goodness of fit; Test-retest reliability is being established and is not yet published; Content validity has been established via an extensive review of the literature; Construct validity—28/29 items demonstrate acceptable goodness of fit statistics using Rasch analysis (Bundy; Linder) |

# Leisure Assessments

| Activity Card Sort (ACS) | |
|---|---|
| **Ages** | Adults with and without cognitive impairment |
| **Purpose** | Originally designed to identify activity level for adults with Alzheimer's Disease; has been used with different populations. Includes Healthy Older Adult version, Institutional version, and Recovering version (Connolly, Law, & MacGuire, 2005) |
| **Format/ Procedure** | 80 photo cards; caregiver or client sorts into categories. Categories vary depending upon version administered; Israeli version has been developed |
| **Psychometric Properties** | Test-retest reliability 0.897 (Baum & Edwards, 2001); Internal consistency for Israeli version: high for IADL (0.82) and cultural activities (0.80) and moderate for low physical activities (0.66) and high physical activities (0.61) (Katz, Karpin, Lak, Furman, & Hartman-Maeir, 2003). Content and construct validity reported (Connolly et al., 2005) |

| Children's Assessment of Participation and Enjoyment (CAPE) | |
|---|---|
| **Ages** | From ages 6 to 21; should be able to sort/categorize (Connolly et al., 2005) |
| **Purpose** | Identify participation in/enjoyment of daily activities |
| **Format/ Procedure** | 55 item instrument; divided into five scales: Recreational, Active Physical, Social, Skill-Based, and Self-Improvement/Educational. Can be categorized into formal and informal activities. Measures participation in five areas: diversity of activity, intensity/frequency, with whom activity occurs, where activity occurs, and enjoyment of activity. Includes two versions: self-administered and interviewer-assisted (Connolly et al.) |
| **Psychometric Properties** | Test-retest reliability ranges from 0.12 to 0.86. Internal consistency ranged from 0.32 to 0.62. Content, construct, and criterion validity are reported (Connolly et al.) |

| Interest Checklist/Activity Checklist | |
|---|---|
| **Ages** | Adolescent to adult |
| **Purpose** | Identify an individual's level of interest in leisure activities |
| **Format/ Procedure** | Original Interest Checklist included 80 items in five categories: Manual Skills, Physical Sports, Social Recreation, ADL, and Cultural/Educational (Matsutsuyu, 1969). Revised and renamed Activity Checklist contains 60 items in four categories: Sports and Physical Tasks, Intellectual and Musical Tasks, Social Tasks, and Fine Manual Tasks and Homemaking (Katz, 1988). Both are self-report instruments with level of interest rating. |
| **Psychometric Properties** | Test retest reliability at three weeks ranged from 0.84 to 0.92 for each category and 0.92 overall (Asher, 1996); internal consistency has not been reported. Testing on content validity has revealed mixed results (Connolly et al., 2005). |

| Leisure Activity Profile (LAP) | |
|---|---|
| **Ages** | Diagnosis of alcoholism |
| **Purpose** | Time use measurement of individuals with alcoholism; identifies dysfunctional patterns of leisure activities related to alcohol use (Mann & Talty, 1990) |
| **Format/ Procedure** | 38 item instrument; 19 related to alcohol consumption. Self-report or interviewer administration. Client reports time spent in activities, with whom activities occur, enjoyment, and alcohol consumption during activities |
| **Psychometric Properties** | Test retest reliability $r = 0.90$ to $r = 0.94$. Internal consistency not reported. Content and construct validity reported (Connolly et al., 2005) |

| Leisure Assessment Inventory | |
|---|---|
| **Ages** | Adults with mental retardation |
| **Purpose** | Measures leisure behavior for adults with mental retardation |
| **Format/ Procedure** | Contains four indices based upon a conceptual definition of leisure: The Leisure Activity Participation Index reflects a person's leisure repertoire and involves 50 picture-cued activity cards; the Leisure Preference and Leisure Interest Indices represent 2 different aspects of choice making to assess the perceived degree of well-being, self-worth, and self-determination experienced during leisure; and the Leisure Constraints Index measures the degree in which internal and external constraints inhibit engagement in new leisure activities. Administered using a structured, three-part interview (Hawkins, Ardovino, & Hsieh, 1998) |
| **Psychometric Properties** | Reliability: Leisure Activity Participation ($r = 0.84$, $p < 0.01$), Leisure Preference ($r = 0.53$, $p < 0.01$), Leisure Interest ($r = 0.77$, $p < 0.01$), and Leisure Constraints ($r = 0.48$, $p < 0.01$); Content validity at $p < 0.01$ for each index |

| Leisure Attitude Scale (LAS) | |
|---|---|
| **Ages** | |
| **Purpose** | To examine leisure attitude |
| **Format/ Procedure** | 36 item instrument; three subscales assessing various aspects of attitude, including cognitive, affective, and behavioral subscales; Elderly version modified from original and includes 26 items measuring desired leisure, perceived leisure, self definition through work or leisure, affinity for leisure, and society's role in leisure planning. Can be administered as an interview or questionnaire (Teaff, N. W. Ernst, & M. Ernst, 1982) |
| **Psychometric Properties** | Overall reliability 0.95; subscales reliability: Cognitive 0.89; Affective 0.90; Behavioral 0.91 (Siegenthaler & O'Dell, 2000) |

| Leisure Boredom Scale (LBS) | |
|---|---|
| **Ages** | Adolescents and young adults |
| **Purpose** | Assess perception of boredom relative to leisure opportunities |
| **Format/ Procedure** | 16-item self-report instrument rating relative to boredom |
| **Psychometric Properties** | Test-retest reliability $r = 0.73$ with 95% confidence interval; Moderate Cohen's Kappa for seven items (0.41-0.52); fair for two items (0.32-0.38); Internal consistency reported at 0.85; 0.86, 0.88; Construct validity reported (Connolly et al., 2005). |

| Leisure Competence Measure (LCM) | |
|---|---|
| **Ages** | Adults |
| **Purpose** | Evaluates changes in leisure functioning |
| **Format/ Procedure** | Service provider rating based on observation, interview, and review of records; eight subscales including Leisure Awareness, Leisure Attitude, Leisure Skills, Cultural/Social Behaviors, Interpersonal Skills, Community Integration Skills, Social Contact, and Community Participation. Takes approximately 1 hour to administer |
| **Psychometric Properties** | No test-retest reliability reported; Inter-rater reliability = 0.91 overall and 0.71-0.91 for subscales; Internal consistency—Cronbach's Alpha 0.92; Content validity reported (Connolly et al., 2005) |

| Leisure Diagnostic Battery [1] | |
|---|---|
| **Ages** | Individuals with adapted IQ of 80 and higher; mental age 12 and older; Rancho Los Amigos level of seven and higher; mild to no orientation disability (Connolly et al., 2005) |
| **Purpose** | Identify client's leisure capacity |
| **Format/ Procedure** | Comprised of four assessments: Leisure Attitude Measure (LAM), Leisure Interest Measure (LIM), Leisure Motivation Scale (LMS), and Leisure Satisfaction Measure (LSM). Leisure Attitude Measure assesses leisure attitude on cognitive, affective, and behavioral levels; Leisure Interest Measure assesses interest in eight areas: physical, outdoor, mechanical, artistic, service, social, cultural, and reading. Leisure Motivation Scale includes 48 item Full Scale and 32 item Short Scale measuring client motivation; Leisure Satisfaction Measure assesses six satisfaction subscales: psychological, educational, social, relaxation, physiological, and aesthetic. Self report instruments |
| **Psychometric Properties** | Test-retest not reported. Internal consistency: LAM: 0.89-0.94; LIM: 0.87 overall, poor internal reliability in artistic domain, acceptable in all others; LMS: Authors report strong internal reliability (Beard & Ragheb, 1983); LSM: overall reliability 0.93; Content validity reported for all four assessments; Construct validity reported for LAM and LSM; Criterion validity reported for LAM (Connolly et al.) |

| Leisure Diagnostic Battery [2] | |
|---|---|
| **Ages** | One version for youth with disabilities; one for adults |
| **Purpose** | Assess perception of freedom and barriers to participation in leisure |
| **Format/ Procedure** | 147 item Full Forms (A and C; youth and adults, respectively) related to control, competence, needs, playfulness, barriers, and knowledge. 25-item Short Form (B). Both forms are self-report instruments. |
| **Psychometric Properties** | Test retest (Form A) 0.72. Internal consistency 0.83 to 0.94 (Form A), 0.89 to 0.94 (Form B), and 0.90 to 0.96 (Form C). Content and construct validity reported for Form A (Connolly et al., 2005) |

| Leisure Satisfaction Scale (LSS) | |
|---|---|
| **Ages** | Adults |
| **Purpose** | To examine leisure satisfaction and the extent in which individuals perceive their needs are being met through participation in leisure activities |
| **Format/ Procedure** | Self report measure; Original version: 51 item instrument; six subscales assessing satisfaction, including Psychological, Educational, Social, Relaxational, Physiological, and Aesthetic subscales; Short Form: 24 item instrument; same six subscales as original version |
| **Psychometric Properties** | Test-retest reliability not reported; One study reports reliability at 0.96 (Siegenthaler & O'Dell, 2000); Internal consistency ranged from 0.86 to 0.92 for subtest and overall 0.96 (original version) and 0.93 (short form). Content validity reported (Connolly et al., 2005) |

| Preferences for Activities of Children (PAC) | |
|---|---|
| **Ages** | From ages 6 to 21; should be able to sort/categorize (Connolly et al., 2005) |
| **Purpose** | Identify activity preferences |
| **Format/ Procedure** | 55 item instrument; five activity scales: Recreational, Active Physical, Social, Skill-Based, and Self-Improvement/Educational in two domains: formal and informal activities. Can be self administered or interviewer-assisted (Connolly et al.) |
| **Psychometric Properties** | Test-retest reliability not reported; Intenal consistency ranged from 0.67 to 0.84. Content validity reported; Construct validity related to participation outcome variables ($r < 0.01$); correlations with CAPE ranged from 0.22 to 0.61 (Connolly et al.) |

# References


Asher, I. E. (1996). *Occupational therapy assessment tools: An annotated index* (2nd ed.). Bethesda, MD: AOTA Press.

Baum, C. M., & Edwards, D. (2001). *Activity card sort*. St. Louis, MO: Washington University at St. Louis.

Beard, J. G., & Ragheb, M. G. (1983). Measuring leisure motivation. *Journal of Leisure Research, 15*(3), 219-228.

Behnke, C. J., & Menarchek-Fetkovich, M. M. (1984). Examining the reliability and validity of the Play History. *American Journal of Occupational Therapy, 38*(2), 94-100.

Bundy, A. C. (2005). Measuring play performance. In M. Law, C. Baum, & W. Dunn (Eds.), *Measuring occupational performance: Supporting best practice in occupational therapy* (2nd ed., pp. 129-150). Thorofare, NJ: SLACK Incorporated.

Connolly, K., Law, M., & MacGuire, B. (2005). Measuring leisure performance. In M. Law, W. Dunn, & C. Baum (Eds.), *Measuring occupational performance: Supporting best practice in occupational therapy* (2nd ed., pp. 249-276). Thorofare, NJ: SLACK Incorporated.

Fantuzzo, J. W., & Hampton, V. R. (2000). Penn Interactive Peer Play Scale: A parent and teacher rating system for young children. In K. Gitlin-Weiner, S. Sandgrund, & C. Schaefer (Eds.), *Play diagnosis and assessment* (2nd ed., pp. 599-620). New York, NY: John Wiley & Sons.

Hawkins, B. A., Ardovino, P., & Hsieh, C. (1998). Validity and reliability of the Leisure Assessment Inventory. *Mental Retardation, 36*(4), 303-313.

Katz, N. (1988). Interest checklist: A factor analytical study. *Occupational Therapy in Mental Health, 8*(1), 45-55.

Katz, N., Karpin, H., Lak, A., Furman, T., & Hartman-Maeir, A. (2003). Participation in occupational performance: Reliability and validity of the Activity Card Sort. *Occupational Therapy Journal of Research, 23*(1), 10-17.

Kelly-Vance, L., & Ryalls, B. O. (2005). A systematic, reliable approach to play assessment in preschoolers. *School Psychology International, 26*(4), 398-412.

Linder, T. (2000). Transdisciplinary play-based assessment. In K. Gitlin-Weiner, S. Sandgrund, & C. Schaefer (Eds.), *Play diagnosis and assessment* (2nd ed., pp. 139-166). New York, NY: John Wiley & Sons.

Mann, W. C., & Talty, P. (1990). Leisure Activity Profile: Measuring use of leisure time by persons with alcoholism. *Occupational Therapy in Mental Health, 10*(4), 31-41.

Matsutsuyu, J. S. (1969). The Interest Checklist. *American Journal of Occupational Therapy, 23*, 323-328.

Power, T. J., & Radcliffe, J. (2000). Assessing the cognitive ability of infants and toddlers through play: The Symbolic Play Test. In K. Gitlin-Weiner, A. Sandgrund, & C. Schaefer (Eds.), *Play diagnosis and assessment* (2nd ed., pp. 58-79). New York, NY: John Wiley & Sons.

Rodger, S., & Ziviani, J. (1999). Play-based occupational therapy. *International Journal of Disability, Development, and Education, 46*(3), 337-365.

Siegenthaler, K. L., & O'Dell, I. (2000). Leisure attitude, leisure satisfaction, and perceived freedom in leisure within family dyads. *Leisure Sciences, 22*(4), 281-296.

Stagnitti, K. (2004). Understanding play: The implications for play assessment. *Australian Occupational Therapy Journal, 51*, 3-12.

Sturgess, J. L. (1997). Current trends in assessing children's play. *British Journal of Occupational Therapy, 60*(9), 410-414.

Swindells, D., & Stagnitti, K. (2006). Pretend play and parents' view of social competence: The construct validity of the Child-Initiated Pretend Play Assessment. *Australian Occupational Therapy Journal, 53*, 314-324.

Taylor, K. M., Menarchek-Fetkovich, M., & Day, C. (2000). The Play History interview. In K. Gitlin-Weiner, S. Sandgrund, & C. Schaefer (Eds.), *Play diagnosis and assessment* (2nd ed., pp. 114-138). New York, NY: John Wiley & Sons.

Teaff, J. D., Ernst, N. W., & Ernst, M. (1982). Elderly Leisure Attitude Scale. In D. J. Mangen & W. A. Peterson (Eds.), *Research instruments in social gerontology: Vol. 2. Social roles and social participation* (pp. 498-499; 535-537). Minneapolis, MN: University of Minnesota Press.

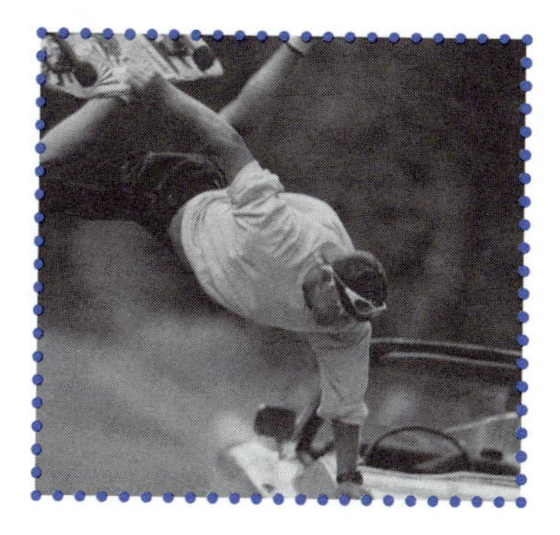

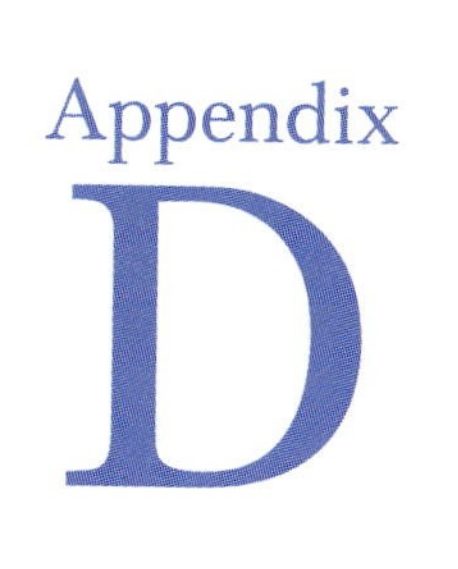

# Appendix D

# INTERVENTION PLAN OUTLINE

# Intervention Plan

Client's Name:
Age:
Date of Plan:
How long will sessions be? Where? When?:

Diagnosis:

Background information:

Precautions:

Strengths and weaknesses:

Goals and objectives:

Frame of Reference:

- Principles of the frame of reference that will be used to design intervention:
- Rationale for using frame of reference:
- Evidence to support using frame of reference with this type of client:

Sample Activity selection:

Progression of activities—how will they be graded and adapted?:

Equipment needs:

Safety concerns:

Describe the role of the occupational therapy practitioner according to the frame of reference:

Describe what is expected of the client:

Other:

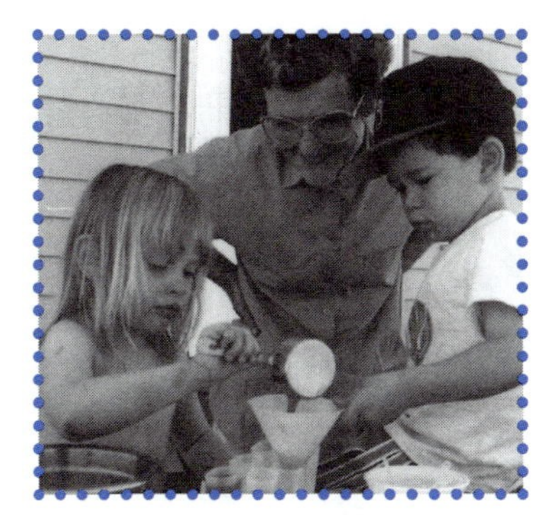

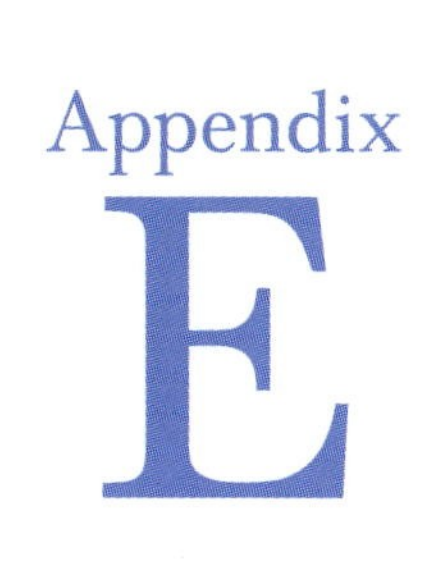

Appendix E

# Sample of an IEP

*Barbara J. Steva, MS, OTR/L*

**SAU/School/Grade or CDS Placement:** RSU #1

Date IEP Sent to Parent: 6-10-08

## INDIVIDUALIZED EDUCATION PROGRAM (IEP)

### 1. CHILD INFORMATION

Child's Name: Suzanne Phillips

Date of Birth/Age: 6/5/2001/ 6 yo

School/Grade: Towne Elementary School

Parent Information: Sharon and Robert Phillips, 21 Turner Road, Harrison, Maine, 02111

State Agency Client: Yes ☐ No ☐

Date of Meeting: 5-11-08

Effective Date of IEP: 5-12-08 to 5-11-09

Date of Annual IEP Review: 5-09

Date of Re-evaluation: 5-09

Date(s) of Amended IEP:

Case Manager: Indira Nehru

### 2. DISABILITY: (MUSER) VII.2

- ☐ Autism
- ☐ Developmental Delay (ages 3-5)
- ☐ Hearing Impairment
- ☐ Other Health Impairment
- ☐ Specific Learning Disability
- ☐ Deaf-Blindness
- ☐ Developmental Delay (Kindergarten)
- ☒ Mental Retardation
- ☐ Orthopedic Impairment
- ☐ Traumatic Brain Injury
- ☐ Deafness
- ☐ Emotional Disturbance
- ☒ Multiple Disabilities (list concomitant disabilities)
- ☐ Speech or Language Impairment
- ☐ Visual Impairment (Including Blindness)

### 3. CONSIDERATIONS

**In developing each child's IEP, the IEP Team must consider-**

**A.** The strengths of child:

Susanne is very motivated and determined. She is willing to attempt anything physically or non-physically challenged, despite her disabilities. She also has a strength in communication, whereas her speech has improved beyond what anyone could have ever imagined. She is very determined to get her message across and wants to do well in school.

**B.** The concerns of parents for enhancing the education of their child:

Suzanne's mother is concerned about the pacing of the 1st grade classroom and if Suzanne will keep up. She is an advocate for Suzanne's independence in and out of school.

**C.** Results of the initial evaluation or most recent evaluation of the child:
Suzanne's 3-year review is due in the Spring 2009. Suzanne participated in the end-of-the-year Kindergarten test, including the Phonological Awareness Skills Test (PAST), Letter identification, and number reasoning.

**D.** Academic, developmental, and functional needs of the child:
Suzanne requires redirection in order to maintain her focus on the task and to have directions repeated as she may not have caught them the first time. She also requires the use of a slant board to help keep the task in her line of vision, as well as assistance maneuvering around some school facilities such as tight quarters or unfamiliar surroundings, uneven terrain, or around new furniture. Suzanne has a visual impairment, although it has not been determined as to how severe the impairment is at this time.

Suzanne demonstrates the need for improvements in academic, developmental, and functional areas. These have been addressed in the goals of this plan.

## Consideration of Special Factors: The IEP team must-

**E.** In the case of a child whose behavior impedes the child's learning or that of others, consider the use of positive behavioral interventions and supports and other strategies to address the behavior:

Check if not needed ☒ **If needed, indicate where it is addressed in the IEP.**

**F.** In the case of a child with limited English proficiency, consider the language needs of the child as those needs relate to the child's IEP

Check if not needed ☒ **If needed, indicate where the need is addressed in the IEP.**

**G.** In the case of a child who is blind or visually impaired, provide for instruction in Braille and the use of Braille unless the IEP Team determines, after an evaluation of the child's reading and writing skills, needs, and appropriate reading and writing media (including an evaluation of the child's future needs for instruction in Braille or the use of Braille), that instruction in Braille or the use of Braille is not appropriate for the child.

Check if not needed ☒ **If needed, indicate where the need is addressed in the IEP.**

**H.** Consider the communication needs of the child, and in the case of a child who is deaf or hard of hearing, consider the child's language and communication needs, opportunities for direct communication with peers and professional personnel in the child's language and communication mode, academic level, and full range of needs including opportunities for direct instruction in the child's language and communication mode.

Check if not needed ☐ **If needed, indicate where the need is addressed in the IEP.** Experiences communication needs—will be met through the goals in Section 9, 10, and 11 of this document.

**I.** Consider whether the child needs assistive technology devices and services.

Check if not needed ☐ **If needed, indicate where the need is addressed in the IEP.** At this time, Suzanne does not qualify for the use of assistive technology due to her cognitive ability. This is something the team will have to reconsider in the future.

## 4. PRESENT LEVEL OF ACADEMIC AND FUNCTIONAL PERFORMANCE

A statement of Present levels of academic achievement and functional performance:
*Math: Suzanne can currently count to 83, read random numbers up to 10, generate an ABAB pattern, and consistently recognize the penny.
*Reading: Suzanne can identify all 26 uppercase letters, 22 lowercase letters, and 22 sounds, give 24 corresponding words beginning with letters, and say whether two words rhyme.
*Writing: Suzanne can write most of the letters in her first name consistently, but her vision and fine motor skills impact the legibility.
*Suzanne moves at a much slower pace physically. It is unknown at this time how much Suzanne is able to see or how well, therefore impacting her stability and movement around the school.

*Occupational Therapy: Suzanne demonstrates mild difficulty coordinating both sides of her body to perform gross and fine motor tasks. Her diminished visual abilities also impact her success in these areas. Suzanne is writing 4/5 letters of her first name independently, but continues to struggle with spatial placement of these.
*Speech and Language Therapy: Suzanne demonstrates low tone in her lips and tongue, which affects articulation, mastication, and a sustained closed mouth posture at rest. She incorrectly articulates /th, r, r-blends/. Jaw instability impacts mastication. Velopharyngeal insufficiency affects resonance. Suzanne correctly uses pronouns, copulas, and helping verbs "am/is/are," WH-questions, interrogative reversal question forms, and regular plural in conversation.
*Physical Therapy: Suzanne currently loses her balance when walking on uneven terrain and has difficulty with single-leg balance activities, poor gait mechanics and safety, and decreased lower extremity core strength and lower extremity flexibility.

How the child's disability affects the child's involvement and progress in the general education curriculum, or for preschool children, as appropriate, how the disability affects the child's participation in appropriate activities:

All of the above academic, social, and developmental areas give us knowledge that Suzanne would have a difficult time with grade-level curriculum work

## 5. ANNUAL GOAL(S)

Measurable annual goals including academic and functional goals designed to meet the child's needs that result from the child's disability to enable the child to be involved in and make progress in the general education curriculum; and meet each of the child's other educational needs that result from the child's disability and how the child's progress toward meeting the annual goals will be measured.
*(For children in grades 9-12 the IEP shall reflect the individual goals to successfully meet the content standards of the system of Learning Results in addition to any other diploma requirements applicable to all secondary school children*

| Measurable Annual Goal | How Goal will be Measured | **PROGRESS 11/08 | 1/09 | 4/09 | 6/09 |
|---|---|---|---|---|---|
| 1. By 5/11/09, given specially designed instruction in appropriate behavior skills, Suzanne will follow directions the first time asked, and take care of herself 80% (20%, 40%, 60%) of the time | 1-4. observation, daily work and informal assessments | 1. **2** | | | |
| 2. By 5/10/09, given specially designed math instruction, Suzanne will count by 5's and 10's, will read and write numbers up to 20, will name all 4 coins and their values, and will tell time to the hour 80% of the time | | 2. **2** | | | |
| 3. By 5/10/09, given specially designed instruction in reading, Suzanne will increase reading readiness skills by being able to produce rhymes and work with phonemes 80% (20%, 40%, 60%) of the time | | 3. **1** | | | |
| 4. By 5/10/09, given specially designed instruction in writing, Suzanne will be able to write her first and last name and form all 26 uppercase letters 80% (20%, 40%, 60%) of the time | | 4. **2** | | | |
| 5. Given direct occupational therapy intervention and consultation to staff, Suzanne will demonstrate improved fine motor manipulation to within one year of her developmental age by 5/09 | 5-6. clinical data collection, observation, informal assessment, and work samples | 5. **2** | | | |
| 6. Given direct occupational therapy intervention, Suzanne will demonstrate improved bilateral hand skills and visual motor skills to within one year of her chronological age by 5/09 | | 6. **2** | | | |
| 7. Suzanne will improve her range of motion, balance, coordination, gross motor skills, gait mechanics, and safety awareness in order to fully participate in her academic program at her highest functional level as measured by physical therapy observation quarterly by 5/09 | 7. Physical therapist observation | 7. **2** | | | |

| | | |
|---|---|---|
| 8. By 5/10/2009, Suzanne will engage in appropriate group activities (play, academics, classroom, discussion, etc) 80% of the time | 8. daily data collection | 8. **1** |
| 9. Given a variety of oral motor exercises, Suzanne will demonstrate improved oral motor strength, respiration, and resonance on 80% of measures by 5/09 | 9-11. clinical data collection and informal assessment | 9. **2** |
| 10. Given a variety of therapeutic activities, Suzanne's expressive language skills will improve. She will use verbs with regular and irregular past tense, simple future verb tense, prepositional phrases, and complex sentences with early developing conjunctions in conversation on 4 out of 5 measures by 5/09 | | 10. **2** |
| 11. Suzanne will correctly articulate /r/ in all positions of words, words with initial /r-blends/, and /th/ in the initial position of words in conversational speech on 80% of measures by 5/09 | | 11. **2** |

**1 = Goal Met** **2 = Adequate Progress** **3 = Limited Progress** **4 = No Progress** **5 = Not Started**

Include a statement to parents of when periodic reports on the progress their child is making toward meeting the annual goals below.

Parents will receive a copy of this IEP showing their child's progress in meeting her goals on a quarterly basis to correspond with the issuance of report cards.

## 6. SHORT-TERM OBJECTIVES

Only for children with disabilities who take alternate assessments aligned to alternate achievement standards, a description of benchmarks or short-term objectives:

**SHORT TERM OBJECTIVES**

Given.... Child will.... As measured by.... By when....

| | 11/08 | 1/09 | 4/09 | 6/09 |
|---|---|---|---|---|
| 1a. By 5/11/09, given specially designed instruction in appropriate behavior skills, Suzanne will follow directions the first time asked 80% (20%, 40%, 60%) of the time as measured by daily data collection. | 1a. **1** | | | |
| 1b. By 5/11/09, given specially designed instruction in appropriate behavior skills, Suzanne will take care of herself 80% (20%, 40%, 60%) of the time as measured by daily data collection | 1b. **2** | | | |
| 2a. Given specially designed instruction in math, Suzanne will count by 5's and 10's 80% (20%, 40%, 60%) of the time as measured by daily work and informal assessments | 2a. **2** | | | |
| 2b. Given specially designed instruction in math, Suzanne will read numbers up to twenty 80% (20%, 40%, 60%) of the time as measured by daily work and informal assessments | 2b. **2** | | | |
| 2c. Given specially designed instruction in math, Suzanne will identify and give the value to all 4 coins 80% (20%, 40%, 60%) of the time as measured by daily work and informal assessments | 2c. **2** | | | |
| 3a. By 5/10/09, given specially designed instruction in reading, Suzanne will produce rhymes 80% (20%, 40%, 60%) of the time as measured by daily work and informal assessments | 3a. **1** | | | |
| 3b. By 5/10/09, given specially designed instruction in reading, Suzanne will isolate ending sounds 80% (20%, 40%, 60%) of the time as measured by daily work and informal assessments | 3b. **1** | | | |
| 4a. By 5/10/09, given specially designed instruction in writing, Suzanne will be able to write her first and last name 80% (20%, 40%, 60%) of the time as measured by daily work and informal assessments | 4a. **2** | | | |

| | |
|---|---|
| 5a. Given therapeutic activities to strengthen the intrinsic muscles of the hands, Suzanne will demonstrate adequate hand strength to maintain a 3- or 4-finger pencil grip with thumb opposed and web space open when writing or coloring for 30 seconds (11/08), 45 seconds (1/09), 1 minute (4/09), and 1½ minutes (5/09) 80% of trials | 5a. **1** |
| 5b. Given therapeutic activities to strengthen intrinsic hand muscles, Suzanne will demonstrate improved muscle control as seen by the ability to maintain her pencil within a ½-inch straight line (11/08), ½-inch curved line (1/09), ¼-inch curved line (4/09), and ¼-inch zigzag line (5/09) with no more than 1 deviation along a 10-inch length 80% of trials | 5b. **2** |
| 6a. Given direct occupational therapy intervention, Suzanne will demonstrate improved visual motor skills as seen by the ability to spontaneously form 6/26 (11/08), 13/26 (1/09), 19/26 (4/09), and 26/26 (5/09) uppercase letters, and numbers 1-20 (5/09) 80% of trials | 6a. **1** |
| 6b. Given direct occupational therapy and consultation to staff, Suzanne will spontaneously form a square (11/08), triangle (1/09), and diamond (4/09) 80% of trials | 6b. **1** |
| 6c. Given direct occupational therapy intervention, Suzanne will demonstrate improved bilateral hand skills and visual motor skills as seen by the ability to cut a 6-inch circle (11/08), 4-inch triangle (1/09), and 10-inch zigzag line (4/09) along a ¼-inch guideline 80% with no more than two deviations from the line | 6c. **1** |
| 7a. Suzanne will improve her balance and gait mechanics/safety by the ability to completely step over four 2-inch objects 3/5 trials by 11/08, four 4-inch objects 3/5 trials by 1/09, four 4-inch objects 5/5 trials by 4/09, and six 4-inch objects 5/5 trials by 5/09 | 7a. **1** |
| 7b. Demonstrate bilateral UE coordination and hand/eye coordination through the ability to catch a tennis ball with hands only thrown from 5 feet away 3/5 trials by 11/08, thrown from 5 feet away 5/5 trials by 1/09, thrown from 10 feet away 3/5 trials by 4/09, and thrown from 10 feet away 5/5 trials by 5/09 | 7b. **2** |
| 7c. Suzanne will maintain proper speed and safety with gait in the school and on the playground by the ability to keep her eyes/head up and in an upright posture with minimal cuing | 7c. **4** |
| 8a. By 5/11/09, given a group setting, Suzanne will make remarks relevant to the topic of conversation 80% (20%, 40%, 60%) of the time as measured by daily data collection | 8a. **1** |
| 8b. By 5/11/09, given direct instruction, Suzanne will ask permission when wanting to give or receive physical contact (e.g., hug) 80% (20%, 40%, 60%) of the time as measured by daily data collection | 8b. **1** |
| 9a. Given a straw hierarchy to improve labial, strength Suzanne will drink 1/4 cup of honey-thick liquids through a medium-diameter straw 4/5 trials by 11/08, drink ½ cup of honey-thick liquids through a narrow-diameter straw 4/5 trials by 1/09, drink ¼ cup of pudding-thick liquids through a medium-diameter straw by 4/5 trials 04/09, and drink ½ cup of pudding-thick liquids through a narrow-diameter straw by 4/5 trials 05/09 | 9a. **2** |
| 10a. Given a model, Suzanne will produce verbs with irregular past tense form in simple sentences on 4/5 measures by 11/08 | 10a. **2** |
| 10b. Given a model, Suzanne will produce sentences using prepositional phrases on 4/5 measures by 1/09 | 10b. **2** |
| 10c. Given a model, Suzanne will produce complex sentences using the conjunctions "because, if, when" on 4/5 measures by 4/09 | 10c. **3** |
| 11a. Given visual cues and a model , Suzanne will correctly articulate /r/ in all positions of words on 80% of measures in 3 consecutive sessions at the spontaneous word level by 11/08, at the phrase level by 1/09, at the sentence level by 4/09, and in conversation by 5/09 | 11a. **1** |

| | |
|---|---|
| 11b. Given visual cues and a model, Suzanne will correctly articulate /r-blends/ in the initial position of words on 80% of measures in 3 consecutive sessions at the spontaneous word level by 1/09, at the sentence level by 4/09, and in conversation by 5/09 | 11b. **1** |
| 11c. Given visual cues and a model, Suzanne will correctly articulate /th/ in the initial position of words on 80% of measures in 3 consecutive sessions at the imitative word level by 11/08, at the spontaneous word level by 1/09, at the sentence level by 4/09, and in conversation by 5/09 | 11c. **2** |

**1 = Objective Met** **2 = Adequate Progress** **3 = Objective Not Taught** **4 = Inadequate Progress**

## 7. SPECIAL EDUCATION AND RELATED SERVICES

| Special Education Services | Position Responsible | Location | Frequency | Duration<br>Beginning/Ending Date |
|---|---|---|---|---|
| Specially Designed Instruction | Special Education Teacher | Special Education Setting | 5 hours daily | 5/12/08 to 6/15/08<br>9/01/08 to 5/11/09 |
| Consultation | | | | |
| Tutorial Services | | | | |
| Extended School Year Services | Special Education Teacher | Special Education Setting | 6 hours weekly | 7/07/08 to 8/08/08 |
| Other | | | | |
| | | | | |

| Related Services | Position Responsible | Location | Frequency | Duration<br>Beginning/Ending Date |
|---|---|---|---|---|
| Speech and Language Services | Speech Pathologist | Special Education Setting | 60 minutes weekly<br><br>30 minutes weekly (ESY) | 5/12/08 to 6/15/08<br>9/01/08 to 5/11/09<br>7/07/08 to 08/08/08 (ESY) |
| Occupational Therapy | Occupational Therapist | Special Education Setting | 60 minutes weekly<br><br>30 minutes weekly (ESY) | 5/12/08 to 6/15/08<br>9/01/08 to 5/11/09<br>7/07/08 to 08/08/08 (ESY) |
| Physical Therapy | Physical Therapist | Special Education Setting | 60 minutes weekly<br><br>30 minutes weekly (ESY) | 5/12/08 to 6/15/08<br>9/01/08 to 5/11/09<br>7/07/08 to 08/08/08 (ESY) |
| Social Work Services | | | | |
| Transportation | | | | |
| Other | | | | |

**8. Supplementary aids and services, based on peer-reviewed research to the extent practicable, to be provided to the child or on behalf of the child and a statement of program modifications or supports for SAU personnel will be provided to enable the child to advance toward attaining the goals, to be involved in and make progress in the general education curriculum and to participate in extracurricular and other nonacademic activities, and to be educated and participate with other children with disabilities and nondisabled children in activities.**

| Supplementary aids, services, modifications, and or supports for SAU personnel. | Position Responsible | Location | Frequency | Duration Beginning /Ending date |
|---|---|---|---|---|

| | | | | |
|---|---|---|---|---|
| Educational Technician | Regular Education Teacher | Regular Education settings | For all social and nonacademic activities | 5/12/08 to 6/15/08<br>9/01/08 to 5/11/09 |
| Educational Technician | Special Education Teacher | Special Education setting | For all math/number activities | 5/12/08 to 6/15/08<br>9/01/08 to 5/11/09 |
| Slant Board | Special Education Teacher | Regular and Special Education settings | For all writing activities | 5/12/08 to 6/15/08<br>9/01/08 to 5/11/09<br>7/07/08 to 08/08/08 (ESY) |

## 9. LEAST RESTRICTIVE ENVIRONMENT

An explanation of the extent, if any, to which the child will not participate with nondisabled children in the regular class and in extracurricular and other nonacademic activities:
Because of the need for individual and small group instruction and compensatory techniques at a slower pace, the intensity and variety of services required preclude the delivery of all educational services in the regular education classroom. Any nonacademic activities can be offered in the same manner for all students with special education support.

## 10. STATE AND DISTRICT WIDE ASSESSMENTS

A statement of any individual appropriate accommodations that are necessary to measure the academic achievement and functional performance of the child on State and district wide assessments:
N/A

If the IEP Team determines that the child shall take an alternate assessment on a particular state- or district-wide assessment of child achievement, a statement of why the child cannot participate in the regular assessment and why the particular assessment selected is appropriate for the child:
N/A

*If this child's IEP does not require Section 11, Secondary Transition and Section 12, Age of Majority, this will be the last page of the IEP.*

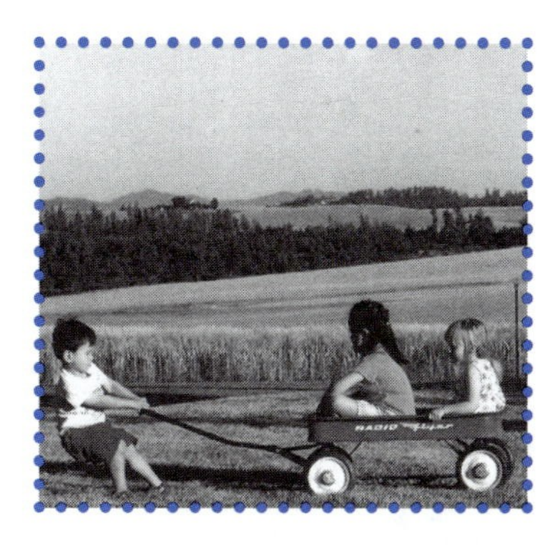

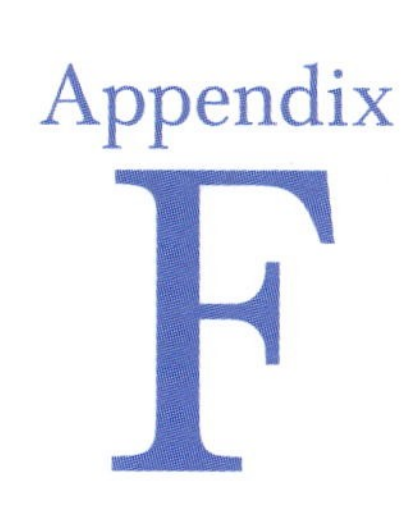

Appendix F

# AOTA's Code of Ethics

*Reproduced with permission from the American Occupational Therapy Association.*

## OCCUPATIONAL THERAPY CODE OF ETHICS (2005)

### PREAMBLE

The American Occupational Therapy Association (AOTA) *Occupational Therapy Code of Ethics* (2005) is a public statement of principles used to promote and maintain high standards of conduct within the profession and is supported by the *Core Values and Attitudes of Occupational Therapy Practice* American Occupational Therapy Association (AOTA, 1993). Members of AOTA are committed to promoting inclusion, diversity, independence, and safety for all recipients in various stages of life, health, and illness and to empower all beneficiaries of occupational therapy. This commitment extends beyond service recipients to include professional colleagues, students, educators, businesses, and the community.

Fundamental to the mission of the occupational therapy profession is the therapeutic use of everyday life activities (occupations) with individuals or groups for the purpose of participation in roles and situations in home, school, workplace, community, and other settings. "Occupational therapy addresses the physical, cognitive, psychosocial, sensory and other aspects of performance in a variety of contexts to support engagement in everyday life activities that affect health, well being and quality of life" (*Definition of Occupational Therapy Practice for the AOTA Model Practice Act*, 2004). Occupational therapy personnel have an ethical responsibility first and foremost to recipients of service as well as to society.

The historical foundation of this Code is based on ethical reasoning surrounding practice and professional issues, as well as empathic reflection regarding these interactions with others. This reflection resulted in the establishment of principles that guide ethical action. Ethical action goes beyond rote following of rules or application of principles; rather it is a manifestation of moral character and mindful reflection. It is a commitment to beneficence for the sake of others, to virtuous practice of artistry and science, to genuinely good behaviors, and to noble acts of courage. It is an empathic way of being among others, which is made every day by all occupational therapy personnel.

The AOTA *Occupational Therapy Code of Ethics* (*2005*) is an aspirational guide to professional conduct when ethical issues surface. Ethical decision making is a process that includes awareness regarding how the outcome will impact occupational therapy clients in all spheres. Applications of Code principles are considered situation-specific and where a conflict exists, occupational therapy personnel will pursue responsible efforts for resolution.

The specific purpose of the AOTA *Occupational Therapy Code of Ethics* (*2005*) is to:

1. Identify and describe the principles supported by the occupational therapy profession

2. Educate the general public and members regarding established principles to which occupational therapy personnel are accountable
3. Socialize occupational therapy personnel new to the practice to expected standards of conduct
4. Assist occupational therapy personnel in recognition and resolution of ethical dilemmas

The AOTA *Occupational Therapy Code of Ethics* (*2005*) defines the set principles that apply to occupational therapy personnel at all levels:

**Principle 1. Occupational therapy personnel shall demonstrate a concern for the safety and well-being of the recipients of their services. (BENEFICENCE)**
**Occupational therapy personnel shall:**

**A.** Provide services in a fair and equitable manner. They shall recognize and appreciate the cultural components of economics, geography, race, ethnicity, religious and political factors, marital status, age, sexual orientation, gender identity, and disability of all recipients of their services.

**B.** Strive to ensure that fees are fair and reasonable and commensurate with services performed. When occupational therapy practitioners set fees, they shall set fees considering institutional, local, state, and federal requirements, and with due regard for the service recipient's ability to pay.

**C.** Make every effort to advocate for recipients to obtain needed services through available means.

**D.** Recognize the responsibility to promote public health and the safety and well-being of individuals, groups, and/or communities.

**Principle 2. Occupational therapy personnel shall take measures to ensure a recipient's safety and avoid imposing or inflicting harm. (NONMALEFICENCE)**
**Occupational therapy personnel shall:**

**A.** Maintain therapeutic relationships that shall not exploit the recipient of services sexually, physically, emotionally, psychologically, financially, socially, or in any other manner.

**B.** Avoid relationships or activities that conflict or interfere with therapeutic professional judgment and objectivity.

**C.** Refrain from any undue influences that may compromise provision of service.

**D.** Exercise professional judgment and critically analyze directives that could result in potential harm before implementation.

**E.** Identify and address personal problems that may adversely impact professional judgment and duties.

**F.** Bring concerns regarding impairment of professional skills of a colleague to the attention of the appropriate authority when or/if attempts to address concerns are unsuccessful.

**Principle 3. Occupational therapy personnel shall respect recipients to assure their rights. (AUTONOMY, CONFIDENTIALITY)**
**Occupational therapy personnel shall:**

**A.** Collaborate with recipients, and if they desire, families, significant others, and/or caregivers in setting goals and priorities throughout the intervention process, including full disclosure of the nature, risk, and potential outcomes of any interventions.

**B.** Obtain informed consent from participants involved in research activities and ensure that they understand potential risks and outcomes.

**C.** Respect the individual's right to refuse professional services or involvement in research or educational activities.

**D.** Protect all privileged confidential forms of written, verbal, and electronic communication gained from educational, practice, research, and investigational activities unless otherwise mandated by local, state, or federal regulations.

**Principle 4. Occupational therapy personnel shall achieve and continually maintain high standards of competence. (DUTY).**
**Occupational therapy personnel shall:**

**A.** Hold the appropriate national, state, or any other requisite credentials for the services they provide.

**B.** Conform to AOTA standards of practice, and official documents.

**C.** Take responsibility for maintaining and documenting competence in practice, education, and research by participating in professional development and educational activities.

**D.** Be competent in all topic areas in which they provide instruction to consumers, peers, and/or students.

**E.** Critically examine available evidence so they may perform their duties on the basis of current information.

**F.** Protect service recipients by ensuring that duties assumed by or assigned to other occupational therapy personnel match credentials, qualifications, experience, and scope of practice.

**G.** Provide appropriate supervision to individuals for whom they have supervisory responsibility in accordance with Association official documents, local, state, and federal or national laws and regulations, and institutional policies and procedures.

**H.** Refer to or consult with other service providers whenever such a referral or consultation would be helpful to the care of the recipient of service. The referral or consultation process shall be done in collaboration with the recipient of service.

**Principle 5. Occupational therapy personnel shall comply with laws and Association policies guiding the profession of occupational therapy. (PROCEDURAL JUSTICE) Occupational therapy personnel shall:**

A. Familiarize themselves with and seek to understand and abide by institutional rules, applicable Association policies; local, state, and federal/national/international laws.

**B.** Be familiar with revisions in those laws and Association policies that apply to the profession of occupational therapy and shall inform employers, employees, and colleagues of those changes.

**C.** Encourage those they supervise in occupational therapy-related activities to adhere to the Code.

**D.** Take reasonable steps to ensure employers are aware of occupational therapy's ethical obligations, as set forth in this Code, and of the implications of those obligations for occupational therapy practice, education, and research.

**E.** Record and report in an accurate and timely manner all information related to professional activities.

**Principle 6. Occupational therapy personnel shall provide accurate information when representing the profession. (VERACITY)**

**Occupational therapy personnel shall:**

**A.** Represent their credentials, qualifications, education, experience, training, and competence accurately. This is of particular importance for those to whom occupational therapy personnel provide their services or with whom occupational therapy personnel have a professional relationship.

**B.** Disclose any professional, personal, financial, business, or volunteer affiliations that may pose a conflict of interest to those with whom they may establish a professional, contractual, or other working relationship.

**C.** Refrain from using or participating in the use of any form of communication that contains false, fraudulent, deceptive, or unfair statements or claims.

**D.** Identify and fully disclose to all appropriate persons errors that compromise recipients' safety.

**E.** Accept responsibility for their professional actions that reduce the public's trust in occupational therapy services and those that perform those services.

**Principle 7. Occupational therapy personnel shall treat colleagues and other professionals with respect, fairness, discretion, and integrity. (FIDELITY)**

**Occupational therapy personnel shall:**

**A.** Preserve, respect, and safeguard confidential information about colleagues and staff, unless otherwise mandated by national, state, or local laws.

**B.** Accurately represent the qualifications, views, contributions, and findings of colleagues.

**C.** Take adequate measures to discourage, prevent, expose, and correct any breaches of the Code and report any breaches of the Code to the appropriate authority.

**D.** Avoid conflicts of interest and conflicts of commitment in employment and volunteer roles.

**E.** Use conflict resolution and/or alternative dispute resolution resources to resolve organizational and interpersonal conflicts.

**F.** Familiarize themselves with established policies and procedures for handling concerns about this Code, including familiarity with national, state, local, district, and territorial procedures for handling ethics complaints. These include policies and procedures created by AOTA, licensing and regulatory bodies, employers, agencies, certification boards, and other organizations having jurisdiction over occupational therapy practice.

*Note*. This *AOTA Occupational Therapy Code of Ethics* is one of three documents that constitute the *Ethics Standards*. The other two are the *Core Values and Attitudes of Occupational Therapy Practice* (1993) and the *Guidelines to the Occupational Therapy Code of Ethics* (2000).

## Glossary

**Autonomy**—The right of an individual to self-determination. The ability to independently act on one's decisions for their own well-being (Beauchamp & Childress, 2001)

**Beneficence**—Doing good for others or bringing about good for them. The duty to confer benefits to others

**Confidentiality**—Not disclosing data or information that should be kept private to prevent harm and to abide by policies, regulations, and laws

**Dilemma**—A situation in which one moral conviction or right action conflicts with another. It exists because there is no one, clear-cut, right answer

**Duty**—Actions required of professionals by society or actions that are self-imposed

**Ethics**—A systematic study of morality (i.e., rules of conduct that are grounded in philosophical principles and theory)

**Fidelity**—Faithfully fulfilling vows and promises, agreements, and discharging fiduciary responsibilities (Beauchamp & Childress, 2001)

**Justice**—Three types of justice are

Compensatory—Making reparation for wrongs that have been done

Distributive justice—The act of distributing goods and burdens among members of society

Procedural justice—Assuring that processes are organized in a fair manner and policies or laws are followed

**Morality**—Personal beliefs regarding values, rules, and principles of what is right or wrong. Morality may be culture-based or culture-driven

**Nonmaleficence**—Not harming or causing harm to be done to oneself or others the duty to ensure that no harm is done

**Veracity**—A duty to tell the truth; avoid deception

### References

American Occupational Therapy Association. (1993). Core values and attitudes of occupational therapy practice. *American Journal of Occupational Therapy, 47*, 1085–1086.

American Occupational Therapy Association. (1998). Guidelines to the occupational therapy code of ethics. *American Journal of Occupational Therapy, 52*, 881–884.

American Occupational Therapy Association. (2004). Association policies. *American Journal of Occupational Therapy, 58*, 694–695.

Beauchamp, T. L., & Childress, J. F. (2001). *Principles of biomedical ethics* (5th ed.). New York: Oxford University Press.

*Definition of Occupational Therapy Practice for the AOTA Model Practice Act* (2004). Retrieved April 9, 2005, from http://www.aota.org/members/area4/docs/defotpractice.pdf

### Authors

The Commission on Standards and Ethics (SEC):
S. Maggie Reitz, PhD, OTR/L, FAOTA, Chairperson
Melba Arnold, MS, OTR/L
Linda Gabriel Franck, PhD, OTR/L
Darryl J. Austin, MS, OT/L
Diane Hill, COTA/L, AP, ROH
Lorie J. McQuade, MEd, CRC
Daryl K. Knox, MD
Deborah Yarett Slater, MS, OT/L, FAOTA, Staff Liaison
With contributions to the Preamble by Suzanne Peloquin, PhD, OTR, FAOTA

Adopted by the Representative Assembly 2005C202

*Note*. This document replaces the 2000 document, *Occupational Therapy Code of Ethics (2000) (American Journal of Occupational Therapy, 54*, 614–616).

Prepared 4/7/2000, revised draft—January 2005, second revision 4/2005 by SEC.

American Occupational Therapy Association. (2005). Occupational therapy code of ethics (2005). *American Journal of Occupational Therapy, 59*, 639–642

| **Guidelines to the *Occupational Therapy Code of Ethics (2005)*** | |
|---|---|
| **Professional Behaviors** | **Principles From Code** |
| **1. Honesty:** ***Professionals must be honest with themselves, must be honest with all whom they come in contact with, and must know their strengths and limitations.*** | |
| **1.1.** In education, research, practice, and leadership roles, individuals must be honest in receiving and disseminating information by providing opportunities for informed consent and for discussion of available options. | Veracity |
| **1.2.** Occupational therapy practitioners must be certain that informed consent has been obtained prior to the initiation of services, including evaluation. If the service recipient cannot give informed consent, the practitioner must be sure that consent has been obtained from the person who is legally responsible for the service recipient. | Autonomy, Veracity |
| **1.3.** Occupational therapy practitioners must be truthful about their individual competencies as well as the competence of those under their supervision. In some cases the therapist may need to refer the client to another professional to assure that the most appropriate services are provided. | Duty, Veracity |
| **1.4.** Referrals to other health care specialists shall be based exclusively on the other provider's competence and ability to provide the needed service. | Beneficence |
| **1.5.** All documentation must accurately reflect the nature and quantity of services provided. | Veracity |
| **1.6.** Occupational therapy practitioners terminate services when they do not meet the needs and goals of the recipient or when services no longer produce a measurable outcome. | Procedural Justice, Beneficence |
| **1.7.** All marketing and advertising must be truthful and carefully presented to avoid misleading the client or the public. | Veracity |
| **1.8.** All occupational therapy personnel shall accurately represent their credentials and roles. | Veracity |
| **1.9.** Occupational therapy personnel shall not use funds for unintended purposes or misappropriate funds. | Duty, Veracity |
| **2. Communication:** *Communication is important in all aspects of occupational therapy. Individuals must be conscientious and truthful in all facets of written, verbal, and electronic communication.* | |
| **2.1.** Occupational therapy personnel do not make deceptive, fraudulent, or misleading statements about the nature of the services they provide or the outcomes that can be expected. | Veracity |

| | |
|---|---|
| **2.2.** Professional contracts for occupational therapy services shall explicitly describe the type and duration of services as well as the duties and responsibilities of all involved parties. | Veracity, Procedural Justice |
| **2.3.** Documentation for reimbursement purposes shall be done in accordance with applicable laws, guidelines, and regulations. | Veracity, Procedural Justice |
| **2.4.** Documentation shall accurately reflect the services delivered and the outcomes. It shall be of the kind and quality that satisfies the scrutiny of peer reviews, legal proceedings, payers, regulatory bodies, and accrediting agencies. | Veracity, Procedural Justice, Duties |
| **2.5.** Occupational therapy personnel must be honest in gathering and giving fact-based information regarding job performance and fieldwork performance. Information given shall be timely and truthful, accurate, and respectful of all parties involved. | Veracity, Fidelity |
| **2.6.** Documentation for supervisory purposes shall accurately reflect the factual components of the interactions and the expected outcomes. | Veracity |
| **2.7.** Occupational therapy personnel must give credit and recognition when using the work of others. | Veracity Procedural Justice |
| **2.8.** Occupational therapy personnel do not fabricate data, falsify information, or plagiarize. | Veracity Procedural Justice |
| **2.9.** Occupational therapy personnel refrain from using biased or derogatory language in written, verbal, and electronic communication about clients, students, research participants, and colleagues. | Nonmaleficence, Fidelity |
| **2.10.** Occupational therapy personnel who provide information through oral and written means shall emphasize that ethical and appropriate service delivery for clients cannot be done without proper individualized evaluations and plans of care. | Beneficence |
| **3. Ensuring the Common Good:** *Occupational therapy personnel are expected to increase awareness of the profession's social responsibilities to help ensure the common good.* | |
| **3.1.** Occupational therapy personnel take steps to make sure that employers are aware of the ethical principles of the profession and occupational therapy personnel's obligation to adhere to those ethical principles. | Duty |
| **3.2.** Occupational therapy personnel shall be diligent stewards of human, financial, and material resources of their employers. They shall refrain from exploiting these resources for personal gain. | Fidelity |
| **3.3.** Occupational therapy personnel should actively work with their employer to prevent discrimination and unfair labor practices. They should also advocate for employees with disabilities to ensure the provision of reasonable accommodations. | Procedural Justice |

| | |
|---|---|
| **3.4.** Occupational therapy personnel should actively participate with their employer in the formulation of policies and procedures. They should do this to ensure that these policies and procedures are legal, in accordance with regulations governing aspects of practice, and consistent with the AOTA *Occupational Therapy Code of Ethics.* | Procedural Justice |
| **3.5.** Occupational therapy personnel in educational settings are responsible for promoting ethical conduct by students, faculty, and fieldwork colleagues. | Duty, Fidelity |
| **3.6.** Occupational therapy personnel involved in or preparing to be involved in research, including education and policy research, need to obtain all necessary approvals prior to initiating research. | Procedural Justice |
| **4. Competence:** *Occupational therapy personnel are expected to work within their areas of competence and to pursue opportunities to update, increase, and expand their competence.* | |
| **4.1.** Occupational therapy personnel developing new areas of competence (skills, techniques, approaches) must engage in appropriate study and training, under appropriate supervision, before incorporating new areas into their practice. | Duty |
| **4.2.** When generally recognized standards do not exist in emerging areas of practice, occupational therapy personnel must take responsible steps to ensure their own competence. | Duty |
| **4.3.** Occupational therapy personnel shall develop an understanding and appreciation for different cultures in order to be able to provide culturally competent service. Culturally competent practitioners are aware of how service delivery can be affected by economic, age, ethnic, racial, geographic, gender, gender identity, religious, and political factors, as well as marital status, sexual orientation, and disability. | Beneficence, Duty |
| **4.4.** In areas where the ability to communicate with the client is limited (e.g., aphasia, different language, literacy), occupational therapy personnel shall take appropriate steps to facilitate meaningful communication and comprehension. | Autonomy |
| **4.5.** Occupational therapy personnel must ensure that skilled occupational therapy interventions or techniques are only performed by qualified persons. | Duty, Beneficence, Nonmaleficence |
| **4.6.** Occupational therapy administrators (academic, research, and clinical) are responsible for ensuring the competence and qualifications of personnel in their employment. | Beneficence, Nonmaleficence |
| **5. Confidential and Protected Information:** *Information that is confidential must remain confidential. This information cannot be shared verbally, electronically, or in writing without appropriate consent. Information must be shared on a need-to-know basis only with those having primary responsibilities for* | |

| | |
|---|---|
| *decision making.* | |
| **5.1.** All occupational therapy personnel shall respect the confidential nature of information gained in any occupational therapy interaction. The only exceptions are when a practitioner or staff member believes that an individual is in serious, foreseeable, or imminent harm. In this instance, laws and regulations require disclosure to appropriate authorities without consent. | Confidentiality |
| **5.2.** Occupational therapy personnel shall respect the clients' and colleagues' right to privacy. | Confidentiality |
| **5.3.** Occupational therapy personnel shall maintain the confidentiality of all verbal, written, electronic, augmentative, and non-verbal communications (e.g., HIPAA). | Confidentiality |
| **6. Conflict of Interest:** *Avoidance of real or perceived conflict of interest is imperative to maintaining the integrity of interactions.* | |
| **6.1.** Occupational therapy personnel shall be alert to and avoid any action that would interfere with the exercise of impartial professional judgment during the delivery of occupational therapy services. | Nonmaleficence |
| **6.2.** Occupational therapy personnel shall not take advantage of or exploit anyone to further their own personal interests. | Nonmaleficence |
| **6.3.** Gifts and remuneration from individuals, agencies, or companies must be reported in accordance with employer policies as well as state and federal guidelines. | Veracity, Procedural Justice |
| **6.4.** Occupational therapy personnel shall not accept obligations or duties that may compete with or be in conflict with their duties to their employers. | Veracity, Fidelity |
| **6.5.** Occupational therapy personnel shall not use their position or the knowledge gained from their position in such a way that knowingly gives rise to real or perceived conflict of interest between themselves and their employers, other association members or bodies, and/or other organizations. | Veracity, Fidelity |
| **7. Impaired Practitioner:** *Occupational therapy personnel who cannot competently perform their duties after reasonable accommodation are considered to be impaired. The occupational therapy practitioner's basic duty to students, patients, colleagues, and research subjects is to ensure that no harm is done. It is difficult to report a professional colleague who is impaired. The motive for this action must be to provide for the protection and safety of all, including the person who is impaired.* | |
| **7.1.** Occupational therapy personnel shall be aware of their own personal problems and limitations that may interfere with their ability to perform their job competently. They should know when these problems have the potential for causing harm to clients, colleagues, students, research participants, or others. | Nonmaleficence |
| **7.2.** The individual should seek the appropriate professional help and take steps to | Nonmaleficence |

| | |
|---|---|
| remedy personal problems and limitations that interfere with job performance. | |
| **7.3.** Occupational therapy personnel who believe that a colleague's impairment interferes with safe and effective practice should, when possible, discuss their questions and concerns with the individual and assist their colleague in seeking appropriate help or treatment. | Nonmaleficence |
| **7.4.** When efforts to assist an impaired colleague fail, the occupational therapy practitioner is responsible for reporting the individual to the appropriate authority (e.g., employer, agency, licensing or regulatory board, certification body, professional organization). | Nonmaleficence |
| **8. Sexual Relationships:** *Sexual relationships that occur during any professional interaction are forms of misconduct.* | |
| **8.1.** Because of potential coercion or harm to former clients, students, or research participants, occupational therapy practitioners are responsible for ensuring that the individual with whom they enter into a romantic/sexual relationship has not been coerced or exploited in any way. | Nonmaleficence |
| **8.2.** Sexual relationships with current clients, employees, students, or research participants are not permissible, even if the relationship is consensual. | Nonmaleficence |
| **8.3.** Occupational therapy personnel must not sexually harass any persons. | Nonmaleficence |
| **8.4.** Occupational therapy personnel have full responsibility to set clear and appropriate boundaries in their professional interactions. | Nonmaleficence |
| **9. Payment for Services and Other Financial Arrangements:** *Occupational therapy personnel shall not guarantee or promise specific outcomes for occupational therapy services. Payment for occupational therapy services shall not be contingent on successful outcomes.* | |
| **9.1.** Occupational therapy personnel shall only collect fees legally. Fees shall be fair and reasonable and commensurate with services delivered. | Procedural Justice |
| **9.2.** Occupational therapy personnel do not ordinarily participate in bartering for services because of potential exploitation and conflict of interest. However, such an arrangement may be appropriate if it is not clinically contraindicated, if the relationship is not exploitative, and if bartering is a culturally appropriate custom. | Beneficence |
| **9.3.** Occupational therapy practitioners can render pro bono ("for the good," free of charge) or reduced fee occupational therapy services for selected individuals only when consistent with guidelines of the business/facility, third-party payer or government agency. | Beneficence<br>Procedural Justice |
| **9.4.** Occupational therapy personnel may engage in volunteer activities to improve access to occupational therapy or by providing individual service and expertise to charitable organizations. | Beneficence |

| | |
|---|---|
| **9.5.** Occupational therapy personnel who participate in a business arrangement as owner, stockholder, partner, or employee have an obligation to maintain the ethical principles and standards of the profession. They also shall refrain from working for or doing business with organizations that engage in illegal or unethical business practices (e.g., fraudulent billing). | Procedural Justice |
| **10. Resolving Ethical Issues:** *Occupational therapy personnel should utilize any and all resources available to them to identify and resolve conflicts and/or ethical dilemmas.* | |
| **10.1.** Occupational therapy personnel are obligated to be familiar with the Code and its application to their respective work environments. Occupational therapy practitioners are expected to share the Code with their employer and other employees and colleagues. Lack of familiarity with and knowledge of the Code is not an excuse or a defense against a charge of ethical misconduct. | Duty |
| **10.2.** Occupational therapy personnel who are uncertain of whether a specific action would violate the Code have a responsibility to consult with knowledgeable individuals, ethics committees, or other appropriate authorities. | Duty |
| **10.3.** When conflicts occur in professional organizations, members must clarify the nature of the conflict and, where possible, seek to resolve the conflict in a way that permits the fullest adherence to the *Code.* | Fidelity |
| **10.4.** Occupational therapy personnel shall attempt to resolve perceived violations of the Code within institutions by utilizing internal resources. | Fidelity |
| **10.5.** If the informal resolution is not appropriate or is not effective, the next step is to take action by consultation with or referral to institutional, local, district, territorial, state, or national groups who have jurisdiction over occupational therapy practice. | Fidelity |
| **10.6.** Occupational therapy personnel shall cooperate with ethics committee proceedings and comply with resulting requirements. Failure to cooperate is, in itself, an ethical violation. | Procedural Justice |
| **10.7.** Occupational therapy personnel shall only file formal ethics complaints aimed at protecting the public or promoting professional conduct rather than harming or discrediting a colleague. | Fidelity [Query: also Nonmaleficence?] |

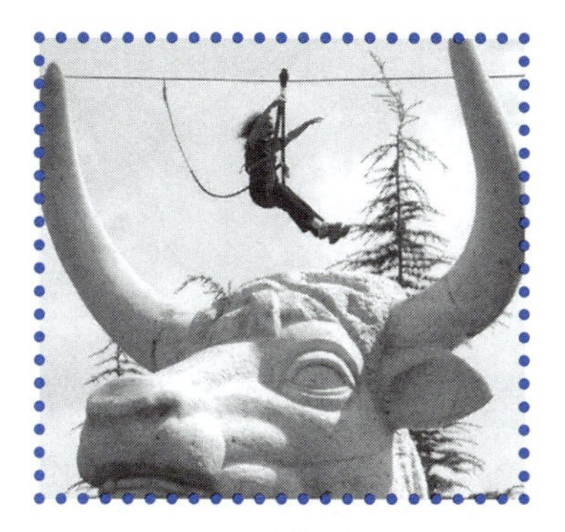

Appendix

# G

# Sample of a Grant Proposal

*Holly St. Onge, MS, OTR/L*

*Completed as a class assignment for Nancy MacRae, MS, OTR/L, FAOTA*

Holly St. Onge, MS, OTR/L
Local Pediatric Clinic
123 School Lane
Somewhere, ME 54321
hstonge@mail.une.edu
207-555-5555

April 23, 2008

Bonnie Jones
Program Manager
US Department of Education
400 Maryland Ave, SW., Rm. 4153
Potomac Center Plaza
Washington, DC 20202-2600

Dear Ms. Jones,

I am writing to you to request that you consider our research project for the grant funded through the Personnel Development to Improve Services and Results for Children with Disabilities Program. I am an occupational therapist working in a pediatric clinic in Maine with children with various disabilities. I am also working with a research group from my alma mater, the University of New England Occupational Therapy Department. We are investigating environmental barriers that limit the educational participation of students with disabilities. In recent studies, students with disabilities report that barriers exist in their physical and social environments, limiting their participation and success in school activities despite federal mandates. According to the research, a significant part of what limits these students are social environmental factors—that is, the attitudes and perceptions of those around them. This includes teachers, school administrators, other school staff, and peers.

We are proposing workshops for education professionals based upon the findings of our study, as well as existing research, to increase awareness of barriers in students' physical and social environments and to decrease the impact of and the actual presence of environmental barriers in schools, which will increase educational participation and academic success. We also plan to collect data and report on the effectiveness of this type of workshop so that these workshops may be replicated in other regions of the country. Our goal is to provide workshops for 100 school districts and to help them develop and implement strategies for changing their physical and social school environments.

Please review our proposal and consider supporting our workshops. The proposed workshops and research support the University of New England's and its occupational therapy department's mission statements and long-terms goals, as well as Healthy People 2010, No Child Left Behind, and IDEA 2004. Enclosed you will find our proposal, résumés, supporting letters, and a budget detailing the fund we have already secured as well as the funds we are requesting from your program. Thank you for your time and consideration.

Sincerely,

Holly St. Onge, MS, OTR/L

# Executive Summary

A research group from the University of New England (UNE) Occupational Therapy Department is requesting funds from the Personnel Development to Improve Services and Results for Children with Disabilities Program to help fund workshops and a research study regarding educational participation of students with disabilities and the barriers they encounter in their physical and social environments. This population faces challenges primarily due to a lack of understanding and knowledge of education professionals regarding adaptations and modifications to activities and curricula. Studies show students are frequently either completely excluded or pushed beyond their abilities due to these reasons. The group aims to provide workshops for 100 school districts and conduct follow-up interviews and consultations to help schools make changes to their physical and social environments after attending the workshops. The researchers have already gained funding for their initial study from the American Legion Child Welfare Foundation and Dreyer's Foundation Small Grants and Product Donations, with in-kind services/supplies from UNE and schools participating in the study, for a total of $10,280. For the workshops, the researchers have already funded supplies from Staples Foundation for Learning, with in-kind/donated space and facilities from the schools and UNE. The group is requesting $44,500 from your program to fund the workshops, which will allow the researchers to help the schools develop plans and strategies for changing their school environments as they strive to increase educational participation and decrease barriers for students with disabilities.

## Background

A research group from the occupational therapy department at UNE, comprised of graduate students, a faculty advisor, and an occupational therapist from a local pediatric clinic (also a UNE alumna) are conducting a study regarding the educational participation of students with disabilities and chronic conditions in New England schools. Following completion of this study, the researchers will provide workshops for school personnel in New England aiming to help these professionals develop strategies and plans for implementing changes to the physical and social school environments to improve educational participation for students with disabilities. The goal of this study and workshops is to increase educational participation by increasing the understanding and knowledge base of teachers, therapists, parents, and other school personnel, while also decreasing environmental barriers to participation. The study and workshops will take place in New England with results being disseminated nationally and internationally through publication in scholarly journals and presentations at the American Occupational Therapy Association (AOTA) National Conference.

UNE is a top-ranked, independent university and is the top institution for the education of healthcare professionals in the state of Maine, with recognized programs in osteopathic medicine; health sciences; biological, marine, and environmental sciences; as well as other areas of excellence. The mission of UNE is to provide "a highly integrated learning experience that promotes excellence through interdisciplinary collaboration and innovation in education, research, and service." Some of the core values of the institution include: Health and Wellness, Scholarship and Research, Excellence and Innovation, and Global Community and Diversity, with long-range goals to continue to be the leading provider of healthcare professionals in Maine who value collaborative, patient-centered, and interdisciplinary interventions, as well as to enter the top tier of research institutions, and "through the generation and dissemination of new knowledge, members of the university will seek to solve the major health, environmental, and cultural challenges faced by society." This study and its following workshops honor and match the University of New England's mission and long-term goals. By including graduate students, faculty, and alumni, this study will aid in the education of future healthcare professionals, add to the current research library, and will also help to improve the quality of education and quality of life for students with disabilities and chronic conditions. As part of its mission, the UNE occupational therapy department aims to produce occupational therapists who use their knowledge of the sciences and occupational therapy theories, clinical skills, and clinical and ethical reasoning to provide excellent, occupation-based intervention. Additionally, UNE strives to instill in its occupational therapy graduates an understanding of the importance of taking on leadership roles at the local, state, and national levels as well as the importance of evidence-based practice and continued research to support and further advance the occupational therapy profession. Completing this study and leading the resulting workshops will allow the masters program occupational therapy students to strengthen their own learning by teaching others, gain a better understanding of the United States education system, improve their ability to provide client-centered care, and learn the importance of evidence-based practice, all while helping to improve quality of life, increase educational participation, and decrease environmental barriers.

The faculty advisor, Jane O'Brien, PhD, OTR/L, has over 20 years experience as a clinician (with a pediatric specialty area), researcher, writer, editor, and professor, and will be providing guidance for the graduate students. The primary researcher, Holly St. Onge, MS, OTR/L, is a UNE alumna who has published a research project she completed with her graduate research team, advised by Dr. O'Brien. She has also worked as a graduate teaching assistant and has experience working with children with a variety of disabilities (please see enclosed résumé). The UNE masters program occupational therapy students who will be working on this project will begin in their senior year and continue until the end of their graduate program. Throughout the occupational therapy curriculum, students are trained in the areas of research design, leading group sessions, giving presentations, analyzing the impact of physical and social environments on performance, grading and adapting activities, and knowing the importance of participation in occupations (meaningful daily activities) for increased quality of life. This research group from the UNE occupational therapy program requests your support to provide educational workshops to education professionals throughout New England. Your financial support will allow us to not only complete our initial research project, but to use the results from this study to try and make changes in school environments for students with disabilities.

## Needs Assessment

- Target Population/Justification of Need in Geographic Area
  - Students in New England with disabilities and chronic conditions
    - As of the fall of 2006, 628,902 children were receiving special education or related services in New England region
  - Education professionals including but not limited to teachers, administrators, therapists, and support staff
    - As of the fall of 2006, there were 164,779 teachers in New England, with only 9,922 having training to provide special education and related services

In the fall of 2006, over 6.6 million students, ages 3 to 21 years old, received some form of special educational services in the United States. This number has been steadily increasing while, concurrently, the amount of time these students are spending in regular classrooms is also increasing. Approximately 52% of students with disabilities spend 80% to 100% of their time fully included with typical peers; about 25% spend 40% to 79% of their time in regular classes; 17% spend less than 40% of their time included; and between 2% and 5% do not attend schools with typical peers (i.e., residential facilities, hospitals, home). Students with more and more complex needs are spending more time with typical peers, which creates new learning opportunities for them, as well as new obstacles for teachers, administrators, and parents. School districts have improved the accommodations provided during state testing, which has led to a narrowing of the gap between students with and without disabilities in terms of test scores, and students with disabilities are achieving more academic success due to improved modifications. Students with disabilities still report barriers in their physical and social environments at school that limit their educational participation and academic success.

A review of recent research revealed that students with disabilities and chronic health conditions face similar barriers across cultural and language differences, ages, and healthcare systems, despite federal mandates. During semi-structured interviews, students from four developed nations with a vast array of disabilities reported that there is a general lack of accessibility of the physical school structures; increased obstacles for older students, students with more severe conditions, and students with "invisible" disabilities who constantly have to fight to prove their need for services; and all students reported that factors in their social environment are the most limiting to their participation. While adaptations and modifications in schools have helped increase participation in basic everyday school tasks, for more complex tasks, participation and performance is still inconsistent and more challenging. Teachers are not necessarily trained to work with students with various physical, cognitive, emotional, and behavioral conditions. Teachers are often unaware of either that a student has a condition or how a condition impacts his or her everyday functioning. Teachers' perceptions of students with chronic conditions were investigated, and it was discovered that teachers feel they lack education and training in regard to having children with disabilities and chronic health concerns in the classroom. Teachers reported being open to the students' inclusion, but were concerned about how to handle the child's special needs. To better illustrate this point, examples from recent research are provided. All students reported that social environmental factors—the attitudes and perceptions of others—are the most difficult to overcome. Many students reported actually being sent home early or to a location separate from their peers during certain educational units such as outdoor education or excluded from classes like physical education and art. On the other hand, one student with a cardiopulmonary condition described being forced to run with his peers during physical education class and roughly encouraged to keep going despite becoming cyanotic (turning blue due to a lack of oxygen) and diaphoretic (sweating profusely). Some students reported that the only way they could accompany their classmates on fieldtrips was by being carried by an adult, even at 13 years old. Another issue students faced was an unwillingness of adults to alter or allow changes in the way an activity is performed; the student is simply excluded completely instead of the adult allowing for and taking time to adapt the activity so the student could participate, in even a small way, with his classmates.

Healthy People 2010, as outlined by the US Department of Health and Human Services, has two major goals: to increase quality of life and to eliminate health disparities. Specific focus areas of Health People 2010 include those with cancer, disabilities and secondary conditions, and educational and community-based programs. By supporting this study and its subsequent workshops for education professionals, the goals of Healthy People 2010 will also be supported. Creating and leading these educational workshops for school staff supports the missions of UNE and its occupational therapy department, Health People 2010, and other government programs like No Child Left Behind and IDEA 2004. Due to all of these factors and the evidence provided, we ask you to support our project.

## Proposal

*Goal*: To increase educational participation and success of students with disabilities and chronic conditions in New England

- Objective 1: To provide educational workshops to 100 school districts in New England by June 2011
- Objective 2: To increase awareness of environmental barriers in students' physical and social environments, as well as decrease the impact of and the actual presence of environmental barriers in children's schools and communities

*Strategies*:

- Conduct a research study to examine the types of environmental barriers students with disabilities and chronic conditions in New England face and to hear their perspectives
- Develop posters or multi-media presentations including the results of the study
- Provide workshops to key education professional and school staff
- Collaborate with educational professionals to develop strategies and plans for implementation into the schools and continued education of other school staff

*Outcomes*:

- 100 School Districts will incorporate strategies and student-perspectives discussed at workshops into the physical and social environments and curriculum
- Students with disabilities and chronic conditions will report decreased impact of and presence of environmental (physical and social) barriers during follow-up interviews

*Evaluation*:

- The researchers will distribute surveys at the end of each workshop to gain feedback from school personnel and improve workshops. By reviewing comments and ratings on the surveys, the presenters will be able to modify the presentations to better benefit school staff.

  Surveys will include 10-point likert scales with space for comments in the areas of presentation style, effectiveness of presentation methods, and questions regarding areas of strength and suggestions for improvement. The researchers will read and analyze the surveys following each workshop for common themes, looking for feedback on the strengths of the workshops as well as areas that need improving. This will allow for improvements to be made during the workshop period of the project.

- o The researchers will conduct school visits and phone interviews to a random selection of the schools participating in the study after 6 and 12 months following the workshops to evaluate changes made to the schools as a result of the workshops. By following-up with the schools, the researchers will be able to examine the effectiveness of their workshops as well as offer assistance if a school is having trouble implementing their ideas.
- o The researchers will conduct follow-up interviews 9 months after the workshops with students who participate in the study using the School Setting Interview to analyze how educational participation and school environments have changed following the initial study and workshops. This will allow the researchers to identify if their workshops were effective and if their over-arching goal was achieved in order to increase educational participation and decrease environmental barriers.

The School-Setting Interview (SSI) is a semi-structured interview based upon the Model of Human Occupation and its conceptualization of environment and client-centered practice. It is used to evaluate student-environment fit and identify areas where adjustments are needed to improve the student's ability to participate. The SSI has 16 items, including writing; speaking; remembering things; doing homework; going to art, music, and physical education classes; getting around the classroom; accessing the school; taking breaks; and interacting with staff. It is meant to be a collaborative and interactive time between the student and occupational therapists to discuss environmental supports and barriers as well as strategies for dealing with barriers.

The SSI is well-refined—a third edition was published in 2005—and has a foundation in the strong evidence base of Model of Human Occupation. It also has strong interrater reliability, construct validity, and content validity for varied and heterogeneous samples of students in primary and secondary schools with physical, developmental, emotional, and behavioral conditions. Psychometric studies of the previous edition found the SSI to "[demonstrate] a sensitivity of 0.96 and a specificity of 0.80 for all items."

## Future Funding/Continuation of Program/Sustainability

The researchers will conduct follow-up interviews and distribute surveys to examine the effectiveness of the workshops. During the workshops, the researchers will work with school staff on how to seek grants, fundraising methods, and also low-tech, cost-effective methods of adapting and modifying tasks and equipment. The importance of collaborating with each student will be emphasized. Electronic versions of the presentations will be available so that school staff may take the information back to their colleagues and share what they have learned. Free long-distance consultation will be available to participating schools, along with a list of resources. Each school with staff who attend the workshops will receive a $300 "environmental change-stimulus" to aid in improvements to the school environments after providing the researchers with written plans.

All data collected during and following the workshops will be analyzed, and findings on the effectiveness of the workshops will be submitted for publication in scholarly journals and presentations at national and state-level conferences. This will allow for future research groups from other areas of the country to replicate the study and workshops. Additionally, this will provide evidence to support school-based occupational therapy practice and will be a resource for education professionals.

| Timetable for Completion of Research Study and Workshops | |
|---|---|
| February 2010 | • Submit study results to AOTA for presentation at national conference<br>• Begin to create presentation for workshops<br>• Begin advertising for workshops beginning with schools who participated in the study |
| April 2010 | • Submit research article for publication<br>• Finalize plans for workshops<br>• Begin workshops |
| May 2010 | • Continue workshops |
| June 2011 | • Complete all workshops |
| Sept-Dec 2011 | • Follow school visits and phone interviews to evaluate changes made at schools following workshops |
| Jan-March 2012 | • Begin follow-up interviews with students using School Setting Interview to discuss possible improvements in education participation and environmental barriers |
| April-June 2012 | • Follow-up with schools to discuss results 1 year after workshops |
| June-July 2012 | • Analyze follow-up data, prepare to submit for publication/presentation at conferences |
| Fall 2012 | • Results disseminated via publication and presentations |

| Budget | | | |
|---|---|---|---|
| *Expenses for Workshops* | | *Total Costs* | *Funding Source* |
| Environmental Change-Stimulus (to help schools make changes following attendance of workshops) | $300/school with staff in attendance | $30,000 | Requesting |
| Professional Presenters Jane O'Brien, PhD, OTR/L and Holly St. Onge, MS, OTR/L (for presentation workshops to education professionals following study) | $50/hr | $8,000 | Requesting |
| MSOT Student Presenters | $25/hr | $4,000 | Requesting |
| Travel to each workshop (gas and tolls) | $4.00/gal (gas); average toll $0.75 | $2,500 | Requesting |
| Space/Facilities for workshops | | $0 | In-Kind from schools participating |
| Supplies for Presentations—Posters, Multimedia, handouts, office supplies for activities, etc. | $0.10/pg; $5.99/box markers; $3.79/box pens | $7,000 | Staples Foundation for Learning |
| *Total Cost Of Workshops* | | *$51,500* | |
| AMOUNT REQUESTED from CDFA No. 84.325T | | $44,500 | Requesting |

| Expenses Already Covered By Other Funding Sources | | | |
|---|---|---|---|
| *Expenses for Research Study* | | *Total Costs* | *Funding Source* |
| Occupational therapists participating in study (for time outside of typical schedule, training included) | $50/hr | $3,500 | American Legion Child Welfare Foundation |
| Statistician (UNE Faculty) | $30/hr x 50 hrs | $1,500 | American Legion Child Welfare Foundation |
| Conference fees (registration, travel, etc) | $1,500 | $1,500 | American Legion Child Welfare Foundation |
| Travel for school visits, training sessions (gas and tolls) | $4.00/gal (gas), tolls average $0.75 | $2,500 | American Legion Child Welfare Foundation |
| Refreshments at training sessions | $400 | $400 | Dreyer's Foundation |
| Digital Audio Recorders | $25/ea x 16 | $400 | Dreyer's Foundation |
| Transcription Software | $200 | $200 | Dreyer's Foundation |
| *In-Kind Services/Volunteers* | | *Total Costs* | *Funding Source* |
| UNE graduate students | | $0 | UNE |
| Faculty Advisor (UNE student research group) | $50/hr | $0 | UNE |
| Use of SFA Manual and Rating Scale Guides | $125 | $0 | UNE |
| Space for training/interviews | | $0 | UNE, participating schools |
| Office supplies | $100 | $0 | UNE |
| Photocopies/printing | $0.10/pg = $200 | $0 | UNE |
| Postage | $100 | $0 | UNE |
| Internet/Email Access | $100/month | $0 | UNE |
| School Function Assessment (SFA) Record Forms | $80.00 per 25 books | | UNE |
| School-Setting Interview (SSI) | $40 | | UNE |
| *Total Cost Of Study* | | *$10,280* | |
| | | | |
| Total Costs (study + workshops) | | $61, 780 | |
| AMOUNT REQUESTED from CDFA No. 84.325T | | $44,500 | |

# Appendices

## Appendix A

Clients served (demographic stats)

- Approximately 628,902 students receive special education services of some kind in New England
- Approximately 9,922 school staff (in New England) with training to provide special education or related services (about 6% of total teachers in New England)
- Approximately 164,779 teachers in New England
- School administrator, school-based physical and occupation therapists, speech and language pathologists, social workers, and counselors

## Appendix B

List of other funding sources

- American Legion Child Welfare Foundation
- Dreyer's Foundation Small Grants and Product Donations
- Staples Foundation for Learning
- University of New England

## Appendix C

Biographies of key personnel

- Primary Researcher: Holly St. Onge, MS OTR/L (see enclosed résumé)
- UNE Faculty Advisor: Jane O'Brien, PhD, OTR/L
- UNE Masters Program Occupational Therapy Students: 3 to 5 TBD

## Appendix D

Organization's by-laws

- Mission of University of New England

  "The University of New England provides a highly integrated learning experience that promotes excellence through interdisciplinary collaboration and innovation in education, research, and service."
- Mission of University of New England, Occupational Therapy Department

  "The OT Department's mission for its Entry Level Masters program is to educate occupational therapy students who will use knowledge, skills, and values to provide exemplary occupation-based practice while assuming leadership roles at the local, state, and national levels. For the Post Professional Masters program we add to the mission fostering the development of theory and research to further the validation of the OT profession."

Kimberly Flecken, MSW
Local School District
321 School Lane
Somewhere, ME 54321
kflecken@mail.une.edu
207-555-5555

April 23, 2008

Bonnie Jones
Program Manager
US Department of Education
400 Maryland Ave, SW., Rm. 4153
Potomac Center Plaza
Washington, DC 20202-2600

Dear Ms. Jones,

I am writing in support of the grant proposal submitted by Holly St. Onge, MS, OTR/L and the research group from the University of New England. Their study and its proposed workshops will benefit education professionals and students alike.

I work with students with a variety of disabilities and their families, and frequently, these families are frustrated by the barriers and obstacles they encounter in the education system. Most often these are created by a lack of understanding and education on the impact a disability has on a student or how modifications may be made to increase participation and academic success for each student. It is considered general knowledge that increased participation and academic success lead to improved productivity as adults. If we can support these students while they are in school, they can learn to advocate for themselves and will be contributing members of society.

This group from UNE consists of high-level students, an expert faculty advisor, and a passionate clinician. I support their efforts and know that the workshops and research they produce will be top quality and worth your investment. I ask that you consider their proposal and offer them the financial support they need to have an impact for students throughout New England.

Sincerely,

Kimberly Flecken, MSW

Mickey M. Mouse, PhD
Director of Special Education Services
Local School District
321 School Lane
Somewhere, ME 54321
Mmouse1@disneyworld.com
207-555-5555

April 23, 2008

Bonnie Jones
Program Manager
US Department of Education
400 Maryland Ave, SW., Rm. 4153
Potomac Center Plaza
Washington, DC 20202-2600

Dear Ms. Jones,

I am writing to you in support of the grant proposal submitted by Holly St. Onge, MS, OTR/L and colleagues from the University of New England. They are highly qualified and experienced professionals and students who have a passion and commitment to research and intervention in this area.

Out of the approximately 165,000 teachers in New England, only about 9,922 have any training in providing special education or related services. There were approximately 629,000 students receiving special education services in New England in 2006. These numbers alone indicate that more professionals require training for working with students with disabilities. Classroom teachers learn from experience how to work with students with disabilities, as over 50% of students are now included in regular class for at least 80% of the time, but generally lack specific training for modifying curricula and activities.

I know that I would strongly encourage all of the staff in my district to attend a workshop such as proposed by this research group. They are striving to provide a service and contribute to evidence-based and client-centered services, and I have no doubt that they will be successful with your support. The University of New England produces healthcare professionals with strong research and leadership skills, as well as excellent clinical skills. With this combination, this group has the tools required to be successful.

Please consider this request and the many students and education professionals that will benefit from these workshops and research studies. Thank you for your time and consideration.

Sincerely,

Mickey M. Mouse, PhD

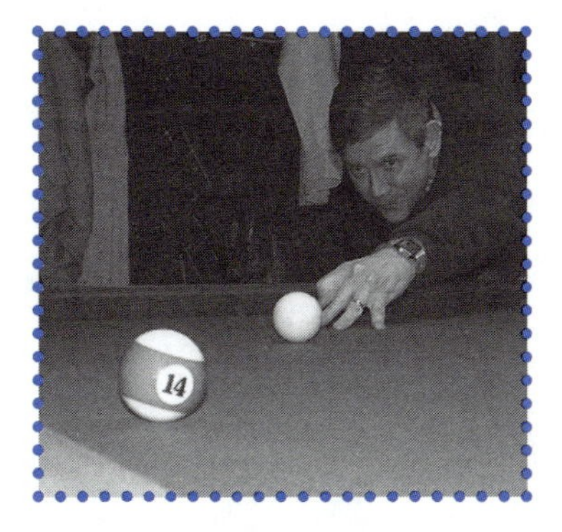

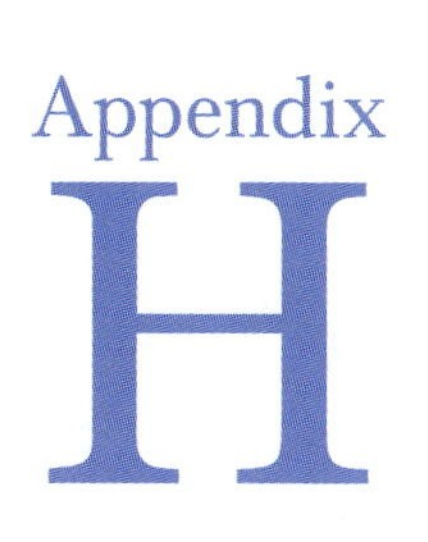

Appendix H

# Procedures for the Enforcement of the NBCOT Candidate/Certificant Code of Conduct

*Reproduced with permission from the National Board of Certification in Occupational Therapy.*

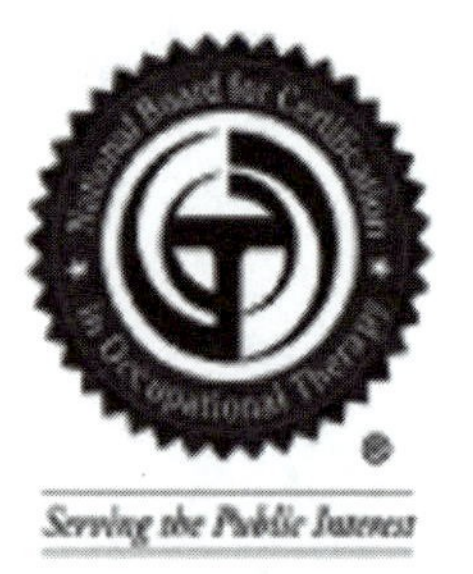


## PROCEDURES FOR THE ENFORCEMENT OF THE NBCOT® CANDIDATE/CERTIFICANT CODE OF CONDUCT

SECTION A. Preamble

In exercising its responsibility for promoting and maintaining standards of professional conduct in the practice of occupational therapy and in order to protect the public from those practitioners whose behavior falls short of these standards, the National Board for Certification in Occupational Therapy, Inc. ("NBCOT®," formerly known as "AOTCB") has adopted a Candidate/Certificant Code of Conduct. The NBCOT has adopted these procedures for resolving issues arising under the Candidate/Certificant Code of Conduct with respect to persons who have been certified by the NBCOT or who have applied for such certification. These procedures are intended to enable the NBCOT, through its Qualifications and Compliance Review Committee ("QCRC"), to act fairly in the performance of its responsibilities to the public as a certifying agency, and to ensure that the rights of candidates and certificants are protected.

SECTION B. Basis for Sanction

A violation of the Candidate/Certificant Code of Conduct provides basis for action and sanction under these Procedures.

SECTION C. Sanctions

1. Violations of the Candidate/Certificant Code of Conduct may result in one or more of the following sanctions:

   a. Ineligibility for certification, which means that an individual is barred from becoming certified by the NBCOT, either indefinitely or for a certain duration.

   b. Reprimand, which means a formal expression of disapproval, which shall be retained in the certificant's file, but shall not be publicly announced.

   c. Censure, which means a formal expression of disapproval which is publicly announced.

   d. Probation, which means continued certification is subject to fulfillment of specified conditions, e.g., monitoring, education, supervision, and/or counseling.

e. Suspension, which means the loss of certification for a certain duration, after which the individual may be required to apply for reinstatement.

f. Revocation, which means permanent loss of certification.

2. All sanctions other than reprimand shall be announced publicly, in accordance with Section D.7. All sanctions other than reprimand shall be disclosed in response to inquiries in accordance with Section D.7.

SECTION D. Qualifications and Compliance Review Procedures

1. Jurisdiction

The NBCOT has jurisdiction over all individuals who have been certified as an OCCUPATIONAL THERAPIST REGISTERED OTR (OTR®) henceforth OTR, or CERTIFIED OCCUPATIONAL THERAPY ASSISTANT COTA (COTA®) henceforth COTA, or who are planning to apply for or have applied for certification, or have applied for Occupational Therapy Eligibility Determination (OTED) to take the NBCOT Certification Examination for OTR. In addition, NBCOT has jurisdiction over all individuals who have applied for an Early Determination Review to determine eligibility to take the Certification Examination for OTR or COTA; Jurisdiction, in this case, is for the limited purpose of acting upon a request for an Early Determination.

2. Initiation of the Process

The QCRC Staff ("Staff") shall initiate the process upon receipt by the QCRC of information indicating that an individual subject to QCRC's jurisdiction may have violated the Candidate/Certificant Code of Conduct. Receipt of such information shall be considered a complaint for the purposes of these procedures, regardless of the source.

3. Staff Investigation and Action

a. Staff shall review all complaints and investigate these complaints, as it deems appropriate.

b. Staff may review any evidence, which it deems appropriate and relevant.

i. If Staff determines that the evidence does not support the allegation(s), no file shall be opened and the complainant shall be notified of the Staff's decision.

ii. If Staff determines that the evidence does support the allegation(s) and decides to investigate, the subject of the complaint as well as the complainant shall be notified. This notification shall be in writing and shall include a description of the complaint and the identity of the complainant. The subject of the complaint shall have thirty (30) days from the date notification is sent to respond in writing to the complaint. The Staff may extend this period up to an additional thirty (30) days upon request, provided sufficient justification for the extension is given.

iii. The subject of a complaint may request voluntary forfeiture of his/her certification. This request must be submitted in writing and can be made while the complaint is either under active investigation or when disciplinary action has been taken by the QCRC but the terms of the sanction remain incomplete.

If the subject applies to regain certification, after voluntary forfeiture, the subject must meet all of the following requirements:

a. submit request to regain certification in writing
b. satisfy current certification examination eligibility requirements (including academic and fieldwork requirements) and
c. re-take and pass the national certification examination

Further, any pending investigation will be resumed upon request to regain certification.

If the subject's certification is voluntarily forfeited, public notice may be given in accordance with Section D. 7 of these procedures.

c. Upon the completion of its investigation, Staff shall either:

i. Dismiss the case due to insufficient evidence, the matter being insufficiently serious, or other reasons as may be warranted. The qualifications and compliance review shall be considered closed at the time such decision is made; or

ii. Propose a settlement agreement.

4. QCRC Review and Decision

Staff shall prepare a case summary of its investigation along with the proposed settlement for the QCRC to consider. The report shall include the basis for Staff's findings, as well as any written responses, or other materials submitted in relation to the investigation of the complaint. Upon review of Staff's investigation, findings, and recommendation, the QCRC may either:

a. Approve the proposed settlement agreement. Upon the subject's acceptance of the settlement, the qualifications and compliance process shall be considered closed. The public notification standards of Section D.5 are applicable if the settlement contains a sanction that warrants such announcement be made; or

b. Reject the proposed settlement. Should the QCRC reject the settlement, it may either instruct Staff with modifications or revisions to the proposed settlement or it may dismiss the case altogether.

Upon notification of the proposed settlement, the subject of the complaint may either:

a. Agree to the proposed settlement and thereby waive his/her right to a hearing; or

b. Not agree to the proposed settlement and request a hearing before the QCRC.

 i. The subject of the complaint may be represented at the hearing by his/her legal counsel, or any other individual of his/her choosing.

 ii. The subject of the complaint shall be solely responsible for all of his/her own expenses related to the hearing. Hearings can be conducted via teleconference call or in person at the sole discretion of the QCRC. Should the subject cancel the hearing, he/she must notify the QCRC of the cancellation no less than five (5) days prior to the hearing date. Should the subject cancel the hearing within five (5) days of the hearing date or not appear at the scheduled hearing, all costs associated with the preparation of the hearing shall be paid by the subject (e.g. court reporting fees, teleconference fees, hearing manual preparation fees).

 iii. The subject of the complaint shall provide the QCRC with any and all materials he/she may wish to include for the hearing no less than ten (10) days prior to the hearing date.

Following the hearing, Staff shall notify (in writing) the complainant and the subject of the complaint of the QCRC's decision within thirty (30) days of the decision. The decision shall take effect immediately unless otherwise provided by the QCRC.

5. Appeals Process

Within thirty (30) days after the notification of the QCRC's decision, any individual(s) sanctioned by the QCRC at the hearing may appeal the hearing decision to the NBCOT Directors. A notice of appeal, which must be in writing and signed by the appealing party, shall be sent by the appealing party to the NBCOT Chairperson in care of the President/Chief Executive Officer. The basis for the appeal shall be fully explained in this notice.

The Chairperson shall form an Appeals Panel within thirty (30) days after receipt of the notice of appeal. The Appeals Panel shall be comprised of three (3) NBCOT Directors and shall include at least one (1) OTR or one (1) COTA and one (1) public member. Members of the QCRC who participated in any aspect of the proceedings related to the complaint shall not serve on the Appeals Panel.

An appeal must relate to evidence, issues and procedures that are part of the record of the QCRC hearing and decision. The appeal may also address the substance of the disciplinary action. However, the Panel may in its discretion consider additional evidence.

Within fifteen (15) days after the notice of appeal is received by the Appeals Panel, the Panel shall either decide the appeal or schedule a hearing.

The Appeals Panel may either:

a. Affirm the QCRC's decision;

b. Deny the QCRC's decision;

c. Refer the case back to the QCRC for further investigation and resolution with full right of appeal; or

d. Modify the decision, but not in a manner that would be more adverse to the subject.

If a hearing is scheduled the appealing party shall be given at least thirty (30) days notice of the hearing. The appealing party may be represented at the hearing by legal counsel or any other individual of his/her choosing. The appealing party shall be solely responsible for all of his/her own expenses related to the hearing. Within fifteen (15) days after the appeals hearing, the Panel shall notify the Chairperson of its decision.

The Chairperson shall promptly notify the appealing party of the Appeals Panel's decision. The decision of the Appeals Panel shall be final.

6. <u>Cooperation with NBCOT Enforcement Procedures</u>

Failure to respond to any aspect of the Enforcement Procedures, will be considered a violation of the Candidate/Certificant Code of Conduct, Principle 2, and is sufficient grounds for the imposition of sanction by the QCRC.

7. <u>Announcement of Sanction</u>

If an individual's certification status is voluntarily forfeited, suspended or revoked, or he/she is censured or placed on probation, occupational therapy state regulatory bodies shall be notified and an announcement included in one or more publications of general circulation to persons engaged or otherwise interested in the profession of occupational therapy. The NBCOT may also disclose its final decision, including ineligibility for certification, to others as it deems appropriate, including, but not limited to, persons inquiring about the status of an individual's certification, employers, third party payers and the general public.

8. <u>Notification</u>

All notifications referred to in these procedures shall be in writing and shall be by confirmation of signature, return receipt mail, unless otherwise indicated. Subjects of complaints who live outside of the U.S. may be given additional time to respond to any notifications they are sent, as determined by the Staff in its discretion.

9. Records and Reports

At the completion of this procedure, all records and reports shall be returned to the Staff. The complete files in the qualifications and compliance review proceedings shall be maintained.

10. Expedited Action

The QCRC Chair may expedite a matter by shortening any notice or response period provided for under these procedures if the responsible party determines in its sole discretion that shortening the period is appropriate in order to protect against the possibility of harm to recipients of occupational therapy services.

In matters where the severity of the allegations and evidence provided warrant such action in order to protect the public, the QCRC may authorize immediate suspension/revocation of certification. The subject will be duly notified of the action and given fifteen (15) days to contest the suspension or revocation.

11. Standard Of Proof

The NBCOT's QCRC and Appeals Panel shall take disciplinary action against an individual only where there is clear and convincing evidence of a violation of the Candidate/Certificant Code of Conduct.

12. Special Accommodations

The NBCOT recognizes the definition of disability as defined by the Americans with Disabilities Act (ADA) and acknowledges the provisions and protections of the Act. The NBCOT shall offer hearings related to qualifications and compliance review or the appeals process in a site and manner, which is architecturally accessible to persons with disabilities or offer alternative arrangements for such individuals.

An individual with a documented disability may request special accommodations for a hearing by providing reasonable advance notice to the NBCOT of his or her disability and of the modifications or aids needed at the hearing at his or her own expense.

13. Amendment to Procedures

These procedures may be amended at any time by the NBCOT Directors.

Revised: October 2008

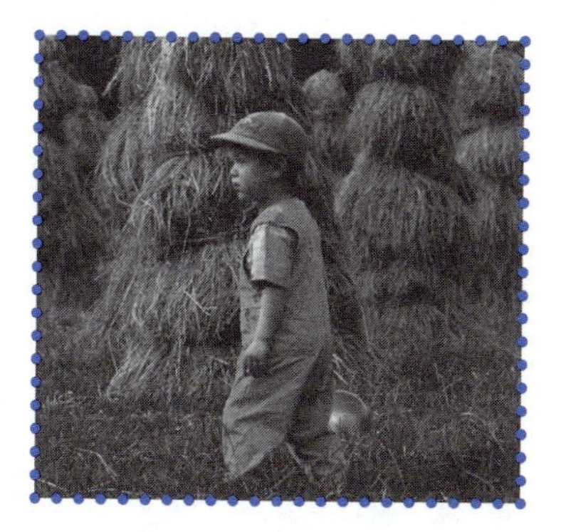

Appendix

# I

# NBCOT Complaint Form

*Reproduced with permission from the National Board of Certification in Occupational Therapy.*

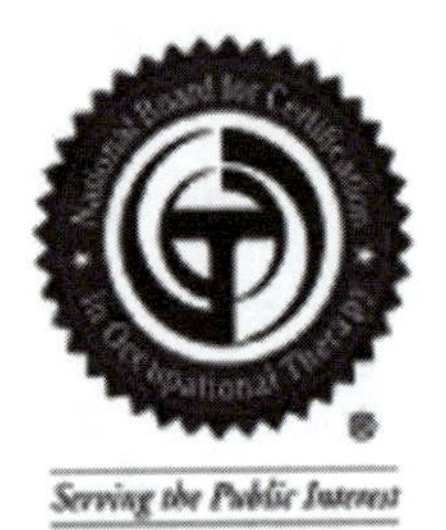


## COMPLAINT FORM

1. **Complaint is filed against:**

**Name:** ______________________ **Telephone:** ____________

**Address:** ______________________ **NBCOT Cert #:** ____________

2. **Person filing complaint (complainant):**

**Name:** ______________________ **Telephone:** ____________

**Address:** ______________________________________

3. **Complainant's relationship with the person against whom the complaint is being filed (e.g., supervisor, co-worker, patient, etc.):**

4. **Summary of complaint (in your own words – who, what, where, when, why, and how): [Use additional sheets if needed].**

5. **Other persons with knowledge of the incident(s) giving rise to this complaint:**

**Name:** ______________________ **Telephone:** ____________

**Address:** ______________________________________

**Name:** ______________________ **Telephone:** ____________

**Address:** ______________________________________

(see reverse side)

6. **Other agencies or organizations you have submitted this complaint to (i.e., state licensing boards, Medicare, AOTA, police or other authorities, etc.):**

7. **State in your own words how this incident(s) relates to the NBCOT's "Candidate/Certificant Code of Conduct" (use additional sheets if needed):**

______________________________________________

______________________________________________

______________________________________________

______________________________________________

______________________________________________

______________________________________________

______________________________________________

______________________________________________

______________________________________________

______________________________________________

______________________________ ______________________

**Complainant Signature** **Date**

(Note: Complete separate form for each complaint or complainant)

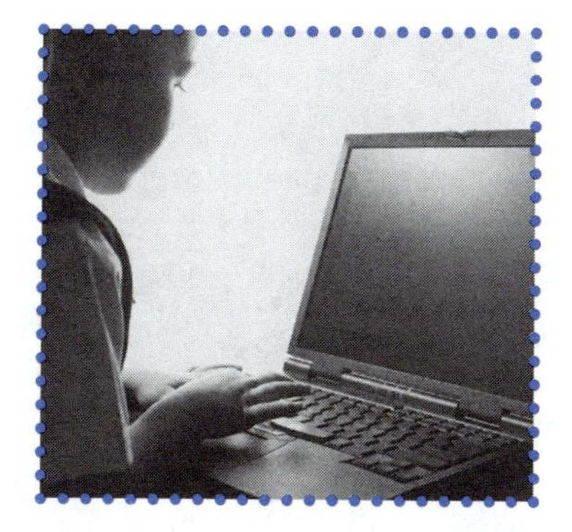

Appendix

# J

# Using Presentation Software Effectively

*William R. Croninger, MA, OTR/L*

# Introduction

Now ubiquitous in education, business, and the military, presentation software such as Microsoft's PowerPoint, Apple Computer's Keynote, or Macromedia Flash has become the defacto standard for delivering lectures (Hanft, 2003). The most common argument for the use of this software is that it allows for simultaneous integration of text and images on the screen. Users also cite the ease in which presentations can be constructed and changed, the belief that students welcome and often even expect material to be presented in this form, and its perceived superiority to "traditional" forms of classroom delivery (Norton, 2004).

The goal of this section is to provide the reader with information on how to make presentations more effective, as well as briefly speak to research on the effectiveness of presentation software. Kupsh (1994) stated that although great speakers, entertainers, and comedians have historically been able to gain and hold the attention of an audience without the use of media, most of us benefit from some level of its use. One must realize, however, that there is no inherent magic in presentation software. It will not automatically make you a better speaker or improve student retention or understanding.

# Organization

One claim often heard is that presentation software helps you organize your lectures better. It can be argued that none of these software products has the power or "intelligence" that would cause this. If your lecture was poorly organized prior to moving it to presentation software, it will remain poorly organized. To put it another way, presentation software is a tool and thus can be used or misused (University of Minnesota, 2006).

In his book *What's the Use of Lectures*, Donald Bligh (2000) speaks of three general means of organizing lectures: hierarchical, problem-centered, and chained.

- *Hierarchical*: In this form, facts are grouped together under their respective headings. Hierarchically arranged presentation software lectures are good for the presentation of facts, particularly when the level of detail and complexity is high. In a kinesiology class, a lecturer might use this form to teach about lever systems in the human body. This strategy has not, however, been found to be an effective method of helping students learn to think critically. Students who received a "lever lecture" delivered in a hierarchical format would still likely experience difficulty analyzing the lever type demonstrated by a specific joint motion.
- *Problem-centered*: Arranged this way, an initial presentation software slide could start with the question, "What class of lever does the elbow joint in extension represent?" The slides that followed might challenge students to identify the information needed to determine a lever classification. The instructor would move forward by providing the information on succeeding slides as a response to the strategies and questions they uncover.
- *Chained*: In a chained lecture, each "link" promotes transition to the next one. Taken together, the entire chain should lead to a stated goal. Bligh notes that although this is one of the more effective forms of lecture, it is likely the most difficult of the three to accomplish. Students generally find it more interesting and easier to stay with the lecture, but only if transitions to the following "link" are clear. He also notes that if a student becomes "lost," he or she will have difficulty regaining the flow.

Suppose a goal is to teach students the process used when forming an impression of a client's cognitive state during the initial evaluation. This topic does not lend itself well to the hierarchical form because an experienced clinician is monitoring a number of different things simultaneously during that first visit. It is not really a problem to be evaluated, thus a problem-centered approach is not necessarily favorable. The teacher/clinician might first draw a set of concentric circles on the board, or display them as a graphic on one page. By showing the students the chain in its entirety, they may be able to form a Gestalt of the overall process. One could then use presentation software to detail the thought process under each link, all the while emphasizing that much of this occurs simultaneously. In this way, students are helped to visualize the chain of logic that followed in determining not only a client's orientation, but their ability to attend, plan, follow verbal directions, recognize, and correct errors. Ultimately, it should be possible to demonstrate how a clinician makes an accurate prediction on a client's ability to live independently.

## Slide Pointers

- An initial slide should state the organization: topic, goals, relevance
- The title of each slide should help the student locate where he or she is in the organizational structure of the lecture. An example might be when talking about the six joints of the shoulder; a slide title will say "Shoulder Joints" for each of the six slides. The joint name will be the first line in the body of its slide.
- Build the slide with transitions, line by line. Do not just throw the entire slide out in front of the students all at once.
- Provide a transition slide when leaving one topic for the next.
- Finish the lecture with a slide that summarizes what students should have learned.

# Effectiveness of Presentation Software

Interestingly enough, there is little research that supports claims using any presentation software results in more effective learning when compared to traditional forms of lecture.

Broadston and Kennedy (2003) found that learning did take place in a graduate measurement course in which they used presentation software. However, since all lectures used Microsoft PowerPoint, no comparison to other methods was possible. Atkins-Sayre, Hopkins, Mohundro, and Sayre (1998) stated that the majority of the 485 student participants in their study felt Microsoft PowerPoint was effective as a "cognitive aid." No attempt was made to compare presentation software to other methods of instruction in terms of retention or learning.

In the situations where student performance was actually measured against traditional methods, Ahmed (1998) and Bartsch and Cobern (2003) found no difference, while Szabo and Hastings (2000) reported that results were more dependent on the "difficulty" of the lecture than on the method in which it was presented. Of particular note in the Bartsch and Cobern study is that there was a significant difference between quiz scores for students who received regular versus expanded presentation software-based lectures. The expanded presentations had audio and images added. Some of the images related directly to the topic, others were clipart that had no relationship to lecture topics. Students felt that the audio and nonrelated clipart were distracters. The lower quiz scores seen in that group would seem to support their impression.

A thorough review of the literature found that students preferred presentation software to blackboard and overhead transparencies. A number of studies found that students felt they were learning more. However, none of the literature reviewed for this paper actually found that lectures delivered by presentation software were demonstrably superior. Is student preference a viable reason for using presentation software over traditional methods? Many individuals have a preference for fast food, and thus an observer might argue what one prefers is not always in line with what might be best. It would seem instructors should consider very carefully whether they should move lectures to presentation software if an evaluation of student learning suggests traditional methods are working.

## Slide Pointers

- Use audio and visual images only if they have a direct relation to the topic, otherwise they are likely to detract from learning.
- Pick a set of fonts and sizes and stick to them! Frequent changes of fonts and text size will only frustrate your viewers.
- Consider the "Rule of Six"—six lines per slide, six words or less in each line. Try to stick with one topic/point per slide (Holzl, 1997).
- Limit the number of colors on any slide to four or less (Holz).

## Instructor Notes

There has been considerable debate as to whether and/or when to provide instructor notes. Bligh (2000) found the research on student notetaking versus handouts "ambiguous." He went on to state that research supports giving notes prior to the lecture. Finally, there would seem to be support for giving the students partial notes that they then complete in class (Annis, 1981). Bligh cautioned that if the instructor wants the notes to actually be read however, they should be an integral part of the course.

## Presentation Software as a Learning Tool

A second common argument for using presentation software is that it can help students build knowledge through the production of presentations on a topic. Perry (2003) argued that creating presentation software presentations can enhance the research process for students. However, no reviewed study found any element in presentation software that would account for this or support this claim.

What is likely to be occurring is a process known as "constructivist" learning. Constructivism holds that individuals learn by integrating new knowledge with old (Sherman & Kurshan, 2005). Constructivist learning is supported by activities that are learner-centered, engaging, and of relevance to the student's major and that involve "action" learning. They are further enhanced by activities that include social interaction, prompt feedback, and a supportive environment. This can certainly be the case with presentation software. However, it in no way is limited to projects involving presentation software.

Students have varied learning styles; learning through the creation of a presentation software presentation may work well for some but not necessarily for others. The following anecdotal observation may be illustrative.

Some years ago, I required students in a kinesiology class to demonstrate mastery of an upper extremity joint through a small group project. The criteria for mastery were speci-fied; the form the project would take was left to the discretion of the students. One group chose the shoulder and decided to "paint" muscles, tendons, ligaments, and bones onto a member of the group. During their oral presentation, one student related that when she watched the paint crack during forearm pronation/supination, she suddenly understood the concept of agonist/antagonist. This young woman needed to "see" that effect to un-derstand the concept. A process utilizing presentation software would not likely have given the same "eureka" experience.

The group in the preceding example learned an additional lesson—the difference between water soluble and insoluble paints. They had used the insoluble variety, and for days thereafter, their "demonstrator" served as a walking reference map to the anatomy of the shoulder.

## Summary

Presentation software has a place in the classroom and boardroom. Practitioners value evidence-based research in their choice of client interventions. In our teaching roles, the teacher/clinician should be equally demanding that new strategies and tools be adopted only when based on research that demonstrates their superiority to other modes of instruction or learning. Presentation software can enhance lectures, but it has not been demonstrated to be superior to traditional forms of lecture. Some students may find that learning is enhanced while constructing a "slideshow" utilizing presentation software. However, the research reviewed did not support the argument that some element of presentation software makes it a superior form of constructivist learning.

# References


Ahmed, C. (1998). PowerPoint versus traditional overheads. Which is more effective for learning? Retrieved March 14, 2006, from http://www.eric.ed.gov/ERICDocs/data/ericdocs2sql/content_storage_01/0000019b/80/17/81/7e.pdf

Annis, L. (1981). Effect of preference for assigned lecture notes on student achievement. *Journal of Educational Research, 74*, 179-182.

Atkins-Syre, W., Hopkins, S., Mohundro, S., & Sayre, W. (1998). Rewards and liabilities of presentation software as an ancillary tool: Prison or paradise? Paper presented at the Annual Meeting of the National Communication Association, November 21-24, 1998.

Bartsch, R. A., & Cobern, K. M. (2003). Effectiveness of PowerPoint presentations in lectures. *Computers & Education, 41*(1), 77-86.

Bligh, D. (2000). *What's the use of lectures.* San Francisco, CA: Jossey-Bass Publishers.

Broadston, P. M., & Kennedy, R. L. (2003). Effectiveness of a graduate measurement course. Retrieved August 18, 2009, from http://eric.ed.gov:80/ERICDocs/data/ericdocs2sql/content_storage_01/0000019b/80/1b/8d/a1.pdf

Hanft, A. (2003). Grist: More power than point. *Inc. Magazine, 25*, 116. Retrieved August 18, 2009, from http://www.inc.com/magazine/20030801/ahanft.html

Holzl, J. (1997). Twelve tips for effective PowerPoint presentations for the technologically challenged. *Medical Teacher, 19*, 175-179.

Kupsh, J. (1994). Visual literacy and multimedia presentations. In Imagery and Visual Literacy: Selected Readings from the Annual Conference of the International Visual Literacy Association (26th, Tempe, AZ, October 12-16, 1994). Retrieved August 19, 2009, from http://eric.ed.gov:80/ERICDocs/data/ericdocs2sql/content_storage_01/0000019b/80/13/b4/52.pdf

Norton, J. M. (2004). Results of a limited survey of PowerPoint usage by UNE faculty... and some additional comments. Paper presented to the faculty of the University of New England. Retrieved January 6, 2006, from http://faculty.une.edu/com/jnorton/PowerPointPresentation/CHPHandout.pdf

Perry, A. (2003). PowerPoint presentations: A creative addition to the research process. *English Journal, 92*(6), 64-69.

Sherman, T. M., & Kunshan, B. L. (2005). Constructing learning using technology to support teaching for understanding. *Leading and Learning with Technology, 35*(5), 10-13.

Szabo, A., & Hastings, N. (2000). Using IT in the undergraduate classroom: Should we replace the blackboard with PowerPoint? *Computers & Education, 35*(3), 175-187.

University of Minnesota, Center for Teaching and Learning. (2006). Active learning with PowerPoint. Retrieved March 17, 2006, from http://www1.umn.edu/ohr/teachlearn/tutorials/powerpoint

# GLOSSARY

## A

**ABA Design**: A single case experimental design where baseline data is measured (A), intervention provided (B), and measurement repeated (A).

**AbleData**: A federally sponsored website that organizes and tracks adaptive tools and provides an overview of a wide range of assistive devices across a wide spectrum of functions.

**Abstract**: Summary of an article or paper containing the most important points of each subsection.

**Activities of Daily Living (ADL)**: An area of occupation; "Activities that are oriented toward taking care of one's own body (adapted from Rogers & Holm, 1994, pp. 181-202). ADL also is referred to as basic activities of daily living (BADL) and personal activities of daily living (PADL). These activities are 'fundamental to living in a social world; they enable basic survival and well-being' (Christiansen & Hammecker, 2001, p. 156)" (AOTA, 2008, p. 631).

**Activity/Activities**: The execution of a task or action by an individual (WHO, 2001); "A term that describes a class of human actions that are goal directed" (AOTA, 2008, p. 669).

**Activity Demands**: Requirements specific to the activity and independent of the person.

**Adaptation**: (As used as an outcome) "The response approach the client makes encountering an occupational challenge. 'This change is implemented when the individual's customary response approaches are found inadequate for producing some degree of mastery over the challenge' (Schultz & Schkade, 1997, p. 474)" (AOTA, 2008, p. 630).

**Adapting**: To make suitable to or fit for a specific use or situation (Dictionary.com); To change something (i.e., the demands of the activity) so that the client is successful.

**Advertisement**: To make something known; To make publicly and generally known; To announce publicly especially by a printed notice or a broadcast; To call public attention to especially by emphasizing desirable qualities so as to arouse a desire to buy or patronize (Merriam-Webster, 2006).

**Advertising**: "A specific communication task to be accomplished with a specific audience in mind in a specific target market during a specific period of time. The advertisement goals are based on achieving one of four aims: to inform, to persuade, to remind, or to reinforce" (Kotler, 2003, p. 312).

**Americans with Disabilities Act (ADA)**: A Federal law that prevents discrimination against individuals with disabilities.

**Analysis of Occupational Performance**: A multi-step process conducted by the occupational therapist. Based on a select model and/or frame(s) of reference, the occupational therapist analyzes the occupational profile in conjunction with other occupational therapist assessments to formulate hypotheses about which factors encourage as well as disrupt the client's successful engagement in occupations and in daily life activities.

**Analysis of Variance (ANOVA)**: A statistical procedure used to measure differences between measurements.

**Annotated Bibliography**: A citation and short summary.

**Applied Research**: Research directed toward the solution of specified practical problems in delineated areas, or to achieve practical goals (Kerlinger, 1979).

**Applied Theory**: The results of applied research, intended to address problems of practical interest.

**Areas of Occupation**: The variety of meaningful activities in which people engage, including the following categories: activities of daily living, instrumental activities of daily living, education, work, play, leisure, and social participation (AOTA, 2008).

**Arts and Crafts Movement**: A transformation of the American lifestyle, created in response to workers and their working environments.

**Aspiration**: The entry of secretions, fluids, food, or any foreign substance below the vocal cords and into the lungs that may result in aspiration pneumonia and may be fatal (AOTA, 2007).

**Assessment**: Specific tools, instruments, or procedures used to obtain data during the evaluative process.

**Assistive Technology**: Devices that augment or extend a user's ability to function in the task environment.

**Associative Level Participation**: Consists of approaching others briefly in verbal or nonverbal interactions.

**Assumptions**: Broad general statements that are taken for granted for the sake of argument.

**Attitude**: Your mindset or outlook.

# B

**Backward Chaining**: A technique that teaches the last part of a task first, thus ensuring success. Once the last part is learned, the next to last part is taught and so on until the entire task is learned.

**Basic Cooperative Level Participation**: Includes selecting longer activities or tasks of mutual interest and following the norms or rules of interaction in play or work.

**Basic Research**: Systematic study to test theory and to understand relations among phenomena without consideration of application of the results (Kerlinger, 1979).

**Bed Mobility**: Safely and effectively moving in bed for comfort, skin integrity, and function.

**Benchmark**: Quantifiable measures of the outcomes of a process used as comparisons to current targets for improvement (Braveman, 2006).

**Body Functions and Structures**: Physiologic and psychological aspects of individual systems, including anatomic parts (WHO, 2001).

**Body Mechanics**: The utilization of appropriate muscles and positions to complete heavy work safely and efficiently (Brookside Associates, 2007).

**Bolus**: Food or liquid in a mass form (AOTA, 2007).

# C

**Care Coordination**: A process that facilitates the linkage of individuals and their families with appropriate services and resources in a coordinated effort to achieve good health.

**Career**: A line of business or a way of making a living.

**Caring**: A set of feelings, attitudes, and actions that convey respect, hope, and care toward others.

**Case Management**: A collaborative process that assesses, plans, implements, coordinates, monitors, and evaluates the options and services required to meet the client's health and human services needs.

**Case Mix Groups (CMGs)**: A term that classifies client discharges into diagnostic categories.

**Certified Occupational Therapy Assistant**: Nonprofessional personnel trained to work alongside registered occupational therapists.

**Client**: A specific person, family of an identified person, or a population who is the recipient of occupational therapy services; The term used to name the entity that receives occupational therapy services. Clients may include: (1) Individuals and other persons relevant to the individual's life including family, caregivers, teachers, employers, and others who may also help or be served indirectly; (2) organizations such as business, industries, or agencies; and (3) populations within a community (Moyers & Dale, 2007; AOTA, 2008).

**Client-Centered Approach**: "An orientation that honors the desires and priorities of clients in designing and implementing interventions (adapted from Dunn, 2000a, p. 4)" (AOTA, 2008, p. 670).

**Client-Centered Care**: Therapeutic interventions where the person who is receiving services has a major role in the decision making regarding his or her care. The practitioner takes a collaborative rather than an authoritative role.

**Client-Centered Practice**: A partnership between a client and therapist that serves to empower a client toward reaching goals of his or her own choosing; "An approach to therapy that supports a respectful partnership between therapists and clients" (Law, Baptiste, & Mills, 1995, p. 256). Client-centered practice includes the following concepts: a) a recognition of each client's unique perspective; b) a shift in power toward the client having more say in defining and directing intervention; c) a shift to an enablement intervention model; d) an understanding of the importance of the influence on intervention of the client's culture, preferences, interests, roles, and environments; e) an understanding of the importance of flexible and dynamic interventions that emphasize learning and problem solving; and f) respect for the client's values regardless of whether shared by the therapist.

**Client Factors**: Functions, structures, spirituality, value, and beliefs required to complete an activity; Those factors residing within the client that may affect performance in areas of occupation. Client factors include values, beliefs, spirituality, body functions, and body structures (AOTA, 2008).

**Clinical Education**: The full scope of application experiences that focus on the development of students' practice skills.

**Clinical Instructor**: On-site supervisor for practical experiences; Assists all parties in recognizing that these individuals are part of the students education thus offering the title of instructor.

**Clinical Pathway**: A method used in health care settings as a way of organizing, evaluating, and limiting variations in expected client care secondary to diagnosis and other client-specific factors.

**Clinical Reasoning**: Complex cognitive process composed of various types of reasoning.

**Cluster Sampling**: When a research collects data from groups of participants.

**Collaboration**: Both parties have their perspectives and beliefs, but individual goals are put aside to do what is best for the situation and the organization, not what is personally best.

**Community Mobility**: Engaging in mobility resulting in successful participation in the community (AOTA, 2008).

**Compensation**: Changing the way a person completes an activity so that they can be successful given their current situation.

**Competencies**: Explicit statements defining specific areas of expertise and are related to effective or superior performance in a job (L. M. Spencer & S. M. Spencer, 1993).

**Compromise**: Both parties work together and each side concedes a portion of their viewpoint in order to arrive at an agreement and to resolve the conflict.

**Concept**: An idea or notion formed by mentally combining characteristics (Reed & Sanderson, 1999).

**Conceptual Models in Occupational Therapy**: Graphic or schematic representations of concepts and assumptions that explain why the profession works as it does (Reed & Sanderson, 1999).

**Concurrent Validity**: A form of criterion-related validity that shows differences between participants at the time of the measure.

**Conditional Reasoning**: Holistic approach to understanding the person, their illness, and intervention.

**Conflict Resolution**: The ability to identify conflict, to understand the various approaches, and to arrive at a resolution that is beneficial to all parties.

**Confounding Variable**: A factor other than the controlled variables that influences the study's results.

**Construct**: Models of assembled relationships between or among two or more concepts (Depoy & Gitlin, 2005).

**Construct Validity**: The relationship of one construct to another such as the relationship of the scores on two different but similar assessments.

**Consultation**: The provision of advice or information; The exchange of ideas with an expert who is called on for professional advice (AOTA, 1994).

**Content Analysis**: Process of analyzing written words as data.

**Contexts**: Environmental factors or social environment that influence a specific client's participation in occupations (AOTA, 2008); The circumstances in which an event occurs; a setting (Dictionary.com); "Refers to a variety of interrelated conditions within and surrounding the client that influence performance. Contexts include cultural, personal, temporal, and virtual" (AOTA, 2008); The multitude of factors that can define the situation in which leadership takes place.

**Continuing Competence**: Refers to an individual's ongoing or lifelong capacity to perform responsibilities as a part of one's professional role performance.

**Continuing Competency**: Focuses on an individual's actual performance in a particular situation according to standard as a part of one's current professional role performance.

**Contractor**: A person who provides services on a contractual basis.

**Control Group**: Participants in an experimental research design who receive no intervention.

**Convenient Sample**: Sample of participants that is easily available to the researcher.

**Correlational Coefficient**: A measurement of the direction and magnitude of a relationship of two variables.

**Counter-Transference**: When one person, usually the therapist, accepts the role the client has placed on him or her.

**Criterion Referenced**: The client's score can be compared to a set of specific skills or skill components of standard performance rather than a normative group.

**Cultural Competence**: A process of gaining self-awareness, knowledge and awareness of others, and skills necessary to interact effectively and sensitively in communicating with diverse groups of people (Wells & Black, 2000).

**Culturally Competent Care**: The process of interacting collaboratively and effectively with culturally diverse clients in order to provide culturally sensitive assessments and interventions.

**Culture**: "Refers to learned behaviors, values, norms, and symbols that are passed from generation to generation within a society" (Loveland, 1999, p. 18).

# D

**DAP Format**: A format for documentation that includes description, assessment, and plan.

**Data**: Any numerical result of research; always plural as in "data are."

**Deep Thermal Agents**: Those procedures or interventions that use a form of energy capable of raising tissue temperature to a depth of up to 5 cm.

**Deglutition**: Consuming of solids or liquids in a normal sensorimotor process (Jenks & Smith, 2006, p. 610).

**Deinstitutionalization**: The closing of mental hospitals and residential institutions, releasing mentally ill clients to the streets.

**Demographics**: "Data related to the size and growth rate of populations in different cities, regions, and nations; age distribution and ethnic mix; educational levels; household patterns; and regional characteristics and movements" (Kotler, 2003, p. 100).

**Dependent Variable**: The variable measured in response to the intervention or independent variable.

**Disability**: Medical and social construct related to the paradox of describing individual capacity (ability and impairment) and community capacity (attitudes and resources) (Finkelstein, 1991).

**Discharge**: The termination of therapy services.

**Discontinuation Note**: A note that summarizes the course of a client's intervention and includes recommendations for the future.

**Disease**: "A disorder with a specific cause and recognizable signs and symptoms; any bodily abnormality or failure to function properly, except that resulting directly from physical injury (Encyclopedia.com, 2008).

**Documentation**: The legal and professional responsibility of recording occupational therapy service delivery and outcomes.

**Driver Rehabilitation**: A form of therapy that focuses on evaluation and intervention in the occupation of driving a vehicle.

**Durable Medical Equipment**: Medically necessary equipment that can be provided to a client to increase safety and independence in the home. Examples include hospital beds, wheelchairs, and walkers. Items as grab bars, reachers, and long-handled sponges are not considered DME. All covered DME requires a physician prescription.

**Dysphagia**: Difficulty with swallowing or the inability to swallow (Jenks & Smith, 2006).

# E

**Eating**: The ability to manipulate and swallow food and liquids (Jenks & Smith, 2006).

**Education**: "Includes activities needed for learning and participating in the environment.

- Formal educational participation—Including the categories of academic (e.g., math, reading, working on a degree), nonacademic (e.g., recess, lunchroom, hallway), extracurricular (e.g., sports, band, cheerleading, dances), and vocational (prevocational and vocational) participation.
- Informal personal educational needs or interests exploration (beyond formal education)—Identifying topics and methods for obtaining topic-related information or skills.
- Informal personal education participation—Participating in classes, programs, and activities that provide instruction/training in identified areas of interest" (AOTA, 2008, p. 632).

**Educational Activities**: Tasks that facilitate learning, such as reading, writing, and math.

**Educator**: A faculty member in an academic setting (AOTA, 2004a).

**Effect Size**: Magnitude of the effect; the strength and magnitude of a relationship between two variables.

**Effective Communication**: The artful interplay between listening and speaking with attention to both verbal and nonverbal communication, coupled with awareness and sensitivity to human diversity.

**Electrotherapeutic Agent**: Those procedures or interventions that are systematically applied to modify specific client factors that may be limiting occupational performance; use electricity and the electromagnetic spectrum to facilitate tissue healing, improve muscle strength and endurance, decrease edema, modulate pain, decrease the inflammatory process and modify the healing process; and are used as an adjunctive method to occupation (Bracciano, 2007).

**Empathy**: A process of reaching for true understanding of the experiences and feelings of another person.

**Enteral Tube Feedings**: Tubes that deliver nutrition directly to the gastrointestinal system (Morris & Klein, 2000).

**Entrepreneur**: Partially or fully self-employed individuals. Includes those in private practice, independent contractors and consultants (AOTA, 2000).

**Environment**: The external physical and social environment that surrounds the client and in which the client's daily life occupations occur.

**Environmental Factors**: Contextual factors extrinsic to the individual, such as the physical, social, and attitudinal environment in which people live and conduct their lives (WHO, 2001).

**Epistemology**: The dynamics of knowing (Hooper, 2006); How we know what we know.

**Ergonomics**: Study of the "fit" between human and environment.

**Error Variance**: The variance left over after all of the studied variance is accounted for.

**Ethical Reasoning**: Making sure one selects the morally justifiable decisions.

**Ethics**: The study of right and wrong conduct as determined by reasonable thought processes.

**Evaluation**: "The process of obtaining and interpreting data necessary for intervention. This includes planning for and documenting the evaluation process and results" (Brayman et al., 2005, p. 663).

**Evidence-Based Occupational Therapy**: Intervention "based on client information and a critical review of relevant research, expert consensus, and past experience" (CAOT, 1999).

**Exceptional Educational Need (EEN)**: Determination that a student exhibits a disability or handicapping condition that prevents educational progress.

**Executive Skills**: High-level cognitive skills that involve planning, problem solving, cognitive flexibility, judgment/insight, and self-monitoring.

**Experience Sampling Method**: The use of an electronic device that randomly beeps throughout the day and requires the subject to record data regarding the quality of experience, associated challenges, and kind of activity in which he or she is engaged.

**External Validity**: The degree to which the study's results can be generalized to another population.

# F

**F-Test**: A statistical measure used in ANOVA.

**Face Validity**: The degree to which experts in the area would agree that a measurement appears to measure what it says it does. Also called *content validity*.

**Feeding**: Setting up, arranging, and bringing food or fluid from a plate or a cup to the mouth (AOTA, 2007).

**Fieldwork Educator**: This individual assists the student integration of classroom knowledge and application to practice. Not permitted to supervise a Level II fieldwork student until they have practiced full-time for one year (ACOTE, 1999).

**FIP Format**: A format of documentation that includes findings, interpretation, and plan.

**Flow Experience**: The way people describe their state of mind when consciousness is harmoniously ordered, and they want to pursue whatever they are doing for its own sake.

**Frame of Reference**: System of compatible concepts from theory which guides a plan of action within a specific occupational therapy domain of concern (Mosey, 1986); A set of ideas, in terms of which other ideas are interpreted or assigned meaning (Dictionary.com). Frames of reference provide intervention guidelines and help practitioners know what to do in practice; provide information on the nature of function/dysfunction, intervention strategies, principles guiding intervention, assessments, and expected outcomes; and define who would benefit from the intervention.

**Framing**: The method through which a player offers cues about how he or she wishes to be treated during play (Bateson, 1972).

**Freedom to Suspend Reality**: The child is able to defer the restrictions of realistic play and use his or her imagination to take on new roles and identities (Bundy, 1997; Rubin, Fein, Vandenberg, 1983); The ability to participate in make-believe activities or pretend play (Bundy, 1997).

**Frequency**: Number of participants who have a specific score.

**Fun**: "That which provides mirth and amusement; enjoyment; playfulness" (Parham & Fazio, 1997, p. 250).

**Function**: The ability to perform meaningful activities and tasks that involve body structure, body functions, activities, and participation (WHO, 2001).

**Functional Mobility**: "Moving from one position to another during performance of every day activities" (AOTA, 2008, p. 631).

# G

**Gastroesophageal Reflux Disease (GERD)**: "Reflux of food, medication, liquids, and gastric juice from the stomach into the esophagus" (AOTA, 2007, p. 698).

**Gastroesophageal Scintigraphy**: Sometimes referred to as a "milk scan," this medical test looks at stomach emptying as well as extent and severity of reflux (Morris & Klein, 2000).

**Gastrostomy Tube (G-tube)**: Bypasses the mouth and is surgically inserted directly into the stomach.

**Goal**: Outcome measure of progress.

**Grading**: Changing aspects of an activity to make it easier or more difficult.

# H

**Health**: "A complete state of physical, mental, and social well-being, and not just the absence of disease or infirmity" (WHO, 1947, p. 29).

**Health Promotion**: Actions or activities that purport to the enhancement of health and well-being.

**Hi-tech**: Devices, often electronic or electric, commonly more expensive and often customized according to the user's needs.

**Holistic Approach**: Perceiving interrelated components as one whole unit that cannot be subdivided into parts.

**Human Factors Engineering**: see *Ergonomics*

**Humanism**: A philosophical approach recognizing the basic goodness of being human and the uniqueness of each individual.

# I

**Ideational Apraxia**: A complete loss of the ability to do a task due to a perceptual disorder.

**Ideomotor Apraxia**: Ability to carry out a task automatically but inability to simulate the task or do it on command due to a perceptual disorder.

**Impairments**: Problems in body function or structure (WHO, 2001).

**Inclusion**: The act of including and providing intervention to students with disabilities in the regular education classroom; Adapting the environment for persons with disabilities to be successful in occupations, roles, and activities with others.

**Independent T-Test**: T-test performed on independent groups of participants' scores to measure differences between the scores.

**Independent Variable**: The variable manipulated; its effects are measured by the dependent variables.

**Individual Education Plan (IEP)**: Written, legal document developed by the individual education team, incorporating the student's strengths and need areas as well as goals and objectives for intervention.

**Instrumental Activities of Daily Living (IADL)**: An area of occupation; "Activities to support daily life within the home and community that often require more complex interactions than self-care used in ADL" (AOTA, 2008, p. 631).

**Interactive Reasoning**: Involves understanding the client as a holistic human being and looking at issues from the client's perspective.

**Interdependence**: Reliance on others.

**Internal Control**: The player is in control of the materials play interactions, and some aspect of the outcome (Bundy, 1997; Connor, Williamson, & Seipp, 1978); The extent to which the child is in control of his or her actions and to some aspects of outcome of the activity (Bundy, 1997).

**Internal Validity**: The degree to which the researcher's conclusions are accurate.

**International Classification of Diseases (ICD-10)**: International framework for coding health conditions including diseases, disorders, and injuries.

**International Classification of Functioning, Disability, and Health (ICF)**: International framework for coding components of health and functioning.

**Intervention Plan**: A collaborative listing of client-oriented actions meant to enhance occupational performance, with specific targeted outcomes, that is based on select models, frames of reference, and evidence.

**Intrinsic Motivation**: What drives a child to participate in an activity for pleasure rather than extrinsic reward (Bundy, 1993); The self-initiation or drive to action that is rewarded by the activity itself, rather than some external reward (Bundy, 1997).

# J

**Jejunostomy Tube**: Placed directly into the jejunum (the central of the three divisions of the small intestine), bypassing the stomach.

**Judgment**: The act of deciding after consideration of alternatives.

**"Just Right" Challenge**: When the challenge of a task does not exceed the abilities to meet the challenge.

# K

**Kinesthesia**: The sense of movement of one's body or part of one's body (e.g., joint or limb) in space.

**Knowledge**: What you know.

# L

**Leadership**: The ability to engage and influence others to facilitate and embrace meaningful change through careful consideration of individual and societal contexts in the embodiment of a shared vision.

**Least Restrictive Environment**: An educational environment most like a regular education classroom; Developing a natural environment that enhances a person's occupational performance in as self-structured a format as possible.

**Legislative Process**: The path through which a bill becomes a law. Involves hearings in Congressional/Statehouse committees, votes by committee members, and if passed, voting on the floor of the legislative body.

**Leisure**: "A nonobligatory activity that is intrinsically motivated and engaged in during discretionary time, that is, time not committed to obligatory occupations such as work, self-care or sleep" (Parham & Fazio, 1997, p. 250).

**Leisure Activities**: "Nonobligatory, discretionary, and intrinsically rewarding activities" (AOTA, 2004b, p. 674).

**Level I Fieldwork**: Introductory practical experiences to expose students to a variety of practice settings.

**Level II Fieldwork**: Practical experiences created to develop competent, entry-level occupational therapists and occupational therapy assistants.

**Lobbyist**: A person who attempts to influence the legislative process by providing information.

**Low-Tech**: Devices that are easily fabricated or obtained.

# M

**Maintenance**: Ensuring continued competency through the use of external devices, templates, or skill retraining, despite expectations of potential or eventual declines in occupational performance.

**Managed Care**: A variety of methods of financing and organizing the delivery of health care in which costs are contained by controlling the provision of services.

**Manager**: An individual often responsible for task-specific functions within an organization.

**Marketing**: "The process of planning and executing the conception, price, promotion and distribution of ideas, goods, and services to create exchanges that satisfy individual and organizational objectives" (Bennett, 1995, p. 21).

**Mature Level Participation**: Combines basic and supportive cooperative participation, focused on task completion and social interaction.

**Mean**: Mathematical average of a set of scores.

**Meaningful Occupation**: A valued activity that contributes to identity, well-being, and quality of life.

**Measures of Central Tendency**: Frequency, mean, mode, median.

**Measures of Variability**: Descriptive statistics of range, variance, and standard deviation.

**Median**: Middle score of a range.

**Meta-Analysis**: Statistical analysis to integrate the results of several studies on one topic.

**Mode**: The most common score in a range.

**Modeling**: Demonstration of behavior.

**Models of Practice**: A set of ideas, in terms of which other ideas are interpreted or assigned meaning which provide an overview of the occupational therapy philosophy and process. Models of Practice help practitioners organize their thinking.

**Monitoring**: The act of observing a client's response to intervention.

**Moral Treatment**: An approach to the treatment of what was called "madness" in the middle to late 19th century that was characterized by an "optimistic view of human nature, and influenced by enlightenment humanism and pietistic evangelicalism... [which at its] core was the belief that if treated like rational beings within a rational environment, the insane would regain their reason" (Lilleleht, 2002, p. 169).

**Moral Treatment Movement**: A theory based on the respect and dignity for all humans and their need to participate in daily occupations.

**Morality**: The accepted standards of right or wrong that direct the conduct of a person or a group.

**Moratorium**: A temporary freeze on the implementation of a piece of legislation.

**Multiple Regression Analysis**: A statistical measure that allows one variable to predict another.

# N

**Narrative Reasoning**: Utilized to learn about the client's life story.

**Nasogastric Tube**: A feeding tube inserted through the oral pharyngeal area supplying liquid nutrition by passing the mouth.

**Natural Environments**: The context in which an individual lives.

**Naturalistic Observation**: Observation of behavior as it occurs naturally without the researcher interfering.

**Neuroscience-Based Treatment**: Founded, primarily, on the idea that "the brain can be studied empirically" (Cohen & Reed, 1995, p. 562). In neuroscience, the brain is considered a dynamic system that includes virtually all of the underlying physiological and neurological processes that support human performance. An understanding of these processes supports the development of occupational therapy models of practice.

**Nonlinear Dynamics**: A framework for analyzing unpredictable, self-organizing systems concerning people and their context.

**Nonverbal Communication**: Communication through eye contact, tone of voice, facial expression, body language, and posture.

**Norm Referenced**: Client scores can be compared to a specific "normative" group utilized during test development.

**NPO (*nil per os*)**: Latin for "nothing by mouth;" no food, liquid or medication is to be given orally (Avery-Smith, 2002).

# O

**Objective**: Building blocks needed to achieve a larger goal.

**Occupation**: Everyday activities and occupations that people find meaningful and purposeful (Moyers & Dale, 2007);

"'Goal-directed pursuits that typically extend over time have meaning to the performance, and involve multiple tasks' (Christiansen, Baum, & Bass-Haugen, 2005, p. 548); 'Daily activities that reflect cultural values, provide structure to living, and meaning to individuals; these activities meet human needs for self-care, enjoyment, and participation in society' (Crepeau, Cohn & Schell, 2003, p. 1031); 'Activities that people engage in throughout their daily lives to fulfill their time and give life meaning. Occupations involve mental abilities and skills, and may or may not have an observable physical dimension' (Hinojosa & Kramer, 1997, p. 865); '[A]ctivities...of everyday life, named, organized, and given value and meaning by individuals and a culture. Occupation is everything people do to occupy themselves, including looking after themselves...enjoying life...and contributing to the social and economic fabric of their communities' (Law, Polatajko, Baptiste, & Townsend, 1997, p. 32); 'A dynamic relationship among an occupational form, a person with a unique developmental structure, subjective meanings and purpose, and the resulting occupational performance' (Nelson & Jepson Thomas, 2003, p. 90); 'Occupations are defined in the science as chunks of daily activity that can be named in the lexicon of the culture' (Zemke & Clark, 1996, p. vii)" (AOTA, 2008, p. 672)

**Occupation-Based**: Refers to providing intervention that includes the actual occupation (activities in which the client engages, in its actual context).

**Occupation-Based Activity**: Activity meaningful to the person, which is conducted in the actual context.

**Occupation-Based Model**: Proposed interaction of person, environment, and occupation that guide the organization of occupational therapy practice (Cole & Tufano, 2008).

**Occupational Justice**: "Justice related to opportunities and resources required for occupational participation sufficient to satisfy personal needs and full citizenship" (Christiansen & Townsend, 2004, p. 278); "To experience meaning and enrichment in one's occupations; to participate in a range of occupations for health and social inclusion; to make choices and share decision-making power in daily life; and to receive equal privileges for diverse participation in occupations (Townsend & Wilcock, 2004)" (AOTA, 2008, p. 630).

**Occupational Performance**: The ability to carry out activities of daily life, including activities of daily living, education, work, play, leisure, and social participation (AOTA, 2008).

**Occupational Performance Model**: A framework for understanding the individual's dynamic experience in daily occupations within the environment (Baum & Law, 1995).

**Occupational Profile**: An initial interview process that may be formal and/or informal. It is meant to reveal the client's personal history, daily living patterns, interests, values, and needs, while highlighting problems from the client's perspective concerning the performance of occupations and daily living activities. At its conclusion, the client is asked to prioritize his goals for occupational therapy intervention; "A summary of the client's occupational history, patterns of daily living, interests, values, and needs" (AOTA, 2008, p. 649).

**Occupational Therapy**: A health and wellness profession enabling people to participate in the everyday activities they want and need to do.

**Occupational Therapy Practitioners**: This term is used to encompass occupational therapists and occupational therapy assistants.

**Outlier**: An extreme score that falls far from the mean score.

# P

***p* Value**: The alpha score of the probability of a type I error.

**Paired T-Test**: T-test performed on paired groups of participants' scores to measure differences between the scores.

**Paradigm**: A shared vision encompassing fundamental assumptions and beliefs, which serves as the cultural core of the profession (Kielhofner, 2004).

**Parallel Level Participation**: Play, activity, or work carried out side by side, without interaction with others present.

**Parenteral Tube Feedings**: Tubes that deliver nutrition via bypassing the gastrointestinal system to deliver nutrition into the bloodstream (Morris & Klein, 2000).

**Participation**: Involvement in life situations and activities that include the capacity to execute and perform tasks (WHO, 2001).

**Partnerships in Health**: Collaborations with individuals and community members that have a central mission to enhance health and well-being.

**Pearson Correlation Coefficient**: The most common measure of relationships between two factors.

**Performance Context**: Environment in which occupational performance occurs, including the physical environment, available resources, sensory input, temporal and societal influences, or the presence or availability of caregivers.

**Performance in Areas of Occupation**: Activities of daily living, instrumental activities of daily living, education, work, play, social participation, leisure, rest, and sleep (AOTA, 2008).

**Performance Patterns**: Habits, roles, and routines providing structure to day-to-day living. Performance patterns also include rituals that can be spiritual, cultural, or societal in nature and give meaning to the client (AOTA, 2008).

**Performance Skills**: Skills needed to participate in areas of occupation including motor, process, and communication/interaction skills (AOTA, 2008); "Observable, concrete goal directed actions clients use to engage in daily life occupations (Fisher, 2006). Performance skills are learned and developed over time, and are situated in context. Multiple aspects such as the context in which the occupation is performed, the specific demands of the activity being attempted, and the client's body functions and structures affect the client's ability to acquire or demonstrate performance skills" (AOTA, 2008, p. 639).

**Personal Factors**: Contextual factors intrinsic to the individual, such as attributes of age, gender, and social status (WHO, 2001).

**Persuade**: To move by argument, entreaty, or expostulation to a belief, position, or course of action; To plead with (Merriam-Webster, 2006).

**Ph Probe**: Medical test used to help identify the amount and severity of gastroesophageal reflux (Morris & Klein, 2000).

**Philosophy**: A fundamental belief (Meyer, 1977).

**Physical Agent Modalities**: Procedures and interventions that are systematically applied to modify specific client factors that may be limiting occupational performance and use various forms of energy in order to modulate pain; modify tissue healing; increase tissue extensibility; modify skin and scar tissue; decrease edema, inflammation, or occupational performance secondary to musculoskeletal or integumentary conditions; and are used as an adjunctive method to occupation (Bracciano, 2008).

**Physical Transfers**: Teaching a client who uses a wheelchair to move from one surface to another.

**Pilot Test**: Trial run of a study to evaluate for problems in future experiments.

**Play**: "Any spontaneous or organized activity that provides enjoyment, entertainment, amusement or diversion" (Parham & Fazio, 1997, p. 252).

**Play Activities**: "Spontaneous and organized activities that promote pleasure, amusement, and diversion" (AOTA, 2004b, p. 674).

**Playfulness**: A play temperament that is comprised of intrinsic motivation, internal control, freedom to suspend reality, and framing; A behavioral or personality trait characterized by flexibility, manifest joy, and spontaneity" (Parham & Fazio, 1997, p. 252).

**Positioning**: The most important first step in the eating and feeding process (Case-Smith & Humphry, 2005; Jenks & Smith, 2006).

**Post Hoc Tests**: Statistical tests used to follow up significant findings.

**Postulate**: A theoretical statement that suggests how two or more concepts are related (Mosey, 1986).

**Practice Skills**: Repetition of an ability to improve the consistency of performance; Components of occupations.

**Practitioner**: Provides occupational therapy services including assessments, interventions, program planning and implementation, discharge planning, and transition planning (AOTA, 2000).

**Pragmatic Reasoning**: Used to understand the practical issues that may have an impact on the situation with the person and family.

**Pragmatism**: A philosophical view that knowledge grows through change and adaptation, and is best gained through practical application and experience (Breines, 1987).

**Preparatory Activity**: Repetitive techniques to get a client ready to perform (e.g., stretching, mental review).

**Pretest Sensitization**: Participants completing the pretest complicates the posttest results.

**Probability**: Likelihood of finding the same results in repeated studies.

**Procedural Reasoning**: Focuses on client performance and diagnosis.

**Profession**: An occupation requiring extensive education or specialized training.

**Professional**: A person engaged in a profession.

**Professional Development**: Ongoing plan to assure practice is current and based on known best practices; a process where one plans and achieves excellence or establishes expertise in seeking a change in responsibilities, or when assuming more complex professional roles.

**Professional Portfolio**: A collection of evidence demonstrating that practice is current and based on known best practices; An archival of one's self-assessment processes, learning plans, evidence of engagement in selected learning methods, reflection on the learning process, and outcomes of the application of learning to practice.

**Promotion**: Advance in station, rank, or honor; To advance (a student) from one grade to the next higher grade; To contribute to the growth or prosperity of, promote international understanding; To help bring (as an enterprise) into being; To present (merchandise) for buyer acceptance through advertising, publicity, or discounting (Merriam-Webster, 2006).

**Proprioception**: The sense of one's body or parts of one's body (e.g., joint or limb) in space.

**Prospective Payment System (PPS)**: Created by the Balanced Budget Act of 1997 as a method for controlling costs. Payment for skilled service is made on a daily rate, chosen based on certain admission criteria indicating an estimated level of need.

**Psychometrics**: The study of psychological and behavioral measurement.

# Q

**Qualitative Research**: Research data collected using words.

**Quality Assessment**: A measure of quality against standards.

**Quality Improvement**: Management philosophy and method for structuring problem solving.

**Quantitative Research**: Research data collected using numbers.

# R

**Range**: Measure of variability between the highest and lowest scores.

**Real Life**: Individuals' description and interpretation of their life.

**Recreation**: Adult play or activities whose purpose is to "regenerate energy to support the worker role" (Glantz & Richman, 2001, p. 249).

**Reductionistic Approach**: Perceiving many individual parts that make up the whole, which may be studied and dealt with separately or interchangeably.

**Referral**: Making a professional judgment to have another occupational therapy specialist, discipline, or facility evaluate the client; The practice of directing an initial request for service or changing the degree and direction of service (Agnes, 1999).

**Reflection**: A useful tool in analyzing thoughts and actions that assists practitioners to justify interventions and gives practitioners the ability to learn from experience.

**Reflective Listening**: A process of listening to both the verbal and emotional content of a speaker and verbalizing both the feelings and attitudes sensed behind the spoken words to the speaker (Davis, 2006).

**Rehabilitation Movement**: Began with a change in the way society viewed those with handicaps to individuals who could become independent and contributing members of the community.

**Related Service**: Services that may be required for a student to benefit from special education. Service providers include occupational therapy, physical therapy, social work, and school health services.

**Reliability**: Accuracy and stability of a measure; The dependability and consistency of a measurement.

**Remediation**: Helping clients regain skills and abilities.

**Researcher**: "Find the process of discovery exhilarating and because they see how it enhances occupational therapy practice" (Kielhofner, 2006).

**Resource Utilization Groups (RUG)**: Categories used in PPS that describe the amount of service clients will need.

# S

**Safety**: Practices that reduce the risk of adverse incidents.

**Sample**: A selection from a population.

**Sampling Error**: The difference between the sample's scores and what the whole population would have scored.

**Scaffolding**: Foundation of prerequisite skills.

**Scientific Reasoning**: Involves the logical thinking about the nature of the client's problems and the optimal course of action in treatment.

**Screening**: The process of gathering and reviewing data with the intent to determine if additional evaluative procedures are warranted.

**Seating Systems**: Selection and utilization of a comfortable, supportive wheelchair or chair seat that encourages symmetry, skin integrity, and occupational performance.

**Self-Assessment**: Provides the means to assess performance, abilities, and skills; to analyze demands and resources of the work environment; to interpret information about clients' outcomes; to reassess current learning goals; and to develop goals and plans for professional growth and continuing competence and competency.

**Simulation**: Creating realistic situations to allow learners to practice and apply skills.

**Site**: Facility offering clinical affiliations to students.

**SOAP Note Format**: Documentation format that includes four parts in documenting a client's intervention: subjective, objective, assessment, and plan.

**Social Participation**: A person's performance of meaningful roles and occupations within preferred social groups such as families, classrooms, work teams, organizations, and communities (Cole & Donohue, in press); Consists of verbal and interpersonal activity interactions among people.

**Standard Deviation**: A measurement of variability, a description of how far from the mean a score is.

**Standard Precautions**: A form of infection control based on the assumption that all bodily substances may transmit infectious diseases.

**Statistical Significance**: The likelihood that the finding is not due to error.

**Suck, Swallow, Breathe Synchrony**: The smooth coordination of sucking, swallowing, and breathing into rhythmic patterns to allow for efficient and effective eating (Case-Smith & Humphry, 2005).

**Superficial Thermal Agent**: Those procedures or interventions that are capable of raising or decreasing the temperature of superficial tissue to a therapeutic level.

**Supervisee**: One who receives direction and undergoes evaluation by a qualified practitioner.

**Supervision**: Direct and evaluate performance.

**Support**: The provision of services that enable clients to achieve maximum occupational performance.

**Supportive Cooperative Level Participation**: Consists of interactions that express feelings and emotions designed to foster social cohesion in a group.

# T

**T-Test**: A statistical measure of the difference between two means.

**Tacit**: Involves learning and skill, but not in a way that can be written down.

**Taxonomy**: A system of classification.

**Technology**: "The branch of knowledge that deals with the creation and use of technical means and their interrelation with life, society, and the environment, drawing upon such subjects as industrial arts, engineering, applied science, and pure science" (Flexner, 1987, p. 1950).

**Test-Retest Reliability**: Consistency of a score of repeated measures over time.

**Theoretical Constructs**: Visible and non-visible ideas and explanations that form into a concept.

**Theory**: Describes, explains, and predicts behavior and/or the relationships between concepts or events.

**Therapeutic Use of Self**: A practitioner's intuitive nature that derives from one's personality traits, self-awareness, and personal experiences; understanding of human behavior; and observations through the use of the five senses. The practitioner makes conscious use of this nature to engage and impact a therapeutic relationship and foster a meaningful experience for the client.

**Transference**: When one person, usually the client, places a role on another, usually the therapist.

**Transition Services**: A results-oriented process that facilitates movement between settings and providers based on changing client needs. This term is most often used in the school setting but is an essential of care coordination across the continuum.

**TriAlliance of Health and Rehabilitation Professions**: "The TriAlliance is the largest constituency of health and rehabilitation professionals representing the professions of occupational therapy, physical therapy, audiology and speech-language pathology. In 1988, informal meetings began among the Presidents and Executive Directors of the American Occupational Therapy Association (AOTA), the American Physical Therapy Association (APTA), and the American Speech-Language-Hearing Association (ASHA)" (APTA, 2000).

**Type I Error**: Finding that the independent variable had an effect when it did not.

**Type II Error**: Finding that the independent variable did not have an effect when it did.

# U

**Universal Design**: Principles that seek to promote access to and use of structures and tools across the lifespan.

**Utilization Review**: A look-over of care/services that were provided in a particular case to ascertain necessity, efficiency, and effectiveness.

# V

**Validity**: Generalizability of a measure to the general population; the extent to which a measurement measures what it is intended to measure.

**Values**: Principles that set a standard of quality or a worthwhile ideal.

**Variability**: The degree to which scores differ from each other.

**Variance**: An index or score of variability that explains the differences between factors.

**Videofluoroscopy**: A primary imaging technique for detailed dynamic assessment of oral, pharyngeal, and upper esophageal phases of a swallow (Arvedson, Brodsky, & Christensen, 2002); also known as *modified barium swallow.*

# W

**Well-being**: The state of being content, comfortable, and satisfied with one's self, relationships, and quality of life.

**Wellness**: A dynamic way of life that involves actions, values, and attitudes that support or improve both health and quality of life (AOTA, 2001).

**Wheelchair Management**: Selection, utilization, and functional mobility of the wheelchair.

**Work**: "Includes activities needed for engaging in remunerative employment or volunteer activities (Mosey, 1996, p. 341):

- *Employment Interests and Pursuits*—Identifying and selecting work opportunities based on assets, limitations, likes, and dislikes relative to work (adapted from Mosey, 1996, p. 342).
- *Employment Seeking and Acquisition*—Identifying and recruiting for job opportunities; completing, submitting, and reviewing appropriate application materials; preparing for interviews; participating in interviews and following up afterward; discussing job benefits; and finalizing negotiations.
- *Job Performance*—Job performance including: work skills and patterns; time management; relationships with co-workers, managers, and customers; creation, production, and distribution of products and services; initiation, sustainment, and completion of work; and compliance with work norms and procedures.
- *Retirement Preparation and Adjustment*—Determining aptitudes, developing interests and skills, and selecting appropriate avocational pursuits.
- *Volunteer Exploration*—Determining community causes, organizations, or opportunities for unpaid 'work' in relationship to personal skills, interests, location, and time available.
- *Volunteer Participation*—Performing unpaid 'work' activities for the benefit of identified selected causes, organizations, or facilities" (AOTA, 2008, p. 632).

# References

Accreditation Council for Occupational Therapy Education. (1999). Standards for an accredited educational program for the occupational therapist. *American Journal of Occupational Therapy, 53*, 575-581.

Agnes, M. (Ed.). (1999). *Webster's new world college dictionary* (4th ed.). New York, NY: Macmillan.

American Occupational Therapy Association. (1994). Occupational Therapy Code of Ethics. *American Journal of Occupational Therapy, 48*, 1037-1038.

American Occupational Therapy Association. (2000). Occupational therapy roles and career exploration and development: A companion guide to the Occupational Therapy Role Documents. In *The reference manual of the official documents of the American Occupational Therapy Association* (8th ed.). Bethesda, MD: Author.

American Occupational Therapy Association. (2001). Position paper: Occupational therapy in the promotion of health and the prevention of disease and disability statement. *American Journal of Occupational Therapy, 55*(6), 656-660.

American Occupational Therapy Association. (2004a). Role competencies for a professional-level occupational therapist faculty member in an academic setting. *American Journal of Occupational Therapy, 58*(6), 649-650.

American Occupational Therapy Association. (2004b). Scope of practice. *American Journal of Occupational Therapy, 58*(6), 673-677.

American Occupational Therapy Association. (2007). Specialized knowledge and skills in eating and feeding for occupational therapy practice. *American Journal of Occupational Therapy, 61*, 686-700.

American Occupational Therapy Association. (2008). Occupational therapy practice framework: Domain and process, second edition. *American Journal of Occupational Therapy, 62*, 625-683.

American Physical Therapy Association. (2000). TriAlliance to explore Medicare alternative payment methods. Retrieved July 19, 2006, from http://www.apta.org/AM/Template.cfm?Section=Home&TEMPLATE=/CM/ContentDisplay.cfm&CONTENTID=30620

Arvedsen, J. C., Brodsky, L., & Christensen, S. (2002). Instrumental evaluation of swallowing. In J. C. Arvedsen & L. Brodsky (Eds.), *Pediatric swallowing and feeding assessment and management* (2nd ed., pp. 341-388). Albany, NY: Singular Publishing Group.

Avery-Smith, W. (2002). Dysphagia. In C. A. Trombly & M. V. Radomski (Eds.), *Occupational therapy for physical dysfunction* (pp. 1091-1109). Philadelphia, PA: Lippincott Williams & Wilkins.

Bateson, G. (1972). Toward a theory of play and fantasy. In G. Bateson (Ed.), *Steps to an ecology of the mind* (pp. 14-20). New York, NY: Bantam.

Baum, C., & Law, M. (1995). Occupational performance: Occupational therapy's definition of function. *American Journal of Occupational Therapy, 49*, 1019.

Bennett, P. D. (Ed.). (1995). *Dictionary of marketing terms* (2nd ed.). Chicago, IL: American Marketing Association.

Bracciano, A. (2008). *Physical agent modalities: Theory and application for the occupational therapist.* Thorofare, NJ: SLACK Incorporated.

Braveman, B. (2006). *Leading & managing occupational therapy services: An evidence-based approach.* Philadelphia, PA: F.A. Davis.

Brayman, S. J., Roley, S. S., Clark, G. F., DeLany, J. V., Garza, E. R., Radomski, M. V., et al. (2005). Standards of practice for occupational therapy. *American Journal of Occupational Therapy, 59*(6), 663-665.

Brookside Associates Multi-Media Edition. (2007). Nursing Fundamentals I. Retrieved August 6, 2009, from http://www.brooksidepress.org/Products/Nursing_Fundamentals_1/Index.htm

Breines, E. (1987). Pragmatism as a foundation for occupational therapy curricula. *American Journal of Occupational Therapy, 47*, 522-525.

Bundy, A. C. (1993). Assessment of play and leisure: Delineation of the problem. *American Journal of Occupational Therapy, 47*, 217-222.

Bundy, A. C. (1997). Play and playfulness: What to look for. In L. D. Parham & L. S. Fazio (Eds.), *Play in occupational therapy for children* (pp. 52-66). St. Louis, MO: Mosby.

Canadian Association of Occupational Therapists. (1999). Joint position statement on evidence-based occupational therapy. Retrieved July 30, 2006, from http://www.caot.ca/default.asp?ChangeID=166&pageID=156

Case-Smith, J., & Humphry, R. (2005). Feeding intervention. In J. Case-Smith (Ed.), *Occupational therapy for children* (5th ed., pp. 481-520). St. Louis, MO: Elsevier Mosby.

Christiansen, C. H., & Townsend, E. A. (2004). *Introduction to occupation: The art and science of living.* Upper Saddle River, NJ: Prentice Hall.

Cohen, H., & Reed, K. L. (1995). The historical development of neuroscience in physical rehabilitation. *American Journal of Occupational Therapy, 50*(7), 561-568.

Cole, M. & Donohue, M. (in press). *Social participation and occupation: In schools, clinics, and communities.* Thorofare, NJ: SLACK Incorporated.

Cole, M., & Tufano, R. (2008). *Applied theories in occupational therapy.* Thorofare, NJ: SLACK Incorporated.

Connor, F. P., Williamson, G. G., & Siepp, J. M. (Eds.). (1978). *Program guide for infants and toddlers with neuromotor and other developmental disabilities.* New York, NY: Teachers College.

Davis, C. M. (2006). *Patient practitioner interaction: An experiential manual for developing the art of health care.* Thorofare, NJ: SLACK Incorporated.

Depoy, E., & Gitlin, L. (2005). *Introduction to research: Understanding and applying multiple strategies* (3rd ed.). New York, NY: Mosby.

Dictionary.com. Retrieved July 24, 2006, from http://dictionary.reference.com

Encyclopedia.com. (2008). Disease. In *Oxford dictionary of nursing*. Oxford University Press. Retrieved August 20, 2009, from http://www.encyclopedia.com/doc/1O62-disease.html

Finkelstein, V. (1991). Disability: An administrative challenge? In M. Oliver (Ed.), *Social work: Disabled people and disabling environments* (pp. 19-39). London, England: Jessica Kingsley.

Flexner, S. B. (Ed.). (1987). *The Random House dictionary of the English language, unabridged* (2nd ed.). New York, NY: Random House.

Glantz, C. H., & Richman, N. (2001). Leisure activities. In L. W. Pedretti & M. B. Early (Eds.), *Occupational therapy practice skills for physical dysfunction* (5th ed., pp. 249-256). St Louis, MO: Mosby.

Hooper, B. (2006). Epistemological transformation in occupational therapy: Educational implications and challenges. *Occupational Therapy Journal of Research, 26*, 15-24.

Jenks, K. N., & Smith, G. (2006). Eating and swallowing. In H. M Pendleton & W. Schultz-Krohn (Eds.), *Pedretti's occupational therapy practice skills for physical dysfunction* (6th ed., pp. 609-645). St. Louis, MO: Mosby.

Kerlinger, F. (1979). *Behavioral research: A conceptual approach*. New York, NY: Holt, Rinehart, & Winston.

Kielhofner, G. (2004). *Conceptual foundations of occupational therapy* (3rd ed.). Philadelphia, PA: F.A. Davis.

Kielhofner, G. (2006). *Research in occupational therapy: Methods of inquiry for enhancing practice*. Philadelphia, PA: F.A. Davis.

Kotler, P. (2003). *A framework for marketing management* (2nd ed.). Upper Saddle River, NJ: Prentice Hall.

Law, M., Baptiste, S., & Mills, J. (1995). Client-centered practice: What does it mean and does it make a difference? *Canadian Journal of Occupational Therapy, 62*, 250-257.

Lilleleht, E. (2002). Progress and power: Exploring the disciplinary connections between moral treatment and psychiatric rehabilitation. *Philosophy, Psychiatry, & Psychology, 9*(2), 167-182.

Loveland, C. A. (1999). The concept of culture. In R. L. Leavitt (Ed.), *Cross-cultural rehabilitation: An international perspective* (pp. 15-24). London, England: Saunders.

Merriam-Webster. (2006). On-line dictionary, 10th ed. Retrieved June 16, 2006, from http://www.merriam-webster.com

Meyer, A. (1977). The philosophy of occupational therapy. *American Journal of Occupational Therapy, 31*, 639-642. (Original work published in 1922).

Morris, S. E., & Klein, M. D. (2000). *Pre-feeding skills: A comprehensive resource for mealtime development* (2nd ed.). Austin, TX: Therapy Skills Builders.

Mosey, A. C. (1986). *Psychosocial components of occupational therapy*. New York, NY: Raven Press.

Moyers, P. A., & Dale, L. M. (2007). *The guide to occupational therapy practice*. Bethesda, MD: AOTA Press.

Parham, L. D., & Fazio, L. S. (1997). *Play in occupational therapy for children*. St. Louis, MO: Mosby.

Reed, K., & Sanderson, S. (1999). *Concepts of occupational therapy* (4th ed.). Baltimore, MD: Lippincott Williams & Wilkins.

Rubin, K. H., Fein, G. G., & Vandenberg, B. (1983). Play. In P. H. Mussen (Ed.), *Handbook of child psychology: Vol. 4. Socialization, personality, and social development* (4th ed., pp. 693-774). New York, NY: Wiley.

Spencer, L. M., & Spencer, S. M. (1993). *Competence at work*. New York, NY: John Wiley and Sons.

Wells, S. A., & Black, R. M. (2000). *Cultural competency for health professionals*. Bethesda, MD: AOTA Press.

World Health Organization. (1947). Constitution of the World Health Organization. *Chronicle for the World Health Organization, 1*(1), 29-40.

World Health Organization (2001). *ICF: International Classification of Functioning, Disability, and Health*. Geneva, Switzerland: Author.

# INDEX